Principles and Practices in Augmentative and Alternative Communication

Principles and Practices in Augmentative and Alternative Communication

Editors

Donald R. Fuller, PhD, CCC-SLP (Ret.), FASHA

Professor and Chair
Department of Communication Sciences and Disorders
The University of Texas Rio Grande Valley
Edinburg, Texas

Lyle L. Lloyd, PhD, CCC-A/SLP, FAAIDD, FASHA, FISAAC

Professor Emeritus (Deceased)
Department of Speech, Language and Hearing Sciences
Purdue University
West Lafayette, Indiana

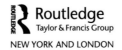

Routledge
Taylor & Francis Group

NEW YORK AND LONDON

Principles and Practices in Augmentative and Alternative Communication includes ancillary materials specifically available for faculty use. Included are PowerPoint Slides. Please visit www.routledge.com/9781630915841 to obtain access.

This book was originally published as Lloyd, L. L., Fuller, D. R., & Arvidson, H. (1997). *Augmentative and alternative communication: A handbook of principles and practices*. Allyn & Bacon.

First published in 2023 by SLACK Incorporated

Published 2024 by Routledge
605 Third Avenue, New York, NY 10158

and by Routledge
4 Park Square, Milton Park, Abingdon, Oxon OX14 4RN

Routledge is an imprint of the Taylor & Francis Group, an informa business

© 2023 Taylor & Francis Group

Cover Artist: Lori Shields

Library of Congress Cataloging-in-Publication Data

Names: Fuller, Donald R, editor. | Lloyd, Lyle L, editor.
Title: Principles and practices in augmentative and alternative
   communication / [edited by] Donald R. Fuller, Lyle L. Lloyd.
Description: Thorofare, NJ : SLACK Incorporated, [2022] | Includes
   bibliographical references and index.
Identifiers: LCCN 2022018469 (print) | ISBN 9781630915841 (hardcover)
Subjects: MESH: Communication Aids for Disabled
Classification: LCC RC428.8 (print) | NLM WL 340.2
   | DDC 616.85/503--dc23/eng/20221115
LC record available at https://lccn.loc.gov/2022018469

ISBN: 9781630915841 (hbk)
ISBN: 9781003525905 (ebk)

DOI: 10.4324/9781003525905

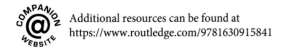

Additional resources can be found at
https://www.routledge.com/9781630915841

DEDICATION

This textbook is dedicated, first and foremost, to individuals around the world who rely upon augmentative and alternative communication (AAC) as their primary mode of communication. Much of what academicians and clinicians have learned about the field has come from interactions with persons who communicate in what many would consider "unconventional" ways.

As I draw ever closer to retirement from more than 3 decades in higher education, there are many people I would like to acknowledge and express my appreciation to for providing me with greater insight into AAC and persons with intellectual, physical, and/or sensory challenges. However, acknowledgment has been given to several of these individuals in the Preface of this book. For those not specifically mentioned, my apologies.

There are two persons to whom I'd like to dedicate this book, as they guided my journey from college student to speech-language pathologist to AAC specialist. Dr. Emilio "Bill" Perez was my major professor for the master's degree at Arkansas State University. It was he who chipped away at the diamond in the rough, forming me into an allied health professional and, generally, a better human being. It was Dr. Perez who encouraged me to go on to earn the doctorate. At that time, I was leaning toward a career as a speech scientist, and I entered Purdue University to pursue advanced study in speech perception and production. Little did I know my choice of career path would change in the space of one semester. My path crossed with that of Dr. Lyle L. Lloyd during his graduate-level course, Non-Speech Communication. My interest quickly changed from speech science to AAC. Dr. Lloyd became more than just a mentor to me—he became a well-respected colleague and friend. Our world will not be the same without him. To Dr. Emilio Perez and "Big Daddy," I simply say, thank you. May you both rest in peace.

I think it would be appropriate to acknowledge two pioneers in the field of AAC who passed on during the production of this book. I developed a collegial relationship and friendship with both individuals while engaged in doctoral study at Purdue University in the mid-1980s. Bruce Baker, inventor of Minspeak and the concept of semantic compaction, was a true gentleman in every sense of the word. David R. Beukelman was a world-renowned scholar on AAC and a colleague and friend I admired greatly. He was also a gentleman in every sense of the word. The AAC community lost two individuals who made a profound influence on the field. Both of them will be missed greatly by the AAC community.

Lastly, but most importantly, I thank my Lord and Savior, Jesus Christ, for my life and life's lessons learned. Ever faithful. Ever true. To Him be the glory, honor, and praise.

—*Donald R. Fuller, PhD, CCC-SLP (Ret.), FASHA*
Professor and Chair
Department of Communication Sciences and Disorders
The University of Texas Rio Grande Valley
Edinburg, Texas

Contents

Part I: Introduction to AAC

Part II: AAC Symbols

Part III: AAC Technology

Part IV: AAC Assessment

Part V: AAC Intervention

Principles and Practices in Augmentative and Alternative Communication includes ancillary materials specifically available for faculty use. Included are PowerPoint Slides. Please visit www.routledge.com/9781630915841 to obtain access.

ABOUT THE EDITORS

Dr. Donald R. Fuller is professor and chair of the Department of Communication Sciences and Disorders at The University of Texas Rio Grande Valley. He earned his Bachelor of Science in Education and Master of Speech Pathology degrees from Arkansas State University and his doctoral degree at Purdue University, where Dr. Lloyd was his major professor and mentor. During his career in higher education, Dr. Fuller assisted in creating a master's degree program in speech-language pathology at Florida International University and was founding chair of the Department of Speech-Language Pathology at Misericordia University. Although Dr. Fuller's passion lies in administration in higher education, he has maintained his interest in augmentative and alternative communication (AAC), publishing several articles and making numerous presentations, primarily involving the iconicity and complexity of aided symbols and theoretical issues in the discipline. He coauthored the 1997 textbook, *Augmentative and Alternative Communication: A Handbook of Principles and Practices* with Dr. Lloyd and Helen Arvidson. Dr. Fuller was elected a fellow of the American Speech-Language-Hearing Association in 1998.

Dr. Lyle L. Lloyd is considered by some to be a father of AAC. His accomplishments in this discipline are detailed in the In Memoriam section of this book. Upon reading the memorial, one will gain considerable understanding of why he is held in such high esteem by the AAC community. Dr. Lloyd earned his Bachelor of Science degree from Eastern Illinois University, his Master of Arts degree from the University of Illinois, and his doctoral degree from the University of Iowa. Dually certified as an audiologist and speech-language pathologist, he served the early part of his career as a clinician and researcher, especially in the area of intellectual disability. His proclivity for research and successful grant writing opened the door to employment at the Parsons State Hospital and Training Center in Kansas and the National Institute of Child Health and Human Development. He held faculty positions at Western Michigan University, Gallaudet College, and Purdue University. During his tenure at Purdue University, Dr. Lloyd mentored nearly 40 doctoral students; many of these former students are now leaders in the field of AAC. Due to his contributions to AAC, special education, and speech-language pathology, Dr. Lloyd earned honors of the American Association on Intellectual and Developmental Disabilities, American Speech-Language-Hearing Association, Council for Exceptional Children, and the International Society for Augmentative and Alternative Communication. Dr. Lloyd passed away February 12, 2020, at age 85 years.

Contributing Authors

Erna Alant, PhD (Chapter 15)
Professor Emeritus of Special Education
Indiana University
Erna Alant Consultancy
Bloomington, Indiana

Meher H. Banajee, PhD, CCC-SLP, FASHA (Chapter 10)
Program Director and Associate Professor
Speech-Language Pathology Program
Communication Disorders Department
School of Allied Health
Louisiana State University
New Orleans, Louisiana

Susan M. Bashinski, EdD (Chapters 8 and 23)
Retired Interim Dean, Graduate School
Professor Emeritus of Special Education
Missouri Western State University
St. Joseph, Missouri
SMBashinski Consultancy
Kansas City, Missouri

Lisa Beccera-Walker, MS, CCC-SLP (Chapter 20)
TEAM MARIO's Voice for Kids Campaign
Edinburg, Texas

Juan Bornman, PhD (Chapter 9)
Center for Augmentative and Alternative Communication
Faculty of Humanities
University of Pretoria
Pretoria, South Africa

Barbara A. Braddock, PhD, CCC-SLP (Chapter 8)
Knights of Columbus Developmental Center
SSM Health Cardinal Glennon Children's Hospital
School of Medicine
St. Louis University
St. Louis, Missouri

Donna R. Brooks, PhD (Chapter 13)
Associate Provost, Academic Affairs
Professor, Communication Sciences and Disorders (Emeritus)
Georgia Southern University—Armstrong Campus
Savannah, Georgia

Janie Cirlot-New, MS (Chapter 10)
Director
T. K. Martin Center for Technology and Disability
Mississippi State University
Starkville, Mississippi

Russell T. Cross, DipCST (Chapter 12)
Language Systems Product Manager
PRC-Saltillo
Wooster, Ohio

Ruth Crutchfield, SLPD (Chapter 19)
Department of Communication Sciences and Disorders
The University of Texas Rio Grande Valley
Edinburg, Texas

Krista Davidson, MS, CCC-SLP (Chapters 10 and 14)
Clinical Associate Professor
Department of Communication Sciences and Disorders
The University of Iowa
Iowa City, Iowa

Aimee Dietz, PhD, CCC-SLP (Chapter 2)
Professor and Chair
Department of Communication Sciences and Disorders
Georgia State University
Atlanta, Georgia

Debora Downey, PhD (Chapter 22)
Iowa Center for Disabilities and Development
The University of Iowa
Iowa City, Iowa

Karen A. Erickson, PhD (Chapter 12)
Yoder Distinguished Professor
Director of the Center for Literacy and Disability Studies
Department of Allied Health Sciences
University of North Carolina at Chapel Hill
Chapel Hill, North Carolina

Lori A. Geist, PhD (Chapter 12)
Assistant Professor
Center for Literacy and Disability Studies
Department of Allied Health Sciences
University of North Carolina at Chapel Hill
Chapel Hill, North Carolina

Lewis Golinker, Esq (Chapter 17)
Director
Assistive Technology Law Center
Ithaca, New York

Michelle L. Gutmann, PhD, CCC-SLP (Chapters 4 and 21)
Clinical Professor
Speech, Language, & Hearing Sciences
Purdue University
West Lafayette, Indiana

Cindy Halloran, BS, OTR/L (Chapter 10)
Director
The Center for AAC and Autism
Wooster, Ohio

John Halloran, MS, CCC-SLP (Chapter 10)
Senior Clinical Associate
The Center for AAC and Autism
Wooster, Ohio

Elizabeth K. Hanson, PhD, CCC-SLP (Chapter 11)
Associate Professor and Clinical Educator
Department of Communication Sciences and Disorders
University of South Dakota
Vermillion, South Dakota

Penny Hatch, PhD (Chapter 12)
Assistant Professor
Center for Literacy and Disability Studies
Department of Allied Health Sciences
University of North Carolina at Chapel Hill
Chapel Hill, North Carolina

Amanda Hettenhausen, MA, CCC-SLP
(Chapters 10 and 14)
Director of Field Operations
PRC-Saltillo
Wooster, Ohio

Richard Hurtig, PhD, FASHA (Chapter 22)
Professor Emeritus
Department of Communication Sciences and Disorders
The University of Iowa
Iowa City, Iowa

Mick Isaacson, PhD (Chapter 1)
School of Arts, Sciences and Education
Ivy Tech Community College
Lafayette, Indiana

Rajinder Koul, PhD, CCC-SLP (Chapter 21)
Houston Harte Centennial Professor
Speech, Language, & Hearing Sciences
The University of Texas at Austin
Austin, Texas

Annette Loring, MA, CCC-SLP (Chapter 10)
Department of Speech and Hearing Sciences
Indiana University
Bloomington, Indiana

John Luna, OTD (Chapter 16)
Department of Occupational Therapy
The University of Texas Rio Grande Valley
Edinburg, Texas

Georgina Lynch, PhD (Chapter 18)
Elson S. Floyd College of Medicine
Department of Speech and Hearing Sciences
Washington State University Health Sciences
Spokane, Washington

Chitrali Mamlekar, PhD, CCC-SLP (Chapter 2)
Assistant Professor
Speech-Language Pathology Department
Misericordia University
Dallas, Pennsylvania

Samuel N. Mathew, PhD (Chapter 23)
Former Executive Director
National Institute of Speech and Hearing
Thiruvananthapuram, Kerala, India
Counselor
Deaf and Hard of Hearing
Division of Vocational Rehabilitation
Wilmington, Delaware

Miechelle McKelvey, PhD (Chapter 11)
Associate Dean and Professor of
Communication Disorders
College of Education
University of Nebraska at Kearney
Kearney, Nebraska

Katrina E. Miller, EdD, CCC-SLP (Chapter 5)
Director
Division of Communication Sciences and Disorders
Shenandoah University
K.E. Miller Enterprises
Leesburg, Virginia

Eliada Pampoulou, PhD (Chapters 3, 6, and 7)
Assistant Professor
Department of Rehabilitation Sciences
Cyprus University of Technology
Limassol, Cyprus

Erin Colone Peabody, MA (Chapter 15)
Department of Speech, Language and Hearing Sciences
Indiana University
Bloomington, Indiana

Vineetha S. Philip, PhD (Chapter 23)
Department of Audiology and Speech-Language Pathology
National Institute of Speech and Hearing
Thiruvananthapuram, Kerala, India

Jack Ruelas, OTR (Chapter 16)
Department of Occupational Therapy
The University of Texas Rio Grande Valley
Edinburg, Texas

Sayda E. Ruelas, MPT (Chapter 16)
Physical Therapy Assistant Program
Nursing and Allied Health Campus
South Texas College
McAllen, Texas

Lin Sun, MA (Chapters 10 and 15)
Department of Curriculum and Instruction
School of Education
Indiana University
Bloomington, Indiana

Gail M. Van Tatenhove, PA, MS, CCC-SLP (Chapter 18)
Private Practice
Orlando, Florida

Annalu Waller, PhD (Chapter 9)
Department of Computing
School of Science and Engineering
University of Dundee
Dundee, Scotland

Kristy S. E. Weissling, SLPD, CCC-SLP (Chapter 11)
Professor of Practice, SLP On-Campus Clinic Coordinator,
and SLP Program Director
Department of Special Education and
Communication Disorders
College of Education and Human Sciences
University of Nebraska–Lincoln
Lincoln, Nebraska

Shirley Wells, DrPH (Chapter 16)
Department of Occupational Therapy
The University of Texas Rio Grande Valley
Edinburg, Texas

Oliver Wendt, PhD (Chapter 2)
Department of Inclusive Education
College of Human Sciences
University of Potsdam
Potsdam, Brandenburg, Germany
Center for Families
Purdue University
West Lafayette, Indiana

PREFACE

What a difference a couple decades make! It is likely many of you reading this book are not aware that some of the content bound within these pages first appeared in 1997 as the textbook, *Augmentative and Alternative Communication: A Handbook of Principles and Practices*, published by Allyn and Bacon. At the time Lyle L. Lloyd, Helen Arvidson, and I coedited the book, we knew the field of augmentative and alternative communication (AAC) was changing, but we could not predict just how much the field would change in the decades that followed. We made one critical mistake, especially for the chapters that addressed technology: We included the actual voice output communication aids—an old term for what we now call speech-generating devices—that were available at the time of the book's publication. Within the span of a couple years, those chapters were outdated. With each passing year, the technology continued to advance—from the dedicated devices of the 1990s eventually to tablet and smartphone technology. Computer software morphed into applications, or "apps." As the years continued to pass, our book became even more archaic as literacy became more of a focus of AAC and new intervention approaches were developed. The book languished throughout the remainder of its run, and for good reason.

When the original book first reached the market, Lyle, Helen, and I thought we had finally created what would be the first true general textbook on AAC. There had been other books before ours—Silverman, Musselwhite and St. Louis, and Blackstone were among the first, with Beukelman and Mirenda and Glennen and DeCoste being among the "second generation" books on AAC—but in our minds, the first generation books did not cover AAC in the breadth and depth we felt was needed. The second-generation books on the market at the time were all very good, but we felt their strengths emphasized more the needs of specific populations and were not meant to be general textbooks on AAC, per se. Hence, Lyle, Helen, and I felt *Augmentative and Alternative Communication: A Handbook of Principles and Practices* arguably represented the first true general purpose textbook in the field. When the book finally ceased publication, Lyle and I decided to regain the rights to the book, update it, and publish it as a new textbook. We brought in some of the brightest academicians and clinicians around the world (see Contributing Authors) to assist in putting together what we were determined would be the finest general textbook on AAC on the market. Upon recruiting our contributors, we asked that they simply update the chapters from the original textbook. Lyle and I made a slight miscalculation: The field of AAC had changed so dramatically over the 20 years since publication of the original textbook, the majority of chapters were not only outdated but woefully so to the point practically a complete rewrite was necessary. The book you are holding in your hands today is the result of a concerted effort on the part of more than 40 people to write a book with the latest information on AAC available to date—or at least as up to date as possible considering the field is evolving quicker than any textbook could possibly keep up!

Enter our friend technology. At least some form of the technology currently evolving in the field of AAC will assist in keeping the contents of this book as updated as possible. Unlike the original textbook, this one has auxiliary materials that may be useful to faculty and students alike, such as PowerPoint files for each of the chapters instructors can use as is or modify according to their needs and preferences. Possibly the largest glossary of AAC terminology in the world is in this textbook. In addition, with future advancements in the field, we have the tools in place to provide updated information between the first and (hopefully) future editions of this book. Not only is this book available in the traditional hard copy format, but an e-book version has also been developed that is more interactive than the hard copy version. The idea is to make information about AAC, its evolution, and its scope as accessible as possible for the reader who is learning about this incredible field for the first time.

Note this textbook consists of five major parts with each part housing a number of chapters related to a specific topic. The first part is an introduction to AAC and presents general information (e.g., viewing AAC from various perspectives, terminological issues), a history of the field, the AAC model (with updated classifications of symbols and technology), and professional and multicultural issues in AAC. The second part introduces AAC symbols. It starts with an overview of AAC symbols in general and then proceeds to comprehensive discussions of aided AAC symbols, followed by unaided symbols. The third part discusses AAC technology with limited mention of specific products. The first of the two chapters in this part discusses the background, features, and principles of AAC technology, while the second provides a discussion of technological applications the reader may consider as the field of AAC assistive technology continues to evolve. The fourth part presents the components of AAC assessment—general assessment principles, vocabulary selection, symbol selection, and finally, the prescription of AAC technology. The final part is the largest of all the parts and addresses AAC intervention. The chapters in this part present the different components of the intervention process: (a) principles of intervention; (b) seating, positioning, and communication; (c) funding of speech-generating devices; (d) intervention for persons with developmental disabilities; (e) using AAC as an approach to promote literacy; (f) communication-based approaches to the management of challenging behavior; (g) intervention for persons with acquired disorders; (h) AAC in acute care settings; and finally, (i) AAC approaches for persons with sensory impairments. I am confident the reader will find this textbook to be the authoritative compendium of the full breadth and depth of AAC.

Before introducing the team of academics and clinical practitioners who contributed to this textbook, I feel there are certain acknowledgments that are in order. When I started my doctoral studies at Purdue University in 1983, it was arguably the first institution of higher education in the United States to offer a standalone course on AAC. As a student during that time, I considered myself to be among the first generation of academics who received *formal training* in AAC but the third generation of AAC experts.

It is always very difficult to acknowledge people who have contributed significantly to the field, as it is inevitable I'll likely leave out a number of persons who are worthy of acknowledgment. That said, the first generation paved the way for what eventually would become AAC at a time when very little was known about the field—in fact, there was no field! Persons such as Richard Schiefelbusch, William Stokoe, and Franklin Silverman come to mind immediately. From this first generation came the second generation of AAC experts—individuals not specifically trained in AAC but who, through early advocacy, study, and research, began to create an independent discipline that originally went by the names "nonvocal," "nonverbal," and "nonspeech" communication. The AAC community owes a debt of gratitude to such luminaries as Bruce Baker, David Beukelman, John Bonvillian, Faith Carlson, Ailsa Cregan, Macalyne Fristoe, Lewis Golinker, Richard Hurtig, Lyle L. Lloyd, Shirley McNaughton, Caroline Musselwhite, Barry Romich, Richard Steele, Gregg Vanderheiden, Beverly Vicker, Stephen von Tetzchner, and Ronnie Wilbur.

I would also like to take this opportunity to acknowledge a number of third-generation AAC specialists who have further advanced the field of AAC—persons whom I consider my contemporaries: Stephen Calculator, Sharon Glennen, Carol Goossens', Jeff Higginbotham, Rajinder Koul, Janice Light, Filip Loncke, Pat Mirenda, Mark Mizuko, Joe Reichle, Mary Ann Romski, Ralf Schlosser, Rose Sevcik, Howard Shane, Jeff Sigafoos, Hans van Balkom, and Kathryn Yorkston.

Now, the fourth generation of persons committed to the field of AAC is upon us. As the AAC family tree keeps branching out, I'll unfortunately have to dispense with naming specific individuals, but know your work is making a huge difference in the lives of persons who rely on or may benefit from AAC as their primary means of communication.

I would like to take this time to introduce to the reader the long list of academicians, advocates, and clinicians who contributed to the publication of this textbook. I cannot emphasize this strongly enough, but had it not been for the assistance of the contributors listed on the previous pages, Lyle and I never would have been able to accomplish what we set out to do a few years ago. The expertise and commitment from the 43 professionals who contributed to this book has made it what I consider an exhaustive, well-rounded, and authoritative source of information on AAC as it exists today.

This textbook was submitted to the publisher just weeks before the outbreak of the COVID-19 pandemic. At the time of submission, Lyle L. Lloyd was experiencing signs of cognitive decline that sometimes come with advanced age. I had hoped Lyle would have lived long enough to see this textbook published, but it was just not to be. With his passing, I had a greater purpose for publishing this book that extended beyond providing the most comprehensive and current information on AAC. As it turns out, this textbook represents Lyle's "swan song"—the culmination of a long career of sustained and significant contributions to the field of AAC. The completion of this textbook is my personal tribute to a man who not only instilled within me a deep love for AAC and persons who must rely on it for communication but who also taught me by example to be a better human being. Thank you, "Big Daddy." I owe my career and all the positive things that came with it to you.

—*Donald R. Fuller, PhD, CCC-SLP (Ret.), FASHA*
Professor and Chair
Department of Communication Sciences and Disorders
The University of Texas Rio Grande Valley
Edinburg, Texas

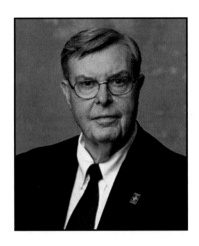

In Memoriam

Lyle L. Lloyd, PhD, CCC-A/SLP, FAAIDD, FASHA, FISAAC

He was not a member of the Corps of Volunteers for Northwest Discovery led by Lewis and Clark in the early 1800s. He was not a crew member of Apollo 11, as Neil Armstrong uttered those famous words "… one giant leap for mankind." He never explored the depths of the world's oceans aboard Jacques Cousteau's *Calypso*. However, it cannot be denied that Lyle L. Lloyd was a pioneer. In fact, some would argue he was the father of augmentative and alternative communication (AAC), although he was not alone in establishing the field. On February 12, 2020, the AAC community lost one of its founders. He lived a good, long life having passed on at age 85 years. He made every minute of his adult life meaningful with a singularity of purpose—to enhance the lives of persons with disabilities.

Lyle's story is far too consequential to be summed up in a couple paragraphs. To truly appreciate Lyle's life's work—his education, early career, involvement in the creation of AAC, contributions to training the next generations of practitioners and scientists, and his never-ending love and devotion to and advocacy for persons who require AAC to communicate to their fullest potential—one must understand the significance of the contributions he made to the field of AAC specifically and to the fields of special education and speech-language pathology peripherally as a result of his pioneering work in AAC. He was a Titan of Titans.

Relatively little is known about Lyle's childhood or his life growing up. He tended to keep his early years to himself, even to those closest to him. Despite this, one gets the impression Lyle had a drive for excellence that started early in his life. He wanted to make a difference in the world and he was going to find a way to do it.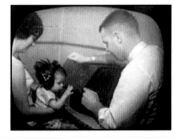

His early years aside, the story of Lyle's career began during his years as a student in higher education. He earned a Bachelor of Science degree in speech-language pathology and physical education at Eastern Illinois University in 1956 at age 22 years. A second major in physical education may seem strange to some, but one thing few people knew about Lyle was the fact he was on the football team at Eastern Illinois. Three years later, Lyle earned the Master of Arts degree in hearing and speech disorders with a minor in special education at the University of Illinois. He became dually certified in audiology and speech-language pathology and practiced both professions. His early career included service as a public school speech-language pathologist in Moweaqua, Illinois (1959-1962), an instructor in the Department of Speech Pathology and Audiology at the University of Iowa (1959-1962), an audiologist at the Constance Brown Hearing and Speech Center and an audiology instructor in the speech clinic at Western Michigan University in Kalamazoo (1962-1964), and a research associate at the Bureau of Child Research, University of Kansas, and director of audiology in the Speech and Hearing Department at Parsons State Hospital and Training Center (1964-1966). It was during these later years Lyle engaged in doctoral study at the University of Iowa. In 1965, he earned a PhD degree in audiology and speech pathology with emphasis on intellectual disability. As it shall be reinforced later in this memoriam, the seeds appeared to be firmly planted for a career involving persons with intellectual and developmental disabilities while he was in college earning his master's and doctoral degrees.

Upon conferral of the doctoral degree, Lyle was hired as an associate professor and chair of the Department of Audiology and Speech at Gallaudet College in Washington, DC (1966-1969). From there, Lyle accepted the position of health science administrator for communication disorders, National Institute of Child Health and Human Development, an office within the National Institutes of Health in Bethesda, Maryland. He held that position from 1969 until 1977.

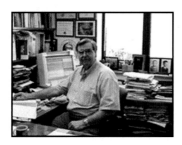

Having a background in audiology, special education, and speech-language pathology focused on persons with intellectual and developmental disabilities, as well as a penchant for procuring federal grants, Lyle was primed for what was to be his most significant contribution to the field of disability rehabilitation. In 1977, he was asked to join the faculty of Purdue University, initially as an associate professor in audiology and speech sciences (now known as speech, language, and hearing sciences). In the early 1980s, Lyle was tasked with building a special education program in the Purdue School of Humanities, Social Sciences, and Education, and served as its director. The Special Education program became part of the Department of Educational Studies and the School of Humanities, Social Sciences, and Education became the College of Education. From there Lyle held a dual appointment as full professor in special education and speech, language, and hearing sciences until his retirement in 2011. In recognition of his exemplary grant writing record, Lyle was appointed assistant director of Sponsored Programs Services within Purdue's Office of the Executive Vice President for Research and Partnerships (1988-1997). Upon retirement from Purdue, Lyle served as an adjunct professor of special education at Indiana University (2011-2017).

It was during his early years at Purdue University when what first had been called "nonspeech communication" evolved into AAC. However, it should be noted that even before nonspeech communication began to coalesce into a unified discipline, Lyle was already engaging in activities that one day would be considered pioneering work in nonspeech communication. Perhaps the most notable of these was the publication of two seminal books that, to some degree, paved the way for nonspeech communication and eventually AAC: (1) *Audiometry for the Retarded: With Implications for the Difficult-to-Test* (with R. T. Fulton, 1969) and (2) *Communication Assessment and Intervention Strategies* (1976). Lyle was a visionary. He understood the early history of what eventually would become AAC, he perceived where rehabilitation for persons with disabilities was headed, and because of his knowledge and affable nature, he developed long-term relationships with many of the earliest academicians and practitioners in rehabilitation for persons with disabilities. As nonspeech communication evolved and developed into a formal discipline, Lyle was there providing his insights and ideas.

Lyle and Macalyne Fristoe developed the first university course in AAC soon upon their arrival at Purdue University in the fall of 1977. Lyle was clearly one of a small number of people who rose to the forefront of the development of AAC as its own discipline. He began to procure professional preparation grants for special education and speech-language pathology doctoral study in AAC. In addition to these federal grants, Lyle assisted doctoral students in procuring competitive internal grants to fund their dissertation research. Two of Lyle's earliest doctoral students of note are Carol Goossens', a master practitioner in AAC, and Judith Page, former chair of the Council on Academic Accreditation and former president of the American Speech-Language-Hearing Association (ASHA).

The watershed years for AAC were 1982 to 1983. At the Second International Conference on Nonspeech Communication in 1982, an ad hoc committee, the Organization Action Committee, was formed to investigate the need to develop nonspeech communication as an independent discipline. In 1983, the committee suggested the founding of the International Society for Augmentative and Alternative Communication (ISAAC). Lyle was a member of that committee and as a result became one of the founding members of ISAAC and one of its charter members of the Board of Directors (1983-1986). The formal, interdisciplinary field of AAC was born. Within 2 years of ISAAC's founding, the society established the first international, interdisciplinary journal devoted entirely to AAC, *Augmentative and Alternative Communication*. Lyle served as the journal's editor from 1986 until 1993. During his tenure as editor, Lyle established the *Augmentative and Alternative Communication* Editorial Awards, which continue to this day.

Throughout the 1980s, Purdue University's program in AAC was rivaled only by the program at the University of Nebraska under David Beukelman. David and Lyle developed a wonderful collegial but competitive relationship that drove each other to greater heights in the development of the AAC movement, especially in terms of its research base and scholarly body of knowledge. Lyle's productivity at Purdue University was beyond impressive. Most of his scholarly work in AAC was conducted and published with doctoral (and in some cases, master's) students. This was a conscious effort on his part, as he wanted to develop the next generation of researchers to continue building the knowledge base of the field. Lyle's research and scholarly activity during his time at Purdue University included 99 peer-reviewed journal articles in 29 of the most prestigious national and international journals in audiology, AAC, psycholinguistics, rehabilitation, special education, and speech-language pathology; 28 conference abstracts, proceedings, or reports; 25 book chapters or updated editions of chapters; and 17 books or newer editions of books. One book particularly was directly related to AAC.

Lyle was senior editor (with Helen Arvidson and myself as junior editors) of the textbook *Augmentative and Alternative Communication: A Handbook of Principles and Practices* (1997). Three weeks before his passing, he and I submitted a complete manuscript for what may likely be the most comprehensive textbook in AAC ever to be published. This book is Lyle's final contribution to the field he loved so much.

In addition to his publications, Lyle gave more than 100 oral and poster presentations at the national level at numerous conferences and conventions, such as ASHA, the American Association on Intellectual and Developmental Disabilities, the Council for Exceptional Children, and the Clinical AAC Research Conference. In addition to his national presentations, Lyle made over 75 presentations at international conferences, such as the Biennial Conference of ISAAC, Congress of the International Association for the Scientific Study of Intellectual Disability, and Congress of the International Association of Logopedics and Phoniatrics.

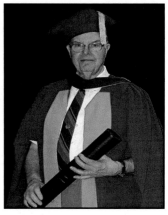

Lyle's presentations did not stop at just international and national professional meetings. His expertise and knowledge were sought by both American and foreign universities. For example, in the United States, he provided invited lectures at Hofstra University, Howard University, Oklahoma State University, Syracuse University, University of Alabama, University of New Mexico, University of Notre Dame, and University of Vermont. Internationally, Lyle was invited to give presentations at institutions of higher education and other facilities in Canada, China, England, France, Germany, Ireland, Portugal, Scotland, South Africa, Spain, Sweden, Switzerland, Taiwan, The Netherlands, United Arab Emirates, and Wales. Most noteworthy was the relationship Lyle had with the Centre for Augmentative and Alternative Communication at the University of Pretoria (South Africa). Not only did Lyle travel there many times to give lectures, but he was invited to serve as an external member for approximately 15 doctoral dissertation committees. His strong collaborative relationship with this institution culminated in Lyle being conferred an honorary doctorate in 2006.

As previously mentioned, Lyle was a prolific grant writer. While on faculty at Purdue University, Lyle had 39 research and scholarly activity grants funded from such agencies as the National Institutes of Health, National Science Foundation, Office of Special Education Programs, and Office of Special Education and Rehabilitative Services. In addition, he successfully wrote 19 external personnel preparation grants and 10 internal grants to support the research of his doctoral students. He was awarded four international travel grants and one grant through the South African Human Sciences Council.

Lyle's service contributions are far too numerous to list, so only positions of leadership and activities of considerable significance are mentioned here: (1) Founding Member of SIG #12: AAC of ASHA; (2) President of the District of Columbia Speech and Hearing Association; (3) Governor, President, Vice President, and Treasurer of the Council for Exceptional Children; (4) President, Senior Vice President, and Secretary-Treasurer of the Purdue University Chapter of The Society of Sigma Xi; (5) Founding Member, Charter Member of the Board of Directors, Vice President for Publications, Member of the Executive Committee of ISAAC; (6) Chair and Vice-Chair of the Speech-Language Pathology and Audiology Professional Specialty Group of the Rehabilitation Engineering and Assistive Technology Society of North America; (7) Founding Member of the United States Society for Augmentative and Alternative Communication; and (8) Founding Member of the Indiana Chapter of the United States Society for Augmentative and Alternative Communication. Lyle also provided professional consultation services for agencies, institutions, and organizations in 13 states in the United States and seven foreign nations. He was an expert witness on intellectual disability and deafness in Jane Doe v. District of Columbia et al. (1987-1988), served as a reviewer for the Office of Special Education and Rehabilitative Services grants for 20 years between 1988 and 2008, and provided peer reviews for eight ASHA position papers, guidelines, and technical reports on such topics as AAC, intellectual and developmental disabilities, facilitated communication, assistive technology in the schools, AAC knowledge and skills, and the speech-language pathology scope of practice. Lyle was instrumental in the decision of the Council on Academic Accreditation and Council for Clinical Certification to change "communication modalities" to "augmentative and alternative communication" as one of the Big 9 areas of clinical practice for preprofessional education in speech-language pathology in the United States. Finally, Lyle helped establish the Edwin and Esther Prentke AAC Distinguished Lecture in 1997.

Throughout his career, Lyle received several honors and accolades. He was a Fellow of the American Association on Intellectual and Developmental Disabilities, ASHA, and ISAAC. He earned Honors of ASHA and Council for Exceptional Children Division for Children with Communication Disorders. Lyle earned the President's Award from ISAAC twice and its Distinguished Service Award once. He earned ASHA's Certificate of Appreciation four times. He was a Fulbright-Hays Senior Research Scholar in 1984 and earned a National Institutes of Health Travel Award in 1985. Lyle was awarded the first Distinguished Alumni Award from the Department of Communication Disorders at Eastern Illinois University. He was chosen Outstanding Graduate Faculty Mentor, College of Education at Purdue University in 2006. Finally, Lyle was appointed to the position of Distinguished Professor (2003-2005) and then was conferred an Honorary Doctorate (2006) from the University of Pretoria.

Over the course of his 34 years at Purdue University, Lyle mentored 39 doctoral students. Of considerable note was the fact that many of his doctoral students were international students (at least 10, and the actual number may be even higher). Lyle was a very strong advocate for training the next generation of AAC researchers both nationally and internationally. Some of his former doctoral students are now among the premiere researchers in the field (e.g., Rajinder Koul,

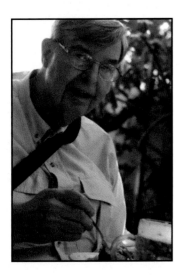

Ralf Schlosser), master practitioners/educators (e.g., Carol Goossens'), and inventors/ entrepreneurs (e.g., Ravi Nigam, Oliver Wendt). Several either served or are currently serving as administrators in higher education (e.g., Kathleen Kangas, Rajinder Koul, Judith Page, Ralf Schlosser, myself). These individuals and many others not mentioned here are carrying on Lyle's legacy and are developing the next generation of AAC academicians and practitioners. Lyle's influence on the AAC community will be felt for a very long time.

What can people say of another person's life once they have passed over into eternity? Perhaps the ultimate question is, "What was their legacy?" In other words, did they change the world for the better during their short existence? For Lyle L. Lloyd, the answer to that question is crystal clear. Lyle departed this world leaving a legacy that will live on as long as human beings continue to face the challenges of disability. Lyle loved humanity; he loved imparting knowledge to his students, to other professionals, and to those in positions of authority to affect change benefitting persons with disabilities. He loved the movement he helped to create and loved watching it evolve from a loosely bound entity into a highly organized discipline that transcends professional boundaries. He loved life, his family, his profession. Just as he played the game of football as a young college student, in his professional life, he left it all out on the field.

No doubt, 50 years from now after most of us have left this world and newer generations carry on the practice of speech-language pathology, the name Lyle L. Lloyd will be among the pantheon of significant change agents of the field, along with luminaries such as Sara Stinchfield, Lee Edward Travis, Charles Van Riper, and Robert West.

With deepest gratitude from all of us who knew you and from those whose lives you changed for the better who never may have known you: Farewell, Lyle L. Lloyd!

—*Donald R. Fuller, PhD, CCC-SLP (Ret.), FASHA*
Professor and Chair
Department of Communication Sciences and Disorders
The University of Texas Rio Grande Valley
Edinburg, Texas

Part I
Introduction to AAC

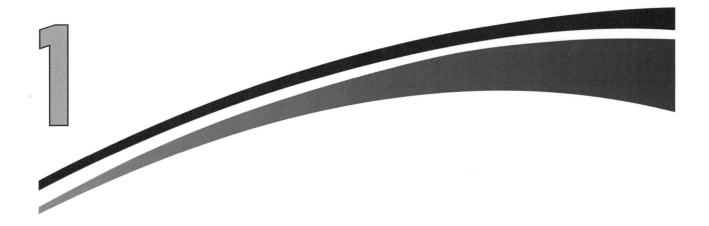

Introduction and Overview

*Donald R. Fuller, PhD; Mick Isaacson, PhD;
and Lyle L. Lloyd, PhD*

MYTH

1. **Augmentative and alternative communication (AAC)** is only used by people who cannot communicate effectively by means of speech.
2. The primary goal of communication is to express wants and needs.
3. Using AAC will prevent or delay speech development.
4. We should wait to use AAC until a person is ready for it.
5. We should not overwhelm the AAC user with access to too many symbols.
6. Somebody who has a **speech-generating device (SGD)** should use it all the time.
7. An AAC system should be a goal for all people who are nonspeaking.

REALITY

1. AAC can be used by a wide variety of communicators. Many augment verbal communication with gestures, facial expressions, and so forth. AAC is not only used by people who do not have functional speech but is also useful for children with delayed speech development and is becoming more commonly used with people who are learning a second language.

2. For most, expressing wants and needs is secondary to social expression. One way to think of this is to put oneself into the position of a person who uses AAC. If you could only say three things, would they be, "I need to go to the toilet," "I'm hungry," and "I'm thirsty," or would they be, "Hi, how are you?" "Can we talk?" and "I love you"? This is not to say that being able to control your environment is not important, but it may not be the most important thing an individual who uses AAC wishes to convey.

3. Studies show that the use of AAC may improve speech development (Silverman, 1995), and it can be argued that it may improve language development as well. It should be noted that even the most sophisticated SGD cannot be as efficient as natural speech.

(continued)

INTRODUCTION

It often has been said that communication is the essence of life. One can see it when an individual glances or gestures to share feelings with a family member or lectures to a large audience. These two major purposes of communication—socialization and information transfer—can be accomplished

Fuller, D. R., & Lloyd, L. L. *Principles and Practices in
Augmentative and Alternative Communication* (pp. 3-28).
© 2023 Taylor & Francis Group.

> ## REALITY (CONTINUED)
>
> 4. Anybody can use AAC. We do not wait to communicate verbally with a typical child until they are ready to talk; rather, we surround them with a wealth of language. The same can be said for a child who uses AAC. We should not wait to introduce other methods of communication until they are ready to use them; rather, we should surround them with a wealth of language (verbally, gesturally, or symbolically based).
>
> 5. We should provide more symbols than a child can use at one time. Again, if we look at typically developing children, they have access to all the sounds of their language by 6 months of age. They use them appropriately when they are able to. The same can be said for symbol communication. If a child is not provided with more symbols than those to which they have mastered, they will not have the opportunity to practice new symbols in a natural progression.
>
> 6. SGDs are often vital components of a person's AAC system. It is true that they should have access to their device all the time (or almost all the time), but there are times when it is not practical or necessary. For example, using an SGD in the bath is not a good idea. Communication by its nature is multimodal; for example, there are many people who use SGDs in most situations, but not at home with their family.
>
> 7. The goal is to have functional communication. An AAC system may be a useful tool for that purpose. This distinction, while subtle, can help tremendously toward setting appropriate goals for a student.

by individuals with a wide range of abilities and disabilities, not only through natural speech and writing, but also through AAC. In recent years, AAC—the supplementation or replacement of natural speech and/or writing—has allowed many individuals with disabilities to more fully realize their potential.

AAC is described in this text as being a process. The term is also used to refer to the transdisciplinary field that uses a variety of symbols, strategies, technologies, and techniques to assist people who are unable to meet their communication needs through natural speech and/or writing. The defining characteristic that places all these symbols, strategies, technologies, and techniques under the category of AAC is that they are not essential for most able-bodied individuals to meet their communication needs of daily life (i.e., for able-bodied people, speech is the primary mode of communication; other modes of communication may be used by these individuals but are not essential, as in most situations, speech alone will suffice).

In general, AAC symbols and techniques may be divided into two broad categories—**aided communication** and **unaided communication** (Lloyd & Fuller, 1986). Aided communication involves use of some external device or equipment that may range from very simple handmade materials, such as a picture board or wallet, to highly complex electronic devices that produce computer-generated speech. Unaided communication requires no additional pieces of equipment; the individual's own body is used to communicate. One of the most common examples of unaided AAC is manual signing. Gesturing, miming, pointing, and eye gazing are also unaided means of communication.

AAC PERSPECTIVES

AAC may be viewed from many perspectives, including those of persons who use AAC, as well as assessment, etiological, historic, intervention, legal and ethical, psychological, technological, theoretical, transdisciplinary, and visionary. These perspectives are not mutually exclusive but are rather interconnected and interrelated. This chapter provides an overview of each of these perspectives. Because of its overriding importance, the perspective of the user is used throughout the entire textbook.

Etiological Perspectives of Persons Who Use AAC

A number of individuals who use AAC and who have been recipients of professional services have provided access to their viewpoints (e.g., Creech, 1992; Sienkiewicz-Mercer & Kaplan, 1989). These reports have important, although sometimes painful, messages regarding communication. Huer and Lloyd (1990) found that frustration was a particularly common theme expressed by persons who use or must rely on AAC. Frustration seems to be very common among individuals with severe communication disabilities.

> I can remember those silent years when my mind was overflowing with questions that were not being answered: remembering the want to verbalize my thoughts, dreams, and hopes, and desiring to share and grow in my world. Life began turning into a room with many windows and a door without a key. (Marshall, 1990, p. 5)

According to Huer and Lloyd (1990), concerns expressed about professional services included lack of knowledge about severe disabilities and lack of concern or respect for the client as an individual, including the practices of educational, medical, and speech-language pathology professionals. Most of the users who commented on their devices reported that the devices themselves were valuable, but they continued to believe that communication, not the use of the device, is the key.

> I had a few speech teachers. Every speech teacher had their own way of doing things. I was confused. One would say do it this way and another would say do it another way. The last speech teacher I had in elementary school said, 'Okay it's time for a Canon,' but the one I had before she came said, 'Use speech.' . . .
>
> [T]he speech teacher did ask me if I liked it [the Canon] and I said, 'No,' but she said, 'Hang in there; it's not going to be overnight.' Most of the time nobody asked. And, if they did, it didn't seem to make them change anything. (Dawn, in Smith-Lewis & Ford, 1987, pp. 15-16)

AAC interventions offer valuable options for persons with severe disabilities when individual strengths and needs are carefully assessed and appropriate goals are established. Understanding the etiology of communication disorders is basic to the provision of AAC services. Significant differences exist; for example, between goals developed for children whose communication disorders result from congenital conditions and goals developed for adults who have acquired communication disorders (e.g., AAC options may become broader in the former case but more limited in the latter). These differences relate to a variety of aspects, such as the relationship of caregivers to AAC users. Parents often take the major role in directly providing or arranging care and services for their children with congenital conditions, whereas spouses and/or adult children often take the major role in providing or arranging care and services for individuals with acquired disorders, especially later in life. Service providers must be sensitive to the impact these different relationships can have on the intervention process and use different approaches, as appropriate, with the different caregivers who will be facilitating the communication of AAC users.

Whether a condition is congenital or acquired may affect a user's level of acceptance or resistance to AAC intervention. Providing functional and motivational intervention is enough to engage some individuals in interactions that will quite naturally lead to improved communication, but may not engage others. Individuals with acquired, progressive disorders, for example, may be dealing with psychological and emotional factors that challenge intervention. Individuals with progressive diseases, such as multiple sclerosis or Parkinson's disease, may not realize the need to develop AAC skills until the disease has progressed to the point that learning new ways to communicate requires more energy and effort than they can expend. Providing services for individuals with acquired, nonprogressive conditions, such as traumatic brain injury, that affect language and memory skills still poses different challenges and underscores the importance of knowing and respecting individual needs and desires.

Individuals with little or no functional speech usually have related impairments in language, memory, cognition, hearing, vision, and/or motor skills that must be carefully assessed and addressed. Intervention must be approached with a clear understanding of individual strengths and needs. However, individuals do not live in a vacuum. Needs will be influenced by the environments in which individuals live and the people with whom they interact. These influences must be considered carefully if intervention is to be effective.

The perspective of AAC users is of paramount importance in the provision of AAC services. Their needs and desires regarding the direction of the intervention process should be respected. Their rights should be protected. The **American Speech-Language-Hearing Association** approved guidelines developed by the National Joint Committee for the Communication Needs of Persons with Severe Disabilities (Brady et al., 2016), which included a Communication Bill of Rights consisting of 15 rights designed to enhance the ability of individuals to affect conditions of their own existence through communication. This Communication Bill of Rights can be seen in Figure 1-1.

Historic Perspectives

The importance for researchers and clinicians/educators to have a solid historic perspective of their field should not be underestimated. AAC is a maturing and rapidly advancing transdisciplinary field with roots in a number of different scientific and technical fields, but it is an independent professional and scholarly field that has emerged with its own **models**, **classification systems**, and research base.

The second editor of this textbook was active in the early development of the field and had a long-standing interest in its historic perspective. He and others contributed to the literature on this historic perspective (e.g., Galyas et al., 1993; Lloyd, 1986, 1993; Lloyd & Karlan, 1984; McNaughton, 1990; Vanderheiden & Yoder, 1986; Zangari et al., 1994). Chapter 2 discusses the historic perspective in greater detail.

Theoretical Perspectives

Establishing a Framework for AAC

The theoretical perspective of AAC will be discussed in greater depth in Chapter 3. For now, this perspective evolved from an understanding of the human communication model proposed by Sanders (1976, 1982). Minor adjustments, such as the **AAC processes and interface** modifications proposed by Lloyd and colleagues (1990), are based on a classification system using aided and unaided as the starting point of the classification structure (see also Lloyd & Fuller, 1986). This structure is applicable to the **means to represent**, the **means to select**, and the **means to transmit**, which in turn has implications for the interaction process and the important transmission and communication environments of the Lloyd and colleagues (1990) AAC model.

Use of the aided vs. unaided taxonomy was further developed by Fuller and colleagues (1992) with subordinate classification dimensions of static vs. dynamic, iconic vs. opaque, and set vs. system aspects of AAC symbols as the means to represent (i.e., symbols). In the latter part of this chapter we will discuss the need for changes to this classification scheme due to the evolution of the AAC field over the past few decades.

Educational/Clinical Theory

AAC emerged from clinical/educational practice (with little or no research base) out of the need to provide services for individuals who had not benefited from traditional speech therapy. In the 1970s, after anecdotal reports of success with AAC strategies and techniques began to appear, interest in

National Joint Committee for the Communication Needs of Persons
With Severe Disabilities (NJC)

COMMUNICATION BILL OF RIGHTS

All people with a disability of any extent or severity have a basic right to affect, through communication, the conditions of their existence. Beyond this general right, a number of specific communication rights should be ensured in all daily interactions and interventions involving persons who have severe disabilities. To participate fully in communication interactions, each person has these fundamental communication rights:

1.   The right to interact socially, maintain social closeness, and build relationships

2.   The right to request desired objects, actions, events, and people

3.   The right to refuse or reject undesired objects, actions, events, or choices

4.   The right to express personal preferences and feelings

5.   The right to make choices from meaningful alternatives

6.   The right to make comments and share opinions

7.   The right to ask for and give information, including information about changes in routine and environment

8.   The right to be informed about people and events in one's life

9.   The right to access interventions and supports that improve communication

10. The right to have communication and acts acknowledged and responded to even when the desired outcome cannot be realized

11. The right to have access to functioning AAC (augmentative and alternative communication) and other AT (assistive technology) services and devices at all times

12. The right to access environmental contexts, interactions, and opportunities that promote participation as full communication partners with other people, including peers

13. The right to be treated with dignity and addressed with respect and courtesy

14. The right to be addressed directly and not be spoken for or talked about in the third person while present

15. The right to have clear, meaningful, and culturally and linguistically appropriate communications

Figure 1-1. The 2016 Communication Bill of Rights. (Reproduced with permission from Brady, N. C., Bruce, S., Goldman, A., Erickson, K., Mineo, B., Ogletree, B. T., Paul, D., Romski, M. A., Sevcik, R., Siegel, E., Schoonover, J., Snell, M., Sylvester, L., & Wilkinson, K. [2016]. Communication services and supports for individuals with severe disabilities: Guidance for assessment and intervention. *American Journal on Intellectual and Developmental Disabilities, 121*[2], 121-138.)

understanding why AAC was successful when more traditional approaches failed became more widespread. Fristoe and Lloyd (1979a) hypothesized 16 factors and characteristics that could account for the facilitative effects reported in the literature. These factors, identified more from clinical/educational observation than research, are based on consideration of AAC as both a stimulus mode and a response medium. Lloyd and Karlan (1984) modified and arranged these factors and characteristics into six groups with general descriptors added for conceptual clarity. With minor rewording

(to update terminology), Lloyd and Kangas (1994) summarized the underlying factors and characteristics of AAC as follows:

1.   *General simplification of input.* The information presented to the individual when in an AAC form is simplified in both context and manner of presentation. This simplification, which presumably facilitates processing and hence understanding of communicative messages, is accomplished in two ways:

A. *Verbiage (noise) is reduced.* When speech and AAC symbols are simultaneously presented, irrelevant or parenthetical words or comments are eliminated from the clinician's speech. AAC allows one to "get to the heart" of the message. For example, in using **aided language stimulation** with a child who is learning to use AAC, the clinician might point to symbols for YOU, HUNGRY, and EAT and say, "You look hungry. Would you like to eat lunch now?" The learner then concentrates on the meaning of the symbols without regard to grammatical correctness.

B. *Rate is adjustable.* When AAC symbols, such as manual signs or graphic symbols, are presented simultaneously with speech, the rate of presentation is slowed, allowing more processing time. Even the most experienced users of manual sign, for example, slow their rate when signing and speaking so it can be expected that trainers who are less experienced with AAC symbol use would slow their presentation rate even more.

2. *Response production advantages.* Four advantages have been identified that relate to the training of expressive language responding and actual production:

A. *Pressure for speech is removed.* It is apparent with some persons with **autism spectrum disorder** or other **developmental disabilities**—especially those capable of some limited, though often barely intelligible, speech production—that parents or others exert great pressure on them to speak. Because expected performance may exceed capacity or readiness to produce speech, the pressure may become detrimental to further speech and language development. AAC symbols provide alternative modes by which messages can be sent, thus relieving the pressure on speech production.

B. *Physical demands are decreased.* The motor acts necessary to produce a response with AAC are far less complex than those required for spoken responding. With unaided symbols, the motor coordination required for manual sign or gestural production, while seemingly complex, is still far simpler than that required for phonation and articulation. Aided symbols, because they are typically graphic and not produced at the time of the response, require only a means to select (i.e., they require an indicating response, not a producing response).

C. *Physical manipulation of the response is possible.* Just as difficulty of response production is decreased when AAC symbols are employed, so is the difficulty of actual physical manipulation by the trainer. Although it is possible to physically guide the individual in producing an oral response, it is quite arduous. The far greater ability of the trainer to physically guide either the formation of manual or gestural responses or the selection of graphic symbols undoubtedly adds greatly to more rapid acquisition of AAC as compared to speech.

D. *Clinician's observation of shaping is facilitated.* With the exception of synthetic speech, the visual modality in which AAC symbols occurs facilitates the trainer's judgment of how close attempts at response production are coming to criterion. Analysis of the characteristics and topography of approximations to desired production requires far less training and technical background than an analysis of oral responses.

3. *Advantages for individuals with severe intellectual impairment.* For individuals exhibiting severe intellectual deficits, use of AAC symbols has some particular features or consequences that might contribute to the acquisition of AAC. Two of these include:

A. *Vocabulary is limited and functional.* The vocabulary is kept small, often as a consequence of training trainers and parents to use and understand the symbol forms. Lexical items selected for representation with AAC symbols are more broadly functional to the user, such as "drink," "play," "no," and "more." In this fashion, conceptual rather than syntactic learning is emphasized.

B. *Individual's attention is easier to maintain.* With visually presented and produced symbols (e.g., graphic symbols, manual signs), evaluation and hence maintenance of attention can be done through assessment of eye contact or direction of gaze. Visible evaluation of attention to auditory/oral symbols is considerably more difficult if not impossible.

4. *Receptive language/auditory processing advantages.* The employment of AAC symbols has direct advantageous effects on the comprehension of language and auditory processing, which in turn affects comprehension of communicative messages. The two apparent causes for these effects reflect different levels of comprehension and include the following:

A. *Structure of language input is simplified.* When AAC symbols are presented concurrently with spoken symbols, the full syntactic structure of the spoken message is often not represented by the AAC symbols. The AAC symbols often represent only the semantically relevant or meaningful information in the message, thus highlighting what is crucial to comprehend.

B. *Auditory short-term memory and/or auditory processing problems are minimized.* Because of their visual modality, AAC symbols may bypass the auditory modality and thus eliminate any particularly pronounced auditory processing deficits that may exist.

5. *Stimulus processing/stimulus association advantages.* Again, because they are produced or displayed primarily in the visual modality, AAC symbols in communication have certain advantages for the processing of visual symbol stimuli or for the development of associations between visual symbols and their referents. These include the following:

A. *Figure-ground differential is enhanced.* The visual nature of most symbols may help to differentiate the figure from the ground with respect to the communicatively salient information from the contextual background. Auditory symbols may not be as easy to differentiate from the ambient background of noise.

B. *Stimulus consistency is optimized.* Visual symbols appear to have greater consistency in representation and production than do auditory/oral symbols (e.g., most graphic symbols are static and permanent whereas the acoustic signal of speech is ever-changing). With manual signs or gestures, especially at slow rates, contextual or coproduction influences are minimal compared with speech where contextual and coarticulatory influences may greatly affect what the listener perceives as the same or different phonemes or words. Certainly, aided symbols have an even greater consistency because they are selected rather than formed (with the exception of handwritten symbols) on each occasion.

C. *Temporal duration is greater.* The temporal duration of the presentation of most AAC symbols is greater than that occurring for natural speech symbols with the exception of synthetic speech and tactile analogs of speech. This duration can be adjusted to be even longer without altering what the individual perceives to be the form of the stimulus. This is a special advantage for individuals who require greater orientation, perception, and processing time for stimulus presentations. The presentation of AAC symbols can be adjusted easily without loss of relevance or information value. Graphic symbols have the added advantage of permanency in contrast to acoustic/auditory symbols.

D. *Modality consistency is facilitated.* A unimodal rather than cross-modal relationship exists between most AAC symbols and visual referents. Being visual in modality, AAC symbols are more easily associated with visual referents than are speech symbols, which exist in a separate (i.e., oral/auditory) modality. Learning that a symbol represents a referent may be easier when both exist in the same stimulus mode (i.e., the object and the symbol for that object are both visual). In addition, the temporal characteristics of the stimulus and referent can be more easily matched when the relationship is unimodal.

6. *Symbolic representational advantages.* Another aspect of symbols that can help to explain the facilitative effects AAC symbols have on communication development is the amount and type of information conveyed within the symbol itself and the use to which it is put. Two possibilities follow:

A. *Supplemental representation is possible.* When used simultaneously with speech, AAC symbols supplement the representational input of the speech symbols. Anecdotal reports indicate this supplementation has led, with some individuals, to accelerated development of both speech comprehension and production. The success of this supplementation is possibly the result of a type of representation found within certain AAC symbols themselves.

B. *Visual representation is possible.* AAC symbols, such as photographs, graphic symbols, and certain manual signs among others, contain visual representations of the referents within the symbols. This representational characteristic has been referred to as **iconicity**; the iconicity of symbols varies but where greater iconicity exists, meaning, memory, and/or concept visualization can be facilitated (Lloyd & Kangas, 1994, pp. 630-634).

Clinicians and educators should consider factors such as these in selecting AAC assessment and intervention strategies and evaluating outcomes, remembering that the preceding factors are based primarily on clinical/educational observation with limited research, none of the hypothesized factors is applicable to every AAC user, and more applied and basic research to test these hypothesized factors (i.e., careful empirical investigation) is needed to establish the role and relative contribution of each factor. Although more is known now than when Fristoe and Lloyd (1979a) hypothesized these factors—especially about iconicity—establishing the relative contributions of the factors and the relationships among them would clarify greatly the directions that could be taken in developing facilitative AAC strategies and techniques.

Psychological Perspective

AAC is focused on improving communication, which involves processing of information. There are many factors that may impact communicative information processing. Developing an understanding of the processes that may be involved in communication and parameters that may influence these processes will provide AAC professionals with knowledge that should increase their capacity for improving communication. This section addresses cognitive information processing and other basic psychological issues that may be important for improving AAC.

Communication and Information Processing

A communicative interaction typically involves information processing consisting of reception of information through the senses, transport of the sensory information to higher-level cognitive processing areas of the brain, processing of the information received by the higher level cognitive areas, and the output of a response.

Cognitive information processing is often portrayed as occurring in stages. An early stage theory was proposed by Atkinson and Shiffrin (1968). The essence of their model is shown in Figure 1-2. Information flows from the external sensory environment to a *sensory* memory stage and then to a short-term memory stage. Conscious processing and motor responses are believed to occur in short-term memory. Processing might also involve connections with long-term memory.

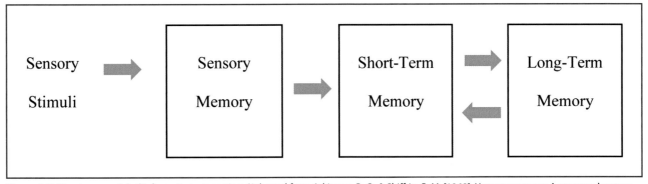

Figure 1-2. The stage model of information processing. (Adapted from Atkinson, R. C., & Shiffrin, R. M. [1968]. Human memory: A proposed system and its control processes. In K. W. Spence & J. T. Spence [Eds.], *The psychology of learning and motivation* [Vol. 2, pp. 89–195]. Academic Press.)

Information flow between short-term and long-term memory is two-way. As shown in Figure 1-2, information can flow from short-term memory into long-term memory or in the reverse direction from long-term memory to short-term memory. The process of putting information into long-term memory is a storage process that is sometimes known as **encoding**. Getting information out of long-term memory and into short-term memory is a retrieval process called **decoding**. Long-term memory content is believed to last a lifetime.

The Atkinson and Shiffrin (1968) model served as the foundation for subsequent models, such as the working memory model proposed by Baddeley and Hitch (1974), who believed that the Atkinson and Shiffrin model was too simplistic. They added details primarily to the short-term component. Subsequent updates to their model retain the major aspects of the 1974 iteration. A brief overview of the major changes made by Baddeley and Hitch (1974) is summarized in Table 1-1. In their model, short-term memory is known as working memory, which has been expanded to include two memory stores: a **phonological store** and a **visual-spatial store**. The phonological store is believed to work with spoken and written material that is in a phonological or verbal form. An articulatory control process that rehearses verbal information in the phonological store was also proposed. Information in a visual and/or spatial form is processed in the visual-spatial store. This store may play a role in navigation. The central executive was another major feature that was added. In short, according to the model, the central executive controls the processes occurring in working memory. For example, it is believed to be involved in the allocation of resources to the phonological and visual-spatial stores.

Characteristics of the Stages

Sensory Memory. Sensory stimuli enter into a sensory memory (sometimes known as a sensory buffer or register). If attention is focused on content in the sensory memory, then it may be transported to the next stage, short-term or working memory. Decay is an important characteristic of sensory memory. The decay rate for sensory memory is very short (only a few seconds at most). *Information in sensory*

TABLE 1-1

Modifications Made by Baddeley and Hitch (1974) to the Atkinson and Shiffrin (1968) Cognitive Information Processing Model

1. Short-term memory is now known as working memory, presumably because processing in the form of cognitive or mental work is occuring in this stage.

2. The addition of two finite capacity storage systems (i.e., a phonological store and a visual-spatial store).

3. The addition of an articulatory control mechanism for the rehearsal of verbal information.

4. The addition of the central executive that controls processing and allocation of resources.

memory must make it to the next stage of short-term memory before it decays. Focused attention on the content in sensory memory is believed to facilitate transport to the next stage, short-term memory.

Short-Term Memory. This memory is sometimes known as active memory probably because it is believed to involve conscious active processing of information. This memory has a finite capacity. Similar to the sensory buffers, information in short-term memory will also decay but it will take longer to do so. An important feature of short-term memory is rehearsal, which is an active process involving repeating content over and over. *Rehearsal is important for preventing decay.*

Working Memory. In the Baddeley and Hitch (1974) model, short-term memory is known as working memory. The Baddeley and Hitch model expanded short-term memory to include two finite memory stores that are particular for the type of information that is stored: a phonological store and a visual-spatial store. They also added a feature called the central executive that is supposed to control processing within the working memory, such as allocation of resources to the phonological and visual-spatial stores. These additions to short-term memory are summarized next.

1. *The phonological store.* This component of short-term memory deals primarily with spoken or written material as added by Baddeley and Hitch (1974). An articulartory control process is used to manipulate information in the phonological store. Rehearsal of verbal material is a common articulatory control process that involves an active process of repeating content over and over. Reheasal is a process that refreshes information and keeps it from decaying. In addition, rehearsal is believed to be involved in the storage of information in long-term memory. This process may be linked to the internal dialog or inner voice that seems to be a part of our active conscious stream of thought. Rehearsal is believed to keep verbal information from fading from memory and may play a role in long-term storage. This store and processes may be related to speech perception and production.

2. *The visual-spatial store.* This memory is believed to contain information concerning visual images and spatial relationships. This store is believed to be important for construction of mental maps and navigation.

3. *The central executive.* This component has been delegated to control the allocation of resources to both short-term stores (phonological and visual-spatial), in addition to other processing issues, such as directing attention to content in the sensory buffers. Despite having a central role in controlling short-term information storage and processing, this component is one of the least understood aspects of the memory system.

Long-Term Memory. This memory store is believed to last a lifetime. Processing of information does not occur within this store. Information within this store needs to be retrieved into the short-term working store for it to be involved in active cognitive processes.

Potentially Important Issues

Attention and Transport From Sensory to Short-Term Working Memory. Attention to stimuli in sensory memory is believed to be important for transportation to the next stage of processing, short-term memory. Transport to the short-term memory stage may be critical for conscious awareness and processing. As communication involves conscious information processing, it is important for communicative content to be transported into this stage.

AAC Implications

It is important to understand characteristics of AAC stimuli and associated processing issues that may direct attention. Such an understanding may be valuable for the development of AAC stimuli and strategies that maximize transport from the sensory memory stage to the short-term memory stage.

Cognitive Load. Capacity issues are a potential concern for information processing, particularly those involving the short-term working memory stage. Cognitive load can be conceived as the amount of strain that is exerted on memory processing components by the content being processed.

AAC Implications

The short-term memory load of AAC stimuli is an under-researched area in AAC. Processing may deteriorate as capacity limitations are approached. Hence, AAC should attempt to minimize cognitive load. This could have a positive influence on communicative information processing. Overlearning is a procedure that may promote the development of automaticity and reduce cognitive load.

Overlearning and Automaticity. Practicing a task even after achieving a performance criterion of 100% accuracy is known as overlearning. Automaticity is a state in which a task can be performed with little or no conscious processing. This type of processing is believed to exert little influence on the memory systems involved in cognitive processes and may contribute to communicative fluency.

AAC Implications

It may be beneficial for AAC professionals to develop and implement overlearning paradigms to enhance AAC fluency. Examples of overlearning are the use of drill and practice procedures with flash cards to promote overlearning of basic math facts or referents for pictorial renderings of objects, concepts, etc. It should be relatively easy to develop overlearning procedures for AAC stimuli. For example, many people enjoy competing against themselves. An overlearning procedure could be used as the basis for self-competition. Once a stable level of 100% accuracy has been achieved, the procedure could be switched to emphasize both accuracy and speed. With each successive trial, the objective would be to achieve an accurate score with a faster response than the previous trial. With some ingenuity and computer expertise, it should be possible to develop computerized programs to increase speed and fluency.

AAC Selection Techniques and Cognitive Load. Short-term memory (also known as working memory) is believed to have a finite capacity. It is unclear as to the load AAC imposes on capacity. Reducing load may facilitate communicative processes.

AAC Implications

Because of capacity limitations, AAC professionals should strive to use AAC stimuli and techniques that place the smallest load on processing as possible. This includes all aspects of processing, not just stimulus properties. To illustrate, different techniques exist for the selection of AAC stimuli. The load imposed on the processing system may depend on the selection technique. Research (e.g., Wagner & Jackson, 2006) indicates memory for graphic symbols is poorer with selection techniques that use scanning compared to selection techniques that use direct selection. For additional details on selection techniques, please see Chapter 9. More research concerning how AAC influences memory and processing is needed.

Cognitive Representations of AAC Stimuli. According to the Baddeley and Hitch (1974) model, short-term working memory includes two types of store. One is for visual-spatial information and the other is for phonological information. It is unclear as to the form taken by AAC stimuli when they enter working memory. To illustrate, many types of AAC use graphic pictorial representations for words and concepts. Are these types of AAC processed in the visual-spatial or the phonological component?

AAC Implications

A better understanding of the cognitive representations of AAC could be instrumental for improving the communicative efficaciousness of AAC stimuli. A potential research project that addresses the above question arises from the *word length effect* in which memory is better for shorter words compared to longer words (Baddeley et al., 1975). This phenomenon has been attributed to longer words taking up more of the capacity of the phonological component of short-term working memory than shorter words. A similar finding with picture-based AAC symbols would be consistent with the notion that picture-based symbols might be processed as verbal or phonological material.

Rehearsal. A conscious process in which verbal information is repeated over and over is known as *rehearsal*. This process keeps information from fading from memory and may be involved in long-term storage.

AAC Implications

It is difficult to imagine how visually based pictorial information found in AAC could be rehearsed; however, sign language involves visual-spatial stimuli and presumably a similar procedure could be developed for rehearsing visual-spatial–based AAC, such as picture-based symbols. Perhaps a procedure in which the imaginary silhouette of pictures were drawn in the air could be used to develop rehearsal strategies for pictorial AAC. For example, Blissymbols are composed of basic elements that often form representaions of referents. Informal observations (Isaacson, 2017) suggest that less complex Blissymbols can be named when they are "air-drawn" in the visual field of an observer. Repetitive air-drawn basic shapes or silhouettes of symbols could act as a rehearsal mechanism for visually based material. Please note that the aforementioned tracing procedure was only mentioned to spur creative thought processes. It has not been empirically tested and should not be considered as efficacious until it has been tested. For additional information on natural sign languages, please see Chapter 8.

The Visual-Spatial Short-Term Store. This store is characterized by memory representations that incorporate visual and spatial dimensions. While it is unclear as to the extent that picture-based AAC is processed within this store, research (Wagner & Shaffer, 2015) indicates that the visual-spatial dimension may play a role in memory of picture communication symbols.

AAC Implications

The AAC field should examine this store with the objective of exploiting the characteristics of this store for reducing processing demands and facilitating memory for AAC stimuli. Symbols used in AAC could be arranged or grouped according to meaningful categories. The spatial arrangements could create spatial-based memories (something akin to mental maps) that might facilitate memory for the items within the spatial arrangement. In addition, as discussed in a following section, Organizational Structure and Cues, the use of organizational structure has been shown to impact memory and could be offered as an alternative explanation for the potential facilitative effects of spatial arrangements. Although the underlying mechanisms that facilitate cognitive processes may not be clearly delineated by research, this should not inhibit the AAC professional from using research to facilitate AAC outcomes.

Long-Term Storage and Retrieval. It is unclear as to the processes that facilitate long-term storage and retrieval of AAC stimuli. A better understanding of AAC storage and retrieval processes may help AAC professionals develop effective strategies for this stage of the communication process. Learning involves processes in which information is stored in long-term memory and retrieval processes that bring information stored in long-term memory into short-term memory.

Generative Processes in Memory. The procedures involved in the learning or storage of information may influence retrieval from long-term storage. Active involvement in the construction of learning content may facilitate memory retrieval processes. Memory researchers have demonstrated enhanced memory when the learner is involved in the construction of the to-be-learned content (Bertsch et al., 2007; Jacoby, 1978; Slamecka & Graf, 1978). This has become known as the **generation effect**. Memory for the relationship between graphic symbols and their referents has been found to be enhanced with teaching procedures that incorporate the generation effect (Isaacson & Lloyd, 2013).

AAC Implications

AAC professionals should develop and conduct additional research on teaching strategies that facilitate memory processes for AAC, such as the generation of to-be-learned material. This could involve maximizing the degree to which users of AAC are involved in the development and/or selection of AAC material. This may improve memory for symbol-to-referent relationships. AAC professionals should not limit their efforts to the generation effect. They should acquire a thorough understanding of knowledge arising from the cognitive memory sciences and should conduct research to determine if such knowledge has any applicability for improving AAC.

Organizational Structure and Cues. Retrieving information from long-term memory is important for conscious active processing. Categories can help to organize or structure information such that they act as cues that may enhance retrieval processes (Bower et al., 1969; Heller et al., 1996; Wortman & Greenberg, 1971). Organizing AAC content into categories may enhance communication by improving retrieval processes.

AAC Implications

As the organizational structure of AAC stimuli may impact AAC processing and issues concerned with communication, it is important for the AAC professional to understand these issues and to structure AAC content accordingly.

Psychophysics and Communication

Psychophysics is concerned with the relationship between physical properties of the stimulus and sensory/perceptual functioning (Kingdom & Prins, 2016). Communicative stimuli need to have enough physical energy to be detectable and to be differentiated from each other. Communicative content also needs to be differentiated from irrelevant stimuli (sometimes called noise or distractors). It is important that communicative information be easily perceived as the targeted stimuli. This section focuses on psychophysical measures that may have relevance for AAC.

Thresholds. Thresholds and related concepts concerning stimulus detection are frequently used in psychophysics. They also have potential relevance for AAC. Following are those that have considerable importance for AAC:

1. *The absolute threshold.* This threshold is concerned with characteristics that make the stimulus reliably detectable. For example, consider a visual stimulus that signals that a group of symbols are active. The visual signal must be of a sufficient intensity for the receiver to detect it reliably.

AAC Implications

Communication would be ineffective if the signals were not perceptible because they were below the threshold for detection.

2. *The difference threshold.* This threshold is concerned with the detection of differences between or among stimuli.

AAC Implications

Effective communication requires that different stimuli be perceptually distinct. Imagine the confusion that would ensue if auditory signals were sufficiently similar that the difference was not readily discernible.

3. *Weber's law.* Detecting the difference between two stimuli depends on a percentage difference rather than a constant amount. To illustrate, adding one light bulb to a group of 10 may produce a detectable difference in brightness. However, adding one light bulb to a group of 100 may not be sufficient to produce a detectable difference.

AAC Implications

Regarding AAC, consider a visual signal that is detectable in a dimly lit room. When that signal occurs in a room with regular light conditions, it may need a boost of one hypothetical unit to remain detectable. However, when it is taken out into the sunlight, it may need a boost of 100 or more units to remain detectable. In short, Weber's law addresses changes in ambient conditions and those factors necessary for maintaining detectability. The AAC professional should be aware of the impact of ambient conditions and may need to incorporate technology/strategies into a client's AAC that compensate for changes in ambient conditions.

4. *Stimulus salience.* Frequently the target content of AAC symbols occurs amid a myriad of background stimuli. It is important for the target to be easily perceived and recognized as the major content and for the background not to contribute to ambiguity. For example, some picture-based AAC may present the target stimulus or symbol along with background stimuli, such as a schoolhouse (the intended target) with trees and mountains (background or context).

AAC Implications

Some AAC users may have a propensity to focus on contextual information rather than the actual target (this may be more of an issue for some cultures relative to others; see Influences of Culture on Information Processing section). Hence, developing and selecting AAC with appropriate degrees of stimulus salience should be a concern for the AAC professional.

Processing of Information as a Function of Disability Type

Conscious processing of information is believed to be a function of short-term working memory. Some theories have added components to short-term memory that focus on phonological and visual-spatial processes (Baddeley & Hitch, 1974). While the nature of the content to be processed may influence the components that are active, individual differences may also play a role. For example, Temple Grandin (2006), an individual who was diagnosed as having autism spectrum disorder, reports that she perceives and thinks about the world primarily through visually based processes, such as pictures.

AAC Implications

It is unclear as to whether Grandin's way of processing extends to others who have autism spectrum disorder, but it does bring attention to the possibility that some individuals with AAC needs may have unique ways of processing information and thinking about the world. It also underscores the need for AAC professionals to take these differences into account when developing AAC for their clients.

Multisensory AAC

Reports from NASA's Ames Research Center (Spirkovska, 2005) and other researchers in the field of aviation (Fuchs et al., 2008) describe the use of multisensory stimuli to improve information processing. Specifically, they address the use of tactile stimuli to improve processing of information in other senses. The use of tactile stimuli in AAC has potential value (Isaacson & Lloyd, 2015); however, it is an area of AAC that has not been abundantly researched.

AAC Implications

There are many ways in which tactile stimuli could be used to improve AAC. For example, tactile cues could be used to direct attention to the salient aspect of AAC symbols. AAC professionals need to increase research efforts in this underutilized but potentially advantageous area.

Applying Learning Across Different Contexts

Generalization. Not all situations that an individual encounters will be identical. This creates a scenario in which application of learning across different contexts is beneficial for functioning. It is important for the individual to be able to apply knowledge learned in one situation to other situations. The application of knowledge across situations is known as **generalization**. The capacity of an individual who has a disability to generalize learning across different situations may depend on the individual's specific disability. Individuals with intellectual disabilities frequently have difficulty with generalization, and the use of remedial strategies to promote generalization may be needed for individuals with this type of disability (Hughes, 1991; Stokes & Baer, 1977).

AAC Implications

It is important for the AAC professional to determine if a particular client has the capacity to generalize AAC and to develop remedial procedures to promote generalization if needed.

Influences of Culture on Information Processing

Experiential factors, such as culture, may influence the processing of stimuli. For example, research indicates that western cultures focus on objects in the foreground or focal targets. In contrast, eastern Asian cultures are more likely to attend to context. These cultural differences in attention appear in a study by Masuda and Nisbett (2001) in which American and Japanese participants were asked to describe underwater scenes. Descriptions of the American participants were more likely to be focused on the focal targets while descriptions of the Japanese participants were more likely to be focused on the context. Because information processing is believed to depend on attentional processes that facilitate the transport of content from sensory memory to working memory, these cultural differences have implications for the development and selection of graphic symbols that maximize attentional focus and transport to the next stage of processing.

The study by Masuda and Nisbett (2001) found cultural differences that presumably occur early in the sequence of information processing (i.e., attentional focus). However, research by Morris and Peng (1994) provides evidence that cultural differences may also influence processing at a higher cognitive level. These researchers showed both American and Chinese participants visual images of a school of fish in which one fish was not in the school. After seeing the images, the participants were asked to explain why the one fish was not in the school. Responses from the American participants tended to emphasize individualistic themes, such as exerting independence. In contrast, responses from the Chinese participants were focused on themes emphasizing collective aspects of the group, such as not fitting in with the group.

AAC Implications

Cultural differences in processing of stimuli are important considerations for the AAC professional because the selection and/or development of the most efficacious symbols may depend upon the cultural background of the AAC client.

Understanding the Relationship Between Pictures and Referents

Match-to-Sample. Graphic AAC symbols frequently use pictorial representation for the words they represent (i.e., their referents). Sidman (1994, 2009) describes a match-to-sample procedure that he used to test whether an individual understands the relationship between symbols and referents. In short, this procedure presents target stimuli in one form with the objective of pointing to the other form from a group of foils (i.e., incorrect responses). For example, in a visual-only condition, participants might be shown a picture of a car and be expected to choose the printed word "car" selected from a group of incorrect word foils to indicate they understood the picture/referent relationship.

Individuals with intellectual disabilities who were institutionalized were found to have difficulty with match-to-sample tasks (Sidman, 1994, 2009). According to Sidman, this was because these individuals had never learned to read nor sit still and make basic discriminations, such as line curvatures or line orientation that occurs in letters—the rudiments of words. Once these individuals were trained to sit still and make basic discriminations, they were trained on a match-to-sample task, including a modification that introduced a spoken rendering of the target. In this condition, a spoken rendering of the target was presented and the participant was to choose the visual rendering that matched the spoken rendering. For example, if the auditory stimulus was the spoken rendering of the word "car," then the correct visual match was either a pictorial representation of a car or a visual rendering of the letters that form the word that matches the spoken auditory stimulus (for this example, the letters C, A, and R). Sidman found that participants who were trained on the auditory-to-visual matching condition but not on a visual-to-visual matching condition were now able to perform the visual-to-visual matching even though they had never been trained on this condition. These findings are consistent with the notion that the memory trace originating from auditory-to-visual and visual-to-visual input may overlap or involve an underlying mechanism that supports equivalence between different input modalities.

This is an area that would benefit from additional research. It would be beneficial to have corroborating evidence for transference between the stores for picture-based AAC. Specifically, as the number of words that are capable of being active in the phonological store may depend on word length, it might be beneficial to understand how the referents associated with picture-based AAC influence the capacity of the phonological store. Such knowledge could be instrumental in the choice of referents. For example, the words "car" and "vehicle" have similar meanings; however, "car" might be a more efficient referent choice in regards to capacity issues because it is shorter and presumably would take up less capacity in the phonological store.

Moreover, as graphic picture representations are frequently used in AAC, it may be beneficial for the AAC user to have or to be able to form an association between graphic renderings and their referents. It is noteworthy that Sidman used a technique that taught the association between visual and spoken renderings with his participants with intellectual disabilities. This may be important because the working memory model includes a phonological store in which verbal or spoken renderings are repeated through a cognitive articulatory process. The association with spoken content may allow the individual to maximize use of pre-existing information-processing structures. Hence, it is important for the AAC professional to be able to determine the capacity of their clients to form such associations and to be knowledgeable of research techniques that may be useful in facilitating such associations.

> ## AAC Implications
>
> One implication is that potential users of AAC may not have the prerequisite skills to use the AAC that is being considered for them and that the AAC professional may need to develop assessment and training procedures for the necessary skills. Another implication concerns the potential equivalence between memory representations. Remember that the working memory model includes two short term stores: a phonological store and a visual-spatial store. As previously discussed, it is unclear as to the short-term store that picture-based AAC might use. Sidman's evidence on equivalence is consistent with the notion that transference between the two stores might occur with picture-based AAC.

Determining an AAC Vocabulary

It is probably not viable to create an AAC vocabulary that approximates the volume of words found in the typical dictionary. As a tangent, it should be mentioned that Blissymbolics has a feature that allows the creation of words and meaning through the combination of basic elements. This feature allows vocabulary expansion and may contribute to the development of creativity. Blissymbols could be a viable AAC choice for some AAC users, particularly for those who show evidence of high levels of creativity.

Moe and colleagues (1982) described a procedure that was used to record spoken words occurring in a naturalistic classroom setting for first graders. From these recordings, word counts were performed, giving the researchers an estimate of the words that are frequently used by first graders. AAC professionals should consider using a procedure similar to that of Moe and colleagues (1982) to develop AAC vocabularies to guide them in choosing vocabularies for their clients. Chapter 12 contains additional information about AAC vocabulary.

> ## AAC Implications
>
> Communication may be enhanced by developing an AAC vocabulary that hones in on the specific needs of the individual ACC user. Hence, it is important for AAC professionals to understand the issues concerning AAC selection and to develop appropriate vocabularies for their clients.

The Self

How one perceives one's self appears to play a role in motivation. For example, self-confidence in one's ability to perform specific activities appears to be related to one's motivation or inclination to engage in those activities (Isaacson et al., 2016). Likewise, developing a sense of self-confidence in one's capacity to use AAC may play an important role in motivation and persistence to use AAC. Moreover, stigma is frequently associated with disability and may contribute to a poor perception of one's self (Jahoda et al., 2010) and possible demotivation to use AAC. Developing self-confidence in the use of AAC may help to reduce self-perceptions of stigma associated with disability and may contribute to communicative competence in regards to the use of AAC.

> ## AAC Implications
>
> Professionals involved in the teaching and acquisition of skills for using AAC should assure that the AAC user has the skills for competently using their AAC. This should increase self-confidence in the user concerning their capacity to communicate using their AAC and should increase motivation to use their AAC and their communicative capacity and competence. It is also possible that communicative competence and capacity may increase the perception of others in regards to disability, which may lessen stigma associated with disability.

Plasticity and Development

The capacity to be molded or shaped is known as plasticity. Language development appears to show plasticity. Children with congenital brain damage are much more likely to acquire language functioning within the range of normal compared to individuals with similar brain damage acquired at a later stage of life (Bates, 1999). These age-related differences in functioning are ascribed to a greater degree of plasticity within the neural substrates at earlier rather than later stages of development.

> ## AAC Implications
>
> AAC may be more successful if implemented at an early age and the AAC professional may need to use different AAC depending on the age at which the need for AAC occurred. Training concerning the use of AAC may take longer for later onset communication disabilities.

Technology Perspectives

The technology perspective is extremely important in AAC. Unfortunately, it is related to a common misconception in the field. Many administrators and clinicians/educators think that AAC and **assistive technology** are synonymous; that is, assistive technology and AAC are two terms for the same thing. Additionally, confusions and concerns related to similarities and differences between AAC and assistive technology often arise. One should remember that AAC is a process, while assistive technology refers to the tools (e.g., SGDs) used to assist individuals with functions and activities. There is an overlap of the AAC process and assistive technology tools, but they are not synonymous. Figure 1-3 provides an illustration of the relationship between AAC and assistive technology. It should be noted that the figure shows visual and hearing (i.e., sensory) prostheses are related to AAC but are not typically thought of as AAC. Chapters 3 and 23 will provide a discussion of the inclusion of sensory technology for receptive communication purposes.

Figure 1-3 illustrates AAC frequently involves the use of assistive technology, but there is much more to AAC than assistive technology. Conversely, there is more to assistive technology (e.g., mobility aids and devices, environmental control devices) than just communication devices. AAC should not be considered a subset or a specialty of assistive technology. A speech-generating or non–speech-generating communication device very likely will be one of the more crucial tools in aided communication. However, an AAC system should include both **aided** *and* **unaided** means to represent, means to select, and means to transmit. In other words, the use of assistive technology is typically only a small part of an overall AAC system. Finally, to further drive home the point that assistive technology and AAC are not synonymous, surveys about the use of technology suggest that communication by AAC users is predominantly *unaided* (e.g., gestures, speech, or even vocalizations of limited intelligibility; Burd et al., 1988; Matas et al., 1985).

Some aspects of job accommodation (e.g., computer access for communication) may overlap with AAC, but many other devices and structure modifications would not be considered part of AAC. Other types of assistive technology, such as mobility orthoses/prostheses, are not part of AAC *per se*. However, in some cases, wheelchairs, walkers, and crutches may be used to transport or hold assistive communication devices, and therefore, indirectly may be considered a part of AAC.

A related misconception about AAC and assistive technology is that providing an assistive communicative device solves the communication problem. Without appropriate training and backup support, most assistive devices are of little or no value. Lack of training and support often result in expensive devices not being used and ultimately ending up on shelves. It is as if nothing has been learned from colleagues in audiology about another type of assistive device:

the hearing aid. Just as one cannot give a hearing aid to an individual and expect to solve a hearing problem, one cannot give an assistive communication device to an individual and expect to solve an expressive communication problem. Valentic (1991) said that AAC and assistive technology are an ongoing journey.

> Making wise use of the technology which is now available is also absolutely essential for a person like me to be able to continue on through high school in a regular class setting. Electric wheelchair, laptop computer, voice synthesizer, ultralight computers are some examples of the modern technology I have been using in recent years . . . Once the decision about my education was made by myself and my parents, plans for how to manage that education were soon underway, and still are today as I complete high school and head for college. We have a formula; as problems present themselves, solutions are sought, and at times, we have learned that you never give up, just keep on trying. (Valentic, 1991, p. 9)

Assessment Perspectives

Although one may not develop the knowledge and skills to be a specialist in AAC, one can expect at some time during their career they will most likely work with individuals with **complex communication needs** (CCN) who may benefit from AAC. This necessitates knowledge of some basic principles of assessment, including AAC as a team process involving planning and implementing interventions for present and future communication needs, a knowledge of the entire gamut of available technology, and assessing communication needs with partners in the individual's social network (Fishman, 2011). The assessment must also include developing a **capability profile** and using **feature matching** to select appropriate components of the AAC system. Assessment must be considered an ongoing process throughout the lifespan of the individual who uses AAC.

Assessment and evaluation are critical to developing an appropriate intervention plan. Knowing what questions to ask, why they should be asked, how to ask them, who to ask, when to ask, and where to ask are the essence of assessment. Knowing how to interpret and when to use the answers to the questions *are* the essence of evaluation. AAC assessment should be field-based (i.e., involving assessment in natural environments), extensive (i.e., including multiple natural environments and communication partners), transdisciplinary (i.e., involving **role release** and collaboration across disciplines), and ongoing (i.e., involving as many assessment sessions as appropriate and also follow-up). Assessment of existing communication abilities and related cognitive, motor, and sensory domains is important, as is the understanding of the etiology of communication disabilities. Especially crucial are assessment and evaluation of auditory, visual, and motor

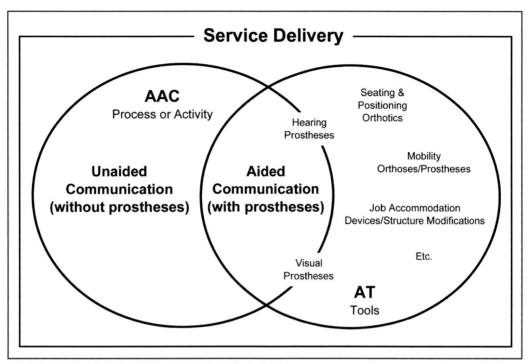

Figure 1-3. The relationship between AAC and assistive technology.

abilities because they are the means to represent (symbols), select, and transmit messages in AAC approaches. Also, AAC users have a high probability of having sensory and/or motor impairments. A combination of the primary impairment (e.g., aphasia, cerebral palsy, intellectual impairment) and concomitant sensory and/or motor impairments results in a disability that is greater than one would expect from the sum of these individual impairments. In addition to discussion of the critical roles of these impairments in the assessment unit of this text (Chapters 11 through 14), motor impairments are discussed in Chapters 16, 18, and 21 and sensory impairments are discussed more thoroughly in Chapter 23.

Team Approach

One of the most basic premises of AAC assessment is that it should involve a team approach. The diversity and complexity of issues involved in AAC require knowledge and skill from many individuals and disciplines. The specific services required by any particular individual with little or no functional speech will vary, but individuals who might typically be on an assessment team for a school child are the child, occupational therapist, paraprofessional, parents, teacher, special educator, and speech-language pathologist. Depending on the specific needs of the child, such individuals as an audiologist, personal aide, physical therapist, psychologist, rehabilitation engineer, social worker, or vision specialist may also be included on the assessment team.

Field-Based Assessment

To provide a true picture of the strengths and needs of AAC users, assessment should be conducted in natural environments. What an individual can do in a testing situation in an isolated, unfamiliar location may not give an accurate indication of communication strengths and needs. Direct observation, video recordings, and interviews in familiar environments with familiar communication partners provide important information about an individual's functional communication abilities.

Standardized and Norm-Referenced Tests

Standardized and norm-referenced tests are sometimes used during the assessment process, but use of these types of tests may not be appropriate for persons who use or rely on AAC. For example, the responses required by a standardized assessment of cognitive, receptive, and/or expressive language abilities most likely will need to be adapted for AAC users (e.g., giving a pointing instead of oral response). Similarly, stimulus materials may need to be presented in nonstandard ways (e.g., enlarged and/or arranged from left to right instead of in a matrix or within cells for the purpose of facilitating visual perception) that can adversely affect the norms of the test. AAC users may also express different fatigue factors than typical individuals of the normative group. The norms provided for standardized and norm-referenced tests will not be valid if modifications have to be made. Test results may give some index of performance level, but they should not be reported as normed scores. A description of any modifications made for the administration of a test must be included in the reporting of results and caution must be used in the interpretation of scores. However, standardized and norm-referenced tests need not be completely discarded because of these limitations. They can provide important information, but criterion-referenced tests are often preferred.

Criterion-Referenced Assessment

Some areas take considerable time to assess because of the extent of information that must be gathered to begin a particular intervention. However, it is not always necessary to gather the most extensive information. Criteria-based assessment, which includes criterion-referenced tests, may be more appropriate. In criteria-based assessment, the clinician does not attempt to determine an individual's ability to use specific symbol sets/systems, specific switches or other technology, and levels of functioning, but rather attempts only to discover whether the skills are sufficient to support a particular AAC strategy. That is, the clinician or educator might not need to complete assessment of fine motor skills to determine whether they are sufficient to make use of manual signing. Although many initial speech and language assessments can be completed within 3 to 6 hours, the initial AAC assessment rarely can be completed within 1 day.

Criteria-based assessment is more appropriate than norm-referenced assessment for clients who may be expected to show changes as various communication interventions are implemented. Individuals with congenital impairments may never have been successful in most communication interactions, and the introduction of a strategy that provides success may have a rather dramatic impact on the further development of language and communication skills. Similarly, many clients with acquired disabilities can also be expected to show changes over time. As previously discussed, some individuals may show patterns of improvement; that is, the level of disability may actually diminish over time. Individuals with progressive disabilities, on the other hand, may develop more severe disabilities. Criteria-based assessment may be more sensitive to these changes and may lead more quickly to decisions to vary or change AAC intervention strategies.

Capability Profile

For most areas of speech and language assessment, the clinician is interested in obtaining maximal assessment; that is, to determine a capability profile that accurately details a person's level of functioning in various important domains. However, in AAC, it is often more effective to operate from a criteria-based approach (Beukelman & Light, 2020; Beukelman & Mirenda, 2013; Yorkston & Karlan, 1986). The abilities of many AAC users are extremely difficult to assess, but time must be taken to assess them properly. Assessment may require a long time because the diagnostic procedures might be extremely tiring for the individual, who may need to take many breaks. Reducing the assessment for those

aspects that will determine possible intervention strategies can both benefit the AAC user and make the clinician or educator more efficient. Assessment and intervention are very much intertwined and usually continue simultaneously. Thus, one could expect that the more extensive maximal assessment type of information would be gathered over a longer time during intervention.

Feature Matching

Once strengths and needs have been assessed and goals have been developed, feature matching should be employed to select components for an appropriate AAC system. Needs and goals that are determined by assessing abilities in natural environments with a variety of communication partners should be outlined and prioritized. Specific aided and unaided approaches should then be evaluated. For example, if an individual with cognitive impairment has good motor control, gestures or manual signs might be considered. If an individual has high cognitive abilities but limited motor control, an SGD with switch access might be considered. AAC systems and communication approaches are different from those used by typical speakers and must be well-matched to the real communication needs of individuals and their environments. Feature matching is critical in the assessment process presented in this text (see Chapters 9, 11, 13, and 14).

Follow-Up

Regardless of the assessment model employed, follow-up is an important component of the assessment process. Abilities and disabilities, as well as communication needs of individuals, change over time. As individuals become successful with one communication approach, new or additional approaches should be considered. Ongoing assessment and reassessment of AAC systems and intervention plans will be needed.

Intervention Perspectives

AAC intervention often begins with the development of goals to expand a repertoire of communication behaviors, develop intentional and symbolic abilities, and/or increase participation in daily routines (Kangas & Lloyd, 1988). Some authors have suggested that AAC intervention should not be initiated until certain levels of cognitive functioning, social skills, and receptive language have been reached (Owens & House, 1984) or until a gap between receptive and expressive language has been demonstrated (Chapman & Miller, 1980). However, evidence to support this prerequisite approach has been based mainly on observations of typically developing children and not on research with children with disabilities. More recently, clinicians and educators have challenged a prerequisite approach, suggesting that intervention can be effective for individuals exhibiting a wide range of skill levels related to both congenital and acquired disabilities.

Several models of service delivery are described in the literature. The **unidisciplinary model** typically includes one professional who is primarily responsible for providing services to improve communication skills. Although this model has been effective with individuals with poor articulation, stuttering, or language delays, one service provider is unlikely to be effective in meeting the many needs of individuals with little or no functional speech. Individuals with sensory, motor, cognitive, and language impairments typically require services from specialists in many fields.

The **multidisciplinary team model** involves the provision of services from many disciplines, including audiology, career counseling, computer science, medicine, occupational therapy, ophthalmology, physical therapy, general and special education, social work, and speech-language pathology. Specialists may provide specific expertise and strategies to meet an individual's needs; however, intervention may become disjointed and fragmented rather than coherent and holistic (Beukelman & Light, 2020; Beukelman & Mirenda, 2013). When individuals with severe communication disabilities are removed from their natural environments to obtain services in the environments of each specialist, the danger of fragmentation is very real.

The **interdisciplinary team model** involves more disciplines and provides for a greater exchange and sharing of information. Specialists may meet on a regular basis to determine goals and discuss intervention strategies. In this model, specialists have access to a variety of perspectives that allows them to better understand the implications of the impairments and disabilities that affect communication. Intervention planning includes consultation and collaboration.

However, AAC services typically require more than sharing, collaborating, and implementing. The success of AAC intervention depends on the coordination and offering of services, not just between disciplines, but across disciplines. The **transdisciplinary team model** involves individuals and professionals from different disciplines sharing knowledge and ideas as they work together to provide services through cotreatment that focuses not on the specific disabilities of an individual but on an individual as a whole. The hallmark characteristic of the transdisciplinary team is role release (i.e., the sharing of information and function across disciplines). Divisions between disciplines become less distinct. A more thorough discussion of team approaches can be found throughout the assessment and intervention chapters in this textbook.

Intervention is based on the development and prioritization of long-range goals and objectives. Exactly what these goals will be, however, depend on an individual's specific needs and expectations. AAC needs may not be readily apparent in individuals with neurogenic progressive diseases, such as amyotrophic lateral sclerosis, multiple sclerosis, or Parkinson's disease (Beukelman & Garrett, 1988). Intervention for these individuals will focus on changing needs that can be expected to increase. Intervention for individuals with short-term neurogenic diseases, such as Guillain-Barré syndrome, will focus on immediate needs that can be expected to diminish.

Intervention typically focuses on developing skills that will enhance participation and independence in the environments in which individuals are expected to function. Specific intervention strategies are discussed in Chapters 18 and 21. An individual with a congenital condition, such as cerebral palsy, or an acquired condition, such as traumatic brain injury, may be expected to begin or return to active participation in society. Goals for such integration will come from several sources (e.g., individuals with disabilities, communication partners, and professionals) and will vary widely with respect to individual needs and different environments. Intervention for an individual who is always with caregivers in a familiar setting will certainly differ from the program designed for an individual who is learning to function more independently in home, school, work, and community environments. The transdisciplinary model can be effective in meeting these goals of integration.

Transdisciplinary and Integrated Perspectives

The transdisciplinary team approach that incorporates collaboration and promotes role release is basic to AAC assessment and intervention. It allows professionals with knowledge and expertise in a variety of disciplines to work together to share information that is known and to develop new ideas and strategies to improve the communication skills of individuals with little or no functional speech. Although improvement in functional communication often appears as a goal, this goal should not be interpreted as being an end but rather as being the means to an end. Individual AAC users have their own ideas as to what ends or outcomes are important to them. For many, the desired end or outcome is acceptance.

> We people with disabilities have historically been separated from the rest of society. This practice of segregation has often been justified as the best to serve our special needs. But the practice has had a very serious consequence. It has taught people in the community that people with disabilities are not part of the community. It has caused them to believe that the exclusion of people with disabilities is the natural order of things, which obviously works against us, as we struggle to be accepted …
>
> The best way to build acceptance is to de-emphasize the idea that our disabilities are the most important difference between us and other individuals. People should be treated equally, regardless of their level of ability. All children should go to school with their age mates from their neighborhood. (Sienkiewicz-Mercer, 1995)

Inclusion into general education classrooms is one way in which individuals can gain acceptance into a group of their peers. However, if the inclusion is only physical, it may do little or nothing to facilitate real acceptance. Unless academic participation and integration is carefully planned, AAC users can feel excluded even in the presence of physical inclusion. Like assessment and intervention, inclusion must be carefully designed to meet individual needs and should be encouraged to the optimal extent that is beneficial.

> Acceptance is not something that can happen overnight. Negative attitudes can be overcome, but we have to be patient, and we have to work together. (Sienkiewicz-Mercer, 1995)

The ability to effectively communicate is critical to achieving integration and inclusion for individuals with severe disabilities. Like typically speaking individuals, AAC users often want to enjoy a sense of community with others. This is difficult to achieve without effective communication. Improving the communication skills of AAC users is often the focus when working toward integration and inclusion, but this should not be the only focus. Improving the communication skills of communication partners is also important and should not be overlooked.

Legal and Ethical Perspectives

Legal and ethical issues arise in the field of AAC as they do in any field of service delivery. However, these issues can be particularly complicated when they involve individuals with little or no functional speech whose messages are typically not sent as completely or received as accurately as messages of typically speaking individuals. Administrators and researchers, as well as clinicians, educators, and others who work with persons who use or must rely on AAC, must understand and be able to appropriately deal with the legal and ethical issues that affect the lives of AAC users.

Two seminal laws set the stage for what would eventually become the discipline of AAC. These were Section 504 of the Rehabilitation Act (PL 93-112, 1973) and the Education for All Handicapped Children Act (PL 94-142, 1975). Section 504 of the Rehabilitation Act extended civil rights to persons with disabilities and provided opportunities for children and adults with disabilities in the areas of education and employment, among others, and mandated reasonable accommodations for persons with disabilities. The Education for All Handicapped Children Act required all public schools that accepted federal funds to provide equal access to a free and appropriate public education within the least restricted environment. The concept of **mainstreaming** resulted from this latter piece of legislation.

The 2016 Communication Bill of Rights (see Figure 1-1) outlines a number of rights designed to facilitate an AAC user's impact on the environment. These rights reflect a social mandate to improve communication and increase participation in social, educational, and vocational settings.

However, AAC users have more than just social mandates behind them. Early broad-based civil rights legislation that laid the groundwork to protect the rights of all individuals has special implications for individuals with severe disabilities. The Americans with Disabilities Act (ADA; PL 101-336, 1990) assigns responsibility and outlines more specifics related to providing services for individuals with disabilities. In 2008, Congress passed and President George W. Bush signed into law the ADA Amendments (PL 110-325, 2008). In short, this law broadened the scope of the term "disability" as it pertained to the original ADA. It included activities not expressly stipulated in the ADA (PL 101-336, 1990), such as reading, concentrating and thinking, and major bodily functions, including immune system and neurological disorders. However, the law also stipulated that an individual may not be eligible for protections if the disability is temporary, spanning 6 months or less.

A comprehensive review of relevant legislation for the prescription of SGDs appears in Chapter 17. Other pertinent laws may appear throughout a number of chapters in this textbook.

Legislation provides a solid base on which to develop programs to meet the needs of individuals with little or no functional speech. Different interpretations contribute to variation in the particulars of providing a free and appropriate public education, but the mandate is clear. Administrators and service providers must be secure in the knowledge of their responsibilities in carrying out such legal mandates. However, they must also be secure in handling the many ethical issues that may arise as they work to implement legislation. Professional organizations provide codes of ethics, but these are typically general guidelines. Administrators and service providers must be prepared to follow not only these general guidelines but also know how to comply with specific ethical rules and regulations.

One ethical issue that has received considerable attention involves the interpretation of messages conveyed by AAC users. Because of the nature of AAC, service providers are often called on to interpret messages whether through repeating more intelligibly what they believe the AAC user has said or by interpreting the symbols to which the AAC user appears to be gazing or pointing. Interpreters must be vigilant in guarding against injecting subjective thoughts that would bias an AAC user's message in any way.

A second ethical issue involves confidentiality. Professionals who work with persons who use AAC must be above reproach. Information that is obtained from persons who use AAC can only be shared when permission is granted. This information may be spoken communication, written documents, and/or any type of recorded media.

A third ethical issue concerns the dissemination of written messages. Persons who use AAC may send spoken messages through SGDs, but they may also send a considerable number of nonspoken messages through computers, tablets, smartphones, and printers. Service providers must be sensitive to the wishes of persons who use AAC regarding the distribution of these permanent messages that endure. AAC users should be secure in knowing that their messages are not indiscriminately distributed to individuals for whom they were not intended.

Visionary Perspectives

AAC has many dimensions that must be viewed from many perspectives. New challenges emerge as more and more individuals become involved as both users and providers of AAC services. Progress has been made in the brief history of the field by the provision of means of communication that were not previously available. Individuals have always had the means to use unaided communication modes, such as gesturing and signing, but these modes are limited by the number of communication partners who can interpret the messages. Advancements in technology (e.g., tablet and smartphone technology, apps) have revolutionized the field of AAC over the last couple decades. Powerful communication devices have become more compact, lighter, more functional, and more user-friendly in terms of improved storage and retrieval systems, memory, and voice output. The area of technology has advanced so rapidly that our way of classifying it must change. A proposed technology classification system that includes both expressive *and* receptive communication will be highlighted in Chapter 3.

Advances in ergonomics and the development of sophisticated switches and software have done much to facilitate operational competence. However, relatively little improvement has been made in improving social competence. AAC users can store and retrieve large amounts of text and graphics for oral presentation and written documents, but efficiency in online, real-time interactive communication is still lacking. Communication partners are often reluctant to engage in true interactive communication with AAC users because of the time it takes to generate spontaneous messages.

As in most areas of endeavor, funding has been—and will most likely continue to be—a factor that influences the future directions of AAC. Funding of assistive technology has improved dramatically over the last couple decades. However, funding for the research that forms the very foundation of the field is necessary but seems to fluctuate significantly from year to year. Funding for personnel preparation, training programs for service providers and individual AAC users who need systems, and educational support must not be forgotten, especially as managed care has become the norm.

Funding alone cannot meet the challenge of achieving communicative competence. Human factors must also be in place. Communication is complex. Achieving competence requires the cooperation, collaboration, and creativity of AAC users and other members of their transdisciplinary teams. Providing AAC users with opportunities to become more functional, spontaneous communicators as they move toward becoming independent, participating individuals in

society is a challenge that will carry the field into the future. Technological advances in the area of biomedicine and engineering are on the cusp of introducing AAC to a brave new world.

BASIC HUMAN COMMUNICATION MODEL

This textbook is based on a broad view of human communication. It is organized around the basic human communication model of a sender and a receiver, both of whom bring to the process experience and physical, psychological, social, cognitive, and linguistic abilities. Communication involves the transmission of a message by a sender to a receiver who may or may not respond. It is also generally considered to be an interactive process between at least two communicators, with the sender and receiver reversing roles. The initial receiver becomes the sender, and the initial sender becomes the receiver. Figure 1-4 provides a simplified illustration of the human communication model. It should be noted this model is a simplified illustration of the communication process; a more thorough model will be presented and explained in Chapter 3.

AAC may be viewed as a broad or robust communication model including a sender who has the intention of communicating (e.g., a message), a receiver who is engaged in an interaction with the sender, a set or system of symbols to represent messages (e.g., feelings, requests, information), a channel through which one sends a message (e.g., acoustic, optic, vibratory), the broader contexts or environments in which the communication act is taking place, and complex feedback systems within (endogenous) and between (exogenous) individuals (Lloyd et al., 1990). The success of communication depends on many factors, including the degree to which the sender and receiver share common linguistic and non-linguistic symbols, their cultural backgrounds, and their experience and skill in combining symbols. Communication involves linguistic (verbal) symbols, which are typically spoken or written, and non-linguistic (nonverbal) symbols, such as gestures, facial expressions, and hand movements. Individuals with functional natural speech frequently augment their spoken communication with non-linguistic (nonverbal) communication. Likewise, AAC users tend to use a variety of both linguistic and non-linguistic forms of communication (Basil & Ruiz, 1985; Liberoff, 1992; Lloyd & Fuller, 1986; Lloyd et al., 1990; van Balkom & Welle Donker-Gimbrere, 1985; Vanderheiden & Lloyd, 1986).

Lloyd and colleagues (1990) proposed that the AAC model should be based on a robust human communication model and not be considered categorically different. In essence, the only differences involve the AAC processes and interfaces: the means to represent the message (symbols), the means to select symbols or messages, and the means to transmit a message. Some individuals suggest that AAC requires a different model, and one such alternate model will

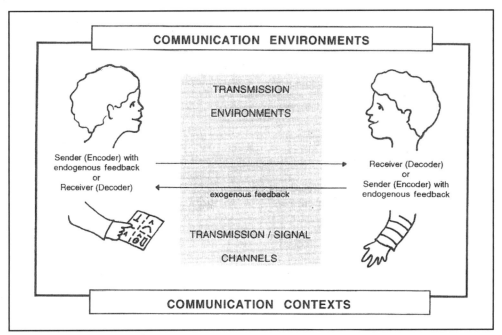

Figure 1-4. Basic elements of the human communication model.

be presented in Chapter 3. However, the overarching framework for which this entire textbook is organized and presented conforms to the AAC model proposed by Lloyd and colleagues (1990).

AAC may be viewed as a process composed of three aspects: (1) means to represent an idea, (2) means to select the representation of the idea, and (3) means to transmit the representation of the idea (Lloyd et al., 1990). Each of these three aspects may be aided or unaided (Lloyd & Fuller, 1986; Lloyd et al., 1990). Although the three aspects are discussed sequentially, they do not necessarily occur in this order. They are typically interactive and frequently occur concurrently. They are discussed in more detail in Chapter 3.

A robust communication model involves two types of environments: **transmission environments** (often referred to as **transmission/signal channels**) and **communication environments** (often referred to as **communication contexts**). These multiple environments must be considered in applying the human communication model to individuals with little or no functional speech. The application of the human communication model to AAC is an important aspect of the theoretical and fundamental perspective previously discussed.

Communication typically involves a dyad (i.e., two individuals interacting). However, in a group situation, the particular individuals engaged in a communication dyad at any one time typically change as conversation shifts. In an even more robust communication model, more than two people are involved in the interaction.

A significant part of communication involves language that includes the symbols or tokens (e.g., printed words, manual signs, spoken words) to represent a message and the rules or logic for combining the symbols (e.g., grammar, syntax). Human communication also includes non-linguistic (e.g., pictures, gestures) and paralinguistic (e.g., prosody) forms.

NATURE AND PURPOSES OF COMMUNICATION

Nature of Communication

Human communication is **multimodal**. Most frequently it involves the auditory and visual channels, but it may also involve the tactile channel as well. Most people use multimodal communication (Vanderheiden & Lloyd, 1986). People speak to convey thoughts, but even when speaking, senders typically use not only the speech mechanism but also the face, hands, arms, and other body parts to convey messages. Additional meaning is conveyed by facial expressions, gestures (e.g., pointing to the coffee mug one wants), tone of voice, and even posture. A typical speaker uses not only speech but also gestures, writing, typing, and audio and/or video recordings (e.g., digitally recorded voicemail). In the span of a single hour, a teacher might speak, write on a whiteboard, show pictures or diagrams using an opaque projector or computer software (such as Microsoft PowerPoint), and point to a map or wall chart. Communication receivers typically use eyes, ears, and touch receptors to receive messages but may also use olfactory cells and taste buds.

There are numerous examples of multimodal communication. People switch easily from one mode to another and combine modes within a single situation. They select the modes of communication that will be most effective and efficient in a given situation for a given listener. For example, one might write a note to a spouse that ends with the words "I love you," but draw a heart to express the same idea to a 3-year-old child. People also select the mode that will best set the tone to achieve specific goals. One might be content to rely only on speech when having a casual chat with an employer, but when discussing a specific idea to improve business, one might choose to put an idea in writing so that an employer will attend to it as a serious proposal.

Users of AAC systems should be viewed as multimodal communicators. Their communication systems should include both aided and unaided modes and strategies. They should include both the communication modes they have developed naturally without formal intervention and those modes, strategies, and techniques that can be facilitated or taught by clinicians or educators. A variety of techniques may be needed to address a varied audience. For example, a person who uses manual sign with familiar listeners would need some other approach to communicate with store clerks or bank tellers who have no knowledge of signing. In addition, an individual who uses an SGD must also have a backup system available for times when the device is broken or the battery needs charging.

Viewing an AAC user as a multimodal communicator implies whatever communication mode the individual chooses should be respected and accepted. Clinicians and educators, in their enthusiasm to teach what they view as more effective communication modes, sometimes refuse to accept simpler, more effective modes. For example, they might put "yes" and "no" on an individual's communication device. When the student attempts to answer a question by nodding or shaking the head, the clinician or educator might respond with, "Use your device to tell me." This is unnecessary because the clinician or educator probably understands the gesture. Users report incidents such as this to be very frustrating (Huer & Lloyd, 1988a, 1998b), and they may have the inadvertent, negative effect of causing students to become discouraged about even trying to communicate.

Purposes of Communication

Light (1988) outlined four purposes that can be accomplished during communicative interactions: (1) communication of needs/wants, (2) information transfer, (3) social closeness, and (4) social etiquette. Communicating needs/wants involves regulation of a partner's behavior to the extent that the sender of the message can obtain something or cause something to happen. In information transfer, the emphasis is on the content of the message. In communication for social closeness, the emphasis is not on the content of the message but rather the establishment, maintenance, and/or development of an interpersonal relationship. Social etiquette can be accomplished through the use of polite social conventions, such as, "Nice to see you" and "Thank you very much."

More generally, communication may be used for information transfer, socialization, or a combination thereof. However, in addition to face-to-face communication, one should consider aspects of communication such as those that relate to online or real-time interaction and recorded or stored messages. Success of communication is strongly related to the match between the sender and receiver, especially their means to represent their messages (i.e., symbols or tokens).

Communicative Competence

Communicative competence is an important concept of the human communication perspective. Competence should be considered within the framework of communication. According to Light (1989), four distinct competencies contribute to overall communicative competence. These are **linguistic competence**, **operational competence**, **social competence**, and **strategic competence**. These four were summarized further by Lloyd and Kangas (1994).

Linguistic Competence

Linguistic competence refers to knowledge of the language or linguistic code. According to Chomsky (1965), linguistic competence refers to the internal abilities of the individual and includes everything the person knows about the language and how the units can be combined. Light (1989) points out that for the AAC user, linguistic competence may include knowledge of both the native language used in the environment (e.g., English or Spanish) and special AAC symbols (e.g., Blissymbolics, modified orthography).

Operational Competence

Operational competence is a unique concern of AAC, especially for aided communication. Operational competence refers to the user's ability to manage the specific devices or techniques that are used in the communication process. This might include the ability to turn a device on or off, adjust the volume, operate a scanning system, and so on. This is, perhaps, the competence that most people focus on first when communicating with a person who uses AAC, mainly because it represents an aspect of AAC that is different from typical spoken communication.

Social Competence

Social competence refers to the broad communication skills addressed by sociolinguistics (Hymes, 1971). This includes discourse strategies, interaction functions, and pragmatic adjustments to context. Examples of abilities that relate to social competence include maintaining a topic, using transitions to change topics, adjusting the type of language used to the ability of the listener, gaining someone's attention before giving information, and giving appropriate indications of maintaining interest and/or understanding the communication partner. Social competence may be a serious issue that is easily overlooked for a person who uses AAC. It is not unusual for AAC approaches to be introduced to an individual who has had extremely limited communication abilities for many years. Social competence abilities that are developed quite naturally for typically developing children may be problematic for persons who use AAC simply because they have not experienced successful communication to facilitate these abilities.

Strategic Competence

Strategic competence (defined by Canale, 1983) refers to adapted strategies that are called into play when there is some breakdown in the communication process. Examples include asking for additional information, recognizing when the listener has not understood, and repeating or changing a message to clarify an error. As pointed out by Light (1989), this is especially important for persons who use AAC. AAC approaches remain imperfect replacements for the ability to use speech easily and effectively. There are probably a greater number of difficulties and barriers to achieving efficient communication when AAC strategies are being used. The ability to adjust and respond to these problems will be crucial to the overall success of an AAC user.

THE RESEARCH DILEMMA

An overarching theme of this section is that communication involves information processing and that factors that may influence such processing are major concerns for the development and implementation of AAC. The rationale for using this theme is to provide AAC professionals with a framework within which to conceptualize and think about processes that may influence communication and to use this knowledge to improve the efficacy of AAC that they might use with their own clients and to advance the AAC field.

Research is important for advancing the field of AAC. Professionals in AAC should have a strong background in basic applied statistics and research design. They should use this knowledge to conduct research on the efficacy of the AAC strategies they use. In addition, they should disseminate the findings from their research so that others can benefit from their research efforts.

It is important for AAC professionals to stay abreast of new findings within their field. Unbiased dissemination of research is important for the achievement of this objective. Hence, the AAC field needs to provide the means for these professionals to disseminate their research in a manner that is unbiased.

Rosenthal (1979) coined the term the **file drawer effect** to refer to the bias to publish research showing statistically significant differences and for researchers to put research that does not show statistically significant differences in their file cabinets without publication and to eventually forget about them. Evidence indicates the file drawer effect

is a real phenomenon that may be increasing in prevalence (Pautasso, 2010). Publication bias creates many potential problems (Fanelli, 2012; Matosin et al., 2014), including biases in meta-analyses and potential faulty conclusions concerning an area of study. In regards to the AAC field, bias may contribute to misinformation concerning the efficacy of AAC treatments and the selection of AAC based on erroneous efficacy data. Researchers from the field of psychology have recognized the potential biases that arise from the predisposition of publishers to publish research that finds statistical significance and have created a publication known as the *Journal of Articles in Support of the Null Hypothesis*. This publication is for research in the area of psychology that does not find statistically significant differences. Perhaps the AAC field should develop a similar journal for AAC research.

The tendency to publish research that finds statistical significance may create a bias in the topics that researchers choose to study (Matosin et al., 2014). This is probably exacerbated by the mentality in academia that has given rise to the notion of "publish or perish." This mentality may contribute to researchers selecting those topics that have a high probability of finding statistical significance. Such a mentality may stifle creativity and may stunt the growth of a field. This mentality is not conducive to expanding the research base of a field. It is important for AAC professionals to understand the negative ramifications of such a mentality and to have an open and creative mindset in regards to AAC research.

It is also important for AAC professionals to understand research-based terminology that is frequently misunderstood. **Statistical significance** is one term that has the potential for being misunderstood. The term refers to the probability of whether or not a difference is due to chance. It does not address the significance of a research finding in regards to the importance of the difference. Rather, it only refers to a probability statement concerning a numerical difference. A solid understanding of statistics and research should help AAC professionals understand confusing terminology they may encounter in professional journals.

TERMINOLOGICAL ISSUES

There have been dramatic changes in AAC over the last couple decades. Chief among them include the appropriate terminology to use for referring to persons who use or can benefit from AAC and terminology related to the rapid proliferation of symbols and advancement of technology in the field. As the discipline of AAC continues on its evolutionary path, terminology must keep up with these changes. In the sections that follow, we will briefly discuss the need for terminology used in the field to keep up with its rapid evolutionary trajectory.

What Should We Call Persons Who Use and Can Benefit From AAC?

One issue not without its controversy is the term persons who do not use or rely on AAC refer to persons who do use or can benefit from AAC. Over the last several decades, a wide range of terms were used to describe these individuals, but each term had its own drawbacks. Without going through an exhaustive list of terms that have been used in the past, we will highlight just a couple of them. In the early years of AAC, the field was referred to as "nonspeech communication." Persons who used nonspeech communication were naturally referred to as "nonspeaking individuals." The inherent flaw in this term is the fact that not all people who use AAC are nonspeaking. In fact, many individuals who use AAC have at least some rudimentary speech abilities—just not sufficient enough to meet their daily communication needs. Another term used in the past was "nonverbal." The word "verbal" implies linguistic or language ability. To say a person is nonverbal is to say they have no linguistic ability at all. This is simply not true because we know a very large segment of the AAC community does indeed have sufficient, if not excellent, language skills. As a final example, the term "nonvocal" was used by some professionals to describe people who use AAC. To be vocal means to be able to use the larynx and vocal tract to produce and modify an acoustic signal. Describing persons who use AAC as nonvocal implies they have the inability to produce any type of acoustic output. Once again, this is not true of a number of persons who use AAC. If a person who uses AAC has some speech ability, then they are also vocal. Those who cannot produce speech might have the ability to produce various vocal sounds, like groans, grunts, laughs, moans, and sighs, which can be used for communicative purposes. These acoustic phenomena are indeed vocal and can be used as part of an AAC system (e.g., to catch a potential communication partner's attention, to protest, or to indicate a "yes" and "no" response).

Eventually, terminology became more direct. The terms "AAC user" and "individual (or person) who uses AAC" came into vogue. For many persons with and without disabilities, "AAC user" has two problems. First, it doesn't use **person-first terminology**. Second, for some it carries a negative connotation in much the same way as "drug user" does. A variant of "AAC user" is "person (or individual) who uses AAC." This term solves the issue of person-first terminology but still may carry a negative connotation for some.

The latest term used to describe people who require or may benefit from AAC is "person (or individual) with complex communication needs." The term "complex communication needs" originated in Australia around 2000 to 2001 as a term to replace "severe communication impairment" as part of the then Victorian State Government's initiative to fund supports for people who were nonspeaking—adults in particular. A workshop was conducted and led by people in Disability Services, Department of Human Services. The Communication Aids Users Society (now Communication Rights Australia), a group of users of AAC in Victoria, objected to the term, and others—such as Teresa Iacono—expressed concern with its ambiguity, as even able-bodied people have CCN. Despite objections, the term was adopted formally as part of policy on disabilities and then eventually found broader use in Australia.

At about the same time or shortly thereafter, through consultation of its Executive Committee, the International Society for Augmentative and Alternative Communication (ISAAC) suggested its use. Susan Balandin, president of ISAAC at the time, provided a definition for CCN in a message from the president in the ISAAC Bulletin. Balandin (2002) stated, "Some people have [CCN] associated with a wide range of physical, sensory, and environmental causes, which restrict/limit their ability to participate independently in society. They and their communication partners may benefit from using AAC methods either temporarily or permanently." (p. 2) During her tenure as editor of *Augmentative and Alternative Communication*, Iacono (2002) wrote an editorial entitled, "Words," and noted the term had been adopted after consultation among ISAAC Board members in reference to the World Health Organization's (2001) International Classification of Functioning, Disability and Health classification system. From that point, ISAAC's peer-reviewed professional journal *Augmentative and Alternative Communication* adopted "persons with complex communication needs" as the official term for persons who rely on or may benefit from AAC (Iacono, 2019).

On the surface, the term "persons with complex communication needs" seems to be adequate in describing people who must rely upon or may benefit from AAC. However, as previously noted, one drawback to the term is it can be used to describe persons *without* disabilities. Consider all the various forms and media in which we send and receive information every day—emails, private messages, radio, social media, television, text messages, typing, or writing. There are so many different ways we communicate on a daily basis. Communication is a complex process and, in these modern times, the platforms we have at our disposal to communicate are just as complex.

To go even further, many professionals (especially speech-language pathologists) would argue that many disorders of speech and/or language are complex, and as a result of these disorders, persons exhibiting them have CCN. Who could argue that a person who stutters does not have a complex communication disorder (to this day we still do not know what causes it!), and therefore, a person who stutters has a CCN? The same could be said for a host of communication disorders—apraxia of speech, paradoxical vocal fold movement disorder, and spasmodic dysphonia, to name a few. Under greater scrutiny, "CCN" seems ambiguous.

TABLE 1-2

Preferred Terminology by Role to Describe Persons Who Use AAC According to a December 2018 Straw Poll

TERM	AAC USER		PARAPROFESSIONAL		PARENT OR OTHER FAMILY		PROFESSIONAL	
	#	%	#	%	#	%	#	%
AAC communicator	0	0.0%	0	0.0%	0	0.0%	1	0.8%
AAC user	13	65.0%	3	100.0%	37	82.2%	52	40.6%
Augmented communicator	2	10.0%	0	0.0%	0	0.0%	3	2.3%
Complex communicator	0	0.0%	0	0.0%	0	0.0%	1	0.8%
Person who uses AAC	4	20.0%	0	0.0%	4	8.9%	32	25.0%
Person with CCN	1	5.0%	0	0.0%	4	8.9%	35	27.3%
Other	0	0.0%	0	0.0%	0	0.0%	4	3.1%
Total	20		3		45		128	

Respondents could choose only one response.

AAC = augmentative and alternative communication; CCN = complex communication needs.

Note that in the foregoing discussion, it was never mentioned how *persons who use AAC* would like to be referred. This begs the question: Has anyone ever consulted persons with severe communication impairments, their caregivers, or professionals who work with them as to the terminology *they* prefer? A review of the current literature does not seem to provide evidence this has ever happened.

Due to the lack of information on the preferences of persons who use AAC, a nonscientific straw poll was conducted in December 2018 on a blog related to AAC to determine the preferences of persons who use AAC, their families, paraprofessionals, and professionals (Fuller, 2019a). A total of 196 self-selected respondents provided a forced-choice response to the question, "In writing about AAC in the general sense (not in reference to a specific individual but rather in a textbook or article), which terminology do you usually prefer?" Results of the analysis can be found in Table 1-2. It was quite surprising that for all four groups (AAC users, paraprofessionals, parents or other family, and professionals) the term "AAC user" was most preferred. For all groups, except professionals, this term was clearly the term of choice with "person who uses AAC" coming in as the second most preferred term. Only for professionals (and perhaps to a lesser extent, family members) was the term "person with complex communication needs" considered an acceptable term to describe persons who use or may benefit from AAC. Of even greater surprise was the respondents' answer to a question regarding preference in terms of identity-first (e.g., "AAC user") or person-first (e.g., "individuals who use AAC") terminology (Table 1-3). Persons who use AAC

and paraprofessionals preferred **identity-first terminology**, professionals preferred person-first terminology, and family members had no particular preference but leaned more toward identity-first terminology. Apparently, persons who use AAC and paraprofessionals and, to a lesser extent, family members, are not as insistent on political correctness as professionals who work with persons exhibiting severe communication impairments!

One must keep in mind two important points: (1) this was not a scientific, controlled study, and (2) respondents were self-selecting. It is not known if the results would have changed considerably had a more scientific study been conducted with individuals who most likely did not participate (e.g., persons confined to hospital beds due to acute health issues, persons who were not members of the blog from which the poll was taken). That said, what can we conclude from this straw poll? First, it is quite clear that an international, scientific survey needs to be conducted to once and for all answer the question as to how persons who use or may benefit from AAC prefer to be referred. Second, the term "complex communication needs" is an acceptable term to use to describe persons with severe communication impairments, but so is "person (or individual) who uses AAC" and "AAC user." The take-away from this discussion is that when describing persons with severe communication impairments, any terminology that is used in a respectful and dignified manner should be acceptable. Therefore, throughout this textbook, the reader is likely to encounter a range of terms used to describe persons in the AAC community.

TABLE 1-3

Preference by Role Toward Person- or Identity-First Terminology to Describe Persons Who Use AAC According to a December 2018 Straw Poll

TERM	AAC USER		PARAPROFESSIONAL		PARENT OR OTHER FAMILY		PROFESSIONAL	
	#	%	#	%	#	%	#	%
Identify-first terminology	16	80.0%	3	100.0%	15	33.3%	16	12.6%
No preference	4	20.0%	0	0.0%	17	37.8%	39	30.7%
Person-first terminology	0	0.0%	0	0.0%	13	28.9%	72	56.7%
Total	20		3		45		127*	

*One professional did not respond to this question.

The Need to Rethink the Classification of AAC Symbols

There has been an explosion in the proliferation of symbols in AAC over the last decade, especially in the number and variety of aided symbols. With the advent of tablet and smartphone technology, entrepreneurs and creative clinicians learned to develop AAC applications (apps) that use a variety of symbols. These symbols range from proprietary sets or systems (i.e., symbols created by an app designer for monetary gain) to already-existing symbols licensed from a secondary source, to traditional orthography (i.e., the letters of the alphabet). Some apps—and by extension the symbols they utilize—are more complex and sophisticated than others. Added to the number of symbol sets and systems that have existed for years, it may be time to revisit the AAC symbol taxonomy proposed by Lloyd and Fuller (1986) and Fuller and colleagues (1992). The current taxonomic classification of symbols with its superordinate dichotomy of aided vs. unaided and subordinate classifications of static vs. dynamic, iconic vs. opaque, and set vs. system appears to be antiquated in light of the proliferation of a wide range of symbols over the last several years. In Chapter 3, Pampoulou and Fuller (2021) will propose the replacement of the current symbol taxonomy with a continuum of symbol classification primarily based on the degree of linguistic structure a particular corpus of symbols possesses. The degree of linguistic structure is determined by a set of interrelated variables that the authors argue have greater clinical relevance than the current taxonomic classification system.

The Need to Rethink the Classification of Technology

Not only has there been an explosion in the proliferation of symbols over the past decade, but the area of technology—especially communication technology—has evolved to the point that is difficult to classify technology simply as being aided or unaided, high technology, low technology, or no technology. Several of these terms have also become archaic and no longer useful for describing the development of technology, including tablet and smartphone technology, the development of AAC apps with or without synthetic speech output, and the recent development and refinement of artificial intelligence. We are truly living in a brave new world when it comes to AAC technology. In Chapter 3, Fuller and Pampoulou (2022) will suggest a communication technology taxonomy that not only classifies current technology but considers potential advancements in the biomedical and engineering fields. The proposed taxonomy also considers for the first time *receptive* communication (Fuller, 2019b; Fuller & Pampoulou, 2022). People who work in the field of AAC have become accustomed to thinking of AAC as expressive communication only. The AAC model proposed by Lloyd and colleagues (1990) clearly shows that AAC, like natural communication, is a two-way street where there must be a message sender and message receiver. The focus up until now has been on the AAC user as the message *sender*. What if the person who uses AAC also has a sensory impairment (e.g., auditory, visual, or both) that impedes their ability to comprehend communication? Should not rehabilitation professionals consider the receptive options that are available to ameliorate the AAC user's diminished ability to understand messages? A proposed communication technology taxonomy presented in Chapter 3 will address this issue.

SUMMARY

The ability to communicate with others is one of the most important human assets. AAC provides options that may replace or support conventional means of communication for individuals who experience severe communication disabilities. The two broad categories of AAC are aided and unaided. Aided strategies involve some external device or equipment, whereas unaided communication is accomplished with the individual's own body. The many aided and unaided strategies and techniques differ from conventional communication because they often use different means to represent, select, and transmit messages. Selection of appropriate AAC strategies requires careful assessment of an individual's abilities and environmental communication needs, and this is best accomplished with a team approach. The goals of AAC intervention should be to enhance the individual's communicative competence in the context of current and future home, school, work, and community settings. When AAC interventions are carried out with the needs and the perspective of the AAC user as a central focus, basic human rights are respected and new opportunities and life choices are made possible.

STUDY QUESTIONS

1. Name at least three aided and three unaided means of communication, not necessarily used by persons who rely on AAC, but also used typically by persons who are able to produce natural speech.

2. Name at least four reasons why AAC intervention strategies tend to be more effective for persons with severe communication impairments when more traditional speech and language approaches are not effective.

3. Elaborate on the significance of five perspectives presented in this chapter.

4. Describe the components of the broad communication model.

5. Explain the meaning of multimodal communication and give examples.

6. Describe the four areas of communicative competence and the role of each in online, real-time communication.

7. Please summarize the generation effect. As an AAC professional, how might you use the generation effect to improve the memory of your clients for their AAC? What would you do to share your findings with other AAC professionals?

8. Please summarize how organizational structure could be used to facilitate memory for AAC. What would you do to share your findings with other AAC professionals?

9. The working memory model includes two storage systems that may be involved in the processing of information. Describe these two storage systems and why a better understanding of how graphic AAC stimuli might be rendered and processed within these two systems and may be beneficial to the development of graphic AAC.

10. Describe the file drawer effect. What are some negative ramifications of this effect? What are some possible solutions for reducing bias that may arise from this effect?

11. Please clarify the differences between "statistically significant" findings and "findings of significance."

12. Discuss why the use of a consistent terminology is important in the field of AAC and why terminology should be revisited periodically.

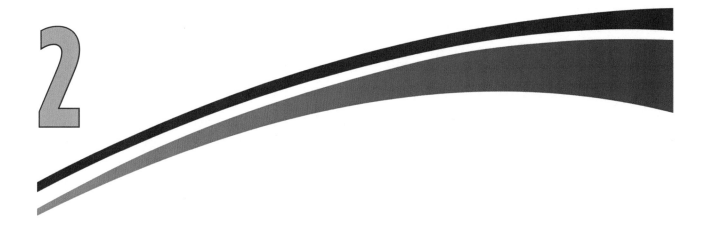

History and Evolution of AAC

Chitrali Mamlekar, PhD; Aimee Dietz, PhD;
Oliver Wendt, PhD; and Lyle L. Lloyd, PhD

MYTH

1. Augmentative and alternative communication (AAC) was not used until the second half of the 20th century.

2. AAC is a separate field of its own that functions independently to meet the needs of individuals with severe communication disabilities.

3. AAC services have always been supported by research.

4. AAC should be a "last resort" for people with complex communication needs (CCN), both those with developmental and acquired disorders, only used when other interventions have failed and no further options are left.

5. There are candidacy criteria that individuals with severe communication disorders must meet to qualify for provision of AAC services. These may include functioning at a certain cognitive level or chronological age, as well as exhibiting the ability to physically point to a device or display.

REALITY

1. AAC developed as a field in the second half of the 20th century, but reports of the use of AAC date back to ancient times.

2. The field of AAC is transdisciplinary, drawing from the expertise of many professions.

3. AAC services grew out of the need to improve the communication skills of individuals with little or no functional speech and was not initially guided by research. Now, however, research provides a broad knowledge base for the field.

4. The literature documents improved speech and language development and recovery via AAC. For these reasons, AAC should be implemented early on in the treatment process to promote communication while supporting speech and language development or recovery. AAC should be considered the standard of care for treating persons with CCN.

5. Everyone is able to communicate in some manner. In fact, communication occurs on a continuum and AAC must be adapted according to individual needs.

Fuller, D. R., & Lloyd, L. L. *Principles and Practices in*
Augmentative and Alternative Communication (pp. 29-38).
© 2023 Taylor & Francis Group.

Awareness and Potential of People With Communication Disabilities

Legislation That Opened the Door to AAC

Organizations run by and developed for people with disabilities have existed since at least the 1800s and included groups, such as disabled veterans (Gerber, 2003), American Psychiatric Association for people with mental illness (Mora, 1997), and the Columbia Institution for the Instruction of the Deaf and Dumb and the Blind (Armstrong, 2014), among others. However, that number seemed to explode in the 1900s. The League of the Physically Handicapped was organized in the 1930s to help people fight for employment during the Great Depression (Longmore & Goldberger, 2000). In the 1940s, a group of psychiatric patients came together to form We Are Not Alone (Pelka, 1997), which supported patients with their transition from hospital to community. During the 1950s and 1960s, there was a noticeable shift in the United States in terms of a general increased understanding of and sensitivity to the needs of individuals with disabilities (Frank & Glied, 2006). World War II and the Vietnam War (Sturken, 1997) were central to these changes, with many veterans developing acquired communication and physical disabilities (Hardy, 1983). To address the needs of this population, clinicians were challenged to create alternatives to provide them rehabilitation services for speech and language impairments, cognitive challenges, and interventions that focused on re-training skills required to complete activities of daily living (Howard & Hatfield, 2018). Moreover, veterans required rehabilitation to be fitted for prosthetic legs and to learn how to walk with their prostheses (Cutson & Bongiorni, 1996). Following World War II, the media increasingly shared information about the experiences and lives of people with disabilities (Axline, 1964), which prompted legislation to mandate services for these individuals.

Under the leadership of President John F. Kennedy, public awareness regarding the significant needs of individuals with cognitive impairment was brought to the forefront of discussion via the President's Panel on Mental Retardation, now called the President's Committee for People with Intellectual Disabilities (Sherrill, 2010). This group was responsible for gathering data about how people actually view cognitive impairment and asked the citizens of the United States their opinion on how to effectively include people with intellectual disabilities into a community that welcomes and sustains them. Through this work, the President's Committee enhanced public awareness of cognitive impairments, which seems to have prompted increased civil rights activity and thus set the stage for increased advocacy and legislation for decades to come.

The aforementioned sociopolitical events led to the discovery of the linguistic nature of American Sign Language, which helped raise public awareness of people's communication needs, as well as emergence of a disability rights movement in the 1970s. Sociopolitical events such as these generated substantial interest in AAC (Gambier & Gottlieb, 2001); by the 1980s, AAC became an area of professional specialization and the American Speech-Language-Hearing Association (ASHA) recognized it as an area of practice (ASHA, 2016c). Although increased social awareness had a positive impact on the emergence of AAC as a set of potentially life-changing strategies for people with CCN (Light & McNaughton, 2012a), AAC was still viewed as a last resort for people with CCN, reserved for situations where all other interventions had failed to develop speech and language in children (Romski & Sevcik, 2005) or recover speech and language in adults (Weissling & Prentice, 2010). In 1986, this issue was addressed by the newly developed National Joint Committee for the Communication Needs of Persons with Severe Disabilities (NJC; 1992). The specific purpose of the NJC is to advocate for people who have significant communication needs, particularly in people with intellectual disability (ASHA, 1992). However, Brady and colleagues (2016) mentioned that the Communication Bill of Rights of 1992 and 2016 is certainly relevant to those with acquired communication challenges as well. In particular, item 11 of the 2016 Communication Bill of Rights (Brady et al., 2016) states that each person has "… the right to have access to functioning AAC and other AT [assistive technology] services and devices at all times" (p. 123). In 2015, the NJC stated three goals of the revised Bill of Rights: (1) advocate for AAC support services, (2) promote opportunities for including individuals who require AAC in decision-making processes, and (3) increase social acceptance of AAC. Since then, significant changes have occurred in assessment, goal selection, interventions to improve communication, interventions to improve environmental supports for communication, and service delivery.

Increased social awareness also influenced the educational policies and practices that affected educators and students with disabilities. It has been estimated that only 5% of all students with a disability complete primary school (Peters, 2003). Even when students with disabilities attend school, they may encounter a curriculum that has not been adapted to their needs (Peters, 2003). The educational policies listed next facilitated a paradigm shift from seeing disability as a clinical and social welfare issue toward recognizing that disability is a fundamental human rights issue and that addressing the development goals of persons with disabilities is necessary to meeting overall global development goals. These educational laws provide a legal framework for all issues related to the lives of people with disabilities and are the basis for children with disabilities receiving education in an inclusive setting and with the support needed to succeed.

Educational Law

Four seminal laws that protect the rights of education for people with disabilities are Section 504 of the Rehabilitation Act, the Individuals with Disabilities Education Act (IDEA), the Technology-Related Assistance Act (Tech Act), and the Americans with Disabilities Act (ADA). A brief history of each act is provided below.

Section 504 of the Rehabilitation Act

In 1973, Section 504 of the Rehabilitation Act became the first disability civil rights law to be sanctioned in the United States. According to this act, people with disabilities should not be discriminated against for reasons related to their disabilities. This act also established the basis for enactment of the ADA years later. Section 504 works together with the ADA and IDEA to protect children and adults with disabilities from exclusion and unequal treatment in schools, jobs, and the community. These laws prevent institutions of higher education from using technology that is inaccessible to individuals with disabilities unless the institutions provide accommodations or modifications that would permit an individual with a disability to use the technology in an equally effective manner. Under Section 504, students with disabilities can be placed in the regular classroom; this ensures that related services are provided.

Individuals with Disabilities Education Act

In 1975, President Gerald Ford signed the Education for All Handicapped Children Act, now known as the IDEA (Yell et al., 1998). This law mandated that all states must provide equal access to education for children with disabilities in order to receive money from the federal government (Beukelman & Mirenda, 1998; Zangari et al., 1994). Though this law did not specifically mention AAC, the legislation guaranteed students receive a free and appropriate education, and children with CCN require AAC to achieve this goal. As such, the landmark IDEA facilitated the provision of AAC services to children (Vanderheiden & Yoder, 1986) via individualized family service plans for children birth to 2 years and individualized education plans for children ages 3 to 21 years (Committee on Children with Disability, 1992). With the passage of this legislation, a generation of students previously denied access to educational services entered the nation's public schools.

Technology-Related Assistance Act

The Tech Act was passed in 1988 and was reauthorized in 1994 and 1998 (Assistive Technology Act of 1998, 29 U.S.C. 3001). This legislation authorized funding to increase awareness of the power of assistive technology to improve the lives of people with disabilities (Assistive Technology Act of 2004, 29 U.S.C. 3002). More specifically, the Tech Act is designed to allow people with disabilities to actively participate in school (including postsecondary level), work, community living, and recreational activities (Assistive Technology Act of 2004). The Tech Act also supports states in assisting and strengthening their ability to address the AAC needs of individuals with disabilities. Moreover, the act also offers federal funds to assist states in developing consumer-responsive systems of access to AAC services (Assistive Technology Act of 2004).

Americans with Disabilities Act

President George H. W. Bush signed ADA in 1990. This was the nation's first comprehensive civil rights law addressing the needs of people with disabilities by prohibiting discrimination in employment, public services, public accommodations, and telecommunications. ADA requires schools and employers to provide reasonable accommodations to people with disabilities that will enable them to perform the essential functions of school or jobs. Providing a reasonable accommodation to a person with a disability can include the acquisition or modification of equipment or assistive devices. Technology has played an important role in offering people with disabilities AAC strategies they can use in the work or school setting.

Professional Organizations

The following are national and international professional and advocacy organizations that have had a major impact on the development of the AAC field. The overarching purpose of each organization, as well as its impact on AAC, is summarized in the following sections.

American Speech-Language-Hearing Association

ASHA is the national credentialing body for more than 223,000 speech-language pathologists in the United States and has the vision of "… making effective communication a human right, accessible and achievable for all" (ASHA, 2022). As a part of its mission for advancing science and setting professional standards, ASHA has recognized AAC as a part of the scope of practice for speech-language pathologists since 1980 (ASHA, 2016c). In 1992, ASHA formed Special Interest Group 12 (SIG 12: AAC; formerly Special Interest Division, or SID). SIG 12 is a group dedicated to improving the quality and availability of AAC services to consumers throughout the lifespan, promoting clinically relevant research, and educating current and future professionals. This group has been pivotal in increasing the visibility and importance of AAC, including the training of speech-language pathologists to be proficient in AAC service provision.

ASHA primarily supports the development of competent speech-language pathologists; however, ASHA also certainly provides powerful advocacy for people with communication disorders as part of its mission. There are several AAC-focused organizations that more directly support the needs and rights of people who use AAC, as well as their family members. These AAC-focused organizations also serve as a platform for professionals and AAC companies to disseminate research and share the latest developments in technology. A brief overview of the major players in this arena is given below.

International Society for Augmentative and Alternative Communication

The Blissymbolics Communication Institute and the Ontario Institute for Studies in Education (University of Toronto) held international conferences on nonspeech communication in Toronto in 1980 and 1982. This led to the landmark development of an international organization later to be known as the International Society for Augmentative and Alternative Communication (ISAAC). ISAAC actively promotes consumer involvement and improves access to AAC services through the dissemination of research in the AAC field. Since its beginning in 1983, ISAAC has been a dominant force in the AAC world (Light & McNaughton, 2012a; Yoder & Kraat, 1993). In fact, as the field has expanded, so has ISAAC's membership. As of the last documented report, ISAAC now includes more than 3,600 members in 62 countries (ISAAC, 2013).

Rehabilitation Engineering and Assistive Technology Society of North America

The Rehabilitation Engineering and Assistive Technology Society of North America (RESNA) was established in 1979 and acts as a nonprofit organization that provides funds to conduct research in the field of assistive technology, specifically in the area of systems change and service delivery. RESNA also advances the AAC field by offering certification, continuing education, and professional development for clinicians who work in this niche area. The AAC Special Interest Group of RESNA was established in 1988 and focuses on assistive technology and aided AAC approaches (RESNA, 2019).

Self-Advocacy Organizations

During the 1980s, people who used AAC began to take more initiative in improving the availability and quality of AAC services by forming self-advocacy organizations, such as Hear Our Voices (Dybwad & Bersani, 1996). More recently, AAC users have used the internet to network by subscribing to listservs, such as the Augmented Communicators Online Users' Group. The main goals of these support groups are to link families to other parent support groups and volunteer services, identify and access resources, and prepare individuals who use AAC to meet their present and future communication needs.

RESEARCH DISSEMINATION

Journals

During the mid-to-late 1970s, print information about the field of AAC experienced a period of exponential growth. A base of systematic research began to emerge with the increased occurrence of articles in refereed journals, such as the *American Journal of Occupational Therapy*, *American Journal on Mental Retardation* (now *American Journal on Intellectual and Developmental Disabilities*), *British Journal of Disorders of Communication*, *The British Journal of Mental Subnormality*, *Journal of Applied Behavior Analysis*, *Journal of Autism and Developmental Disabilities*, *Journal of Speech and Hearing Disorders* (now *Journal of Speech, Language and Hearing Research*) and *Mental Retardation* (now *Intellectual and Developmental Disabilities*). For example, ISAAC has supported numerous activities that represent major contributions to the AAC field, chief among them a biannual international conference and a professional, peer-reviewed journal, *Augmentative and Alternative Communication*.

With the proliferation of venues in which to disseminate information, professionals in one part of the world began reading what was happening in other regions. One comprehensive report that came to be regarded as an influential international addition to the knowledge base of AAC was published by the Swedish Institute for the Handicapped in the 1970s, *Technical Aids for the Speech-Impaired: An International Survey on Research and Development Projects*. This report provided a comprehensive compilation of information on the research and development of AAC in different parts of the world up to that time (Lundman, 1978). The report led to further cooperation, collaboration, and dissemination of information related to professional and technological developments in AAC; it was supported by the International Project on Communication Aids for the Speech Impaired (Zangari et al., 1994). The circulation of newsletters describing the use of AAC strategies also contributed to the spread of information about AAC, as did the publication of books and book chapters, and eventually, internet websites and blogs.

In 2010, ASHA's SIG 12 (then named SID 12) introduced *Perspectives on Augmentative and Alternative Communication*, a quarterly publication that has emerged as a major source of practical information. In January 2019, this publication merged with the newsletters of the other ASHA SIGs to create a peer-reviewed journal entitled, *Perspectives of the ASHA Special Interest Groups*.

Books

In the 1970s, the first books on language and communication with two or more chapters dedicated to AAC appeared (Lloyd, 1976; Schiefelbusch & Lloyd, 1974). The chapters were focused primarily on teaching supplementary communication skills using AAC to students with severe communication disorders. Reviews and textbooks devoted entirely to AAC also began to appear (Copeland, 1974; Schiefelbusch, 1977; Vanderheiden & Harris-Vanderheiden, 1976; Vicker, 1974). The materials in the books provided initial information for clinicians who sought to serve individuals with severe communication impairments. For example, some of the early books provided an introduction to AAC symbols, strategies, and devices. Goldberg and Fenton (1960) were the first to reference aided AAC systems in their book *Aids for the Severely Handicapped* (Copeland, 1974); one section was devoted to methods of communication for people with communication disorders. This text was an especially useful resource for professionals in rehabilitation programs who worked with individuals with cerebral palsy. The book, *Non-vocal Communication Techniques and Aids for the Severely Physically Handicapped* (Vanderheiden & Harris-Vanderheiden, 1976) and the chapter on communication systems and their components (Vanderheiden & Lloyd, 1986) served as resources and focused on early AAC devices that tended to be heavy, nonportable pieces of equipment. In addition to addressing limited mobility, the primary AAC strategy relied on alphabet spelling that limited applicability to populations with at least a relatively intact language system. Recognizing the limitations of the current AAC options, the authors also pointed out that such devices had limited use for nonspeaking individuals in the real world—even for those who were literate. For these reasons, there was a call for documentation of the clinical implementation of AAC strategies (e.g., Fristoe, 1975; Silverman et al., 1978; Vicker, 1974).

Today there is a wide range of books dedicated to AAC across the age span. *Augmentative and Alternative Communication: Supporting Children and Adults with Complex Communication Needs* has been through five editions (Beukelman & Light, 2020; Beukelman & Mirenda, 1998, 2002, 2005, 2013) and is a mainstay among books on AAC interventions and technologies. There are also several companion-type books on AAC that provide current information on various AAC technologies for specific populations and approaches. For example, *Augmentative and Alternative Communication: An Interactive Clinical Casebook* (McCarthy & Dietz, 2015) features a collection of case studies that incorporate AAC assessment and intervention in different settings across the lifespan. Likewise, *What Every Speech-Language Pathologist/Audiologist Should Know about Alternative and Augmentative Communication* (Binger et al., 2010) is a

supplemental book that provides information on tools for AAC assessment or candidacy. Finally, *Assistive Technology: Principles and Applications for Communication Disorders and Special Education* (Wendt et al., 2011) is a book that provides information on current rehabilitation strategies, available assistive technologies, and resources to supplement AAC assessment and intervention.

With the establishment of the AAC field came the need to standardize terms that could facilitate the international and transdisciplinary development of the field (Lloyd & Kangas, 1988). Lloyd (1985) proposed the standardization of a glossary of terms and concepts used in AAC (a work that was more than 35 years in the making but is now one of the supplemental materials for this textbook).

In fact, Lloyd was the first to recommend integrating the terms "augmentative communication" and "alternative communication," which were being used simultaneously but separately in the literature. Lloyd noted, "… using both terms can become awkward in many communication situations …" (1985, p. 66). A second article by Lloyd and Fuller (1986) proposed a stronger emphasis on the issue of taxonomy for AAC. As a result, an ISAAC terminology committee was formed in March 1988 with the purpose of standardizing terms used to represent nonverbal communication systems, development of guidelines, policies and recommendations, and a discussion of evolving issues within the field (Lloyd & Blischak, 1992; Lloyd & Kangas, 1988). This committee took into consideration the recommendations proposed by the journal *Augmentative and Alternative Communication*, which established itself as the premiere journal in this emerging, new field.

Thus, the 1980s marked an era of AAC specialization. As more professionals began to know about and implement AAC, professional organizations and universities began to respond. The following section reflects on professional preparation and the multidisciplinary nature of the field.

PROFESSIONAL PREPARATION

During the academic year 1977-1978, Marquette University, Purdue University, and the University of Wisconsin were the first universities to offer a course on AAC. Considering the multidisciplinary nature of AAC, the course at Purdue University was offered to students in special education, audiology, and speech-language pathology. Greg Vanderheiden and his colleagues at the Trace Research & Development Center at the University of Wisconsin were influential in using technology with individuals with severe communication impairments, and they developed workshops to introduce AAC technology to professionals in the United States (Borden et al., 1993). To this day, the Trace Research & Development Center continues to provide training on rehabilitation engineering and assistive technology

(Vanderheiden & Treviranus, 2011). Presently, almost all communication disorders or speech-language pathology academic programs in the United States offer at least one course with primary content in AAC, and some universities offer more than one course on AAC (Johnson & Prebor, 2019; Ratcliff et al., 2008).

By the 1980s, AAC was established as an independent field, and in 1989, ASHA outlined nine specific roles and responsibilities concerning the knowledge base and competencies that are appropriate for speech-language pathologists who provide AAC services:

1. Identification of appropriate AAC clients

2. Determination of appropriate AAC systems for clients that can be used to promote communication

3. Development of intervention/management plans for clients aimed at achieving and establishing "maximal functional communication"

4. Implementation of the intervention plans

5. Evaluation of the intervention outcome

6. Evaluation of new AAC technology, strategies, techniques, and symbols

7. Advocacy for AAC clients

8. Provision of in-service training to professionals and AAC users

9. Coordination of AAC services (ASHA, 1991)

Beukelman and Cumley (1992) proposed that professional preparation in AAC must occur at a minimum of three levels to meet the challenges posed by a fast-growing field: (1) preprofessional preparation, (2) advanced preparation, and (3) special preparation. They proposed that preprofessional preparation should serve to familiarize people with basic issues related to AAC. This includes training future clinicians to engage in direct services with individuals using AAC while receiving supervision from skilled mentors. Individuals training to be primary service providers (e.g., teachers, rehabilitation professionals) should also receive advanced training (Koul & Lloyd, 1994). Finally, a special level of preparation is needed for persons who intend to serve as AAC specialists and consultants at a regional, state, or national level. The advanced and special levels of preparation would necessitate continuing education programs because of rapid developments in the AAC field. Additionally, for programs focused on preprofessional and in-service training, an AAC assessment framework is required as it offers a way to provide focused instructions. Instructors may customize the materials and training as per specific roles assumed by an individual in the assessment process. For instance, instruction and training on AAC assessment for general practice clinicians would involve different methods and content than those used by AAC clinical specialists.

AAC Technology: Then and Now

Although AAC was recognized as an independent field in the 1980s, recent advances in research concerning assessment, treatment, rehabilitation, and education of people who use AAC systems has contributed to further development of the field (Light & McNaughton, 2012b; Mirenda, 1998; Zangari et al., 1994). Reference to the use of manual signs by individuals who are deaf dates back to the works of Plato (Levinson, 1967). Additional documentation of the use of manual sign alphabets and sign systems appeared during the Middle Ages (Bulwer, 1644; Dixon, 1890; Savage et al., 1981; Stokoe, 1960). However, the use of manual signs extended beyond individuals who were deaf. Benedictine monks who had taken vows of silence communicated through manual signs (Chaves & Solar, 1974); this strategy was also common among individuals with cognitive impairments during the 1800s (Bonvillian & Miller, 1995). Gestural communication was also used among individuals from different cultures to facilitate communication across languages (Skelly, 1979).

Then came the aided AAC system. Aided systems require an external communication book, device, or display. Examples of aided systems include the use of picture communication boards (Figure 2-1) and speech-generating devices (SGDs; Beukelman & Mirenda, 1998; Miller & Allaire, 1987). The most remarkable change in AAC has been the upsurge in the availability and capabilities of technology. The arrival of the microcomputer led to the development of user-friendly communication devices with sophisticated voice output (an early electronic aid, the Vocaid, can be seen in Figure 2-2). These advances led to more sophisticated communication options and further promoted the development of the AAC field. The following section provides background information on the technological advancements in AAC, as well as important milestones leading to the growth of the field.

AAC Debuts (1950 to 1980)

President John F. Kennedy's 1961 Panel on Mental Retardation provided the public with insight into the problems and needs of individuals with cognitive impairments. According to Caves and colleagues (2002), the first published reference to aided AAC systems was in a book by Goldberg and Fenton (1960). This text served as a guide to the development and use of non–speech-generating conversation boards for individuals with cerebral palsy. Since this early reference to nonelectronic communication boards, there have been significant developments resulting in a large array of aided and unaided AAC systems.

It was during the 1970s that Blissymbols were first introduced in Canada as a means of communication for children with cerebral palsy who were unable to effectively use

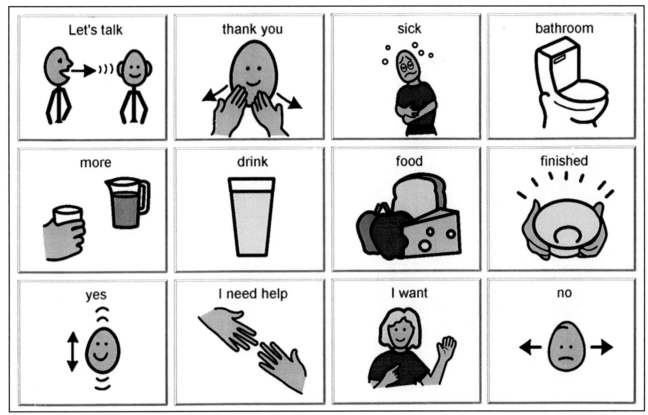

Figure 2-1. Non–speech-generating communication board using Picture Communication Symbols. (Courtesy of University of Central Florida Research Lab on AAC and Autism.)

traditional orthography to communicate. This innovative symbol system was implemented in 1971 in an educational program at the Holland Bloorview Kids Rehabilitation Hospital (formerly called the Hugh MacMillan Medical Centre; Kates & McNaughton, 1975).

While much of the early development of AAC focused on children with severe communication impairments, American Indian Hand Talk (Amer-Ind) was developed by Skelly (1979) for an adult with an acquired loss of speech due to glossectomy. Based on the hand signals in use for centuries by Native Americans, Skelly and her colleagues systematized this approach for use with individuals who experienced severe motor speech disorders (Skelly et al., 1975). Amer-Ind gestures are centered on concepts rather than words and reflect concrete ideas in contrast to other manual communication systems. Amer-Ind has no required grammatical or structural rules (Skelly, 1979) and is more intelligible (i.e., iconic) to untrained viewers (Duncan & Silverman, 1977).

AAC Grows Up (1980 to 2000)

Since the 1980s, technological advances have facilitated a continued interest in using computerized applications to enhance communication for populations of individuals with CCN (Vanderheiden, 2003). Many of the earliest technologies (e.g., AutoCom) took the designs of nonelectronic

communication boards and computerized them with available technology. Over time, increased research and development resulted in a broad array of SGDs made available to individuals with CCN from a range of assistive technology manufacturers (Hourcade et al., 2004; Shane et al., 2012). Despite variations in specifics, in many ways the designs of these SGDs uniformly conformed to the designs of the original nonelectronic communication displays (i.e., grid-based layouts of AAC graphic symbols).

Improvements in computer technology including the development of better voice synthesis and improved computer graphics led to a greater variety of user-friendly AAC devices (Beukelman & Mirenda, 1998; Zangari et al., 1994). In 1939, Homer Dudley introduced the first speech synthesizer named VODER (Voice Operating Demonstrator) at the New York World's Fair (Flanagan, 1972). In 1981, a sophisticated voicing source called the Klattalk system was introduced by Dennis Klatt (Klatt, 1987). In the late 1970s and early 1980s, a significant number of commercial text-to-speech and speech synthesis products were introduced (Klatt, 1987). In 1980, Texas Instruments introduced the Speak-n-Spell synthesizer based on linear prediction coding (Schroeder, 1993). In particular, improved speech synthesis technologies made augmentative and alternative communication services more accessible for individuals with severe disabilities (Romski et al., 1988).

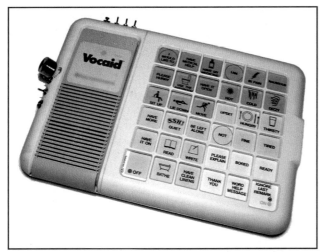

Figure 2-2. Vocaid SGD. (Retrieved from https://www.flickr.com/photos/wwiggins/1616149.)

AAC devices offer synthesized and/or digitized (or recorded) speech output (Drager et al., 2010). Qualitatively, digitized speech sounds more natural than synthesized speech, as it is a time-sampled reproduction of actual human speech. Both digitized and synthesized devices produce speech that is highly intelligible to the listener (Rupprecht et al., 1995). Digitized voice output devices, such as the IntroTalker by the Prentke Romich Company and the McCaw by Zygo, were graphic in nature, making them more usable by people who were unable to read or write (Zangari et al., 1994).

In addition to voice output features, access methods have also changed considerably over the years. The earliest microcomputer interfaces consisted of simple switches. Switches evolved from simple buttons to pneumatic (i.e., "sip-and-puff") and head-position (i.e., mercury) switches. The head mouse (Figure 2-3) was an early computer interface that went beyond the typical switches seen at the time. Eventually, eye-tracking access became a useful alternative for individuals with physical limitations over their hand movements. Eye-tracking devices trace the movement of one's eyes and allow users to navigate through the web and AAC systems (Figure 2-4). An example of a system working with electro-oculography signals for a computer mouse substitution is Eagle Eyes developed at Boston College by DiMattia and Gips (Majaranta & Räihä, 2002).

Technology is not always the ideal AAC solution for people with CCN. As such, unaided and non–speech-generating strategies remained the most frequently used methods throughout the 20th century. Even those who use SGDs often relied on multimodal communication approaches and supplemented communication with non–speech-generating or unaided strategies (Miller & Allaire, 1987).

Historically, the choice of communication system often was based on the belief that individuals with severe physical disabilities would benefit most from aided systems whereas persons with severe cognitive disabilities with lesser levels of physical disability should use unaided systems. This principle changed with the recognition that the combination of aided and unaided communication systems yielded substantially enhanced communicative power (Musselwhite & St. Louis, 1988). Musselwhite and St. Louis' findings helped to create a paradigm shift in how AAC treatment is administered. For example, a person with amyotrophic lateral sclerosis may use an aided system with eye gaze when communicating novel information to their physician or when communicating via social media, but use unaided strategies, such as simple gestures, when interacting with family, especially at the end of the day when they are fatigued (Morris et al., 2013). Likewise, a child may rely more on an aided system during the school day in the classroom but communicate via unaided techniques, such as gesture and vocalizations, in the evening with parents or on the playground when a device is not available (Binger et al., 2008). These examples illustrate the importance of developing a multimodal system for people with CCN.

AAC Establishment (2000 to 2010)

In recent years, efforts to enhance communication access have extended beyond traditional AAC systems to include the use of partner-listening strategies (e.g., Kagan et al., 2001; Hustad et al., 2011) and communication assistants who translate messages communicated via AAC much as sign language interpreters translate between oral speech and a sign language. Ongoing research and development expanded the range of AAC options available, including new symbol sets (Roche et al., 2014), interface designs (Dietz et al., 2006; Dietz et al., 2013), selection techniques (Light & Drager, 2007), and output (Hux et al., 2017).

In the past, a small number of AAC manufacturers developed, produced, and supported a comparatively small number of dedicated AAC SGDs (DeRuyter et al., 2007). More recently, the field has witnessed the explosion of mobile technologies (e.g., touchscreen phones and tablets, such as the Apple iPad) with a wide range of software applications (i.e., apps), including those intended to support communication (McNaughton & Light, 2013; Rehabilitation Engineering Research Center on Communication Enhancement, 2011). One of the first full-featured AAC apps for iOS, named Proloquo2Go, was developed by AssistiveWare in 2009. Proloquo2Go supports text-based and symbol-based communication and benefits children and adults in developing literacy skills. It also includes ExpressivePower, which allows personalization of the app to include natural intonation or prerecorded expressions and sounds. The following section highlights the significance of this boom in mobile technology.

Mobile Technology Boom (2010 to Present)

The landscape of technology began to change in 2008 with the opening of the Apple App Store with the modest number of 552 apps being made available for download. As of 2019, 1.8 million apps were available through the Apple

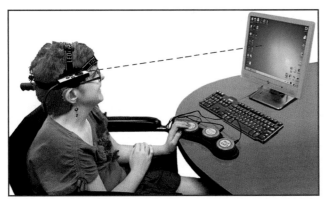

Figure 2-3. An individual using a head mouse ("air mouse") on a stationary personal computer. (Reproduced with permission from Air Mouse. Enabling Devices. 800-832-8697. enablingdevices.com/)

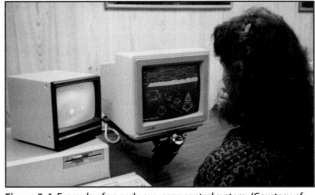

Figure 2-4. Example of an early eye-gaze control system. (Courtesy of LC Technologies, Inc./eyegaze.com.)

store! Such advances are not limited to Apple; the Google Play Store, Amazon, and independent app developers also contribute significantly to the potential of the app market. These developments contributed substantially to the field of AAC. Seemingly overnight, communication apps became affordable for download onto portable devices that people with CCN and their families hoped would be the answer to their AAC needs. An example of an Apple-based iPad AAC app can be seen in Figure 2-5.

Today, rather than going through a lengthy evaluation and funding process, a prospective AAC user can obtain a communication app ranging from no cost to $200 that can be downloaded readily onto a device they may already own. This provides the person with CCN and their family a greater sense of control and participation in the process of communicating with others (Kagan, 1998).

On many levels, the potential of these new opportunities is exciting; however, technology in and of itself cannot adequately address the complex needs of people who require AAC. The mobile technology boom created complicated scenarios of families bringing prepurchased technology to speech-language therapy appointments and asking the clinician to "make this work" for their loved one. As a profession, we had to respond—and quickly—to this dilemma (Light & McNaughton, 2013); we cannot sit idle. We must continue to educate people on the role of speech-language pathologists in helping to personalize AAC systems through the assessment process and to provide appropriate instruction during treatment to ensure success (Beukelman & Ray, 2010; Binger et al., 2010; Costello et al., 2010; Dietz et al., 2012; Lund et al., 2017).

AAC AND LIFE PARTICIPATION

Assessment procedures have significantly improved over the last several decades. Not so long ago it was necessary for individuals to establish candidacy as an AAC user and to later demonstrate the need for the use of an AAC system (Dietz et al., 2012; Hourcade et al., 2004). These criteria essentially involved a double-edged sword. On the one hand, as

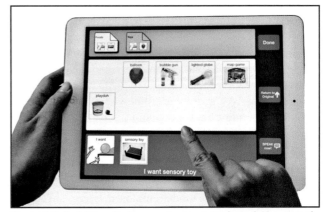

Figure 2-5. An AAC application running on an Apple iPad. (Courtesy of University of Central Florida Research Lab on AAC and Autism.)

reviewed by Rowland and Schweigert (2003), children have been excluded from AAC services because they fail to demonstrate so-called "prerequisite skills" that were thought necessary to successful AAC communication—many of which were cognitive in nature, including Piagetian constructs like means-end play or object permanence (Hourcade et al., 2004; Romski & Sevcik, 2005). Children who did not meet the candidacy criteria were not considered able to benefit from AAC intervention, and thus, were explicitly denied those services. However, another aspect of the eligibility issue involved children with some existing or potential speech skills. In part because of the concern discussed earlier that AAC implementation might impede speech development, AAC was perceived as a "last resort" approach implemented only when it appeared that spoken communication might not ever be able to fully serve the range of an individual's communication needs. This meant young children with severe communication support needs often did not receive AAC intervention until they were older, and of course, correspondingly more delayed. In both cases, the result has been to restrict access to functional communication modes. Moreover, due to medical advances, children with significant communication disabilities who require AAC are living longer (Balandin & Morgan, 2001), thus increasing even more the prevalence of individuals who require AAC. Similarly, older adults (i.e., 65 years of age and older) are more likely to experience concomitant sensory perceptual, motor, cognitive, and language impairments (Segalman, 2011) and may require AAC supports to communicate their needs.

Unfortunately, the use of candidacy criteria, like cognitive level or chronological age, as the basis for exclusion from services can still be seen in practice (Wilkinson & Hennig, 2007), even though it has been explicitly rejected by ASHA (ASHA, 2004b, 2005) and NJC (2002, 2003). In its place is the understanding that AAC reflects a continuum of communication that can range from simple unaided gestures or vocalizations to sophisticated aided technologies that employ eye tracking. AAC intervention goals for someone who is not yet ready for symbolic communication should be designed to reflect the person's current abilities while bearing in mind what may be needed in the future (Binger & Light, 2007). For example, a child's short-term AAC goals may include using aided modes to establish and maintain simple turn-taking routines (e.g., peekaboo games), while long-term goals include more advanced symbolic behavior (e.g., increased classroom participation using their AAC device). Similarly, a short-term AAC goal for an adult with fluent aphasia may include expanding their communication notebook to provide them with vocabulary to establish the communication contexts (e.g., people in their family, food, feelings) for the communication partner (Lasker, 2008) and to help reduce jargon/mazes (Dietz et al., 2018).

A contemporary model employed largely throughout the last 2 decades aligns most closely with the Participation Model (Beukelman & Light, 2020; Beukelman & Mirenda, 1998, 2005; Hourcade et al., 2004). Using the Participation Model, the individual's communication access and opportunity barriers are assessed to plan intervention for now and the future (Beukelman & Light, 2020). The Participation Model stresses the need to identify participation patterns, barriers, and specific communication needs for individuals with CCN. The model highlights opportunity and access barriers that may be common factors for both adults and children with communication challenges (Higginbotham et al., 2007). Opportunity barriers may include the skills and knowledge of AAC facilitators (e.g., teachers or caregivers) to support full participation. On the other hand, access barriers relate to limitations imposed by AAC systems or the individual skills and characteristics of people who use AAC. Access barriers may be influenced by an individual's physical and motor limitations, capacity for decision making, or sensory perceptual skills. Beukelman and Light (2020) encourage AAC stakeholders to recognize opportunity and access barriers as they plan current and future assessment and intervention tasks. Speech-language pathologists, along with families and professional teams, should develop and implement individualized intervention plans. Although each intervention plan or program is unique based on each individual's needs, the ultimate goal of AAC intervention is to facilitate effective and successful communication between the person with AAC needs and their communication partners (ASHA, 1992).

SUMMARY

The field of AAC has developed to the point that individuals with a variety of communication disabilities are benefiting from AAC services more than ever before. Today, AAC services are offered by members of transdisciplinary teams at home, at school, in the workplace, in medical settings, and in extended care facilities. The development of improved educational strategies, increased availability of assistive communication devices, increased opportunities for academic and professional preparation of service providers, and increased educational opportunities for individuals with communication disabilities have all played roles in bringing the field of AAC to where it is today.

Research serves as the foundation for the development and implementation of AAC programs. Over the past 3 decades, AAC has emerged as a field backed by a strong evidence base. For over a decade, current technological advances have shaped AAC intervention by fostering the integration of language restoration and compensation philosophies. The end goal of AAC research is to provide effective and efficient interventions, strategies, and technologies to help individuals whose natural speech is not functional to actively participate in their daily activities. Today, AAC researchers are attempting to gather critical evidence on the effectiveness of brain-computer interfaces to support communication in individuals with CCN. The subsequent chapters in this textbook will help the reader understand how to navigate the maze of technological options, personalization, and intervention strategies required to achieve this goal.

STUDY QUESTIONS

1. List four seminal federal laws that laid the foundation for the development of the AAC field.

2. Name three major organizations that serve AAC practitioners, researchers, and consumers.

3. When and where did the first AAC personnel preparation programs emerge?

4. Discuss at least three major computer applications that were incorporated into modern AAC devices.

5. Describe at least three major changes to the provision of AAC through the mobile technology boom.

6. What must practitioners continue to advocate for in terms of incorporating mobile technology into AAC interventions?

7. Name at least two major challenges the AAC field needs to address in the future.

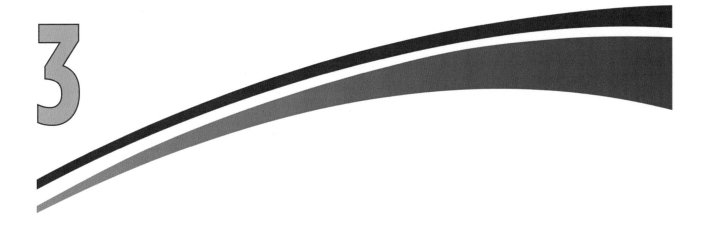

AAC Models and Classification Systems

Donald R. Fuller, PhD; Eliada Pampoulou, PhD;
and Lyle L. Lloyd, PhD

MYTH

1. Models and classification systems are important only for researchers and theorists to understand. As an educator/clinician, models and taxonomies have no relevance to my daily practice.

REALITY

1. Models and classification systems help not only researchers and theorists to conceptualize the issues that are important and in need of empirical investigation, but they also help educators and clinicians see how various components of a process or entity fit together and relate to each other. It is only through a complete understanding of a process and its interrelated components that an educator or clinician can truly provide the best possible services to their clients.

INTRODUCTION

One of the definitions for model in the Merriam-Webster (n.d.) online dictionary is "a description or analogy used to help visualize something … that cannot be directly observed." The operative words in this definition are "description" and "visualize." A model is typically a construction based on one's current understanding of how a particular phenomenon operates; that is, a model is simply a description or visualization of how something operates or exists. Human relationships can include economics, psychology, or any other system in which humans are an integral part, including **communication**. Communication is an extremely complex phenomenon that is not fully understood to this day. As such, the best one can do is offer a theory for how communication within the human species takes place. To assist in visualizing or conceptualizing all the various aspects that make up communication, a model can be employed based on current knowledge of the process. Lloyd and colleagues (1990) identified several benefits of constructing a model for augmentative and alternative communication (AAC). A model allows for the formulation of questions and hypotheses about the individual aspects of AAC and how the individual aspects

Fuller, D. R., & Lloyd, L. L. *Principles and Practices in*
Augmentative and Alternative Communication (pp. 39-61).
© 2023 Taylor & Francis Group.

interrelate. From this, systematic quantitative and qualitative research can be designed to address the questions and hypotheses. In the short term, research affords the opportunity to adjust the model, if necessary, to reflect new knowledge. In turn, the expansion of the knowledge base through research ultimately allows for the development of effective assessment and intervention strategies. Another benefit of a model is that it provides structure to the knowledge base. At the same time, the relationships between and among various fields can be better conceptualized through the use of a model. This is especially important for AAC, which can be described as a field of fields that includes audiology, medicine, occupational therapy, physical therapy, rehabilitation engineering, social work, special education, speech-language pathology, and other professions.

With the vast amount of information that exists in the field of AAC, it is not only beneficial but also necessary to conceptualize the AAC process by developing a model based on current theory. This model will serve as the basis for organizing and presenting the information concerning AAC for the remainder of this textbook. However, before presenting the model, the reader may be in a better position to understand the complex process of AAC if a brief background discussion on the evolution of communication models in general is provided. Therefore, the following section examines a representative number of models that have come from information processing, speech production, and communication. From this discussion, the reader should be able to see a direct relationship between these fields and AAC.

COMMUNICATION MODELS: A HISTORIC PERSPECTIVE

The process of human communication has been conceptualized by several individuals over the past 8 decades (Berko et al., 1977; Fairbanks, 1954; Sanders, 1971, 1976, 1982; Shannon & Weaver, 1949). Each model presented in this section is based on a different orientation or school of thought, but they all share similar aspects. The model proposed by Shannon and Weaver (1949) was developed to illustrate general information processing and not necessarily communication *per se*, although human communication could be considered a form of information processing. The key aspects or elements of their model include a source, **message**, transmitter, signal channel, receiver, and destination. In human speech communication, the source represents the individual's brain where the message (i.e., the idea to be transmitted) is formulated. The message is sent through the transmitter (i.e., the speech mechanism) as an acoustic signal. This signal channel may or may not include noise. Eventually, the signal is perceived by the receiver (i.e., the listener's ear) and then interpreted at the destination (i.e., the listener's brain). This model does not consider the give and take of communication but simply describes a single message being conveyed from **sender** to **receiver**.

Fairbanks (1954) presented a model to describe speech production that for most individuals is their primary mode of communication. As such, his model is not concerned with communication but instead with how speech is produced. This does not lessen the impact of his model because it provides a rather detailed account of at least one half of the communication process (i.e., the sender). A unique feature of the Fairbanks model is that it is a closed-loop or servo-system, meaning that ongoing **feedback** is an integral part of the model. In essence, the signal (i.e., the message that is to be conveyed by speech) is stored in a controller unit, then sent through an effector unit (i.e., the speech mechanism), where it is finally sent out as an acoustic signal. The unique feature of this model is the sensor unit, which is responsible for comparing the signal that went out to the message that was intended. According to this model, the hearing mechanism is the chief anatomical structure responsible for receiving feedback, with the output acoustic signal being fed back to the hearing mechanism through air and bone conduction. Other sensors are also responsible for the feedback mechanism (e.g., tactile and kinesthetic receptors of the individual speech organs). Feedback has direct implications for AAC, as iterated by Lloyd and colleagues (1990):

> Speech, or any communication output, is self-corrective in most senders. This is possible because the sender is able to constantly monitor the output via various forms of feedback (e.g., auditory, tactile, visual) and adjust such output according to a preconceived standard based on previous experience. If the sender lacks the experience or receives distorted sensory feedback, there may be a serious deterioration in communication effectiveness. In AAC, message distortions may be related to the nature of the input or output system used (e.g., poor visual acuity and hearing impairment). Furthermore, such sensory distortions may alter perception of the environment and result in inappropriate understanding and interaction with that environment. This may have serious implications for the individual's cognitive and social development. In AAC, distortions in sensory feedback may result because of the significant variations in the form and/or latency of the feedback. For example, synthesized speech provides no proprioceptive or kinesthetic feedback and may be substantially delayed, as compared with the instantaneous feedback of the output of the vocal mechanism. (p. 182)

Clearly, an AAC model should include some form of feedback mechanism.

The model proposed by Berko and colleagues (1977) attempts to describe how such variables as attitudes, experiences, and physical states enter into the process of communication. According to their model, two communicators (i.e., a source and a receiver) convey information and ideas to one another through a communication environment that may or may not be superimposed by a noise component (either internally or externally generated). In this sense, their model is similar to the model proposed by Shannon and Weaver (1949). The uniqueness of the part intangible variables play in communication sets this model apart from the others. The source communicator's (i.e., sender's) attention is first aroused by an idea or a need to communicate. The sender then chooses to communicate a message by using language symbols. Memory and past experiences are used to govern the selection of language symbols for encoding the message. The sender's message is then tempered by the sender's attitudes, physical state, and expectations. The message is sent through a channel within the communication environment and is received by the receiver communicator. This person's attention is aroused by aural stimuli or the need to communicate. The message is received in distorted form due to the introduction of the noise component. The receiver communicator must then rely on memory and past experiences to decode the message. The information is then stored and the receiver communicator offers feedback to the source communicator.

Sanders (1971, 1976, 1982) proposed a model that included aspects from the models of Fairbanks (1954) and Berko and colleagues (1977). It addressed the complexity of interaction between a sender and receiver within a communication environment and also addressed the issue of feedback. It is, however, a much more widely expanded model of communication because it describes in greater detail the sender and receiver. The message encoding and decoding processes are also explained in more detail. A key component of the Sanders model is the multimodal description of message sending and receiving. Irrespective of disability, most individuals do not rely solely on speech as a means of communication. Some may rely on facial expressions, gestures, and posture and movement in addition to speech. The use of symbols (please see Chapters 6 through 8 for a full discussion of symbols) is also a possibility when speech or gestures fail to get the message across (e.g., when two persons of differing languages attempt to communicate). As such, communication tends to be a multimodal phenomenon. This is especially important for AAC because any and all modalities (e.g., gesturing, pointing, speaking, writing) must be manipulated to maximize the probability of successful communication. An AAC model should therefore include a multimodal component.

The reader who is interested in a more thorough discussion of these models is encouraged to locate the original papers (Berko et al., 1977; Fairbanks, 1954; Sanders, 1971, 1976, 1982; Shannon & Weaver, 1949). In addition, a compendium of these models can be found in the article by Lloyd and colleagues (1990). We will return to components of some of these historic models when we discuss the comprehensive AAC model proposed by Lloyd and colleagues (1990).

EXAMPLES OF AAC MODELS

In this section, the reader will be introduced to two models of AAC. The first model views AAC from a broader perspective—that is, the entire AAC process from a bird's eye view, so to speak. The second model—and the one that was developed 30 years ago but is still considered the best description of how the process of AAC works—is a view of AAC from a comprehensive perspective.

Viewing AAC From a Broad Perspective

Any model that views the overall process of AAC without going into considerable detail about its individual components can be considered to view AAC from a broad perspective. One such model was proposed by Golinker in 2019 (Figure 3-1). In this model, AAC is seen as taking the form of two types of strategies: unaided and aided (Lloyd & Fuller, 1986). Any type of symbol, strategy, or access method that only requires the parts of one's natural body are unaided. For example, gestures and manual signs are unaided. Pointing to symbols with a finger or using eye gaze to select symbols from a display are examples of unaided selection methods. It would be logical to assume that aided strategies require some type of device or instrument that is not part of the natural human body. Any type of graphic symbols (including traditional orthography—the letters of the alphabet) are aided because the symbols have to be stored on some type of display. In the case of traditional orthography, the most common aided means of reading words is via a book or magazine. These are external to the body; therefore, the symbols and the manner in which information is sent or received is also aided. If an individual who uses AAC requires the use of a head wand to point to symbols on a display, then the means of selecting symbols is aided. As can be seen from the Golinker model, aided strategies also include non–voice-output aids and voice-output aids. The foregoing examples of aided symbols, selection methods, and transmission methods are all non–voice-output aids. Voice-output aids, as the term implies, are devices that produce synthetic speech output. These are also aided, as the device that produces speech output is external to the natural body. Voice-output aids can produce either digitized (e.g., prerecorded) words and messages or synthesized messages (e.g., devices that produce speech using an algorithm according to the words the user types) or a hybrid form of speech output that uses both digitized and synthesized messages. This is AAC in a nutshell. Note that there is no detail beyond these very basic components.

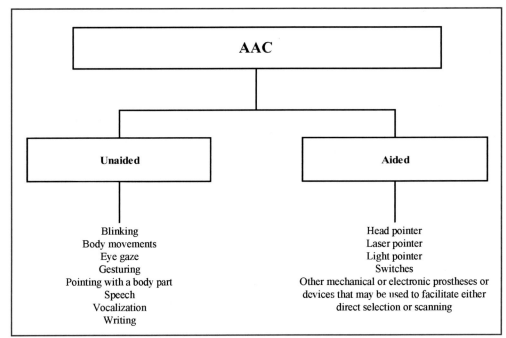

Figure 3-1. Golinker model of AAC from a broad perspective.

The Participation Model

Although the Participation Model (Beukelman & Light, 2020; Beukelman & Mirenda, 2013) appears to be related more to service delivery than the components of AAC per se, for a well-rounded discussion of AAC models, it bears mentioning. The Participation Model consists of three stages: (1) the identification of participation patterns and communication needs of individuals with complex communication needs (CCN), (2) the planning and implementation of intervention for immediate and anticipated future needs, and (3) evaluation of the effectiveness of intervention.

Subsumed under the first stage of the model is the identification of barriers that prevent active participation. This includes the assessment of barriers to opportunity and access. Opportunity barriers include policies, practices, attitudes, and lack of facilitator knowledge and skills that prevent the potential AAC user from taking an active part in communication. Access barriers are determined through a thorough assessment of the individual's current communication abilities and include access potential to increase natural abilities, to make environmental adaptations, and to utilize AAC systems and devices.

The second stage is intervention. Once a thorough assessment of barriers to opportunity and access has been conducted, intervention is planned and executed with a goal toward reducing or eliminating barriers that prevent the potential user from being an active participant in the communication process. It is at this stage that what is commonly identified as AAC intervention takes place. Opportunity and access barriers are addressed within the context of intervention, not only considering immediate needs but potential

future needs as well. The intervention process includes not only the AAC user but persons who may be tasked with the responsibility of facilitating communication in the person with CCN.

The final stage of the Participation Model involves the evaluation of effectiveness of AAC intervention. It is this third stage where the clinician or educator asks, "Is the AAC user actively participating in the communication process?" If the answer to this question is yes, periodic follow-up is essential. As with all humans, the communication needs and environments of AAC users change with time. This question is not one-off. It should be repeated periodically to ensure the AAC user continues to participate actively and effectively in communication without barriers impeding them. If the answer to the question is no, the entire process of assessment of communication needs and barriers and the introduction of effective intervention strategies is repeated.

The discussion provided here only touches upon the Participation Model without going into the intricate details of what is included in the entire process. The interested reader is referred to Beukelman and Mirenda (2013) or Beukelman and Light (2020) for a more detailed presentation and explanation of the Participation Model.

Viewing AAC From a Comprehensive Perspective

The Lloyd and colleagues (1990) AAC model is a more comprehensive model. It considers components from the preceding discussion on historic models that share several aspects of general communication and information

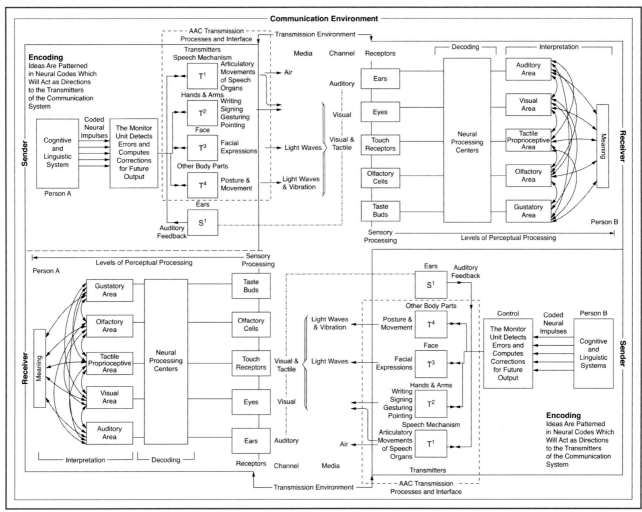

Figure 3-2. AAC model. (Reproduced with permission from Lloyd, L. L., Quist, R., & Windsor, J. [1990]. A proposed augmentative and alternative communication model. *Augmentative and Alternative Communication, 6*[3], 172-183. https://doi.org/10.1080/07434619012331275444)

processing. These components include the sender, message, receiver, feedback, and communication environment (Lloyd et al., 1990). Successful communication must have at least two individuals—a sender of an idea and a receiver of that idea. In addition, communication implies that a message is being transmitted. This message is transmitted and the communicators exchange ideas within a communication environment, which may have noise components (internally and/or externally generated). Finally, feedback—both internal (e.g., auditory through bone conduction and kinesthetic) and external (e.g., auditory through air conduction, visual, and linguistic and non-linguistic indicators that the message has been understood)—is a crucial component of the communication process. Communication is a multimodal process. Speech is not the only mode by which ideas are transmitted. Facial expression, gestures, pointing, and writing are also legitimate means of conveying information. Typically, several of these tend to be transmitted simultaneously. For persons with disabilities, a multimodal approach to communication is essential and an AAC model should contain all these components.

The Lloyd and colleagues (1990) AAC model is illustrated in Figure 3-2 and takes into consideration all these aspects. This model is an expansion of the Sanders (1971, 1976, 1982) model of general communication with modifications made to reflect what occurs during the AAC process. Lloyd and colleagues (1990) argued that an AAC model could be subsumed under a general communication model instead of being designed as a categorically different entity for three reasons. First, AAC is typically an intentional, symbol-based, and rule-governed form of communication consisting of a message being transmitted from a sender to a receiver within a communication environment with appropriate feedback being given. Second, a model based on general communication lends itself to direct observation and comparison between AAC and other forms of communication (e.g., animal communication, spoken communication, and other forms of human communication between individuals with and without disabilities). Finally, AAC is an interactive process between communicators, one of whom may not have a communication impairment. In other words, communication often takes place between an AAC user and a person without a disability. An AAC model must consider these facts.

In Figure 3-2, the key elements of a general communication model are the sender, message, transmitter, communication environment, receiver, and feedback (both endogenous and exogenous). Lloyd and colleagues (1990) added the communication environment to the Sanders model. The communication process is influenced by different communication environments. Recognition of this is critical for effective AAC intervention. Therefore, clinicians and educators must consider the communication environment as a critical part of the AAC process. With this addition, what Sanders referred to as the environment was retitled the transmission environment or transmission/signal channels for the AAC model (see Figure 3-2). Whereas the communication environment includes the people, places, and contexts in which communication is taking place, the transmission environment is the actual propagating medium or signal environment. The transmission environment is typically air for conducting light and/or sound waves, but it could be some other medium, such as water. In other words, there are two different types of environments (i.e., communication and transmission) and each has multiple possibilities.

Another addition was the AAC **transmission processes** and AAC **interface** component, which will be explained in more detail later. For purposes of discussion, the process of AAC will be described in terms of the sender being an AAC user. However, keep in mind that in the natural environment, either the sender, receiver, or both may be using AAC.

If one looks closely at the AAC model in Figure 3-2, they would notice that the bottom half is just a reversal of the upper half. This illustrates the back-and-forth nature of communication. The upper half of Figure 3-2 shows a typical scenario between two communicators in which the sender is using AAC. Person A (the sender) forms an idea to be communicated. Coded neural impulses are generated via the sender's cognitive and linguistic systems. These impulses pass through a monitor unit that detects errors and makes corrections for future output (a form of endogenous feedback). Coded impulses then drive any one or number of the transmitters (e.g., speech mechanism, hands and arms, face, and other body parts) to encode the message. If the speech mechanism is driven, the output will be speech via the articulatory movements of the speech organs. If the hands and arms are driven, the output could be pointing, gesturing, manual signing, or writing. Facial expressions will be generated if the muscles of the face are activated. Finally, other body parts (e.g., shoulders, legs) when driven will assist in generating communication through posture and movement. Any one or all of these modes of communication may be in operation at a given time. The output message then passes through the transmission environment (e.g., speech as an acoustic signal or sound vibration waves and manual signs as a visual signal or light waves) to Person B's receptors (i.e., ears, eyes, touch receptors) where sensory processing takes place. Simultaneous with this process, Person A's ears may be receiving auditory feedback, either endogenously from within self (e.g., bone conduction), exogenously from air

conduction, from Person B, or from some other source in the communication environment. The sensory organs of Person B transduce the incoming signal(s) where the information is decoded at neural processing centers. The message is interpreted in the various somatic areas of the brain (e.g., auditory, proprioceptive, tactile, visual), and meaning is finally achieved.

As previously stated, the lower half of Figure 3-2 is simply a reversal of the upper half. That is, the two communicators have changed places so that Person B is now the sender and Person A is the receiver of a message. The process of general communication is thereby described. Keep in mind that this is only a superficial discussion that does not adequately describe the true complexity of AAC.

Housed within the AAC transmission processes are three important components: the means to represent (symbol), the means to select a symbol, and the means to transmit a symbol or message. Although these processes can equally describe how persons without disabilities transmit information via different modalities, the main focus of this part of the model describes how persons with severe communication disabilities may form, select, and transmit messages. Because speech is typically not sufficient to meet these individuals' daily communication needs, they may have to rely on other forms of communication, such as graphic (printed) symbols or words, gestures, manual signs, or other types of symbols.

Symbols used for AAC are typically categorized as either **aided symbols** or **unaided symbols**. In keeping with the definitions proposed by Lloyd and Fuller (1986), aided symbols require some type of external assistance, aid, or device (e.g., communication board, electronic aid, or paper and pencil) to produce a message. On the other hand, unaided symbols require nothing external to the user's body to produce a message. The aided/unaided dichotomy can also be used to describe the selection and transmission of symbols.

At this point, the AAC transmission process will be described more fully (Figure 3-3). First, the user must formulate a message and then choose symbols to represent that message. As already stated, symbols can be classified as either aided or unaided. This is not to imply that a typical AAC user will be using symbols from only one of the two domains. To the contrary, an effective AAC communicator will in all likelihood be communicating using symbols that are both aided and unaided.

Second, once the symbols are chosen to represent the various concepts to be communicated, they must be selected from the pool of all symbols available to the AAC user. If the AAC user chooses to use unaided symbols, the means to select will also be unaided. For example, if the user is communicating with American Indian Hand Talk (Amer-Ind) gestures, the selection of the symbols will be by hand(s) and arm(s). On the other hand, if the AAC user is communicating with aided symbols, the means to select those symbols can be either aided or unaided. Consider the individual who communicates with Picture Communication Symbols (PCS). In unaided selection, the user has the motor ability to use an

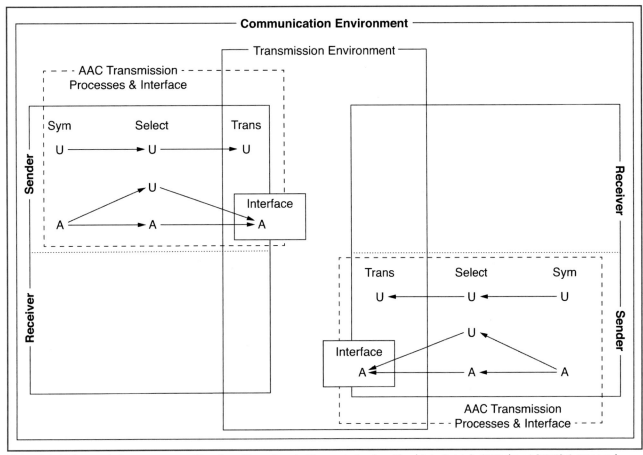

Figure 3-3. AAC transmission processes and interface. (Reproduced with permission from Lloyd, L. L., Quist, R., & Windsor, J. [1990]. A proposed augmentative and alternative communication model. *Augmentative and Alternative Communication, 6*[3], 172-183. https://doi.org/10.1080/0743461 9012331275444)

eye, finger, or hand to point to the symbols on a communication board. Because the user is selecting the symbols with body parts (in this case, the eye, finger, or hand), the means to select is unaided. However, suppose that the user does not possess adequate motor control to use their eye, finger, or any other body part. The only consistent motor control the user possesses is adequate head movement. Obviously this user will not be able to select PCS directly through body parts. However, if the user is fitted with a head stick or light pointer, the ability to point to the symbols on the communication board can be achieved. Because a device is being used to select symbols, the means to select in this case is aided.

Once the symbols are chosen and selected, the message is transmitted through some means. Once again, if the AAC user communicates with unaided symbols, both the means to select and the means to transmit will be unaided. In this case, the individual is considered to be directly transmitting the message through the movements of body parts. Direct transmission is classified as an unaided means to transmit.

When a person uses aided AAC symbols, those symbols must be displayed on some type of aid, device, or display. This can include anything from simple communication boards to wallets, booklets, **E-TRAN** (eye transfer) boards, and tablet or smartphone apps. Because some type of external aid or

device is required to display aided symbols, the means to transmit is always aided if the symbols are aided, regardless of whether the means to select is aided or unaided. Therefore, for the two examples with PCS symbols above the means to transmit is aided, even though in one case, the individual had the ability to directly select symbol choices.

The Lloyd and colleagues (1990) AAC model is a broad multimodal model that accounts for the major aspects of AAC. The degree of communication and miscommunication is directly related to the match or mismatch of the sender and receiver. In general, communication is more effective and efficient when the sender and receiver are more closely matched on cognitive ability, culture and experience, linguistic competence, motivation, interest, perceptual skills, and abilities.

This model can be used as a framework to aid in understanding which communication modes will be selected. External factors that influence communication and the interactive nature of communication are key aspects of the model. The formulation of a message and the selection of modes are influenced by the way communication partners perceive each other's abilities. In the communication process, the communicative intent or function is more important than the form. Communicators are driven by seeking relevance in the message (Sperber & Wilson, 1986).

Relevance has been considered crucial in discussions of AAC models (von Tetzchner et al., 1996). While the Lloyd and colleagues (1990) AAC model is robust in its multimodality and consideration of environmental and external factors, it does not elaborate on the internal cognitive and linguistic systems, nor does it explain how neuroprocessing centers encode and decode messages. Psycholinguists have proposed models, such as Levelt's blueprint for the speaker, that account for underlying communication processes (Levelt, 1993). However, Levelt's model focuses only on spoken language and does not account for the multimodal nature of AAC. Loncke and colleagues (1997) have extended Levelt's model to account for both linguistic and non-linguistic communication in various modes. An AAC model considers more than just spoken language.

With an AAC model in place, it is now time to focus more fully on describing an AAC classification system for symbols (i.e., the means to represent), selection techniques (i.e., the means to select), and transmission modes (i.e., the means to transmit).

Classification Systems for the Means to Represent, Select, and Transmit

By definition, **taxonomy** is the science of classification. Humans tend to categorize and group things in their environment to enhance memory, storage, and retrieval. In AAC, a system of classification not only provides for the organization of various symbols, selection techniques, and modes of transmission, but also provides insight into how these phenomena interact. Taxonomy affords the opportunity to make direct comparisons between and among symbols, selection techniques, and modes of transmission.

In the discussion of the Lloyd and colleagues (1990) AAC model, the communication environment was described. Housed within this environment are the AAC transmission processes and interface (refer back to Figure 3-3). The AAC transmission processes include the means to represent, the means to select that representation, and the means to transmit the message. Recall that in each case, the aided/unaided dichotomy was used to classify these processes. In essence, a simple taxonomy was described for the means to represent, select, and transmit. More specifically, a superordinate level (i.e., aided vs. unaided) was described for each of the three AAC transmission processes.

However, over the 30 years since a symbol taxonomy was proposed, there has been a significant proliferation of aided symbols (the number of unaided symbols has remained relatively the same over the same time period), primarily due to the advent of tablet and smartphone technology and the development of literally hundreds of AAC apps (Pampoulou & Fuller, 2021). Similarly, over the past couple decades, there has been a technological explosion in the field. The variety of technological options has blurred the lines between the traditionally used terms **high technology** and **low technology**.

The astute observer may have recognized during the discussion of the AAC model that the focus was exclusively on *expressive* communication; the model did not elaborate on *receptive* communication. Although the failure to discuss receptive communication does not negate any part of the AAC model, it is time educators, clinicians, and researchers consider receptive communication, especially in cases where the person(s) who use(s) AAC to communicate expressively may also have sensory impairments. This lack of consideration for receptive communication, as well as the fact that terms such as high and low technology have become obsolete and clinically irrelevant, necessitates a rethinking of how the means to transmit (i.e., the technology) should be classified. Similarly, the taxonomy for the means to represent (i.e., AAC symbols) has always been flawed (as will become apparent in the following discussion), as some of the levels within the taxonomy are not truly dichotomous as all levels of a taxonomy should be. For this reason, perhaps it is also time to consider a more effective and clinically relevant manner of classifying the means to represent.

All that said, the next section of this chapter will focus on the three components of the AAC transmission processes and interface. For the means to represent and transmit, we will first discuss the traditional manner in which these processes have been classified but will then propose a new and more meaningful way to classify these processes. As the reader shall see, a discussion of the means to select will be rather brief by comparison to discussions of the other two processes.

The Means to Represent

The Traditional View

Of the three AAC transmission processes, the means to represent has received the most attention (Fuller et al., 1992; Lloyd & Fuller, 1986; Lloyd et al., 1990). Examples of the various AAC symbols as classified under the aided/unaided dichotomy show the original superordinate taxonomic level as proposed by Lloyd and Fuller (1986). However, for the means to represent, Fuller and colleagues (1992) proposed further subordinate levels. These levels, along with the original superordinate level of aided vs. unaided, are illustrated in Figure 3-4. These subordinate taxonomic levels include **static** vs. **dynamic**, **iconic** vs. **opaque**, and **symbol set** vs. **symbol system**.

Vanderheiden and Lloyd (1986) defined static symbols as being permanent and enduring. These symbols do not require any movement or change to express meaning. Conversely, dynamic symbols are not permanent and enduring and do require movement or change to convey meaning. This level is immediately subordinate (i.e., the secondary taxonomic level) to the aided vs. unaided superordinate level. The tertiary level of the symbol taxonomy is iconic vs. opaque (Fuller et al., 1992). Symbols that have some degree of visual relationship to the concepts (i.e., referents) they represent are

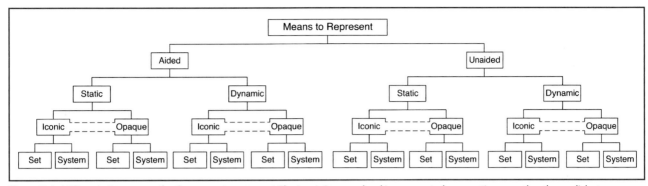

Figure 3-4. AAC symbol taxonomy for the means to represent. The iconic/opaque level is represented as a continuum rather than a dichotomy because there is considerable overlap between translucent symbols and transparent and opaque symbols. (Reproduced with permission from Fuller, D., Lloyd, L. L., & Schlosser, R. [1992]. Further development of an augmentative and alternative communication symbol taxonomy. *Augmentative and Alternative Communication, 8*[1], 67-74. https://doi.org/10.1080/07434619212331276053)

iconic. To the contrary, symbols that have very little, if any, visual relationship to their referents (and therefore tend to be arbitrary representations) are opaque. The final (i.e., quaternary) taxonomic level for the means to represent is the set vs. system distinction (Fuller et al., 1992). Symbol sets are simply collections of symbols in which each symbol has one or more specified meanings. Although sets can be expanded to some small degree, they have no specified rules for expansion. Examples of aided symbol sets include pictures or images, emojis, and Yerkish lexigrams (Romski et al., 1985; Rumbaugh, 1977). Unaided symbols, such as yes/no gestures or other common gestures, are also sets. Symbol systems, on the other hand, have formal rules and internal logic for the creation of new symbols so that vocabulary is virtually unlimited. Examples of aided symbol systems are Blissymbolics (Bliss, 1965; McNaughton, 1976, 1985; Wood et al., 1992) and Sigsymbols (Cregan, 1982; Cregan & Lloyd, 1990). American Sign Language and British Sign Language are examples of unaided systems that have their own syntactic and morphological structures. Signed English and the Paget Gorman Sign System do not have their own syntactic structures but are still considered systems because they mimic the syntax of English (i.e., subject-verb-object). To an even lesser degree, Amer-Ind gestures (Skelly, 1979) have a means for expansion called **agglutination**, but this expansion capability is very limited; therefore, Amer-Ind is on the cusp of being a true symbol system.

Typically, symbol sets represent concrete referents better than abstract referents while symbol systems represent both equally well, thus providing greater **representational range**. The set vs. system classification is a true dichotomy, clearly dividing AAC symbols into mutually exclusive groups. Aided symbols are discussed in greater detail in Chapter 7, and unaided symbols are more thoroughly discussed in Chapter 8.

Although all symbols used for AAC can be classified according to this taxonomy, there are inherent problems with a couple of the taxonomic levels. With the rapid proliferation of new symbols, the issue with the secondary (i.e., static vs. dynamic) and tertiary (i.e., iconic vs. opaque) levels is even more problematic. Neither of these levels is a true dichotomy

and this should be a requirement for any taxonomy. Take the static vs. dynamic classification as an example. The letters of the American manual alphabet (i.e., fingerspelling) are *predominantly* but not exclusively static. Two of the fingerspelling symbols ("j" and "z") require movement in order for meaning to be conveyed; therefore, these two symbols are dynamic, whereas the other 24 symbols are static. By the same token, the iconic vs. opaque classification is also problematic. In any given symbol set or system, there are a number of symbols that look like their referents, or the meaning between symbol and referent is understood when the two appear together. However, there are likely going to be a number of opaque symbols within a given set or system where the symbols are arbitrarily assigned meaning. The meanings of these symbols must be learned, as they are not intuitive. Any clinically relevant taxonomy should have levels that are all true dichotomies, meaning they are mutually exclusive so that *all* symbols in a given set or system fall into one of the two categories. Separate from the issue of lack of mutual exclusivity, with so many new symbols becoming available each year, this symbol taxonomy may very well have come to the end of its useful life.

The Means to Represent From a More Clinically Relevant Perspective

A number of aided and unaided AAC symbols have inherent linguistic capacity, which is dependent in large part on the existence of internal logic within the corpus. When a corpus has clearly defined rules that are generative, this allows the user to create new meanings (Alant et al., 2006; Fuller et al., 1997; Vanderheiden & Lloyd, 1986). The more sophisticated these rules, the greater the flexibility for expanding the vocabulary beyond the initial finite number of symbols (i.e., **expansion capability**). Inevitably, this allows the user to express a wide range of ideas and concepts, thus providing some graphic symbol systems an excellent representational range (Fuller & Lloyd, 1997b). Although representational range has not been clearly defined in the existing literature, Pampoulou and Fuller (2021) contend it appears

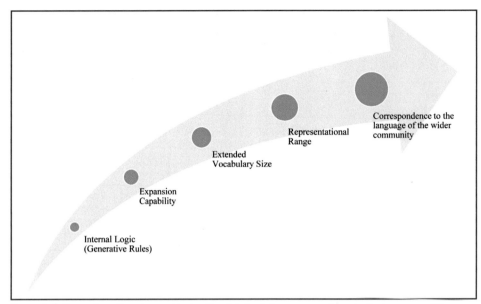

Figure 3-5. Illustration of how internal logic ultimately leads to correspondence to the language of the wider community—a hallmark of a symbol system.

reasonable that the greater number of concepts or meanings that can be expressed over a wide range of communication contexts (and representing not only the here and now but past and future as well), the larger this range, and hence, the closer the symbol system corresponds to the language of the wider (i.e., oral) community (Figure 3-5). These terms are defined in Table 3-1.

This relation is widely discussed in the existing AAC literature under the notion of the symbol set vs. system dichotomy. Symbol sets are those whose corpuses include symbols that do not have any specific rules to allow for expansion of the number of symbols beyond the original corpus (Wasson et al., 1997). In contrast, "[s]ymbol systems include rules or a logic for the development of symbols not already represented in the system" (Vanderheiden & Lloyd, 1986, p. 71). One symbol system that has received considerable attention in the AAC literature is Blissymbolics (Fuller, 1988; Mirenda & Locke, 1989; Rajaram et al., 2012; Smith, 2006; Venkatagiri, 2002). Despite the fact that the Fuller and colleagues (1992) dichotomy clearly defines the distinction between a symbol set and system, it fails to include those corpuses that fall between these two categories. It is for this reason and the reasons described in the preceding section related to the taxonomic levels static vs. dynamic and iconic vs. opaque that Pampoulou and Fuller (2021) proposed there should be a shift away from the old quaternary symbol *taxonomy* toward a quaternary *continuum* of AAC symbols.

According to Pampoulou and Fuller (2021), the available range of symbol corpuses can be classified initially into three broad categories, namely *non-linguistic, pre-linguistic,* and *linguistic.* Their classification in this manner is based primarily on the internal logic of the corpus, which inevitably—as shown in Figure 3-5—determines their expansion capability, extended vocabulary size, representational range, and ultimately, greater correspondence to the wider community language.

Table 3-2 provides the components of a quaternary continuum of AAC symbols as opposed to the archaic taxonomic system (Pampoulou & Fuller, 2021). The classification scheme proposed in Table 3-2 was developed by conducting a literature review on aided symbol taxonomy (Fuller & Lloyd, 1997a; Fuller et al., 1992; Lloyd & Fuller, 1986) and symbol selection considerations (Fuller & Lloyd, 1997b; Goodenough-Trepagnier, 1981; Jones & Cregan, 1986; Kiernan et al., 1982; Lloyd & Karlan, 1983, 1984; Musselwhite, 1982; Musselwhite & St. Louis, 1988; Nietupski & Hamre-Nietupski, 1979; Silverman, 1995; Vanderheiden & Harris-Vanderheiden, 1976; Vanderheiden & Lloyd, 1986; Yoder, 1980) and then synthesizing the information from the two topic areas.

By examining the foregoing body of knowledge, the reader can see immediately that research on the characteristics of symbols has been relatively sparse in recent years. These older studies represent what we have known about symbol characteristics going back as far as 4 decades ago. Fortunately, however, much of what we have learned over the past 40 years still applies today. In addition to relying on the current published knowledge base, the authors also took into account their considerable knowledge and expertise in the field, especially in the area of AAC symbols and their characteristics.

As indicated in Table 3-2, the quaternary continuum starts with simple **symbol groups** and moves toward linguistic symbol systems. The table provides a proposed continuum of symbol classification that takes into consideration the absence, partial presence, or presence of internal logic (i.e., generative rules) with its concomitant effects on expansion capability, extended vocabulary size, representational range, and correspondence to language of the wider community. In referring back to Figure 3-5, the reader can see that there is a directly proportional effect from internal logic to extended

TABLE 3-1

Definitions of Variables Related to the Differentiation Between Symbol Sets and Systems

Internal logic	The presence and sophistication of generative rules within a group of symbols that allows for expansion of symbols beyond the original number provided
	Categorized as absent, limited, defined but unsophisticated, or sophisticated
Expansion capability	The degree of vocabulary expansion beyond an initial group of symbols as a result of varying degrees of internal logic
	Categorized as none, minimal, limited, or unlimited
Vocabulary size	The number of symbols within a particular collection
	There are two types of vocabulary size: initial and extended
	For symbol sets and systems, extended vocabulary size is dependent upon the degree of internal logic and expansion capability
	Categorized as none, small, larger, or unlimited
Representational range	The degree to which symbols represent the morphological, semantic, and syntactic components of spoken and/or written language
	The greater the extended vocabulary size, the more likely representational range will be greater
	Categorized as very limited, narrow, broader than a symbol set, or unlimited
Correspondence to the language of the larger community	The degree to which a symbol system corresponds to the components of the natural language of the broader (i.e., persons without disabilities) community
	Categorized as poor, fair, good, or excellent

Reproduced with permission from Pampoulou, E., & Fuller, D. R. (2021). Introduction of a new AAC symbol classification system: The multidimensional quaternary symbol continuum (MQSC). *Journal of Enabling Technologies, 15*(4), 252-267.

TABLE 3-2

A Quaternary Continuum of the Means to Represent Based on Certain Characteristics

CHARACTERISTICS	NON-LINGUISTIC	PRE-LINGUISTIC		LINGUISTIC
	Symbol Group	*Symbol Set*	*Transitionary Symbol System*	*Linguistic Symbol System*
Initial vocabulary size	Small	Variable	Variable	Variable
Internal logic (i.e., generative rules)	Absent	Limited	Defined but unsophisticated	Sophisticated
Expansion capability	None	Minimal	Limited	Unlimited
Extended vocabulary size	None	Small	Larger than symbol set	Unlimited
Representational range	Very limited	Narrow	Broader than symbol set	Unlimited
Correspondence to the language of the larger community	Poor	Fair	Good	Excellent

Reproduced with permission from Pampoulou, E., & Fuller, D. R. (2021). Introduction of a new AAC symbol classification system: The multidimensional quaternary symbol continuum (MQSC). *Journal of Enabling Technologies, 15*(4), 252-267.

vocabulary size via expansion capability. With a greater degree of internal logic (i.e., clearly established and conventionalized rules) comes the potential for greater expansion capability (i.e., the collection of symbols possess more mobility to expand beyond the original symbols in the collection). The result of a greater degree of expansion capability is an expanded vocabulary representing a wider representational range (i.e., the ability of the symbols to represent more closely the morphological, semantic, and syntactic components of spoken or written language), resulting in greater correspondence to the oral and written language of the broader community. The following paragraphs describe each of the four classifications of symbols across the quaternary symbol continuum and are summarized in Table 3-2 according to the amount, degree, or sophistication of each of the characteristics that determines whether symbols are non-linguistic (i.e., symbol collections), pre-linguistic (i.e., symbol sets or transitionary linguistic systems), or linguistic (i.e., linguistic symbol systems).

It should be noted in the sections below, the classification of symbols as non-linguistic, pre-linguistic, or linguistic will be discussed in reference to aided AAC symbols. Table 3-3 provides examples of aided symbols within each of these three categories, as well as additional considerations, such as physical and design attributes. These are also discussed more in-depth in Chapters 6, 7, and 8. The six design attributes include:

1. Object
2. Pictorial
3. Line drawing
4. Phonemic- or phonetic-based
5. Alphabet-based
6. Vocal

The four physical characteristics of aided AAC symbols include:

1. Two-dimensional
2. Three-dimensional
3. Animated
4. Acoustic

While studying Table 3-2, the reader is encouraged not only to become familiar with the large number of aided symbols that are available but their classification along the quaternary continuum, as well as their physical and design attributes (see Table 3-3). These multiple dimensions have clinical implications that will be discussed toward the end of this chapter.

A separate discussion of unaided symbols will be provided after a discussion of aided symbols. A slightly modified classification system will be discussed for unaided symbols (Table 3-4). Unaided symbols are classified along the same quaternary continuum but are not classified according to physical attributes, as all unaided symbols share the same physical attribute—manual production. However, there are seven design attributes for unaided symbols, including:

1. Gestural
2. Sign languages
3. Pedagogical sign systems
4. Tactile or vibrotactile
5. Phonemic- or phonetic-based
6. Alphabet-based
7. Vocal

The Quaternary Continuum of AAC Symbols

Characteristics of Non-Linguistic Symbols With Examples. Non-linguistic symbols are those that, as the title suggests, do not possess any inherent linguistic characteristics (see Table 3-2). Due to their non-linguistic nature, a grouping of similar symbols falling into this category is referred to as a *group* of symbols instead of a corpus. Lacking internal logic and expansion capability, end-users cannot generate additional symbols beyond the original collection. Instead, expansion of the number of symbols in the collection is dependent upon whether or not the developer(s) or designer(s) of the collection choose(s) to create more symbols. Generally, symbol groups usually possess a relatively small number of functional symbols. Examples of groups of aided symbols include three-dimensional symbols (e.g., objects, miniature objects, tangible or textured symbols), as well as two-dimensional photographs, simple pictures, emojis, and Microsoft ClipArt.

Within the last decade, there has been a proliferation of individuals and companies that have developed apps for communication purposes. Many of these tend to consist of small collections of symbols either as photographs, pictures, and/or line drawings. These would then be considered non-linguistic symbol collections. Note from Table 3-2 that the physical attributes of aided symbols can be three-dimensional (e.g., objects, tangible or textured symbols) or two-dimensional (i.e., any type of aided symbol that is graphic in nature). The design attributes of non-linguistic symbols include object, pictorial, or line drawing.

Characteristics of Pre-Linguistic and Linguistic Symbols. As the terms imply, these symbols have an inherent linguistic characteristic in the form of internal logic that allows users to create new symbols beyond the original corpus. As shown in Table 3-3, for pre-linguistic and linguistic symbols, internal logic (and with it, expansion capability, extended vocabulary size, representational range, and correspondence to the language of the wider community) may be limited (i.e., symbol set), more defined but unsophisticated (i.e., transitionary symbol system), or—at the most advanced level—sophisticated to the degree that unlimited communication is possible (i.e., linguistic symbol system). The physical attribute of all pre-linguistic and linguistic corpuses of symbols is two-dimensional, but the design attributes are line drawing, phonemically or phonetically based, alphabet-based, and electronically generated.

TABLE 3-3

Categorization of Aided AAC Symbols Using the Quaternary Continuum Along With Physical and Design Attributes

PHYSICAL ATTRIBUTES		LINGUISTIC CHARACTERISTICS				DESIGN ATTRIBUTES
		Non-Linguistic	*Pre-Linguistic*		*Linguistic*	
		Symbol group	Symbol set	Transitionary symbol system	Linguistic symbol system	
	Three-dimensional	Real objects Miniature objects Tangible and textured symbols				Object
	Two-dimensional	Photographs Pictures or images Microsoft ClipArt Self-created or proprietary emojis				Pictorial
	Two-dimensional	Small corpuses of line drawings created by parents, specialists, etc.	Core picture vocabulary DynaSyms Imagine symbols Lingraphica concept-images Mulberry Symbols ParticiPics Pics for PECS Pictograms Simple rebus SymbolStix Talking Mats	Makaton PCS Widgit Symbols	Blissymbolics Cyberglyphs PICSYMS Picture English Sigsymbols	Line drawing
					Complex rebus Phonetic alphabets Visual phonics	Phonemic- or phonetic-based
					Graphic representations of fingerspelling Modified orthography Morse code Traditional orthography	Alphabet-based
	Three-dimensional				Braille	

(continued)

TABLE 3-3 (CONTINUED)

Categorization of Aided AAC Symbols Using the Quaternary Continuum Along With Physical and Design Attributes

		LINGUISTIC CHARACTERISTICS					
		Non-Linguistic	*Pre-Linguistic*		*Linguistic*		
		Symbol group	Symbol set	Transitionary symbol system	Linguistic symbol system		
PHYSICAL ATTRIBUTES	Animated	Animated graphics Autism Language Program Library of International Picture Symbols	Some DynaSyms symbols Some Pictogram symbols			Pictorial	**DESIGN ATTRIBUTES**
	Acoustic				Synthetic speech	Vocal	

PCS = Picture Communication Symbols; PECS = Picture Exchange Communication System.

Reproduced with permission from Pampoulou, E., & Fuller, D. R. (2021). Introduction of a new AAC symbol classification system: The multidimensional quaternary symbol continuum (MQSC). *Journal of Enabling Technologies, 15*(4), 252-267.

A Closer Examination of Pre-Linguistic Symbols. "Pre-linguistic symbols possess inherent linguistic characteristics but only partially in the form of limited rudimentary generative rules that allow minimal expansion capabilty, and therefore, a small extended vocabulary (these can be thought of as approaches or strategies)" (Pampoulou & Fuller, 2021, p. 261). There are two types of pre-linguistic symbols. The simpler type of pre-linguistic symbols (symbol set) includes corpuses of symbols that have at least some limited degree of internal logic. However, this internal logic is more a function of the intelligence, creativity, or ingenuity of the person who uses AAC. In other words, it is the person who uses AAC who develops simple strategies or rules for expanding the size of the vocabulary. Whatever limited internal logic exists increases expansion capability to a minimal degree, resulting in a small but extended vocabulary beyond the initial corpus, which in turn may increase representational range to some degree. Symbol corpuses that fit this description are referred to as *pre-linguistic symbol sets*. Symbol sets are classified as exclusively two-dimensional line drawings, with some being animated.

On the other hand, the more complex type of pre-linguistic symbols includes symbol corpuses where there is an inherently defined but unsophisticated degree of internal logic built into the corpus (Pampoulou & Fuller, 2021). This also results in a limited degree of expansion capability but not quite as limited as pre-linguistic symbol sets. Because internal logic is somewhat better defined and expansion capability is greater, yet still limited, the result is a relatively larger vocabulary size and a somewhat broader representational range than for pre-linguistic symbols. Symbol corpuses that meet these criteria for the more complex type are referred to as pre-linguistic *transitionary symbol systems*. Interestingly, despite their higher level along the continuum, transitionary symbol systems are similar to symbol sets in that they are exclusively two-dimensional line drawings.

- A Further Discussion of Symbol Sets With Examples
  - ○ A symbol set is a group of similarly developed symbols initially consisting of a fixed number of symbols representing a finite initial vocabulary. The number of initial symbols may vary considerably from set to

TABLE 3-4

Categorization of Unaided AAC Symbols Using the Quaternary Continuum Along With Design Attributes

LINGUISTIC CHARACTERISTICS					DESIGN ATTRIBUTES
Non-Linguistic	Pre-Linguistic		Linguistic		
Symbol group	Symbol set	Transitory symbol system	Linguistic symbol system		
Idiosyncratic gestures Pantomime Pointing Yes/no gestures	Generally understood gestures	Amer-Ind		Gestural	
		International Sign Language (Gestuno)	American Sign Language British Sign Language Other sign languages	Sign languages	
	Makaton Manually coded English PGSS	SEE-I SEE-II Signed English		Pedagogical sign systems	
Vibrotactile codes			Tadoma	Tactile or vibrotactile	
			Cued speech Danish mouth-hand system	Phonemic- or phonetic-based	
			Gestural Morse code Manual alphabet	Alphabet-based	
Vocalizations			Natural speech	Vocal	

Amer-Ind = American Indian Hand Talk; SEE-I = Seeing Essential English; SEE-II = Signing Exact English; PGSS = Paget Gorman Sign System.

Reproduced with permission from Pampoulou, E., & Fuller, D. R. (2021). Introduction of a new AAC symbol classification system: The multidimensional quaternary symbol continuum (MQSC). *Journal of Enabling Technologies, 15*(4), 252-267.

set. A symbol set is characterized primarily by limited internal logic. For example, there may be some strategies to allow the AAC user to form a limited number of symbols beyond the original set, but these strategies typically are the result of the ingenuity or creativity of the AAC user, as opposed to being offered by the developer of the symbol set. This could include such strategies as symbols for "opposite of" or "sounds like" and/or the inclusion of a number of simple morphological markers (e.g., "-ed," to represent past tense, or "-s" to represent plural and possession) developed by the AAC user to change the basic meanings of some vocabulary items. For the most part though, expansion capability is minimal at best (i.e., the AAC user's vocabulary may expand beyond the original set but not considerably) and representational range is relatively narrow (i.e., the AAC user must rely primarily on concrete concepts with possibly a small number of more abstract concepts). Although the AAC user has the ability to modify the size of the set depending on their ingenuity, symbol sets by and large are similar to symbol collections in that the primary manner of increasing vocabulary size is by having someone create more symbols as needs dictate—in the case of symbol groups, this is accomplished by the symbol developer; in the case of symbol sets, expansion is most likely accomplished by the AAC user without relying on the symbol developer to create new symbols. Due to limited internal logic, the number of symbols in a symbol set will remain relatively limited as well. That said, the fact that a symbol set has at least some limited internal logic places it in a completely different category than a symbol group. Because their limited internal logic and minimal expansion capability results in at least a slightly larger vocabulary, the symbols within a symbol set mark the lower end of pre-linguistic symbols (i.e., they allow for at least a minimal degree of expansion capability resulting in a slightly wider representational range, thereby allowing the AAC user to communicate in a manner than is more sophisticated than through a symbol group but less so for transitionary or linguistic symbol systems).

○ Symbols within a symbol set might be used in conjunction with non–speech-output technology, such as communication boards, E-TRANs, or tablet or smartphone apps without speech output. These means to transmit only allow for a limited number of simple messages with some limited novel messages. Symbol sets can also be used in conjunction with speech-generating software or apps. However, although the technology may be more sophisticated, the flexibility to produce a message that is linguistically complex is limited primarily by the constraints of the symbol set. For symbol sets whose initial vocabulary size is large (e.g., Pics for Picture Exchange Communication System [PECS]), this limitation is not as pronounced. As large as the Pics for PECS vocabulary is, there are no rules for expansion beyond the initial vocabulary.

○ Examples of aided pre-linguistic symbol sets, which are described in greater detail in Chapter 7, are Pictograms (formerly Pictogram Ideogram Communication), Pics for PECS (Pyramid Educational Consultants), SymbolStix (News-2-You, Inc), Mulberry Symbols, and ParticiPics, among others.

- A Further Discussion of Transitionary Symbol Systems With Examples
  ○ It is at the level of transitionary symbol systems that we begin to see a greater focus on internal logic. The initial number of symbols can vary from a small collection to hundreds of symbols. Transitionary symbol systems have developer-defined rules for creating new symbols beyond the original set, but the expansion rules tend to be somewhat rudimentary and not sufficiently developed to allow for unlimited expansion capability; although, there is some degree of expansion capability due to the rules that do exist. This allows the transitionary symbol system to have a larger representational range than either symbol groups or symbol sets. However, since expansion capability is limited, the person with CCN still must rely primarily on the communication of their ideas by using the existing vocabulary. Persons who can use transitionary symbol systems are even more likely than persons who use symbol sets to take advantage of traditional orthography to fill in the gaps in communication. However, it is not whether or to what degree a person with CCN can use the letters of

the alphabet that determines how symbols are classified. To repeat, the key is internal logic and how this one variable allows for a larger vocabulary, greater expansion capability, and closer correspondence to the language of the wider community.

○ Because of the defined but somewhat unsophisticated internal logic that exists in transitionary symbol systems, the user is able to expand vocabulary and representational range to at least a greater degree than for symbol groups or symbol sets, placing transitionary symbol systems at an even more advanced level of pre-linguistic communication than symbol sets.

○ Examples of transitionary symbol systems are Widgit Symbols and Makaton. Despite the fact persons with CCN and clinicians do not have total flexibility to create new symbols, a relatively small number of new symbols can be generated based on the rudimentary rules that exist in these transitionary symbol systems. Makaton and Widgit Symbols both utilize grammatical markers to communicate the nuances of language. For example, both of these transitionary symbol systems include an arrow that indicates the tense of the word play—a left-pointing arrow signifies a past action while a right-pointing arrow signifies a future action. For Makaton symbols, internally developed morphological markers, such as "-ed'" or "-ing," may be placed typically after the root symbol. By comparison, for Widgit Symbols, markers—such as one, two, or three exclamation points—are used to indicate an adjective or adverb, its comparative, and its superlative (e.g., "!" = good; "!!" = better; "!!!" = best). These basic rules allow the user to create new symbols when necessary (e.g., when the person with CCN wants to change present tense "play" to regular past tense "played" or the comparative "higher" to the superlative "highest"). The reader must understand the subtle difference between symbol sets and transitionary symbol systems in regard to internal logic. One may have noticed the ability to include simple morphological markers in both symbol sets and transitionary symbol systems. However, note that for transitionary symbol systems, grammatical markers *are included*; it is not up to the AAC user's own ingenuity or creativity to develop morphological markers as a strategy for increasing vocabulary. For pre-linguistic symbol sets, on the other hand, expansion of vocabulary by using simple morphological markers depends on the intelligence, ingenuity, and creativity of the AAC user. With transitionary symbol systems, morphological markers and other simple rules for expanding vocabulary are built into the system.

○ Vanderheiden and Lloyd (1986) argued that symbol sets (by comparison to symbol systems) do not have rules for generating new symbols (and therefore, vocabulary) beyond the limitations of the original collection of symbols. The quaternary continuum expands upon Vanderheiden and Lloyd's definition of symbol set by making a distinction between simple corpora of symbols without linguistic characteristics to more linguistically based symbols. This shift starts with the proposed definition of symbol sets (i.e., persons with intact cognitive skills may have the ability to develop strategies for utilizing symbols in a more quasilinguistic manner), and hence, by the new definition, symbol sets are referred to as less complex pre-linguistic symbols. With transitionary symbol systems, a rudimentary internal logic is built in, making it easier to communicate at a higher linguistic level. However, transitionary linguistic symbols do not possess the sophistication of the highest level of symbols; hence, the symbols at this point along the continuum are referred to as pre-linguistic transitionary symbol systems. For transitionary symbol systems, defined but unsophisticated internal logic allows for limited expansion capability that results in the development of a relatively larger expanded vocabulary, and with it, a slightly broader representational range of concepts and ideas. However, since internal logic is relatively rudimentary, transitionary symbol systems tend to lack true linguistic characteristics in their internal logic, expansion capability, extended vocabulary size, representational range, and correspondence to the language of the larger community.

Characteristics of Linguistic Symbols With Examples. The most sophisticated type of aided symbols is the linguistic symbol system. Linguistic symbol systems may have an initial vocabulary that can range from small to very large. However, original vocabulary size is not what sets this level apart from the other levels on the quaternary continuum. Linguistic symbol systems are unique in that they have sophisticated internal logic—rules so comprehensive that the full range of language may be realized. The sophistication of the internal logic results in virtually unlimited expansion capability, nearly the entire lexicon, and the broadest representational range. Aided linguistic symbol systems may be viewed as the visual equivalents of auditory-vocal or acoustic symbols, such as spoken words whether produced by natural or synthetic speech. Linguistic symbol systems are similar to spoken symbols because of their ability to be *segmented*, thereby allowing for maximum communication based on a finite set of sub-symbol components—symbols representing individual speech sounds or alphabetic letters to form words (Smith, 2006).

It is not surprising then that symbol systems that serve as an analog to oral or written language are members of this level of classification. Traditional orthography or any of its analogs (e.g., Braille, aided Morse code) are examples. Nu-Vu-Cue (which uses an E-TRAN to display the cues of hand-cued speech) and graphic representations of the sounds of a language (e.g., the characters of the Initial Teaching Alphabet or International Phonetic Alphabet) would also be classified as linguistic symbol systems. Analogs of traditional orthography (e.g., Braille, Morse code, or phonetic alphabets) are sometimes referred to as *modified orthography*. Finally, not all linguistic symbol systems are traditional or modified orthographically based. Blissymbols is a linguistic symbol system, as there are very clear rules governing how basic elements are combined to form a practically infinite number of composite symbols. The same is true for Sigsymbols. This system has fairly detailed rules for creating symbols beyond the original vocabulary, similarly to PICSYMS. For example, there are special elements used consistently to depict concepts related to spatial prepositions (e.g., "in," "on," "under," "between"). Likewise, Sigsymbols uses a "blob" to represent the unspecified thing (or "it" pronoun). At first glance, it would appear Sigsymbols would be classified as transitionary. However, upon closer inspection, one will find Sigsymbols, whose concepts cannot be depicted readily using pictographs or ideographs, are sign-linked (i.e., the salient features of the production of manual signs are depicted within many of the Sigsymbols), thereby further strengthening this system's internal logic and placing it within the classification of linguistic symbol systems.

In summary, the sophisticated nature of the internal logic that exists with linguistic symbol systems allows for unlimited expansion capability, vocabulary, and representational range—the very elements that distinguish systems from sets, as defined by Vanderheiden and Lloyd (1986) nearly 40 years ago. As far as classification beyond the quaternary continuum is concerned, linguistic symbol systems are the most robust of all symbols. They range from two-dimensional line drawings (e.g., Blissymbols) and phonemic-/phonetic-based symbols (e.g., phonetic alphabets), to alphabet-based and electronically generated acoustic symbols (e.g., synthetic speech). Interestingly enough, alphabet-based linguistic symbols can either be two-dimensional (e.g., traditional orthography) or three-dimensional (e.g., Braille).

Classifying Unaided Symbols Using the Quaternary Continuum

To this point, we have only discussed the quaternary continuum as it relates to aided AAC symbols. However, the basic quaternary continuum can also be applied to unaided symbols with the exception that all unaided symbols share the physical attribute of manual production. However, their design attributes are many: gestural, sign languages, pedagogical sign systems, tactile or vibrotactile, phonemic- or phonetic-based, alphabet-based, and vocal (see Table 3-4).

Symbol group includes the design attributes of gestural (e.g., pantomime, pointing, yes/no gestures) and tactile or vibrotactile (e.g., vibrotactile codes). Symbol set also includes two design attributes: (1) gestural (e.g., generally understood gestures) and (2) pedagogical (e.g., manually coded English or what is also referred to as Pidgin Signed English [where manual signs from a sign language are produced in subject-verb-object English word order], Makaton, Paget Gorman Sign System). Three design attributes comprise transitional symbol system: (1) gestural (e.g., Amer-Ind), (2) sign languages (e.g., International Sign Language, the current term for what used to be called Gestuno), and (3) pedagogical sign systems (e.g., Seeing Essential English, Signing Exact English, and Signed English). Finally, linguistic symbol system is the most robust of all in terms of design attributes. Five of the seven design attributes are represented by the wide array of unaided linguistic symbol system options. These include: (1) sign languages (i.e., any natural sign language used by the Deaf community, such as American Sign Language, British Sign Language, Chinese Sign Language, Russian Sign Language), (2) tactile or vibrotactile (e.g., Tadoma), (3) phonemic- or phonetic-based (e.g., hand-cued speech), (4) alphabet-based (e.g., fingerspelling, gestural Morse code), and (5) vocal (e.g., natural speech). Many of these unaided symbol sets and systems will be discussed in Chapter 8 of this textbook.

The Means to Select

The taxonomy for the means to select is the simplest of the three AAC transmission processes. Only one level is needed to effectively classify the means to select. As mentioned in an earlier section of this chapter, the aided vs. unaided classification is all that is necessary for classifying all the different means of symbol selection (Fuller & Lloyd, 1997a; Fuller & Pampoulou, 2022). Keep in mind the aided vs. unaided distinction is a true dichotomy.

Recall that the means to select describes how the AAC user chooses the symbols they wish to convey to a communication partner. If symbols are aided, the means to transmit will also be aided (because the symbols must be stored or displayed on a device that is external to the natural human body). However, the means to select for aided symbols can be either aided or unaided. If the person who uses AAC has the ability to select symbols with their own body parts (e.g., pointing with a finger, hand, or foot; eye gaze) then the means to select is unaided. However, if the person with CCN does not possess the motoric ability to choose symbols via their body parts, then a device, such as a head wand, light pointer, or some type of switch in the case of electronic devices, is external to the body and the means to select in this case is then aided.

The Means to Transmit

The Traditional View

The final transmission process is the means to transmit. The means to transmit can be aided or unaided. Any time the AAC user's system consists of unaided symbols (e.g., fingerspelling, gestures, manual signs), the means to select *and* the means to transmit will both be unaided as well. It makes perfect sense that if a person with CCN uses unaided symbols (which are produced by natural body parts), the means of selecting the symbols and the means of transmitting a message are also going to be unaided. Therefore, we will not focus on the unaided means to transmit in this section. Instead, our focus will be on the aided means to transmit.

The aided means to transmit traditionally has been classified as simply aided vs. unaided. As mentioned before, if the person who uses AAC communicates with unaided symbols, transmission is going to be through natural body parts making the means to transmit unaided. However, if the AAC user must store or display symbols on some type of device external to the body (e.g., a communication board or a speech-generating device [SGD]), the means to transmit will always be aided. The means to select may be either aided or unaided, but the means to transmit will always be aided due to the fact a device external to the body must be used (Fuller & Lloyd, 1997a).

The Means to Transmit From a More Clinically Relevant Perspective

At the time of writing this chapter, the authors were unaware of any attempt in the last 30 years to classify technology used in AAC. Before our discussion about a clinically relevant taxonomy for technology, the reader must understand that AAC technology is more than just SGDs. In fact, SGDs are just one of many types of assistive technology. Assistive technology also includes mobility devices (i.e., wheelchairs and walkers), alerting devices (i.e., flashing lights instead of an audible sound for deaf individuals when a doorbell is pressed), environmental control devices (i.e., electronic devices that will turn lights on and off, turn on the television and adjust the volume), and ergonomic devices for work or other activities (i.e., an **expanded keyboard** or **keyboard emulator** to allow a person with a physical impairment to interface with a computer, bypassing the computer's keyboard where the keys may be too small to access). Communication devices also fall under the broader category of assistive technology. Since the topic of the textbook is augmentative and alternative *communication*, we will focus the discussion of this section on communication aids and devices. The reader will gain some exposure to other assistive technology in Chapter 16 on seating, positioning, and communication.

In terms of communication aids and devices, Fuller and Lloyd (1997a) proposed using the aided vs. unaided dichotomy to classify the means to transmit. Aided means to transmit messages include communication boards, books, cards, charts, vests, or wallets; E-TRAN boards; simple electric or electronic scanning devices, such as clock scanners; calendar boxes with scanning capability; and paper and pen or pencil. Unaided means to transmit would involve direct transmission through body parts, such as the arms, face, hands, and/or vocal tract. However, the use of the terms aided and unaided really do not capture the full range of technological options. In the early to mid-1980s, the terms "high technology" and "low technology" caught on and have been used ever since. At one time, these two terms represented a true dichotomy, but with the proliferation of varied technology over the last couple decades, the line between high and low technology has become less clear.

Years ago, any type of device that used a microcomputer chip was considered high technology. However, in current times, would one call a smartphone or tablet that uses a simple communication app without speech output high technology? Some may, but some may not. As technology continues to advance, the line between high and low technology will eventually be obliterated. Over the last half decade, biomedical engineers and scientists developed a wireless implantable device that sent electrical signals to the spinal cords of people who could not stand up or walk due to spinal cord trauma. Within a week, a number of the patients were able to walk with supports. Cochlear implants have been available for approximately 40 years. In addition to cochlear implants, now biomedical scientists are developing brainstem implants to bypass the inner ear and cochlear nerve. Just within the last couple years, neural implants and artificial intelligence were beginning to be used to develop an implantable device that will "read" a person's thoughts and convert them into speech production!

In the case of implants, would these be considered aided or unaided devices? One could make an argument for either classification, especially if the term "unaided" is modified to include any transplanted device that is meant to be as integral a part of the human body as one's own body parts. Using the strict sense of the definition of "unaided," implants would not fall under this classification. However, consider that the broadened definition of "unaided" provides a compelling argument for classifying implants as unaided devices.

In the area of aided technology, Starkey recently introduced the Livio AI, a hearing aid that uses artificial intelligence. This device not only serves as a digital hearing aid, but also translates several spoken languages into the user's ears, monitors vital functions like heart rate, and automatically adjusts to the environment the wearer is in. In Chapter 1, there was a brief section on the visionary perspective of AAC. With what's going on in the fields of biomedicine and engineering today, who knows what the future will bring? The day has already arrived where fully implantable electrodes and artificial intelligence are being combined to read a person's mind and then send signals directly to the larynx and articulators to actually produce natural speech. This area of biomedical engineering could be refined, perfected, and placed on the market within our lifetimes.

With the rapid advances occurring in the field of communication technology, the blurring of the terms high and low technology may indicate these terms are ready to be sent to the dustbin of history. They certainly do not have clinically relevant implications, as most medical insurance or other payment or reimbursement sources do not make a distinction between high and low technology (at least not in the United States). The terms **dedicated communication device** and **nondedicated communication device** are also going the way of the dinosaur because they are beginning to

hold little clinical relevance. It has become quite clear that the field of AAC needs a new way of classifying communication technology—one that is meaningful, especially in terms of reimbursement issues (Fuller & Pampoulou, 2022). Such a new taxonomy is offered as Figure 3-6. The astute observer will realize right away that the superordinate level of classification is *expressive* vs. *receptive*. As was mentioned earlier in this chapter, up until now, the field of AAC has been focused on expressive communication; after all, that is the primary purpose of AAC—to get the person with a severe communication impairment expressing their wants, needs, desires, and other information. However, the AAC model proposed by Lloyd and colleagues (1990) also has a receptive component, but almost without exception, most of us have always thought of the receiver of the message produced by a person who uses AAC being an individual without any type of impairment. This is certainly true in many cases, but there are also cases when the sender and/or the receiver of an AAC-encoded message has a sensory impairment, such as a hearing loss, visual impairment, or both (referred to as **dual sensory impairment**). Sensory impairments and their implications for AAC will be discussed more thoroughly in Chapter 23 of this textbook, but for now, our focus is on receptive communication as it relates to a comprehensive communication technology taxonomy. Please note in Figure 3-6 that part of the figure is blue while some of it is red. The blue components of the taxonomy represent technology that exists and is in use today. Those parts in red indicate technology currently under development or potential future technology. One will note right away that the red rectangles are *unaided*. So far, the authors of this chapter are unaware of any unaided technology, whether that technology is receptive or expressive. In fact, as mentioned before, for there to truly exist unaided technology, the definition of "unaided" would have to be modified somewhat.

For purposes of this discussion and for potential future technology, unaided is redefined as anything that requires only the natural parts of the human body *or are completely and totally implanted in such a way that for all intents and purposes, they become part of the natural human body*. Such technology already exists, just not in AAC—dental implants and knee (or other joint) replacements, to name a couple. Once implanted, these essentially become part of the human body and cannot be removed without considerable difficulty. Cochlear implants come close, but there is part of the implant that can be detached from the body. Therefore, cochlear implants (and auditory brainstem implants, for that matter) have not gotten to the point that they can be fully and totally implanted in the human body. The future? There may come a day when these devices become totally and irreversibly implantable. Other fully implantable devices may also be developed over the next few decades.

Now we redirect our attention more closely to Figure 3-6. The superordinate taxonomic level is expressive vs. receptive. The secondary level of classification is aided vs. unaided. There already exists both expressive and receptive

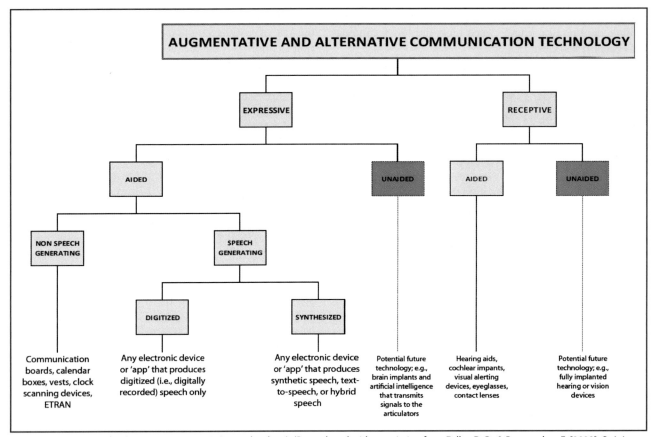

Figure 3-6. Taxonomy for the means to transmit (i.e., technology). (Reproduced with permission from Fuller, D. R., & Pampoulou, E. [2022]. Opinion: Revisiting the means to select and transmit of the AAC model. *Journal of Enabling Technologies, 16*[1], 321-339.)

aided technology. On the receptive aided side, there is no further classification beyond the secondary level. Receptive aided technology includes hearing aids, cochlear or auditory brainstem implants, auditory alerting devices, eyeglasses, contact lenses, and visual alerting devices. Many of these devices are covered either partially or totally by health insurance. On the receptive unaided side, we have yet to see technology to put under this classification; however, the future most likely will bring fully implanted auditory and/or visual devices that would be classified as unaided as long as those of us in the AAC field agree that completely implanted AAC devices are unaided (precedent has been set by dental implants and knee replacements; who could argue these are not part of the person's body who has them?).

The expressive side of the technology taxonomy is more clinically relevant at the present time, and especially for the secondary classification of aided. Note that there are tertiary and quaternary levels of classification for expressive aided communication technology. At least in the United States, the tertiary level is non–speech-generating vs. speech-generating. This has direct clinical relevance especially in terms of medical insurance coverage, including Medicare. Very few, if any, third-party payers will fund non-SGDs. These devices for the

most part, are essentially what we have traditionally called low technology. Communication boards, E-TRAN boards, and simple electronic clock- or linear-scanning devices are all non–speech-generating. Naturally, SGDs produce synthetic speech output, and these are the devices most likely to be funded through third-party payers, including Medicare. The quaternary level applies to the speech-generating side only. SGDs produce either synthesized or digitized speech. Synthesized speech includes text-to-speech and hybrid (both digitized and synthesized speech) options. Digitized speech is simply digitally recorded speech in much the same way as music is digitally recorded on compact discs. For the expressive unaided classification, no further levels exist. As is true for the receptive side, to date there are no expressive unaided options, but in the future, there very well could come a day when fully implanted devices are used to signal the vocal folds to start and stop vibrating, as well as make adjustments to pitch and vocal intensity. Fully implanted electrodes and artificial intelligence may be used in tandem to one day read one's thoughts and convert that to vocalizations and movements of the articulators. If and when that day does come, the technology taxonomy in Figure 3-6 will be able to accommodate such advances in biomedical engineering.

CLINICAL IMPLICATIONS OF THE USE OF CLASSIFICATION SYSTEMS FOR THE MEANS TO REPRESENT, SELECT, AND TRANSMIT

To recapitulate, the AAC model developed by Lloyd and colleagues (1990) includes both expressive and receptive components. It also includes the AAC transmission processes and interface. The AAC transmission and interface includes three interdependent and almost simultaneously occurring elements: the means to represent, the means to select, and the means to transmit. The means to represent for persons with CCN involves symbols, whether they use unaided, aided, or both. If the symbols are unaided, the means to select and means to transmit will also be unaided. If the symbols are aided, the means to transmit will also be aided but the means to select may be unaided or aided.

We now have classification systems for all three of these transmission processes. For the means to represent, we have a multidimensional quaternary continuum that ranges from symbol groups to linguistic symbol systems. In addition, our symbols can be further classified according to their physical and design characteristics (for aided symbols) and their design characteristics only for unaided symbols. For the means to select, we have a simple single-level dichotomy—aided vs. unaided. Finally, for the means to transmit, we have a technology taxonomy that takes into consideration both expressive and receptive communication. For now, only the secondary classification of aided is active; the secondary classification of unaided is waiting for a time when technology will advance to the point that this particular level accommodates newly developed unaided technology.

There are two examples of receptive unaided communication that come to the authors' minds; they are not technology but rather methods or strategies. These are Tadoma and fingerspelling and/or signing into the cupped hands of a person who has a dual sensory impairment. In both these cases, the message receiver is engaged in unaided receptive communication. Certainly the technology is not far behind. Receptive aided technology is nothing new to any of us—devices to improve hearing and visual acuity and orientation, alerting devices, etc. For the early part of the 21st century, we have finally developed a comprehensive classification system for the three primary components of AAC: (1) the symbols, (2) the methods of selecting those symbols, and (3) the means to transmit messages using the symbols chosen. How can classification systems be used to make sound clinical decisions? Consider the following case studies.

Case Study 1

You are working in a regular classroom with a 7-year-old child who has a severe to profound hearing impairment. His visual skills are intact. His language output is currently limited, but he has the potential to develop language skills, as his cognitive skills are within normal limits for a child his age. The child is very active and loves to play on the playground and socialize as much as he can at lunchtime or at home given his hearing impairment. He has good gross and fine motor skills. His expressive vocabulary appears to be limited, but no one really knows for sure because of his inability to communicate effectively with others. With just this information, what might be some of our options in terms of the means to represent, select, and transmit? Also, what receptive options do we have for this young boy?

One Potential Solution

Whatever AAC system we develop for him, we want to make sure it is multimodal. Starting with the means to represent (i.e., symbols), what are his options? We do not know the extent of his vocabulary because of such limited output. However, we do know he has no intellectual impairment. Since we do not know the extent of his expressive communication ability, we could start with a less sophisticated type of symbol set just to see how well he communicates without the added pressure of having to learn the components of language (e.g., morphology, semantics, syntax) right away. On the aided side, we could start with a pre-linguistic symbol set first just to see how he takes to it. If it proves to be too difficult for him, we could back down to a symbol group option. If he takes to the pre-linguistic symbols right away, we could assist him in developing some strategies of his own to communicate ideas that are not in his display of symbols. If successful, we could then introduce him to one of the transitional symbol systems, which will provide even more language structure. Once he seems to have mastered that and it appears he has excellent potential to develop language skills, we can move him to a linguistic symbol system. An alternate approach would be to start him at the transitional symbol system level first (perhaps Widgit Symbols, so he can understand the concept of morphology)—especially if we think he will succeed fairly quickly—then move him up to the linguistic symbol system level. At this highest level, we may want to consider modified orthography or a phonetic alphabet before transitioning him to traditional orthography or just going straight to traditional orthography if he appears ready to learn without the intermediate step. On the unaided side, the same principle applies. Symbol groups are likely going to be too simple for him, so perhaps we should start at the pre-linguistic symbol set or transitionary symbol system level.

Some of our options could be manually coded English (especially teaching him manual signs or sign approximations that correspond to the vocabulary he is using with his aided symbols) or a transitory symbol system, like Amer-Ind, or a pedagogical sign system, such as Signed English, where he can learn the concepts of segmentation and English syntax. Assuming he masters this level, we would then want to move him up to an unaided linguistic symbol system that corresponds to his aided system as much as possible. For example, if he is using the letters of the alphabet to spell words, perhaps introducing him to fingerspelling might be an option on the unaided side. Of course, we would want to integrate his own natural vocalizations as much as possible into his communication repertoire. Simultaneous to or perhaps slightly ahead of his development of expressive communication, we would want to address his receptive needs. Having a severe to profound hearing loss would require hearing aids or a cochlear implant if he is a good candidate for such a device. With at least some degree of restored hearing, our ability to bring him along expressively stands a much better chance.

Back to the expressive side of communication—we have the symbols. What will be the means to select? Since he has good gross and fine motor skills and he is a pretty active boy, we would probably want his display to be as small and unobtrusive as possible with the potential to include a fairly large vocabulary eventually. Obviously, we are going to provide an unaided means to select. Since he has good motor skills, he will simply be asked to point to the symbols to form messages when appropriate.

That leaves the means to transmit. Since he is so active and has good motor skills, perhaps the best technology option at this time would be a non-SGD, such as a communication book or wallet. Vocabulary can be organized in the manner that is most optimal for him finding the symbols he wants with little effort. Given his hearing impairment—even with some improvement with hearing aids or a cochlear implant—SGDs would likely not be an option at least in the initial stages. Should his residual hearing be enough for him to develop sufficient speech discrimination skills, then a speech-generation option may be a potential possibility. In his case, if he ever got to the point of being able to use an SGD, you would most likely want to use either digitized or hybrid speech output, as they sound more natural and clearer than the robotic sound of synthesized speech. Remember that in addition to the technological option for his aided system, he also has an unaided option to use in environments when he does not have ready access to his aided symbol display (or SGD, if he ever got to that point). Naturally, we would want to continually assess his receptive and expressive communication to ensure he is at the right level and is continuing to make progress in his communication and academic skills. Keep in mind that there is a very thin line between assessment and intervention. It is difficult to tell where one ends and the other begins. In fact, you are likely to be engaged in both simultaneously.

Case Study 2

You are working in a hospice setting. One of your patients is a 54-year-old woman who has late stage amyotrophic lateral sclerosis (ALS). Her motor activity is practically nonexistent with the exception she still has the ability to fixate on an object and track its movement with her eyes. She was a junior high school teacher and is fully literate. She knows she does not have much more time to live, so one of her primary concerns is getting her affairs in order with her family (her immediate family of husband and two grown children, a male and a female, as well as her extended family of parents, two sisters, and a brother-in-law). Her auditory and visual skills are intact, although she may fatigue easily.

One Potential Solution

It is evident that her motor skills have diminished rapidly over the last few months. She is still completely in control of her cognitive and mental faculties. She is completely literate. As for the means to represent, on the aided side, we will present her two options, both of them involving the highest level of symbols—linguistic symbol systems. Since she knows how to read, the obvious choice would be traditional orthography. As for the means to transmit, we want to give her two options. One option is to be used when she is sitting up and has a tray on which a tablet with an app that uses traditional orthography and speech output can rest (at this late stage in her life, the purchase of an expensive SGD would be inappropriate). Her second, non–speech-generating option would be a communication board with words and phrases on it, spaced apart enough so that she can discriminate words, phrases, and sentences easily.

The biggest key to this woman's AAC system is going to be the *means to select*. All she has left is consistent eye gaze and movement. The tablet should be outfitted with eye-gaze access so she can find words and choose them by fixating on them for a couple seconds. Ideally, to speed up the communication process, it may be advantageous to have word prediction software installed along with speech output. Once she has chosen a word, she can either store it while she is forming a complete sentence or speak each word individually as she completes them. The non–speech-generating option also has traditional orthography. Ideally, the 26 letters of the alphabet would be on the display so she can spell out words. Vocabulary words should be customized to her hospice stay and to getting her affairs in order, among more pleasant topics. Since she cannot select the words herself, she will require an aide to use the communication board. The aide would use a row-column approach. The aide would start with the first row and ask, "Is what you want to say in this row?" The patient can respond "yes" by directing her eye gaze upward or "no" by directing her eye gaze downward. The aide would go column by column in each row until the patient indicated the word, phrase, or sentence she wanted. Another way to speed up communication would be to use a frequency of use strategy where the words, phrases, and sentences she uses most often are placed in the most optimal position of the communication board where she can indicate her choices much quicker than having to wait row to row, column to column. Finally, although we would love to be able to offer her an unaided option (e.g., simple gestures) to communicate when she does not have access to either of her aided devices, her lack of motor ability will preclude any type of unaided expressive communication option. Since it does not appear she is having any issues related to sensory abilities and communication, we can forgo any type of receptive communication options at this time. As in all cases, the patient should be evaluated on a continual basis to ensure she has the right technology and vocabulary to allow her to communicate as efficiently as possible. Adjustments should be made as necessary.

In both cases, you may not have realized it, but you used the quaternary symbol continuum. The decisions you made regarding the school-aged child were based on what you considered to be the appropriate point on the continuum to provide symbols. Adjustments could then be made by moving up or down the continuum. With the adult with ALS, because of her intact intellectual skills and her literacy, you knew right away the only clear option would be to use what she's already accustomed to using—traditional orthography. Her intellectual and linguistic skills led you directly to the highest level on the continuum.

The child's and adult's means to transmit (i.e., the technology) were also based upon the communication technology taxonomy we discussed in this chapter. Considering the child's circumstances, you appropriately chose something durable, compact, and inexpensive for expressive communication—a non-SGD, at least in the initial stages of intervention. You backed up his aided symbols with appropriate unaided symbols that required only his body parts to transmit. For the adult, knowing she had limited motor ability, you knew her transmission options were limited. An SGD was appropriate but not an expensive dedicated device. Tablet and app technology was a more appropriate choice. You also provided a non–speech-generating option for the means to transmit. This is always a good idea, as there will likely be times when her SGD may not be available to her (e.g., a dead battery, a bug in the app software, need for repair or replacement of the tablet, communicating in certain environments where an SGD may not be effective).

Having good motor skills, the child's means to select in both cases (unaided and aided symbols) was appropriately unaided. You already knew that if the symbols are unaided, the means to select and transmit would also be unaided. Since he's using an unaided approach to choose unaided symbols, it makes perfect sense to use those same skills to access his means to transmit messages using unaided symbols. In the case of our ALS patient, with eye fixation and tracking the only motor abilities she has left, it was clear that for expressive communication the only way she would be able to access her non-SGD and SGD options was through eye gaze. An unaided expressive communication option was not appropriate, given her poor motor skills.

Finally, you took the appropriate steps in each case in terms of receptive communication. Since the child had an uncorrected severe to profound hearing loss, some type of auditory amplification system was necessary. A hearing aid could be tried first. If that does not provide enough gain, a cochlear implant may be a better option for the child. The adult with ALS had no sensory issues affecting her ability to understand or produce language. Therefore, there was no need to explore auditory or visual sensory options.

SUMMARY

Any AAC situation can be described in rather striking detail, as can be seen from the preceding examples. With the AAC model in place, the overall process of communication and the symbols, selection techniques, and modes of transmission can be described thoroughly to allow clinicians, educators, and researchers to gain insight into the complexity of AAC. The symbol classification continuum provides the structure for the systematic classification of symbols so important to the process of symbol selection. The classification of the means to select and transmit will likewise provide the framework for Chapters 9 and 10 on technology. In fact, the AAC model and classification systems presented in this chapter will serve as the framework for the remainder of this textbook. The reader's attention is now turned toward professional issues in AAC—the last remaining topic of this first unit of the textbook.

STUDY QUESTIONS

1. What are some of the communication models proposed over the past several decades? What are the similarities and differences among the older models?

2. Briefly describe the major components of AAC models that view the discipline from a macro to a comprehensive level.

3. Briefly describe the AAC transmission processes and interface.

4. For the means to represent, describe the classification system. Assign at least four symbol sets or systems at the appropriate point along the classification system's continuum.

5. What are some aided means to select symbols? What are some unaided means?

6. Briefly describe the classification system for AAC technology. Think of two specific forms of technology that would fall appropriately under each classification within the technology taxonomy.

7. Briefly describe how the AAC model and classification systems for the means to represent, select, and transmit can inform decision making in regard to the provision of appropriate AAC systems for persons with CCN.

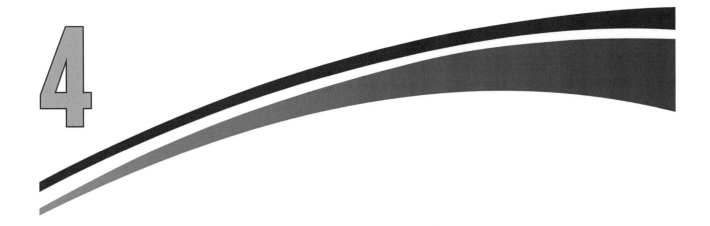

Professional Issues in AAC

Michelle L. Gutmann, PhD
and Lyle L. Lloyd, PhD

MYTH	**REALITY**
1. There are no professional issues unique to the practice of augmentative and alternative communication (AAC).	1. There are professional issues unique to AAC, particularly since the practice of AAC can involve the prescription of communication devices, commonly referred to as speech-generating devices (SGDs).
2. A graduate school curriculum with direct coursework and/or clinical practicum in AAC is not essential to provide enough background for students to address the full range of AAC needs that their clients or patients may have.	2. Skill acquisition in AAC is deliberate and time-intensive. Students must be taught the theoretical underpinnings of AAC, its research base, and how to apply AAC clinically to diseases and disorders across the lifespan.
3. The proliferation of mobile tablets and apps has all but eliminated the need for dedicated AAC assessment and intervention.	3. The proliferation of mobile tablets and apps has altered the landscape of AAC assessment and intervention but has in no way obviated the need for dedicated and skilled AAC assessment and intervention.

Fuller, D. R., & Lloyd, L. L. *Principles and Practices in Augmentative and Alternative Communication* (pp. 63-68).

Professional Issues Related to Education in AAC

American Speech-Language-Hearing Association Terminology

In 2005, the American Speech-Language-Hearing Association (ASHA) Certification Standards (see the evolution of these standards at https://www.asha.org/certification/CCC_history/) transitioned to competencies related to knowledge and skills. Nine primary areas of clinical practice were identified (referred to as the "Big 9"), and originally, AAC was subsumed within the "communication modalities" area of practice. By 2014, the wording of this area of practice changed from "communication modalities" to "augmentative and alternative communication" to more accurately reflect the intent of the certification standards. This change in the specificity of the wording reflected the intent to better prepare graduates of speech-language pathology programs for work with people who need AAC by way of both coursework and clinical experience. This may have spawned change in the existence and consistency of pre-service training in AAC.

Pre-Service Training

Pre-service training in AAC has been a topic of interest in the literature spanning 25 years (Costigan & Light, 2010a; Johnson & Prebor, 2019; Koul & Lloyd, 1994; Ratcliff & Beukelman, 1995; Ratcliff et al., 2008). Research indicates that pre-service training in AAC is subject to significant variability across academic programs. However, following the 2005 change in ASHA's Standards of Practice, a positive trend in the research emerged with respect to programs offering at least one course in AAC, although only half of respondents indicated that the course was mandatory. Further, in programs where courses were mandatory, faculty with expertise in AAC did not always teach these courses (Ratcliff et al., 2008).

Johnson and Prebor (2019) reported two major improvements since the last published review in 2008. The first improvement was an increase in the number of academic programs that offered pre-service training in the form of a graduate course in AAC. The second improvement was that AAC courses increasingly were being taught by faculty members with specific expertise in AAC. In some programs, additional advanced AAC coursework was offered and taught by faculty with AAC expertise.

Despite this positive news, Johnson and Prebor (2019) cautioned that many students graduate without adequate clinical training in AAC. This means that students may have completed coursework in AAC but needed continued education and experience to be prepared to meet the AAC needs of

their clients and patients. Given the broad scope of potential AAC intervention for persons with disorders as diverse as amyotrophic lateral sclerosis (ALS), aphasia, autism, cerebral palsy, and Down syndrome, the need for pre-service training becomes increasingly important. AAC coursework and clinical experience should be part of all graduate students' experiences. Without pre-service training in AAC, students may graduate not having had exposure to any AAC tools, techniques, and strategies that are applicable across the lifespan for people who have severe communication disorders. This is particularly problematic because the necessity of providing assessment for and implementation of AAC occurs across educational, health care, and home care settings, at least one of which is where many new graduates will be employed.

Enthusiasm about the Johnson and Prebor (2019) findings should be tempered with "on-the-ground" reality. Although positive momentum is welcome, AAC remains an area of practice that is still opaque to many clinicians. Students need more, not less, instruction on how to provide assessment and intervention to people who require AAC. To that end, graduate programs must continue to offer AAC coursework, make an AAC course mandatory, and supplement coursework with guided and varied clinical experiences to the greatest extent possible (e.g., Gutmann, 2016; Senner & Baud, 2016).

Professional Issues Related to Clinical Function in AAC

AAC clinical function may take place in a variety of settings—clinic, home, hospital, or school. Across settings, professionals must be prepared to provide assessment, intervention, and education to all stakeholders regarding all available AAC options that will best meet a client's needs. It is incumbent on clinicians to provide unbiased services across settings by maintaining the objectivity that professionalism demands and adhering to the highest possible standards of practice.

Interprofessional Practice

By its very nature, the practice of AAC is an example of **interprofessional practice** in action. AAC often requires the combined input of multiple professionals and disciplines to provide the best possible communication options for an individual who uses AAC. ASHA uses the terminology "interprofessional collaborative practice" to refer to members of two or more professions associated with education, health, or social interaction, engaged in learning with, from, and about each other (Craddock et al., 2006, as cited in ASHA's Scope of Practice in Speech-Language Pathology, 2016c). The literature indicates that it is most common for people who need AAC to be seen by a team of professionals, often led by the speech-language pathologist, to address needs, such as access, education, seating and positioning, and vision, among others (Alant, 2017a; Beukelman, Garrett, et al., 2007; Beukelman & Light, 2020).

In addition to the speech-language pathologist, other professionals may include but are not limited to audiologists, biomedical engineers, occupational therapists, physiatrists, physical therapists, rehabilitation engineers, respiratory therapists, social workers, special educators, teachers, technologists, and vision specialists. Often these professionals work together to assess and implement AAC solutions for a given client. In some settings, a core group of professionals (e.g., occupational therapist, physical therapist, speech-language pathologist) routinely work together when seeing clients who require AAC. In other settings, the team may be constituted as needs and personnel allow.

Mentorship in AAC

One aspect of clinical function in AAC that deserves attention is mentorship for new graduates and/or clinicians who are new to AAC. Given that expertise in AAC is gained over time with repeated exposure to clients who have a variety of AAC needs, a well-defined mentorship program or system is needed. This type of mentorship may be started during a clinical fellowship experience and beyond, or may be part of a programmatic plan at any time during employment. At present, there is no formalized AAC mentorship program through national organizations. Individual employers may offer various levels of mentorship in AAC. Going forward, further development of mentorship programs in AAC will continue to be important to address the ongoing need for clinician training. Further, more formalized mentoring programs in AAC may extend the current reach of existing services and build clinical capacity in AAC.

Technological Advances and AAC

Technological advances have provided new options for people who need and/or use AAC. The proliferation of mobile tablets and the AAC applications (i.e., apps) that run on them have created a technological revolution (McNaughton & Light, 2013). This revolution has rejuvenated the visibility of AAC in the public domain.

Media personalities, such as Steve Gleason—a former football player for the New Orleans Saints—have used their celebrity to shine a light on access to SGDs for people with ALS and other neurodegenerative diseases. Heightening public awareness of AAC is an outgrowth of this phenomenon. Indeed, The Gleason Act, enacted in 2015 (Vitter, 2015) and replaced in 2018 by The Steve Gleason Enduring Voice Act (Larson et al., 2017), permanently enshrines the changes to Medicare funding of SGDs for people with neurodegenerative diseases. This provision means that Medicare will continue to fund SGDs for people with ALS (and other diseases) regardless of the care setting, even if the person has had an SGD less than a year. Further, this act provides coverage for the accessories needed to allow SGDs to work most efficiently to meet the user's needs. The Steve Gleason Enduring Voice Act of 2018 is one example of how technological advances support the development and acquisition of urgently needed communication options for communicatively vulnerable populations who need it, as well as stands as an example of how technological advances can effect legislative changes.

Further technology advances continue to expand options for alternate access. Research and development of new and more refined access options continues such that previously unfathomable access solutions have become reality. Eye tracking is now widely available as an access option. New switches that leverage materials science, such as the NeuroNode (Control Bionics), or those that provide one portal that supports multiple options for access, such as the Noddle (Voxello), are now available. An active area of research in terms of alternate access for AAC is **brain-computer interfaces** (BCIs). Although a thorough discussion of BCIs is beyond the scope of this chapter, it is important to mention them in the context of alternate access since this is an active area of research. BCIs "… are assistive technology interfaces that directly interpret brain activity to enable a person to control (another) technology. In AAC applications, a BCI can be conceptualized as a system of four basic components: sensors to record brain activity, signal analysis methods to extract desired control signals from the brain activity, communication rate enhancement techniques to improve the efficiency of each selection, and the output that results from the process, often on a display" (Huggins & Kovacs, 2018, p. 13). At present, use of BCIs as modes of access for people with neurodegenerative diseases is extremely limited and still largely confined to use in research settings or protocols (e.g., the RSVP Keyboard [Oregon Health & Science University] BCI; Fried-Oken et al., 2015). Neurodegenerative conditions themselves may present challenges for the use of BCIs since both physical and cognitive status may change with disease progression and may influence one's ability to use a BCI. More research is required to determine what type(s) of BCIs will support continued access to AAC systems in the face of intellectual and/or physical deterioration and how to provide the user with the most robust communication options.

Telepractice and Tele-AAC

ASHA defines **telepractice** as "… the application of telecommunications technology to the delivery of speech-language pathology and audiology professional services at a distance by linking clinician to client or clinician to clinician for assessment, intervention, and/or consultation" (ASHA, n.d.h). Telepractice services may be **synchronous** (i.e., interactive, in real time), or **asynchronous** (i.e., use recorded data, such as video, images, or voice recordings, that are sent to the remote clinician), also referred to as "store-and-forward."

There are also hybrid approaches in which some combination of synchronous and asynchronous service delivery is used to provide optimal services. Decisions concerning which type of telepractice services to use should be decided on a case-by-case basis by a clinician who is well-versed in telepractice.

Telepractice offers much to the profession of speech-language pathology and is gaining traction as one of many modes of service delivery across a variety of disorders (e.g., Boisvert et al., 2012; Burns et al., 2016; Cherney & van Vuuren, 2012; Coyle, 2012; Hall et al., 2013). Although the body of literature supporting the implementation of telepractice as both feasible and effective across various disorders continues to grow, issues related to the environments in which it is practiced, the need for secure and constant internet access and connectivity, regulation at the state and national levels, and licensure continue to challenge widespread adoption and implementation of telepractice (Cason & Cohn, 2014). For speech-language pathologists in the United States, the lack of licensure portability across state lines is a telehealth practice constraint.

On April 28, 2021, Representative Mike Thompson (D-CA) introduced H. R. 2903, and the following day, Senator Brian Schatz (D-HI) introduced S. 1512, the Creating Opportunities Now for Necessary and Effective Care Technologies Health Act of 2021. Although first introduced in 2016, this legislation may become a reality due to health care service delivery issues created by the COVID-19 pandemic. As this legislation is complex, the reader is referred to the face sheet at https://www.cchpca.org/2021/05/CONNECT-Act-Fact-Sheetfinal.pdf. At the time this book went to press, H. R. 2903 and S. 1512 were both in committee. The interested reader should keep in mind that H. R. 2903 and S. 1512 may have passed the appropriate committees, reconciled, passed by Congress, and signed into law by the president by the time this book is published.

Telepractice is a broad term that subsumes the provision of skilled speech-language pathology services to a broad range of clients across environments. The term **tele-AAC** was introduced by the Tele-AAC Working Group of the 2012 Research Symposium of the International Society for Augmentative and Alternative Communication to refer to "a unique cross-disciplinary clinical service delivery model that requires expertise in both telepractice and AAC systems" (Anderson et al., 2012). The tele-AAC resolution was an early attempt to begin describing and codifying practical and research needs in AAC. To summarize the more detailed document, key elements of the resolution were that the person who uses AAC should identify their circle of communication partners and tele-AAC should address the needs of those communication partners, opportunities and constraints of tele-AAC should be investigated and articulated, institutions of higher education and professional organizations should provide training in tele-AAC, and people who use AAC should be involved in research and development of valid measures of tele-AAC effectiveness (Anderson et al., 2012).

Practitioners have defined tele-AAC as the use of telepractice to provide services to individuals using AAC (Hall & Boisvert, 2014; Hall et al., 2019). In its broadest scope, tele-AAC refers to the provision of AAC services to people that need them and the education of clinicians and other stakeholders in AAC. Tele-AAC holds much promise for the broader AAC community in terms of the avenues it opens for education, building professional capacity, and extending the reach of AAC services to people who may otherwise not be able to access them.

In addition to the technological infrastructure necessary to support telepractice, tele-AAC requires additional equipment, and in some cases, personnel. In terms of equipment, tele-AAC may require the clinician to have a duplicate of the client's AAC system and a way for the clinician to view the screen of the client's device. This may require extra hardware (e.g., various cameras and flexible mounts), as well as duplicate systems. This need may introduce further complexity into a tele-AAC scenario. However, research indicates that use of a trained person, sometimes referred to as an **e-helper** or **onsite facilitator**, may offset some of the complexity. An e-helper is someone knowledgeable about the AAC system (i.e., access method, mount, system) who can support the client during a tele-AAC session (for a fuller discussion of tele-AAC and its many constituent parts and aspects, the reader is referred to Hall et al., 2019).

Importantly, the promise of tele-AAC is that it offers much to the field of AAC. It can help build clinical capacity by being used in a consultative way to provide a programmatic approach to educating clinicians to gain competence and expertise in AAC. In this way, clinical expertise is shared over time and distance so more clinicians can provide AAC services. Tele-AAC furthers the reach of clinicians who provide AAC service by supporting access to those services to people who may not be able to physically access them due to geography, transportation, inclement weather, logistics, or some combination of these factors.

Ethics in AAC

Ethical practice is central to all clinical, educational, and research endeavors. In the United States and Canada, clinicians are governed by ASHA's Code of Ethics (2016b) and must adhere to them for assessment and intervention. With respect to assessment, not all centers or agencies, either in health care or in education, are equipped for all contingencies in terms of technological options. For this reason, speech-language pathologists may find themselves contacting vendors or representatives to request loaner device(s) prior to an assessment. Vendors or representatives may loan equipment to clinicians or they may request to demonstrate it during the assessment. Depending on the situation, either may be appropriate. It is particularly important to establish how this situation will be handled *a priori*. Clarification of roles and boundaries of how and when a vendor may participate in an AAC assessment is critical. This is especially important where the vendor may have a speech and language background (e.g., a baccalaureate degree in communication sciences and disorders) or may be a certified speech-language pathologist who has decided to work as a vendor. The critical variable is that the clinician, not the vendor, maintains stewardship of the assessment and any decisions made.

In a similar vein, there are situations where a vendor may be providing a demonstration of their product in the absence of clinical input. This may happen when access to a clinician knowledgeable about AAC is not available or when a potential client does not know where to turn given their needs. For instance, a person recently diagnosed with ALS may read online that many people who have ALS require AAC. In a proactive effort to meet anticipated needs, the person may search for options in their community prior to a referral or completion of a comprehensive assessment. The individual with ALS may contact a vendor or a number of vendors to view available options. A vendor is in the business of selling products. To this end, the vendor may inform the person they should seek an AAC assessment and/or that a given product may be insurance-eligible. On the other hand, the vendor may not inform the individual with ALS of these facts. If the individual with ALS likes the product(s) demonstrated, they may make arrangement for purchase of a given option with payment out-of-pocket. This scenario is dangerous because (1) the person may be unaware there are other options available, (2) their physical status may change over time, (3) a system that is suitable at one point in time may not be suitable at a later point in time, and (4) a clinician should be conducting an AAC assessment. As previously noted for the case of neurodegenerative disease, some clients and/or their families may buy commercially available technology that meets an existing need on the advice or recommendation of well-meaning salespeople, advertisements, and/or information online. Although seemingly expedient at the outset, doing so may compromise care as the disease progresses without affiliations with licensed professionals who can provide expert care and guidance with respect to AAC needs.

In a related vein, clinicians are ethically bound to demonstrate technology and have a client try as many potential options as possible, not just the options with which they are most familiar and/or habitually prescribe. This may require requesting loaners and educating oneself about new options as they become available.

Another ethical issue in AAC includes the use of **facilitated communication**. This method was popularized during the early 1990s for use with people with autism (e.g., Biklen et al., 1992; Crossley & Remington-Gurney, 1992). Facilitated communication was highly controversial when it was introduced as an AAC option. Many of its opponents referred to the use of facilitated communication as "the Ouija Board effect." On the other hand, proponents lauded it as a breakthrough in communication options for people with autism. Scientific research demonstrated a lack of validity that facilitated communication promoted authentic communication authored by the communicator. Rather, evidence suggested messages were authored by facilitators instead of the clients themselves (e.g., Schlosser et al., 2014; Shane & Kearns, 1994) and that the method was not valid. ASHA updated its statement on the use of facilitated communication to indicate that it is "... a discredited technique that should not be used. There is no scientific evidence of the validity of facilitated communication, and there is extensive scientific evidence—produced over several decades and across several countries—that messages are authored by the 'facilitator' rather than the person with a disability. Furthermore, there is extensive evidence of harms related to the use of [facilitated communication]" (ASHA, 2018b).

Another ethical issue similar to facilitated communication is the use of the Rapid Prompting Method (RPM; Mukhopadhyay, 2018; also Mukhopadhyay, 2008 as cited in ASHA's Position Statement on Rapid Prompting Method [2018b]), which has recently gained exposure, also used with persons with autism. RPM is similar to facilitated communication in that both are facilitator-dependent techniques (i.e., techniques that involve the person with the disability being dependent upon a facilitator to presumably produce their messages by their direction [Tostanoski et al., 2014, as cited in ASHA's Position Statement on Rapid Prompting Method {ASHA, 2018b}]). These techniques reportedly are designed to provide access to alphabet/letter/word boards or SGDs for communication or education. In RPM, the instructor or facilitator holds the alphabet board or keyboard and provides repeated verbal, auditory, visual, and/or tactile prompts. ASHA's position statement on RPM concludes that, "RPM is not recommended because of prompt dependency and the lack of scientific validity. Furthermore, information obtained through the use of RPM should not be assumed to be the communication of the person with a disability" (ASHA, 2018c).

SUMMARY

Professional issues related to clinical and educational endeavors in AAC derive from a myriad of factors associated with current and evolving technology, the heterogeneity of the populations who require or may benefit from AAC, preprofessional preparation and ongoing educational needs of professionals who provide AAC services, and the need for ongoing research in the field to continue to improve the tools, techniques, and training that comprise the AAC enterprise. ASHA's Code of Ethics (2016b) provides a mandatory ethical framework that guides students and governs clinician conduct. ASHA has provided clear guidance by way of position statements concerning the use of facilitated communication and RPM. ASHA supports the proposed Creating Opportunities Now for Necessary and Effective Care Technologies Health Act of 2021, which may provide portability of speech-language pathology licensure across state lines, thus opening previously blocked options for speech-language pathologists to conduct telepractice. As a part of telepractice, tele-AAC is a burgeoning enterprise that has the potential to build professional capacity in AAC and to extend the reach of AAC services previously precluded by factors, such as geographical distance, lack of transportation, travel time and expense, and ill health.

Recent technological advances have created AAC options, such as mobile tablets and AAC apps, that are now commercially available. Greater commercial availability underscores the need for professional guidance in their use across settings and populations. Judicious application of ASHA's Code of Ethics (or the codes of ethics of professional organizations in other countries) holds the most promise for optimizing the impact of AAC across clinical and educational settings.

STUDY QUESTIONS

1. Identify and discuss two professional issues related to the clinical application of AAC.

2. Identify and discuss two changes noted in the most recent review of pre-service training in AAC.

3. Define tele-AAC and describe why it is unique. What are some of the obstacles that may affect how tele-AAC can be implemented?

5

Cultural and Linguistic Diversity and AAC

Katrina E. Miller, EdD

MYTH

1. Traditional speech and language assessment procedures are appropriate for use with culturally and linguistically diverse augmentative and alternative communication (AAC) users.
2. The definition of what constitutes a disability is universal.
3. Successful AAC assessment and intervention require only a speech-language pathologist and an AAC user.

REALITY

1. To obtain the most valuable information during an AAC assessment, it is important to incorporate a variety of components, including file review, interview, observation, and dynamic assessment. AAC assessment should be family-focused and consider cultural and/or linguistic differences that may be present.
2. What is viewed as a disability or a difference varies across the society in which a person lives. A family's view of what may or may not constitute a disability may be culturally bound. A definition of disability can also be impacted by an individual's social or supernatural belief systems.
3. Successful AAC assessment and intervention must incorporate a collaborative model. This includes interdisciplinary and transdisciplinary models. Understanding cultural and/or linguistic differences and incorporating the client's family in assessment, symbol and technology selection, and intervention is crucial for successful AAC use.

INTRODUCTION

It would be irresponsible to discuss AAC without discussing the role culture plays in every aspect of AAC use. The cultures to which persons who rely on AAC belong are just as diverse as individual needs of AAC users. Similarly, it is imperative for speech-language pathologists and other practitioners who provide AAC intervention services to be culturally responsive. In order to be a culturally responsive practitioner, one must provide services that are aligned with their client's values and beliefs (Mindel & John, 2021).

Since AAC practitioners are working with more culturally and linguistically diverse clientele than in previous years, an examination of relevant cultural and professional topics is needed (Mindel & John, 2021). While the American

Fuller, D. R., & Lloyd, L. L. *Principles and Practices in Augmentative and Alternative Communication* (pp. 69-74).
© 2023 Taylor & Francis Group.

Speech-Language-Hearing Association provides assistance for speech-language pathologists to understand the roles culture and cultural linguistics play within their scope of professional practice, integrating these components (i.e., research, clinical experience and scientific evidence, caregiver and client perspective) into practice may be challenging but is mandatory (American Speech-Language-Hearing Association, 2005).

This chapter provides an overview of culturally responsive practice with AAC users. The sections that follow will explore culture and AAC in terms of changing demographics, theory and discussion of cultural differences, cultural attitudes toward disability, and clinical issues in AAC assessment and intervention.

CULTURE AND AAC

Changing Demographics

The racial and ethnic demographics of the United States are changing. Recent census data indicate 53.8% of children under age 5 years are from ethnic backgrounds other than western European, White, or Caucasian groups (Hyter & Salas-Provance, 2019). The combined population of First Nation/Native American, African-American, Asian, Hispanic, and Pacific Islander individuals is expected to rise to over 60% of the total U.S. population by 2060; these racial and ethnic groups comprised just 38% of the U.S. population in 2017 (Hyter & Salas-Provance, 2019).

While English is currently the predominant language spoken in the United States, there are more than 350 languages spoken in U.S. households (Hyter & Salas-Provance, 2019). Of these 350 languages, approximately 10% of them are spoken by at least 100,000 persons over the age of 5 years. Finally, data from the 2019 U.S. Census Bureau American Community Survey reports that 23% of children aged 5 to 17 years speak a language other than English.

Limited demographic data estimate that approximately 12% of preschoolers enrolled in special education in the United States have complex communication needs (CCN) that necessitate the provision of AAC services (Pope et al., 2022). Furthermore, an increasing number of these children are from homes where a language other than English or along with English is spoken (King et al., 2022). Combine this with the disproportionate rates of culturally and linguistically diverse students placed in special education programs (Mindel, 2020), and one can see the importance of culturally responsive AAC assessment and intervention practices.

Understanding the diverse racial and ethnic makeup of our country helps professionals to better plan and prepare themselves for appropriate therapeutic interventions and also assist universities with their program curriculum designs. Data indicate the importance and need to equip communication disorder professionals with the tools needed.

Theory and Discussion of Cultural Differences

The definition of culture often depends on the person you are asking or the institution providing a response. The definition of culture can be as complex as "… the collective programming of the mind that distinguishes the members of one group or category of people from others" (Hofstede, 2011, p. 8) or as simple as "my family traditions." Regardless of the definition one utilizes, culture is learned, transmitted socially, and based on beliefs, attitudes, and value systems (Hyter & Salas-Provance, 2019). Another crucial piece is that culture assists in the development through which an individual views themselves and the world. Culture defines a person and is all-inclusive. Therefore, an individual's culture must be considered during the assessment and intervention process for AAC users.

Battle (2012) argues that understanding another's culture is a continuous process. Much of the literature on multiculturalism uses the term **cultural competence** to describe an individual's ability to cross cultural boundaries and understand differences based on cultural background. In order to be an effective clinician, the journey to competence is ongoing. In addition, being able to understand one's individual biases is a necessary component toward developing cultural competence (Battle, 2012; Hyter & Salas-Provance, 2019).

Another key factor to cultural competence is understanding culture-bound and language-bound variables (Battle, 2012). Understanding these variables and how they intersect with culture will assist the practitioner in the assessment, intervention, and training of persons with CCN from culturally and linguistically diverse backgrounds. While understanding these variables is important, implementing cultural knowledge may be uncomfortable when clients are from cultural groups different from their providers (Leslie et al., 2021). Being aware of these differences serves as a starting point for culturally responsive practice.

Hofstede (2011), a psychologist, developed six dimensions of natural cultures:

1. Power distance
2. Uncertainty avoidance
3. Individualism/collectivism
4. Masculinity/femininity
5. Long-/short-term orientation
6. Indulgence/restraint

Extensive research was conducted across cultures and countries to assess the validity of these dimensions. Similarly, Battle (2012) mentions the importance of individual and group variables within a culture and discusses these variables and their differences within cultural groups. Battle's variables include individualism and collectivism, power distance, time orientation, and verbal/nonverbal communication dimensions. A number of these variables are discussed later in light of AAC intervention.

When viewing individualism, emphasis is placed on the freedom of the individual, while collectivism focuses on the needs of the group (Battle, 2012; Hofstede, 2011). As examples, cultures from western European heritages support individualism while persons from Arab, Asian, African, and Hispanic heritages support more of a collectivist viewpoint (Battle, 2012).

Power distance variables concentrate on the relationships between people of different social status. For example, individuals in high power distance cultures do not question their superiors, while persons from low power distance cultures do not necessarily accept superiors' orders. In light of this cultural variable, attitudes regarding following through with therapeutic recommendations may be viewed differently if the clinician and client are from two different power distance systems (Battle, 2012). Power distance variables can also include male and female relationships. Hofstede (2011) further describes this variable as the understanding that members of an organization recognize power is distributed unequally.

Time orientation is different across cultures, with nonwestern cultures being more focused on the past while western cultures are more future-oriented (Battle, 2012). In Hofstede's model (2011), short-term orientation is seen in cultures that view life events that occurred in the past as more relevant, while cultures with long-term orientation view life events occurring in the future as more important. Time orientation is central to understanding how long-term goals may not appear as relevant as short-term goals across cultures (Battle, 2012). This can be challenging when AAC practitioners are a part of the mainstream cultural group or do not understand the time orientation dynamic.

Finally, verbal and nonverbal communication can be quite different across cultural boundaries (Battle, 2012). Nonverbal communication includes transmission of messages or information by means other than words, such as kinesics or the use of body movements (e.g., facial expressions, head positioning, and eye contact that differs across cultures). The use of personal space or proxemics is important to consider in order to avoid offending others, especially during communication exchanges (Hyter & Salas-Provance, 2019). Other paralanguage variables that may hinder communication include silence, vocal loudness, and voice inflection (Battle, 2012).

Verbal communication (e.g., pragmatics and semantics) can be a language barrier (Battle, 2012). The manner in which language is used can interfere with the communication process. In order to be a culturally responsive practitioner, one should understand the role these variables and others play when addressing AAC needs. One must keep in mind that understanding these cultural differences will not solve all issues concerning culture and AAC use but is part of the tools needed to be an effective service provider.

When speech-language pathologists and other practitioners consider AAC for their clients, it is imperative several factors are taken into consideration. In addition to the type and severity of the client's impairment, the AAC professional must consider age, gender, health, occupation, and socioeconomic status. Each of these variables has distinctive characteristics along with different levels of importance across societal groups. It is an error to assume all people of color have the same life experiences, and therefore, one type of AAC intervention will be effective for every individual in a particular ethnic or racial group.

Cultural Attitudes Toward Disability

Attitudes regarding disability and AAC intervention can be deeply rooted in culture. This is particularly true since culture and language interact and impact so many areas of expression, including conversation styles, pragmatics, and paralinguistics (Leslie et al., 2021; Mindel & John, 2021). The origins of disabilities can be viewed through a variety of cultural lenses, including but not limited to supernatural, social, and individual (Mindel & John, 2021). When a culture believes that the person's disability is a result of supernatural origins, the disability is a reflection of sin and should be accepted. A disability of social origin reflects poorly on the family or community and is viewed as shameful. Finally, when the belief that the disability's origin is individual, the person with the disability is responsible for their recovery and must help themselves (Mindel & John, 2021).

While being aware of values and beliefs that may be a part of a racial or ethnic group is important, the first approach to understanding attitudes toward disabilities is self-inquiry (Soto, 2018). Self-inquiry allows a culturally responsive practitioner to collaborate with families and other professionals to assure the practice is inclusive of their values and belief systems. It also provides the professional an opportunity to explore any biases or misinformation they have regarding a particular racial or ethnic group.

AAC practices tend to veer toward privileged members of mainstream communities (Hyter & Salas-Provance 2019; Mindel, 2020). Communication difficulties of a person who has CCN may not be the only reason a person is marginalized (Soto, 2018). This is important to remember, so that a culturally responsive AAC practitioner will consider all the covert factors that may affect their clients. Factors such as socioeconomic levels, race, ethnicity, and learning English as a second language may also contribute to a client's marginalization. While no one can know all the different cultural norms and languages of the individuals they treat, professionals can agree to collaborate with others, including communities, to make their practices as welcoming and supportive as possible (Soto, 2018).

CLINICAL ISSUES:
AAC ASSESSMENT AND INTERVENTION

The goal of AAC assessment and intervention is to improve access to communication for persons with CCN. The variety of strategies and approaches to assessment with culturally and linguistically diverse populations across disorders are well documented in the communication sciences and disorders literature (Hyter & Salas-Provance, 2019). To further complicate matters, barriers to AAC access and service provision has impacted confidence levels of speech-language pathologists in this area of practice (King et al., 2022). This section is designed to provide a brief overview of topics to consider when designing AAC assessment and intervention strategies in light of multicultural issues.

Assessment Issues

The procedures for AAC assessment may not be as clear as a classic speech and language assessment for communication disorders professionals. AAC assessments are a dynamic process, utilizing observations and standardized test results (Mindel & John, 2021). When preparing for an AAC assessment, one should keep in mind that 70% of children with CCN have an associated diagnosis of developmental delay or autism spectrum disorder (Pope et al., 2022). It should also be noted that increasing evidence suggests that barriers to effective clinical and educational services, including delays in diagnosis, are intensified for African-American children and other children of color (Pope et al., 2022). This fact stresses the importance that health care providers should listen to the concerns of parents in order to avoid racially biased care. Listening to parental concerns is imperative since the first step to an AAC assessment is the referral. Factors that may further delay the referral process include a lack of exposure to AAC, cultural attitudes toward the disability, linguistic barriers, and availability of services (Mindel & John, 2021).

Initial research findings further suggest that racial inequity in school-based intervention services extends through secondary school (Pope et al., 2022). While this issue will not be solved through the current discussion, being aware of potential inequities will allow the AAC practitioner to view assessment through a variety of lenses. It is also believed that this will assist AAC providers in being effective advocates for their clients regardless of their ethnicity or racial backgrounds.

The goal for the AAC practitioner is to conduct an appropriate assessment, design a suitable AAC system, and develop goals appropriate for intervention (Mindel, 2020). In order to gather the most relevant and useful information, the examiner must be prepared to utilize alternative methods for an AAC assessment. These components can include but should not be limited to review of records or client files, observations (in a variety of environments with several communication partners, if possible), family and caregiver interviews, and input from other professionals (e.g., regular or special education teachers, physicians, social workers). A form of interviewing that has allowed patients and families to participate in the decision-making process is called motivational interviewing (Leslie et al., 2021). Motivational interviewing encompasses a recognition of cultural differences and adapts interviewing techniques to include those differences. Assessments should be conducted in the child's native language when possible. Interviews and interactions with family members should be completed with interpreters when appropriate and in welcoming environments.

Standardized Testing

While standardized testing will be an important component of an AAC assessment, it is crucial the examiner remember that most standardized tests are normed on White monolingual English-speaking populations. This fact can make most of these assessment tools inappropriate for culturally and linguistically diverse populations (Mindel & John, 2021). Incorporating standardized speech and language tests normed on the population with which the culturally and linguistically diverse child identifies will provide useful information. Using these diagnostic methods in isolation will not provide a true picture of the individual's communication abilities (Mindel & John, 2021).

Hyter and Salas-Provance (2019) identify several methods of adapting standardized testing to gather the maximum amount of useful information during an assessment. Such alternative methods include using criterion-referenced tests, modifying norm-referenced tests (e.g., varying prompts, extending time on test items, using more than allotted practice items), and measuring processing ability vs. language knowledge.

Observations

Observations are an important part of an AAC assessment and can be structured or unstructured. It is important that observations be done in a variety of environments (e.g., home, school, workplace) and with several communication partners. These partners should include peers and family members (Mindel, 2020). If observation in the home environment is not an option, the AAC practitioner can request that the caregiver record a brief video (Mindel & John, 2021). AAC practitioners should be aware of a potential cultural mismatch between families and the examiner to avoid miscommunication and to assist in the development of the most appropriate intervention plan (Mindel, 2020). Observations can start in virtually any environment. Information recorded during an observation should include differences in interactions with peers vs. family members and others, languages that may be used and in which settings, and pragmatics. Observations can serve as important components of the assessment and intervention process.

Dynamic Assessment

Dynamic assessment has been used for numerous years and is a way to distinguish a communication difference from a disorder (Hyter & Salas-Provance, 2019; Mindel & John, 2021). There are several ways to organize the information gathered during dynamic assessment. Mindel and John (2021) refer to three methods of dynamic assessment, including (1) testing limits, (2) graduated prompting, and (3) test-teach-retest. Testing limits can be used during norm-referenced testing and include using alternative instructions and providing feedback during prompts. Graduated prompting, which encompasses the use of hierarchical and predetermined prompts, can also be part of dynamic assessment. Finally, the test-teach-retest format relies on the modification of standardized test results but will provide useful qualitative information.

Hyter and Salas-Provance (2019) recommend different methods to gather useful information. One approach is the SWOT method, where the professional processes the client's *s*trengths, *w*eaknesses, *o*pportunities, and *t*hreats. The GRASP (i.e., *g*ather, *r*eview, *a*sk, *s*ee, and *p*roceed) and RIOT (i.e., *r*eview, *i*nterview, *o*bserve, and *t*est) methods can serve as alternative methods of assessment. The reader is referred to Hyter and Salas-Provance (2019) for a deeper discussion of these methods of dynamic assessment.

Interviewing

To receive the maximum amount of information during the interview process, a culturally responsive examiner will remember the cultural variables previously discussed in this chapter. It is imperative the examiner be mindful of cultural practices, including power variables, communication styles, and linguistic barriers. An ethnographic interview style may be the most appropriate way to gather information. Ethnographic interview style is rooted in social research and follows a qualitative method (Hyter & Salas-Provance, 2019). Ethnographic interviews incorporate descriptive questions and are designed to be engaging and are recommended with culturally and linguistically diverse populations (Hyter & Salas-Provance, 2019; Mindel & John, 2021). While a general checklist can also be used during the interview process, it may not yield as much information with persons who exhibit cultural and/or linguistic diversity. Ethnographic interviews use open-ended questions, ask for examples, and provide summaries to allow opportunity for correction (Mindel, 2020).

Use of Interpreters

Ideal assessment and intervention with culturally and linguistically diverse families are undoubtedly enhanced with the use of interpreters (Mindel & John, 2021). This is especially true when the family's primary language differs from that of the examiner. Most school and health care systems have a pool of interpreters assigned to their organizations. Professionals who utilize interpreters mention the importance of incorporating debriefing time following assessment or intervention sessions (Battle, 2012; Mindel, 2020). This debriefing time allows for an exchange of information—especially cultural variables—that can be valuable to the examiner. Hyter and Salas-Provance (2019) emphasize the importance of an interpreter not merely being a speaker of the examiner's and examinee's languages but also being sure that appropriate educational or medical vocabulary be expected from the professional interpreter. Battle (2012) provides a clear definition of interpretation as "… the transmission of information from one language to another, while translation references … written transmission" (p. 264). When no other options are available, peers or cultural liaisons may prove to be invaluable (Battle, 2012; Mindel & John, 2021) in assisting the examiner in gathering useful information.

Intervention Issues

With assessment completed, or in many cases while assessment is ongoing, the AAC practitioner begins to direct their attention to developing and implementing an AAC system and its associated technology. Continued relationship building with family and communication partners is still crucial during the intervention process (Mindel & John, 2021). Attention to the client's cultural beliefs, practices, and values is necessary at this stage, particularly since symbol selection is tied to vocabulary and language use. Soto (2012) categorizes several barriers that may arise during the AAC implementation process. These barriers include insistence on the use of mainstream American English, cultural and linguistic barriers between professionals on the AAC team and culturally and linguistically diverse clients and their families, poor culturally relevant vocabulary, culturally inappropriate aided and/or unaided symbols, and lack of family-centered AAC training.

Another barrier that is important to mention at this stage is the cost of AAC devices. A study conducted by Brock and Thomas (2021) on the effectiveness of aided AAC modeling for Belizean children identified economic factors that may impact intervention outcomes. These factors are not unique to Belize and can be reflected in the United States and elsewhere, where wealth inequality tends to exist. Speech-generating device abandonment tends to be a common issue, so assuring cultural appropriateness during the prescription of technology is an important success factor (Mindel, 2020). Finally, sufficient access to AAC intervention should be noted, particularly among underserved and underrepresented populations (Pope et al., 2022). These are intervention issues that may affect successful use of AAC in culturally and linguistically diverse populations. Being aware of these issues ahead of time helps the practitioner be better able to meet the needs of their culturally and linguistically diverse clients.

Training Communication Partners

The time to begin family and caregiver training is at the referral stage. Including family members and other important stakeholders helps the AAC assessment and intervention process to be more effective. Stakeholders are persons who have an active role in the success of the client's AAC use. These persons not only include peers and persons from educational environments but can and should extend to family and community members as well (Mindel & John, 2021). As previously mentioned, being aware of personal biases and having a base knowledge of the client's cultural beliefs assist with the success of a family-centered approach to intervention.

The family-centered approach provides culturally inclusive collaboration among stakeholders in multiple environments (Mindel & John, 2021). This collaboration allows for the most beneficial vocabulary and symbols to be identified along with the most appropriate pragmatic use. By including family in this process, AAC practitioners are able to identify and use items and methods that already may be effective within the home environment. This partnership also ensures that the person using an AAC system has partners to communicate.

Battle (2012) provides several guidelines to assist the AAC practitioner in implementing culturally relevant intervention. These guidelines include being flexible with scheduling, being flexible with the selection of materials, presenting clear objectives, using multiple levels of questions, and using methods and procedures that do not violate the cultural norms of the client. In the same light, Mindel and John (2021) provide suggestions for building team partnerships when working with AAC clients. These suggestions include being clear with communication, being calm and curious, being culturally informed, being culturally deferential, and being a responsive listener.

The main objective for communication partner training is to assist the AAC user in the development of their communication skills (Mindel & John, 2021). One should not forget the importance of siblings as communication partners. When providing training for communication partners, find ways to prevent families from becoming overwhelmed. Use simple vocabulary while identifying communication opportunities and provide information in small increments (Mindel & John, 2021).

SUMMARY

While implementing AAC assessment and intervention with culturally and linguistically diverse populations, several factors need to be considered. The changing demographics of the United States require a culturally responsive approach to AAC assessment and intervention. These diverse populations encompass not only students who are English language learners but who also have CCN.

When working with persons who must rely on AAC, one must understand not only their own cultural biases but also the AAC user's and family's cultural attitudes toward disability and AAC use. This chapter further discussed assessment and intervention challenges that may be encountered with AAC users from culturally and linguistically diverse backgrounds. Assessment and intervention strategies were discussed for culturally and linguistically diverse populations along with the training necessary for the AAC user's communication partners.

It should be noted that while this chapter addressed cultural and linguistic diversity and AAC in general, more specific information regarding cultural and linguistic diversity is also included in several of the other chapters of this textbook.

STUDY QUESTIONS

1. List the components of a dynamic assessment in light of an AAC user who is a member of a nonmainstream cultural group.
2. Identify and discuss two cultural variables that may make AAC assessment or intervention challenging.
3. Discuss how the changing demographics of the United States may impact AAC users.
4. Identify and discuss tips for working with interpreters, persons with CCN, and their families.
5. Discuss how cultural views on disability can affect AAC intervention.

Part II
AAC Symbols

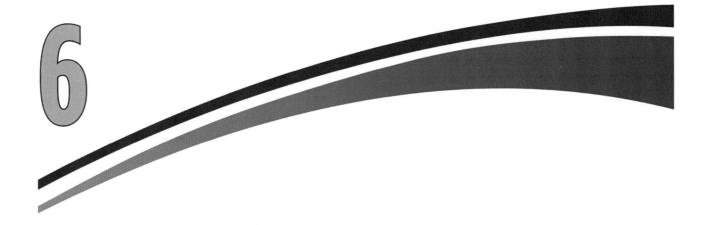

6

Introduction to AAC Symbols

Eliada Pampoulou, PhD
and Donald R. Fuller, PhD

MYTH

1. If you encourage a child to use augmentative and alternative forms of communication, such as signs and/or photographs/pictures, that child will never develop speech.

2. The person must have certain prerequisites (i.e., a certain level of cognitive skills) to be able to use augmentative and alternative communication (AAC) symbols for their communication needs.

3. Individuals with complex communication needs should use unaided symbols, such as manual signs, rather than aided symbols, such as pictures or Blissymbols.

REALITY

1. There is no evidence that the use of AAC prevents the development of speech. To the contrary, there are many reports of individuals who failed to develop speech until they became successful communicators through the use of these types of communication.

2. Everyone is capable of using AAC symbols to communicate regardless of the level of their cognitive (or other) skills. A comprehensive AAC assessment can identify the skills of the individual so clinicians can decide upon the best options for that person to communicate their needs and thoughts with others.

3. A host of impairments can prevent a person from speaking clearly. Many of these involve only the motor production of speech with the ability to understand speech and to think clearly remaining intact. Some of these people might also have motor difficulties, and thus, the use of unaided forms of communication is difficult, if not impossible, for them. In this and many other cases, the use of aided forms of communication (e.g., line drawings, photographs) would be more beneficial because there are many ways to access them (e.g., direct selection, scanning).

INTRODUCTION

Communication is defined as the exchange of thoughts and ideas between at least two people. As was explained in Chapter 3, during this interaction, both the sender and the receiver focus on a common topic and, through a dynamic process, share their thoughts and perspectives. Through

Fuller, D. R., & Lloyd, L. L. *Principles and Practices in*
Augmentative and Alternative Communication (pp. 77-81).

communication exchanges, people are capable of requesting something they wish to have, rejecting something they do not want, or commenting about something they saw on TV, for example. This interaction is such a dynamic process that both parties use a variety of forms to communicate, such as eye contact, facial expressions, gestures, pointing, and speech. Decades of linguistic research on various areas of communication have shown quite convincingly that the characteristics of genuine human communication and language are, to some extent, universal and form part of each individual's biological endowment. A close look at the characteristics of human communication and language in general will provide a better understanding of the characteristics of symbols that can be used in AAC. Hence, one could argue that the organization of AAC—and the communication modes within it—should as much as possible follow these general principles of human communication and language. While the linguistic and communication capacities of AAC users may be restricted in some ways, there is no reason to assume they consist of substantially different elements than those for communicators without disabilities. Hence, before discussing some basic characteristics of AAC symbols, there needs to be consideration of some of the most basic features of natural languages and human communication.

Human Communication, Natural Languages, and AAC Symbols

Humans communicate with each other to convey their thoughts and ideas to their communication partners. Human communication is inherent and its expression starts from the very beginning of life. Communication between parents and their baby (and especially the mother and baby) is essential for the continuous development of the baby's communication skills. The baby looks at their mother during communication attempts for socialization and as an expression of their needs. For instance, the baby's crying is different when they are hungry, tired of being alone, wishes to seek interaction, or is sick or in pain. Very often, the message receiver—who in this case is the mother—learns to recognize the different ways their baby cries and to act accordingly. Toddlers in their second year of life communicate mainly via gestures and vocalizations when expressing their wishes. Even when speech is gradually developing, gestures remain the main form of communication (Anderson & Shames, 2013). Moreover, even in later years, children communicate using gestures, as well as eye contact, facial expressions, and body language. In fact, these forms of communication remain throughout our lives, but not to the same extent as in our childhood. It is thus very appropriate that these forms of communication are also used within the AAC field for people to communicate and compensate for the lack of intelligible speech production. Unaided forms of communication, such as facial expressions (e.g., smiling or frowning), gesturing "yes" or "no," and pointing to a desired object are all forms of communication used in human interaction, whether speech is present or not.

Human communication is based on natural human language, a conventional system of arbitrary symbols and grammatical rules to combine the symbols into larger units (e.g., phrases, clauses, sentences) to convey meaning (Anderson & Shames, 2013). A natural language is one that has evolved from social interaction between human beings, that is, it has not been expressly invented. Spoken languages are natural languages.

Sign languages used by the Deaf are also the result of natural development. Because of hearing loss, these individuals are often hindered in their communication through spoken language, but the adaptational powers of humans have resulted in the evolution of sign languages well-suited for the sensory impairment of deafness. For persons who are deaf, sign language is an alternative means of communication to speech production. Sign languages are languages in a different modality; they are not oral-aural like spoken languages but are instead produced in the manual-visual channel mainly with the hands and perceived by vision. Deaf children acquire a sign language as their first language, and the course and pace of this acquisition are much the same as for the acquisition of a spoken language (Newport & Meier, 1985).

Sign languages are nonvocal but are verbal forms of communication. The term verbal should be equated with linguistic (or language) ability, not with speech per se. In the AAC field, sign language is categorized as an unaided form of communication because the person does not require anything separate from their body to communicate. Sign languages are linguistic systems. In human social interaction, natural languages transmitted through the oral modality (i.e., spoken) are the benchmark by which all other forms of communication are compared. For persons with cognitive and/or physical impairments, modes other than oral communication may have to be used. These are often judged by communication partners in comparison to spoken communication. An AAC system designed for an individual with a severe communication disability should approximate spoken, natural language as closely as possible in terms of the symbols used, its representational range (and hence, linguistic capacity), and the rate of message transmission.

SYMBOL TERMINOLOGY

It is widely accepted that common and concise terminology used by professionals can lead to efficient communication. An absence of common terminology can lead to confusion and miscommunication among professionals supporting people who might benefit from AAC (Lloyd & Blischak, 1992). For instance, Pampoulou (2015, 2017) found that professionals often refer to different terms when they mention symbols and the available corpuses of symbols. This leads inevitably to misunderstandings among practitioners, researchers, and symbol developers who all have some vested interest in AAC symbols. It is thus essential that we establish terminology that will be used in this chapter and throughout this textbook.

It is important to first refer to the etymological definition of "symbols," as well as to definitions given in more recent dictionaries. The specific term originates from the Greek word σύμβολον, which comes from συμβάλλω (i.e., "to throw together"; Skeat, 1958). This means that based on some convention, a symbol represents something else, and hence, a symbol can be "… a token, pledge, a sign by which one infers a thing" (Skeat, 1958, p. 537). In the *Concise Oxford English Dictionary*, a symbol is "… a thing conventionally regarded as typifying, representing, or recalling something, especially an idea or quality" (Thompson, 1995, p. 1411). Hence, a symbol is something that represents something else (i.e., a referent, as discussed later).

In the field of semiotics, two of its leaders—Ferdinand de Saussure and Charles Sanders Peirce—also focused on the relation previously mentioned. Saussure and Peirce refer to linguistic signs as the relationship between the signifier and the signified, where the former denotes the mental concept someone has in their mind and the signified sound pattern. The nature of this relation is dependent on social and cultural conventions, as accepted by all members of a linguistic community (Chandler, 2002). According to Chandler (2002), while for Saussure and Peirce the term "sign" relates to language (more specifically the speech and writing people use to connect a mental concept with its sound pattern [i.e., the psychological impression of a sound]), the "signified" can also take other forms, such as material items (e.g., tree and paper). As Chandler (2002, pp. 18-19) comments, "The signifier is now commonly interpreted as the material (or physical) form of the sign—it is something which can be seen, heard, touched, smelled, or tasted" [sic]. Thus, based on Saussure's dyadic model, the sign is the relationship that exists between the signifier (i.e., mental concept) and the signified (i.e., acoustic pattern, materials).

For Peirce (1931), "[a] sign, or representamen, is something which stands to somebody for something in some respect or capacity" (vol. 2, p. 228). Similarly, in the discipline of AAC, a symbol (the sign in semiotics) represents a referent (the object in semiotics). While it can be posited under both definitions (AAC and semiotics), there is a dual relation because the symbol (or sign) represents something else (the referent or object). This is not the case with Peirce (1931), as he adds a third element: the interpretant. The interpretant is the "sense-making" (Chandler, 2002), or in other words, the idea, that is evoked in the mind, which happens because "[t]he sign opens up the object so that it (the object) can spawn a thought" (Corrington, 1993, p. 148). Thus, the relation between the sign and the object creates the interpretant. For Peirce, the interpretant (the idea evoked or the thought) is important because "[t]he meaning of a sign is not contained within it, but arises in its interpretation" (Chandler, 2002, p. 35). However, the interpretant depends on the "… interpreter—though Peirce doesn't feature that term in his triad" (Chandler, 2002, p. 35).

Within the AAC community, symbols are "… used to represent objects, actions, relationships, etc." (Fristoe & Lloyd, 1980, p. 402). Lloyd and Blischak (1992) stated that a "… symbol refers to a representation to a referent" (p. 107). Hence, within the field of AAC, symbols are defined as things used to represent referents. Although the AAC definition of symbol does not include the interpretant or the interpreter (i.e., the person who interprets), both elements are important in AAC research. For instance, the literature surrounding iconicity focuses on a person's previous experiences with symbols among other things (Sevcik et al., 1991). In this chapter, it will be argued that the notion of interpretant is vital, and as such, must be included in the definition of symbols. According to Pampoulou (2017), AAC symbols reflect "… the interpretation that a person has for the relation that exists between a symbol and its referent" (p. 98). The interpretation is vital because without an interpretant, the relationship between a symbol and its referent does not exist. In the AAC field, the interpretant is flexible and changes according to the needs of the person who uses symbols, whereas in other disciplines or with other types of symbols (e.g., acoustic), it is fixed and does not change (Smith, 2006). For example, in AAC, a two-dimensional symbol of an apple on a communication board can have a number of meanings depending on the needs or interpretation of the person who uses graphic symbols to communicate. The symbol for apple might represent an actual apple but could also be used by the communicator to represent fruit in general, the color red, or messages, such as, "I am hungry" or "I want an apple." Similarly, three-dimensional symbols might also possess multiple meanings. For instance, cup as a real object or miniature might represent an actual cup, the concept of coffee, or messages, such as, "I want coffee" or "I am thirsty." According to the needs and/or cognitive skills of the end-user, AAC symbols can hold multiple relationships to their referents and these relationships are more fluid and flexible than for other existing symbols, such as spoken (i.e., acoustic) ones. As Smith (2006) asserts, people with complex communication needs have various vocabulary constraints, so to improve their communication interactions, it may be necessary that symbols have alternate interpretations in addition to their primary or more obvious interpretations. Therefore, when focusing on the terminology of symbols, it is vital that the focus shifts beyond the symbol and its referent to include the relationship that exists between the two (the interpretant), taking into account the person's skills and needs (the interpreter). Hence, it is proposed that symbols are *the interpretation a person has for the relation that exists between a symbol and its referent.* It should be noted that the term symbols is typically used generically to refer to all symbols regardless of whether they are part of a set or system. A **symbol corpus**, on the other hand, is a collection of symbols that all share the same design characteristics.

Other terms to describe symbols widely found in the AAC literature are **spoken**, **graphic**, and **manual** and are partly dependent upon the modality that is being used. That is, "[w]hile spoken symbols are conveyed through the auditory-vocal modality, graphic and manual symbols are conveyed through the visual modality" (Fristoe & Lloyd, 1979a, p. 402). One example of spoken symbols is natural speech, which is conveyed through the vocal modality whereby it involves "the use of systematized vocalizations to express verbal symbols or words" (Ricks & Wing, 1975, p. 193). Graphic symbols are printed symbols, such as pictures and line drawings, conveyed through the visual modality. Manual symbols also typically are conveyed via the visual modality (Lloyd & Blischak, 1992) and can include pointing, gestures (such as yes and no), pantomime, eye blink codes, and manual signs. Spoken, graphic, and manual symbols can also be classified under the traditional dichotomy of aided vs. unaided symbols, which is the next topic.

AAC Symbols:
The Means to Represent

The AAC model presented in Chapter 3 described AAC as a process composed of three components: (1) means to represent, (2) means to select, and (3) means to transmit. Each of these three aspects may be aided or unaided. While these three components are usually discussed separately, they are typically interactive and occur concurrently.

Of primary importance to this and the following two chapters is the means to represent, including the aided and unaided symbols that are used to convey messages by persons with severe communication disabilities. The aided vs. unaided dichotomy is the superordinate (i.e., primary) level of an AAC symbol taxonomy proposed by Lloyd and Fuller (1986) and its application is still useful today. According to Lloyd and Fuller (1986), "[t]his dichotomy is based upon production demands of the symbol ..." (p. 168). More specifically, unaided symbols are those that convey meaning without the need for any aids or devices external to the body, such as a pen and paper or symbol display of some sort (Fuller et al., 1992; Lloyd & Fuller, 1986). Examples of unaided symbols include vocalizations, natural speech, eye blink codes, gestures, manual signs, sign languages, and manual-sign based approaches, such as Makaton (Fuller et al., 1992; Lloyd & Fuller, 1986). Table 3-4 (in Chapter 3) provides many examples of unaided symbols and a more in-depth discussion of these symbols is provided in Chapter 8.

On the other hand, aided symbols "... refer to those symbols that require some type of external assistance, or an aid or device (e.g., paper, pencil, pictures, charts, communication boards, and in some cases, electronic devices) for production" (Lloyd & Fuller, 1986, p. 168). Examples of aided symbols are real or miniature objects, photographs, pictures, traditional orthography, and graphic symbol corpuses, many of which are described in greater detail in Chapter 7 (also see Table 3-3, see Chapter 3). Aided symbols are those where the person needs something separate from their body to support communication interactions, which might be due to a physical disability. For instance, many people with cerebral palsy do not possess the physical capacity required to sign, and thus, aided symbols are often used to support their communication interactions.

Aided and unaided symbols have their own unique characteristics, and it is imperative clinicians understand these characteristics in deciding which symbols are more appropriate for their AAC users and the communication partners who support them. **Total communication** is desired and recommended, whereby all the different modalities (e.g., auditory, manual, oral, tactile, and visual) are used with both aided and unaided symbols to support the AAC user in communication. For example, a person with aphasia might use different forms of communication, such as eye contact, pointing to a desired object, and a tablet to show photos of family members, depending on their skills. On the other hand, a person with cerebral palsy might use eye contact to catch the attention of another person, gestures for specific vocabulary, and a communication book for more complex interaction. The decisions clinicians must make to match a potential AAC user to an effective means to communicate require that they have a good understanding of the aided and unaided symbol options that are available and the characteristics these symbols possess. In the following section, the characteristics of aided and unaided symbols are briefly discussed.

General Characteristics of Aided
and Unaided AAC Symbols

Research on the characteristics of aided and unaided symbols has been relatively sparse the last few years, as the focus has shifted to the use of technology in the AAC field. At the same time, symbols—especially aided ones—have been developing at a rapid pace due to the same technological advancements (Pampoulou, 2017; Pampoulou & Fuller, 2021). As a result, clinicians are faced with the difficult task of choosing the most appropriate collection of symbols for their AAC users by incorporating evidence-based practice where a relative paucity of research is available to support their choices (Pampoulou, 2017; Pampoulou & Fuller, 2020, 2021). In this section, the focus is on two characteristics shared by aided and unaided symbols: the presence or absence of linguistic characteristics and segmentation capability.

One of the key characteristics of both aided and unaided symbols is the potential capability of a corpus to represent language. This potential capability is linked to the presence or absence of **linguistic characteristics** inherent to a corpus of symbols. More specifically, as it was explained in detail in Chapter 3, corpuses of symbols that possess a high degree of internal logic (i.e., clearly established and conventionalized rules) also have better expansion capability (i.e., the ability to create additional symbols beyond the original collection), thus allowing for the development of a larger vocabulary than was provided in the original corpus. The net result is a wider representational range (i.e., the ability of the symbols to represent more closely the morphological, semantic, and syntactic components of spoken and written language). This relationship among linguistic characteristics is illustrated in Figure 3-5. As language and literacy have become a primary focus of AAC in recent years, classification of symbols according to the degree of their inherent linguistic characteristics may be more clinically meaningful than using the older symbol classification system composed of a superordinate (i.e., aided vs. unaided) and three subordinate (i.e., static vs. dynamic, iconic vs. opaque, set vs. system) levels. It is for this reason that Pampoulou and Fuller (2021) proposed a new classification of symbols that should be perceived as a quaternary continuum that includes:

- Non-linguistic symbols
- Pre-linguistic symbols, which are further classified as:
  - Symbol sets
  - Transitionary symbol systems
- Linguistic symbols

The primary characteristic that distinguishes each point along the continuum is the degree of inherent logic within each corpus. Another characteristic directly related to these linguistic characteristics is whether **segmentation** of symbols is possible. Segmentation is often related to the creativity referred to by Noam Chomsky, which focuses on the fact that a number of restricted segments are capable of having multiple combinatorial possibilities in such a way that they create new meanings (Smith, 2006). AAC symbols "… vary in their potential for segmentation" (Smith, 2006, p. 152). Some examples of aided corpuses of symbols that possess segmentation capability, and thus, can produce symbols having novel meanings are Blissymbols, expanded or complex rebus, Visual Phonics, traditional orthography (the 26 letters of the alphabet), and to a lesser extent, Sigsymbols. Sign languages and traditional orthography–based manual symbols (e.g., fingerspelling and gestural Morse code) and, to a lesser extent, some pedagogical sign systems, are examples of unaided corpuses that possess segmentation capability. All these linguistic symbol systems are structured in a way that, once the rules for expansion have been learned, the user can create a virtually infinite number of messages.

In other corpuses of symbols, this segmentation is not present. For instance, Picture Communication Symbols (Tobii Dynavox) have a fixed number of symbols, and there are no rules that can allow the creation of new ones (Smith, 2006). Similarly, simple gestures do not possess segmentation capability. Although, in some cases, non- or pre-linguistic symbol corpuses may be relatively large, there is no potential to expand vocabulary beyond the original corpus. Linguistic symbols have both segmentation ability and the inherent logic that allows for virtually unlimited expansion of the original vocabulary.

There are other characteristics besides inherent linguistic structure and segmentation capability that are specific to aided or unaided symbols. These will be discussed in greater detail in Chapters 7 (aided symbols) and 8 (unaided symbols).

SUMMARY

In this chapter, a broad overview of aided and unaided AAC symbol sets and systems has been provided. Following a brief discussion on symbol use in natural languages, specialized symbols for AAC were introduced, then the focus shifted to establishing a common terminology when referring to symbols. Finally, characteristics common to both aided and unaided symbols were presented to prepare the reader for the following two chapters that explicitly focus on a broader discussion of aided (Chapter 7) and unaided (Chapter 8) symbols.

STUDY QUESTIONS

1. Define "natural language."
2. Explain how the natural development of communication is linked to AAC.
3. Briefly discuss the terminology that has been used to describe and categorize AAC symbols.
4. Define and elaborate on "linguistic characteristics" and "segmentation capability."

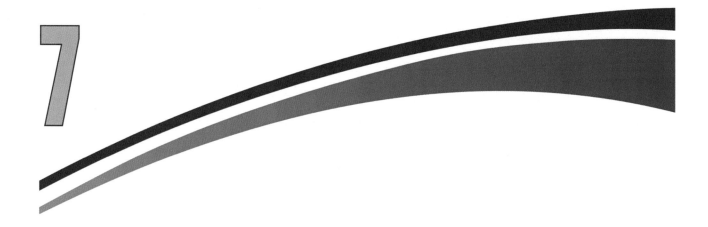

Aided AAC Symbols and Their Characteristics

Eliada Pampoulou, PhD
and Donald R. Fuller, PhD

MYTH

1. All augmentative and alternative communication (AAC) aided symbols (e.g., objects, photographs, synthetic speech) are the same.
2. The use of unaided symbols (e.g., gestures and manual signs) is always preferred to the use of aided symbols.
3. Aided symbols are limited in their capacity to represent linguistic characteristics.

REALITY

1. There are many aided and unaided symbol sets and systems available for use with persons who use AAC. These symbols are as different from one another as people. Some symbols are object-based. Some are picture-based and some are alphabet-based. Others are phonemically or phonically based, while others are logographic. Finally, some aided symbols are produced electronically through vibrotactile and/or acoustic modes. It is clear that symbols are very different from one another. The educator/clinician must be able to recognize and appreciate these differences and what their implications are for use with persons having severe communication impairments.
2. Aided symbols possess some characteristics that may be more beneficial to a person with complex communication needs (CCN) than unaided symbols. For example, most aided symbols are permanent and enduring, which means the cognitive demand they place on the user in terms of recall memory is less than for unaided symbols. Similarly, unaided symbols by and large tend to be more physically demanding than aided symbols. The appropriate symbols for a specific individual have to be carefully matched to that individual's abilities.

(continued)

INTRODUCTION

The focus of this chapter is on three-dimensional objects and two-dimensional graphic symbols conveyed through the visual channel. Their difference when compared to manual symbols is that object-based and graphic symbols are aided while manual symbols are unaided. The term "aided symbols" was chosen for this discussion to reinforce the

Fuller, D. R., & Lloyd, L. L. *Principles and Practices in Augmentative and Alternative Communication* (pp. 83-133).
© 2023 Taylor & Francis Group.

REALITY (CONTINUED)

3. The linguistic capacity inherent in aided symbols varies. Some corpuses of symbols have limited linguistic capacity whereas others have developer-defined rules for creating new symbols beyond the original corpus, but the expansion rules tend to be somewhat rudimentary and not sufficiently developed to allow for virtually unlimited expansion capability. There are also corpuses of symbols that are unique because of their sophisticated internal logic, and thereby, the full range of language may be realized, leading to unlimited communication.

superordinate classification of symbols proposed by Lloyd and Fuller (1986). The corpuses of aided symbols currently available are characterized by multidimensional components illustrated in Table 7-1; these being:

- Linguistic capacity
- Physical characteristics (dimensionality)
- Design characteristics

As discussed in-depth in Chapter 3, aided symbols are based primarily on their linguistic characteristics, which can be categorized as non-linguistic, pre-linguistic, and linguistic (see Table 7-1; the term "quaternary" comes from the fact that one of the three linguistic levels—pre-linguistic—includes two types). This particular characteristic is directly related to the inherent linguistic structure of a corpus of symbols, and hence, to their level of correspondence to spoken and written language (Pampoulou & Fuller, 2021).

A second way to categorize symbols is based on their physical characteristics, which refers to whether the symbols are acoustic, animated, two-dimensional, or three-dimensional. Hence, based on their physical properties, aided symbols can be classified according to three broad categories:

- Acoustic symbols—those produced as synthetic speech through speech-generating devices (SGDs)
- Animated—symbols that require movement to assist in conveying meaning
- Three-dimensional—object-based symbols
- Two-dimensional—symbols categorized as static (i.e., those that do not include movement) and kinetic (i.e., those in which movement or animation is one of their key elements)

The third categorization, which focuses on the design attributes of aided symbols, concerns the manner in which symbols are designed, such as objects, pictures, line drawings, or alphabet-based symbols to list a few examples.

THE QUATERNARY CONTINUUM: AIDED AAC SYMBOLS BASED ON THEIR LINGUISTIC CHARACTERISTICS

One of the primary purposes of aided AAC symbols is to serve the needs of people with CCN who have the capacity for developing or retaining speech and/or literacy. For this reason, these symbols are designed and used in such a way that they represent language. As was discussed in Chapter 6, graphic symbols have the capacity to represent different meanings depending on the person's needs and skills (Smith, 2006). For instance, a symbol for apple might represent the actual fruit, "I am hungry," or the color red. The focus here is on the inherent linguistic structure that corpuses have, which primarily derives from the way they are designed and not to the meaning assigned to them by end-users. As explained in Chapter 3, a number of AAC symbols have inherent linguistic capacity that allows them, based on the internal logic built into the corpus of symbols, to create new symbols that do not exist in the initial corpus. In this way, symbols with new meanings are created. Symbols so designed have greater expansion capability. This provides more flexibility for the user to communicate with their peers.

Before introducing the reader to the large number of aided AAC symbols that are available, it should be noted here that three of them are highly related to each other, as they were created by the same individual over the course of several years. These corpuses of symbols are classified differently—and thereby, do not appear in this chapter in succession or chronological order—which may make it confusing for the reader. Figure 7-1 summarizes the commonalities and differences among these three symbol corpuses—DynaSyms (Poppin & Co.), PICSYMS Categorical Dictionary (Baggeboda Press), and Piclish (i.e., Picture English).

We now turn our attention to a large host of available aided symbol corpuses categorized along the quaternary classification developed by Pampoulou and Fuller (2021), including non-linguistic, pre-linguistic, and linguistic symbols. In the sections that follow, we will provide the reader with detailed information about the aided symbols that are currently available for use with AAC systems.

Non-Linguistic Symbols

Symbol Groups

In this lowest classification of aided symbols, the symbols hold little, if any, inherent linguistic characteristics, and therefore, are referred to simply as symbol groups. As explained in Chapter 3, these symbol corpuses lack internal logic and expansion capability as well. Hence, a person with complex communication difficulties can communicate only with the symbols that exist within the original collection.

TABLE 7-1

Categorization of Aided AAC Symbols Using the Quaternary Continuum Along With Physical and Design Characteristics

NON-LINGUISTIC SYMBOLS

Symbol Groups

Three-Dimensional	Two-Dimensional	Animated
Object	Pictorial	
• Miniature objects • Real objects • Tangible and textured symbols	• Microsoft ClipArt • Photographs • Pictures	• Animated graphics • Autism Language Program • Library of International Picture Symbols

PRE-LINGUISTIC SYMBOLS

Symbol Sets		*Transitionary Symbol Systems*
Two-Dimensional	Animated	Two-Dimensional
Line Drawings	Pictorial	Line Drawings
• DynaSyms • Imagine symbols • Lingraphica concept-images • Mulberry Symbols • ParticiPics • Pics for PECS • Pictograms • Simple rebus symbols • SymbolStix • Talking Mats	• Some DynaSyms • Some Pictograms	• Makaton • PCS • Widgit Symbols

LINGUISTIC SYMBOLS

Linguistic Symbol Systems

Two-Dimensional			Acoustic
Alphabet-Based Symbols	Phonemic-/Phonetic-Based Symbols	Line Drawings	Electronically Generated Symbols
• Aided representations of fingerspelling • Braille • Modified orthography • Morse code • Traditional orthography	• Complex rebus • Phonetic alphabets • Visual Phonics	• Blissymbolics • CyberGlyphs • Piclish • PICSYMS • Sigsymbol-elaborated words • Sigsymbols	• Synthetic speech

PCS = Picture Communication Symbols; PECS = Picture Exchange Communication System.

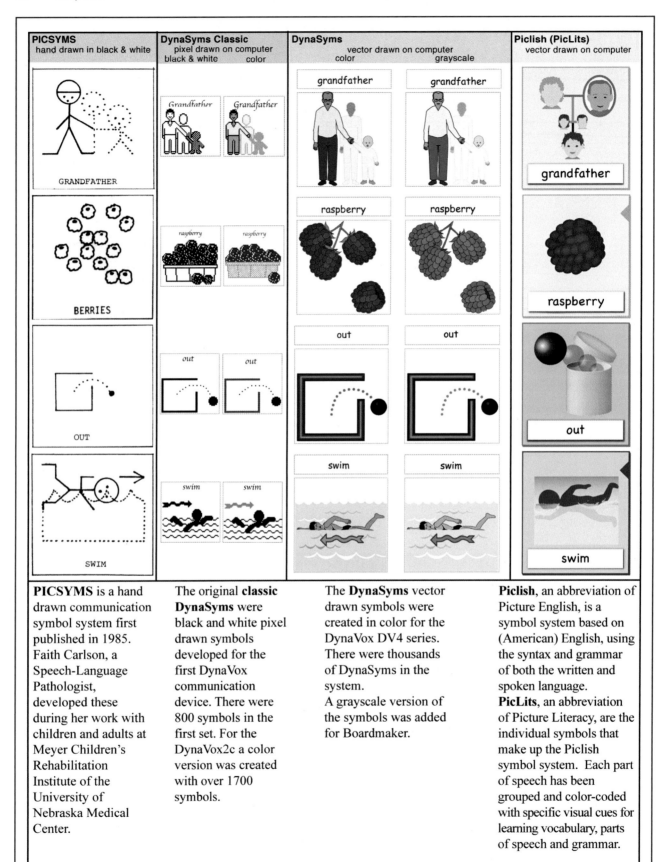

PICSYMS is a hand drawn communication symbol system first published in 1985. Faith Carlson, a Speech-Language Pathologist, developed these during her work with children and adults at Meyer Children's Rehabilitation Institute of the University of Nebraska Medical Center.

The original **classic DynaSyms** were black and white pixel drawn symbols developed for the first DynaVox communication device. There were 800 symbols in the first set. For the DynaVox2c a color version was created with over 1700 symbols.

The **DynaSyms** vector drawn symbols were created in color for the DynaVox DV4 series. There were thousands of DynaSyms in the system.
A grayscale version of the symbols was added for Boardmaker.

Piclish, an abbreviation of Picture English, is a symbol system based on (American) English, using the syntax and grammar of both the written and spoken language.
PicLits, an abbreviation of Picture Literacy, are the individual symbols that make up the Piclish symbol system. Each part of speech has been grouped and color-coded with specific visual cues for learning vocabulary, parts of speech and grammar.

Figure 7-1. Three symbol corpuses created by Faith Carlson: PICSYMS, DynaSyms, and PicLits. (Reproduced with permission from Faith Carlson.)

These symbols are often free of charge and are usually available online (e.g., photographs, emojis, Microsoft ClipArt) or within a communication product (e.g., an app) that is free or has a low cost compared to other products that use more linguistically based symbols (e.g., Picture Communication Symbols [PCS], traditional orthography, Widgit Symbols).

Our initial focus is on three-dimensional symbols, as these are distinct from two-dimensional symbols by an extra dimension, namely depth. **Three-dimensional symbols** are often object-based symbols and include real objects, miniature objects, and tangible and textured symbols.

Three-Dimensional Symbols

Real Objects. Real (or whole) objects and miniature objects are classified as tangible symbols (Rowland & Schweigert, 1989a) and can be manipulated for communication purposes (Roche et al., 2014). They can be an effective choice for individuals who are beginning to communicate, as well as for persons with cognitive, physical, and/or sensory impairments (Beukelman & Light, 2020; Musselwhite & St. Louis, 1988; Parker et al., 2010; Rowland & Schweigert, 1989a, 1989b, 1990). Trief (2007) found that people who have multiple disabilities and visual impairment may use whole objects as part of their communication interaction with others. For persons with cognitive impairments, the similarity of object symbols to their concrete referents makes them a powerful means of communication, especially because real objects place low memory demands on the user (Roche et al., 2014) and are iconic by comparison to other aided symbols, such as two-dimensional symbols (Mirenda & Locke, 1989). The additional three-dimensional nature of objects allows them to be easily manipulated by persons with visual impairments. The major drawback for real objects is their size. For some concepts (e.g., chair, bed), the use of real objects would be impractical. The size of objects then limits the number that can be transported or displayed at a given time. Because of this, miniature objects may be a more viable means of representation.

Miniature Objects. Miniature objects (and parts of whole objects) must be matched carefully to the potential communicator's impairments and abilities. One should be cautious when choosing miniature objects, as they may not be as representative of the real object or concept for a particular individual as the clinician or other communication partners might expect (Vanderheiden & Lloyd, 1986). Mirenda and Locke (1989) noted that for some persons with cognitive impairments, two-dimensional representations may be more easily recognizable than miniature objects.

A second caution concerns tactile discrimination. Some individuals with visual impairments may experience difficulty understanding the miniature of an object is being used to represent the real object because the two in all likelihood will not provide the same tactile feedback (Beukelman & Light, 2020; Beukelman & Mirenda, 1992). A few examples about how miniature objects need to be carefully chosen can

be drawn by the study of Lund and Troha (2008). For their participant, these investigators successfully used a marble covered by masking tape to represent a computer mouse, a piece of plastic with rice in it that sounded similar to the preferred toy of the individual participating in the study, and a cloth to represent a pillow. Thereby, when choosing miniature objects, the shape of the object is important but also auditory feedback and other cues can help the person recognize it. On the whole, miniature objects have been found to be a viable means of representation for persons having cognitive (Mirenda & Locke, 1989), physical (Landman & Schaeffler, 1986), and sensory impairments (Lund & Troha, 2008; Rowland & Schweigert, 1989a, 1989b, 1990), including dual sensory impairment.

Tangible and Textured Symbols. Tangible symbols can be either two- or three-dimensional and must be permanent, easily discriminated tactilely, highly iconic, and easy to manipulate. Shape and texture are important properties of tangible symbols. Symbols that use textures to represent referents are known as textured symbols. Symbols can either be directly or arbitrarily associated with their referents. In the former case, a small square of sandpaper may represent sandpaper or wood working. In the latter case, that same small sandpaper square may represent an animal, such as a dog or cat. Tangible symbols also include raised line drawings that can be felt by persons with visual impairments (Edman, 1991; Garrett, 1986). Case studies by Locke and Mirenda (1988) and Murray-Branch and colleagues (1991) have shown that tangible symbols can be used effectively with persons having singular or multiple sensory deficits, as well as severe cognitive impairment.

Assuming a symbol user is capable of moving from objects (e.g., real and miniature objects) to higher levels of representation, a pairing process may be used to help that individual generalize from objects to pictures (Van Tatenhove, 1979). Objects are typically matched with symbols that have a higher level of representation (e.g., Makaton or PCS) and then are gradually faded so that the two-dimensional symbols remain. Goossens' and Crain (1986) also suggested another strategy involving the use of object pictures to provide a transition from objects to a higher level of representation. In this strategy, a cross-section of the object is mounted on a surface, resulting in a three-dimensional picture. This picture then evolves so that the height of the raised picture is gradually decreased. Eventually, the individual transitions to a flat surface (i.e., two-dimensional symbols).

Two-Dimensional Symbols

Two-dimensional symbols possess the dimensions of height and width but not depth. Due to their physical characteristics, and hence, their ease and efficiency of use for persons with CCN, two-dimensional symbols have received plenty of attention by both clinicians and developers, especially symbols that were systematically developed to serve communication.

The genesis of the systematic development of two-dimensional symbols to facilitate communication in the AAC field dates back to the late 1940s with the vision of a man wishing to bring peace to the world through a common graphic language. That man was Charles Bliss, his self-published book was entitled *Semantography*, and his symbols came to be known as Blissymbols. Naturally, these symbols were not used originally as an AAC system. It was not until 1971 that a Canadian educator, Shirley McNaughton, discovered the second edition of *Semantography* (Bliss, 1965) and realized the potential Blissymbols had for bridging the gap between pre-linguistic and linguistic behavior in her children with physical impairments (Blissymbols will be discussed later in greater detail). The 1970s saw the first era of aided symbol proliferation. Although many of the symbols developed at that time were simple non-linguistic collections, a small number of pre-linguistic and linguistic symbols were also developed. These higher-level symbols sparked the phenomenon of using symbols for supporting people with CCN in conveying their thoughts and ideas to others and in developing their literacy skills, thereby opening up the world of access to oral and written information.

The consequent use of two-dimensional graphic symbols started as a non–speech-generating approach where speech-language pathologists and related professionals started using these symbols in graphic displays, such as flashcards and communication boards. For those who practiced from the 1970s and into the 1990s, it is widely known that during this early era, considerable time was spent by clinicians and educators copying, coloring, cutting, formatting, and pasting symbols to create communication displays to house the symbols. Concurrent advances in technology eventually led to the development of computer software to assist clinicians and educators in organizing and copying entire symbol displays (the first of these may have been Boardmaker, created in 1989 using Mayer-Johnson's PCS). Table 7-2 provides a summary of the development and proliferation of aided two-dimensional symbols over the past several decades.

As can be seen in Table 7-2, in the 1980s, a second era of growth occurred in the number of corpuses of graphic symbols being developed. This can perhaps be attributed in part to the advancement of technology in the field of AAC, such as the use of graphic symbols in devices that produced synthesized speech for communication purposes (Pampoulou, 2015). In the early 1980s, Bruce Baker created Minspeak symbols, semantically based symbols used on communication devices manufactured by the Prentke Romich Company. Although originally not developed to serve as symbols on electronic AAC devices, the first set of approximately 700 PCS was published in 1980; these symbols continued to expand in number throughout the 1980s and into the 1990s.

In the 1990s, the development of corpuses of graphic symbols stagnated somewhat, but a third era of symbol development was established early in the 21st century. This third era could be attributed to several reasons (Pampoulou & Fuller, 2020, 2021). First, due to the rapid advancement of

technology, aided symbols could be used not only on personal computers but also on electronic tablets and mobile smartphones. As a consequence of the greater flexibility and wide range of devices for their storage and retrieval, the demand for new aided symbols proliferated at a much faster rate than in the past. A second reason—commercial interest—resulted in the rapid proliferation of AAC apps for tablets and smartphones. The creators or developers of some of these apps entered into licensing agreements with already-established symbol owners (e.g., PCS symbols changed hands from Mayer-Johnson to Dynavox and finally to the Swedish-based Tobii Group; PCS symbols have been licensed for use with many currently available AAC apps). On the other hand, many apps have been developed with their own proprietary symbols.

There are advantages and disadvantages associated with the rapid development of technology. On the positive side is the flexibility of options that technological advancements provide. On the negative side is the desire by many app developers to avoid copyright issues and/or keep the cost of their products accessible to end-user, which may create a potentially negative side effect of symbol corpuses being poorly developed or insufficient in number to support the needs of AAC users in a comprehensive manner. Table 7-3 provides a list of available applications that use a number of different AAC aided symbols.

The AAC field continues to evolve and consequently new AAC approaches and methods are being developed in order to effectively meet the needs and skills of people with CCN. For instance, the Talking Mats method was developed by a group of AAC specialists at Stirling University in the United Kingdom to assist people with communication difficulties to understand and express their own views about issues that concerned them (Cameron & Matthews, 2017; Murphy, 2000; Murphy & Cameron, 2008). The Talking Mats method and its symbols were completed in 2013 initially to support people with aphasia but were later adapted for people with Alzheimer's disease and other populations with communication difficulties, such as dementia (Murphy & Oliver, 2013) and Huntington's disease (Ferm et al., 2010). AAC specialists around the world recognize the efficiency and usefulness of these symbols for different populations of AAC users, as well as other purposes (Pampoulou, 2016; Pampoulou & Fuller, 2020, 2021).

For the remainder of this chapter, the evolution of AAC aided symbols purposefully developed to serve AAC communication needs is explained in detail. However, as ClipArt, photographs, pictures, and emojis are also used in AAC even though they were not developed for this purpose, a discussion about these symbols is also provided.

Microsoft ClipArt. ClipArt consists of colorful or black and white images or "clips" that illustrate objects or scenes of everyday life (Figure 7-2). These are stored under particular categories depending on what they represent. Each clip is matched with a keyword. Hence, if a person is searching for a word on Microsoft's Design Gallery (https://www.clipart.

TABLE 7-2

Chronological History of Collections of Graphic Symbols

YEAR	COLLECTION	KEY PERSON OR DEVELOPER	WEBSITE	ORIGINAL PURPOSE OR INTENT
1949 1965	Blissymbols	Charles Bliss	www.blissymbolics.org	Symbols developed as an attempt to establish a universal language
1968	Rebus symbols	Vanderbilt University		Symbols used with the *Peabody Rebus Reading Program*
1971	Blissymbols	Shirley McNaughton	www.blissymbolics.org	Symbols adapted for use with children with disabilities
1976	Rebus symbols	Judy van Oosterom		Symbols used in England for educational purposes at Saint Reeds Thomas School
1980	Pictograms	Subhas Maharaj	www.pictogram.se/	Symbols developed to support AAC
1980	Widgit Symbols	Kathleen Devereux and Judy van Oosterom	www.widgit.com	Symbols designed for access within the school setting
1982	Sigsymbols	Ailsa Cregan		Symbols designed as a multimodal system
1984	Makaton	Margaret Walker, Kathy Johnston, and Tony Cornforth	www.makaton.org	Symbols developed for the Makaton Vocabulary Development Project
1985	PCS	Roxana Johnson	www.mayer-johnson.com	Symbols designed for face-to-face interaction between symbol user and communication partners
1988	BeTa symbols	Specialists in The Netherlands	www.betasymbols.com	Symbols developed to support students in special schools
1990	Bonnington Symbols	Tom Orr	www.tomorraccessibility.co.uk	Symbols designed to provide accessible information
1990	DynaSyms	Faith Carlson, for DynaVox	www.languagesymbols.com/dynasyms.html	Symbols created using PICSYMS principles for use on DynaVox SGDs
1998	Beeldlezen symbols	Stichting Beeldlezen		Symbols to be used with persons with disabilities
2001	SymbolStix	News-2-You	www.n2y.com	Symbols designed to be used for an online newspaper
2002	Widgit Symbols	B. Rae	www.widgit.com	Symbols redesigned and extended to include older learners with literacy needs
2004	Sclera symbols	B. Serrien	www.sclera.be/	Symbols designed to support adults in a day care center
2006	Arasaac symbols	Sergio Palao	www.arasaac.org	Symbols designed as part of a project funded by the government of Aragon, Spain to support AAC

(continued)

TABLE 7-2 (CONTINUED)
Chronological History of Collections of Graphic Symbols

YEAR	COLLECTION	KEY PERSON OR DEVELOPER	WEBSITE	ORIGINAL PURPOSE OR INTENT
2006	Mulberry Symbols	Paxton Crafts Charitable Trust	www.opensymbols.org/ repositories/mulberry	Symbols used to provide users a collection of graphic symbols at no cost
2006	SeeSense symbols	Sensory Software	https://grids. thinksmartbox.com	Symbols designed for use with Grid2 software
2008	Clarity symbols	Prentke Romich Company	www.liberator.co.uk/ clarity-symbols	Symbols designed for use with the Liberator for literacy and communication
2012	Piclish	Tease the Easel	www.languagesymbols. com	Symbols used as a communication and language acquisition tool
2013	Talking Mats symbols	Talking Mats Ltd	www.talkingmats.com	Symbols created by a group of speech-language pathologists in the United Kingdom for basic communication

AAC = augmentative and alternative communication; PCS = Picture Communication Symbols; SGD = speech-generating device.

TABLE 7-3
The Use of Aided AAC Symbols in Tablet and Smartphone Applications

APPLICATION	AIDED AAC SYMBOLS		
	Non-Linguistic Symbols	Pre-Linguistic Symbols	Linguistic Symbols
AAC Speech Communicator is a generic, easy-to-learn communication tool for anyone with speech disabilities. It forms grammatically correct sentences when a series of pictograms are clicked and then speaks them aloud (text-to-speech). Because of the pictograms, this tool is especially good for children or those who have limited reading and writing abilities.		Arasaac	
Alexicom AAC and Elements apps are applications for people who use AAC to communicate. They can also be available via switch and scanning options.	Photographs ClipArt	PCS SymbolStix	
Avaz is an AAC app intended to support communication for nonspeaking children. It benefits children with ASD, cerebral palsy, intellectual disability, Down syndrome, etc.		SymbolStix	
Clicker Communicator is a child-friendly AAC app that gives a voice to learners with speech and language difficulties. It has been specifically designed to support communication within the classroom.	CrickPix Library	SymbolStix Widgit PCS	

(continued)

TABLE 7-3 (CONTINUED)
The Use of Aided AAC Symbols in Tablet and Smartphone Applications

APPLICATION	AIDED AAC SYMBOLS		
	Non-Linguistic Symbols	*Pre-Linguistic Symbols*	*Linguistic Symbols*
CoughDrop is an app that aims to bring out the voices of those with CCN through powerful open-source technology that easily adapts to the individual and supports everyone around them trying to help them succeed.	Flickr Public domain images Pixaby	Open symbols (i.e., a repository with open-licensed symbols) LessonPix images	
GoTalk Now is a customizable AAC app that integrates the simplicity of GoTalk devices and the dynamic abilities of an iPad.	Photographs Go Talk Image Library	SymbolStix PCS MetaCom Widgit Symbols	
Grid 3 and Grid for iPad is a user-friendly application for people with CCN for their communication and educational needs.		Widgit Symbols PCS SymbolStix Metacom for Germany Arasaac for Portugal BeTa	Blissymbols
HelpTalk app is directed at people unable to communicate fluently orally or through writing with health professionals, family, or any other person.	Emojis	http://www.helptalk.mobi	
LAMP Words for Life is a language system and an adaptation of Unity. It offers core and fringe vocabulary and grammar so the nonspeaking individual can independently communicate with speech output or copy text into other programs. It was designed to support the LAMP approach, which is a strategy initially developed to teach language and communication to individuals with ASD, but it can also be applied to other individuals with developmental language disabilities.		Minspeak	
LetMeTalk is a free AAC talker app for Android that supports communication in all areas of life, and therefore, providing a voice for everyone. It was first intended to help children with ASD but is used by several other groups today as well.	Photos Pictures	Arassac	
Proloquo2Go is a symbol-supported communication app to promote language development and grow communication skills from beginning to advanced communicators.		SymbolStix	
TouchChat is a full-featured communication solution for individuals who have difficulty using their natural voice. TouchChat is designed for individuals with ASD, Down syndrome, ALS, apraxia, stroke, or other conditions that affect a person's ability to use natural speech.	Photographs	SymbolStix	

AAC = augmentative and alternative communication; ALS = amyotrophic lateral sclerosis; ASD = autism spectrum disorder; LAMP = Language Acquisition through Motor Planning.

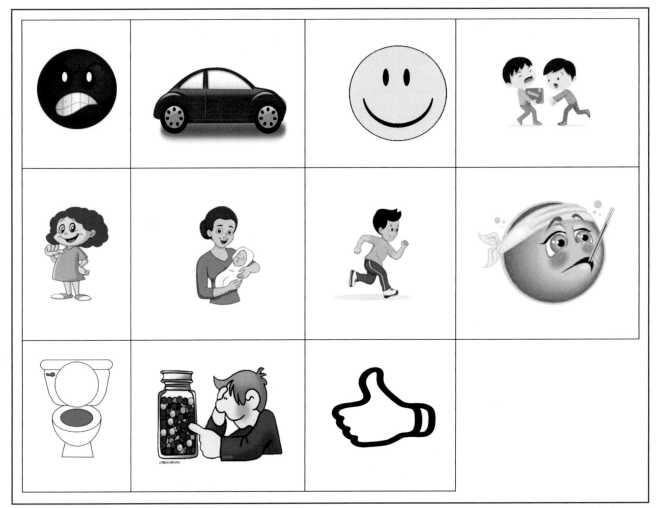

Figure 7-2. A representative sample of Microsoft ClipArt. From left to right, top to bottom: angry, car, happy, help, I/me, mother, run, sick, toilet, want, and yes. (Reproduced from Microsoft.)

com) or even the Google or DuckDuckGo search engines, they may come up with a large collection of clips. The style of clips may be different, but the majority of them seek to portray an object as it is in its true form. On the other hand, more abstract concepts are not as easily illustrated. Moreover, a number of clips may be based upon the illustrator's personal concept of abstract ideas, and thus, many clips may then not be universally appropriate (Dillon, 2006). In a study conducted by Rose and colleagues (2003), brochures focusing on health issues were modified in such a way that they were aphasia-friendly. One interesting finding is that, although these modified brochures assisted people with aphasia to access written information, half of them rejected the symbols. Stigmatization and the feeling of lack of respect were the main complaints for their rejection of the ClipArt images that were used. Similar findings were also found in another research project conducted by Brennan and colleagues (2005) in which symbols were obtained by ClipArt and images from an online search (i.e., Google Image Search). Therefore, Clipart (and any like corpus of symbols) must be used with caution, taking always into consideration the end-user's needs and preferences (Pampoulou, 2017; Pampoulou & Fuller, 2020).

Photographs. In the past, good quality photographs could be obtained from any number of sources, such as catalogs, children's picture dictionaries, magazines, picture books, travel aids, and other printed media (Mirenda, 1985). In more recent years, electronic photographs have been made possible with digital cameras, smartphones or tablets, and other devices. Photographs can then be shared easily with others via different modes, such as text messaging or social media (e.g., Facebook, Twitter). Almost all apps designed for AAC include the feature of digital photography; these symbols in many cases are imported into an AAC communication display within the app. Photographs, either color or black and white, can be modified easily with the support of editing tools that are typically included in the technology used. For instance, many smartphones allow users to modify their photos, such as changing the color or hue or cropping a photograph to focus on a smaller aspect of the photograph.

Only few AAC systems are composed of photographs exclusively. Typically, photographs are used as more realistic representations of important entities in the user's life (e.g., specific people with whom the user comes into daily contact or specific possessions that the user requests frequently).

However, developers of speech-generating AAC systems may, in their attempt to keep down the cost of their software or app, use small collections of prefabricated or public domain photographs to allow users to customize their AAC system to some degree while having the ability to add a number of their own symbols. In other cases, the use of specific photographs in an AAC system is fundamental, as end-users may face difficulty in recognizing more complex symbols, such as those that appear typically in transitionary symbol or linguistic symbol systems (these are discussed in more detail below). For instance, apps—such as PhotoTalk, CoCreation, and Lingraphica—allow for digital photography because these products have been specifically designed to serve the needs and skills of people with aphasia (Brown & Thiessen, 2018).

In terms of production of photographs, Reichle and colleagues (1991) suggest that the addition of contextual information is very important. Whatever contextual information is required to allow the user to understand the photograph should be included in the photograph. On the other hand, Detheridge and Detheridge (2002) suggest that, in some cases (e.g., when the end-user has a cognitive or visual processing impairment), contextual information can confuse the end-user as to the meaning of the photograph (i.e., the end-user may not be able to discriminate the referent from contextual information in the photograph). It might then be the case that there are no universal rules in terms of how to take the best photographs for end-users and that the criteria depend upon the end-user's needs and skills. Most would agree that to the extent possible, the end-user should take their own photographs they wish to have included in their AAC system. Brown and colleagues (2010) found that photographs people with aphasia take tend to be effective for their communication needs; being customized, photographs can facilitate conversational interactions between end-users and their communication partners. Brown and Thiessen (2018) focus on a number of characteristics that one should take into consideration when taking photographs for communication purposes for individuals with aphasia. These include image type, amount of depicted content and context, engagement, and image presentation or layout. Here, it may be argued that including people with CCN in the design of their AAC system (such as taking their own photographs) can actually minimize potential abandonment of their system (Pampoulou, 2018).

Dixon (1981) reported that persons with severe disabilities had less difficulty in associating color photographs with their referents if the figure was cut out as opposed to remaining intact. Mirenda and Locke (1989) determined that for their sample of persons with intellectual impairments, color photographs were matched with somewhat better accuracy to their referents than black-and-white photos of the same referents. Sevcik and Romski (1986) found that their subjects with cognitive impairment were able to more accurately match black and white photographs to their referents than line drawings. The findings for the latter two studies would seem to suggest a symbol hierarchy for persons with cognitive impairments: color photographs, black-and-white photographs, and finally line drawings. However, this hierarchy should be viewed with caution because of the paucity of research in this area.

In terms of vocabulary representation, photographs are typically used to represent concrete referents, such as people, objects, places, and easily depicted verbs, among other activities (Beukelman & Mirenda, 2013). They are less effective when one attempts to use them to represent more complex verbs and modifiers (Vinson, 2001). It is for this reason that in the categorization of aided AAC symbols using the quaternary continuum, photographs are categorized as nonlinguistic symbols under the category of *symbol collections*. They do not possess internal logic that can allow the user to create new symbols beyond the original corpus.

Pictures. Pictures (or images) are aided symbols used for decades for speech and language therapy purposes. In fact, there are numerous resources for speech and language therapy that are picture-based. Clinicians often use these in their sessions, but they are not necessarily oriented toward AAC. It should be noted that, while photographs and pictures are similar materials, for the former, a camera is used to provide the image, but for the latter, some drawing skills may be necessary (Jones & Cregan, 1986). However, as technology continues to quickly evolve, drawing skills by hand may no longer be necessary, as a number of software packages and smartphone and tablet apps provide electronic drawing options. In addition, current options, such as scanning, printing, emailing, and texting, allow pictures to be easily disseminated to colleagues, parents, and others.

Core Picture Vocabulary. This collection comprises a relatively small corpus of symbols (approximately 160 color line drawings) depicting mostly concrete referents, including basic nouns, simple verbs, and adjectives. Because of their limited vocabulary, they are typically not used exclusively as part of an AAC system but rather are used to augment symbols from other aided sets and/or systems. Don Johnston Incorporated was at one time the copyright owner of this symbol set, but as of the writing of this textbook, it is not clear if the symbols have a new copyright owner or have gone into the public domain. Due to issues in trying to determine the copyright holder, we cannot provide any images of these symbols here. Although it is not clear if these are the original Core Picture Vocabulary, a line of print products called "AAC—Core Vocabulary" can be purchased on the Teachers Pay Teachers website (https://www.teacherspayteachers.com/Browse/Search:core%20vocabulary).

Emojis. Emojis are graphic symbols that depict several categories ranging from smiley faces to more specific concepts and ideas, such as food, animals, country flags, shapes, everyday objects, modes of transportation, activities, and many more (Novak et al., 2015; Riordan, 2017). However, the meaning of an emoji may change depending on the culture of the user. For this reason, the recipient could potentially misinterpret a message (Hurlburt, 2018). Recently, the use

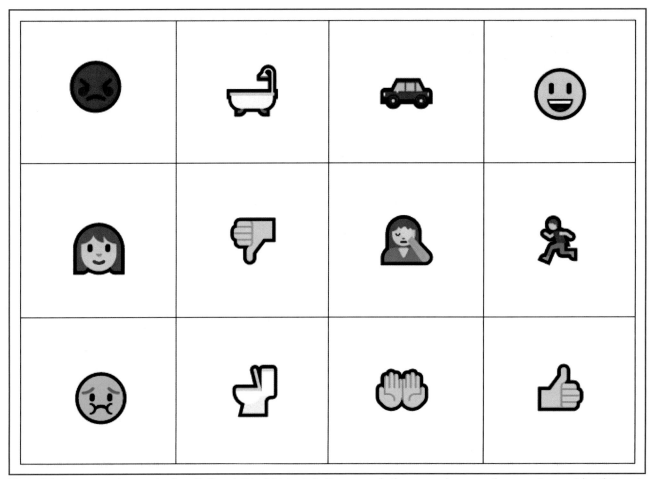

Figure 7-3. A representative sample of emojis. From left to right, top to bottom: angry, bathroom, car, happy, mother, no, pain, run, sick, toilet, want, and yes. (Reproduced from Microsoft.)

of emojis has rapidly increased in online communication, especially through social networking platforms, with their role being to clarify or enhance the meaning of written text when the writer wants to express feelings or emotions, metaphors, implied information, or even irony (Kaye et al., 2017; Niediek, 2016; Weissman & Tanner, 2018). There is currently very little research on the use of emojis for AAC purposes. Paterson (2017) suggested that due to the growing use of social media worldwide, future research should focus on their usefulness for improving the communication of people with acquired conditions. Paterson asserted it should be easier for people to communicate with emojis through social media if they have had previous experience with them. Thus, it could be argued if researchers find this way of communication functional, emojis could possibly be integrated into speech therapy training sessions, including their use in AAC systems. Examples of emojis can be found in Figure 7-3.

Animated Symbols

Animated symbols are two-dimensional symbols that require movement to assist in conveying meaning. Change in size, rotation, and transfer from one point to another are some of the features that such symbols may have, and thus,

are considered to be more dynamic compared to static ones (Jagaroo & Wilkinson, 2008). However, unlike static symbols, they can only be displayed on speech-generating technology and cannot be printed out. For this reason, animated symbols are most likely to be found in AAC software or apps, or some SGDs. Currently, a multitude of software and apps that include such symbols can be easily downloaded on mobile devices, tablets, or laptops and can be used in different contexts. This saves time, as clinicians and families do not need to print, cut, or laminate these symbols (Shane et al., 2012).

The Autism Language Program, Animated Graphics (AAG), Pictograms, DynaSyms, and the Library of International Picture Symbols are some symbol sets and systems that include animated symbols (Fujisawa et al., 2011; Jagaroo & Wilkinson, 2008; Schlosser et al., 2011; Schlosser et al., 2014).

AAG is a set of 114 animated symbols that was introduced by the Center for Communication Enhancement at Boston Children's Hospital in 2009. The symbols illustrate action verbs and prepositions. They were created to enhance the use of difficult-to-learn concepts by individuals with autism. According to Shane and colleagues (2012), some individuals with autism can interpret the meaning of a symbol only if it is animated. In 2012, the AAG symbol set was extended with the addition of approximately 250 new symbols and was renamed Visual Communication Symbol Set. The new symbol set includes not only verbs and prepositions but adjectives as well. Moreover, environmental sounds have been embedded to improve the recognition of verbs.

Over the last decade, research on the potential use of animated symbols for AAC purposes has been conducted (Fujisawa et al., 2011; Mineo et al., 2008; Schlosser et al., 2011; Schlosser et al., 2014). Specifically, in a study by Mineo and colleagues (2008), typically developing preschool children were asked to identify the spoken target word among four symbols that were presented on a computer screen. Symbols that represented actions were effectively identified when they were animated. Also, older children were found to perform better than younger ones in pointing out the correct symbol. In a different study, Schlosser and colleagues (2011) evaluated the performance of 32 AAG static and animated symbols that depicted verbs or prepositions. The symbols were compared in terms of their transparency, name agreement, and identification. The results showed that animated symbols were slightly more identifiable than static ones among 4- and 5-year-old children, whereas 3-year-old children performed better with static symbols. Also, verbs were more easily identifiable than prepositions regardless of whether they were animated. In a similar study by Schlosser and colleagues (2014), animation was found to improve the identification of the targeted symbol but not the naming of it. This is because it is generally an easier task to identify the correct answer if a small number of possible stimuli are given. Moreover, animation was found to increase accuracy in identifying and naming symbols that represent verbs, but this was not so for prepositions.

A limitation of the studies discussed above is that the use of animated symbols was evaluated with typically developing children who are not candidate users of AAC. In contrast, Fujisawa and colleagues (2011) wanted to ascertain whether animation would improve the naming of 16 symbols by 16 students with intellectual disabilities. The chronological age of the participating students (11 to 18 years of age) did not match the age of their linguistic development (38 to 91 months). The symbols examined in this study were animated or static and represented action verbs. The static form of all symbols was taught to the students before the experimental stage and they then divided into four groups. One group served as the control group. The rest of the participants were first asked to name the static symbols presented. Then, for those who had answered incorrectly, the animated symbol of the same action was presented and they were asked to name it. The results showed that the naming of symbols was improved when animation was added. Moreover, animation was found to improve the naming of symbols by students whose linguistic-developmental age was lower. According to the aforementioned studies, the use of animated symbols can be effective for some parts of speech, such as verbs. Hence, more investigation is warranted in order to improve our understanding about their full capacity of use in the AAC field.

Pre-Linguistic Symbols

Pre-linguistic symbols, as the term implies, are symbols that have at least a limited degree of inherent linguistic capacity in the form of internal logic that allows for the creation of new symbols. However, this linguistic capacity exists to a lesser degree in pre-linguistic symbols than linguistic ones and is not sufficient to allow an AAC user to express virtually any thought or idea.

Pre-linguistic symbols have two subcategories, namely *symbol sets* and *transitionary symbol systems*. Chapter 3 provided in-depth discussion about the characteristics of each of the two and why these are identified as two different categories. In this chapter, it is important to recall that these symbols possess some linguistic characteristics in that they provide the user with some internal rules that allow for expansion capability, but these are limited in that the user does not have the flexibility to create unlimited new symbols. Of the two, transitionary symbol systems have a greater degree of internal logic, and hence, greater expansion capability and wider representational range. However, for the purpose of classification, transitionary symbol systems are technically symbol sets with a shift toward greater linguistic capacity, just not on the same level as true symbol systems—hence the term "transitionary."

As also elucidated in Chapter 3, a symbol set is a group of symbols representing a finite vocabulary, and yet, the number of initial symbols may vary considerably from set to set. The key characteristic of symbol sets is that they have limited internal logic, and thus, there is limited expansion capability and representational range. Symbol sets may be used to access vocabulary on SGDs and may be found in other products aimed at keeping the cost low or even free. The sections that follow present and discuss a number of pre-linguistic symbols, starting with symbol sets and then shifting to transitionary symbol systems.

Symbol Sets

Symbol sets are lower-level pre-linguistic symbols that have rudimentary internal logic. This allows for some limited expansion beyond the original corpus of symbols. All symbol sets possess the physical attribute of two-dimensionality with just a couple of sets possessing the physical attribute of animation. In terms of design attributes, all symbol sets are comprised of line drawings; however, the animated symbols in some symbol sets are pictorial.

Two-Dimensional Symbols

DynaSyms. Faith Carlson's first symbols, PICSYMS, were created to be easily drawn by hand during face-to-face interaction with children with CCN. PICSYMS are discussed later in this chapter. As speech-generating technology started to become more sophisticated, a number of manufacturers needed to find symbol corpuses to use with their devices to

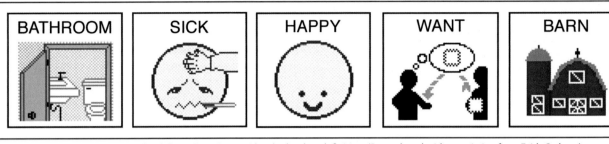

Figure 7-4. A representative sample of classic DynaSyms with color but low definition. (Reproduced with permission from Faith Carlson.)

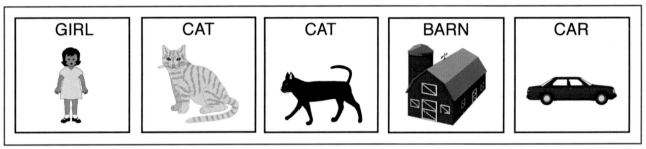

Figure 7-5. DynaSyms with color and high definition (i.e., vector images). (Reproduced with permission from Faith Carlson.)

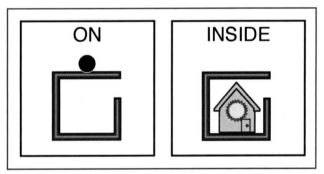

Figure 7-6. DynaSyms depicting positional prepositions. (Reproduced with permission from Faith Carlson.)

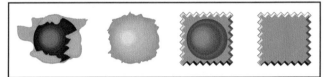

Figure 7-7. Development of the unspecified pronoun "it" (i.e., the "thing" symbol). (Reproduced with permission from Faith Carlson.)

access vocabulary. Carlson developed a new symbol system for speech-generating technology that followed the same symbol language principles as PICSYMS but visually adapted to the way drawings were created at the time using a computer paint program. DynaSyms were created as bitmap images 52 by 62 pixels in order to have the largest number of symbols possible for the memory capacity of the original Dynavox SGD. They were first created in black and white, but when flat screens began to utilize color, the symbols were recreated in color (Figure 7-4). A number of DynaSyms symbols utilized animation. In 1988, DynaSyms for Boardmaker was made available. This software allowed for a library of 3,300 color DynaSyms to be generated by computer.

As memory capacity for microcomputers became greater, DynaSyms were revised as vector images (Figure 7-5). This provided for sharper looking images with more detail. DynaSyms symbols are not just a group of pictures or visual symbols but a visual language system organized semantically with strategies for picturing concepts with categories having common shapes and colors. As a result, the system can be

used to create materials for children who are just acquiring language. It also can be used as a visual tool for retraining or re-establishing language skills after illness or injury for both children and adults.

Thousands of DynaSyms were created and made available on Dynavox devices. Since many individuals using Dynavox were not able to spell or search for symbols in alphabetical order, the symbols could be accessed by category. Within the DynaSyms corpus symbols for things, people and animals are simple pictures. Objects that have varying shapes or colors are symbolized by one and sometimes more representations. The colors of object symbols vary. Position symbols are blue or black and are represented by a box with an open side; circles and other objects are used to represent the position relative to the box (Figure 7-6).

Individuals using DynaSyms are able to recognize categories by common shapes and colors when searching. Abstract concepts, such as "thing," are represented abstractly. The "jagged-edged thing" symbol is a stylized version of paper crumpled around an object (Figure 7-7). The concept of thing (as well as object, item, or noun) can be introduced by using a piece of paper to crumple around objects or use a thing-shaped cutout placed over a picture of something, such as a ball. As seen in Figure 7-8, amounts are represented by gray domino or tumbler shapes; hands and dots

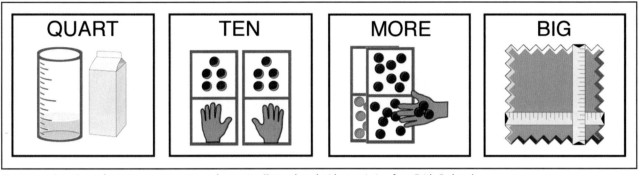

Figure 7-8. DynaSyms depicting amount, size, and quantity. (Reproduced with permission from Faith Carlson.)

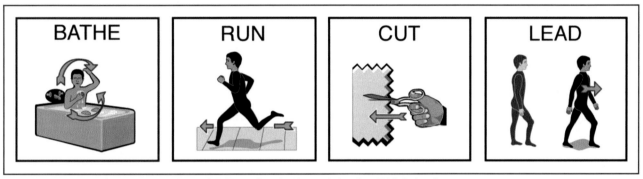

Figure 7-9. DynaSyms depicting action (i.e., verbs). (Reproduced with permission from Faith Carlson.)

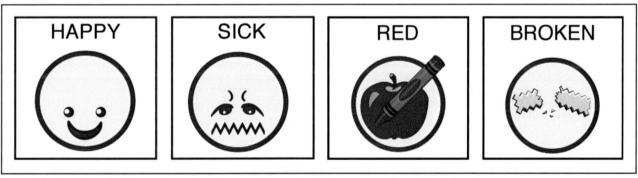

Figure 7-10. DynaSyms depicting attributes (i.e., adjectives). (Reproduced with permission from Faith Carlson.)

indicate the specific amount. Size symbols use a gray jagged thing symbol and yellow measuring tape. Actions are drawn in green and black. This is taken from the green that represents go on traffic lights. People and objects performing the actions are wearing black for consistency within the action category (Figure 7-9). Attribute, feeling, and color symbols have a large circular shape containing facial expressions or objects representative of the concept. Attribute colors are red and yellow (Figure 7-10).

Preceding are just a few examples of the categories or groups of symbols within the DynaSyms system. Because it is a semantically based system, it is possible to use DynaSyms in other languages with the addition of a few symbols unique to the chosen language, such as German or Spanish. As of the writing of this textbook, DynaSyms are no longer available on the open market but can be obtained by contacting the author, Faith Carlson.

Imagine Symbols. Imagine symbols were created in 2010 by a team of individuals from four different companies coming together to make a set of symbols that could be readily utilized with their products. The team was responsible for developing a corpus of symbols that could be used by teens and adults for everyday communication. Two of the four companies, Attainment Company and Saltillo Corporation (now PRC-Saltillo), continue their work with the symbols to this day. The symbols in the Imagine Symbol Directory published by Attainment Company in 2010 were readily available for no charge for individual, noncommercial use via a website that was functional at that time. Currently, requests for Imagine symbols are fielded directly by Attainment Company. There are currently approximately 4,000 symbols, and these are freely available with their products.

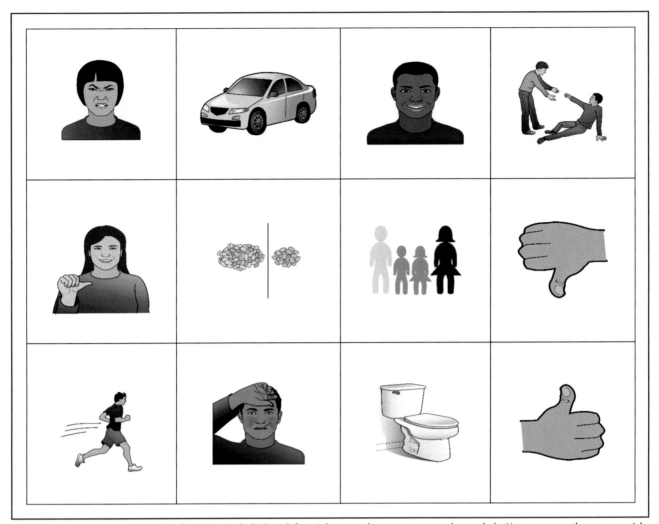

Figure 7-11. A representative sample of Imagine symbols. From left to right, top to bottom: angry, car, happy, help, I/me, more, mother, no, run, sick, toilet, and yes. (Reproduced with permission from Attainment Company, Inc.)

The development of Imagine symbols was based on feedback by different team members, such as assistive technology specialists, consumers, educators, occupational therapists, parents, and speech-language pathologists from three different English-speaking countries. Each symbol was field-tested among individuals with varying ability levels to ensure that the symbol either conveyed the intended meaning or could be taught via a systematic method to the individuals who use them. The ultimate goal was to develop symbols that could be easily learned by people with cognitive and/or other disabilities. For this reason, different principles were developed during their design, such as shading a specific part of a symbol to elicit a word or using color to draw attention to the salient information in the symbol. Additionally, the symbols use consistent elements to help users identify the intended vocabulary word. For example, the same icon is used in the symbols for a variety of community buildings. Examples of Imagine symbols can be found in Figure 7-11.

Lingraphica Concept-Images. Examples of Lingraphica concept-images can be found in Figure 7-12. The symbols were developed between 1984 and 1990 as part of the Computerized Visual Input Communication system, an intervention program for persons with aphasia. Lingraphica concept-images serve as the vocabulary access system for the Lingraphica SGD designed by the Tolfa Corporation (Richard Steele, personal communication, 2018). They number approximately 2,100 concept-images or icons. Research and development was conducted by a host of professionals, including specialists in computer science, linguistics, neurology, psychology, and speech-language pathology at the Veterans Affairs Palo Alto Health Care System.

Each icon can be assigned up to nine different concepts (e.g., couch, loveseat, recliner, rocking chair, sofa), that allows the symbols to be personalized to the individual end-user. Approximately 15% of the symbols are dynamic; these include mostly verbs and prepositions. The Lingraphica SGD uses Macintosh-based hardware, and vocabulary is accessed through dynamic displays. The entire system uses spoken and printed words, icons, and text processing. The U.S. Food and Drug Administration views the Lingraphica SGD as a medical device, which means it can only be dispensed by physician prescription. As can be seen with the depiction

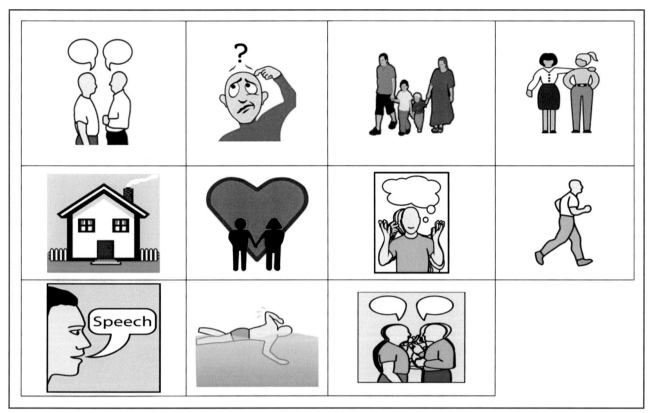

Figure 7-12. A representative sample of Lingraphica concept-images. From left to right, top to bottom: communication, confused, family, friend, house, love, remember, runner, speech exercises, swim, and talk. (The images for "remember" and "talk" are animated; therefore, the multiple lines in the animation exist as if the symbol was photographed at a specific instant.) (Reproduced with permission from Richard Steele.)

of the concepts "remember" and "talk" in Figure 7-12, it is more difficult to depict animation using two-dimensional symbols. Lingraphica concept-images are flexibly customizable, interactive, and highly stimulating, allowing for a range of human-computer user interactions available by design in association with each icon. The reader is referred to https://www.aphasia.com/ where educational videos are available for interested parties.

Mulberry Symbols. The Mulberry Symbols Project was originated by Garry Paxton in 2003 with the symbols getting their name from the Mulberry Trust, which financed the first 2 years of the project. Mulberry Symbols were developed over the next 3 years until 2007 by the Paxton Crafts Charitable Trust (United Kingdom) who then transferred copyright over to Steve Lee in 2018.

The aim was to develop a symbol corpus that was free of cost, and in fact, these symbols are free to use based on the Creative Commons license terms. This is to encourage individuals, such as parents, who might have the skills to create symbol-based software products but who lack a symbol resource to incorporate into their software or application. Hence, their license agreement means that developers can freely incorporate Mulberry Symbols into their work, distribute them, and even modify them in order to create their own derivatives.

The symbols were designed by a talented graphic artist with experience in AAC (see Figure 7-13 for examples). During their development, many members of the American Speech-Language-Hearing Association's AAC Special Interest Group became volunteer reviewers who reviewed and commented on each of the symbols until no further changes were deemed needed; only then were they published on the Straight Street website. The design of the symbols was led by the principle that they are applicable across a range of ages, including adult populations. One of the key elements of this particular corpus of symbols is its modifiers, which can potentially help individuals in categorizing the symbols. In Figure 7-14, examples of the different modifiers used are shown and explained.

ParticiPics. ParticiPics are symbols (i.e., pictographic images) initially created in 1996 by the Aphasia Institute, a Canadian community-based center focusing on helping people with aphasia. The first person responsible for illustration and design of these symbols was the graphic artist, Carmela Simone. Dr. Aura Kagan, executive director and director of applied research and education at the Aphasia Institute, has been leading the ParticiPics team for their ongoing development the last several years.

ParticiPics symbols were designed primarily to serve the needs of people with aphasia who, due to the difficulties they face, find it challenging to express their needs and thoughts with others. These symbols can also be used with other people

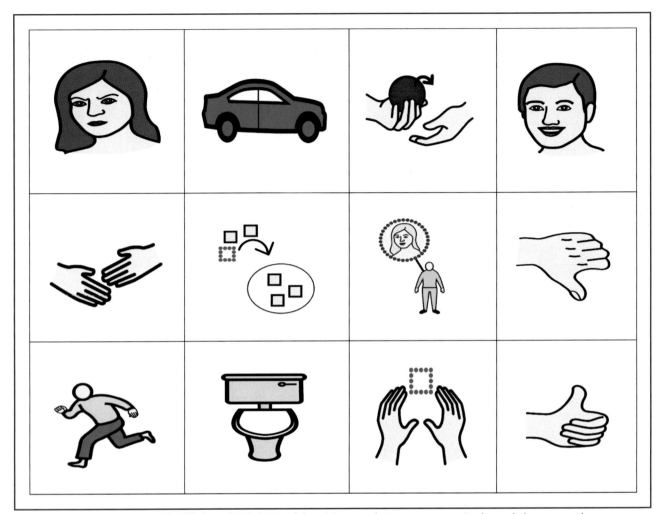

Figure 7-13. A representative sample of Mulberry Symbols. From left to right, top to bottom: angry, car, give, happy, help, more, mother, no, run, toilet, want, and yes. (© Steve Lee 2018/2019. This work is licensed under the Creative Commons Attribution—ShareAlike 2.0 UK; England & Wales License. Mulberry Symbols may be accessed at https://mulberrysymbols.org.)

who have CCN and who need pictographic images to express themselves. Due to their core purpose to support adults with aphasia, ParticiPics design features are tailored for adults, being simplified drawings with a neutral affect and gender non-specificity. They are available in black and white, as they are most easily readable in this way. ParticiPics symbols are freely available and can be downloaded from the Aphasia Institute (www.aphasia.ca/participics). In addition, the Aphasia Institute has a large bank of symbol resources specifically developed to serve the communication needs of people with aphasia. Examples of these symbols can be viewed in Figure 7-15.

Pics for Picture Exchange Communication System. The Pics for Picture Exchange Communication System (PECS) symbol corpus was started with only 151 symbols. They were based originally on the most commonly used symbols and were compiled over several years by tracking the symbol vocabulary development of hundreds of new PECS users. Over the years, the number of symbols has been expanded to the point where there are currently over 3,000 symbols. The Pics for PECS corpus of symbols was initially directed toward younger learners and it had many symbols for toys, but with time, the vocabulary was expanded and

now covers a wide range, hence making it appropriate for all ages. Pics for PECS now includes symbols for action words, activities, associated items for activities, daily routines, and job tasks. The design of the symbols remains consistent, developing symbols in a generic manner such that they can be combined with attributes for making precise requests (e.g., "I want big red block") and comments ("I see four monkeys"). Pics for PECS are used on an international scale and are available in multiple languages. They allow for changing of referents (i.e., meanings) for symbols in case someone wants to assign different meanings to the symbols.

The Pics for PECS corpus can be used for a wide range of purposes. For instance, the symbols can be used to create printed communication boards, schedules, literacy activities, visual supports, and overlays for SGDs. A compact disc is available that currently includes more than 3,400 symbols and instructions for use. Figure 7-16 illustrates some examples of Pics for PECS symbols. Symbols for referents, such as "I" and "me," are not included because, when teaching pronouns during the application of the PECS method, these are represented by actual photographs of the student.

Example of Symbols	Description
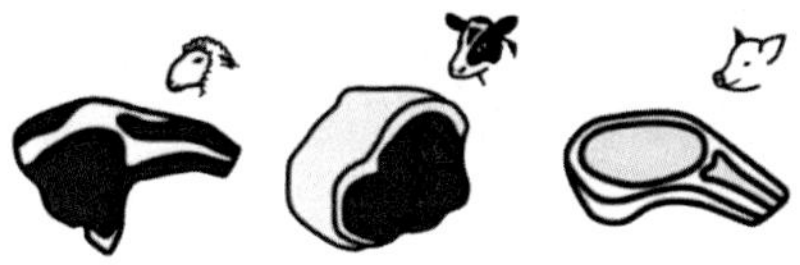	**Categories** The modifier at the top right in some symbols indicates the type of meat the symbol represents.
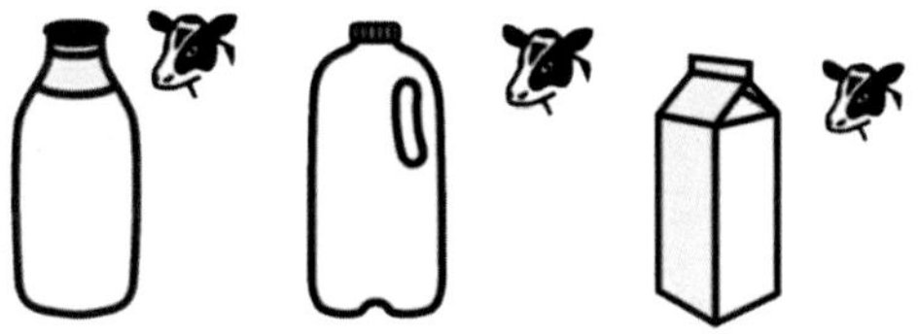	**Categories** These three symbols are for milk. The small image of a cow's head in the top right is the modifier, which helps to bring semantic clarity to the symbol. The symbols show "milk bottle," "2-liter milk container" and "milk carton." Similarly, the symbol for carton can be modified (e.g., with an image of an orange creates the symbol for "carton of orange juice").
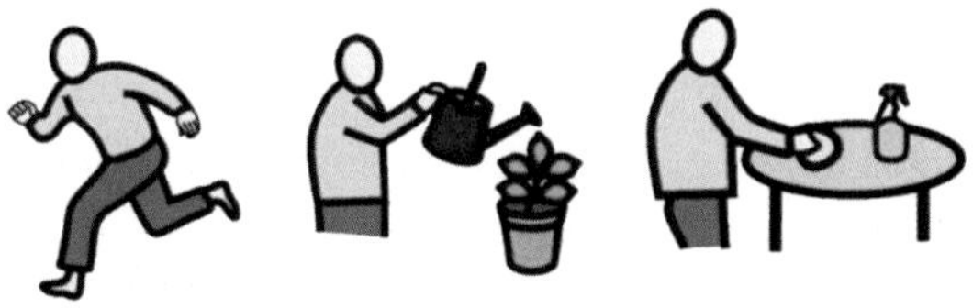	**Verbs** As shown here, the blue clothing indicates verbs.

Figure 7-14. Explanation of the modifiers used in Mulberry Symbols. (© Steve Lee 2018/2019. This work is licensed under the Creative Commons Attribution—ShareAlike 2.0 UK; England & Wales License. Mulberry Symbols may be accessed at https://mulberrysymbols.org.)

Pictograms. The Pictogram corpus was designed originally for persons with cognitive and/or physical impairments. Originally called Pictogram Ideogram Communication (PIC), these symbols were created in Canada by Subhas Maharaj in 1980. The symbols were created purposefully with a reverse image (i.e., white-on-black instead of black-on-white) presumably to enhance figure-ground discrimination, and hence, to make the symbols more visually salient (Figure 7-17). However, several studies have indicated that a white-on-black background is not necessarily more visually salient than a black-on-white background (Bloomberg, 1984;

Blyden, 1989; Campbell & Lloyd, 1986; Cooper & Fuller, 1994; Meador et al., 1984). Nonetheless, Pictograms have been used successfully with persons having severe/profound impairments (Leonhart & Maharaj, 1979; Reichle & Yoder, 1985) and autism (Reichle & Brown, 1986). Translucency studies have been conducted using Pictograms. Bloomberg and colleagues (1990), in a study of adults with average cognitive and physical abilities, found that Pictograms were more translucent than Blissymbols although less translucent than rebus symbols and PCS. Leonhart and Maharaj (1979) determined that with no prior training, short-term acquisition

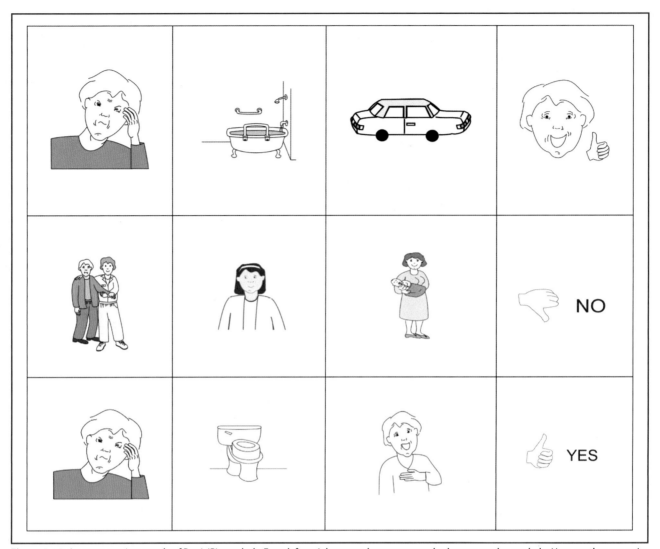

Figure 7-15. A representative sample of ParticiPic symbols. From left to right, top to bottom: angry, bathroom, car, happy, help, i/me, mother, no, pain, toilet, want, and yes. (© Aphasia Institute. The pictographic images are the intellectual property of the Aphasia Institute and are used with permission.)

was quicker for Pictograms than Blissymbols for adults with severe and profound cognitive impairments. These data seem to indicate that Pictograms are relatively iconic and easy to learn.

Pictograms are currently available in a number of countries in Scandinavia and northern Europe with perhaps the symbols being used more often in Sweden than anywhere else. What started as a small corpus of 400 symbols has since expanded to more than 2,000, and the white figure can be colored as long as the black background remains (Falck, 2001). To use Pictograms, permission must be sought through the Swedish Institute for Special Needs Education.

It is worth mentioning here that evidence shows professionals often use the term "pictogram" when they refer to graphic symbols in general. This leads inevitably to confusion and misunderstanding during communication (Pampoulou, 2015, 2017a). Many individuals in the AAC field use the terms "pictogram" (or "pictograph") and "symbol" interchangeably. However, in the professional literature, the two

terms are used with a clear distinction, as symbols are not limited to just pictographs but also can include objects, photographs, pictures, line drawings, or orthographic characters. On the other hand, by strict definition, pictograms refer only to pictures or pictorial representations of concepts.

The original name of Pictograms (i.e., PIC) was in fact a better term for this corpus, as many of the symbols are ideographs (i.e., symbols that depict more abstract referents). Nonetheless, the term "pictogram" is used on many websites in reference to a number of graphic symbol corpuses instead of individual graphic symbols. Similarly, the term "pictogram" is used in other fields outside AAC. In developing signage for airports, highways, and other public facilities, "pictograph" or "pictogram" is used to refer to symbols found in our daily lives (i.e., airport and highway signs, restroom doors) because of their realistic design. As is evident in this discussion, use of the term "pictogram" in AAC seems to be somewhat ambiguous with there being no clear consensus of the term's meaning (Pampoulou, 2015, 2017a). One should

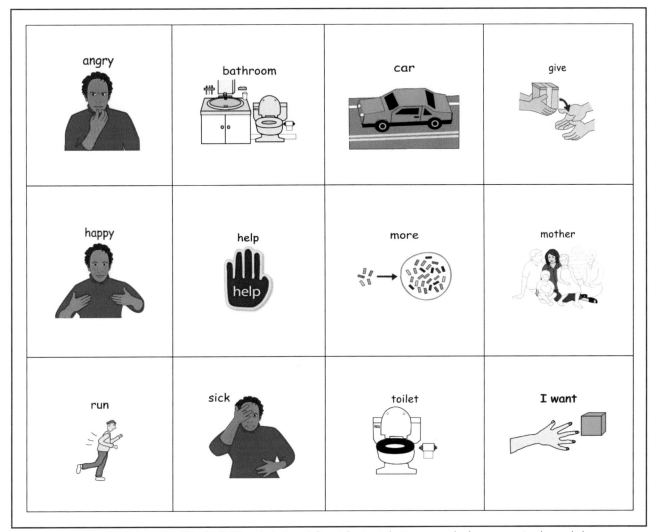

Figure 7-16. A representative sample of Pics for PECS symbols. From left to right, top to bottom: angry, bathroom, car, give, happy, help, more, mother, run, sick, toilet, and I want. (Images used with permission from Pyramid Educational Consultants [(www.pecs.com]. All rights reserved.)

be very clear when using the term "pictograms," as in one case it is referring to this particular corpus of symbols but in other cases the term may be used to refer to symbols in general, such as pictograms vs. ideograms.

Simple Rebus Symbols. By definition, a rebus is a puzzle consisting of pictures and alphabetic letters that are combined to form a word (e.g., a picture of an ear with "h+" placed immediately before it denotes the word "hear"; this is referred to as the rebus principle). Rebuses have been around for centuries; in the Middle Ages, they were used as heraldic emblems that included a pictorial representation of, or pun on, the name of the bearer.

Centuries later, Woodcock (1965) edited *The Rebus Reading Series* as the first part of a series of books for teaching reading to children with cognitive impairment (see also Clark et al., 1974; Clark & Woodcock, 1976; Woodcock, 1968; Woodcock et al., 1968). *The Rebus Reading Series*, and eventually the *Peabody Rebus Reading Program*, utilized the rebus principle for the purpose of reading instruction. In the formative years of AAC when few aided symbols were available,

some clinicians and educators simply borrowed the graphic rebus symbols from the reading program for use on communication boards (Vanderheiden & Lloyd, 1986) but did not take advantage of the full potential of the rebus principle. When just the graphic symbols from *The Rebus Reading Series* are used (and not the rebus principle), one has a set of predominantly iconic pictures. This is referred to as *simple rebus* and is the focus of the discussion here.

Later in this chapter, we will return to rebus symbols when we discuss alphabet-based and phonically based symbols. In this case, the symbols from *The Rebus Reading Series* and letters of the alphabet are used to convey a wide range of ideas and are referred to as "complex rebus."

Figure 7-18 provides a number of examples of simple rebus symbols. There are three types of simple rebus symbols: (1) iconic symbols, which depict objects and actions; (2) relational symbols, which typically depict locations or directions; and (3) opaque symbols, which are somewhat arbitrarily assigned meaning. To avoid some of the more arbitrary rebuses and to make them more appropriate for persons with

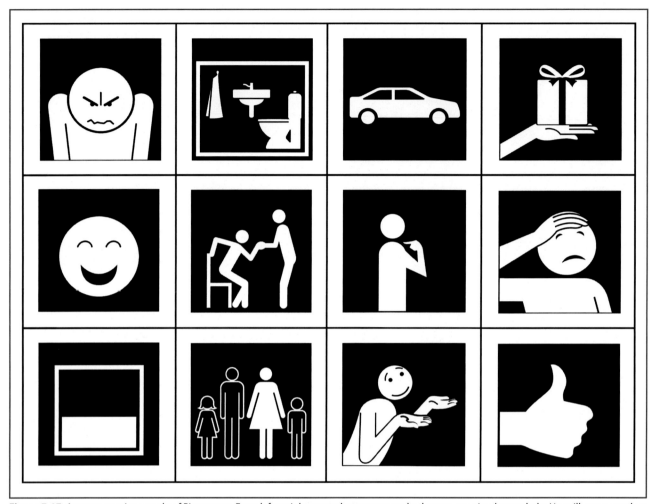

Figure 7-17. A representative sample of Pictograms. From left to right, top to bottom: angry, bathroom, car, give, happy, help, I/me, ill, more, mother, want, and yes. (Reproduced with permission from Specialpedagogiska Skolmyndigheten.)

cognitive impairments, educators in the United Kingdom have developed other pictographic sets of rebus symbols (e.g., Chapman, 1982; Devereux & van Oosterom, 1984; Jones, 1979; Jones, 1972, 1976; van Oosterom & Devereux, 1982, 1985; Walker et al., 1985). Clark and colleagues (1974) have made similar revisions in the United States. Although *The Rebus Reading Series* went out of print years ago, simple rebus symbols can still be found today.

SymbolStix. SymbolStix is an American symbol set designed in 2001 by a family-run business called News-2-You for use in its internet weekly newspaper and online curriculum, *Unique Learning System*. The newspaper began as a weekly classroom project where the text was symbol-supported for easier access by beginning readers and pupils with special educational needs. Currently, SymbolStix symbols are also designed to support access to language, literacy, and general communication for all ages of people. Examples of SymbolStix can be found in Figure 7-19. The set consists of approximately 11,000 symbols that can be designed in color or black and white and claims to be the only symbol set with the capability to change skin tones digitally on the SymbolStix PRIME platform.

Activities and people are depicted as lively, vibrant stick figures drawn in a manner to create stick figures with an attitude. Generic people are depicted as stick figures with no gender, age, or culturally specific attributes. This allows learners to focus on the concepts portrayed to prevent distraction or misunderstanding. The set also includes a range of culturally-significant images, such as actors, athletes, historical figures, politicians, and popular fictional characters. SymbolStix can be used in conjunction with reading and writing software, more specifically Clicker, to support writing or to create a powerful communication aid.

SymbolStix has been found to be effective in adapting lessons and making them more accessible for students with intellectual disabilities. Particularly, Evmenova and colleagues (2017) used SymbolStix to caption educational videos shown in class. The same symbols were later used by students to answer questions about the video they had seen. This adaptation resulted in improved performance for all students who were assessed.

Talking Mats. Talking Mats symbols were designed as a result of the Talking Mats framework developed by a group of researchers at Stirling University in the United Kingdom in order to support people with communication difficulties to understand and express their views on an issue of their concern (Cameron & Matthews, 2017). Created by speech-language pathologists with the support of comic artist, Adam Murphy, Talking Mats symbols were developed in 2013 and copyrighted to Adam Murphy and assigned to Talking Mats Ltd. The leading criteria for the design of these symbols are that they should promote understanding and thinking and not act as a distraction to the user (Cameron & Matthews, 2017). Therefore, these symbols are unique in the sense that they:

- Are both attractive and engaging
- Are simple but represent concepts clearly
- Distinguish between concrete and abstract concepts
- Show the full body, not stick figures
- Are acceptable in terms of age and ethnicity
- Are balanced between males and females
- Provide additional visual clues within topics to support understanding (Cameron & Matthews, 2017)

As shown in Figure 7-20, the design of Talking Mats symbols is based more on the concepts they intend to convey rather than on vocabulary *per se*. More specifically, the concepts represented by the symbols were developed in collaboration with different specialists in the educational and health care fields focusing on specific topics and concepts rather than on a list of vocabulary words. For instance, the symbols are developed using two key frameworks: (1) the World Health Organization International Classification of Functioning, Disability and Health, particularly aimed at adults, and (2) Getting It Right for Every Child (Petit et al., 2016), which, along with the World Health Organization International Classification of Functioning, Disability and Health, is aimed at children and young people (Joan Murphy, personal communication, 2018).

Transitionary Symbol Systems

While transitional symbol systems still fall under the classification of pre-linguistic symbols, these symbols have developer-defined rules for creating new ones beyond the original corpus, but the expansion rules tend to be somewhat rudimentary and not sufficiently developed to allow for unlimited expansion capability, although there is limited expansion capability due to the rules that do exist. It is for this reason that transitionary symbol systems have a larger representational range compared to the previously discussed corpuses of symbols. Compared to linguistic symbol systems, expansion capability of transitionary symbol systems is not as comprehensive in allowing symbol users to communicate freely all their ideas and thoughts with their communication partners. Next are some examples of transitionary symbol systems. These can also be identified and compared with the other corpuses of symbols listed in Table 7-1. All transitional symbol systems possess the physical attribute of two-dimensionality and the design attribute of line drawings.

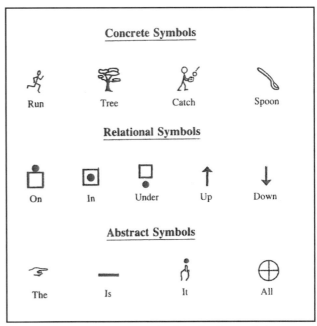

Figure 7-18. A representative sample of simple rebus symbols. (Adapted from Clark, C. R., & Woodcock, R. W. [1976]. Graphic systems of communication. In L. L. Lloyd [Ed.], *Communication assessment and intervention strategies* [pp. 549-605]. University Park Press.)

Two-Dimensional Symbols

Makaton Symbols. During the 1980s, The Makaton Charity developed a symbol corpus to be used in conjunction with manual signing to enhance people's communication (Walker et al., 1985). Symbols have certain properties that support language and literacy development in people with communication difficulties, and they have been found to capture and hold people's attention when they are presented to support spoken communication. Studies suggest visual information provided by symbols is easier to process than just having aural information. As shown in Figure 7-21, Makaton's symbols have been designed to be simple, pictographic, easy to draw, and reflect language themes. In appearance, they are black line drawings easy to interpret, as they look like what they represent and can be easily drawn on white boards with markers during free-flowing spontaneous communication. Drawing and interpreting symbols is easier to achieve because there are certain language themes that are reflected in their appearance (e.g., drawing a circle around "lady" changes its meaning to "mother"). Similarly, one can change a noun into a verb by having a person in the symbol (e.g., one can change "a shower" to "take a shower" by adding a person in the "a shower" symbol).

The selection of symbols is made after a thorough assessment of each user's functional communication needs, interests, learning goals, and literacy skills. Based on these aspects, users can be introduced to symbols in a variety of ways for adding value to the quality of their interactions. The size of the symbol can be adapted to each individual user depending on their visual scanning and processing abilities.

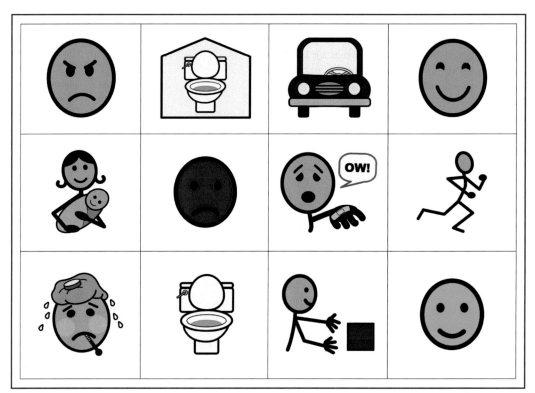

Figure 7-19. A representative sample of SymbolStix symbols. From left to right, top to bottom: angry, bathroom, car, happy, mother, no, pain, run, sick, toilet, want, and yes. (© 2020 n2y, LLC. All rights reserved. Used with permission. www.n2y.com.)

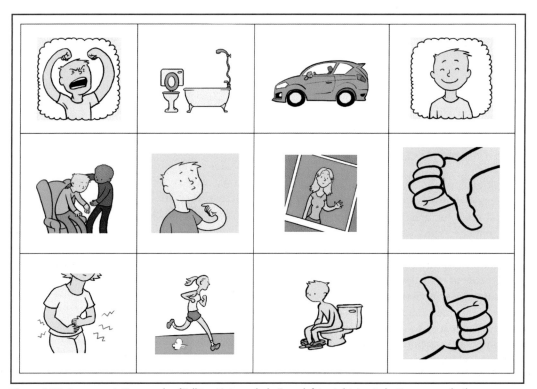

Figure 7-20. A representative sample of Talking Mats symbols. From left to right, top to bottom: angry, bathroom, car, happy, help, I/me, mother, no, pain, run, toilet, and yes. (Reproduced with permission from Talking Mats.)

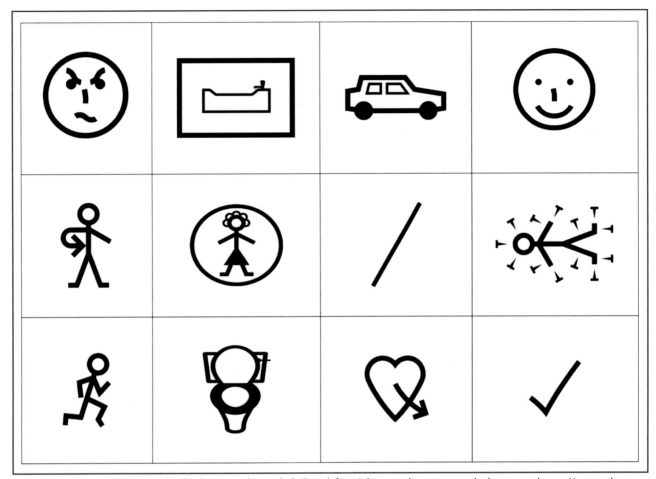

Figure 7-21. A representative sample of Makaton graphic symbols. From left to right, top to bottom: angry, bathroom, car, happy, I/me, mother, no, pain, run, toilet, want, and yes. (Reproduced with permission from Makaton Charity. The copyright in the Makaton Symbol and Sign graphics is owned by The Makaton Charity [Registered Charity 1119819 and Registered Company No. 06280108]. The Makaton graphics used within this book are based on British Sign Language and are only suitable for U. K. Makaton. If you buy this book out of the United Kingdom, please be advised that the Makaton graphics may not be suitable to use within the country of origin.)

Makaton aided AAC symbols have also been used on core vocabulary boards—either non–speech-generating or speech-generating—for producing sentences relating to specific functional and motivating activities. The MyChoicePad app for the iPad, developed in the United Kingdom, has 4,500 signs and symbols that are used in this way. When used with an SGD, it provides voice output for the sentences that a person can construct using the core vocabulary on a grid relating to an activity. The app has a facility for seeing videos of the signs for all the core vocabulary and some resource vocabulary. Similarly, other texts can be made more accessible to people with literacy difficulties, such as booklets, leaflets, poems, stories, songs, etc. (see The Makaton Charity resources of texts that have been translated into symbols).

Based on a survey conducted by Abbott and Lucey (2005), it was discovered that the most common symbol sets in the United Kingdom special schools are PCS, Makaton, and Widgit Symbols. More recent literature illustrates similar results. Pampoulou (2015) found that Makaton is one of the most common corpuses of symbols used in inclusive

primary schools in England and Cyprus and is used by a range of professionals, such as speech-language pathologists, teachers, and teaching assistants. Participants also commented that they use both aided graphic symbols and sign language, something that was not a surprise taking into consideration these symbols are part of a multimodal communication program for which instructors need to attend training workshops offered by The Makaton Charity.

Picture Communication Symbols. Another popular corpus developed in the 1980s is PCS. In the United States, speech-language pathologist Roxana Johnson created these graphic symbols to support face-to-face communication with cognitively impaired teenagers with whom she was working (Johnson, 1985). The primary objectives of PCS were that they should:

- Be easily learnable
- Be appropriate for all age levels
- Consist of simple, clear drawings for visual clarity
- Be relatively inexpensive and readily reproducible on copying machines

- Be easily separated into categories of symbols so potential users need only use the appropriate symbols
- Be available in standardized sizes for easy placement in standardized grids

Many of the symbols are quite complex in their appearance, so hand-drawing may not be an option (Musselwhite & St. Louis, 1988).

PCS symbols are mostly pictographic, having a smaller proportion of ideographic symbols. For some concepts that are too abstract to depict by pictographs or ideographs, the English word is simply used. Although traditional orthography (or the alphabet) is used to simply spell out words that cannot be depicted by symbols, PCS offers no rules for the formation of new symbols, thereby making PCS nongenerative (Whitley, 1985). As such, PCS is classified as a symbol set.

There are in total five different types of PCS symbols—*Classic* (Figure 7-22), *ThinLine* (Figure 7-23), *High Contrast* (Figure 7-24), *In-Context*, and *Persona*. The design of PCS Classic symbols is clear and concise, comprising thick lines, bright colors, egg-shaped heads, and an uncluttered appearance. PCS ThinLine symbols are more realistic, being designed with thinner lines and natural colors. Due to their design, they are often more appealing to teenagers and adults than the Classic version of the symbols. PCS High Contrast symbols, as their name implies, are designed with bright colors and minimal details and can be used effectively by people with cortical visual impairments. Their design is based on PCS Classic symbols, but High Contrast symbols have black backgrounds (see Figure 7-24 for examples). PCS In-Context symbols are designed specifically for communication purposes for adult populations in different daily living situations, and their design is based on the PCS ThinLine style.

PCS remains as one of the most commonly used aided symbol sets in the world, as the developers have kept up with the latest technology over the decades. What started out as a set of approximately 700 symbols has grown to approximately 5,000; with a supplemented general-purpose addendum and country-specific libraries, the total number of PCS symbols exceeds 37,000 representing over 40 different languages.

The first technological advancement for PCS symbols was the creation of the computer software program Boardmaker in 1989. Since then, Boardmaker has been extended to Boardmaker Plus!, which allows the clinician or educator to create interactive books, worksheets, schedules, and learning games with the use of animation, sound, and/or video; and Boardmaker Studio, which allows the clinician or educator to import, edit, and modify their Boardmaker and Boardmaker Plus! creations. The technology has also developed over the years, from floppy discs and compact discs in the earlier years to the internet and now Cloud technology. For instance, in 2008, the company initially launched a free activity sharing site called AdaptedLearning.com, which can now be found as https://goboardmaker.com/, with members approaching half a million. Boardmaker has become a

mechanism for Tobii Dynavox (the current copyright owner of PCS symbols) to deliver new symbols on a weekly basis, which means that the PCS library is continuously growing. It is worth mentioning the integration of the PCS picture dictionary with Microsoft's Immersive Reader. In this way, people can benefit greatly from the use of visual stimuli, as written text can also be illustrated using PCS symbols. With the additional support of auditory feedback, readers have at their disposal a variety of ways to access written text.

PCS has been used effectively with individuals exhibiting autism (Rotholz et al., 1989), cerebral palsy (Goossens', 1989), and cognitive impairments (Mirenda & Santogrossi, 1985). Musselwhite and St. Louis (1988) suggest that PCS is also appropriate for use with persons with aphasia, apraxia, and those undergoing postoperative vocal rest, although no known research has been conducted with these populations.

PCS has not been devoid of research scrutiny, as the set has been included in several studies. In a study involving 3 year olds with average cognitive abilities, Mizuko (1987) found that symbols from PCS were more transparent than PICSYMS and Blissymbols. Mirenda and Locke (1989) determined that PCS was more transparent than Blissymbols for persons with cognitive impairments. Adults with cognitive impairments found PCS and PICSYMS equally transparent and easy to recall (Mizuko & Reichle, 1989). Bloomberg and colleagues (1990) compared translucency across five aided symbol sets and systems including PCS. For the five symbol sets and systems studied, Bloomberg and colleagues (1990) learned that undergraduate college students found PCS and rebus symbols to be the most translucent symbols followed by Pictograms, PICSYMS, and Blissymbols. Tsai (2013) reported that the transparency of PCS is generally higher compared to Gus Communication Symbols among adults without known disabilities and of different age groups. However, the results suggested that accuracy of identifying correct symbols was related to chronological age.

Studies of the iconicity of PCS in languages other than English have shown mixed results. PCS symbols proved to be iconic for persons whose primary language was Mandarin and Mexican-Spanish (Huer, 2000), but iconicity did not appear to be a factor for typically developing Afrikaans- and Zulu-speaking children (Basson & Alant, 2005; Haupt & Alant, 2002). Finally, Dada and colleagues (2013) suggested that culture, spoken language, second language use, intellectual disability, and linguistic skills play a significant role in recognizing PCS. The authors noted mixed results when they compared the use of 16 symbols with students who had mild intellectual disability, English as an additional language, and who were coming from different backgrounds. Nevertheless, the iconicity of PCS was found to be relatively high among this population (i.e., approximately 75% accuracy in correctly identifying PCS symbols). These studies indicated that although PCS symbols are generally iconic, the degree of iconicity appears to be culturally constrained (Nigam, 2003).

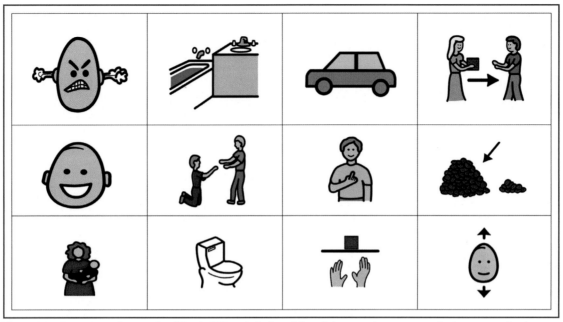

Figure 7-22. A representative sample of Classic PCS symbols. From left to right, top to bottom: angry, bathroom, car, give, happy, help, I/me, more, mother, toilet, want, and yes. (PCS is a trademark of Tobii Dynavox LLC. All rights reserved worldwide. Used with permission.)

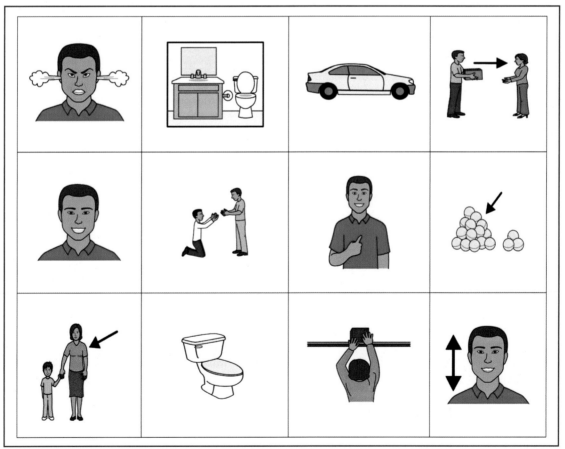

Figure 7-23. A representative sample of ThinLine PCS symbols. From left to right, top to bottom: angry, bathroom, car, give, happy, help, I/me, more, mother, toilet, want, and yes. (PCS is a trademark of Tobii Dynavox LLC. All rights reserved worldwide. Used with permission.)

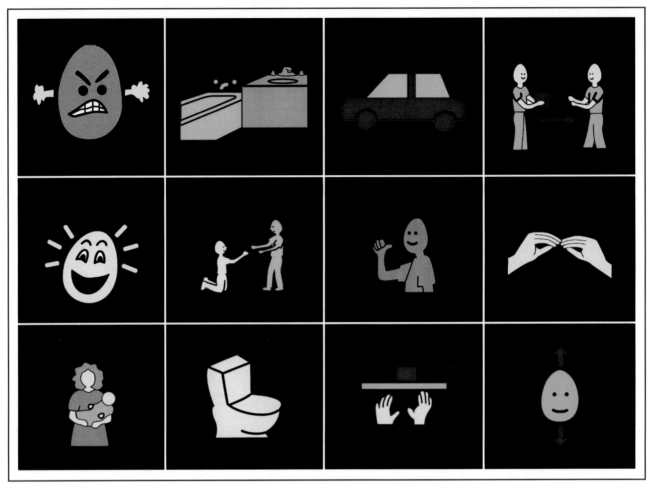

Figure 7-24. A representative sample of High Contrast PCS symbols. From left to right, top to bottom: angry, bathroom, car, give, happy, help, I/me, more, mother, toilet, want, and yes. (PCS is a trademark of Tobii Dynavox LLC. All rights reserved worldwide. Used with permission.)

As mentioned earlier, the PCS corpus is used widely in the United States but also in several other countries of the world. For example, Abbott and Lucey (2005) and Pampoulou (2017) found that PCS symbols are one of the three most common corpuses of symbols used in the United Kingdom. Figure 7-25 shows some examples of how PCS symbols are used in a kindergarten in the United Kingdom as a visual program. The PCS symbols at the top left show the different activity choices children have, while the upper right PCS symbols illustrate children's choices of how their daily program will develop. The bottom PCS symbols illustrate a visual timetable of the routine that a child should follow when washing hands. This is but one example of the use of PCS outside the United States.

Widgit Symbols. Widgit Symbols (Figure 7-26) were initially derived from the rebus corpus as part of the *Peabody Rebus Reading Program* developed in the United States in the 1960s. During the 1970s and 1980s, rebus symbols were initially used at Rees Thomas Special School, Cambridgeshire, in the United Kingdom by Judy Van Oosterom and Kathleen Devereux in order to support language development of pupils with moderate or severe learning disabilities. In the

mid-1990s, teachers Tina and Mike Detheridge, with the support of Judy van Oosteroom, continued developing the specific corpus, and in the year 2000, Widgit Symbols acquired the copyright of the rebus symbol collection. This enabled them to set up the Widgit Symbol Development Project, a 2-year project to redevelop the corpus in order to further improve its linguistic components (Detheridge & Detheridge, 2002). Figure 7-27 shows a small number of key principles that govern the linguistic components that characterize this corpus.

To be more specific, different options of symbols were designed to represent words that carry meanings that apply differently in different settings, such as work in an office, manual work, or simply to imply work as a noun. Actually, the specific design of symbols has proven to be vital for people who fall on the spectrum of autism and need specific information to understand language (Wellington & Wellington, 2002). Additionally, the specific corpus includes a number of rules so users can understand and generalize the meaning of different concepts. For example, in Figure 7-27, rooms are included in a box (illustrating the rooms in a building). Standard buildings, such as libraries and clinics,

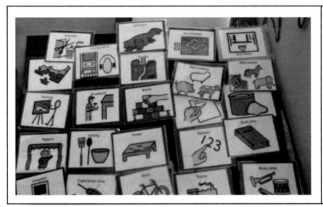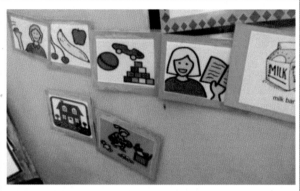

Figure 7-25. An illustration of PCS used in U.K. schools. (PCS is a trademark of Tobii Dynavox LLC. All rights reserved worldwide. Used with permission.)

are designed as houses, whereas the design differs for larger buildings, such as hospitals. Grammatical markers are also included within this corpus of symbols. As shown in Figure 7-27, arrows indicate the tense of action symbols and plurals are indicated by the double plus sign.

The teaching of Widgit Symbols focuses on an approach where the user learns the rules that govern the symbols so knowledge can be applied to understanding novel symbols. For instance, the red ball in Figure 7-27 shows the preposition that the symbol represents. The color red is used to show a feature or relationship, such as foreground to background. Personal pronouns are illustrated in the hand of the figure by having an arrow point to the person. On the other hand, a small filled circle design represents possessive pronouns. People in Widgit Symbols are represented in different ways, following the rule that the figure of the person shows the relationship with the concept that needs to be conveyed (see example in Figure 7-27). For instance, the jobs people do are represented by a person plus qualifying elements. In conveying different meanings attached to family members, a circle represents the concept of belonging. "Mother" is a woman in a circle, and "wife" has a heart attached. "Girlfriend" includes the heart but not a circle. Step relations are indicated by a dashed circle.

The Widgit Symbols corpus was initially designed in black and white with the belief that color may impede the learning and understanding of symbols. However, since 2002, the symbols have been available in color. In fact, Widgits Symbols' generating software, SymWriter, allows users to create symbol resources in black and white or color (Pampoulou, 2015). In 2005, a subset of Widgit Symbols was designed for people with visual impairments. In terms of the thickness of lines used in its images, Widgit Symbols were traditionally designed as thin line drawings in order to avoid visual clutter when used for literacy purposes (Pampoulou & Detheridge, 2007). In 2009, the original thin line Widgit Symbols were redesigned with thicker (i.e., medium thick) lines but not as thick as the lines designed specifically for people with visual impairment. The new lines of medium

thickness are easier to see and print than the original thin lines. Thick lines are used in Widgit Symbols for people with visual impairment to allow for the drawing of more complex images (symbols representing real things, like specific buildings or people, tend to be relatively complex).

The Widgit Symbols corpus is under constant development in order to meet the needs of professionals and users alike. As one of the most commonly used corpuses of symbols in the United Kingdom (Abbott & Lucey, 2005; Pampoulou, 2015), Widgit Symbols appear to be in a continuous state of development to accommodate the broader vocabulary needs of people who use these symbols. To address the needs of clinicians and users alike, in 2013, the company released The Widgit Health Symbols with an updated version of these symbols developed in 2018. To accommodate health-related vocabulary, a new, more human-like body style was developed for the health symbols. That said, it should be stated that the original purpose of Widgit Symbols has been language and learning rather than face-to-face communication; regardless of continuous changes, the overall design of this transitionary symbol system remains faithful to its original intent.

Linguistic Symbols

As explained in detail in Chapter 3, linguistic symbols are the most sophisticated level of aided symbols. These corpuses are the most advanced due to their sophisticated and comprehensive internal logic that allows virtually unlimited expansion capability, that is, there are no limitations in terms of creating new symbols. Symbol systems are organized according to four design attributes and three physical attributes. The physical attributes include acoustic, three-dimensional, and two-dimensional. Design attributes include alphabet-based, electronically generated, line drawings, and phonemic-/phonetic-based symbols. In the sections that follow, symbol systems will be organized and presented according to their *design* attributes.

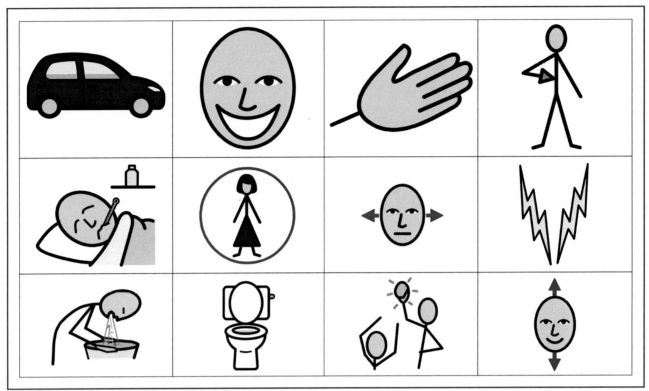

Figure 7-26. A representative sample of Widgit Symbols. From left to right, top to bottom: car, happy, help, I/me, ill, mother, no, pain, sick, toilet, want, and yes. (Widgit Symbols © Widgit Software, 2002-2019. www.widgit.com)

Linguistic Symbol Systems

Alphabet-Based Symbols

Shifting one's attention to alphabet-based symbols (the reader is also urged to see Table 7-1), it is reasonable to assume many alphabet-based symbol corpuses are symbol systems because they allow unlimited communication and promote literacy skills. Although many alphabet systems exist worldwide, discussion in this textbook is limited to the English alphabet (referred to as traditional orthography) and modified orthographies based on English.

From a technical standpoint, alphabet systems could be thought of as a form of augmentative communication, that is, they augment the spoken language of the able-bodied community by providing a permanent record that can be referred to at a later time. Alphabet-based systems somewhat mimic the spoken language of the community, so they are open-ended and extremely powerful in expansion capability. These systems include aided representations of the manual alphabet (also referred to as fingerspelling), Braille, modified orthography, Morse code (when used as an aided approach), and traditional orthography. With the exception of modified orthography, these systems tend to be opaque. For example, the letters D, O, and G, when combined se-quentially, produce the word "dog," which, in turn, is used to represent the house pet that barks. However, the spelled out word "dog" does not look in any way, shape, or form like the corresponding animal; hence, traditional orthography is primarily opaque

with the exception of a small set of iconic words known as onomatopoeia (i.e., words that sound like the referents they describe, such as "meow," "zip," or "cuckoo").

Descendants of traditional orthography where sub-characters (e.g., the dits and dahs of Morse code or the raised dots of Braille) or handshapes (e.g., fingerspelling) are also *predominantly* opaque (e.g., a small number of fingerspelling characters, such as the letters C, D, and O are iconic). The exception is a modified orthographic approach known as accentuation, embedding, or embellishment, which was designed for the purpose of making traditional orthography (or other graphic symbols) more iconic.

Aided Representations of Fingerspelling. Aided representations of fingerspelling (Figure 7-28) allow for display permanence of the individual finger configurations that make up the letters of the alphabet. Because aided representations of fingerspelling are simply graphic depictions of unaided fingerspelling, the symbols can be combined in a virtually unlimited number of ways to express any thought. Therefore, aided representations of fingerspelling have an excellent expansion capability and a wide representational range. Printed fingerspelling cards and other print media are quite common and can be easily obtained. Of course, to use a printed fingerspelling chart effectively, the sender must know how to spell and the receiver must know how to read. Animated fingerspelling (whether by computer, electronic glove, or robotic hand) is also an aided representation of fingerspelling.

Example of Symbols	Description
work work work water water water water water saw saw saw	**Alternative Meanings** There are alternative symbols for the different meanings of words: Office work, manual work, job.
book library book shop librarian librarians health clinic hospital doctor doctors	**Schematic Approach** The corpus includes a number of standard elements that, when learned, will help the reader to understand new symbols and concepts independently.
sleep slept apple apples good better best	**Grammatical Markers** A '←' indicates past tense, '+' indicates plurals, and '!' indicates comparatives.
in on behind middle foreground background	**Prepositions** The red ball shows position by its relationship with other objects. Where the ball is not appropriate, the color red is still used to show position.
he his she hers you your	**Pronouns** Personal pronouns are illustrated by the hand of one human figure having an arrowhead pointing to the target person. On the other hand, a small filled circle design represents the possessive pronoun instead of the arrowhead.
man father boyfriend husband baker plumber dentist vet	**People** The jobs that people do are represented by a person plus qualifying elements. In conveying different meanings attached to family members, the circle represents the notion of belonging.

Figure 7-27. A representative sample of Widgit Symbols illustrating internal logic. (Widgit Symbols © Widgit Software, 2002-2019, www.widgit.com)

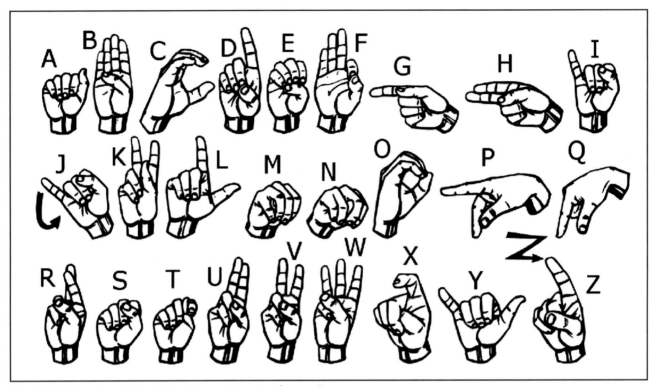

Figure 7-28. Illustrations of the alphabetic letters in American fingerspelling.

Braille. The Braille system is actually one step removed from traditional orthography in that a series of raised dots are used to represent letters, which in turn are combined to form words to represent referents in the language (such an arrangement is referred to as an analog of traditional orthography). Invented by Louis Braille in 1824, the system is not an AAC system *per se*; it allows persons with visual or dual sensory impairments to read English by feeling the encoded letters. Braille characters consist of six-dot matrices of two columns and three rows (Figure 7-29). For example, for the letter A, only the dot in row 1, column 1 is raised. The letter Z is represented by raised dots in row 1, column 1; row 2, column 2; and row 3, columns 1 and 2. A variety of raised dot configurations make up the other alphabet letters, parts of words, and in some cases whole words (e.g., "for" and "please"). There are three grades of Braille. Grade 1 contains no contractions so that all words must be spelled out. Grade 2 uses some contractions, which increases the rate of reading. Grade 3 is essentially a shorthand form. Of the three, Grade 2 is used most commonly in the United States (Beukelman & Light, 2020). Braille has other applications besides as a means of reading English. It can be used as a music code, a Nemeth code (for using scientific notation in mathematics), and a computer code (Beukelman & Light, 2020). Microcomputer-based devices exist that automatically translate fully spelled-out text into Braille and Braille into regular text using traditional orthography (Vanderheiden & Lloyd, 1986). Since the Americans with Disabilities Act, Braille is seen now by the general community with greater regularity (e.g., in elevators, on candy and soda machines, at bank ATM machines).

Modified Orthography. Modified orthography involves accentuation, embedding, and embellishment of alphabetic letters or whole words to make the letters or words more iconic. This approach was developed out of the problems experienced by many non- or pre-literate individuals in trying to decipher the traditional orthography system.

Basically, the letters in words or whole words are modified or embellished to make them more visually salient or representative of their referents (Figure 7-30). There are several examples of modified orthography (e.g., Blischak & McDaniel, 1995; Devereux & van Oosterom, 1984; Fuchs & Fuchs, 1984; Hoogeveen et al., 1989; Jeffree, 1981; Marko, 1967; Tabe & Jackson, 1989; Wendon, 1979). Some of these approaches are still in use but a number of them no longer enjoy mainstream use. Regardless, a number of modified orthography approaches are presented here to give the reader a better understanding of how traditional orthography can be modified—at least in the early stages of literacy development—to make letters and words more clearly visually representative of their referents.

Bannatyne (1968) described an approach in which such strategies as color coding of vowel phonemes is used to accentuate words. The *Diacritical Marking System* (Fry, 1964) and *Symbol Accentuation* (Miller, 1967, 1968; Miller & Miller, 1968, 1971) approaches use accentuation or embellishment of words to make them more visually resemble the referents the words depict (e.g., the word "cold" may be embellished by having icicles dangle off the letters or the word "look" may have dots in the center of the two O letters to make them look like eyes).

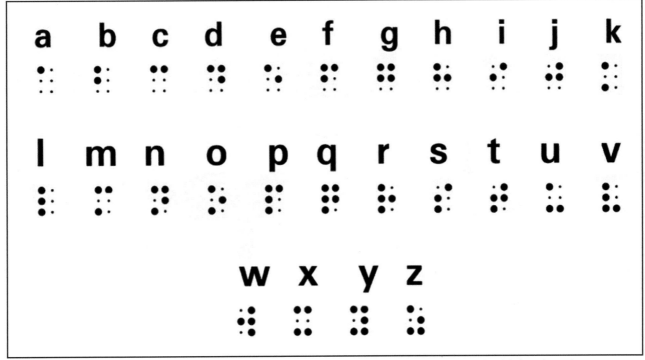

Figure 7-29. Illustrations of the alphabetic letters in Braille. (The larger dots are the raised parts that comprise the alphabetic letters.)

Modified orthography is similar to the embellishment of other graphic symbols (e.g., *Picture Your Bliss* for Blissymbols). As the learner understands the word or symbol with embellishments, the embellishments are faded until only the alphabetic letters or symbol and corresponding word remain.

Morse Code. International Morse code is also based on traditional orthography and is an analog of it. In this case, a series of dots (called dits) and dashes (called dahs) are used to represent the alphabet letters, numerals, punctuation, and transmission signals (e.g., "error," "wait," "end"). The reader may remember being exposed to Morse code or even recall the familiar "••• --- •••" for SOS. When used with a Morse code emulator that provides full access to standard computer software, the dits and dahs can be signified by either the activation of two different switches or by different periods of delay in the activation of a single switch. Most often, Morse code is not used as an AAC system *per se* but rather is used with speech-generating technology that has Morse code input capability. In these cases, Morse code is an aided system. Morse code can also be used in unaided communication, as discussed in Chapter 8. See Figure 7-31 for the Morse code characters that comprise the English alphabet.

Traditional Orthography. English traditional orthography is based on the Roman alphabet of 26 letters. Traditional orthography primarily serves as an augmentation to spoken language for persons without disabilities. In AAC systems, traditional orthography can be used in a variety of ways. For example, each of the 26 individual letters can be placed on a communication board or other display or device so the user can spell out words by pointing to or otherwise accessing the individual letters. This may be the only AAC system for some people, whereas for most others, it may be only part of a system that includes other symbols. In addition to the 26 individual letters, common letter combination sequences (e.g., *-ly, -ed, -ing, th, ph, ck*) can be displayed to speed up the rate of communication (e.g., see the WRITE approach by Goodenough-Trepagnier et al., 1982). Either alone or in combination with letters and letter sequences, words and phrases can be displayed to improve the rate of communication even more (Beukelman et al., 1985).

Traditional orthography is used typically with other aided symbols as well. For example, word glosses (i.e., the spelled out word equals the referents that the symbols are representing) usually appear with other graphic symbols (e.g., Blissymbols, PCS, Pictograms, Sigsymbols) when they are displayed on a communication board or other aid or device. Traditional orthography is also an integral part of complex rebus, as will be discussed in a later section of this chapter. When the alphabet is used as part or all of a communication system, the letters may appear in the QWERTY keyboard arrangement (especially for electronic devices), but the letters may also be arranged alphabetically from A to Z or in the order of the most commonly used to the least commonly used letters (the American game show "Wheel of Fortune" is familiar with this strategy). For some individuals, a display of all 26 alphabet letters may be used to spell out entire words, whereas for those with dysarthria (e.g., hypokinetic dysarthria seen in Parkinson's disease) or apraxia of speech, the letters may be used to assist the individual in gaining better intelligibility of speech. In this case, an individual with dysarthria or apraxia typically points to the letter that

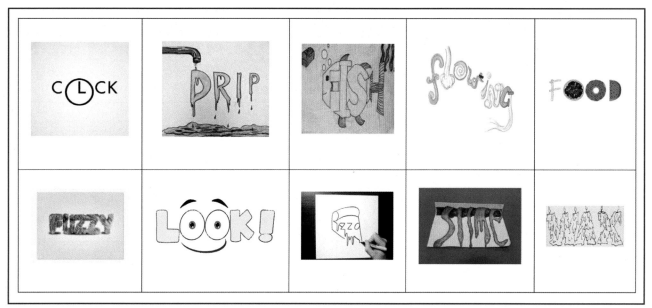

Figure 7-30. Examples of modified orthography (also known as word or symbol accentuation, enhancement, or embellishment).

corresponds to the first letter of each word they are speaking (Beukelman & Yorkston, 1977). This naturally slows down their rate of speech, thereby improving intelligibility while at the same time providing cues to the communication partner as to the words that are being spoken (i.e., each word begins with the letter to which the end-user points).

Not surprisingly, research involving the learnability of traditional orthography has been relatively unfavorable. By comparison to other graphic symbol sets and systems (e.g., Blissymbols, PCS, Pictograms, PICSYMS, and rebus symbols), traditional orthography consistently has been found to be the least iconic and most difficult to acquire over the short term (Briggs, 1983; Clark, 1977, 1981; Clark et al., 1974; Kuntz, 1975; Mirenda & Locke, 1989; Romski et al., 1985; Woodcock, 1968).

To use traditional orthography to its fullest advantage, the user must know how to spell and read. In addition, there is not a one-to-one correspondence between letters of the alphabet and the sounds that are made by those letters. For example, two letters are sometimes required to represent a single sound (e.g., *ph* sounds like /f/; *ck* sounds like /k/). Similarly, at least one alphabetic letter represents more than one sound (e.g., C can sound like either /k/ or /s/) depending on the context, and at least one letter is sounded out by two adjoining sounds (i.e., the letter X makes the sound /ks/). This lack of a one-to-one relationship between letter and sound may create problems for some individuals when learning to read or write. The lack of iconicity of most of the letters of the graphic alphabet only exacerbates the problem. Because of these problems, modified orthography (i.e., accentuation, embedding, or enhancement), or phonemic- or phonic-based systems (see the following) may be an alternative or bridge to traditional orthography.

Phonemic-/Phonetic-Based Symbols

Phonemic- or phonetic-based symbols are similar to traditional orthography in that they consist of a finite number of characters that can be combined systematically to produce words. Unlike traditional orthography, where a single letter can represent more than one sound (e.g., the letter C can represent the /s/ sound, as in "re*c*eive", or the /k/ sound as in "*c*ake") or a combination of letters can represent a single sound (e.g., the letters TH can be sounded out as either /θ/ or /ð/), phonemic- or phonetic-based symbols are designed so that each character represents a specific sound. In this way, there is a one-to-one relationship between character and sound, unlike traditional orthography.

Rather than serve as an analog to traditional orthography, phonemic- or phonic-based symbols are direct analogs to the *acoustic signal of speech*. That is, the symbols of these systems are related to the sound of spoken language. Recall that a major shortcoming of traditional orthography is that there is not a one-to-one relationship between letter and sound. Phonemic- or phonetic-based symbols serve to map onto the sound system, thereby improving the relationship between symbol and sound. As referenced in Table 7-1, examples of phonemic- or phonetic-based symbols are complex rebus (i.e., use of the full power of the rebus principle), Visual Phonics, and phonetic alphabets.

Complex Rebus. The history of rebus symbols (as part of the *Peabody Rebus Reading Program*) was covered in the section on non-linguistic symbols. It should be kept in mind that only the graphic symbols that comprised the *Peabody Rebus Reading Program* are classified as non-linguistic. When the full power of the *Peabody Rebus Reading Program* is utilized (i.e., the creation of concepts by combining symbols, such as "chalk" and "board" equals "chalkboard", or most often by adding or subtracting letters of the alphabet,

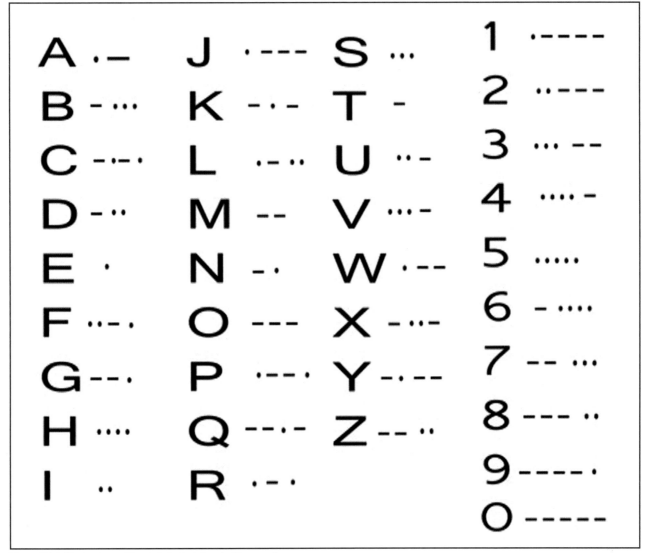

Figure 7-31. Illustrations of the alphabetic letters in Morse code.

such as "spout" minus "s" equals "pout" or "st" and "ring" equals "string"), rebus symbols become a linguistic symbol system (Figure 7-32). It should be noted that complex rebus is seldom, if ever, used as a sole means of communication; however, there is nothing preventing a clinician or educator from utilizing the rebus principle to transition a pre-literate AAC user to traditional orthography or other linguistic symbol system.

Because complex rebus relies on the sounds of words and not on words *per se*, the potential user must have adequate sound-blending skills to use the system effectively. The expansion of rebus using letters and rhyming is "… limited to the level of language and cognitive development of the user" (Vanderheiden & Lloyd, 1986, p. 107).

Regarding their use in the United Kingdom, complex rebus symbols were initially used at the Saint Reeds Thomas School by Judy Van Oosterom and Kathleen Devereux to help students who had moderate or severe learning disabilities learn to read and write, although with some adaptations

to some of the more arbitrary rebus symbols (Devereux & van Oosterom, 1984). In the 1980s, the initial rebus corpus morphed into two corpuses of graphic symbols, Makaton and Widgit Symbols. To this day Makaton and Widgit Symbols share approximately the same 350 symbols from the original rebus corpus (Pampoulou, 2015).

Phonetic Alphabets. Current and former students of speech-language pathology may recall (for better or worse!) learning phonetic transcription using the International Phonetic Alphabet (IPA). Because of the lack of a one-to-one relationship between letter and sound in traditional orthography, the IPA and other phonetic alphabets, such as the Fonetic English Alphabet, Goldman-Lynch Sounds and Symbols, Initial Teaching Alphabet (ITA), Ten-Vowel Alphabet, and UNIFON, were created to provide systematic and unambiguous pronunciation of English words (Downing, 1963, 1970; Downing & Jones, 1966; Goldman & Lynch, 1971; Malone, 1962; Matthews, 1966; Rohner, 1966).

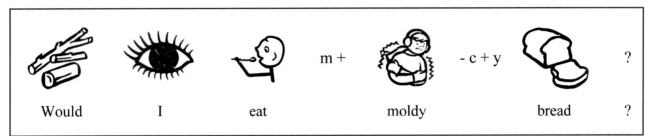

Figure 7-32. Use of the rebus principle in complex rebus: "Would I eat moldy bread?"

For example, in the IPA, the Greek symbol theta (/θ/) is used to represent the voiceless "th" sound (e.g., "breath," "thimble," and "toothbrush"), while the symbol eth (/ð/) is used to represent the voiced "th" sound (e.g., "breathe," "mother," and "these"). Likewise, the IPA character /k/ is always used to denote the "k" sound, as in the words "block," "cat," "Iraq," and "kiss," regardless of the letter or letters used as an analog to that sound. This allows each *sound* in the English language (or any other language for that matter) to be represented by a single symbol. In addition to the IPA, one of the best-known phonetic alphabets is the ITA (see Figures 7-33A and 7-33B for examples of the IPA and ITA character sets, respectively).

To enhance the rate of message transmission, phonetic characters can be chunked together into the most commonly occurring sound blends (e.g., chunking the "k" and "r" together into "kr" to represent the sound blend in "Christmas" or "crispy"). Goodenough-Trepagnier and Prather (1981) describe such a method (known as SPEEC), which is similar to the WRITE approach—the chunking of letters in traditional orthography. A French form of chunking phonetic characters is called Par le si la b.

Persons who use phonetic alphabets exclusively or as part of a communication system must have a good internalized phonetic record of the sounds of language. In some cases, phonetic alphabets may be used as a means of input for SGDs. In this case, the number of potential communication partners may be practically unlimited. However, if the individual uses a phonetic alphabet as *the* means of output, the size of the potential audience may be reduced, as most people are not familiar with phonetic alphabets. Potential communication partners would have to be taught the phonetic alphabet in use.

Visual Phonics. Visual Phonics (Figure 7-34) transcends the aided and unaided symbol domains and is therefore multimodal. Created by the International Communication Learning Institute in 1982, Visual Phonics consists of 45 hand movements that look and feel like speech sounds. This part of the system is *unaided*. The *aided* portion consists of graphic symbols that resemble the hand in action along with pictures that are related to the hand movements.

Visual Phonics has been used successfully with a wide variety of populations, including preschool and elementary-aged children without disabilities (i.e., as instruction for reading); individuals with autism, Down syndrome, and other cognitive, physical, and hearing impairments; and persons with learning disabilities and articulation disorders caused by cerebrovascular accident (Amend, 1987; International Communication Learning Institute, 1986). Initially, Visual Phonics had hand movements and written symbols for only the speech sounds of English. In 2017, hand movements and written symbols were developed for most of the sounds identified by the IPA. This makes Visual Phonics internationally useful with all the aforementioned populations, as well as with second-language learners.

Line Drawings

Blissymbolics. One of the first corpuses of graphic symbols still used today is Blissymbolics. The founder of Blissymbolics, Charles Bliss, was born in Austria near the Russian border. He recognized early the misunderstandings that could result when people do not share a common language. His father was an optician and electrician, and Bliss himself became a chemical engineer. Through his own and his father's work, he was exposed to the logic and symbols used in these fields. As a result of World War II, Bliss left Europe and resided in China where he was intrigued by the ideographic system of Chinese writing. During the 1930s, the political climate in Europe had reinforced in Bliss the idea that all the strife in the world was due to the lack of a common language. He began to formulate a graphic system of communication that would transcend spoken languages. The influence of his father's and his own profession, as well as the logic of the Chinese system of writing, was clearly evident in the international communication system he called "semantography" (which in Greek means "a meaningful writing"). His system was not widely accepted by the scientific community, so he published his own work in the book, *Semantography* (Bliss, 1949, 1965). He continued perfecting his communication system despite little support from the scientific or political communities. At some point after the war, Bliss immigrated to Australia where he continued his work over 2 decades hoping for the day it would be accepted as an international communication system.

In 1971, Shirley McNaughton, an educator working at the Holland Bloorview Kids Rehabilitation Hospital in Toronto, discovered his system while working with an interdisciplinary team that was mandated to assist students with severe physical impairments to communicate. The team began teaching Blissymbols to children aged 4 to 6 years and immediately

THE INTERNATIONAL PHONETIC ALPHABET (revised to 2015)

CONSONANTS (PULMONIC)   © 2015 IPA

	Bilabial	Labiodental	Dental	Alveolar	Postalveolar	Retroflex	Palatal	Velar	Uvular	Pharyngeal	Glottal
Plosive	p b			t d		ʈ ɖ	c ɟ	k g	q ɢ		ʔ
Nasal	m	ɱ		n		ɳ	ɲ	ŋ	N		
Trill	ʙ			r					R		
Tap or Flap		ⱱ		ɾ		ɽ					
Fricative	ɸ β	f v	θ ð	s z	ʃ ʒ	ʂ ʐ	ç ʝ	x ɣ	χ ʁ	ħ ʕ	h ɦ
Lateral fricative				ɬ ɮ							
Approximant		ʋ		ɹ		ɻ	j	ɰ			
Lateral approximant				l		ɭ	ʎ	L			

Symbols to the right in a cell are voiced, to the left are voiceless. Shaded areas denote articulations judged impossible.

CONSONANTS (NON-PULMONIC)

Clicks		Voiced implosives		Ejectives	
ʘ	Bilabial	ɓ	Bilabial	ʼ	Examples:
ǀ	Dental	ɗ	Dental/alveolar	pʼ	Bilabial
ǃ	(Post)alveolar	ʄ	Palatal	tʼ	Dental/alveolar
ǂ	Palatoalveolar	ɠ	Velar	kʼ	Velar
ǁ	Alveolar lateral	ʛ	Uvular	sʼ	Alveolar fricative

OTHER SYMBOLS

ʍ Voiceless labial-velar fricative   ɕ ʑ Alveolo-palatal fricatives

w Voiced labial-velar approximant   ɺ Voiced alveolar lateral flap

ɥ Voiced labial-palatal approximant   ɧ Simultaneous ʃ and x

ʜ Voiceless epiglottal fricative

ʢ Voiced epiglottal fricative   Affricates and double articulations can be represented by two symbols joined by a tie bar if necessary.   t͡s k͡p

ʡ Epiglottal plosive

VOWELS

Where symbols appear in pairs, the one to the right represents a rounded vowel.

SUPRASEGMENTALS

ˈ	Primary stress	ˌfoʊnəˈtɪʃən
ˌ	Secondary stress	
ː	Long	eː
ˑ	Half-long	eˑ
̆	Extra-short	ĕ
ǀ	Minor (foot) group	
‖	Major (intonation) group	
.	Syllable break	ɹi.ækt
‿	Linking (absence of a break)	

DIACRITICS   Some diacritics may be placed above a symbol with a descender, e.g. ŋ̊

Voiceless	n̥ d̥	Breathy voiced	b̤ a̤	Dental	t̪ d̪
Voiced	s̬ t̬	Creaky voiced	b̰ a̰	Apical	t̺ d̺
Aspirated	tʰ dʰ	Linguolabial	t̼ d̼	Laminal	t̻ d̻
More rounded	ɔ̹	Labialized	tʷ dʷ	Nasalized	ẽ
Less rounded	ɔ̜	Palatalized	tʲ dʲ	Nasal release	dⁿ
Advanced	u̟	Velarized	tˠ dˠ	Lateral release	dˡ
Retracted	e̠	Pharyngealized	tˤ dˤ	No audible release	d̚
Centralized	ë	Velarized or pharyngealized	ɫ		
Mid-centralized	ẽ	Raised	e̝ (ɹ̝ = voiced alveolar fricative)		
Syllabic	n̩	Lowered	e̞ (β̞ = voiced bilabial approximant)		
Non-syllabic	e̯	Advanced Tongue Root	e̘		
Rhoticity	ɚ a˞	Retracted Tongue Root	e̙		

TONES AND WORD ACCENTS

LEVEL			CONTOUR		
e̋ or ˥	Extra high		ě or ˩˥	Rising	
é ˦	High		ê ˥˩	Falling	
ē ˧	Mid		e᷄ ˧˥	High rising	
è ˨	Low		e᷅ ˩˧	Low rising	
ȅ ˩	Extra low		e᷈ ˧˩˧	Rising-falling	
↓ Downstep			↗ Global rise		
↑ Upstep			↘ Global fall		

Figure 7-33A. The IPA. (Reproduced with permission from IPA Chart, http://www.internationalphoneticassociation.org/content/ipa-chart, available under a Creative Commons Attribution-Sharealike 3.0 Unported License. Copyright 2015 International Phonetic Association.)

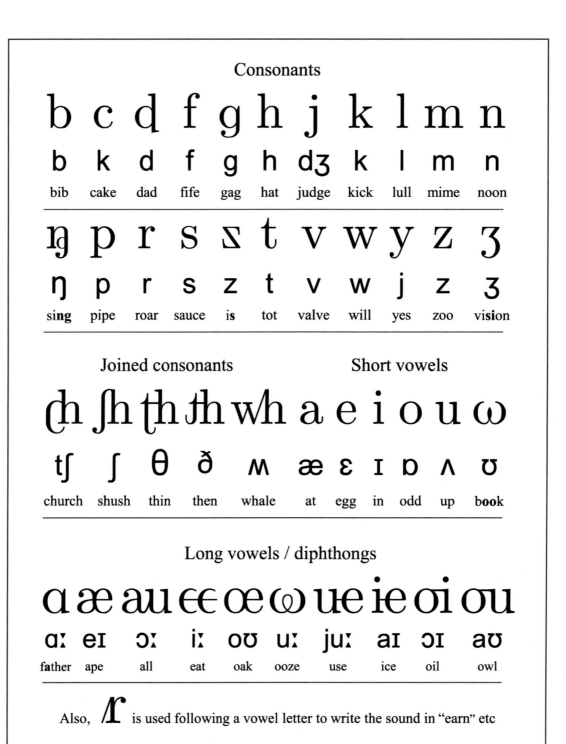

Figure 7-33B. The ITA. (By AnonMoos - Own work [Original text: Self-made graphic, created from scratch based on fonts and publicly-available information], Public Domain, https://commons.wikimedia.org/w/index.php?curid=12094872)

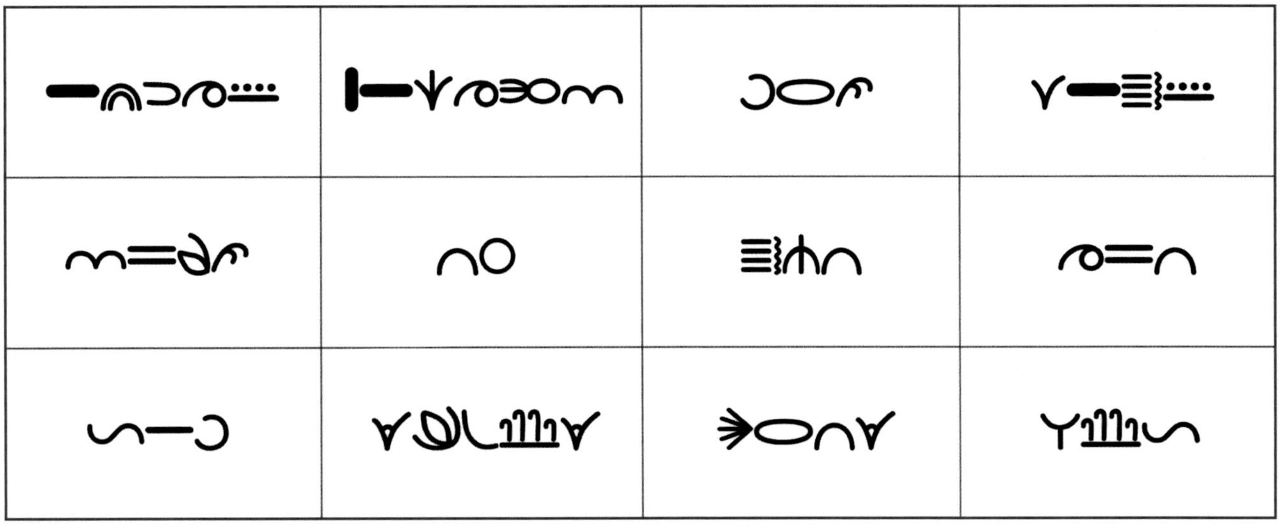

Figure 7-34. A representative sample of Visual Phonics. (Reproduced with permission from the International Communication Learning Institute.)

recognized the potential the symbols possessed as a communication system for persons with physical disabilities (Kates & McNaughton, 1975). The team members contacted Bliss and told him of the success of his system with the children in Canada. Although he had always envisioned his system as an international means of communication, he eventually came to realize that Blissymbolics could make an important contribution to the lives of individuals with speech impairments.

The Blissymbolics Communication Institute (now known as Blissymbolics Communication International) was established in Toronto in 1975. Bliss gave this organization a perpetual, worldwide (with the exception of Australia) exclusive license to his copyright for supporting the use of the system by persons with communication, language, and learning difficulties. In 1982, the Blissymbolics Communication Institute was entrusted with the worldwide authority and responsibility for Blissymbolics through a legal agreement with Bliss. Based on the performance of the Blissymbolics Communication Institute from 1982 through 2000, and again in 2007, this agreement was reaffirmed and expanded to include all applications (e.g., computer and internet applications, international communication) by the Semantography Trust.

Use of Blissymbolics has expanded from Canada to 33 countries around the globe. In the existing literature, Blissymbols is categorized as a linguistic symbol system due to its sophisticated structure and systematic rules to allow users to communicate unlimited ideas and thoughts with others (Pampoulou & Fuller, 2021; Smith, 2006). It is a semantic graphic language composed of more than 5,000 authorized symbols—Bliss-characters and Bliss-words—which when used based on the system's sophisticated rules, the individual can in fact communicate with anybody across the globe, as Blissymbols is an international graphic language.

In terms of their design, Blissymbols are line drawings, and like Chinese, are developed as a graphic language. Thereby, Blissymbols have all features of a language, such as vocabulary, morphology, and syntax and can be used both in verbal and written form. Blissymbols are designed on the meaning of a concept and those included in the Bliss-word are the most distinctive features of the concept (pictorial, functional, or scientific). This in fact is linguistically educational when teaching Blissymbolics for the purpose of AAC. Furthermore, the structure of Blissymbolics allows AAC learners to explore word formation themselves, which is something typically developing children do around 3 to 5 years of age (Jennische & Zetterlund, 2015). Due to its flexibility, Blissymbolics is used with individuals with CCN, but it can also support others for language learning.

The corpus of Blissymbolics has a finite number of graphic symbols (at one time referred to as semantic elements), and with the use of indicators and different strategies, the user can produce unlimited messages. For instance, the combination of symbols "water" and "chair" result in the symbol "toilet" (Figure 7-35). Another example is the referent "mother," for which the symbol is a woman with the primary function to protect the child. In most other collections of graphic symbols, this segmentation is not present. For instance, PCS has a fixed number of symbols, and there are no rules that can allow the creation of new ones (Pampoulou, 2015; Smith, 2006). Figure 7-35 shows the derivations of Blissymbols of a number of different referents that were also used as examples in the other corpuses of symbols in this chapter. Further information and learning about the structure of Blissymbolics is available at https://media.medfarm.uu.se/play/kanal/409.

CyberGlyphs. CyberGlyphs (originally Jet Era Glyphs) were conceived in the early 1960s (Zavalani, 1995) for a similar purpose as Blissymbolics, that is, as a means of communication between people who do not share a common language. More recently, these symbols have been used to some small degree by persons with severe communication disabilities. The symbols are semantically based in much the same way as Blissymbols, but unlike them, CyberGlyphs are intended to be hand-drawn (see Figure 7-36 for an example of the

Bliss-Words With All Meanings	Derivation	Component Parts	Comments
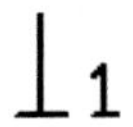 ⊥1 I,me,myself	First person, person number one.	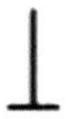 ⊥ 1 Person Number 1	Compare with second person pronoun: 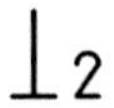 ⊥2 you
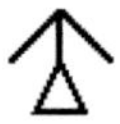 🔺 mother,mom,mommy,mum	Mother is a woman with the primary function to protect her child.	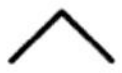 ⌃ △ Protection 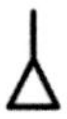 Woman	The shape of a roof has the abstract meaning of protection. Compare with father. 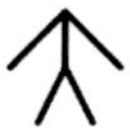 ⋀ father
+!! yes-(exclamatory)	Positive with exclamation.	+! positive ! Exclamation mark, intensity	Compare with "no." Exclamation mark: when following another symbol, it enhances meaning in a qualitative way.
—!! no-(exclamatory)	Negative with exclamation.	—! negative ! Exclamation mark, intensity	Compare with "yes."
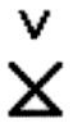 ˅ X more	Small multiplication meaning "much", can also be used to express comparative and superlative form of an adjective. The 'V' indicator denotes "descriptive word class"	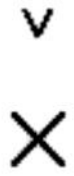 ˅ X much,many,very — reference line	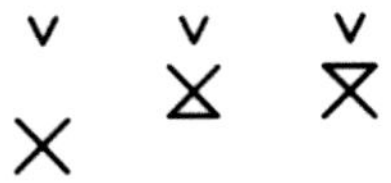 ˅ ˅ ˅ X X̿ X̄ much/many more most Comparative and superlative examples

Figure 7-35. A representative sample of Blissymbols. (Blissymbolics: © C.K. Bliss 1949. © Blissymbolics Communication International, 1982. Bliss-characters and Bliss-words used herein conform to the Blissymbolics Communication Institute Authorized Vocabulary as published by Blissymbolics Communication Institute, 1982-2022. For more information see www. blissymbolics.org.) (continued)

car,automobile,motor_vehicle	Pictograph of a car, but in accordance with the gloss and spoken word "car," it does not depict a specific kind of car.		Pictograph: The symbol depicts a simple outline shape of its referent.
bathroom,washroom	A room for bathing.	⌐ **room** ⌣ **bath**	room: ceiling, wall, floor bath: ⌣ container ~ water
toilet	A chair with water.	⊢ **chair** ~ **water**	Pictograph: The symbol depicts a simple outline shape of its referent.
happy, glad	A feeling of up; here with the descriptive indicator "V" (an adjective).	♡ **feeling** ↑ **up**	A heart has the abstract meaning of feeling, thus all Bliss-words for feelings start with a heart as the classifier.
angry, mad	Much feeling of opposition, being against + descriptive indicator, adjective.	V × **much** ♡ **feeling** 《 **opposition** V **descriptive indicator, adjective**	Opposition: Two arrowheads pointing back, against something, showing opposition to something.

Figure 7-35 (continued). A representative sample of Blissymbols. (Blissymbolics: © C.K. Bliss 1949. © Blissymbolics Communication International, 1982. Bliss-characters and Bliss-words used herein conform to the Blissymbolics Communication Institute Authorized Vocabulary as published by Blissymbolics Communication Institute, 1982-2022. For more information see www.blissymbolics.org.) (continued)

∨ ∧ sick,ill	A lying body with legs bent in pain. Descriptive indicator, adjective.		Pictograph: The symbol depicts a simple outline shape of its referent.
♡∧ pain,suffering	A feeling resulting from sickness.		Heart for feeling, plus sickness.
Λ̂ help,aid,assist,serve,support-(to)	Support being given to a person + action indicator, a verb.	Λ help ⊥ person ∧ action indicator	Pictographic, showing support to keep person upright.
Λ̂ →ǀ run,jog-(to)	Legs and feet + fast moving + action indicator, verb.	∧ legs and feet →! quickness	"Legs and·feet" symbol is pictographic, moving forward *quickly*, to run. Verb indicator appears over the classifier (usually the first) element. Adverb, "quickly" is inferred.
♡̂ ≀ want,desire-(to)	A feeling of burning with desire for something + action indicator, verb.	≀ fire ≀̂ burn-(to)	A flame, pictographic.
⬆̂ give,offer,provide-(to)	The container represents something (concrete or abstract) that one has. For "give," the arrow shows the direction out of the container + action indicator, verb.	⊍ container ↑ up	Contrast "give" with "get:" ⬇̂ get,acquire,receive-(to) For "get," the arrow points down into the container.

Figure 7-35 (continued). A representative sample of Blissymbols. (Blissymbolics: © C.K. Bliss 1949. © Blissymbolics Communication International, 1982. Bliss-characters and Bliss-words used herein conform to the Blissymbolics Communication Institute Authorized Vocabulary as published by Blissymbolics Communication Institute, 1982-2022. For more information see www.blissymbolics.org.)

recurring element "money" in all concepts related to money). The system is composed predominately of pictographs with a smaller proportion of ideographs and arbitrary symbols. A number of basic rules govern the production and use of CyberGlyphs making the system logical and expandable. Abstract thought in addition to concrete ideas can be represented by the symbols. Syntactic structure for CyberGlyphs has been adapted to the syntactic structure of English.

Piclish. Piclish (from "Picture English") is a symbol system based on American English, using the grammar of both written and spoken language. Each part of speech (e.g., adjectives, adverbs, articles, conjunctions, interjections, nouns, prepositions, pronouns, and verbs) has been grouped and color-coded with specific visual cues for learning vocabulary, parts of speech, and grammar.

PicLits, an abbreviation of Picture Literacy, are the individual symbols that make up the Piclish symbol system, which was created as a communication and language acquisition tool. Each symbol has two components: a form and a drawing. The form is color-coded for each part of speech (see examples in Figure 7-37). Drawings within the forms represent the meaning of the word and a label is provided within the text box to promote reading and to interpret the symbols for those who can read (Figure 7-38). Grammar markers are placed toward the outer edges of a number of the symbols. Each part of speech has a set of grammatical markers that make it possible to make nouns plural, conjugate verbs, etc. In Figure 7-38, see the marker of a triangle to indicate the irregular verb "get" and the marker of a gauge to indicate a comparative in the adverb "faster."

A brown bag represents an unspecified object or thing (i.e., the brown bag is used in PicLits when the object or thing is not specified). For example, note the symbol for "get" in Figure 7-38. The concept "get" means to actively receive something. The word "get" is not associated with a single object or thing but can be used in association with many objects or things (e.g., "get a job," "get my slippers," "get the ball"). Since "get" can apply to many objects or things, "get" utilizes the object symbol to indicate "get an object" or "get something." The symbol for the specific object or thing that is gotten appears immediately after the symbol for "get."

PicLits related to amounts and numbers use beads like those on an abacus (see "two" in Figure 7-38). The grammar marker for plural incorporates a double set of beads like those in the amount symbol "two" (Figure 7-39). The plural form of nouns is designated by this grammar marker that appears in the upper right-hand corner of the form. Plural nouns are also represented by two or more of the items within the PicLit's drawing area of the form. The multiple items make it easier for beginning communicators to learn about plurals, and the beads provide a consistent cue as individuals advance in their language skills. The possessive grammar marker is a hand grasping or possessing a ball. The possessive grammar marker appears in the lower right area of the form (see Figure 7-39).

PicLits verb forms are green with dark green figure(s) or object(s) in the drawing. The color green was selected because of the action "go" on traffic lights. When the context requires other symbols or parts of symbols for clarification, the colors of the symbol from which it was derived are used (Figure 7-40). When conjugating verbs in Piclish, two symbol changes occur. The *past tense* symbol of a PicLits verb appears as a figure or object in outline form to show an action has previously occurred. The remaining tense changes are in the form of grammatical markers (Figure 7-41). Prepositions are represented by gold-colored containers and maroon balls. Faded balls are used to represent both the position and the act of getting into that position (see the symbol "in" in Figure 7-42).

Symbols for all parts of speech, as well as the grammatical variations, have been created, and an instruction guide for expanding the system is available. PicLits symbols have been thoughtfully developed for use by all age groups and a wide range of learning styles and abilities. To fully represent English, Piclish appears to be very complicated; however, it can be used in a basic manner for those just starting out. Piclish can be used by individuals simply using single words, as well as those using full sentences (Figure 7-43).

Symbols can be added to the system within a drawing program in conjunction with the instruction and guidebooks developed for Piclish. PicLits can be animated for teaching concepts, such as "in" or "out" and "on" or "off." New noun PicLits can also be created by placing photos on the noun form and using the appropriate grammar markers.

PICSYMS. Faith Carlson did not start out to develop an AAC symbol system. Carlson had been using simple drawings while working with speaking children who had a variety of speech and language difficulties. In the 1960s, she began to work with a child who was unable to speak, read, or write and had limited motor skills. However, the child was able to draw, so student and clinician communicated with each other through simple drawings. As Carlson encountered more children with similar problems in her work, she began to develop communication boards and notebooks with cut out pictures and drawings. As other people requested symbols and pictures, Carlson formalized the systems she created following five guidelines. These guidelines include:

1. The system should be dynamic so it can change as the communicator advances or as spoken and written language changes.

2. The system needs to maintain the rules of spoken and written language.

3. Symbols should be interpreted for communication between partners in their language using a written label or spoken output.

4. Symbols need to look like what they mean.

5. The system or individual symbols need to be revised as the medium on which they are displayed advances.

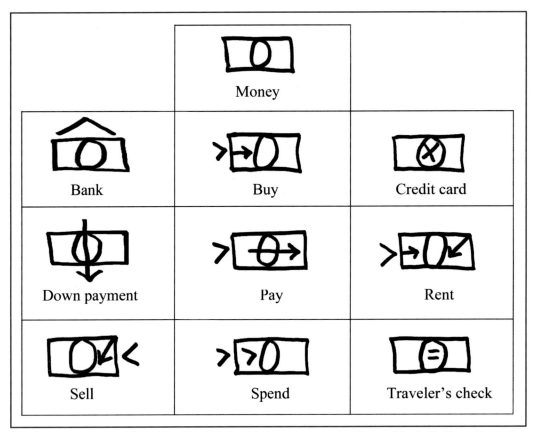

Figure 7-36. A representative sample of CyberGlyphs with the money-recurring element. (Created by Tomor Zavalani; rights currently owned by Claire and Rudy Zavalani. Used by permission.)

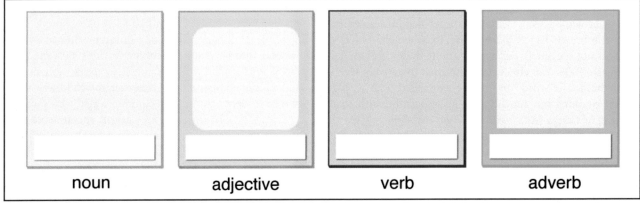

Figure 7-37. Color-coded part-of-speech boxes used in Piclish. (Reproduced with permission from Faith Carlson.)

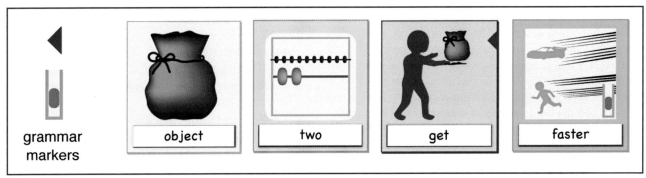

Figure 7-38. Irregular past tense and comparative grammatical markers in Piclish. (Reproduced with permission from Faith Carlson.)

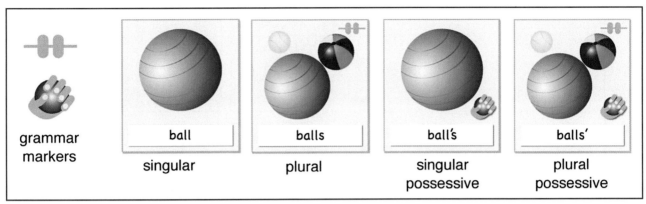

Figure 7-39. Plural and possessive grammatical markers used in Piclish. (Reproduced with permission from Faith Carlson.)

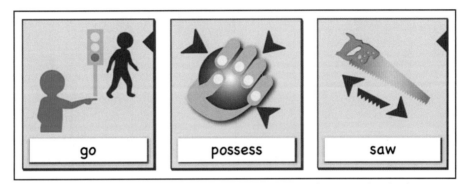

Figure 7-40. Using the same symbol form for derivative symbols in Piclish. (Reproduced with permission from Faith Carlson.)

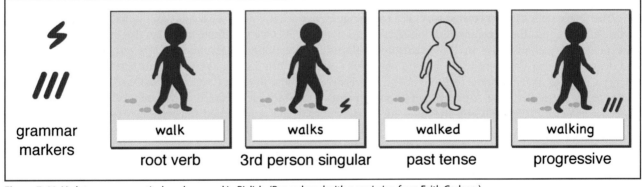

Figure 7-41. Verb tense grammatical markers used in Piclish. (Reproduced with permission from Faith Carlson.)

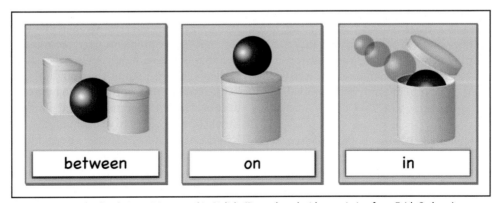

Figure 7-42. A sample of prepositions used in Piclish. (Reproduced with permission from Faith Carlson.)

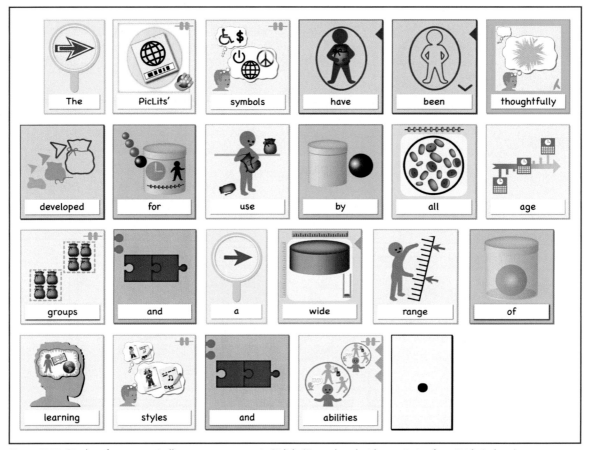

Figure 7-43. Display of a grammatically accurate sentence in Piclish. (Reproduced with permission from Faith Carlson.)

The first system Carlson created was PICSYMS (Figure 7-44). It is a hand-drawn communication symbol system first published in book form in 1985. Carlson developed the symbols during her work with children and adults at Meyer Children's Rehabilitation Institute of the University of Nebraska Medical Center. A paperbound book presents language rules for PICSYMS. Categories of words are drawn in a specific fashion to better define the words in the category (e.g., for symbols involving humans, the people appear as stick figures with all solid lines). People used in action symbols were a combination of solid or dotted lines with an arrow showing the direction of the action (see Figure 7-44).

PICSYMS have a degree of expansion capability in that parents, teachers, and others can create new symbols within the guidelines set forth in the book. Many adults do not have confidence in their drawing skills; therefore, the book has instructions for creating new symbols for the system using a pen or pencil and paper with a grid if necessary (see Figure 7-44). This makes it possible to instantly add a symbol/word using minimal drawing skills whenever a new concept is encountered.

Sigsymbol-Elaborated Words. Some children with language delay or cognitive impairment struggle to recognize printed or written words, which severely hinders their mastery of reading skills. However, it has been established that items presented in picture format can be encoded more

effectively than text, and so, improve retention (Hazamy, 2009). One technique that takes this into account and assists recognition is elaboration of text with some aspect of a picture (also known as symbol enhancement or symbol accentuation; Jones & Cregan 1986). Once a student has learned to label a pictorialized word, symbol elaboration has done its job and can be faded and eventually removed.

Pictorialization is not always straightforward, so extension of vocabulary by this technique may be inhibited. Notably, pictures may be impractical or restrictive as to situation due to the abstract nature of many referents. In such a context, Sigsymbol-elaborated words (SEWs) offer an approach that is more than serviceable as a substitute for conventional pictorial enhancement (Figure 7-45). If Sigsymbols are already familiar, ideographic elaboration poses few comprehension problems once the meaningful features are pointed out. The same applies to elaboration with sign-linked Sigsymbols, when stimulating physical activity also should be involved as part of the learning process. On their introduction, SEW elaborations based on familiar Sigsymbols should be penciled onto written or printed text (the red color is optional according to a user's needs but does reinforce the cue) to be faded as appropriate.

No clinician or teacher needs a course in sign language to use elaborated text. A simple hand or finger position or movement can be devised to represent a particular word.

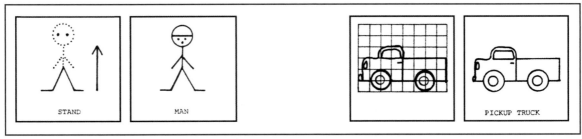

Figure 7-44. A representative sample of PICSYMS. (Reproduced with permission from Faith Carlson.)

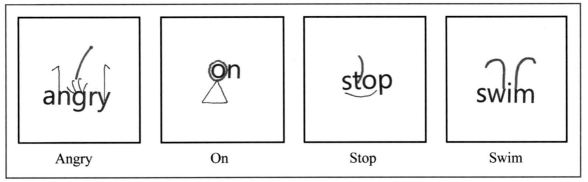

Figure 7-45. SEWs. The elements of the four Sigsymbols pictured in Figures 7-47 and 7-48, later familiarized to the would-be reader, elaborating the cognate printed words to provide meaning-cues during the learning process. (Reproduced with permission from Ailsa Cregan.)

This invented sign can then—with the help of the system's design guidelines, as previously noted—be transformed into a Sigsymbol for on-the-spot word elaboration to assist early reading.

It should be noted that SEWs are no longer mass marketed. However, any interested party—AAC users, family members, or professionals—may contact the creator of these symbols, Ailsa Cregan, for more information and assistance.

Sigsymbols. Developed by Ailsa Cregan in the United Kingdom in the early 1980s, Sigsymbols comprise a system of graphic symbols developed in the context of teaching a small group of adolescents with severe cognitive impairment. Some members of the group could use a few single spoken words but did not form sentences. All were institutionalized, so socialization was relevant in parallel with fostering communication. To render participation sociably enjoyable, Sigsymbols were shown to the students on sturdy 3-inch square cards, available to be handled by all in a variety of learning games and activities (Cregan, 1990).

Sigsymbols differ from many other aided systems, having not been conceived as an actual communication system but rather as a teaching tool serving to promote speech step by step. The first step in which a limited number of symbols is introduced at any one time focuses essentially on comprehension (Sevcik 2006; Sevcik et al., 2018). To broaden and deepen students' understanding, meaning is supplemented by the presentation of objects, pictures, mime, and gesture (Vogt & Kauschke, 2017). An accompanying focus is symbol recognition, assisted by growing familiarity and comprehension.

At the introduction of each symbol, its spoken-word label should be frequently repeated by the teacher. Meanwhile, the nontransitory nature of the graphic symbols facilitates various modes of repetition and review to maximize retention.

The second teaching step focuses on the introduction of manual signs when each one should be demonstrated along with the Sigsymbol for the same referent. Signs should be accompanied by the spoken word. Students cued by Sigsymbols are encouraged—and helped if necessary—to make the signs themselves. This active physical involvement in the context of the familiar symbol acts as a further aid to memory (Dandashi et al., 2015). At this stage, learning games, such as Sigsymbol Lotto, involve graphic symbols with manual signs and words spoken by the teacher.

The third teaching step stresses use of spoken words by the student. The aim is that a familiar sign prompted by a symbol card or used spontaneously should serve as a self-produced portable cue. The involvement of signing parallels the way gesture plays a crucial part in early language development, paving the way for future language development (Iverson & Goldin-Meadow, 2005).

Once the second and third steps are attained, the lower levels gradually become redundant. However, their use should be discontinued only if a student group as a whole is no longer reliant on them.

With the aim of promoting easy comprehension and retention, Sigsymbols evolved as a hybrid system in which the most basic strategy was the use of pictographic Sigsymbols (Figure 7-46). The blob in the "give" symbol represents the

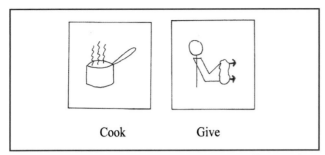

Figure 7-46. Pictographic Sigsymbols. Cook: represented by a simple-to-draw object, readily related to cooking. Give: depiction of an unspecified object (represented by the "blob") being given away in the direction of the red arrows. (Reproduced with permission from Ailsa Cregan.)

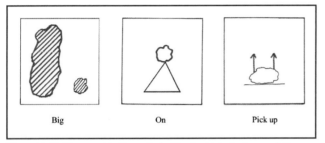

Figure 7-47. Ideographic Sigsymbols. Big: the blobs indicate relative sizes. The red color is the meaning-signifier of the Sigsymbol. Each blob represents an unspecified object (cf. Figure 7-46, Give). On: the position of the red blob relative to the triangle indicates the meaning. (The triangle has a natural orientation, apex upwards.) Pick up: the red arrows indicate the upward movement of the blob as it is picked up. (Reproduced with permission from Ailsa Cregan.)

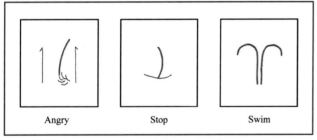

Figure 7-48. Sign-linked Sigsymbols. Angry: the black clawed hand depicts the initial position of the right hand in front of the signer's body, prior to its upward movement as indicated by the red line. Stop: the black line represents the flat left hand in horizontal position. The red line represents the flat right hand after it has moved to land edge-on onto the left hand. Swim: the red lines indicate the movement of the hands as in breast stroke; the hands themselves are not represented. (Reproduced with permission from Ailsa Cregan.)

thing being given without restricting it to a specific item. Ideographic Sigsymbols employ blobs in a similar way, as in some adjectives, positional prepositions and verbs of action (Figure 7-47). In the Sigsymbol "on," the blob is colored red to highlight its meaningful role. It is shown in relation to a triangle, chosen to enhance meaning as it has a natural orientation with its apex pointing upward. In the Sigsymbol "pick up," the arrows pointing upward from the blob are colored red to stress movement and direction. Red is also used to highlight the salient aspect of a polar adjective, while its

black contrast presents the opposite for comparison (e.g., the red blob in the symbol "big" is not big in an absolute sense, but its bigness is clear in relation to a smaller black blob within the compass of the symbol). Sigsymbol design is flexible, allowing modifications to suit the user, the situation, or the preference of an instructor. Thus, an alternative design for "pick up" might show a stick figure in the process of picking up a blob.

The most innovative feature of the whole system is the inclusion of sign-linked Sigsymbols, which are an integral part of its role as a teaching tool (Figure 7-48). In fact, the word "Sigsymbol" is a shortened form of "sign-symbol." This derives from the third type of graphic symbol whose linkage is with the sign language used by the Deaf community of the region (e.g., British Sign Language in the United Kingdom; American Sign Language in the United States). Sign-linked symbols can also be designed at will to match personally chosen signs or signs from another region or country. The precise design and extent of currently available vocabulary as it appears in the manual *Sigsymbols: American Edition* (Cregan & Lloyd, 1990) is not sacrosanct, whereas all-important is the system's functionality for the population involved.

Sign-linkage is a form of concretization of an abstract concept or for any referents difficult to represent using a pictograph or ideograph. A sign-linked symbol does not set out to be a complete and faithful representation of a manual sign—each one is an approximation of a greater or lesser part of that sign, sufficiently distinctive not to be easily confused with other Sigsymbols. Brief design guidelines are as follows:

- Simplified, schematized hand or finger representations are designed from descriptions/illustrations in a manual of signs
- When drawn in black, the symbols show initial position(s) of the hands and/or fingers when making a sign
- Representation in red of hands and fingers indicates their final position after movement within the sign
- Red line(s) indicate a movement trace, sometimes (as in "swim" in Figure 7-48) in the absence of any hand representation

It should be noted that Sigsymbols are no longer available on the open market. However, one may obtain the finite corpus of symbols and rules for generating new symbols by contacting the creator of Sigsymbols, Ailsa Cregan.

Electronically Generated Symbols

As the term implies, symbols classified in this manner are acoustic, generated either by digitally recorded or synthesized speech. Therefore, synthetic speech is the only symbol system that is included under this category.

Synthetic Speech. Synthetic speech is any type of electronically produced speech, whether digitally recorded, generated by text-to-speech, or a combination of the two. As natural speech is the gold standard by which all other AAC symbols are compared (especially in terms of rate of transmission), one goal of AAC intervention is to provide a system of communication that not only meets the AAC user's communication needs but also allows them to communicate at a rate that is as close as possible to the rate of communication employed by others (natural speech is produced at a rate of approximately 175 to 180 words per minute). Most AAC systems fall far short of a natural rate of production because of sensory, physical, or other impairments on the part of the individual with CCN. Nevertheless, all things considered, synthetic speech is the gold standard by which all other aided symbols are compared.

In the majority of cases, synthetic speech is part of an individual's AAC system by virtue of the fact the speech is being produced by an SGD. However, for individuals who use SGDs, there should always be other aided options, as well as unaided options, for communication when environment or other circumstances do not allow for the use of synthetic speech. Some individuals who use AAC may not be able to use an SGD, so other aided and unaided options should be made available to them.

CHARACTERISTICS OF AIDED AAC SYMBOLS

Physical Characteristics

Regarding the *physical characteristics* of aided symbols, these can be grouped into three broad categories: two-dimensional, three-dimensional, and acoustic. As the name suggests, three-dimensional symbols have three dimensions (height x width x depth) and are object-based symbols.

Two-dimensional symbols possess the dimensions of height and width but not depth. They are sometimes referred to as flat symbols, but in this chapter, we refer to them as two-dimensional. Two-dimensional symbols can be subcategorized into static (i.e., those that do not require movement to convey meaning) and kinetic or animated (i.e., movement or animation is one of their key characteristics).

The third and last category based on physical characteristics are acoustic symbols—those produced by synthetic speech on SGDs. Although they are acoustic, these symbols are aided because the person needs a device separate from their body to be able to access the synthetic speech and communicate with others. Animated may be considered by some to be a fourth category of physical characteristics for aided symbols.

Design Characteristics

Another important aspect of AAC aided symbols is their *design characteristics*, which are very much influenced by their physical properties. Based on the design attributes of symbols, these can be categorized as alphabet-based, electronically based, line drawing–based, object-based, phonemic- or phonetic-based, and pictorially based.

In terms of their design attributes, objects are easy to distinguish from the other categories of symbols. Pictorial and line-drawing symbols are similar in that they are two-dimensional. However, as the term denotes, pictorial symbols are more pictographic and less ideographic or arbitrary. Their ability to represent language is limited, and as Vinson (2001) states, while photographs can be used as symbols for nouns, representation is not as effective for verbs and modifiers. On the other hand, line drawings are also pictorial but to a lesser degree (with a higher degree of ideographic and arbitrary symbols), and for this reason, they are capable of representing a wider range of vocabulary.

As mentioned previously, design attributes of aided AAC symbols also include alphabet-based, electronically based, and phonemic- or phonetic-based symbols. Alphabet-based symbols use either the letters of the alphabet or variants of the alphabet (i.e., dits and dahs, raised dots). Modified orthography can also be alphabet-based. Electronically based symbols are sounds, words, phrases, and sentences produced by synthetic speech. Finally, phonemic- or phonetic-based symbols are based on the *sounds* of a language instead of alphabetic letters. Their distinguishing characteristic is the one-to-one correspondence between phonemic or phonetic characters and the speech sounds of a language.

Perceptual Characteristics

Iconicity

Iconicity is one of the most well-investigated characteristics of symbols and refers to the degree to which a symbol resembles its referent or some aspect of it. Iconicity actually can be represented as a continuum with transparent and opaque symbols at opposite poles. Transparent symbols have a strong visual resemblance to their referents, and hence, the viewer can easily recognize them (Fuller, 1997). On the other hand, opaque symbols have no visual relationship between the symbol and its referent, and thus, the viewer must learn and memorize the relationship that exists between the two (Fuller & Lloyd, 1991). Translucent symbols fall between, and to some extent, overlap the two aforementioned extremes, where the relationship between the symbol and its referent can be understood when the person realizes the rules or the convention that exists between the two (Fuller & Lloyd, 1991).

One important work in the field of AAC was conducted by Mirenda and Locke (1989) who explored the iconicity of different types of symbols in 40 nonspeaking individuals with autism and mild to severe intellectual impairment. Eleven aided sets and systems (black and white photographs, Blissymbols, identical colored photographs, miniature objects, nonidentical colored photographs, nonidentical objects, PCS, PICSYMS, rebus, Self-Talk, written words) were compared according to their transparency. Results indicated real objects were more readily recognized than any of the other symbols, and Blissymbols and written words were more difficult than any of the other symbols.

Iconicity has also been found to be one of the key characteristics speech-language pathologists take into consideration when choosing the most appropriate corpus of symbols for their users (Pampoulou, 2006, 2015, 2017a; Pampoulou & Fuller, 2020). However, it should be noted that iconicity is inconsistent and changes across different word categories (Mizuko & Reichle, 1989). For example, Bloomberg and colleagues (1990) found that among the five collections of graphic symbols they studied, nouns were the most translucent items whereas verbs proved to be more translucent than modifiers for rebus, PCS, and PIC symbols. In contrast, for the Blissymbols and PICSYMS symbol corpuses, findings suggested that translucency is equivalent for both verbs and modifiers. It also has been contended that nouns are more concrete referents in comparison with other word types, such as verbs or even abstract nouns (Schlosser & Sigafoos, 2002) in that they can be easily depicted in symbol form, and thus, are easier to understand than other parts of speech, such as verbs (Simone, 1995).

It should be noted that despite the fact iconicity was well researched in the 1980s and 1990s, there has been somewhat a stagnation of inquiry into the topic in recent years. It is important this type of research be continued, as evidence shows iconicity is one of the key characteristics to which speech-language pathologists focus during the process of choosing the most appropriate symbols for their users. Also, there has been virtual nonstop development of new corpuses of AAC symbols over the past couple decades; iconicity has not yet been investigated for these new symbol corpuses.

Complexity

Complexity as a characteristic of AAC aided symbols is not an easy term to define because, through the years, it has been defined in several different ways. For instance, Silverman (1995) defined it as the relation of figure information to the background of a symbol. Thus, complexity can be related to the sophistication of a graphic symbol; the more information contained within it, the greater the complexity of the symbol. For instance, some photographs might be relatively complex because they include considerable visual information. Imagine a photograph of someone reading a book at a desk while a library full of books is in the background. This photograph easily can have more than one meaning, such as "library," "reading," and "studying," to name a few. Complexity can also refer to the number of semantic elements or strokes required to produce symbols (Fuller & Lloyd, 1987; Luftig & Bersani, 1985). However, from a practical point of view, this cannot be used as the operational definition of complexity because the majority of graphic symbols do not lend themselves well to the counting of strokes and very few are composed of semantic elements. At the present time, a clear, unambiguous definition for complexity has not been developed; therefore, it is not fully understood how complexity affects the acquisition and retention of aided AAC symbols.

Perceptual Distinctness

Another characteristic of aided symbols is **perceptual distinctness**, which refers to the degree to which a symbol seems obviously different and distinct from others within a given symbol corpus. According to Lloyd (1997), this characteristic is important when learning new vocabulary. For instance, for opposites—such as hot vs. cold and clean vs. dirty—it is important to have perceptual distinctness among the symbols to facilitate acquisition, retention, and retrieval. Note the Blissymbol for "happy" in the middle of Figure 7-35. The Blissymbol for "sad" differs from "happy" only in the orientation of the arrow (the arrow points downward for "sad"). These two symbols would not be considered perceptually distinct.

Degree of Ambiguity

The degree of ambiguity pertains to the number of concepts a single symbol can represent. Symbols with more ambiguity represent a larger number of distinct concepts (Lloyd, 1997). This flexibility of ambiguity can prove beneficial for some individuals who use individual symbols to communicate a number of different meanings. While the degree of ambiguity can be determined by the relationship between a symbol and its referent, it can also be altered based on the interpretation that the interpretant gives to this relationship. As was discussed in Chapter 6, the meaning of symbols depends on the interpretation the interpretant gives to the relation that exists between a symbol and its referent (Pampoulou, 2017a).

Size

The size of symbols is also important, as changes in size can denote different meanings. Physical size refers to the physical, measurable dimensions of a symbol which is often important for individuals with visual impairments. Vocabulary size refers to the size of the original lexicon the symbol corpus represents. Corpuses of symbols that have generative rules provide for the expansion of vocabulary beyond the original corpus, and it is this variable that determines what constitutes a symbol collection or set from a symbol system. One should keep in mind there is a trade off between symbol size and the number of symbols that can appear on a display. Fewer symbols can be displayed at a time if the symbols are large as opposed to smaller.

It is important to highlight how the different characteristics of currently available corpuses of symbols play a vital role when it comes to the difficult task speech-language pathologists often face when choosing the most appropriate corpus(es) for their clients who require AAC for communication (Pampoulou, 2017). As Pampoulou and Fuller (2020) have noted, the majority of existing literature surrounding symbol characteristics has focused on iconicity. Despite the fact that iconicity plays a major role when it comes to the learnability and retention of symbols, more recent evidence shows that other factors are equally important when it comes to choosing the most appropriate symbols for end-users (Pampoulou, 2006, 2015, 2017; Pampoulou & Fuller, 2020). The process of choosing the most suitable corpus(es) of symbols is crucial, as it has a considerable impact on end-users in terms of addressing their linguistic needs and capacities in a way that allows them to communicate to their fullest capacity (Pampoulou & Fuller, 2020).

A New Age for Studying Aided AAC Symbol Characteristics

Pampoulou and Fuller (2020) investigated the characteristics of corpuses of symbols speech-language pathologists in Texas and Cyprus consider when choosing the most appropriate corpus(es) of two-dimensional symbols, such as Blissymbols, Makaton, or PCS, for their clients or patients. These investigators initially conducted an online survey with multiple-choice answers in which they included a number of potential characteristics of aided symbols. Most of the participants indicated that when they choose the most appropriate corpus of symbols for their client or patient, they focus on symbol characteristics, such as correspondence to the oral language of the general community, their design (e.g., simple line drawings by contrast to pictorial graphic symbols), ease of learning, vocabulary size (i.e., the size of the original lexicon the graphic symbol corpus represents), and the availability of specific vocabulary for the person's needs (e.g., activities of daily living, curriculum, work). Pampoulou and Fuller (2020) probed the influence of additional factors that could eventually influence the decision of speech-language pathologists regarding which corpus(es) of aided symbols to choose for their clients. These additional characteristics were categorized as environmental (i.e., how physical setting affects symbol use), financial (i.e., available funding), and technological (i.e., the availability of symbol-generating software). These findings align with the outcomes of another research project conducted in the United Kingdom and Cyprus (Pampoulou, 2017b). It would not be inaccurate to claim that speech-language pathologists in different parts of the world are influenced by similar factors when faced with the process of choosing the most appropriate corpus(es) of symbols for their AAC users. Perhaps a new era is dawning in AAC where clinicians and researchers begin to dig down deeper into the characteristics of aided symbols that influence their acquisition, retention, and retrieval.

SUMMARY

Aided AAC symbols can be distinctly different in terms of their linguistic and physical characteristics, as well as their design attributes. For clinicians working with people with CCN, it is vital they are familiar with these characteristics in order to be able to identify and choose the most appropriate corpus(es) of symbols for their clients or patients who use AAC. In this chapter, aided AAC symbols were presented and described primarily based on their linguistic characteristics because they are used for the purpose of communication. The level of communication interaction is dependent upon the degree to which a corpus of symbols allows for vocabulary expansion and correspondence to the oral and written language of the larger community. As has been posited in this chapter, linguistic characteristics of different corpuses of symbols can be viewed from a quaternary continuum perspective, starting with non-linguistic symbols and moving on to pre-linguistic and finally linguistic ones. Generally speaking, as one moves from non-linguistic to linguistic communication, symbol corpuses become increasingly more flexible in terms of internal logic, expansion capability, a larger resulting lexicon, and greater representational range. Naturally, linguistic symbol systems more closely parallel the oral and written language of the larger community than symbols having lesser linguistic characteristics. The chapter concluded with a brief discussion of aided symbol characteristics, including iconicity, complexity, perceptual distinctness, degree of ambiguity, and size (both physical size of symbols and vocabulary size represented by a given symbol corpus), with a view toward more systematic studies on how symbol characteristics can best be used to facilitate communication and literacy.

STUDY QUESTIONS

1. Briefly describe one object-based symbol set.
2. Briefly describe one pictorial-based symbol set that does not have linguistic characteristics.
3. Briefly describe one symbol system that does have linguistic characteristics.
4. Briefly describe aided representation of fingerspelling.
5. Briefly describe one alphabet-based system besides traditional orthography.
6. Briefly describe one phonemic- or phonic-based system.
7. Briefly discuss characteristics of aided AAC symbols. What are the implications for individuals with severe communication impairments?

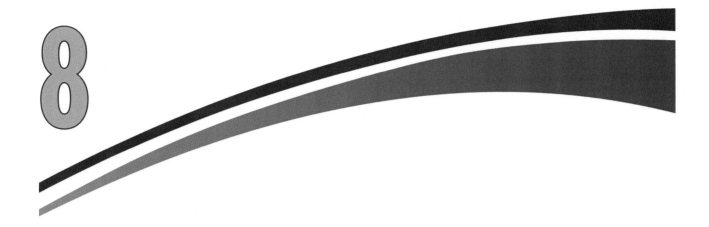

8

Unaided AAC Components

Susan M. Bashinski, EdD and Barbara A. Braddock, PhD
With contributions from Lyle L. Lloyd, PhD

<table>
<tr><td>

MYTH

1. Unaided forms of augmentative and alternative communication (AAC) are generally straightforward. The only legitimate, effective unaided AAC systems are the various manual sign language systems utilized around the world.

</td><td>

REALITY

1. Unaided communication systems vary widely in levels of sophistication and complexity. Authentic, meaningful unaided communication systems take many modes, ranging from idiosyncratic nonsymbolic forms, to deictic and representational gestures, to a multiplicity of educational sign systems and very abstract linguistic forms. It is only through an understanding of the full range of legitimate unaided communication types that educators and speech-language pathologists can effectively work with interprofessional teams to build appropriate multimodal systems of communication for the individuals with whom they work.

</td></tr>
</table>

INTRODUCTION TO UNAIDED AUGMENTATIVE COMMUNICATION COMPONENTS

Unaided communication requires nothing external to the communicator's body (as a whole or one or more of its parts) to be used for the purpose of expression. The vocal tract, mouth, tongue, lips, and respiratory system are crucial for production of vocalizations and natural speech. Hands, arms, facial expressions, body posture, pointing, physical action, and movement are important for gestures and manual signs; additionally, changes in muscle tone, rate of respiration, eye contact, and gaze, as well as gross body movements, may be utilized for unconventional unaided communication expression.

The following sections of this chapter will provide the historical and theoretical background of sign languages and other unaided systems of communication; explain the rationale for the exclusion of formal sign languages from this

Fuller, D. R., & Lloyd, L. L. *Principles and Practices in Augmentative and Alternative Communication* (pp. 135-169).

chapter; present the benefits of multimodal communication and the use of unaided AAC to augment natural speech; discuss the basic characteristics of many various systems of unaided communication, including earlier intervention with infants and toddlers in the use of AAC; suggest a classification and categorization approach for unaided communication signals and symbols; and discuss the challenges and benefits of successfully implementing unaided AAC programming with individuals who experience significant communication delay or disorder.

Differentiation From Aided AAC

Simply stated, what sets "aided" augmentative communication elements (i.e., those discussed in Chapter 7 of this book) apart from "unaided" communication components is that aided AAC involves "… the use of aids external to the communicator's body" (Loncke, 2014, p. 4).

The aided component could involve a learner who functions primarily at a **nonsymbolic** level (discussed later in this chapter) *utilizing another person's body* to express a communicative message. Examples might include a young child or learner with limited mobility *reaching out to grab the pant leg of another person* as they walk by (to communicate, "Hey, I'm here; pay attention to me") or an individual *taking the arm of a communication partner* and walking them to the refrigerator or snack cabinet to communicate, "I'm hungry and want a snack." Some individuals in the field of AAC do not view the above two italicized examples as aided communication. However, strictly defined, "[a]ided communication involves modes that are not part of the individual's own body" (Reichle et al., 2002, p. 30). In the italicized examples, the individual utilizes another person's clothing or body for the purpose of communication. "Unaided communication modes refer to methods of communication that do not involve additional equipment (e.g., speech, facial expressions, body language, gestures, sign language, sign systems)" (Johnston et al., 2012, p. 26). Examples of aided communication include use of objects, low tech communication boards, topic boards, textural or tactile symbols, and any of the wide variety of speech-generating devices (SGDs)—accessed through any means.

Clarification of the Parameters of Unaided AAC

It bears repeating that unaided communication involves *nothing external to the communicator's body* for successful conveyance of a communication expression. Unaided communication expressions may take many forms, including the individual's entire body, one or more of its parts, and vocalizations and natural speech. As will be developed in subsequent sections of this chapter, a comprehensive view of unaided communication includes both nonsymbolic (i.e., non-linguistic or pre-linguistic) and linguistic forms

(Loncke, 2014). The classification of unaided symbols, according to the multidimensional quaternary symbol continuum model as proposed by Pampoulou and Fuller (2020), is presented in Table 3-4.

HISTORICAL AND THEORETICAL BACKGROUND OF UNAIDED AAC COMPONENTS

The use of unaided communication is not a recent phenomenon. Even before fingerspelling was introduced by Juan Pablo Bonet in the 17th century for use in the instruction of children who were deaf, the manual alphabet (hand alphabet) was reportedly already in use (Savage et al., 1981). In the second half of the 18th century, manual signing was considered to be the key to educating deaf children in France; its use spread over several countries of Europe and into North America in subsequent decades. The term "manual sign" referred to the elements of either naturally developed sign systems and/or fingerspelling. That is, manual sign was the visual-gestural equivalent of words in spoken and written language.

Although records indicate that small Deaf communities existed before the second half of the 18th century, the establishment of schools for deaf children at the end of that century was a catalyst in the development of Deaf communities. The discovery of signing as a powerful tool to convey information had led to dramatic changes in the way deaf individuals were perceived by the educational and academic community. Previously, deafness had been equated with impossibility of education and inaccessibility to human language and culture (Lane, 1984).

However, in the second half of the 19th century, signing was largely abandoned throughout Europe and in many United States schools for deaf children. The assumption that use of manual sign was linguistically inferior to spoken language had gained widespread support, as was the belief that manual sign interfered with the acquisition of speech. At the Congress of Milan in 1880, educators of the Deaf proclaimed that the so-called oral method was the only viable way of educating deaf children. Sign language was considered to be harmful to the objectives of spoken language acquisition and social integration into the world of people who were hearing and communicating through speaking.

However, regardless of prevalent educational policy, many individuals who were deaf continued to use signing as their vernacular language. In the United States, a special situation continued to exist at Gallaudet College (now Gallaudet University) in Washington, D.C. Gallaudet is well-known as a liberal arts college founded in 1864 to provide higher education for students who experience hearing loss. The policy of this university has always supported the use of manual sign as the primary teaching approach for deaf individuals throughout the United States.

Reconfirmation of Manual Sign Language as a True Language

Although signing never completely disappeared from the education of deaf children, it was the discovery of the full linguistic nature of signs and sign languages (Stokoe, 1960) that resulted in a significant breakthrough regarding the status of manual sign language. Gradually, educators in programs for students with hearing impairments felt pressure to reconsider the basic premises on which curricula and teaching methods were built, leading to the reintroduction of signing in schools and educational programs.

Negative assumptions regarding manual signing significantly shifted only during the last few decades of the 20th century as major changes regarding theoretical perspectives of language structure, language acquisition, and communication development became well recognized. One of the more significant changes was the acknowledgement that language competence is different from language performance (Chomsky, 1965; Pinker, 1994), which fostered the idea that the connection between internal language capacity and salient observable language behaviors might allow for variation. Hence, contrary to former beliefs, researchers began to ask whether the primary expressive modality of a language could be something other than speech. It was concluded that manual sign languages evolved over centuries by individuals who experienced congenital profound hearing loss or acquired this degree of loss pre-lingually—just as children learning spoken languages have done.

If this were true, manual sign communication within Deaf communities could, and should, be regarded as genuine, unique languages—equal in status and power to spoken language but different in form. The first primary generation of sign language research demonstrated that this indeed was the case. In their publication *The Signs of Language* (1979), Klima and Bellugi depicted American Sign Language (ASL) as a visual communication system with its own phonological and morphosyntactical rules. The rejection of manual sign on the basis of its "non-linguistic" nature was demonstrated to be based on myth. Today, the full linguistic nature of the sign languages of Deaf communities is no longer a matter of debate (e.g., Ahlgren et al., 1994; Faurot et al., 2000; Klima & Bellugi, 1979). In fact, nearly as many sign languages exist around the world as do oral languages (Table 8-1).

Explanation Regarding Exclusion of Sign Language From This Chapter

This chapter has purposefully not provided an in-depth discussion of sign languages for reasons cited in the section Reconfirmation of Manual Sign Language as a True Language (earlier in this chapter). In their respective countries, the sign languages utilized by the Deaf community (e.g., ASL, Belgian Sign Language, British Sign Language, Dutch Sign Language) stand on their own as genuine, unique, legitimate languages. These sign languages do not "augment" the language spoken in a given country.

True sign languages (in contrast to educational/pedagogical sign systems) are visual communication systems with their own phonological and morphosyntactical rules, each of which maintains an intimate relationship with the culture of the country/region where it is utilized. Since sign languages are *not* viewed as an augmentation to the language of a given country (Loncke, 2014), they will not be explored in detail in this chapter. Using manual signs to augment oral communication in a native tongue is totally different than using manual signs within the context of ASL (or the native sign language of another country) as elements of the unique language it is. That said, sign languages are classified as unaided linguistic symbol systems.

POWER OF MULTIMODAL COMMUNICATION

Multimodal communication is more the rule than the exception. Especially when a given situation makes both visual and auditory reception possible, as in most face-to-face interactions, communication partners tend to frequently combine speech, gestures, pointing, and handling of objects. The majority of such communication exchanges are, in fact, multimodal (Mirenda, 1999). Multimodal functioning is highly natural. Generally, communication partners are sensitive in selecting appropriate modes of communication to ensure maximum successful information exchange (Lloyd & Kangas, 1994), thus making communication more efficient and enhancing understanding (Sigafoos & Drasgow, 2001).

Scholars increasingly have found that when speech communication is not readily accessible for any number of reasons, other modalities (e.g., aided and unaided communication forms) can assume many of the linguistic functions that speech serves in individuals who are typically developing. Unaided communication is frequently combined with aided communication. For example, some hearing children with characteristics of autism may be better at processing linguistic and non-linguistic symbols if these are presented visually. An AAC user of an SGD (see Chapters 7, 10, and 14) may combine electronic speech production with eye gazing, gestures, pointing, and/or vocalizations. These examples illustrate that though a person may have trouble understanding and producing speech, they are nevertheless able to acquire language if presented via another modality (e.g., manual signs, traditional orthography, or other graphic symbols). Particularly in the case of an individual for whom it is not clear whether an aided or unaided augmented system of communication might be most effective, use of a multimodal system offers the distinct advantage of "covering all the bases" (Beukelman & Mirenda, 2013; Reichle et al., 1991). For

TABLE 8-1
A Sampling of World Sign Languages

COUNTRY	SIGN LANGUAGE	SAMPLE CHARACTERISTICS
Australia	Auslan	Two-handed manual alphabet and fingerspelling
Belgium	Flemish Sign Language	One-handed alphabet
Canada (most of the country)	ASL	Large number of initialized signs One-handed alphabet
Canada (Québec)	Langue des Signes Québécoise	One-handed alphabet
China	Chinese Sign Language	One-handed alphabet Unrelated to Taiwanese Sign Language
France	French Sign Language	Large number of initialized signs One-handed alphabet
Hong Kong	Hong Kong Sign Language	Makes no use of initialized signs No manual alphabet, no fingerspelling
India	Indian Sign Language	Several commonalities with ASL Standardized grammar throughout the country
Mexico	Mexican Sign Language	Initialized signs more fully integrated into the sign language than most (Faurot et al., 2000) More common use of initialized signs than most
Nepal	Nepali Sign Language	Initialized signs more fully integrated into the sign language than most
The Netherlands	Dutch Sign Language Nederlandse Gebarentaal	Not officially recognized
Pakistan	Indo-Pakistani Sign Language	Far fewer initialized signs than most Two-handed manual alphabet
Sweden	*Svenskt teckenspråk* (Swedish Sign Language)	One-handed manual alphabet Self-created language; does not stem from any other
Taiwan	Taiwanese Sign Language	Makes no use of initialized signs No manual alphabet, no fingerspelling
United Kingdom	British Sign Language	Two-handed manual alphabet and fingerspelling Official sign language in England, Scotland, and the European Union Not mutually intelligible with users of ASL
United States	ASL	Large number of initialized signs "… not primarily a pedagogical language" (Beukelman & Mirenda, 2013, p. 49) One-handed alphabet

ASL = American Sign Language.

effective and efficient communication, individuals with autism spectrum disorder (ASD) have been observed to make use of multimodal communication to include both aided and unaided AAC, often depending on context and availability of aided AAC (Sigafoos & Drasgow, 2001).

Even after linguistic development has matured to mastery of signed or spoken language use, unaided communication modes—particularly gestures—remain important in communication exchanges. Speakers often use gestures to represent real-world actions to complement and even

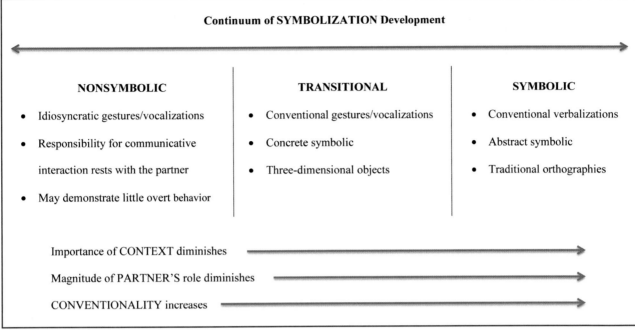

Figure 8-1. Symbolization development. (Reproduced with permission from S. M. Bashinski. [2011]. Assessment of prelinguistic communication of individuals with CHARGE. In T. S. Hartshorne, M. A. Hefner, S. L. H. Davenport, & J. W. Thelin [Eds.], *CHARGE Syndrome* [pp. 278-281]. Plural Publishing, Inc.)

add information to speech. Speakers who seek to emphasize a point may use more pronounced gesturing. Also, when speakers struggle with a message, gesturing will often increase; in other words, use of gestures tends to enhance speech that requires support for successful message expression. Kimura (1990) has proposed a model that assumes gesture and speech production have a common underlying neuromotor basis. McNeill (1985, 1992, 1993) stresses that gesture and speech function in a complementary and redundant way.

Generally, research shows that speech and gestures break down together in individuals with communication disabilities (see Glosser et al., 1986; Graziano & Gullberg, 2018; McNeill, 1992). This reciprocal relationship between gestures and speech illustrates well the multimodal nature of communication.

SYMBOLIC COMMUNICATION

The ability to communicate symbolically involves **representational thinking skill**—the ability to comprehend that one thing stands for/refers to something else. This involves the ability to hold a representation of something in mind when it is not present in the here (i.e., space) and now (i.e., time). Representational thinking involves the concept of "distancing," a construct developed by prominent psychologists Werner and Kaplan (1988). Symbolic communication requires a learner's ability to use representations that do not resemble a referent in order to communicate about someone or something in a different place and/or time (i.e., a distancing between referent and representation [Bruce, 2005]).

Recent Knowledge of Symbolic Communication

Since the publication of the previous version of this textbook in 1997, a multitude of new knowledge and evidence-based practice has emerged in regard to the validity and criticality of nonsymbolic (i.e., **presymbolic**) communication. Since the time the field of AAC first was recognized as a unique applied discipline, it was never questioned that AAC interventions could be beneficial for individuals who had already acquired symbolic language skills. Though it has taken some time for wider acceptance of the importance of recognizing individuals' nonsymbolic communicative signals and augmenting individuals' receptive and expressive communication skills at the nonsymbolic level in order to facilitate further communication development (Branson & Demchak, 2009; Kangas & Lloyd, 1988; Loncke, 2014; Romski & Sevcik, 2005), this is the predominant perspective today.

Emergence of Symbolization Ability

Symbolization ability, the skill to understand that one thing can meaningfully refer to something else, evolves over time. The manner in which unaided communication forms are used varies tremendously and covers the full range of nonsymbolic expressions through abstract, fully symbolic communication elements (Figure 8-1). Different authors and researchers cite varying numbers of stages of symbolization development. In this chapter, three primary levels are discussed.

TABLE 8-2
Categories and Characteristics of Unaided Communication

CATEGORY	CHARACTERISTICS	USE
Nonsymbolic (Presymbolic)		
PCAs	Nonconventional vocalizations, movements, changes in bodily function	Expression
Touch	Touch cues made on the individual's body to alert them as to what is about to happen	Comprehension
Deictic gestures	Reaching, giving, showing, or pointing—in any form	Expression
Transitional Symbolic		
Representational gestures	Conventional pictorial or emblematic gestures learned as a part of one's culture	Comprehension and expression
Symbolic		
Simultaneous communication	Simultaneous presentation of natural speech and manual sign	Comprehension
Pedagogical sign systems	Manual signs produced to follow English syntactic and morphological rules and word components	Comprehension and expression
Other linguistic systems	Alphabet-based systems, phonemic-based symbols	Comprehension and expression
Tactile communication	Manual signs made coactively, hand-under-hand, in contact with AAC user	Comprehension and expression

AAC = augmentative and alternative communication; PCA = potential communicative act.

At the nonsymbolic (i.e., presymbolic) level, potential unaided communicative signals might involve a change in the individual's level of alertness or affect, a variety of body movements, or **idiosyncratic** gestures or body posturing (Sigafoos et al., 2000). Idiosyncratic gestures are gestures that have been created by an individual or through the interaction between an individual and the environment. Gestures have a naturally augmentative and sometimes an alternative function in communication among persons without disabilities, as well as persons with disabilities. Though it is the responsibility of the individual's partner to ensure a successful communicative interaction at this level, the context in which the nonsymbolic signal occurs is critical to the partner's derivation of meaning (Bashinski, 2014b).

At the transitional (concrete symbolic) level, an individual's communication may involve jargon and variation of inflection in his vocalizations. The unaided forms the individual will begin to use include conventional gestures, such as pointing, and acting on a partner or an object in various ways (Watt et al., 2006). The individual will begin to incorporate some aided communication forms (e.g., textures, tangibles) as the communication becomes more concretely linked to referents available in that context (Bashinski, 2014b).

As symbolic ability becomes fully developed, the individual will incorporate abstract, conventional, unaided communicative forms, such as fingerspelling, conventional manual signs, or tactile signs, in their communication repertoire. Young children learn that words, gestures, and signs

have meaning, and they learn to play in pretend (i.e., symbolic) ways. Through conventionalization, the individual's communicative gestures and signs become understandable by a wider audience (Brady et al., 2004).

The achievement of symbolic ability relates to major advances in social communication and cognition. Transition from one stage of symbolization ability to the next does not occur overnight. Development of skills in symbolization emerges over time, at different rates with familiar/unfamiliar partners and in familiar/unfamiliar environments. It is important to remember that some individuals might never develop abstract symbolic ability. For this reason, it is critical to consider potential communicative acts (PCAs), as discussed later in this chapter.

MAJOR CATEGORIES AND CHARACTERISTICS OF UNAIDED AUGMENTATIVE COMMUNICATION COMPONENTS

Unaided communication components encompass not only a wide variety of categories of communication forms but also exemplify a wide array of characteristics that cover the full range of non-linguistic (i.e., nonsymbolic/presymbolic) through highly abstract linguistic forms (see Table 8-2, compared with the unaided symbols in Table 3-4).

Presymbolic Unaided Communication

At the presymbolic level of communication, many of the individual's signals that are interpreted as communicative are idiosyncratic in form. Idiosyncratic actions, movements, and/or sounds are recognized only by communication partners who are familiar with the individual (e.g., throwing the remote control to say, "Change the channel!"; biting the palm of one's own hand to communicate, "It's way too loud in here for me!"; or vocalizing "unh" for "no" and shrieking for "yes"). Individuals with presymbolic communication may have very little or no functional speech; nevertheless, these sorts of idiosyncratic signals can be highly useful with frequent communication partners in familiar environments (Vanderheiden & Lloyd, 1986).

Some individuals largely produce PCAs and remain nonsymbolic (i.e., presymbolic/pre-linguistic) communicators throughout their lifetimes, while others go on to develop symbolic, intentional communication.

Nonsymbolic communication behavior in some clinical populations is described in the literature, including individuals who experience trisomy 13 and trisomy 18 (Braddock et al., 2012; Liang et al., 2013), CHARGE syndrome (Bashinski, 2015a, 2021; Peltokorpi & Huttunen, 2008; Thelin & Fussner, 2005), Rett syndrome (Grether, 2015), Angelman syndrome (Calculator, 2002), ASD (Watt et al., 2006; Wetherby, 2014), and persons with dual sensory impairment (DSI; Bruce & Bashinski, 2017; Dammeyer, 2012; see also Chapter 23 of this textbook).

Additionally, communicative functions expressed by children's pre-linguistic gestures inform assessment and intervention practices. Profiling pre-linguistic gesture development in young children with little natural speech can enhance assessment and intervention practices (Brady & Bashinski, 2008; Crais et al., 2009). Children demonstrating typical development use pre-linguistic gestures for communicative functions to meet basic needs, including behavioral regulation (e.g., request action or object, protest), social interaction (e.g., request a social routine, request comfort, greet, call, show off, request permission), and joint attention (e.g., request information, comment about an object, action, or person; Beukelman & Mirenda, 2013; Loncke, 2014; Machado, 2016). By 15 months of age in typical development, all three communicative functions are used consistently with a variety of means (Crais et al., 2004).

In many ways, gestural communication is one of the earliest spontaneously developing unaided communication forms (Wetherby, 2014). Before the onset of linguistic development, young children use gestures in symbol formation when they communicate and interact with their environment. Delayed gestural development can sometimes indicate delayed language development (Thal & Tobias, 1992; Wetherby, 2014). Because of its crucial role in development, the use of gesture has very strong potential for use as unaided communication either within gestural symbol sets or as a point of departure for developing linguistic communication through manual signs, graphic symbols, and/or speech (Miller et al., 2011).

Potential Communicative Acts

The phrase "**potential communicative act**" is used here to refer to any behavior that another person interprets as meaningful and may include a range of behaviors, such as changes in respiration, body movement, vocalization, eye gaze, facial expression, and/or problem behavior (Sigafoos et al., 2000), as well as few words and AAC symbols. Communicative gestures are defined as actions produced with the intent to communicate, mostly involving the fingers, hands, and arms, but can include full body movements, such as jumping to refer to a frog, or facial movements, such as lip smacking to refer to eating (Iverson & Thal, 1998).

Given that infants communicate all kinds of information without being aware of it, communicative intervention with individuals who experience severe communication disability should also be guided by this reality. Sigafoos and colleagues (2000) have described this phenomenon as PCAs. PCAs often include idiosyncratic behaviors or other behaviors that are interpreted by caregivers as meaningful in a particular context. For example, an individual may vocalize and move the mouth to indicate, "I'm thirsty." The phrase "potential communicative acts" is helpful because it places a focus on communication and values both nonintentional and intentional communication. To gather important data about PCAs, clinicians and educators work closely with familiar caregivers to determine those behaviors that should be considered potentially communicative (see Table 8-3 for examples).

A careful analysis of potential communicative behaviors provides insight into the types of behaviors that caregivers interpret as pragmatically meaningful in everyday environments (Braddock et al., 2012). Further, a dynamic assessment approach is often useful for clinicians, educators, and caregivers to consider if an individual's small repertoire of meaningful behaviors can be extended (Snell, 2002). This is done by carefully introducing new symbols while considering communicative contexts to foster more effective communication at a nonsymbolic level.

In trisomy 13 and 18, individuals of varied ages were found to produce informal behavior in coordinated ways in the absence of natural speech (Braddock et al., 2012). For example, one individual vocalized and pushed a toy away during a communication temptation task with an examiner over several trials. Given the persistence and coordination of behaviors, the examiner inferred that the individual did not want to participate in play with her. A follow-up study indicated that individuals with trisomy 13 and trisomy 18 mostly produced PCAs categorized as body movement followed by

TABLE 8-3
Examples of Potential Communicative Acts

PCA	EXAMPLE
Expressive Communication	
Body movement	Individual takes another's hand to lead them to a door; communication partner infers that they want to "go."
Change in respiration	Individual breathes at a faster rate when playing a game; communication partner infers they are happy.
Eye gaze	Individual looks at their communication partner in play; communication partner infers that they are interested in playing with that particular item.
Facial expression	Individual frowns when they are asked to stop an activity; communication partner infers that they want the activity to continue.
Challenging behavior	Individual bangs their head when a preferred toy is removed; communication partner infers that they want to keep the toy.
Vocalization	Individual vocalizes when food is provided; communication partner infers that they like the food choice.
Receptive Communication—Touch Cues	
Tap learner's ankle twice	"It's time to put on your ankle-foot orthotic."
Touch back of learner's right hand	"Relax. I am here. You are safe."
PCA = potential communicative act.	

vocalization and facial expression (Liang et al., 2013). Still some individuals produced a few symbolic communicative behaviors. About one-half of the participants sampled were reported by caregivers to produce at least one spoken word, gesture, or manual sign, or use picture communication. In other words, caregivers relied primarily on PCAs when communicating with individuals with trisomy 13 and trisomy 18 because AAC usage and speech skills were very limited.

The communication profiles of individuals with CHARGE syndrome vary tremendously due to the incredibly broad spectrum of the complex characteristics of this condition (Miller et al., 2011). CHARGE syndrome affects potentially nearly every major body system: auditory, behavioral, cardiac, cognitive, digestive, endocrine, genitourinary, immunologic, neurological, olfactory, renal, and visual. Every feature of CHARGE varies from severe to total absence in individuals diagnosed with this condition (Hartshorne

et al., 2021). The acronym "CHARGE" was first coined in 1981 when a group of physicians proposed it to identify a newly recognized cluster of anatomic and physiologic features (Hefner, 1999). At that time, the condition was named "CHARGE association," with each of the selected letters referring to what *at that time* were believed to be the condition's primary identifying features.

In 1981, the letters C-H-A-R-G-E referenced the following:

- C: **Coloboma**, which appears like a cleft or gap in one of the structures of the eye that may or may not cause vision loss (e.g., colobomas in the retina or optic nerve are associated with varying degrees of vision loss)
- H: Heart defects
- A: **Atresia of the choanae**, also referred to as choanal atresia, which refers to blockage of the nasal passages
- R: General delay (i.e., "retardation") of the individual's growth and development
- G: Genitourinary abnormalities, including reduced hormone production that delays puberty or makes this developmental process incomplete; external features of genital abnormalities present more in males than females
- E: Abnormalities of the outer, middle, and/or inner ear that may affect one or both sides of the body; inner ear abnormalities not only affect the cochlea and auditory nerve resulting in hearing loss but also the semicircular canals, which cause vestibular system and balance problems

Diagnostic criteria for CHARGE were revised by a board of physicians in 1998, reprioritizing the symptomology believed to most directly point to a diagnosis of CHARGE syndrome. Coloboma, atresia of the choanae, and ear abnormalities remain as three of the primary features of this syndrome, though heart defects (H), growth delay (i.e., "retardation"; R), and genitourinary abnormalities (G) are identified as less specific to a diagnosis of CHARGE syndrome today—though they continue to be recognized as significant symptoms. "These features are no longer used in making a diagnosis of CHARGE syndrome, but we're not changing the name" (CHARGE Syndrome Foundation, 2019, para. 4).

"Though communication profiles vary tremendously from individual to individual, it is generally accepted that development of both receptive and expressive communication abilities is delayed, in at least some areas, in all persons who experience [CHARGE syndrome]" (Bashinski, 2021, p. 353). Professionals who work with individuals who have CHARGE syndrome are well-advised to recognize the potential communicative value of all overt behaviors. Parents/guardians of individuals with CHARGE syndrome frequently report noncompliant behavior as communication (Miller et al., 2011).

Only limited research describing the communication skills of individuals who have CHARGE syndrome has been published in the extant literature base (Bashinski, 2015a; Miller et al., 2011; Peltokorpi & Huttunen, 2008; Smith et al., 2010). However, it is projected that approximately 60% of individuals with CHARGE syndrome do eventually develop symbolic language skills (Miller et al., 2011; Swanson, 2011). Said another way, approximately 40% of individuals with CHARGE syndrome continue to rely primarily on non-symbolic communication forms throughout their lifetimes. The majority of individuals who have CHARGE syndrome continue to develop new communication skills beyond the critical age that typical language learners do. Even in the cases of individuals with CHARGE syndrome who do acquire symbolic communication skills, it is not unusual for these individuals to require lengthier periods of time to process language, and many engage in repetitive or ritualistic talk (Bruce et al., 2018).

Enhanced Natural Gestures

Many individuals who experience Angelman syndrome continue to rely on use of manual signs, though these are often modified from conventional presentations. Even so, this reliance on sign is viewed as surprising given the high frequency of athetoid movements associated with this condition and the concomitant lack of motor control individuals generally experience. To address the resulting reality that unfamiliar communication partners are often unable to interpret the signs used by individuals with Angelman syndrome, the value of manual sign communication is generally limited.

To address this need, Calculator (2002) introduced the **enhanced natural gestures** (ENGs) approach as an alternative to manual sign. "Unlike signs, ENGs consist of intentional gestures individuals are already using, sometimes as natural gestures. As such, ENGs require minimal instruction. Unlike signs and natural gestures, all ENGs are screened to verify their ease of interpretation by others" (Calculator, 2015, p. 109). Subsequent to Calculator's initial suggestion of the ENG approach, additional research has been conducted to evaluate its efficacy. In a study by Calculator and Diaz-Caneja Sela (2014), the ease with which untrained, unfamiliar partners were able to successfully interpret enhanced natural gestures was validated. Even so, the lack of information regarding evidence-based strategies for communication instruction with individuals who experience Angelman syndrome is severely lacking (Calculator, 2015).

EMERGENCE OF COMMUNICATIVE INTENTIONALITY ABILITY

The intentionality with which unaided communication forms are used varies tremendously and covers the full range from **nonintentional**, to intentional behavior (that is *not* intentionally communicative), to overt behaviors that are intentionally employed for the purpose of communication, which transitions to conventionality, and finally, to fully intentional, symbolic behaviors intentionally employed for the purpose of communication (Table 3-4 and Figure 8-2). Different authors and researchers cite varying numbers of stages of communicative intentionality development. In this chapter, three primary levels are discussed (intentionality, described here, should not be confused with the continuum of linguistic levels presented in Table 3-4).

At the nonintentional level, the individual's behavior is *neither* intentional *nor* intentionally communicative. The individual's overt, unaided behaviors might be reflexive, apparently random, or driven by their internal behavioral state(s). For all intents and purposes, the individual's communication at this level is one-way communication; the individual's partner must interpret their behavior as communicative at this level (Bashinski, 2014a; Loncke, 2014).

At the transitional level, the individual's overt, unaided behaviors *become intentional*, and as such, can be understood as meaningful in a given context. However, some degree of interpretation is still likely required of the individual's communication partner since the individual's behavior is still *not yet intentionally communicative* (Bashinski, 2014a). As the individual's gestures/vocalizations transition to become more conventional, the communication partner's responsibility for success of communication diminishes. Communicative context also becomes less critically important.

As communication becomes fully **intentional**, the individual's unaided, overt behaviors are both intentional *and* intentionally communicative. In social interactions with others, young children become more intentional or directed in their communication by coordinating eye gaze with gestures, vocalizations, and/or words. At this stage of communication development, the individual is using their behavior for the purpose of having an impact on or affecting another person.

A clearly defining characteristic of intentional communication is the directing of that particular behavior toward a communicative partner (Bates et al., 1979; Warren & Yoder, 1998). The achievement of communicative intentionality relates to major advances in social communication and cognition. However, it is important to remember that some individuals might never achieve this skill over their lifetimes.

GESTURES

As a review, gestures are defined as actions produced primarily with the fingers, hands, and arms (i.e., upper extremities) but can include facial features and full body movements (Iverson & Thal, 1998). Even before first words are expected, very young children use nonspeech communication when interacting with others, communicating with their caregivers through crying, smiling, and a variety of other behaviors. Gestures can be selected from culturally developed conventions, or they can be created/selected by one or more communication partners. Throughout the prelinguistic period, young children are socially interacting with caregivers and learning about the world around them, which contributes to the formation of a strong foundation for later

Continuum of COMMUNICATIVE INTENTIONALITY Development		
⟷		
NONINTENTIONAL **(Perlocutionary)**	**TRANSITIONAL** **(Illocutionary)**	**INTENTIONAL** **(Locutionary)**
• Reflexive behavior • Random behavior • Behavior state	• Behavior is intentional • Behavior is *not* intentionally communicative • Behavior is meaningful *in context*	• Behavior is intentional • Behavior *is* intentionally communicative • Deliberate pursuit of goal *and* means to obtain goal • Behavior is used to affect partner
(Partner must *interpret* behavior)	(Some degree of partner interpretation may be involved)	

Figure 8-2. Communicative intentionality development. (Reproduced with permission from S. M. Bashinski. [2011]. Assessment of prelinguistic communication of individuals with CHARGE. In T. S. Hartshorne, M. A. Hefner, S. L. H. Davenport, & J. W. Thelin [Eds.], *CHARGE Syndrome* [pp. 278-281]. Plural Publishing, Inc.)

communication and language development and includes the emergence of a number of gestural forms (Bashinski, 2012; Tomasello, 1988; Wetherby, 2014). It is for these reasons among others, that gestures must be critically considered as essential elements of unaided AAC. A significant percentage of individuals who experience various syndromic or other developmental disabilities are unlikely to demonstrate communicative development beyond a nonsymbolic level. Even with individuals from these groups who will eventually develop symbolic communication skills, augmenting their instruction with unaided receptive and expressive gestural strategies has been demonstrated to be effective in furthering their progress (Brady et al., 2004; Loncke, 2014; Sigafoos & Mirenda, 2002).

Increased interest and research into children with or at risk for ASD has provided new knowledge about gesture understanding and use. Spontaneous or natural gesture use is routinely examined in children at risk for ASD. Central to the *Diagnostic and Statistical Manual, Fifth Edition* (American Psychiatric Association, 2013) criteria for ASD are deficits in the understanding and use of gesture. The FIRST WORDS Project (2014) has documented that young children produce a variety of gesture types or use unaided AAC before first words are spoken. These researchers found that young children add about two new communicative gestures per month to their repertoires between 9 and 16 months of age, reaching to levels of about 16 communicative gestures by 16 months of age (Wetherby, 2014). The lack of gesture communication is

considered one of the first "red flags" or warnings of possible ASD in very young children (i.e., lack of pointing or showing to share attention with another person). A body of research into pre-linguistic and minimally verbal communicators on the autism spectrum supports using typical development as a predictable pathway to aid in assessment and intervention (Keen et al., 2016).

For individuals with little natural speech and risk for ASD, clinicians examine types of gestures used, communicative function, and intentional rate (with and without coordinated vocalizations or speech), among other indicators. One instrument, the *Autism Diagnostic Observation Schedule, Second Edition* (Lord et al., 2012), places a high priority on the synchrony or coordination of gesture production with coordinated eye gaze, facial expression, and/or vocalizations/verbalizations.

Over time, as gesture production becomes more synchronized with directed vocalizations/verbalizations and eye gaze, unaided communication behaviors typically become both more symbolic and more intentionally communicative (i.e., words and gestures; Bates, 1976; Bates et al., 1979). It is important to recall that during approximately the first 2 years of life, development of symbolization ability and communicative intentionality are considered pivotal growth-related achievements (see Figures 8-1 and 8-2). However, it should not be inferred that the three stages of each of these two developmental continua overlay one another exactly; this is not the case.

In fluent communicators who have developed skills at the symbolic level, spontaneous gesture may be classified by type. McNeill (1992) described five gestural categories:

1. Iconic (also known as descriptive gesture): Gestures that depict a pictorial quality of the intended referent in terms of size, shape, or direction of movement
2. **Metaphoric**: Gestures that refer to images of abstraction or a referent that is not easily depicted
3. **Deictic**: Gestures that single out a referent from other possible ones, such as pointing out
4. Beats (also known as **emphatic** gestures): Gestures produced using biphasic up and down or side to side movement of the hands, to mark time with speech, and/or provide emphasis to co-occurring words
5. Conventional (also known as **emblematic** gestures): Gestures that are shared by a wider audience and uniquely learned within a given culture, such as waving good-bye or producing the "OK" sign with the index finger and thumb (for English language users)

Various researchers describe gesture types in a number of different ways. One of the more common categorizations of gestural forms was offered by Iverson and Thal (1998). These researchers described typically developing young children's earliest gestural forms as deictic gestures that single out a referent from other possible ones and **representational** (or descriptive and conventional) gesture types.

Deictic Gestures

Deictic gestures (Table 8-4) are used to establish reference by calling attention to or indicating an object, action, or person. Some of the earliest types of deictic gestures to emerge may be present in typical development at approximately 7 to 9 months of age (Crais et al., 2004). These early occurring deictic gestures are often produced by touching an object or communication partner and may be dependent on context and/or tied to routines, as seen in a child reaching with hands up to indicate the desire to be picked up by another or pushing an object or a caregiver's hand away to protest.

Around 8 to 14 months of age, children demonstrating typical development produce more advanced deictic gesture types, such as giving, showing, requesting (reaching), and/or pointing (Bates, 1976; Bates et al., 1979; Wetherby, 2014). For example, showing an object to another person to share attention may serve the same communicative function as pointing out, yet occurs with the object in hand. Showing involves holding up an object in the communication partner's line of vision while giving involves the release of the object. A pointing gesture may take many different forms (e.g., open-hand [whole hand] pointing, eye pointing, foot pointing, tapping with fingers, and touching the index fingers to an object of interest) but generally can be described in one of two categories—a **contact gesture** or a **distal gesture** (McLean et al., 1991).

TABLE 8-4
Examples of Deictic Gestures

DEICTIC GESTURE	EXAMPLES
Contact pointing	Conventionally, an individual extends an isolated finger (or thumb) and points out object of interest; gesture is directed to their communication partner with coordinated eye gaze. However, pointing may also include eye pointing or pointing with the foot, elbow, or other body part over which the individual possesses volitional control.
Distal pointing	Individual extends isolated finger (or thumb) and points to an out-of-reach object while coordinating eye gaze and/or directing vocalization to their communication partner. Pointing may also include eye pointing or pointing with the foot, elbow, or other body part over which the individual has volitional control.
Giving object	Individual places a toy car in their communication partner's hand to direct attention to it.
Reaching for object	Individual directs a reach gesture to their communicative partner to signal "cracker" from other possible snacks.
Showing object	Individual holds up a block for communication partner to see, but does not release object, to directly reference the object of interest.

A contact gesture involves just that with a communicative partner—touch or contact. In contrast, a distal gesture establishes reference with a communication partner to a person or item of interest that is some distance away. The emergence of a distal point with an isolated index finger (or thumb) extended to an out-of-reach referent suggests that the individual is developing symbolic communication; however, literature on the use of gestures by individuals with significant intellectual disability cites it is the function of the distal gesture and not the distal form itself that is indicative of a more advanced level of communication development (McLaughlin & Cascella, 2008; McLean et al., 1999).

BASIC CHARACTERISTICS OF UNAIDED SYMBOLIC COMMUNICATION

Some fundamental characteristics of unaided symbols are related to the general properties of human language; others are only relevant within the context of AAC. The type and importance of a wide range of characteristics varies considerably both between and within manual symbol sets and signing systems. For example, characteristics such as handshape and physical complexity differ from one unaided symbol corpus to another.

Naturalness

Many symbols develop in a natural way as part of the human inclination toward communication. The origin of several signs in various sign languages is nothing more than the conventionalizing of a gesture that has adopted the formal characteristics of manual signs. Mylander and Goldin-Meadow (1991) showed how idiosyncratic gestures tend to develop similar features as sign languages, including rules for sign formation, sign order, and sign combination. Complex symbol systems, such as spoken or sign languages, have never been designed in an artificial way. Natural languages strongly indicate that humans have an enormous capacity for developing communication symbol sets and systems (Loncke, 2014). The capacity of managing sets of symbols is mostly reflected by the enormity of the lexical content of the average natural language user. It has been estimated that a person can handle an internal lexicon of at least 50,000 elements. Additionally, individuals use the generative power of combination rules in a number of various ways to produce derived and inflected words, compound words, phrases, sentences, and discourse in highly creative respects.

Symbols and symbol sets can also be contrived, primarily as explicit agreements between two or more people, but also as artificial designs (e.g., **Paget-Gorman Sign System**, cued speech). Many pedagogical sign and manually coded systems borrow a majority of manual signs from true sign languages, though borrowed signs are often modified through a process of **initialization**. Initialization involves the use of handshapes from the origin country's manual alphabet (if that country's sign language includes one; not all do) to create meaningful manual signs. Frequently, initialized signs are developed through use of the first letter of their translation of a spoken word from the country's local oral language to establish a family of signs with related meanings. The individual letter handshapes are used to make the same movement pattern (e.g., C for "class," F for "family," G for "group," S for "society," T for "team"; both hands held close together then drawn apart and around to the front of the body, in respective letter handshape).

Conventionality

Because of the arbitrary nature of words, in principle, any form can convey any meaning. However, to be able to successfully communicate with one another, communication partners must use the same form to refer to the same semantic content. If not, communication will fail. All relationships between form and meaning of words rest on tacit conventions between the users of the same system of communication—whether augmented or not. This also holds true for iconic manual signs. For example, whereas the sign for "cat" in Signed English is a representation of a cat's whiskers, a different visual feature could have been selected for an iconic representation of this animal (e.g., the form of a cat's tail or its manner of walking). However, this sign referring to a cat's whiskers has become conventionalized.

Conventionalized manual signs often reflect the culture of the country/region from which they emerge. Examples of this phenomenon can be drawn from two different true sign languages: in ASL, the sign for "pig" is made with the downturned prone hand placed under the chin, illustrating a pig's snout digging into a trough, while in Belgian Sign Language, "pig" is made with the top of the extended index finger touching the side of the neck, illustrating the typical way of stabbing a pig when it is slaughtered. Though these examples are drawn from true sign languages, the manual signs themselves may be transferred to use in other unaided augmented communication systems.

TYPES OF SYMBOLIC UNAIDED COMMUNICATION

As noted previously, unaided communication requires nothing external to the communicator's body for the purpose of formulating an expression. *Symbolic* unaided communication involves the representational thinking skill—the ability to hold an image of something in mind when the person, place, object, or activity is removed in space and/or time. Nonsymbolic (i.e., non-linguistic) unaided communication types (e.g., acoustic and visual) are contrasted with various symbolic unaided AAC symbols that are linguistic (e.g., acoustic, visual, and tactile), as seen in Table 8-5 along with brief explanations or examples of each. These symbolic unaided communication types are discussed in the following sections.

The reader will note that the classification system utilized to organize much of the content of this chapter is *different from the official quaternary continuum* proposed in Table 3-4. However, it is important to note that the categorization presented in Table 8-5 is defensible because it includes another dimension of unaided communication elements that is *not* captured in the official quaternary classification system—in particular, the acoustic, visual, and tactile elemental nature of unaided AAC components. The reader is encouraged to take note of the striking similarities between the information, as presented in Table 8-5, and the categorization of unaided AAC symbols using the quaternary continuum, as presented in Table 3-4. Essentially, the four linguistic components of the quaternary continuum (see Table 3-4) have been collapsed into nonsymbolic and symbolic components in Table 8-5.

TABLE 8-5

Classification of Unaided Augmentative Communication Elements

CATEGORY	TYPE/FORM	EXPLANATION/EXAMPLES
Nonsymbolic (i.e., non-linguistic)		
Acoustic elements	Cry	Shriek, grunt, sigh
	Vocalization	Any phoneme or phonemic combination
Tactile elements	Idiosyncratic body movements	Unusual actions on own body
		Stereotypy
Visual elements	Idiosyncratic gestures (PCAs)	Turning away from partner (in protest/rejection); rapid increase in breathing rate
	ENGs	Reaching in direction of a cabinet with stored snacks
	Deictic gestures	Child reaching up with hands to indicate the desire to be held
Symbolic (i.e., linguistic)		
Acoustic elements	Natural speech	Verbalizing word(s)
Tactile elements	Tactile sign language	Print-on-palm; braille hand speech; tactile fingerspelling
	Tadoma	
Visual elements	Amer-Ind	Combine gestures BOOK and LOOK to express "reading"
	Representational gestures	Shaking head "no," waving "hello" or "good-bye"
	Simultaneous communication	Concurrent presentation of manual sign and speech
	KWS	Inclusion of only essential signs to accurately express an abbreviated message
	Makaton	Signs for key information-carrying words accompanied with natural, full speech
	MCE	Pidgin Signed English
	PGSS	(United Kingdom) Complete, accurate representation of spoken English with full speech
	Pedagogical sign systems (e.g., SEE-I, SEE-II, Signed English)	Gestural equivalent of spoken language; includes manual signs and variety of affixes
	Fingerspelling (and other alphabet-based systems)	Use of one- or two-handed alphabets to spell message
	Phonemic-based hand-cued systems	Cued speech

Amer-Ind = American Indian Hand Talk; ENG = enhanced natural gesture; KWS = key word signing; MCE = manually coded English; PCA = potential communicative act; PGSS = Paget Gorman Sign System; SEE-I = Seeing Essential English; SEE-II = Signing Exact English.

American Indian Hand Talk

American Indian Hand Talk (Amer-Ind) is essentially a set of gestures loosely based on those created by Native American tribes for their intertribal communication. The impetus for creation of this manual code was to allow tribes with different language systems to cross language barriers and effectively communicate with one another. The earliest record of any extensive standardized vocabulary (which consisted of only 104 signs) dates back to 1823 (Seton, 1918).

By the 1890's, this symbolic communication system came to be known as "Sign Talk" (Seton, 1918); during the 20th century, its label morphed into the abbreviated "Amer-Ind" reference, which is still in use today. Amer-Ind is not regarded as a linguistic system but rather as a collection of signals or labels; frequently, Amer-Ind is referred to as a pictographic transitionary symbol system. Its labels express broader semantic fields than spoken words generally do. Amer-Ind has a limited lexicon of approximately 250 gestures but is expanded through the use of compound forms through a process known as **agglutination**. For example, the expression of

TABLE 8-6
Examples of Representational Gestures

REPRESENTATIONAL GESTURE	EXAMPLES
Conventional or emblematic gestures (e.g., standard gestures learned as part of one's specific culture)	Individual looks at communication partner and waves "good-bye" to indicate time to go. Individual responds to their communication partner by nodding their head up and down to indicate "yes." Individual directs communication to their communication partner by holding up their hand as if to indicate "wait."
Object-related or descriptive gestures (e.g., pictorial-like gestures used to describe the referent)	Individual looks at their communication partner then cups and holds their hands out to indicate size—"so big"—or shape of a ball. Individual looks at communication partner and moves hand and arm along a wave-like trajectory to indicate "swimming."

"reading" involves a combination of the gestures "book" and "look" (Tomkins, 1969), and the communication "I live here" involves "I" plus "house" plus "sit."

Amer-Ind has been adapted for use with and by individuals with communication disabilities (Duncan & Silverman, 1977; Lloyd & Daniloff, 1983). An advantage of Amer-Ind is the low level of motor control required for producing the gestures (i.e., "labels"; Daniloff & Vergara, 1984). Amer-Ind is also considered valuable for use with individuals who, because of intellectual disability, are challenged to store and/or process a large vocabulary, though estimations of transparency vary from more than 80% (Skelly, 1979) to less than 50% (Doherty et al., 1985), somewhat dependent on the individual's cognitive level.

Representational Gestures

Representational gestures (Table 8-6) generally emerge around 12 months of age in young children showing typical development, usually after a few deictic gestures are observed. Young children may show individual variability in the use of representational gestures based on their learning environments (Crais et al., 2004), but all are generally consistent with the child's cultural conventions.

Representational gestures are used to establish reference and indicate specific meaning (Acredolo & Goodwyn, 1988). Representational gestures include both object-related gestures and conventional gesture types. Object-related gestures depict a pictorial quality or describe some feature of the referent, such as cupping the hand to represent "cup" or "drinking" or moving the hand downward to represent "slide" or "sliding." Object-related gestures are considered symbolic when produced without the real object in hand. In contrast, conventional gestures have a standard, shared social meaning and are learned culturally. For example, in North America, young children learn that hand waving indicates "hello" or "good-bye" and nodding the head indicates "yes." Conventional gestures are also referred to as emblematic gestures because their use indicates a symbolic representation of a particular concept or construct rather than an object.

Relationship of Gesture Use to Speech

As previously mentioned, Kimura (1990) proposed a model that assumes gesture and speech production share a common underlying neuromotor basis. The production of natural gestures appears to be triggered by the content of a message in the speech planning process. McNeill (1985, 1992, 1993) stressed that gesturing and speech function in both complementary and redundant ways. Although a gesture is different from the spoken word, both are based on the same underlying thought. In a study conducted in Italy, a clear developmental pattern for the emergence of early actions and gestures was identified (Caselli et al., 2012). Their findings were consistent with studies that investigated various Western languages, "…indicating a common biological and cultural basis" (Caselli et al., 2012, p. 526) between early actions, gestures, and spoken vocabulary. Recent research has demonstrated that speech and gestures break down simultaneously in individuals who experience communication disabilities (Graziano & Gullberg, 2018). Thus, it can be argued logically that facilitating an individual's use of gestures and overall gestural abilities is likely to enhance that individual's continued development toward more conventional forms of symbolic communication.

Bridge to Symbolic Communication

In addition to gestures, an individual's use of other idiosyncratic and nonconventional forms of unaided communication (i.e., PCAs), which are repeatedly interpreted as having communicative value by their communication partners, is very likely to facilitate growth along the continuum of symbolization (Malloy & Bruce, 2008). Repeated interpretation of nonsymbolic, and even unintentional behaviors (i.e., "signals"), might shape intentionality over time as the individual begins to impact their environment and experience the power of communication. Responsive partners' acknowledgement of intentional communicative gestures, whether conventional or nonconventional, shows understanding and increases the likelihood that the individual will develop more symbolic communication abilities (Bashinski, 2015a; Bruce et al., 2008; Wetherby, 2014).

Caselli and her colleagues (2012) demonstrated a relationship between early actions and gestures and spoken vocabulary in both production and comprehension. Their analyses revealed interesting similarities between the related meanings of early actions and gestures with the meanings of early words, whether or not objects were also involved. Utilization of early actions and gestures showed a higher correlation with comprehension than with word production, thus indicating that the transition from early actions and gestures to speech is more likely mediated by word comprehension.

Simultaneous Communication

Despite its negative image among many professionals, some schools and educational service providers continued to use some forms of manual sign as pedagogical tools prior to the rejection of the myth that manual sign was non-linguistic in nature. During the late 1960s and the early 1970s, the use of simultaneous signing and speech in the education of deaf children became widespread in the United States, and later in several European countries. In 1988, Kouri and colleagues demonstrated the effects of simultaneous communication when used with preschoolers who experienced severe disabilities. It is interesting to note that during the period between approximately 2000 and 2010, a noticeable decline in the number of publications regarding manual signing systems appeared in AAC journals (Grove, 2018).

Simultaneous communication, sometimes referred to as total communication, was proposed to expedite the transfer of information for educational purposes, as well as facilitate the acquisition of the structures of spoken language. The simultaneous presentation of manual sign and speech was intended to make spoken language structures more visually transparent, and hence, easier for deaf children to understand and acquire. The term "manual sign" is used to refer to the elements of either naturally developed sign systems and/or fingerspelling. That is, manual sign is the visual-gestural equivalent of words in spoken and written language.

The natural sign languages of Deaf communities were not used for simultaneous communication because the structures of sign language and spoken language are incongruent. Elements of a manual sign language and the spoken language of a particular culture are impossible to simultaneously combine for reasons previously discussed (i.e., the word order in a spoken language sentence is different from the order of manual signs when the sentence is translated in a true sign language).

Therefore, the system referred to as "simultaneous" or "total" communication, which allowed better parallel production and processing of manual sign and speech, emerged. Beginning in the late 1960s, several such systems were developed as pedagogical strategies in an effort to assist learners with significant communication needs to achieve their educational communication goals. "A number of research studies have found that a combined manual sign plus speech intervention is often more effective in establishing production and/or comprehension skills than either mode taught singly" (Beukelman & Mirenda, 2013, p. 48). Though, this is not true in the case of every individual. Some persons have been observed to pay more attention to the manual signs utilized in simultaneous communication situations than to their accompanying speech utterances (Carr et al., 1978).

Key Word Signing

Some researchers view **key word signing** (KWS) as a subset of manually coded English (described in the next section), but the KWS approach is described separately here because it also encompasses standardized intervention packages that include both aided and unaided AAC elements.

KWS is most succinctly described as "telegraphic" manual signing. That is, in KWS, manual signs are utilized to express an abbreviated message by including only those signs required to accurately communicate its essence (Beukelman & Mirenda, 2013; Grove, 2018) instead of coding all lexical elements of the spoken message. KWS is succinct, thereby involving fewer motoric demands (in the case of the individual who is expressing the message) and lesser cognitive demands (in the case of the individual who is receiving the message). The sentence, "Go get your shoes and give them to me, please," could be manually signed in KWS using the key words "get," "shoes," "give," and "me," though the complete sentence would be simultaneously spoken. This example illustrates that KWS very often incorporates simultaneous communication (Bonvillian & Nelson, 1978; Konstantareas, 1984).

KWS has been found to be associated with a change in the rate of spoken language when manual signs and speech are communicated simultaneously. Windsor and Fristoe (1991) demonstrated that KWS results in longer and more predictable pauses during a spoken utterance, thereby forcing the speaker to slow down their rate of speech. This result should benefit message comprehension by individuals who experience intellectual disability.

For some time, speech-language pathologists and educators seemed to favor the use of artificial sign sets or systems. In many regions, these sets and systems are still the main option for hearing individuals who experience significant communication challenges, for whom the utilization of manual communication is considered beneficial. The lexicon of such an approach can be built gradually and controlled in size depending on the needs and progress of the individual. Also, particular vocabulary items can be selected to allow maximum physical and/or cognitive accessibility.

A few KWS systems emerged to meet the specialized needs of a particular region or individuals who experience a particular type of disability. For example, the Duffy system was developed to meet the communicative needs of a group of learners who experienced severe cerebral palsy and related speech disorders (Duffy, 1977). Signalong (Kennard et al., 1992) was developed in the United Kingdom and uses a combination of speech, manual signs, real objects, and expanded descriptions at a level appropriate for the individual's needs. Signalong consists of a core vocabulary of approximately 1,726 concepts, not taught in any specific order but rather introduced as deemed to be incidentally appropriate in real situations.

Makaton

The most widely utilized standard KWS system in AAC intervention is **Makaton** (Grove & Walker, 1990), which is now reported to be in use in more than 40 countries around the world (Walker et al., 2019). Due to research evidence of Makaton's efficacy in both clinical and educational contexts, it can be implemented transnationally and transculturally.

Makaton relies on the combined use of signs and graphic symbols and is therefore appropriately described as a multimodal approach to communication since it employs all sensory modes for enhancing communication (i.e., visual, auditory, and kinesthetic). The purpose of Makaton is to develop a person's spoken output in combination with other AAC supports.

Makaton was initially developed in the United Kingdom by a speech and language therapist, Margaret Walker (1973), from her research with adults and children with intellectual disabilities to assist them to communicate more effectively in daily activities with their various partners. Walker's work resulted in the initial identification of 350 concepts, which were subsequently enlarged to 450 core vocabulary concepts required for basic communication and used in everyday living (e.g., where, what). Additionally, a larger, topic-based, open-ended resource vocabulary is regularly updated to incorporate a broader range of changes in culture, linguistics, and technology (Grove & Walker, 1990; Walker, 1977). Although the largest group of users is individuals who experience intellectual disabilities, the Makaton program is also used by children and adults with attention deficit disorders, ASD, dyspraxia, articulation difficulties, developmental and acquired neurological disorders, and sensory impairments.

The signs used in Makaton are derived from true manual sign languages because these are living languages and include signs that are not artificially contrived. Signs for Makaton are matched to concepts of the core and resource vocabularies from standardized sign languages to avoid confusion for individuals who use Makaton. Only signs for key information-carrying words are signed, and all applications of Makaton are accompanied with natural, full speech.

It is important for communication partners who interact with Makaton users to also learn their system in order to model its use. The Makaton Charity provides resources and a range of training courses and workshops run by qualified tutors for parents, care providers, and professionals to learn and implement the system appropriately. Additional information is available at www.makaton.org. Studies suggest that the role of the interactive partner is crucial in the development and generalization of a user's communication skills. Interactive partners can significantly influence users of unaided AAC, including Makaton, to initiate communication and gain more confidence in expressing their needs, opinions, and feelings.

Manually Coded English

The basic characteristic of manually coded sign systems is their parallelism to spoken English language words; the structure of the manually coded message is derived from speech. Manual codes "… follow English word order and contain specific signs for bound morphemes to signify English verb tenses, adverbs, and function words" (Luetke-Stahlman & Milburn, 1996, p. 30). Most forms of manually coded languages tend to be used in direct face-to-face communication through either simultaneous communication or bimodal speech and manual sign. "In North America, the United Kingdom, Australia, and New Zealand, the most common MCE [manually coded English] system is called contact sign (sometimes referred to as Pidgin Signed English), a blend of a local Deaf sign language and English" (Beukelman & Mirenda, 2013, p. 49).

Advantages of MCE are the provision of a more complete visual picture of elements of a spoken message and their order, as well as closer correspondence with the written elements of the language. Although a comprehensive use of manually coded spoken language has these advantages, it has noteworthy drawbacks as well. The primary disadvantage associated with use of MCE is that, because executing a manual sign takes about twice as much time as does the spoken articulation of a word, combined use of speech and sign is bound to lead to synchronization problems for the signer and/or speaker. Studies show that signers and/or speakers demonstrate variable levels of success in simultaneously signing and speaking the same content in both modalities (Fischer et al., 1991; Maxwell et al., 1991; Wodlinger-Cohen, 1991).

Paget Gorman Sign System

One of the earliest manually coded English systems was the British "A Systematic Sign Language," originated by Richard Paget in the 1930s, and further developed and standardized by Grace Paget and Pierre Gorman. This system later became known as Paget Gorman Sign System (PGSS) and is utilized today in the United Kingdom, Ireland, and Australia (Paget-Gorman Sign System, n.d.).

PGSS was used in several schools for deaf children as a visualization technique for English language structures through the 1960s and 1970s (Kyle & Woll, 1985). Its purpose is to provide a complete and accurate representation of spoken English; signs are always accompanied by speech (Paget-Gorman Sign System, n.d.). The Paget-Gorman system is designed as an educational tool; it is not intended for lifetime use. PGSS supports the development of literacy skills particularly in reading. Current practitioners who use the system simplify the system's elements to be used as prompts for cuing learners regarding not only their language but also their behavior. More than 4,000 signs are included in PGSS (Paget-Gorman Sign System, n.d.).

Pedagogical Sign Systems

These artificial sign systems were designed to provide a gestural equivalent of spoken language. More commonly today, these pedagogical sign systems are referred to as educational sign systems.

Interestingly, the use of manual signs for improving communication in hearing individuals who experienced intellectual disability and communication disorder was introduced as early as 1847 (Bonvillian & Miller, 1995). During the latter part of the 20th century, pedagogical/educational sign systems gained acceptance as a viable instructional approach for teaching deaf children who experienced intellectual disability and/or other additional disabilities (Moores, 1978). The most widely known English-referring pedagogical sign systems are Seeing Essential English (SEE-I; Anthony, 1974), Signing Exact English (SEE-II; Gustason et al., 1980), and Signed English (Bornstein & Saulnier, 1984).

Seeing Essential English

SEE-I was the first of the pedagogical sign systems invented in the United States during the 20th century. It was created by David Anthony, a deaf son of deaf parents who was an experienced teacher of children with deafness. Anthony's purpose in developing this manual sign system was to facilitate acquisition of a high proficiency level of the syntax and grammar of English by children who were deaf. His work was motivated by two primary concerns: first, "[s]everal ASL signs were used to gloss more than one English word with only minor stress and movement variations. That is, 'beauty,' 'beautiful,' and 'beautifully' all used the same sign, as did 'lovely,' 'pretty,' and 'attractive,'" (Luetke-Stahlman & Milburn, 1996, p. 30); second, several single English words were represented by multiple manual signs (e.g., "run"; Luetke-Stahlman & Milburn, 1996).

As an expansion of his 1966 unpublished master's thesis, Anthony worked with a group of members of the Deaf community, teachers, and parents to develop a collection of several thousand signs for English morphemes and words, along with a detailed explanation of SEE-I grammar. Basic English words that did not have a sign in ASL were developed on the basis of ASL pivot words (Luetke-Stahlman & Milburn, 1996). To create an authentic visual-manual representation of spoken English, Anthony and his committee developed signs for a variety of affixes: verb endings (e.g., *-ing, -ed*), comparative adjective markers (e.g., *-er, -est*), adverb markers (e.g., *-ly*), and prefixes (e.g., *non-, un-, re-*), as well as articles.

The primary rule of SEE-I was "… one word, one sign, no matter the 'sense' of the words, since a word has no intrinsic 'sense' until it is put in context with other words to make a statement" (Washburn, 1983, p. 27). Anthony and the other SEE-I authors originated a second rule that "[i]f two out of three characteristics between the spelling of a word, the meaning of a word, and the sound of the word are the same, the words are signed in the same manner" (Luetke-Stahlman & Milburn, 1996, p. 30).

The committee Anthony assembled to teach the first SEE-I classes and continue the development work split into two groups over practical and philosophical differences. In 1971, Anthony published two loose-leaf volumes and the guidelines he initially authored; this system was then formally designated as SEE-I. The remaining members of this committee began to work independently and developed the system now known as SEE-II (Luetke-Stahlman & Milburn, 1996), which is discussed below.

Once popular in the Midwestern United States, SEE-I is rarely used today, likely due to its significant differences from other pedagogical sign systems (Bornstein, 1990). It is sometimes referred to as a morphemic sign system (Luetke-Stahlman & Milburn, 1996).

Signing Exact English

SEE-I and SEE-II have several major characteristics in common:

> Both [*sic*] systems utilize English syntax and grammar, incorporate manual features such as gestures, directionality, use of space, fingerspelling, and words; utilize invented English markers based on English sound and spelling; use one sign for one word, regardless of the meaning conveyed; and are signed literally. SEE I and SEE II differ in that SEE I utilizes signs for all morphemes (prefixes, roots, and suffixes) and some are further divided (e.g., the word 'motor' is signed with two signs). In SEE II each English word is signed differently, and those words for which there are no signs are fingerspelled. (Luetke-Stahlman & Milburn, 1996, p. 31)

Gustason, Pfetzing, and Zawolkow were original members of Anthony's sign system development committee. When they split from his team, they advanced SEE-II (which they refer to as SEE 2) in the early 1970s, citing their main concern as "… the consistent, logical, rational, and practical development of signs to represent as specifically as possible the basic essentials of the English language" (Gustason et al., 1980, p. ix). These authors did not intend for SEE-II to replace ASL; they intended its use to be for teachers of English and families of young children who were deaf, for the purpose of creating an authentic visual-manual representation of spoken English.

SEE-II is based on nine important principles:

1. English should be signed in a manner that is as consistent as possible with how it is spoken or written in order to constitute a language input for the deaf child that will result in [their] mastery of English.

2. A sign should be translatable to only one English equivalent.

3. 'Basic words' are words that can have no more taken away and still form a complete word.

4. 'Complex words' are defined as basic words with the addition of an affix or inflection.

5. Compound words are two or more basic words put together. If the meaning of the words separately is consistent with the meaning of the words together, then and only **then** [emphasis supplied] are they signed as the component words.

6. When a sign already exists in ASL that is clear, unambiguous, and commonly translates to one English word, this sign is retained.

7. When the first letter is added to a basic sign to create synonyms, the basic sign is retained wherever possible as the most commonly used word (i.e., the basic sign is initialized with alphabetic letters to create the synonyms).

8. When more than one marker is added to a word, middle markers may be dropped **if** [emphasis supplied] there is no sacrifice of clarity.

9. While following the above principles, respect needs to be shown for characteristics of visual-gestural communication. (Gustason et al., 1980, pp. xiii-xiv)

Today, the most widely used pedagogical sign systems are SEE-II and Signed English (Luetke-Stahlman & Milburn, 1996).

Signed English

The Signed English system first put forth by Bornstein (1990) is less motorically and linguistically complex than SEE-II, though it is based on the same foundational premise. Signed English was created to model the English language, that is to develop a signing system in which manual signs are utilized to match each spoken word of English. It is intended that Signed English always be used with speech (Bornstein & Saulnier, 1984).

The Signed English pedagogical system utilizes two basic types of manual signs or gestures: actual sign words and what the authors term "sign markers." The majority of signs included in the Signed English lexicon are taken from ASL. In some cases, ASL signs were modified for inclusion in the Signed English vocabulary. In any instance in which two or more ASL signs existed for a given word, Bornstein "… chose the simplest to execute" (Bornstein & Saulnier, 1984, p. x). Therefore, each vocabulary sign in Signed English stands for one and only one English word. No English prefixes or suffixes are included in Signed English. Any time such an affix is required for communication, the developer recommends the affix be fingerspelled. However, when this occurs, the entire word (i.e., the affix plus the root sign) should be fingerspelled (Bornstein & Saulnier, 1984).

In total, 14 sign markers exist in the Signed English system. These are used to enable manual expression of sign vocabulary in the same order as the spoken/written words in an English sentence. Therefore, these "markers" are utilized to code the grammatical elements of English, including plurality, verb tense, possession, and changes in number. Sign markers do not exist for all possible grammatical markers of spoken English but rather only for those used most frequently. The most commonly used sign markers of Signed English include:

- Signed -*s*: regular plural noun (e.g., apples, cats)
- Signing a word twice: irregular plural noun (e.g., children, sheep)
- Signed -*ed*: regular past tense verb (e.g., listened, walked)
- Sweep of right hand to the right: irregular past tense verb (e.g., ate, ran)
- Signed -*s*: third person singular verb (e.g., cries, walks)

The remainder of the 14 Signed English sign markers consist of indices for possessives, parts of speech/sentences, and affixes, including -*ing* is present progressive verb form, -*y* is adjectival form, -*ly* is adverb form, agent (person), agent (thing), -*er* is comparative adjective, -*est* is superlative adjective, and *un-* is to indicate opposite of. Thirteen of the 14 markers are made immediately following the sign the marker is to change; only the marker for opposite (i.e., *un-*) is signed before the vocabulary word it modifies (Bornstein & Saulnier, 1984).

Numerous other principles are incorporated in the pedagogical Signed English system; many of these characterize certain classes of words (e.g., always spell infinitives and function words, show contractions by a twist of the signing hand, form a compound word by combining two base signs). Initialization of signs is frequently used.

Differentiation From Sign Languages

Pedagogical sign systems do not constitute true, unique languages. A pedagogical (i.e., educational) sign system follows the morphology, semantics, and syntax of the spoken language it has been designed to mirror. In most cases, each morpheme and/or spoken word is represented by a manual sign: handshape and/or movement (which are often extracted from an existing natural sign language).

The use of pedagogical sign systems involves manually coding all syntax and grammar elements of the spoken language in some form while following the order of the spoken words. One common variation in English pedagogical signs from ASL is the addition of information to the ASL sign in an attempt to communicate the exact English word intended in a conversation (Miller, 2010).

Pedagogical sign systems utilize the lexicon of the sign language of the national Deaf community (i.e., ASL in the United States), without adopting the sign language's syntactical rules. These systems are elaborated by adding morpheme-referring signs and/or fingerspelling, such as those corresponding to *-s* or *-ing* word endings, noting apostrophes for contractions, adding *-ly* for adverbs, and indicating verb tense markers, to name only a few. The sentence, "Go get your shoes and give them to me, please," would be expressed by use of manual signs/fingerspelled letters in the following order: GO GET YOUR SHOE+S AND GIVE THEM TO ME PLEASE. Another example would be "The boys walked, but the girls were running," which would be signed: THE BOY+S WALK+ED BUT THE GIRL+S WERE RUN+ING. These additions are intended to make the linguistic information conveyed via manual sign more complete in reference to the oral or spoken language of the broader community.

Complete sentences might be simultaneously spoken with the use of educational sign systems, but as noted in regard to the use of MCE systems, the concurrent use of speech and sign leads to synchronization problems for the signer and/or speaker. The addition of signs and fingerspelling to represent morphemes and grammatical markers makes simultaneous communication through sign and speech even more difficult.

Physical Features of Manual Signs

Certain unaided communication symbols, particularly manual signs, have been introduced in clinical and educational settings and individualized education programs because of the physical ease of facilitating their acquisition and production. When introduction of manual signs is considered, the learner's motor skills are one of the primary factors that must be considered. Introduction of signs to any given individual should consider their functionality for that person, as well as reserving the introduction of complex signs until more easily produced and interpreted signs have been mastered (Bornstein & Jordan, 1984). However, it is critical to also bear in mind that "[k]nowledge of the motor development of sign is *not enough* [emphasis provided]. Signs, like spoken words, are only symbols—only overt representations of deeper concepts, experiences, and objects. An imitated gesture does not suddenly have meaning" (Dunn, 1982, p. vii).

The variable of motor ability has been analyzed in several studies, especially in regard to manual signs. The following parameters have been suggested to play a potential role in determining the relative physical ease of production of signs (Dunn, 1982):

- Touch vs. nontouch: Several studies have shown that signs in which one hand comes in contact with the body (e.g., MY, RED) or with the signer's other hand (e.g., FRIEND, ON) are more easily acquired. It is inferred that these symbols allow the individual a higher degree of tactical and kinesthetic control while the manual sign is being produced (Doherty, 1985; Dunn, 1982; Kohl, 1981; Lloyd & Doherty, 1983).

- Visible vs. invisible: A manual sign (or gesture) described as "visible" is one the user can visually monitor while their hands and arms are making the sign (e.g., BOOK, GREEN, MILK). Visual feedback can be an advantage for many individuals, as manual signs made within the communicator's field of vision tend to be more easily produced (Dunn, 1982). This aspect alone provides an argument in favor of the incorporation of unaided elements in an AAC user's communication repertoire as a contrast to speech, which provides exceptionally limited visual feedback (e.g., "cow," "father," "thirsty") via lip and jaw movements and excursion of the larynx.

- One-handed vs. two-handed: In general, one- or two-handedness of a sign alone is not a reliable, direct measure of difficulty involved in producing the sign (Doherty, 1985; Lloyd & Doherty, 1983). Some manual alphabets involve single-hand representations for each letter; others (e.g., British Manual Alphabet) require two hands for production of some letters. Dennis and colleagues (1982) suggest that the important factors are laterality (i.e., unilateral/bilateral), combined with whether or not the midline of the body is crossed. For example, two-handed symmetrical signs (e.g., PERSON, WAIT, WANT) can be more easily produced than a one-handed sign that crosses the body midline (e.g., HOSPITAL, OUR, POLICE).

- Toward midline/body vs. away from midline/body: Movement of a manual sign toward the body or face (e.g., EAT, LOVE, SWEET) is more easily imitated than those that involve movement away from the body or face (e.g., BAD, GIVE, THANKS; Dunn, 1982). For most individuals, the movement involved in the production of a manual sign is more easily imitated than is the more refined characteristic—handshape (Dunn, 1982), which is discussed later.

- One movement vs. two or more movements: Unaided manual sign production varies in the degree of complexity required; many gestures require peripheral movements. The less complicated the required movements are for the expression of a manual sign, the more likely a person who experiences limited motor and/or visual discrimination abilities will be able to learn them.

- Symmetrical vs. asymmetrical: Symmetrical signs are those in which both hands perform the same pattern of movement. The movement of one hand is either the mirror image of the other or both hands reciprocally perform the same pattern. Symmetrical signs (e.g., BIG, PAIN, SHOE) are generally more easily learned and performed than are asymmetrical signs, that is, one hand is dominant and one hand assists (e.g., EARLY, HELP, TOAST; Dunn, 1982), because symmetrical signs require a lower level of neuromotor organization. Symmetrical signing allows the same neuromotor command to be issued to the two sides of the body, whereas asymmetrical signing requires activation of a particular movement for one hand and arm and inhibition of this movement pattern on the other side (Kohl, 1981).

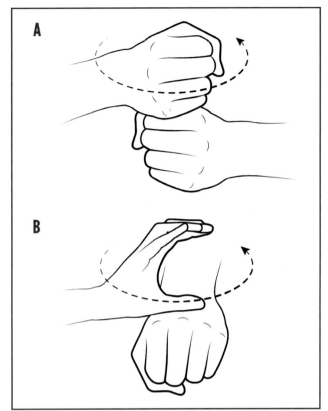

Figure 8-3. Two signs from ASL that are produced in the same location and with the same motion but differ only in handshape. (A) Coffee. (B) Chocolate. (Reproduced with permission from Christopher A. Neal, PhD.)

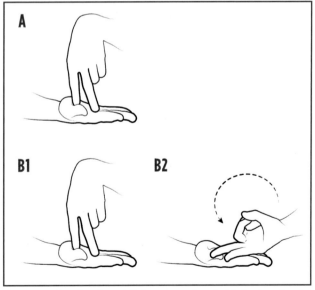

Figure 8-4. Two signs from ASL that are produced with the same hand-shape but differ only in orientation of the dominant hand. (A) Stand. (B1, B2) Fall (verb). (Reproduced with permission from Christopher A. Neal, PhD.)

- Complexity of handshape and/or movement: The configuration of the hand(s) performing a sign is probably the most analyzed parameter of the physical features of manual signs (Boyes-Braem, 1973). Some hand-shapes are more easily performed than others. Six basic handshapes have been distinguished. These include those that young children first learn in a natural way: the flat hand (or B-hand), the O-hand, the fist hand (or A-hand), the index hand, the C-hand, and the spread hand (or 5-hand). Studies of sign perception under visual noise show that sign observers tend to reduce perception of the signal to one of these basic forms (Klima & Bellugi, 1979). Preference for signs with these basic handshapes is recommended in the selection and/or adaptation of manual signs (and even gestures) for individuals who experience motor and/or intellectual disabilities. Logically, the more complex a handshape pattern is (i.e., those different from these six basic handshapes), the more difficult it is to learn (e.g., middle finger isolation—FEELING; thumb and little finger isolation—AIRPLANE; complex finger isolations—PURPLE).

- Maximum topographical dissimilarity: The ability to distinguish between manual signs requires they be recognizably different from one another. The greater the number of physical features shared by manual signs, the more difficult they can be to discriminate. Studies of naturally occurring errors in signing (i.e., "slips of the hands"; Klima & Bellugi, 1979) show that users of manual sign communication sometimes confuse signs that are minimally different from one another. So-called "minimal pairs" of signs have all but one critical feature in common. Figures 8-3 and 8-4 provide two examples of manual sign minimal pairs from ASL. In Figure 8-3, the two signs differ only in handshape. In Figure 8-4 the signs vary only in the orientation of the dominant hand.

Preference for signs that do not involve minimal pairs is recommended in the selection of manual signs for individuals who experience intellectual disabilities and/or difficulties in visual processing and discrimination—not uncommon challenges experienced by many users of AAC. For persons with significant communication disability, the number of manual signs learned might be quite limited. To maximize learnability, teachers and clinicians should select signs based on features, such as handshape, location relative to body, and/or direction of hand movement. Additionally, when teaching manual signs, programming teams must consider the functional utility of the sign to the learner, the representational value of the sign (i.e., its "guess-ability"), and the physical or motor characteristics of the sign (Bornstein & Jordan, 1984).

Iconicity, Concreteness, Abstractness of Representations

Unlike spoken language words, several types of unaided symbols can be processed through other less cognitively demanding ways. For example, many manual signs are considered to have a certain degree of "guess-ability" of meaning—that is, a communication partner who is not familiar with the manual sign is likely to interpret it correctly due to some visually physical resemblance with the sign's referent or an aspect of the referent. The degree to which a manual sign visually resembles its referent is described as iconicity. "*Iconicity* [emphasis supplied] means that the symbol has image-value" (Loncke, 2014, p. 6). Examples of iconic/transparent ASL signs include BABY, which involves laying the two arms atop one another and moving them back and forth as if rocking a baby, and DEER, which is made by placing two numeric 5 hands at the sides of the head to depict a deer's antlers. Iconicity is generally more easily achieved with unaided symbols than with graphic symbols (Loncke, 2014).

Unaided communication symbols vary in the degree to which they allow access to meaning based on visual recognition of the physical form. This results in the representations being classified along a continuum of iconicity; "*[t]ransparency* [emphasis supplied] implies that you can 'look through' the symbol and immediately extract its meaning" (Loncke, 2014, p. 6). This continuum ranges from truly obviously recognizable signs (as previously described), to those that are **translucent**, that is, easily retained/recognized once the relationship between the sign and referent is clearly explained (Lloyd & Blischak, 1992), to signs that are classified as opaque—only arbitrarily related to a referent. Examples of translucent signs are the ASL signs YEAR ("… produced by holding one fist steady while the other fist makes a rotation around it … [w]hen explained that this symbolizes the earth's rotation around the sun" [Loncke, 2014, p. 7]) and DOG (produced by slapping a flat hand against the thigh and snapping the fingers). Opaque manual sign examples include CANADA, PUNISH, and WHEN; these representations simply must be memorized.

Deaf and hearing users of sign languages largely ignore the visual relationship between a manual symbol and its referent while processing. They prefer a more linguistic strategy, which implies that manual sign recognition is based on analyzing the abstract configuration of the location, movement, and other significant parameters of the sign because linguistic processing allows for a more direct and faster lexical decision. Nonetheless, iconicity has been a central issue in the literature about manual signs and other unaided and aided symbols (Doherty, 1985; Fristoe & Lloyd, 1979b; Lloyd & Fuller, 1990; Luftig & Lloyd, 1981). Numerous studies have demonstrated strong evidence that iconic features of manual signs and other unaided symbols can be meaningfully processed through association or visual recognition and increase the accessibility of these by individuals who experience intellectual disability.

Although iconicity generally increases access to the meaning of a symbol through a perceivable relationship between the symbol and its referent, referents might differ in the degree of concreteness. It is recommended that particularly in initial lexicon selection, a programming team select symbols that refer to concrete and highly relevant elements in the daily lives of individuals who experience intellectual disability. However, it is equally important to recognize that abstract concepts can be effectively conveyed through unaided symbols that do not require speech.

Other Linguistic Unaided Symbol Systems

Eye-blink codes can be used for communication purposes. Individuals can learn to use eye blinking to convey a limited number of messages or through mastery of a process known as encoding. Encoding is a technique through which a communicator expresses multiple signals of a singular type that, in combination, specify a desired message. For example, by successively blinking a specified number of times or in a prespecified sequence, the individual could communicate a request for a change in body position or a drink of water. The manner in which the code is represented should be matched to an individual's strengths and abilities (Beukelman & Mirenda, 2013); eye-blinking is but one technique. Similarly, the eyes could be used to encode messages via a display-based code as an aided AAC option. Eye-blink codes are likely to become increasingly more common and important as additional sophisticated human-computer interfaces are perfected for individuals who experience significant physical disabilities (Królak & Strumiłło, 2012).

In special populations, such as head and neck cancer or trauma, other communication systems must be considered. For example, after total laryngectomy to surgically remove the larynx and vocal folds, individuals require an alternative method of communication or voice. Following total laryngectomy, three alaryngeal speech options for communication are routinely provided: an electrolarynx or artificial larynx, tracheoesophageal voice prosthesis (TEP), or **esophageal speech**. Of these three options, esophageal speech is the *unaided* AAC choice because it makes use of the body alone. Nothing in addition to the body is required. However, to master this skill, individuals often require extensive speech-language treatment and ongoing practice.

Esophageal speech involves teaching individuals after total laryngectomy to trap air in the upper esophagus using an injection or inhalation method (for method reviews see Gardner, 1962; Gately, 1971; Weinberg & Bosma, 1970). Upon air expulsion, the pharyngoesophageal segment becomes the vibratory source for sound production. Individuals are encouraged to overarticulate to increase speech intelligibility while expelling air from the upper esophagus. In comparison to laryngeal speakers, individuals producing esophageal speech have a reduced reservoir of air to support longer phrase and sentence production.

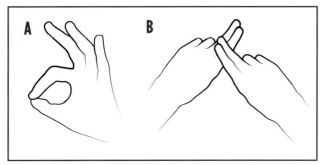

Figure 8-5. Sample elements from one- and two-handed manual alphabets. Each of these illustrations represents the letter F. (A) Shows the handshape for F in the ASL alphabet, which is a one-handed manual alphabet. (B) Represents the handshape for F in the British Manual Alphabet, in which all but one letter (i.e., C) are represented by two-handed configurations. (Reproduced with permission from Christopher A. Neal, PhD.)

In a recent systematic review of 26 available studies, researchers reported that most studies of speech outcomes after total laryngectomy were generally flawed in design and showed weak levels of evidence (van Sluis et al., 2018). Research conclusions indicated that, relative to esophageal speech speakers, TEP-aided speakers had more favorable outcomes in terms of acoustics parameters, fundamental frequency, maximum phonation time, and intensity. Perceptually, relative to esophageal speech and electrolarynx speaker groups, TEP speakers were rated significantly higher on measures of vocal quality and speech intelligibility. Yet, researchers concluded that after total laryngectomy, all speaker groups reported a degree of voice handicap.

Online survey results of individuals after total laryngectomy indicated that no single respondent in the technology device group used just one method of AAC (Childes et al., 2017). Moreover, findings indicated that individuals after total laryngectomy used multimodal unaided communication, including esophageal speech, gestures, and manual signs, as well as a variety of aided AAC options. A few respondents were unable to produce alaryngeal speech to support face-to-face and telephone communications.

Another less commonly used, but valid unaided AAC system, is pantomime, or simply, **mime**. Mime is best described as an elaborated form of gesturing. In general, mime includes the communicator using the whole body as opposed to primarily the face and upper extremities, as is the case in producing gestures and manual sign. Mime involves a more continuous series of actions and movements instead of discrete units, as is typical in a gestural system. For some users and their communication partners, this ongoing "acting out" can prove to be of benefit. For example, some individuals who experience aphasia are sometimes able to communicate through mimed sequences. Finally, mime can be used as an entry point for a communicator who demonstrates transitional symbolic skills before moving toward the use of gestures, manual signs, or other more abstract symbol corpuses.

Alphabet-Based Systems

The use of the *manual alphabet* [emphasis supplied] and all its derivative forms is also a potentially powerful means of alternative linguistic communication … [t]he manual alphabet refers to orthography—which, in turn, is based on spoken language (not sign language). The use of the manual alphabet is often called ***fingerspelling*** [emphasis supplied]. (Loncke, 2014, p. 68)

Fingerspelling dates back to ancient cross-cultural communication techniques (Savage et al., 1981). Used to some degree in the 17th century, fingerspelling techniques became more widely used during the 19th century as teachers at the Rochester School for the Deaf (New York) began to use it in a systematic way for language exposure and teaching with children who were deaf. This use of fingerspelling became known as the Rochester Method (Marschark et al., 2008). Apart from this use in educational programs, fingerspelled words are often intermingled in sequences of manual sign language communication, although more in some sign languages than others.

Several manual alphabets are in use around the world. Most of these differ only minimally, evidenced in a few handshapes. For example, the T in the American manual alphabet is a closed fist with the thumb extruding between the index and middle fingers. Presumably because this hand configuration was considered to be obscene, it has been banned from many European manual alphabets; instead of using a closed fist for the T, the middle, ring, and little fingers are extended. Although the American and several of the European manual alphabets are one-handed, some world sign languages are associated with two-handed manual alphabets (e.g., Australian, British, Pakistani; see Figure 8-5 for an example of one-handed and two-handed individual letter elements).

Morse code utilizes only two basic elements, a dot (i.e., dit) and a dash (i.e., dah). This system's surface-level simplicity is possible because of the underlying conventional combination rules (i.e., combinations of dots and dashes stand for an individual letter) and the underlying use of traditional orthographic rules. For individuals with strong cognitive and orthographic skills, Morse code can easily be utilized as an unaided AAC system. The dits and dahs can be signaled by many different body parts: eye blinking, using gestures or vocalizing, depending on the abilities of the communicator *and* the individual's communication partner(s). Eye-blink Morse code can be done by contrasting short and long eye blinks (i.e., duration of eyelid closure). Gestural Morse code might imply either the production of a single gesture using two durations (e.g., the example immediately preceding) or the production of two different gestures (i.e., an eye blink for the dit and a finger tap for the dah). Analogously, vocal Morse code uses two different forms of the same vocalization type (e.g., high vs. low pitched grunt) or two different vocalization types (e.g., a grunt and an "mmm").

Phonemic- or Phonetic-Based Symbols

Hand-cued systems have been designed primarily to provide greater visualization of speech as few cues are provided during the flow of natural speech in communication. The extra visual cues facilitate the reliability of speechreading. Even experienced speech readers are not able to distinguish voiced and voiceless phoneme pairs (e.g., /d/ and /t/, /b/ and /p/). The principle behind hand cues is to supplement invisible but critical phonological information to clarify a speaker's utterances.

Cued speech involves a linguistic level of access to language. It is a system developed by Cornett (1967) at Gallaudet University in the United States for the purpose of improving the literacy levels of individuals who are deaf (*not* to improve the individual's speech). Cued speech is currently used worldwide for teaching children who experience all levels of hearing loss, as well as others who benefit from visual access to spoken language; in 2006, it was estimated that cued speech had been adapted for use with more than 60 languages and major dialects (Ruberl & Franklin, 2006). The National Cued Speech Association estimates that cued speech adaptations are now utilized with approximately 70 languages (S. Roffe, personal communication, December 19, 2019). The adaptations can vary significantly from the English version since world languages have some phonemic differences from American English (Ruberl & Franklin, 2006). For a person who is deaf, a phoneme refers to a visual representation of an individual building block of manual sign; these are derived from handshape, location, palm orientation, and movement (Ruberl & Franklin, 2006). An overview of the English version of the cued speech system is provided in Figure 8-6. Cued speech may be used alone or in combination with other symbol corpuses. Some researchers suggest that use of a visual, bilingual-bicultural approach to communication programming for learners who experience hearing loss enhances the effectiveness of the cued speech system.

Alegria and colleagues (1992) demonstrated that the frequent use of phoneme-based cueing can facilitate the development of an internalized understanding of a language's phonological system. Contrary to more typical observations, these researchers found that deaf children who have been regularly exposed to cued speech showed improved performance on a series of phonological tests and performed at a higher level on reading tasks. In an earlier study, Périer and colleagues (1990) noted that the use of physical cues to distinguish speech articulations that appeared very similar but were phonemically different helped to establish an improved internalized relationship between phonemes and graphemes for individuals who experience reading disabilities or who are beginning readers. Later studies, including an investigation by Campbell and colleagues (1998) that involved the utilization of cued speech "… as a primary language medium immersing the child in a rich language environment" (p. xi), demonstrated improved receptive phonology and

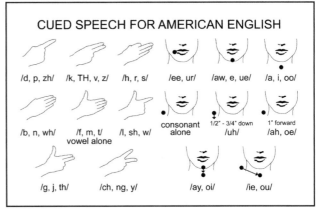

Figure 8-6. Cued Speech for American English. (Reproduced with permission from National Cued Speech Association.)

phonologic discrimination at levels similar to those of children without hearing impairment. It is believed this performance is attributable to the fact that "cued speech delivers *phonological* [emphasis provided], not (transformed) auditory information to the deaf person" (Campbell et al., 1998, p. xi).

Cued speech is but one of many phonemic-based systems used around the world. Other systems used in a variety of European countries include the Assisted Kinemes Alphabet (or Alphabet de Kinemes Assistes), the Danish Mouth-Hand System, and the Borel-Maisonny system.

A comparison of key features of one language-based unaided AAC symbol set/system for each of five primary linguistic levels of access to language is provided in Table 8-7.

Vibrotactile/Tactile Unaided Communication Components

Vibrotactile methods are based on the observation that a portion of spoken information can be experienced through recognition of vibrations from the speaker's vocal folds through an individual's tactile exploration and observation of the speaker. The use of vibrotactile information for teaching receptive communication skills emanates from educational practices with children who experienced severe hearing impairment. The best known vibrotactile communication approach is the **Tadoma method**. In this method, the individual places their thumb on a speaker's lips and fingers along the speaker's jaw. The middle three fingers of the person receiving the communication message rest along the speaker's jaw/chin and the little finger is in contact with the speaker's throat—to pick up vibrations of the speaker's vocal folds. Through these vibrations, the physical contact of the jaw opening and closing and facial expressions, the individual is able to decipher at least a portion of the speaker's spoken words (Reed et al., 1989). Learning to communicate through the Tadoma method is difficult and very time-consuming.

TABLE 8-7
Linguistic Levels of Language-Based Unaided Symbols

UNAIDED SYSTEM	RECEIVER'S PARTICIPATION	LINGUISTIC LEVEL OF ACCESS TO LANGUAGE MODEL	SKILLS REQUIRED OF SENDER
Cued speech	Bottom-up strategy (analytic skills) Short-term memory skills Development of phonologic, morphologic, and syntactic skills	Phonological	The sender must know and be able to identify and sign the phonological elements (i.e., phonological mastery).
Fingerspelling	Bottom-up strategy Facilitation of mental storage of words as written entities Short-term memory skills	Orthographical	The sender must know the orthographic rules and be able to recode spoken language into orthography.
KWS	Top-down strategy Context sensitivity Cognitive skills to process manual signs	Syntactical	The sender must be able to identify the words in the sentence that carry most information.
Signed English	Top-down strategy Short-term memory skills Cognitive skills to process manual signs Development of syntactic skills	Lexical	The sender must be able to access and activate (speak and sign) words and manual signs synchronously.
SEE-II	Combination of low-level elements (morphemes) with lexical units (words) Short-term memory skills Cognitive skills to process manual signs Development of syntactic skills	Morphological	The sender must demonstrate morphological mastery; must be able to access and activate (speak and sign) words and manual signs simultaneously.

KWS = key word signing; SEE-II = Signing Exact English.

A variety of other unaided tactile approaches (e.g., touch cues, signs on body, **co-active signing**, tactile sign language, **print-on-palm**, tactile fingerspelling, **Braille hand speech**, tactile Morse code) are broadly applicable for persons with acquired, developmental, or sensory disabilities (see Chapters 18, 21, and 23 for additional, more detailed information). Particularly in the case of individuals who experience DSI, unaided tactile communication approaches are frequently the forms of choice for augmenting receptive and/or expressive communication. Research suggests that especially in the case of an individual who learns tactile sign after mastering a visual sign system/language (Checchetto et al., 2018), the user is likely to become conversationally competent.

If communication partners are to employ tactile unaided communication strategies, it is critical the individual's programming team evaluate tactile sensitivities and skills. In addition, any time interpersonal touch is going to be involved in an individual's communication system, it is critical that person's cultural mores be taken into account by the team designing the AAC system. These considerations are discussed more thoroughly in Chapter 23.

MOTOR CONSIDERATIONS IN IMPLEMENTING UNAIDED AUGMENTATIVE COMMUNICATION COMPONENTS

Unaided AAC elements, primarily gestures and manual signs, do rely primarily on an individual's control and volitional movement of their upper extremities, though sometimes lower extremities might also be utilized. As previously discussed in this chapter, eye movement (i.e., eye pointing, eye-gaze shift, tracking) is a legitimate form of gesture, though one less conventionalized; therefore, eye gestures are recognized by a narrower range of potential communication partners. In a study that investigated an adaptation of the pre-linguistic milieu teaching model to learners with DSI and additional co-morbid disabilities, Brady and Bashinski (2008) found that learners who experienced significant physical disability demonstrated smaller gains in initiation rate than did participants without motor involvement. These learners did show improvement in communication rate, as well as in the diversity of communicative forms and functions utilized, but all at lower levels than the participants who experienced DSI and intellectual disability without motor impairment.

An individual's overall body control and **vestibular** function are also important considerations since various body positions might be more or less facilitative of the person's ability to express a message through unaided means (vocalization and/or manual sign). Core instability might also interfere with the AAC user's ability to receive and comprehend a message because of preoccupation with trying to maintain one's upright posture, head control, and/or balance. The individual's control of muscle tone and gross motor movements might be indices of what could be the most appropriate type(s) of unaided AAC for implementation.

When implementing AAC components with an individual who experiences significant motor disability, it is likely that a greater number of viable options would be available through aided AAC due to the wide variety of switch types and options for switch placement. Nonetheless, the contributions that facial expressions and controlled movements of any body part (e.g., eyes, elbow, foot) should not be excluded as potentially valuable unaided communication system components.

Basic Neurological and Sensory Considerations

In addition to hand and arm dexterity, facial expression, and overall body balance and vestibular functioning discussed before, an interprofessional team determining the implementation of unaided AAC must also consider other basic areas of ability. Due to the extreme ranges AAC users demonstrate in neurological function (including cognitive ability), visual skills, and hearing abilities, an unaided communication system must be customized for each individual. Obviously, the individual's level of cognition function must be taken into account if a team is to design an appropriate AAC intervention program.

When considering the use of any unaided tactile communication approach for either receptive or expressive communication purposes, the team must identify any severe neurological disability that might affect the individual's ability to perceive touch. If touch cues are to be used to enhance comprehension of communication, it is important to determine the type of touch (i.e., firm or light) the individual

favors, as well as the preferred placement on the individual's body. Tactile sensitivities must be considered. The AAC team should also assess specific ways in which the individual uses touch (e.g., how one's hands are used and for what purposes). Assessment should also be conducted regarding whether or not the individual shows awareness of being touched demonstrates reflexive behavior, and if they attend, alert, recognize, discriminate, and/or comprehend the touch or tactile stimulus.

In addition to considering an individual's basic neurological function, an interprofessional team selecting unaided components for an individual's AAC system must take into account the individual's visual and auditory abilities. Impairment in either or both of these sensory systems unquestionably interferes with accessibility to data from the external world because these are a person's primary information-gathering senses.

In regard to impairment in either hearing or vision, it is most important for team members to be aware of the time in the individual's life at which the impairment(s) onset. Congenital hearing and/or vision loss impact communication and language development very differently than do losses that occur later in an individual's life. The key questions to be asked are: Had the individual developed language prior to the onset of hearing loss? Had the individual developed visual memory prior to the visual impairment?

An individual's visual and auditory abilities can be impaired in a wide variety of ways. Critical considerations an AAC team must make when determining unaided components for the individual's communication system include both the degree(s) and type(s) of impairment in these two sensory systems. Is a sensory loss progressive or static? Regarding vision loss, which particular visual skills are impacted, visual acuity and/or visual field, or does the client exhibit signs of cortical visual impairment? Answers to these questions will have a critical impact on the individual's ability to receive and process gestures and manual signs expressed by a communication partner. If the individual cannot see adequately to receive visual input, comprehension is out of the question.

Regarding hearing impairment, is the loss conductive or sensorineural? Is it bilateral or unilateral? What are the decibel ranges and overall severity of the individual's hearing loss? Is there a central auditory processing disorder? If the individual cannot hear to adequately receive and process vocalizations/verbalizations expressed by a partner or SGD, both receptive and expressive communication abilities are likely to be severely impacted. For an individual who experiences vision and/or hearing loss, understanding concepts through more than one sensory/communicative mode will be imperative. The individual's communication partners should be planning a multimodal AAC system.

For an expanded discussion of these concepts and the ways in which hearing impairment, vision impairment, and DSI impact AAC program planning, please see Chapter 23 of this text.

Sequence of Gestural Development

Three primary principles describe the developmental pattern of individuals' overall motor abilities. First, motor skills mature in a cephalocaudal progression; that is, a person gains control of the head, neck, and trunk before developing motor control of the shoulders, hips, etc. Second, motor abilities develop in a proximal-distal pattern, that is, movements become coordinated in muscles closest to the body's midline until core control is gained. Only then does motor maturation proceed toward the distal parts of the body (e.g., elbows, wrists, fingers). Third, gross motor skills develop before fine motor skills are refined (Dunn, 1982). These principles explain why a particular gesture or movement of a manual sign is more easily imitated than is the refined handshape of a sign. In general terms, AAC teams should bear these developmental principles in mind when attempting to teach children whose motoric systems are immature to imitate the production of manual signs. (These principles also provide the theoretical foundation for the discussion of the Physical Features of Manual Signs that appears earlier in this chapter.)

Illingworth (1967) was among the first to integrate the developmental theories of Gesell, Piaget, and Halverson regarding the development of **prehension** skills. He expressed the view that acquisition of various prehension and motor skills is dependent on the level of maturity of a child's neurological system. Succinctly stated, Illingsworth's position was that "[n]o amount of practice can make a child learn certain prehensile skills until his nervous system is ready for them" (Priest Erhardt, 1974, p. 593). AAC teams considering unaided expressive communication systems for a particular child would be well advised to keep this principle in mind. For children and youth who experience multiple disabilities, and therefore, demonstrate atypical neurologic development, the interprofessional team should strive to balance opportunities to inhibit the individual's interfering reflexes and facilitate typical muscle tone. "To pave the way for the fine coordination of prehension and manipulation, the facilitation techniques should be used within the framework of the sequential process" (Priest Erhardt, 1974, p. 593).

In her 1974 publication, Priest Erhardt included a table of the key features of hand and finger movements in the sequential development of typical prehension skills. Excerpts from this table pertinent to the development of gesturing and manual signing ability are provided in Table 8-8. Teams considering the development and implementation of unaided AAC systems with very young children and youth who experience multiple disabilities might find guidance in this document. Regarding the emergence of conventional gestures in typical development for American culture, the gold standard resource is Wetherby's "16 Gestures by 16 Months" (16by16; 2014). "Development of gestures at 9 to 16 months predicts language 2 years later" (Wetherby, 2014, slide 22).

A research team associated with the FIRST WORDS Project (2014) has documented that young children produce a variety of gesture types or use unaided AAC before first words are spoken. In all, the FIRST WORDS Project team has published information regarding the 16 gestures critical to language learning (Table 8-9) and 16 actions with objects young children should demonstrate by 16 months of age. These skills provide the foundation for future language and literacy learning. Currently in development by FIRST WORDS Project researchers are 16 ideas to communicate for social connectedness, 16 ways to demonstrate cooperation (by managing emotions), and 16 critical-thinking messages. As noted before, it would behoove AAC teams considering unaided AAC intervention with children and youth to strive toward the accomplishment of these basic gestures (to the maximum extent the child's motor abilities will allow) before proceeding to an unaided communication system that requires considerable motoric skill.

IMPLEMENTATION OF UNAIDED AAC PROGRAMMING

Challenges an interprofessional team are likely to encounter when considering the implementation of an unaided AAC system with an individual, along with benefits to be reaped by the individual's mastery of such a system, are discussed in the sections that follow. When determining whether or not an unaided approach is the most appropriate communication system for trial with an individual, the interprofessional team is strongly encouraged to consider the many various types of unaided systems presented in this chapter (e.g., PCAs, ENGs, deictic/representational gestures, simultaneous communication, KWS, Makaton, MCE, PGSS, pedagogical sign systems, coding systems, alphabet-based systems, phonemic-/phonetic-based symbols, vibrotactile/tactile communication methods, *and* formal sign language).

This consideration alone of the many types of unaided systems presented in this chapter constitutes one of the foundational challenges an interprofessional team must face when deciding on an initial unaided AAC system, particularly for a young child. Families report feeling overwhelmed by the large number of choices available when first learning about unaided communication options for their child (Beginnings Board of Directors, 2007).

Challenges

In this section, the more generic types of challenges families and educational teams of children and adults who use unaided AAC systems (i.e., those *not* unique to a particular type of disability or traumatic event) will be discussed. Specific challenges associated with loss of motor skills/control, visual access to unaided AAC, and cultural considerations will be described subsequently.

One of the issues most commonly discussed by users of unaided AAC systems is the challenge of identifying communication partners who understand their unaided

TABLE 8-8

Sequential Levels in the Development of Typical Prehension Skills

AGE (IN WEEKS)	DESCRIPTION OF KEY OBSERVABLE MOTOR BEHAVIORS
20	Raking motion, involving fingers only
	No thumb or palm involvement
	Immediate approach and grasp on sight
24	Palmar grasp
	Still no thumb participation
	Eyes and hands combine in joint actions
28	Whole-hand grasp
	Thumb begins to adduct
	Unilateral approach to objects
	Transfers objects from one hand to the other
32	Inferior scissors grasp (also known as "monkey grasp")
	Thumb is adducted, no opposition
36	Fingers on radial side provide pressure on an object
	Thumb begins to move toward opposition
40	Inferior pincer grasp
	Isolated, poking index finger with inhibition of other four digits
	Beginning of voluntary release
44	Neat pincer or forefinger grasp
	Grasp with slight extension of the wrist
52	Opposition or superior forefinger grasp
	Wrist extended and deviated to ulnar side for efficient prehension skill
	Smooth release for large objects; clumsy release for small objects

This table is adapted to include developmental levels with particular relevance to the development of gesturing and manual signing ability.

Adapted from Priest Erhardt, R. (1974). Sequential levels in development of prehension. *The American Journal of Occupational Therapy, 28,* 592-596.

TABLE 8-9

Sixteen Gestures by Sixteen Months (16by16)

APPROXIMATE AGE (IN MONTHS)	GESTURE DESCRIPTION
9	Give
	Shake head (to indicate "no")
10	Reach
	Raise arms
11	Show
	Wave
12	Point with open hand
	Tap with fingers together
13	Clap
	Blow a kiss
14	Point with index finger
	"Shhh" gesture
15	Head nod
	Thumbs up
	Hand up (to indicate "wait")
16	At least one other symbolic gesture (e.g., high five, shoulder shrug [to indicate "I don't know"], universal peace sign)

Adapted from Wetherby, A. M. (2014, April). *Engaging families of children with developmental disabilities in early detection, early intervention, and prevention.* Keynote presentation at the National Academy of Sciences' Workshop on "Strategies for Scaling Tested and Effective Family-Focused Preventive Interventions to Promote Children's Cognitive, Affective, and Behavioral Health," Washington, DC.

communication and can use it to express messages back to them in order to have a true conversation. This applies not only to the individual's community generally, but sometimes to educational or work environments as well. Even family interactions can prove challenging if an individual uses simultaneous communication, KWS, Makaton, manually coded language, SEE-II, Signed English, or any type of coding system/symbols or formal sign language. In one of the lead author's experiences, teenaged twins in a classroom (at a residential school for the deaf) were crying because they "had to go home for the holidays," and they had no one there with whom they could communicate except for one another.

Interprofessional teams are earnestly requested to try to ensure that family members in particular, but also peers and coworkers, are provided training in how to use elements of the individual's unaided AAC system in order to communicate with them in some meaningful way. Even if communication might be limited, teams should do their best to ensure the AAC user will experience authentic opportunities to communicate with others at home, school, work, and in the community.

Even among high-achieving individuals with typically developed intellectual abilities, feelings of social isolation are often expressed. In particular, children—along with parents on their behalf—mention feelings of social isolation and the difficulties they experience in making and maintaining friendships. In the case of adult unaided AAC users, many individuals express concerns regarding obtaining employment and holding a job. Many aspects of daily living present challenges for unaided AAC users and their families (e.g., placing a food order in a restaurant, communicating with a dentist, making arrangements for car or home repairs). Again, AAC team members are encouraged to consider including the facilitation of social relationships/friendships in therapy interventions at a child's school or an adult's rehabilitation center, etc. as one component of the unaided AAC communication programming intervention.

In the case of a child or adult who has been diagnosed with some type of progressive disabling condition (e.g., Alzheimer's disease, amyotrophic lateral sclerosis, Huntington's disease, Usher syndrome) or who has experienced a traumatic event or closed head injury (with resulting **aphasia**, **apraxia**, or loss of motor/sensory skills), additional concerns and needs are added to the individual's and family's challenges. In the latter case, not only do the individual and family need to deal with the new necessity for an unaided AAC system, they are grieving the loss of the individual's former skills. In the case of an individual diagnosed with a progressive condition, the families and children/teenagers face practical *and* emotional challenges associated with the inevitable loss of skill(s) in the future. The uncertainty of this challenge alone can be paralyzing to an individual and one's family. Added to this is often fear of the unknown, depression, uncertainty, and/or anxiety. Members of an individual's AAC team should never underestimate the impact these emotional challenges might have on an individual's ability and/or interest in learning to use an unaided form of AAC.

Additionally, if an interprofessional team is implementing an unaided AAC program for an individual with a progressive loss of motor, visual, hearing, and/or cognitive skills, the team members must be proactive. While it is critical the team members be sensitive to the feelings the individual and family members are experiencing at any given point in time, the team must be planning the next step to be implemented in the AAC program when the individual's skill levels will no longer support their current unaided system. Take for example the case of an individual with Usher syndrome whose vision is rapidly deteriorating. The team needs to begin transitioning the individual's unaided communication system from a pedagogical sign system to a tactile sign system before the vision loss becomes too great and leaves the individual with no way to effectively communicate.

In the case of children and adults who experience cognitive disabilities in addition to their communication disorder, including those individuals who are experiencing intellectual decline due to dementia or Alzheimer's disease, it is essential the AAC team consider the level of the individual's linguistic understanding. The concreteness/abstractness of the elements in the unaided system is of increased importance in these circumstances. The interprofessional team might need to focus on iconic unaided manual signs and use of deictic or conventional representational gestures for inclusion in the individual's communication system.

Finally, interprofessional teams will find themselves challenged by the need to assess and plan for the manner in which each individual will both receive and express unaided components of the AAC system. The presenting challenge here is exacerbated when a given individual requires different forms of communication for receptive and expressive purposes.

Motor Ability/Control

A message is expressed through a motor plan whether by the oral musculature resulting in speech, by the hands and fingers resulting in manual signs of some nature, or by general body movements resulting in gestures or mime. It is indisputable that an individual's motor skills will in some way influence the ability to effectively utilize unaided AAC for the purposes of expressive communication. Important questions to be asked in this regard include whether or not the disability/condition limits the individual's range of motor actions and/or the nature of voluntary motor actions the individual can independently perform (Loncke, 2014). With this said, it is equally important to point out that an unambiguous causal relationship between the ability to learn manual signs and fine motor skills has never been established (Ogletree, 2010).

Although a majority of literature regarding motor planning and AAC system utilization focuses on aided systems and activation of icon sequences, motor planning and motor skills do affect the efficacy with which various unaided AAC strategies can be used with a given individual. The particular motor characteristics an individual demonstrates will be associated with the location, extent, and level of damage to the brain (Beukelman & Mirenda, 2013).

Both aphasia and apraxia are speech disorders, and both can result from brain injury, hemorrhage, or head trauma—most often to the left side of the brain. Aphasia primarily manifests as an impairment of linguistic capabilities, difficulty expressing language, and/or loss of ability to understand speech. Aphasia "… may affect mainly a single aspect of language use … [m]ore commonly, however, multiple aspects of communication are impaired, while some channels remain accessible for a limited exchange of information" (National Aphasia Association, n.d.a, para. 2). A condition of aphasia will likely impact primarily the types of motoric unaided AAC forms the individual will be able to receive and best comprehend.

Apraxia is a neurological disorder characterized by the inability to perform familiar movements on request. Although the request is comprehended, the individual has typical muscle tone and strength and is willing to perform the movement. Individuals with apraxia "… are usually unable to perform common expressive gestures on request, such as waving good-bye, beckoning, or saluting, or to pantomime drinking, brushing teeth" (National Aphasia Association, n.d.b, para. 1). Apraxia will impact the motor aspects of unaided communication production. An AAC team's knowledge of the individual's disability and/or diagnosis can serve as one important source of data for program planning. It is the responsibility of the AAC team to attempt to determine the remaining function available in each of the channels for the comprehension of motoric unaided AAC and the choice of form(s) of unaided AAC components to be attempted.

In the case of children and youth who experience developmental disability, physical and occupational therapists may contribute ideas about proper body positioning to best promote respiration patterns that will support vocalization. In addition, these professionals can advise AAC teams regarding optimal positions to provide adequate trunk support and head position, freeing the individual to focus on facial, arm, and hand movements for the purposes of expressive communication. An upright, stable body position will also facilitate the individual's ability to physically access a message from a communication partner.

Progressive weakening of muscles and loss of muscle control in conditions, such as amyotrophic lateral sclerosis, muscular dystrophy, and other neurodegenerative diseases that affect nerve cells in the brain and spinal cord will definitely impact the individual's ability to use an unaided AAC system (but also aided AAC components as well; Beukelman & Mirenda, 2013). These individuals will require intensive, ongoing assessment of motor abilities (e.g., bilateral fine motor skills, dexterity, facial expressions, general body movement, and motor control) if they are to remain successful augmented communicators. Interprofessional teams working with individuals who experience a progressive condition must always be planning for the future and preparing the individual for the next step in terms of what might be the most pragmatic approach as motor skills decline. The individual's motor ability to express communication through unaided means will undoubtedly change (as will their ability to access aided system components).

Visual Access to Gesture/Manual Signs

The challenges that confront the families and educational teams of individuals who experience visual impairment vary quite significantly based on the type(s) of loss, severity, and time of onset of the vision loss. The AAC team should prioritize the individual's use of their residual skills in order to visually perceive unaided AAC components. A majority of individuals who experience vision loss will maintain some degree of functional vision; therefore, AAC interventions should focus on strategies for supplementing residual visual skills to enhance communication effectiveness and satisfaction.

Visual access to gestures and manual signs might be influenced by many different variables. Visual accuracy will vary in day and night conditions for some individuals (e.g., those who experience retinitis pigmentosa will experience difficulty seeing at night; Willoughby, 1995). Some individuals with visual impairment will benefit from increased lighting, others will perform optimally in reduced lighting conditions. Some individuals will profit from targeted lighting (i.e., an intensive light focused on the hands of the communication partner or interpreter). Glare from windows or overhead lighting will very likely interfere with an individual's ability to receive and comprehend gestural or signed messages from a partner.

Reduced visual acuity might necessitate a communication partner being in closer proximity to the individual receiving an unaided communication message (i.e., to enable the individual to see the movement and/or handshape delivering the message content). However, in the case of a visual field loss (as opposed to a loss in acuity), the communication partner or interpreter might need to be positioned at a distance from the individual. If an individual retains central vision, the partner or interpreter needs to be further away as the visual field narrows, provided visual acuity remains strong. However, it is important to remember that fingerspelling cannot be enlarged and is difficult to accurately perceive from a distance (Flodin, 2004). If an individual experiences a central field loss and relies on peripheral vision to see, the communication partner or interpreter will need to stand to one side of the AAC user in order for the message to be received. Other determinations related to visual acuity and visual field that an AAC team must make include the size of the gestures/manual signs themselves and the size of the signing area. "Most signs are made within an imaginary rectangle in front of the body—an area extending from the top of the head to the waist and from shoulder to shoulder" (Flodin, 2004, p. 17). Depending on an individual's visual field and acuity, this signing area might need to be reduced in size.

Considerations similar to those made by AAC teams working with individuals who experience progressive loss of motor skills need to be made by interprofessional teams working with individuals who will experience progressive vision loss. The primary example of these is Usher syndrome (types I, II, and III; see Chapter 23 for a full discussion of the continual patterns of decline of vision and/or hearing skills for individuals who have this diagnosis). Usher syndrome type I typically involves a fairly rapid onset of progressive vision loss. No one can predict how a particular child will respond emotionally to their changing vision, how receptive they and the family will be to the introduction of tactile supports for language and learning, or the rate and pattern with which the vision loss will present and proceed. It is the responsibility of the AAC team to help the individual and family prepare for the inevitable change.

Diligent efforts in ongoing assessment are required of AAC teams in order that programs be designed to support continued use of the individual's current sensory abilities to the greatest extent possible while still preparing the individual to use unaided communication forms in the future (albeit with reduced visual skills). The AAC team is obligated to not only plan for the present but to also include long-range plans for transitioning the individual's mode of receptive communication from visual modalities to tactile/vibrotactile communication forms due to a progressive vision loss.

Finally, the impact of vision loss on the ability to receive unaided communication messages presents as a more frequent issue with the older adult population. For individuals who have been AAC users for much of their lifetimes, a clinician will need to bear in mind ways in which a loss of visual acuity will impact an individual's communicative competence.

Cultural Considerations

One important consideration in selecting gestures and symbols is how well they correspond to the community language and communication systems. Various factors are involved. One factor concerns the system's structure—to what degree do the rules used to combine symbols approximate the syntactical rules of the community's language? For example, pedagogical sign systems mirror the structure of spoken and written language, but sign languages typically have a dramatically different structure from the languages of hearing communities around the world. A second factor is the degree to which the guessability and intelligibility of gestures and symbols approximate the community's communication, and therefore, facilitate accessibility to meaning by a non-AAC user. Not only do sign language elements (i.e., manual signs and the manual alphabet) vary from culture to culture, gestures considered to be "conventional" vary from culture to culture as well. Some gesture sets may be very easily understood because they are part of the gestures conventionally used and understood within a culture; on the other hand, the meanings of most manual signs have low guessability for nonsign users. A third factor involves the degree to which the symbols lend themselves to being simultaneously produced and processed with spoken language (i.e., manual sign is often used simultaneously with spoken language). By producing both at the same time, the manual symbols are related systematically with the words of the spoken community language.

A significant number of deaf individuals identify themselves as multicultural—one valued culture is the Deaf/hard of hearing community and the second is the individual's own ethnic heritage. "Groups such as the Black Deaf Advocates and various organizations established by Hispanic, Asian, and American Indian deaf individuals testify to the complex and diverse multicultural identities of deaf Americans, (National Association of State Directors of Special Education, 2006, p. 12).

It is imperative that AAC assessment and intervention teams be aware of the conventions of the individual's culture regarding eye contact, touch, and touch between people of different genders and age groups. This knowledge is critical to culturally responsive education and rehabilitation plans.

Schools might be particularly challenged to consider each learner's unique linguistic and cultural needs and background. Interprofessional school teams "… should take into consideration that immigrant deaf children may know a sign language other than ASL or English and should not be considered as having 'no language' … [t]hese students may need specialized support from a second language perspective" (National Association of State Directors of Special Education, 2006, p. 12).

Benefits

Simply stated, the benefit of AAC intervention is central to quality of life, as well as access to and meaningful participation in activities of everyday living for an individual with significant communication challenges and their family. Other than the treatment of any potentially life-threatening health conditions, communication is consistently identified as the number one priority by families of children who experience significant communication delays or disorders in association with developmental disability (Beukelman & Light, 2020; Hartshorne et al., 2021; Wetherby, 2014; Williams, 2000), as well as individuals with acquired communication disorders and their families (Beukelman & Light, 2020; Pistorius, 2013). For individuals who do not acquire natural speech through the typical development process as young children or who lose such capability later in life due to a syndromic condition, illness, or injury, effective AAC intervention provides the gateway to communicative competence.

Effective AAC intervention does not just fulfill the desires and dreams of an individual and family. All individuals who experience disability to any degree, whether congenital or adventitiously acquired, have a basic right to fully participate in meaningful communication interactions and decision making to the greatest extent they are able and to affect determinations regarding their own lives (Brady et al., 2016). Fifteen specific, fundamental communication rights are articulated in the Brady and colleagues article, which presents the United States National Joint Committee for the Communication Needs of Persons with Severe Disabilities' *Revised Communication Bill of Rights*. Similar position statements have been developed in other countries around the world (e.g., by Communication Rights Australia and an adaptation of the original National Joint Committee for the Communication Needs of Persons with Severe Disabilities work in the United Kingdom in 2012).

A lifelong AAC user himself, Williams (2000) succinctly emphasizes the criticality of this perspective—and the benefits of AAC, both unaided and aided systems:

> The silence of speechlessness is never golden. We all need to communicate and connect with each other—not just in one way, but also in as many ways as possible. It is a basic human need, a basic human right. And much more than this, it is a basic human power. (Williams, 2000, p. 248)

In her hallmark paper in which she first proposed a definition of communicative competence for individuals who use AAC, Light (1989) emphasized the functionality of communication and the adequacy of an individual's knowledge and skills for supporting meaningful interactions. This first definition of communicative competence for users of AAC targeted the integration of knowledge, judgment, and skills in four interrelated domains: linguistic, operational, social, and strategic. Linguistic competence refers to an adequacy of the linguistic codes of not only the particular AAC system but the language spoken in one's community as well. Operational competence entails the user's mastery of the skills required to utilize an AAC system; Light proposed that system operations pertain to not only motor demands necessary for using the system but also to its cognitive and sensory/perceptual demands. Social competence refers to an individual's understanding of turn-taking and other discourse strategies, as well as interaction and communicative functions. Strategic competence entails the AAC user making "… the best of what they do know and can do" (Light, 1989, p. 141) in any given situation, allowing the individual to use compensatory strategies in order to effectively communicate, even if only in a restricted sense.

In 1997, Light wrote that the "… development of communicative competence has been identified as the central goal of [AAC] intervention" (1997a, p. 61). She highlighted the fact that communication goals should change across an individual AAC user's lifespan and emphasized that communicative competence both needs to be and can be learned.

Light (2003) further expanded her original definition and argued that the attainment of communicative competence is influenced not only by the four areas of competence explained previously but also by a variety of environmental barriers and supports and psychosocial factors. Confidence not only in oneself but on the part of family and interprofessional team members can be a major contributor to communicative competence. Confidence can influence motivation and attitude and undergird the resilience many AAC users will need to demonstrate in order to successfully navigate the waters of meaningful communicative interaction due to the challenges and inevitable failures to be encountered along the journey.

In the 25 years since the publication of the proposed draft of communicative competence for individuals who use AAC, significant changes in the AAC field have occurred, including changes in the "… demographics of the population that uses AAC … the scope of communication needs that must be considered … AAC systems that are available; and … expectations for participation by individuals who use AAC" (Light & McNaughton, 2014a, p. 7). However, these researchers concluded that the originally proposed definition:

> … continues to provide a useful framework for this new era of communication. Despite the dramatic changes in the AAC field, the essential goal of intervention has not changed … What has changed dramatically over the past 25 years, however, is how these communication goals are achieved. Whereas 25 years ago, the emphasis of AAC intervention was face-to-face interactions, today the scope of communication needs that must be addressed has exploded. (Light, 1989, p. 11)

AAC users must now be supported to access an ever-expanding variety of information technologies that are an integral part of everyday living and to do so within their own communities (i.e., home, school, work, leisure). Therein lie the benefits of a successfully implemented AAC system: fulfillment of an individual's and family's dreams, affordance of basic human rights and an avenue to self-determined power in one's environments, and the achievement of communicative competence within a variety of contexts in one's own community. These benefits apply particularly to forms of unaided AAC in those cases where personal preference, family interest/support, cognitive skill, financial resources, availability, and a variety of other factors rule out the choice of an aided AAC system for a particular individual.

Analysis of Unaided Features

As discussed in the section Sequence of Gestural Development, the three developmental maturation patterns of typical motor development should be the starting point for an AAC team considering the introduction of an unaided AAC system for a given individual. Individuals with developmental disabilities that impact their motor system (e.g., cerebral palsy, perinatal birth injury, Prader-Willi syndrome) or who experience lessened motor skills later in life due to injury or condition (e.g., multiple sclerosis, muscular dystrophy) should not be ruled out as candidates for an unaided AAC system! However, an AAC team would be well advised to consider these maturation principles when planning the expressive communication mode for an individual who has an immature or impaired motor system.

Priest Erhardt (1974) beseeches AAC teams to remember that "[n]o amount of practice can make a child learn certain prehensile skills until [their] nervous system is ready for them" (p. 593). AAC team members are encouraged to review the sequential levels in the development of typical prehension skills (outlined in Table 8-9), along with the detailed discussion of eight parameters that have been suggested to play a potential role in determining the relative physical ease of performance of individual signs (in the Physical Features of Manual Signs section of this chapter). This information should provide guidance for teams in analyzing the features of unaided AAC elements under consideration and assist them in determining the most appropriate unaided communication type(s) for a particular individual.

As another element in the interprofessional team's decision-making process, the team is encouraged to probe the individual's motor imitation ability. If a gestural system is being considered, provide a model of gross motor movements (e.g., push object away, reach with open palm, wave, point) in an authentic context and see if the individual can or will imitate the movement. The team should also evaluate the accuracy of the imitated movement and the amount of time it took the individual to reproduce it. If an AAC team is "… considering the use of manual signs, [members] should first attempt to teach a few signs that are highly motivating and functional for the person of concern" (Beukelman & Mirenda, 2013, p. 148), and as done in regard to gestures, take note of the accuracy with which the individual reproduces the manual sign and observe to see if the person begins to use the sign independently.

Teachability

The entire area of unaided AAC is premised on the foundational belief that individuals who do not have an effective means of functional communication can be taught to use a variety of unaided communication components. Whether an individual does or does not currently demonstrate abstract symbolic or linguistic ability and intentionality is irrelevant to this claim. For even those individuals who currently function at a nonsymbolic/pre-linguistic level of communication development, AAC teams can facilitate more effective communication interactions.

In the case of individuals who express communication through idiosyncratic behaviors and other nonconventional unaided forms, repeated interpretation of the communicative value of these attempts by communication partners is very likely to facilitate growth along the continuum of symbolization (Bashinski, 2014b; Malloy & Bruce, 2008). Over time, responsive partners' repeated interpretation of nonsymbolic and even unintentional behaviors (i.e., signals) and gestures might also shape intentionality and/or communicative intentionality (Bashinski, 2014a; Bruce et al., 2008). Consistent responses to an individual's potential communication signals facilitates growth in the direction of conventional communication (Sigafoos et al., 2000; Sigafoos & Mirenda, 2002) as the individual begins to impact the environment and experience the power of communication.

When interacting with an individual whose communication abilities are nonsymbolic and unintentional, the responsibility for a successful communicative interaction rests on the individual's partner(s). For growth to occur, it is critical that all members of an individual's AAC team, including family members, respond consistently to the PCAs targeted by the team for shaping into more conventional, intentional expressive signals. One way to accomplish this is through the development and implementation of an expressive signal dictionary (Bashinski, 2015b; Beukelman & Mirenda, 2013; Siegel & Wetherby, 2000; see Table 8-10 for an example). However, an AAC intervention program for a nonsymbolic and unintentional individual would be incomplete without a reciprocal component to target the growth of the AAC user's receptive communication skills. To this end, an AAC team is encouraged to implement a receptive signal (i.e., augmented input) dictionary (Bashinski, 2015b; see Table 8-11 for one example) as a complement to the expressive communication tool. Even with the implementation of these dictionary strategies, some individuals will primarily produce only PCAs and remain nonsymbolic (i.e., presymbolic/pre-linguistic) communicators throughout their lifetimes, though others will go on to develop symbolic, intentional communication.

A number of researchers have documented that individuals can be taught to use communicative gestures (FIRST WORDS Project, 2014; McNcill, 1992; Wetherby, 2014). Loncke (2014) states that gestures are "… an obvious and natural choice to express symbols at a time during development when children are not entirely ready for speech yet" (p. 62). In an investigation designed to teach communicative gestures through an adapted pre-linguistic milieu teaching model, Brady and Bashinski (2008) worked with learners who experienced multiple significant disabilities. These researchers found that all learners showed improvement in communication rate using gestures, as well as diversity of the communicative gestural forms used and functions utilized. Learners who experienced significant physical disabilities demonstrated smaller gains in initiation rate and diversity of gestural forms than did participants without motor involvement.

A motor argument can be made for teaching a person in need of an AAC system to use manual signs. Simply stated, this argument is premised on the fact that production of a manual sign is a motor task more easily accomplished than is speaking. Also, it is possible for members of an AAC team to physically mold the individual's hands and fingers into a desired configuration and assist with any required arm movements in order to produce the desired sign (Loncke, 2014). Such is not possible with regard to speech sounds.

As noted before, when an AAC team is considering the use of manual signs with a potential AAC user, a trial period should be implemented during which team members "… should first attempt to teach a few signs that are highly motivating and functional for the person of concern" (Beukelman & Mirenda, 2013, p. 148). Data should be collected regarding the accuracy with which the individual reproduces the manual sign and whether or not the person begins to use the sign independently. A manual sign unaided AAC system is not likely to be truly functional if an individual does not demonstrate acquisition of signs at a reasonable rate and reproduce them, such that they are readily understood by unfamiliar, as well as familiar, partners (Mirenda, 2003).

As a Supplement in Multimodal AAC Systems

The vast majority of all communication exchanges are, in fact, multimodal (Mirenda, 1999). This is the way mostly everyone communicates most of the time, though in some situations, individuals shift to rely more or less on speech, unaided forms (e.g., gestures, mime, manual signs), and aided forms (e.g., handling of objects, photographs, speech-generating technologies) across familiar/unfamiliar partners and environments. Facile speakers of a native language can sometimes shift across modalities with little effort, though transitioning to use another language (spoken or signed) can result in the speaker shifting to a different unaided or aided communication modality. Speakers often use gestures to represent real-world actions to add information to their spoken message; for example, sometimes to emphasize a point, a speaker might use more pronounced gesturing.

TABLE 8-10

Expressive Signal Dictionary

EACH TIME SUSAN DOES THIS ...	IT WILL BE INTERPRETED TO MEAN THIS ...	SUSAN'S PARTNER WILL DO THIS ...	SUSAN'S PARTNER WILL SAY THIS ...
Leans upper body in the direction of the adult who has entered her space	"Please interact with me; I want to do something with you!"	Give Susan attention—make eye contact and provide touch cue to left forearm	"You want to talk for a little while…"
Makes a high-pitched squeal	"I'm getting stressed—I can't do this!"	Go to her; calmly put one hand on Susan's right shoulder	"I'll help you get the _____," or "I'll help you do the _____."
Hits own left shoulder or chest	"No! I don't want to do that!"	*If request **is** optional*, move away *If request is **not** optional*, take a break for 10 seconds	*If optional*, "You want to do something else." *If not optional*, "Take a break."
Scrapes hand with teeth and/or bites the lower palm of her hand	Susan is feeling some type of major distress (e.g., pain, frustration, fear)	Gently lower Susan's hand, then firmly squeeze both sides of the base of Susan's neck with own two hands	"Relax, I'm here. It will be OK" (using a reassuring tone of voice).
Reaches in the direction of an object (placed on table or her wheelchair tray)	Susan is interested in the object—"I want that…"	*If Susan **may handle** the object*, let her hold it, use it, or explore it *If Susan **may not handle** the object*, assist her to look at it for 15 to 20 seconds, then remove the object	*If Susan **may handle** the object*, "You want the _____." *If Susan **may not handle** the object*, "I'll help you see the _____."

Note: For the purpose of this chapter focused on unaided AAC components, all references to *object* cues have been removed from this example dictionary.

Adapted from Bashinski, S. M. (2015b, March/April). Receptive and expressive dictionaries for students who do not use symbols. *Word of Mouth, 26*(4), 16.

The primary reason that unaided communication components might be used as supplements in multimodal AAC systems is because SGDs are not feasible modes for communication in all settings (e.g., a bathtub, swimming pool) and these will not always be operational (e.g., batteries die, devices malfunction). Non-SGDs, such as calendar boxes, line drawings, or Blissymbol boards, might not always be available either (e.g., when an individual is in bed, in a dark movie theater). For an individual with a large vocabulary, an aided AAC user's lexicon may be limited considerably by using a non–speech-generating or speech-generating display or device; however, emergency and high-frequency words should be available to the individual at all times. How is this accomplished? It is most easily accomplished by helping the primarily aided AAC user learn vocal or other unaided symbols to convey those high priority messages.

AAC users, particularly those who communicate primarily via sign language or another unaided linguistic symbol system, will frequently find it necessary to substitute their expressions when they encounter a partner who does not understand their language or dialect. In these situations, the individual will often shift to the use of pointing, manipulating available objects, or using other gestures conventional to the communication partner. With this change, the AAC user has increased the chances of having a successful communication interaction. The point is that accomplished communicators do whatever it takes to make their communication efforts successful and enhance their partner's understanding (Sigafoos & Drasgow, 2001).

Use of a multimodal system offers the distinct advantage of covering all the bases (Beukelman & Mirenda, 2013) when a team is designing an AAC system for an individual. For a more detailed discussion on this topic, see the section titled Power of Multimodal Communication earlier in this chapter.

TABLE 8-11

Receptive Signal (i.e., Augmented Input) Dictionary

TOUCH CUE	USED TO COMMUNICATE THIS MEANING …	SUSAN'S PARTNER WILL DO OR SAY …	WHAT IS EXPECTED FROM THE LEARNER
Touch to Susan's left forearm	"Hi! I'm here to do some work with you."	Make eye contact as approach, pause, provide TOUCH cue. **SAY:** "Hi, Susan, it's time to do some work."	Reach out with one or both hands in the direction of the person as an indication of her readiness for interaction
Tap two times on Susan's ankle (right and left); repeated for each	"It's time to put on your AFO."	Extend arm and hand, palm up, as target for Susan. **SAY:** "Ready for your AFOs?"	Move the leg (to which cue was given) up, in the direction of the adult's hand
Tap back of Susan's hand (in which she is holding something) with partner's index finger	"I want you to give me the _____."	Extend arm and hand, palm up, as target for Susan. **SAY:** "Give me the _____."	Voluntarily release grasp on the object, giving it to the partner

AFO = ankle foot orthotics.

Note: For the purpose of this chapter focused on unaided AAC components, all references to *object* cues have been removed from this example dictionary.

Adapted from Bashinski, S. M. (2015b, March/April). Receptive and expressive dictionaries for students who do not use symbols. *Word of Mouth, 26*(4), 16.

CONSIDERATIONS FOR SUCCESS IN THE IMPLEMENTATION OF UNAIDED COMPONENTS FOR COMMUNICATION INTERVENTION

First and foremost, the elements of the AAC system being considered for adoption must be acceptable to the potential user, the family (e.g., parents, children, siblings), and other significant individuals (e.g., peers, friends, medical personnel, clergy). These parties will likely serve as the unaided AAC user's primary communication partners; therefore, they must have an understanding and appreciation of the unaided AAC system and be taught ways in which to meaningfully interact with the person who will be using the system for communicative expression. Detailed plans for teaching both the individual who will use the various unaided AAC system components and all their most likely communication partners are critical to the successful implementation of an unaided AAC system. The further removed an unaided system is from the conventional vocalizations and gestures commonly utilized within a given culture, the more essential training becomes for potential communication partners. If the individual does not welcome and embrace both the receptive and expressive types of unaided AAC elements being proposed, achievement of communicative competence is not likely, even if the system is exceptionally well-designed to match the user's needs and abilities.

Next, the achievement of successful unaided AAC implementation should consider the type and extent of the individual's specific language impairment and needs; their motor abilities and challenges, including the presence of any neurogenerative disease; the individual's level of cognitive function and any possible diagnosis of progressive intellectual decline; and the types and degrees of their vision and/or hearing losses, as well as the diagnosis of any condition that will result in a continued loss of sensory abilities.

Insights from the developmental literature provide a rationale for intervening earlier using unaided AAC with infants and toddlers, as well as older individuals with severe communication disability. Under this view, AAC may not be used solely as a primary output mode for communication but rather for a language and communication intervention strategy and/or a tool to augment existing natural speech (Cress & Marvin, 2003; Romski & Sevcik, 2005). This also relates to multimodal communication or the use of all available modes for more efficient and effective communication. For example, unaided AAC can augment available speech (e.g., child points to a cup and vocalizes "ah" to indicate "drink"). Unaided AAC can provide for both an input mode and/or output mode for language and communication (e.g., caregiver produces sign for "drink" then child shakes head "yes" to indicate "I want drink."). Further, unaided AAC can be used as a language intervention strategy (e.g., clinician pairs the spoken word "drink" with manual sign DRINK to teach a child to combine manual sign with vocalization or a close approximation of a spoken word). The developmental literature shows that it is never too early to incorporate AAC into language and communication intervention for young children with a significant communication disability (Romski & Sevcik, 2005). Clinicians and educators must have the knowledge and skills to link AAC to early language and communication development.

For older individuals with significant communication disabilities who function primarily at the pre-linguistic level, unaided and aided AAC approaches may be useful to scaffold more intentional communication. The myth that AAC should be used only as a last resort when all other verbal treatments have failed has now been debunked (Cress & Marvin, 2003; Kangas & Lloyd, 1988; Romski & Sevcik, 2005). Rather, current literature supports the idea that clinicians, educators, and caregivers should introduce AAC to individuals who have severe communication disabilities early in development. See the American Speech-Language-Hearing Association practice portal on AAC for a summary of AAC myths and realities and roles and responsibilities of speech-language pathologists (https://www.asha.org).

Specifically, clinicians and educators working with individuals who function primarily at the pre-linguistic level of communication should assess the effectiveness of existing communication (i.e., modes and communication functions), find the right AAC intervention to make pre-linguistic communication as effective as possible (i.e., consider both unaided and aided AAC) and explore the possibilities to facilitate transition toward linguistic communication (i.e., multimodal communication facilitating speech and AAC use; Loncke, 2014). PCAs and gestures can be noted in an expressive signal dictionary, which can be a useful tool to record the expansion and evolution of an individual's use of various expressive forms. However, implementation of this sort of dictionary would be incomplete without pairing it with a complementary dictionary for augmenting input to the beginning AAC user (see Tables 8-10 and 8-11 for examples).

For individuals who capably use transitional symbol systems or linguistic symbol systems, the AAC team should be engaged in ongoing dynamic assessment with each person to ensure the individual's exposure to new lexical content, function, and more sophisticated forms of expression. The interprofessional team should hold high expectations for each and every unaided AAC user with the ultimate goal of helping the individual achieve comfort and mastery with the unaided system/language to which they aspire. Through data-based decision making and scaffolding of therapy and instruction, no AAC user's articulated goals should be deemed out of reach.

Summary

Augmenting an individual's communication skills through a variety of unaided forms can provide a powerful assist for individuals who experience significant communication disabilities.

Evidence assembled to date in the extant literature base suggests that the use of unaided gestural forms or manual signs does not negatively impact an individual's motivation to speak nor interferes with this ability in any known way. In fact, it has been suggested that the utilization of unaided AAC forms might enhance an individual's development of conventional speech communication (Beukelman & Mirenda, 2013; Loncke, 2014; Millar et al., 1999).

As Light (1997a) so powerfully reminded us more than 2 decades ago, "Communication is the essence of human life." The onus is on AAC team members of all individuals who utilize unaided AAC approaches or unaided AAC elements as components of their multimodal augmented communication systems, to make these individuals' communicative attempts effective realities in authentic, meaningful ways.

Study Questions

1. Describe three key features that differentiate formal sign languages from pedagogical sign language systems (e.g., ASL compared to SEE-I, SEE-II, Signed English).

2. Differentiate unaided and aided AAC symbols. Clarify the parameters of all types and corpuses that are included under the umbrella of unaided AAC.

3. Describe the contributions the partner of a nonsymbolic (i.e., presymbolic) communicator must contribute to ensure a successful communication interaction.

4. Briefly explain the elements involved in an individual's development of communicative intentionality. Be sure to contrast intentional behavior and intentionally communicative behavior.

5. Briefly describe the expectations for the emergence of gestures in the process of typical communication development. Discuss the ways in which gestural development contributes to symbolic language and literacy skills.

6. Consider the many various types of unaided AAC corpuses. Choose at least three of the following and compare and contrast their similarities and differences: PCAs, ENGs, Amer-Ind, KWS, Makaton, PGSS.

7. Select at least three individual manual signs. Analyze each of these manual signs in regard to each of the eight feature categories of manual signs that should be considered by an AAC team when selecting an unaided lexicon for an individual.

8. Choose one of the unaided AAC systems described as a "linguistic unaided symbol system." Describe its features and the aspects of the system by which it qualifies as a symbolic linguistic system.

9. What are some of the challenges associated with the implementation of an unaided AAC system with an individual? What are some of the benefits?

10. Briefly describe the ways in which an AAC team should consider an individual's neurological, sensory, and motor strengths and limitations to inform decision making in regard to the provision of appropriate AAC services for a person with complex communication needs.

Part III
AAC Technology

9

Background, Features, and Principles of AAC Technology

Juan Bornman, PhD; Annalu Waller, PhD;
and Lyle L. Lloyd, PhD

MYTH

1. Access to information and the ability to communicate with a computer will at last close the gap between individuals with and without disabilities.

2. Technology can be used effectively only by individuals with higher cognitive skills; therefore, speech-generating devices (SGDs) are of little value to individuals with intellectual impairments.

3. Such tremendous strides have been made in technology over the last couple decades that SGDs now offer the ultimate solution to meeting the communication needs of individuals with little or no functional speech.

REALITY

1. Many people have suggested that technology will enable individuals with disabilities to function on an equal basis with persons without disabilities. However, since technology serves all people, it is possible that the gap could be widened even further, as technology dramatically increases the productivity of able-bodied individuals. The challenge is to continue to increase the extent to which individuals with disabilities can develop their skills to their full potential, enjoy independence, and participate meaningfully in society.

2. Although it is true that the power of technology includes increased access to vocabulary and often requires cognitive skills to code and retrieve messages, there are many documented cases of the successful use of SGDs by individuals with significant cognitive impairments. With systematic teaching and good environmental support, speech and language have also been facilitated by the auditory feedback provided by devices with voice output (Morin et al., 2018; Rispoli et al., 2010; Romski et al., 2010).

(continued)

Fuller, D. R., & Lloyd, L. L. *Principles and Practices in Augmentative and Alternative Communication* (pp. 173-194).

REALITY (CONTINUED)

3. It is true that the power of technology can provide access to communication for many individuals with severe disabilities (e.g., an individual with quadriplegia can now operate an SGD via eye gaze). However, speech-generating technology is not a panacea. It requires additional cognitive effort on the part of the user and may be limiting in certain environments. In many cases, non-SGDs may be a more appropriate approach.

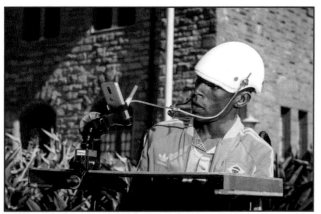

Figure 9-1. "I have a special voice."—France Mngenge, 2012. (Reproduced with permission from Mariki Uitenweerde, EyeScape Photography.)

INTRODUCTION

I would like to tell you about myself. I don't have a voice like other people do, but I can speak. I have a special voice on my laptop that helps me to communicate better with others. With this new voice of mine, I started to feel different because it got my head high and I started to believe in myself. It kept me going and every time when I wake up in the morning, I just can't wait to use my voice. If you have a voice, life is easy because you are free to talk about anything … France Mngenge (2012; Figure 9-1)

The fourth industrial revolution (Schwab, 2016), characterized by cyber-physical systems, has stimulated science and technology advances in areas, such as the internet of things, 3D printing, and advanced robotics and supporting technologies, including artificial intelligence and big data/analytics (Liao et al., 2017). Digital technologies are no longer isolated but are interconnected via the internet, allowing them to go beyond traditional organizational and territorial boundaries, revolutionizing the way in which society functions. This revolution has impacted the augmentative and alternative communication (AAC) field, with the explosion of mobile AAC apps and use of mainstream social media (Hemsley et al., 2017; Hemsley & Murray, 2015; Hynan et al., 2015; Wepener et al., 2019).

Advancements in mainstream mobile devices (e.g., smartphones and tablets) have opened communication opportunities and environments, such as convenient electronic commerce, rapid sharing of information, contact with other cultures, emotional support, and entertainment for all—with 1.85 billion users in 2014, 2.32 billion in 2017, and 2.87 billion in 2020 (Statista, 2017). In terms of AAC technologies, speech-generating systems can be divided into **dedicated communication devices** (i.e., those developed solely for the purpose of communication), and nondedicated devices, such as computers that have been adapted to allow them to function as a communication tool but can also be used for other functions (e.g., navigation and access to the web). Individuals with disabilities, and specifically communication impairments, stand to gain the most from nondedicated mainstream technologies. The 21st century has seen a paradigm shift from expensive, dedicated SGDs to nondedicated, relatively inexpensive devices with the added benefit of being stylish and "cool" (Foley & Ferri, 2012; Meder & Wegner, 2015). In low- and middle-income countries, mainstream mobile devices with dedicated communication apps have become the preferred AAC system for many individuals (Bornman et al., 2016).

HISTORICAL OVERVIEW

Despite the potential of technology, persons who use AAC tend to be passive, seldom initiate interaction by introducing a conversational topic, respond with one-word utterances, and rely on others for transitions (Judge & Townsend, 2013; Waller, 2006). Researchers have pleaded for many years that AAC technology should be user-driven (not manufacturer-driven, as is the case currently) and that incorporating the priorities and preferences of AAC users themselves will improve the design of AAC technologies (Judge & Townsend, 2013; Light et al., 2007; Waller et al., 2005).

There is no doubt that the design of AAC systems have benefited from the fourth industrial revolution. For example, technological advances have resulted in: (a) miniaturization leading to mobile technologies and increased portability; (b) enhanced speech technology leading to improved intelligibility (including a choice of accents) and the concept of voice banking, which uses digitized natural voice to drive speech synthesis; (c) a wider range of physical access, such as touchscreens and eye-gaze technologies; (d) improved displays and access to image capture leading to the use of color, photography, and video in AAC systems (e.g., the use of **hotspots** on **visual scene displays** [VSDs]); and (e) connectivity leading to accessing mobile communications (e.g., texting and social media).

However, despite these revolutionary changes in the broader technology field, the underlying design of AAC systems has not kept up with these exponential changes. Most systems rely on a grid-based paradigm, where users navigate screens containing a fixed set of lexical items (e.g., letters, words, symbols). Mnemonic retrieval codes (e.g., Baker,

1982, 1987) and hierarchical vocabulary organization (used in dynamic screen systems) provide access to prestored words, phrases, and messages. These systems provide pre-literate users with access to spoken language. Literate users can benefit from word prediction to speed up typing rates, but little has changed since the development of early prediction systems, such as the Predictive Adaptive Lexicon system in the 1980s (Swiffen et al., 1987), despite significant advances in mainstream text entry systems driven by the ubiquitous use of small mobile screens for texting and social media (Zhai & Kristensson, 2012).

The World Health Organization (WHO) estimates that the prevalence of disability has increased from approximately 10% in 1970 to about 15% worldwide, which means that more than a billion people are estimated to live with some form of disability (WHO & World Bank, 2011). Of these, 2.2% to 3.8% have a significant disability, which implies that they will benefit from using technology—a staggering 22 to 38 million people! Furthermore, the demographics of those who could benefit from AAC have changed in relation to the increase in the severity and variability of disability (Light & McNaughton, 2014a). Creer and colleagues (2016) report that 0.5% of persons in the United Kingdom (97% of whom have conditions, such as autism, cerebral palsy, dementia, head injury, learning disability, multiple sclerosis and motor neuron disease, Parkinson's disease, or stroke) could benefit from AAC. The increase of severity of physical disability and extended life expectancy suggests that AAC systems need to be more flexible and adaptable.

CURRENT USES OF TECHNOLOGY

Assistive technology has become part of everyday life and is used to help us live, learn, work, and play in a variety of contexts with as many different interaction partners as we choose. The International Classification of Functioning, Disability and Health states that the ultimate goal of assistive technology is to increase independence and participation (WHO, 2001). Technology is used ubiquitously for—among others—online services (e.g., banking); communication purposes (e.g., social media, such as Facebook, LinkedIn, and Twitter, as well as text messaging, picture capturing, and emailing); education and employment (e.g., tablets); entertainment (e.g., books, news, video); environmental control (e.g., using Amazon Alexa and other voice-assistant smart home systems); health and safety (e.g., activating a distress call on a smartphone); mobility (e.g., wheelchairs); navigation (e.g., GPS); and personal organization and cognitive support (e.g., address book, calendar, clock, and customer services, like airport check-in; Bryen et al., 2017; Shane et al., 2012).

Persons with disability can now, through the use of mainstream assistive technology, also log on and order groceries, shop and pay for appliances, research health questions, participate in online discussions, and catch up with friends or make new ones at any time and from anywhere (Bornman

et al., 2016). Despite these benefits, access remains challenging with only 35% of persons with disabilities in North America having access to mainstream mobile devices, compared to 75% of persons without disabilities (Duchastel de Montrouge, 2014).

AAC technology can be regarded as one of the subcategories of assistive technology. In the past, AAC devices were described using a low technology vs. high technology dichotomy. Low technology was seen as inexpensive, simple-to-make, and easy-to-obtain devices, as well as those that require simple equipment and typically referred to communication boards, switch-operated toys, loop tapes, and tape recorders and switches (Cook & Hussey, 1995; Glennen & DeCoste, 1997; Quist & Lloyd, 1997). High technology, on the other hand, referred to sophisticated, usually programmable devices that typically use an integrated circuit (Glennen & DeCoste, 1997; Quist & Lloyd, 1997).

However, the once-clear line between low technology and high technology has blurred over the years—especially over the last decade. For example, tablet technology could be considered low technology if the only use is to serve as a communication board without speech output; however, adding speech output to tablet apps could very well change the tablet into a type of high technology. In this chapter, we propose to not use this archaic dichotomous view, but to rather focus on the technology classification scheme proposed in Chapter 3. For this chapter, the focus is on expressive, aided technology, so for the remainder of this chapter, we will make the distinction between non–speech-generating and speech-generating technology. However, it is imperative to state that non–speech-generating (often self-made and low cost) should not necessarily be viewed as inferior to speech-generating (often more expensive) options (van Niekerk et al., 2017). Considering the diversity of both communication partners and environments, persons who use AAC may well need speech-generating options in some settings and non–speech-generating in others—in fact, non–speech-generating options should be a critical part of all communication systems, in line with the focus on multimodal communication (Bornman, 2011). For example, an 8 year old may use a speech-generating option for academic purposes in the classroom, but a non–speech-generating communication bracelet with symbols for the playground. Furthermore, in a group situation, a non–speech-generating alphabet board might be preferred to ask private, discreet questions (e.g., "I need the bathroom") rather than using an SGD. Non–speech-generating options can also serve as back-ups if and when SGDs break down or need servicing (Quist & Lloyd, 1997).

One of the greatest threats to AAC technology is to regard it as an appliance—similar to a toaster or a coffee maker—something that does not need training to operate it. Nothing could be further from the truth. Owning a violin does not make one a violinist just as owning a bicycle does not make one a cyclist. Neither does owning AAC technology make one a communicator. Although the technology (whether a violin, bicycle, or AAC) has the potential to increase an individual's participation in family life, education, leisure, and ultimately, quality of life, training is required for that to happen. Therefore, AAC technology should be viewed as a tool rather than as an appliance. Despite the rapid growth of available technologies for individuals who require AAC to communicate, concerns have been raised that these technologies may in fact have limited functional use.

Although applied technology offers many benefits, the AAC community is not yet reaping them, and the high rate of abandonment of technology remains a concern (van Niekerk et al., 2017; van Niekerk et al., 2019). Some authors quote an estimated rejection rate of AAC technology as high as 53.3% (Prior et al., 2013). This high rate of rejection is multifaceted but is partly due to the lack of user-centered design in the development of these devices, a poor match between user requirements and technology, and lack of training and knowledge to adapt and configure AAC technology to meet the developmental and changing needs of users and environments in practice (Norrie et al., 2021). Therefore, it is essential to understand the features and types of AAC technology in order to choose systems that will support communication needs and goals of individual users, support users to use the system, and adapt technology for use in different contexts and as the user's requirements change over time.

Feature Matching

When selecting and using AAC technology, we need to identify the requirements of the person who uses AAC, their communication partners, and those who support and maintain the systems. AAC practitioners would generally agree that technology should be able to "level the playing field" for the person, be able to work effectively in cross-settings, be portable to increase accessibility, be easy to maintain, be affordable to replace and/or maintain, and have good and reliable technological support and training. Therefore, feature matching is a continuous process of optimizing technology to adapt to the ever-changing requirements of both individuals and the environments in which they live, learn, and work.

In the AAC field, the important viewpoint of the family, or the "circle of support," has often been emphasized in the selection of devices and subsequent intervention (Blackstone & Hunt Berg, 2003). While it is certainly of paramount importance to consider the family's expectations and preferences, the preferences and perspectives of the person who uses AAC (whether they are a child or an adult) should be considered. Unfortunately, this factor is less often considered, particularly in the case of children, despite the fact this could contribute to their satisfaction and ultimate utilization of the device (van Niekerk et al., 2017).

Furthermore, professionals who provide services to persons who use AAC and their families (both with regards to assessment and intervention) should consider how their own preferences regarding technology and specific AAC devices influence this process. Devices might be selected based on the professional's knowledge, confidence, and preferences rather than on the skills and needs of the user. The well-known

Dutch adage reminds us that, "Unknown is unloved," highlighting the importance of keeping up to date with the latest trends and developments in the field.

Before considering what technology will be appropriate, we need to understand the range of competencies that need to be mastered by the person who uses AAC. This allows us to match systems to the user, which will maximize their opportunities to explore and develop their communication skills as they grow in confidence and ability. Communication does not exist for the sole purpose of making our physical needs known but rather enables individuals to exchange information and to develop social closeness (Light, 1988). Communication of social closeness requires an ability to engage in social etiquette and sharing of personal experience. Such interaction requires the mastery of complex skills across the domains of linguistic, operational, social, and strategic competencies (Light & McNaughton, 2014a). It is too often the case that the person requiring AAC is deemed not to have the intellectual or linguistic ability to use AAC when it is in fact the system that is not designed or set up for the individual's physical and sensory abilities to allow for exploration and skill development.

> Jane was introduced to a linear alphabetic scanning system using a single switch—her first opportunity to independently select letters without facilitated support. A step scan was chosen due to Jane's inability to coordinate pressing the switch when the target letter was automatically highlighted. She was shown a toy tractor and asked to spell the word. Jane pressed the switch to highlight the A and stopped. The teacher remained silent and wrote down an A. Jane stopped at C and with a heavy heart a C was recorded. The teacher was tempted to call the experiment to a halt and question Jane's selection, but Jane persisted and stopped at the O followed by R and then T. And suddenly ... the penny dropped ... and the teacher helped Jane to reorder the letters.

Jane's story provides a tangible example of the inherent dangers if the ability or inability to master the operation of a system is equated to an individual's potential to use technology. In Jane's case, she demonstrated competencies by planning how to select (operational competency) the necessary letters (linguistic competency) in the most efficient way (strategic competency). However, without realizing that her strategy for achieving the task may not have been apparent to others (social competency), Jane's ability to spell was almost missed and the task terminated as the teacher initially assumed that Jane was selecting letters at random.

Communication Competencies

Features of AAC systems should support the development and mastery of competencies, but there should also be an awareness of how AAC technologies place increased demands on users.

Linguistic Competency

Does the technology support the scaffolding of language? Can users "play" (experiment) with new vocabulary? How do users access different aspects of the linguistic code (e.g., written, spoken)? Can the technology adapt as the user develops their linguistic competence, or does the user have to change systems at each developmental stage, often losing access to personalized vocabulary and stories?

Operational Competency

Does the technology minimize the cognitive and physical demands on the user? Is there an awareness of the skills required to recall and retrieve target language? Do the operational demands of the system mask the user's linguistic competency? Do the features of the technology enhance or make it difficult to use? For example, color coding may be an issue if a user has a color deficiency; an older user may be developing an age-related visual impairment; reducing the number of selections to retrieve a favorite story may encourage use of a system.

Social Competency

Waller (2019) reflects on the need for AAC technologies to support a range of communication, from transactional (i.e., the expression of needs and wants, e.g., "I want a drink"; and the communication of instructions, commands, warnings, requests, etc.) to interactional (i.e., phatic, or predictable, communication, like "Hello," "How are you?" and free narrative, like personal and fantasy storytelling and telling jokes) conversation. Does the technology support easy access to these modes of communication, such as making use of a mixture of prestored utterances (transactional and phatic communication) and stories (sequences of utterances)?

Strategic Competency

Does the design of the technology support intuitive use of the system or must the user develop innovative ways to express themselves? Is the design consistent so that users are able to extend their communication skills without having to learn new operational skills? Does the system have different routes to access language, and can it adapt to the individual user's thinking?

Matching Features of Technology With Users

When considering the features of technology, we should address those features that will support the mastery of communication competence and enable persons supporting the use of technology to adapt and maintain the system in order to ensure continued and effective use of the technology. Technology features (Table 9-1) include physical features (e.g., access, voice, physical display, and portability), language features (e.g., the linguistic representation—symbols, images, text; how linguistic items are displayed; and how these are accessed), and support features (e.g., customization and maintenance of the software and hardware).

Feature matching provides a framework for identifying appropriate technology that will meet the needs of the person who uses AAC. However, in a systematic review and qualitative synthesis of the literature, Baxter and colleagues (2012) found that individuals who use AAC tend to rely on non–speech-generating options and abandon the speech-generating options. If technology is truly to support the person's communication, practitioners should be aware of the reasons why technology is abandoned. Factors to be considered include (Judge & Townsend, 2013):

- Simplicity of technology design and ease of use: Usability refers to the ease of use and learnability of technology and depends on how well the system is designed. Given the complexity of communication, the challenge is to strive for simplicity in the design of AAC technology while providing access to the range of communicative needs for a diverse and changing user population. In assessing the usability of AAC technology, practitioners should take into account aspects, such as user freedom and control (i.e., can users access functionality in different ways?), match between the system and the real world (i.e., does the system reflect the user's view of language?), recognition rather than recall (i.e., does the system scaffold language rather than require the user to memorize access codes?), and flexibility and efficiency of use (i.e., does the system change and adapt to different stages and levels of user needs?). See Nielsen and Molich (1990) for 10 heuristics used to assess the usability of software. Reflecting on the usability of AAC technology will better allow engineers and other practitioners to design, develop, and manage systems, thereby increasing appropriate adoption and reducing abandonment of technology (Waller, 2018).

- Reliability: Persons who use AAC complain about devices initially not being set up effectively, inadequate battery life of the devices resulting in batteries going dead, and devices needing repair too often followed by an unnecessarily long length of time taken to repair their AAC systems with a lack of available loan devices when systems are broken and being repaired (Baxter et al., 2012). Effective practices, such as the availability of a device on loan for a trial period during assessment and/or intervention, should be widely incorporated into evidence-based practice (van Niekerk et al., 2019). Technical problems are also a common cause of frustration, particularly with more sophisticated devices.

- Access to a variety of communication functions: Baxter and colleagues (2012) reported that although SGDs are useful for teaching a limited number of communicative functions (e.g., expressing wants and needs, and requesting skills), more research is needed to determine the effectiveness for more complex communication skills, such as exchanging information and social closeness (Morin et al., 2018).

TABLE 9-1
Feature Matching

FEATURE	ASPECTS	SPECIFIC EXAMPLES
Physical Features	Access	**Direct selection:** key guards, head pointer, chin stick, Tongue Drive System, touchscreens (dwell, delay, release options)
		Mouse options: head mouse, alternative mouse, joystick, trackball, vertical wireless mouse
		Eye gaze: activation signal (dwell, blink, switch), feedback (color, cursor style, highlight)
		Switches: movement site interface and positioning principle, different scanning options
		ASR: use of voice or sound to activate technology
		BCI: use of brain signals to activate technology
		Biofeedback: use of physiological information, (e.g., heart rate and galvanic responses to activate technology)
	Voice	**Type of voice:** digitized (recorded) speech, text-to-speech, mixed mode (i.e., hybrid)
		Personalization options: sex, age, pitch, rate
		Language options: English, Spanish, Dutch, bilingual, etc.
		Clarity and volume: built-in or external speakers (e.g., classroom), ability to adjust volume
	Display	**Grid layout:** type of grid, size, spacing, number of options per page
		Navigation buttons: number, placement, consistency
		Visual support: color, font type and size, background color
	Portability	**Size/weight:** important for ambulatory users
		Mounts/stands: ease of use, different locations, ergonomics
		Durability: protective casing, moisture resistant
		Transportability: carrying straps, handles
Linguistic Features	Graphics/symbols	**Level of representation:** photographs, line drawings, graphic symbols (range on iconicity continuum), text
		Type: two-dimensional (graphic-based symbols), three-dimensional (tactile symbols, including object symbols, textured symbols, parts of objects, Braille)
	Language	**Complexity:** beginning communicators to advanced communicators—allow language to grow with the user
		Presentation: activity-based, core-/fringe-based, grid display, VSDs, literacy-based
		Visual display: number of messages per page, layout
Support Features	Customization	**Choice of features:** language, vocabulary, layout, access
		Ease of editing: customization of pages and buttons, "hide" functions, ability to back up data
	Maintenance	**Availability of technical support:** problem-solving in family, availability of repair, loan devices
		Cost: initial cost and funding options, types of warranties, cost of insurance, locations where it will be used and insurance implications, repair costs
		Operational requirements: batteries (cost and availability), charging schedule if rechargeable

ASR = automatic speech recognition; BCI = brain-computer interface; VSD = visual scene display.

- Training and availability of technical support: AAC technology is often viewed as an appliance—technology that can be plugged in and used without adaptation or support (such as a refrigerator or iron). In order to implement and use technology effectively and to reduce abandonment, there is a requirement for ongoing technical support. **Technophobia** is often a barrier to introducing an AAC device. Staff must have training and support to facilitate effective use of technology. Research on abandonment is recognizing the need to support communication partners and instructors. Projects, such as I-ASC (Identifying Appropriate Symbol Communication Aids) for children who are nonspeaking to enhance clinical decision making (https://iasc.mmu.ac.uk/) and ethnographic studies in a special school (Norrie et al., 2018), are highlighting the importance of high-quality support. Even when technology is innovated in collaboration with a wide range of stakeholders and identified by multidisciplinary teams, the adoption of AAC technology depends on a knowledgeable support environment.

- The voice and language produced through technology: The frustration that arises when spelled words are mispronounced by SGDs contributes to device abandonment. This is of particular concern in multilingual, multicultural contexts. Yet, a systematic review by van Niekerk and colleagues (2017) indicated that although the influence of cultural factors form an integral part of different theoretical models, these factors are often not considered in the selection process. Theoretical models include:

  ○ The Assistive Device Selection Framework (Scherer et al., 2007), which illustrates that environmental factors (e.g., cultural and financial priorities, as well as policies and legislation) along with personal factors of both the user and the provider (e.g., their knowledge and expectations) interact together to influence decision making and device selection.

  ○ The Human Activity Assistive Technology model (Cook & Polgar, 2015), which emphasizes human (i.e., the skills and abilities of the person with a disability), activity (i.e., a set of functional tasks to be performed by the person with a disability), context (i.e., the social, cultural, and physical contexts or settings that surround the environment in which the activity must be completed), and assistive technology (i.e., the devices suggested to bridge the gap between the person's abilities and the demands of the environment) factors.

- The decision-making process—family perceptions and support: Persons who use AAC and their families are often not considered during the decision-making process. A considerable amount of clinical reasoning is required to ensure an appropriate match between the person who requires (or uses) AAC, their family, and technology specifications to ensure optimal functioning of the individual within a specific environment. However,

careful consideration of all these aspects could ensure the satisfaction of the person who uses AAC and their family and could limit difficulties and disappointment with the technology during the implementation process (van Niekerk et al., 2019). Therefore, families and practitioners may do well to adopt an eclectic approach in line with multimodal communication (Iacono et al., 2016). Despite the clear importance of the selection process for long-term satisfaction, not much information is available about the reasoning of practitioners regarding their technology selection practices (Friederich et al., 2010), which has clear implications for evidence-based practice.

- Communication rate: Persons who use AAC want technology that is fast and as spontaneous as possible. In practice, communication using AAC tends to be prohibitively slow. Compared to speaking rates of between 125 and 185 words per minute (wpm), aided communication rates fluctuate between 2 wpm (for **scanning** interfaces) and 8 to 10 wpm (for **direct selection**; Swiffin et al., 1987). In practice, many persons who use AAC tend to abandon technology for a faster solution—the human interpreter! However, independent communication must be balanced with reliance on others.

The development and mastery of communicative competencies needed to use AAC technology should be viewed in the context of the Universal Design for Learning (Thunberg et al., 2022). As such, the design of AAC technologies should support the developmental acquisition of skills by providing multiple means of interface design to give users various ways to operate the system (e.g., different scanning options), providing multiple ways of accessing language to provide users the opportunity to demonstrate what they know (e.g., providing access to the alphabet for a symbol user), and minimizing cognitive and physical demands that may reduce the user's motivation to use the system.

FEATURES OF AAC TECHNOLOGY

As technology has developed and diversified, the number of features (functionality) offered by systems has increased. In order to identify appropriate technology that will meet the needs of individual users, practitioners need to understand the different components that make up an AAC technological solution. Table 9-1 provides a structure within which different aspects of AAC technologies can be understood.

Physical Features

Due to the nature of many of the disabilities leading to communication impairment, users of AAC may not be able to use traditional input devices (e.g., keyboards, mice, and touch screens) to interact with AAC technology. Aspects such as portability, screen visibility, and intelligibility of

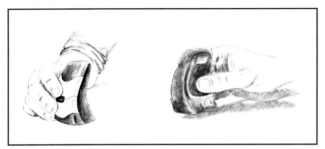

Figure 9-2. Example of an alternate (vertical) mouse.

speech output can also affect the usability of the system. Therefore, the physical features of a system address the input device, the access method (direct or indirect selection), the display (the physical use of the display, including the way in which items are located on the screen), the types of voice output, and the degree of portability.

Input Devices

Input devices provide the physical connection between the user and the system. Conventional input devices include keyboards, touchscreens, and mice. However, such devices require physical dexterity to manipulate them. For some users with restricted movement, a wide range of alternative input solutions are used, including switches, eye gaze, voice, brain-computer interfaces (BCIs), and biofeedback.

Keyboards

A variety of adapted keyboard options are available to literate users, such as enlarged keyboards, miniature keyboards, keyboards with key guards, and one-handed keyboards. In some cases, keyboard labels (e.g., some keys might be marked in a brightly colored label) can act as a visual cue for a person with visual challenges, such as a restricted visual field.

Mice

Different mouse emulators exist; for example, there are smaller mouse options that can help with control and other mouse options that require minimal hand or wrist movement and light touch (Koczur et al., 2015). A range of vertical wireless mouse options that capitalize on an ergonomic relaxed neutral wrist and hand position, as well as on the higher processing abilities of the small muscles and joints of the fingers as opposed to the arm, are commercially available (e.g., the DXT Fingertip Vertical Wireless Mouse [Kinesis Corporation]; City Ergonomics, 2018). These mouse options function with minimal resistance requiring little effort to accomplish effective cursor control. The weighted zinc base also provides vertical stability and enhanced tactile feedback. This type of mouse has precision grip for accurate navigation, as can be seen in Figure 9-2.

A trackball operates as an upside-down mouse, so rather than rolling the ball on the table by sliding the mouse around, the ball is moved directly by the user. The trackball does not need to be held, but the ball only needs to be nudged gently using a hand, chin, elbow, foot, or stick held in the mouth. Buttons are used to select left and right button clicks, as well as supporting click and drag functionality. Moreover, trackballs come in many sizes, including ones that can be operated by a single finger. As a trackball remains in a stationary position on a desk or mounted on a stand, it can be a good option for a person with a limited range of motion.

Touchscreens

A touchscreen is a computer display screen that is also an input device. The screens are sensitive to pressure and a user interacts with the computer by touching graphic symbols (i.e., pictures or words) on the screen using a finger, infrared beam, or a stylus. These screens are not affected by outside elements, such as dust or water. Despite advantages to some individuals (e.g., persons who experience difficulty using keyboards and mice because of physical or cognitive disabilities), touchscreens can present barriers to some persons with physical disabilities who are unable to touch the device, as well as persons with low vision and blindness for whom the device does not provide tangible controls that can be appreciated by sense of touch (Kane et al., 2011). The way in which touchscreens are controlled can be customized to meet the physical abilities of the user (see Access Methods section).

Switches

Switches (Judge & Colven, 2006) are used by persons with complex physical impairments that restrict their ability to access keyboards or touchscreens. They can also provide access for young children or persons who need simple activities. Switches come in different shapes and use different methods of activation. For instance, a "button switch" is pressed and released for activation, while a "sip and puff" switch requires the user to suck (i.e., generate negative pressure) and puff (i.e., generate positive pressure) to operate the switch. Figure 9-3 illustrates a variety of switches available.

More complex switch systems are used when individuals can access more than one switch. These input devices can range from a multiple switch array (e.g., one switch to move and another to select an item) to systems, such as the Tongue Drive System. This minimally invasive wireless device enables individuals with high-level spinal cord injuries to operate a computer (and electric wheelchair) by moving their tongues (Huo & Ghovanloo, 2012). The device is placed in a dental retainer embedded with an array of magnetic sensors that can wirelessly detect the individual's tongue movement using a small magnetic tracer secured on the tongue. It then translates the movements into a set of user-defined commands in real time, which can then be used to communicate with the devices in the individual's environments. In a qualitative 6-week usability study with 21 participants with high-level spinal cord injury, all were satisfied with how the Tongue Drive System performed, and most said that they were able to do more things using this switch than with their current assistive technology (Kim et al., 2014).

Eye Gaze

Recent developments in eye-gaze technology have opened up direct access opportunities for persons with complex physical disabilities (Borgestig et al., 2017; Karlsson et al., 2018). Eye-gaze tracking is a noninvasive technological solution to estimate eye-gaze direction. As natural eye gaze is often used by emerging communicators to make choices, eye-gaze tracking provides a powerfully intuitive way of providing access to technology. In many instances, it has superseded the use of switch access, making direct selection a viable option for a wider group of users. Eye movement alone allows the user to directly select a choice on a visual array. As such, eye gaze provides hands-free access to communication without requiring any further body movement, allowing users to independently navigate their communication program of choice.

However, eye gaze is not a panacea as some individuals with varying eye problems or visual impairment are unable to benefit from such technology. The calibration of eye-gaze systems can be frustrating, and practitioners should be aware of the operational load associated with the mastery of this technology. Unlike other input systems, eye gaze requires users to switch between modes of looking (the natural use of their eyes) and selecting (using their eyes to replicate the actions of a mouse; Light & McNaughton, 2014a).

Automatic Speech Recognition

Voice and sound can be used to control technology. Sound activation can be used as a rudimentary switch while automatic speech recognition (ASR) technology can convert spoken words into text. ASR technology, such as Dragon NaturallySpeaking (Nuance Communications), could be trained to recognize individual speakers and has been used for many years to enable people with consistent speech patterns to operate environmental control systems, software, and word processors. ASR has improved significantly and is now commonly used in many commercial systems, such as Amazon's Alexa. Software algorithms can adapt to improve the accuracy of recognition of the speaker, and research has demonstrated successful use of ASR to recognize unintelligible dysarthric speech (Sriranjani et al., 2015). The system can translate this speech using synthesized speech to output an equivalent message (Hawley et al., 2007).

Brain-Computer Interfaces and Biofeedback

Recent advances using BCIs (Lazarou et al., 2018) and the potential to use biofeedback (Memarian et al., 2014) may offer viable access methods for individuals with conditions, such as locked-in syndrome, and profound multiple

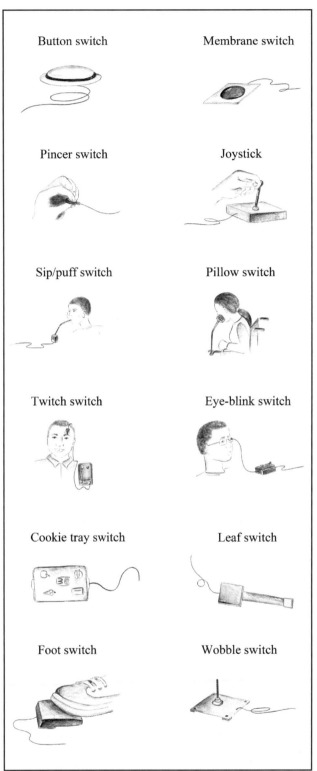

Figure 9-3. Examples of different switches.

disabilities that make it difficult to identify consistent and reliable responses needed to access technology. This technology is in its infancy, requiring sensitive sensors positioned on the skull (often worn as a cap). However, this area of research and development promises to produce viable, robust products in the not-too-distant future.

Selection of the Input Device

The choice of input device will depend on many user-dependent factors. These factors can be considered using the movement, site, interface, and positioning principle (Musselwhite & St. Louis, 1988):

- M: Movement of body part. Does the individual have sufficient dexterity to access a keyboard or touchscreen, or will they need to use alternative access? If a switch is required, a reliable, accurate, easily performed movement must be identified. A voluntary normal movement pattern is preferred to reduce undesired consequences, such as increased muscle tone.

- S: Control site. Identify how the user will access the input device. First consider the hand or upper extremities. If these do not provide reliable and accurate activation, consider the head or lower extremities (knee or foot). Access to a keyboard does not necessarily have to be a finger or the hand but can be the elbow, foot, or head. Take the user's own preferences into consideration as well.

- I: Interface. The type of interface (i.e., the way in which the input device operates) must address the physical and cognitive needs of the user. Consider the following features:

  - *Force*: The degree of pressure needed to activate the input device. Some devices cannot be adjustable, while others may require force on a continuum from light to heavy.
  - *Feedback*: The manner in which the device responds to the user. It is important that users know when activation has been registered. This could be auditory (e.g., a click), visual (e.g., change in colors/shape), tactile (e.g., feel of the key/switch), or vibrotactile (e.g., movement and feel).
  - *Range of movement*: The distance that the activation surface must move in order to activate the input device. For example, how far must a lever switch be moved before an activation is registered?
  - *Amount of play*: The inherent "give," unrelated to the activation.
  - *Size*: The size and height profile of the activation surface. Are the switch or keys large enough to be selected?
  - *Weight*: This aspect requires careful consideration if worn by the user or when it is mounted away from a surface that could have provided support.
  - *Moisture resistance*: If the input device is positioned in the vicinity of the mouth (or if the user drools), or if the person is incontinent and the input device is positioned in the vicinity of the seat, a sealed device should be used.
  - *Safety*: The input device should always be properly earthed and sealed with no sharp edges.
  - *Directionality*: This may range from uni-, to bi-, to multidirectional and is important when considering how the system is operated.
  - *Mounting*: How the device is positioned. The mounting of the input device should facilitate optimum use and stability.

- P: Positioning. Determine the ideal position for optimal, reliable, and effective control by the user. To a large extent, this is dependent on the control site and the specific movement selected. Care must be taken to ensure correct positioning of the device, as small changes in seating or issues, like fatigue, may mean that it will require repositioning. The way input devices are positioned will affect their use. When positioning the device, consideration must be given to the angle of the device; for example, tilting it to make it easier for the user to access. Physical positioning of the user aims to achieve the best possible motor functioning that will allow independent, reliable, and repeated movements. Good posture and use of orthoses can control tremors (e.g., a weight cuff worn on the user's hand) or improve accuracy (e.g., wearing an arm splint).

Customizing and Adapting the Operation of the Input Device

When using input devices, such as computer keyboards, touchscreens, and pointing devices (e.g., a mouse, eye gaze), most operating systems (e.g., Windows, iOS, Android) allow the user to customize the operation of the input device. For example, individuals with minimal movement will require a device that will be able to respond to the slightest movement and recognize it as an activation, or individuals with uncontrolled and involuntary movement (e.g., individuals with ataxia or athetosis) will require a device that does not respond immediately when it is activated, as this might be the result of an uncontrolled movement.

Input devices can be configured in the way in which they are activated:

- Timed activation: The input device will only register an activation when contact is sustained for a specific length of time. This is the most frequently used activation strategy and is particularly important if users have restricted coordination that affects their control in terms of activation and release. This type of activation can be achieved with pressure (e.g., finger pressing down a physical or on-screen key) or by dwelling on an on-screen target (e.g., using eye gaze or an infrared light beam). Unwanted selection of keys is minimized when using a physical keyboard while the user moves across a screen without activating each key.

- Release activation: A selection is activated only when contact is removed. This type of activation helps users with restricted movement who prefer to maintain contact with the device so they can ensure the correct choice is made before selecting it by releasing their hand, finger, etc. from the device.

- Filtered activation: The device filters and dampens random or uncontrolled movements to determine the target activation. The device identifies the target area that has registered the most activity (e.g., the keys that are pressed most often) or where the user fixates (e.g., using eye gaze) for the longest period of time. This activation strategy requires ongoing adaptation in order to provide customized support for a particular individual (this may require time for initial calibration).

Access Methods

All AAC devices are accessed typically by direct selection or scanning. Therefore, physical access to technology must address the selection method (direct or scanning) and the display (how items are located on the screen).

Direct Access

Direct selection is an access method by which a person indicates a desired choice on a communication system directly by pointing with either a body part (i.e., an unaided means to select) or with a device (i.e., an aided means to select) to make a selection. The body part, or the access device, is used to indicate a choice directly. Typically, the index finger would be used for direct selection (mimicking natural pointing), although other body parts may be used equally effectively; for example, eye gaze or a gross hand movement or motion of the elbow or foot. All these are unaided means of making selections. Direct access tools (Figure 9-4) can be used to support direct selection when the user lacks the dexterity required to point. A hand pointer, a head stick (as used by France Mngenge in Figure 9-1), a chin stick, or a laser pointer mounted on the person's head are all tools to support direct selection (all these are aided means to make selections).

Some individuals will be able to use a physical keyboard or on-screen keyboard using a touchscreen. Others will require support to operate pointing devices (e.g., hand pointer, head pointer, metacarpal band) or technological solutions, such as eye gaze or the Tongue Drive System. Direct selection should always be the preferred choice as far as physical access is concerned, as it is the most rapid and efficient form of access, providing the user with a logical, intuitive approach to sending commands to the communication system. It is also easier for the partner to understand the physical access method to assist the user when required while indirect methods may require specific partner training.

Indirect Access

Scanning is a method by which a user selects items when they are unable to do so using a direct physical access method. Scanning makes use of a switch to provide binary (on/off) input to a system that then reacts in a predetermined way (making the use of most switches an aided means to select). For example, when pressing a single-switch message

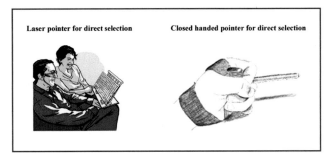

Figure 9-4. Examples of two direct selection tools.

recorder, the device would "speak" the recorded voice message (unaided selection); pressing a switch can also be used to choose a target item when that item is highlighted on a digital display (aided selection). Although scanning is a powerful solution for people with significant physical disabilities, users must master both the operation of the physical switch and the conceptual operation of the scanning system.

When using a switch or multiple switches, each item from which a choice can be made (i.e., the selection set) must be offered to the user for selection. Items (i.e., pictures, symbols, letters, words) are typically scanned by either visually highlighting or speaking the items in some predefined order. The scan typically starts in the top left corner and moves rightward and downward, although some cultural groups may prefer different scan directions (Judge & Townsend, 2013). Auditory scanning provides auditory feedback for each scan and is used primarily with users with visual impairments but can also benefit others. The highlighting of choices can be automated or directed by the user (called step scanning). Care must be taken when choosing a scanning method/layout for individual users. A user with increased muscle tone might tense up in anticipation of activating a switch, and therefore, may benefit from a step scan. The way in which items are scanned influences the speed of communication, but the algorithm (pattern of scanning) may be complex, imposing a high cognitive load on the user requiring both operational and strategic competencies. The simplest scanning method would be a linear scan, where items from the selection set are scanned one after the other. For example, the alphabet could be scanned in order (A, B, C, etc.) until the target letter is chosen. The user would select each letter in turn to spell a word. However, to be *efficient*, items from the selection set can be rearranged (e.g., according to frequency) or grouped (e.g., in rows and columns) in ways to accelerate communication (see Acceleration Techniques: Strategies for Rate Enhancement).

In row/column scanning (Figure 9-5), each row (or column) is highlighted. Once the desired row has been selected, each column within the selected row is highlighted from left to right until the item is encountered and selected.

Partner-assisted scanning (an aided means of selection), a simple scanning solution, can also be used (Bornman, 2011). The communication partner scans the items from the selection set either visually and/or using auditory prompts.

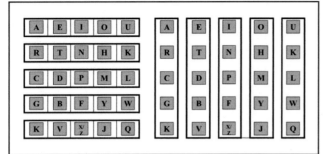

Figure 9-5. Row-column (left) and column-row (right) scanning with vowels in top row and the remaining letters arranged by frequency of occurrence (English). In row-column scanning, all the letters in the first row would be highlighted in some manner. If the desired letter is in this row, the user would activate a switch that would highlight each letter from left to right. If the desired letter is not in this row, the letters in the second row would be highlighted while the letters in the top row would return to their normal state. The user proceeds row by row, indicating by switch that the desired letter is in a particular row. The switch activation then starts the highlighting of individual letters in that row from left to right. When the desired letter is highlighted, the user activates the switch again, which keeps the desired letter highlighted while fading all other letters in that row. Another switch activation will start the process all over again. The same is true for column-row scanning, except the scanning would first proceed column by column and then letter by letter from top to bottom of the chosen column.

In visually prompting, the partner shows or points to the items one by one with a finger or light without verbally labelling the items. Therefore, this technique relies on the visual skills of the person who uses AAC. In auditory prompting, the partner reads the labels out loud for each item (e.g., letters of the alphabet) or a group of items (e.g., foods, drinks, activities, people). This technique relies on the auditory skills of the person who uses AAC. To maximize the support a person may need, a combination of visual and auditory (e.g., showing or pointing to the items while simultaneously reading out loud the labels for each item) is usually used in practice. Figure 9-6 illustrates the three types of partner-assisted scanning. Partner-assisted scanning has been used effectively with emerging communicators: with children who have—among other difficulties—severe motor, communication, and visual impairments (Bayldon et al., 2021; Marshall & Hurtig, 2019), and by adults in intensive care settings or in late stages of degenerative diseases, such as amyotrophic lateral sclerosis (ALS; Beukelman & Light, 2020).

Types of Displays

Most AAC technologies display visual information on a screen. The size of the screen and the definition of the display must be considered, as users may have visual acuity issues or difficulties manipulating small touchscreens. People who use AAC technology often find it difficult to see screens in sunlight, which may restrict their opportunities to communicate.

The manner in which graphic elements (e.g., pictures, symbols, letters, words) are displayed on the communication system should be optimized to the access method (e.g., eye gaze, keyboard, mouse, scanning, touchscreen). For example,

common words might be situated within easy reach of the user or redistributed to provide accurate selection when using eye gaze. Elements can be arranged on a fixed or **dynamic display**.

Fixed Display

In fixed displays (also known as **static displays**), the graphic elements are fixed in a specific location, typically in a grid pattern with rows and columns. Fixed graphic displays can be color-coded, grouping semantic categories together, with a fixed number of symbols being presented at a specific time. In a study with 112 speech-language pathologists with experience in AAC concerning current intervention practices, 83% reported they used grid-based displays most of the time (Thistle & Wilkinson, 2015). The authors hypothesized that it might be because grid-based layouts have been available longer than other methods, resulting in greater awareness and knowledge regarding their use. Grid layouts also facilitate scanning, whether linear or row/column. The number of messages that can be generated is thus dependent upon the number of symbols, which are usually limited (fewer than 100 in the largest displays) because each available item is always visible. In order to expand the range of symbols in a fixed display, some AAC systems utilize multiple, often hierarchical displays to accommodate various communication needs, environments, and listeners (Bruno & Trembath, 2006). In an intervention study using iPad-based SGDs for three children with autism spectrum disorder, the researchers reported that these children could learn to use this system to complete multistep communication sequences that included requesting and social communication functions. They concluded that moving from a static display to a progressive dynamic display appeared to facilitate improved communication (which was maintained during follow-up with an unfamiliar partner), suggesting that there may be some value in reconfiguring the technology to suit the learning characteristics of individual children (Waddington, et al., 2014). Non–speech-generating systems (such as communication books) and many standalone devices use fixed displays.

Dynamic Display

In dynamic displays, the interface (screen display) changes automatically to a new graphic symbol display based on the user's previous selection. For example, if the "toys" symbol is activated, a whole page of different toy options will become available, such as blocks, cars, noise makers, etc. As such, they offer simple, logical choices, making communication faster, easier, and more natural, especially for emerging young communicators. The fact that multiple levels of symbol options (and thus language) is available, not restricting what the user can see at one particular point in time, provides the user access to countless vocabulary options. Similar to fixed displays, dynamic displays are typically also presented in a row-column grid pattern, with the different options available through page linking (Drager et al., 2003). Linking the different pages on dynamic displays can either be done in a dynamic active manner (i.e., each symbol on one page linked to a second page) or in a dynamic passive manner (i.e., two pages of symbols linked by a "go to" symbol). In a participatory research project in which young children were asked to design a communication system, all children suggested multiple pages or screens on their devices to encompass the large number of vocabulary items required (Light et al., 2007). Most SGDs use dynamic displays (Beukelman & Light, 2020). The use of animation for some symbols in an electronic display would also be considered dynamic.

Hybrid Display

In hybrid displays, a fixed display usually is presented with a dynamic component (e.g., indicator lights that highlight items, word prediction on alphabetic displays; Beukelman & Light, 2020). Another example would be to have dynamic hotspots embedded in VSDs that move the display away from the visual scene to a text or grid display (Gevarter et al., 2016). Hybrid displays may be used across the full range of AAC technology types.

Voice

Having a "voice" allows users to view themselves as speakers and increases motivation to communicate, as it enhances effective communication with familiar and unfamiliar partners. Voice output can also be used in different situations; for example, having telephone conversations and communicating with others face-to-face over a distance.

Digitized (Recorded) Speech

Digitized (recorded) speech can be used in absence of literacy skills, as messages can be prestored using any graphic symbols. As messages are prerecorded, the voice output can be age-, sex-, and language-appropriate (specifically in multilingual contexts), and therefore, it allows communication with a variety of communication partners (natural sounding, thus intelligibility is not problematic).

Some of the disadvantages of prerecorded messages are that a person cannot generate their own messages and the devices are relatively expensive (i.e., in terms of the device itself, cost of training, cost of maintenance, and cost of repair). Some devices are also heavy, thus reducing portability.

Text-to-Speech (Synthesized)

As text-to-speech systems are literacy-based, they may enrich and expand the individual's language skills. Typically, these systems have a word prediction functionality that increases access speed and accuracy resulting in fewer communication breakdowns, reduces effort due to fewer keystrokes, and reduces subsequent fatigue. Due to the memory function of these systems, lengthy messages can be prestored (e.g., for delivering speeches). Furthermore, educational possibilities

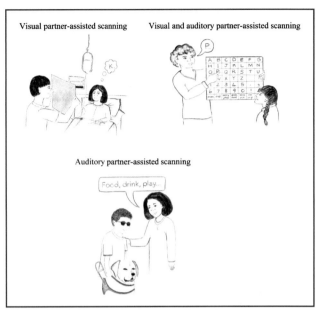

Figure 9-6. Three types of partner-assisted scanning.

are enhanced as academic tasks are expanded, and users can do homework independently. It also increases leisure time activities (e.g., letter writing, playing computer games, and even singing).

Text-to-speech is achieved by using robotic voices that are electronically synthesized, or more recently, by concatenating parts of natural voice recordings. Text-to-speech systems based on concatenated speech units sound more natural and can reflect different accents and age groups. Speech technology is also delivering improved prosody and inflection. Voice-banking is becoming more common, enabling people with degenerative disabilities to use their own voice as a basis for speech synthesis. Unfortunately, text-to-speech options are not available for all languages (e.g., many languages spoken in Africa), and some persons also do not like the quality of voice, stating that it sounds too robotic, although significant strides have been made in this regard over recent years.

Mixed Mode (Hybrid Speech)

AAC technology often allows access to both recorded and synthesized speech. This allows for the production of common and personalized unique messages. It also allows playback of nonspeech sounds, which is advantageous when working with young people, as it encourages early and fun interaction. It is also more natural-sounding, offers several voice options (e.g., adult female, adult male, and child voices), and borrows the best features of digitized speech.

Portability

Portability speaks directly to one of the critical dimensions of communication, as it is concerned with the availability of the person's communication system. With the dawn of mobile technology, the portability of AAC systems was positively influenced (Hornero et al., 2015). One important consideration regarding portability that is often overlooked is the locations in which the technology will be used. A basic rule of thumb applies: the more unique places and situations in which it is used, the more portable it has to be (e.g., a child may need to use a device at home, at school, or on the playground, while someone with a degenerative disease may be in a wheelchair [or bed] permanently, and therefore, not require a device in different locations). In cases where a portable device might not be a high priority, a communication system using a desktop computer can be considered. However, individuals who use less portable technology may need frequent visits to the doctor. Therefore, a laptop or mobile technology device is more portable and will allow the person to travel with the system, enabling critical patient-doctor interaction.

Mobility of the individual is an equally important consideration. Individuals who are ambulatory or partially ambulatory require a device that can be carried around (e.g., in a shoulder bag, around the waist, or on an armband). It must be worn in such a manner that the hands are free, and the technology should be operable with only one hand. As these individuals are not restricted in their access to the environment and to social interactions, their devices must be portable, unobtrusive, and intelligible to all potential communication partners while also keeping the user's preferences in mind. For users who use wheelchairs and have their devices mounted on them, the size of the device is equally important. The device must not be too big or take up so much space on the lap tray that there is not enough space left for anything else, such as a cup of tea. A device that is too big might also make the user feel confined.

Language Features

Language features refer to the ways in which users can generate language using AAC technology. When considering the language features of AAC technology, four different types of AAC technology are described: single-function devices, graphic-based AAC systems, literacy-based AAC systems, and hybrid systems.

Single-Function Devices

AAC technology can offer a single-function device in comparison to more complex software systems, which are programmable and provide a variety of communication functionality alongside other software tools. Single-function devices include those used to attract attention and may include voice recorders and voice amplifiers.

Attention-Getting Devices

Attention-getting devices include general devices without voice output, such as bicycle horns, cow bells, or battery-powered doorbells, as well as single-message voice output devices, such as the BIGmack communicator (AbleNet Inc.;

in this case, attention-getting devices should not be confused with alerting devices used by the Deaf; alerting devices for the Deaf are categorized under the receptive aided side of the AAC technology classification system described in Chapter 3). The sole purpose of these devices is to attract attention specifically for persons with reduced vocal intensity or for individuals with progressive degenerative diseases, such as ALS. For emerging communicators, these devices can be used effectively as a means of teaching cause-and-effect behavior. A message, such as, "Please help me," can be recorded for use in specific situations, such as in the classroom or in hospitals. It is imperative that the person has access to this device in all situations (e.g., in the classroom, at home, when going on an outing), as well as in all different body positions (e.g., standing, sitting, in bed while lying down). It has the added advantage of allowing a person to call for assistance over a distance.

Voice Recorders

Voice recorders, also referred to as digital speakers have the potential to record voice (messages can thus be recorded in any language, which has implications in multiple contexts). Not only can a language-appropriate message be recorded, an age- and gender-appropriate voice can also be used. As digital recorders record natural speech, intelligibility is not negatively affected. These devices are particularly useful for emerging communicators to first experience the power of "having a voice," and as such, enhance effective communication with both familiar and unfamiliar partners while also increasing motivation to communicate. These devices can be used in absence of literacy skills. Graphic symbols (including textured symbols) can be attached to the access switch if multiple switches are used. On the downside, as these devices make use of prerecorded messages, the user cannot generate their own messages. Waller and Black (2012) demonstrate how to extend the use of voice recorders to support story sharing (Grove, 2010) and provide guidelines on how individuals with complex communication needs can be involved in sharing personal experience. Parts of a story sequence are recorded on a multimessage switch allowing a speaking communication partner to provide the scaffolding to share a personal experience.

Voice Amplification

In some cases where a degenerative condition is present, such as ALS or Parkinson's disease, vocal intensity might be affected. In these cases, voice amplifiers, such as the ChatterVox voice amplifier or the Voicette and Mini-Vox (Luminaud), might be effective solutions.

Graphic-Based AAC Systems

Graphic-based systems display collections of single-meaning pictures designed for communication that allow individuals to access prestored linguistic items using a variety of AAC symbols, icons, photographs, and other images, as discussed in Chapter 7. Apart from only considering the type of graphic symbols that will be included, the vocabulary that needs to be presented (i.e., is the concept representable with a graphic symbol?), as well as vocabulary organization, should also be considered (i.e., will symbols be organized according to categories, frequency of use, alphabetically?). Graphic-based AAC systems can take the form of non-SGDs (e.g., communication boards, books, files) or SGDs.

Visual Scene Displays

VSDs describe SGDs in which graphic scenes or photographs are used to provide context for embedded prestored messages. VSDs are personalized and use contextual visual representations, such as photographs and drawings. In VSDs, photographs, pictures, and events against the background in which they occur (e.g., cooking in a kitchen or walking through a park or zoo) are provided to the user in order to provide a rich contextual background (Thistle & Wilkinson, 2015). This creates a shared communication space that can present both generic and highly personal contexts and vocabulary to create meaningful interaction. Recorded audio (e.g., speech/sound) or text is embedded under hotspots within the VSD. When these hotspots are pressed, the prestored audio or computer-generated speech (using text-to-speech technology) is played. VSDs support wide interactive communication, such as using basic communication intent (e.g., requesting, greeting, protesting), as well as basic pragmatic functions (e.g., turn-taking) for a variety of ages and disability groups, including emerging communicators (Olin et al., 2010). VSDs, in the form of apps on tablet devices, have been successfully applied to children and adults with significant cognitive and linguistic disability (Holyfield et al., 2016; Tuthill, 2014; Wilkinson et al., 2012), children with complex communication needs (Drager & Light 2006; Therrien & Light, 2016), individuals on the autism spectrum (Chapin et al., 2018; Ganz et al., 2015; Gevarter et al., 2014), and persons with aphasia (Beukelman et al., 2015; Brock et al., 2017; Dietz et al., 2006; Ulmer et al., 2016). Using approaches, such as just-in-time programming (Holyfield et al., 2019), practitioners can upload photographs into VSD systems and embed linguistic items under hotspots in real time, thereby allowing communication partners to support interactions.

Dynamic Screens

Devices that use dynamic screens provide multilevel message retrieval. Dynamic display devices (Waller, 2009) mirror the use of communication books, which are indexed on the first page. Each screen (or page) is usually organized as a grid. Cells (which can be labeled with icons, images, or text) either connect to a linguistic item that is spoken on selection or to another page. Developers of dynamic screen AAC systems offer a variety of software solutions that provide a structured hierarchy of pages suitable for different stages of language acquisition. These pages are editable but require some training and effort to reprogram (Black et al., 2012).

Semantic Compaction

An alternative to multilevel message retrieval is to encode each linguistic item using a sequence of keystrokes. One such encoding system, semantic compaction (Baker, 1982, 1987), provides a mnemonic multimeaning icon encoding strategy in which each linguistic item is retrieved by activating a sequence of up to three user-chosen icons on a static keyboard consisting of as few as four icons up to a full keyboard of 144 icons. By memorizing the icon code sequences of prestored vocabulary, users can save significantly on keystrokes compared to letter-by-letter typing (Higginbotham, 1992).

Literacy-Based AAC Systems

Although speech output can be accessed through graphic-based interfaces, these systems provide only a finite vocabulary. Unlike graphic-based systems, literacy-based systems allow users to generate novel concepts and ideas using the 26 letters of the alphabet (in the case of English). Individuals with acquired (e.g., locked-in syndrome) or degenerative disabilities (e.g., ALS) resulting in communication impairment tend to retain literacy skills. However, when selecting a literacy-based system, not only should the literacy skills of the user be considered but also that of their communication partners (e.g., primary caregivers; van Niekerk et al., 2019).

Hybrid Systems

In hybrid systems, users have access to text input, as well as using graphics linked to prestored linguistic items. As the ultimate goal is to aim for literacy, it is important that users have access to text. For example, in order to reduce the number of keystrokes (which will ultimately reduce fatigue and increase the rate of communication), some text might be prestored under a single graphic symbol (e.g., personal information can be stored under a "person" symbol). However, if the user then needs to compile a novel, unplanned message, the literacy option is available to construct this new message.

Acceleration Techniques: Strategies for Rate Enhancement

Communicators need to be able to convey their messages as quickly as possible. If speed is not addressed, it may lead to lack of spontaneity in communication. Communication partners often become impatient if they regard waiting for a response as being "too long," resulting in them chatting among themselves while the user is preparing a message. In some cases, well-meaning communication partners try to speed up communication by anticipating the AAC user's messages by guessing the words and messages, often resulting in communication breakdowns that add to interpersonal frustration and further reduce the speed of communication. Moreover, if partners guess what the user is trying to say, they remain in control of the interaction, pushing the AAC user into a passive role of responding to communication and not initiating interaction. Resorting to closed yes/no questions may speed up communication but restricts opportunities to develop communication skills. Having prestored messages that remind the communication partner to wait while the user constructs their message or training users to scaffold and support responses to open-ended questions provides opportunities for users to develop their communicative competencies.

Rate enhancement strategies can be divided into three broad types: (1) layout optimization, (2) expansion of codes, and (3) prediction.

Layout Optimization

When using static displays, items should be arranged according to frequency of use, with the most commonly used items within easy reach (for direct selection) or at the beginning of the scan (for indirect selection). Graphic-based systems require knowledge of the individual's use of the system, while literacy-based systems can make use of general frequency information. Tools are emerging that can automatically optimize scanning grids for individual users by measuring the way the user accesses input devices (e.g., switches) and the user's performance during the scanning process (Koester & Simpson, 2017).

Expansion of Codes

Codes can be expanded into whole words, phrases, or complete messages. Examples of encoding techniques can be found in traditional word processors that offer users the facility to store words or phrases under abbreviation sequences; for example, "ph" could be expanded to "telephone." Autocorrection can support typists by automatically replacing commonly mistyped words (e.g., "teh" with "the"). Phrases, such as "Best wishes," can be stored under a user-defined sequence of keys, such as "BW." Strategies, such as semantic compaction (Baker, 1982, 1987), use a set of icons as a mnemonic system to encode words, phrases, and sentences. Expansion techniques tend to be programmed by the user. Codes must be recalled and can increase cognitive load. Table 9-2 shows the range of expansion techniques using encoding.

Prediction

Three types of prediction, namely language-, word-, and message-prediction, will be described.

Language Prediction

A wide variety of different prediction types exist, including word completion, next-word prediction, linguistic prediction, message prediction, and icon prediction (Dowden, 2016). Message construction can be supported using statistical and syntactic knowledge of written language to predict (anticipate) the next character/word/phrase. Language prediction can result in a reduction in keystrokes or switch activations. Although prediction is usually associated with literacy-based systems, graphic-based systems can be designed with some predictive support. Systems that use encoding, such as semantic compaction, can highlight possible keys that follow a selected sequence. For example, if the "rainbow" icon is activated, all icons that are programmed to follow the rainbow are highlighted (e.g., the "sun" icon to retrieve the word "yellow," the "apple" icon to retrieve the word "red," and the "frog" icon to retrieve the word "green"). Thus, activating rainbow and then sun results in the SGD production of "yellow," rainbow and then apple results in "red," and rainbow and then frog produces the word "green."

Word Prediction

Word prediction (Higginbotham, 1992; Swiffin et al., 1987) was initially developed to assist typists with physical disabilities. It also played an important role in early automatic speech recognition to improve the accuracy of recognizing speech input.

Ironically, word prediction is now available on most mobile devices due to the challenges of typing on a small onscreen keyboard. Text entry has become an important research area for mainstream technology resulting in improved interface design and prediction (e.g., Vertanen et al., 2018). These advances will bring further benefits for persons with physical impairments.

Prediction systems are implemented in different ways. For example, predicted words can be listed below the cursor, or can be displayed in a window above the keyboard (as in Figure 9-7). The number of words predicted can often be adjusted (studies suggest up to five words to reduce the need to visually scan too many options) as can the minimum length of words (users may find it more efficient to ignore short words in order to boost the prediction of longer words).

Prediction can reduce the negative effects of a very slow transmission rate discussed earlier, such as partners becoming bored, starting their own conversations, and guessing what the user wants to say. In the classroom environment, the rate of interaction also impacts time required for academic tasks; prediction assists children to keep up with the rest of the class. Word prediction can benefit children learning to read and write, as well as dyslexic individuals who are able to recognize the target words they wish to type (Newell et al., 1992).

By using prediction techniques, the increase in communication rate is at most 50% (Higginbotham, 1992). There are a myriad of human factors associated with rate of communication, and therefore, the extent to which prediction impacts rate might be underestimated. For example, when considering the number of keystrokes, often only motor abilities are taken into account, thereby minimizing the effects of cognition, visual skills, and timing, to name a few. Five factors should be considered when using word prediction:

TABLE 9-2

Examples of Expansion Techniques That Use Encoding

STRATEGY	CODE	MESSAGE
Letter category encoding	GH	(**G**reetings) **H**ello, how are you?
Salient letter encoding	HH TO	**H**ello, **h**ow are you? Please turn the **T**V **o**n.
Alpha-numeric encoding	G1 G2	Hello, how are you? (arbitrary numbers—shows first greeting stored) Have a good day. (shows second greeting stored)

Iconic encoding (e.g., Semantic Compaction, using the Unity84 Minspeak Application Program)		Hello, how are you?
		
		This utterance can be retrieved in different ways (e.g., as "Hello" and "How are you?" (1) or by generating "Hello," "How," "are you" (2)
		
		1. Retrieving two prestored linguistic items:
		   a. Hello.
		      i. First icon: used for all interjections
		      ii. Second icon: codes communication words
		   b. How are you?
		      i. First icon: used for prestored greetings
		      ii. Second icon: codes the word "you"
		
		2. Retrieving three prestored linguistic items to generate the utterance:
		   a. Hello.
		      i. First icon: used for all interjections
		      ii. Second icon: codes communication words
		   b. How
		      i. First icon: used for all interrogatives
		      ii. Second icon: a rhyming code, as in "ow," "pow," "how"
		   c. are you?
		      i. First icon: the bee is for "to be" verbs and the life preserver around the bee is because "be" is a helper verb
		      ii. Second icon: codes the word "you"

Adapted from Thistle, J. J., & Wilkinson, K. M. (2009). The effects of color cues on typically developing preschoolers' speed of locating a target line drawing: Implications for augmentative and alternative communication display design. *American Journal of Speech-Language Pathology, 18,* 231-240 and Waller, A. (2009). Interpersonal communication. In C. Stephanidis (Ed.), *The universal access handbook.* CRC Press Taylor and Francis Group.

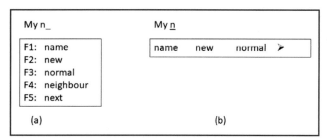

Figure 9-7. Two common prediction displays. (A) Vertical list using function keys to select a word. (B) Horizontal list using touchscreen/mouse selection and providing further predictions by selecting arrow buttons.

1. The linguistic cost (average number of selections needed to communicate a word)

2. Length (average number of motor acts required for each selection)

3. Time (average time per motor act)

4. Cognitive processing time and load involved in deciding which selections are necessary

5. Simple prediction support can be based on predicting frequently occurring words

Providing quick access to the first 100 words has a much greater impact on speed than providing access to the next 100 words; therefore, using the most frequently used words is a prediction technique. However, this assumes commonality across users. Some software can adapt to the way users type; therefore, prediction reflects the individual user's most frequently used words. Software can also "learn" new words typed by the user. Although this is an effective strategy, it can become problematic if the user has poor spelling skills, as the program learns misspelled words.

Some prediction methods consider word length. Predicting longer words obviously reduces rate more substantially than predicting shorter words. As prediction also requires fewer keystrokes to produce a message, fatigue is reduced. Furthermore, prediction also decreases the amount of time needed to prepare messages, minimizing the gap between input and output.

Message Prediction

Word prediction incurs an extra cognitive load for the user that might be attributable to the visual scanning it requires or to the fact that it might be more intuitive to type. Even when word prediction is used, communication rates seldom reach 20 words per minute. This aspect remains demoralizing when one considers that typical speech rates vary between 125 to 185 words per minute. One way to approach natural speech rates is by storing whole phrases, sentences, and paragraphs in AAC systems, which can be made available to the person using prediction based on context-appropriate prediction and rules of pragmatics or by structuring the content appropriately. Utterance-based/pragmatic-based prediction allows up to 64 wpm (Todman et al., 2008).

Context-aware systems are relatively new (Dominowska, 2002; Kane et al., 2012) and use information, such as location and knowledge of the partner, to improve prediction. Location information (i.e., automatically using GPS or manually by user input) has been used to present topic vocabulary, such as what would be needed when placing an order in a café (Dye et al., 1998).

To conclude, faster communication (i.e., increases in rate) has positive effects, such as the partner not having to wait for messages to be compiled, less communication breakdowns, less interpersonal frustration, and more opportunities for interaction.

TOP TEN TECHNOLOGY MANTRAS

The features for an ideal communication device (considering the whole technology continuum) are incorporated into the following discussion of the top 10 mantras (see Table 9-3 for a summary list). It is also interesting to note that many of these principles are intrinsically linked with the reasons mentioned earlier as to why devices are abandoned.

1. *Technology should contribute to the AAC user's full range of communication functions.* Although SGDs can be effective in summoning help from a distance, as well as facilitating the understanding of a message, vocalizations, gestures, or communication boards can be equally effective in communicating basic needs. A simple buzzer can be very effective for gaining attention. **Integrated systems** (e.g., mobile phones, tablets, and computers with AAC apps), on the other hand, provide users with more options than communication, such as gaming, educational programming, drawing, information systems, and word processing. However, the law of parsimony (which states that things should be as simple as possible) should also be considered. Figure 9-8 illustrates an extreme violation of the law of parsimony. Because technological advances are so ubiquitous and excite the imagination, one is tempted to consider elaborate systems for use with AAC users. A comprehensive multimodal system that includes unaided forms of communication should be considered to ensure that the goals of communication are met. The more elaborate the technology system, the more frequent and serious drawbacks it may have, such as cost, excessive equipment to attach or transport, and potential for breakdown during use. Whatever combination of approaches are selected, the user is encouraged to use all modes of communication to achieve the greatest flexibility in communication. A laptray on a wheelchair with communication symbols displayed on it, for example, may serve as a communication board, a food tray, and a game board.

2. *Technology should be compatible with other aspects of the AAC user's life.* If the person who uses AAC is mobile, the system should be portable. If the person is restricted to specific positions, the communication system should be easily

TABLE 9-3

Top Ten Technology Mantras

1. Technology should contribute to the AAC user's full range of communication functions.

2. Technology should be compatible with other aspects of the AAC user's life.

3. Technology should also consider the communication partner's needs, abilities (e.g., literacy skills), and requirements.

4. Technology should be usable in all environments and physical positions.

5. Technology should not restrict the topic or the scope of communication.

6. Technology should enhance the effectiveness of the AAC user's communication.

7. Technology should allow and foster the AAC user's development (e.g., skills in device usage, motor abilities, and language).

8. Technology should be acceptable and motivating for the user and significant others.

9. Technology should be affordable.

10. Technology should be easily maintained and repaired.

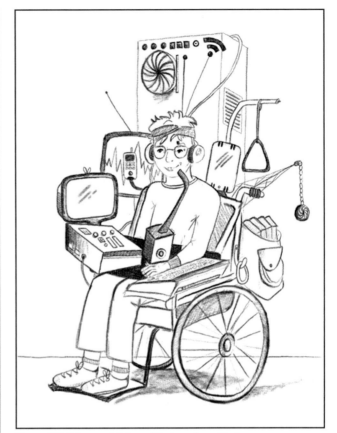

Figure 9-8. Extreme violation of the law of parsimony.

accessible to reduce fatigue. The system should be placed to encourage its use for communication and other functions, such as environmental control. Mounting a device on a wheelchair is a particularly demanding task because of the need to allow free access to a food tray and power controls and to avoid too many controls (e.g., communication aid, environmental control, steering, and speed of wheelchair). As impressive as such an arrangement might be, the communication system should never interfere with other life functions. The more accessible the device and more easily operated, the more the AAC user will be encouraged to integrate it within typical living patterns.

3. *Technology should consider the communication partner's needs, abilities (e.g., literacy skills), and requirements.* Although SGDs allow communication over a distance, aspects, such as confidentiality, should also be considered, particularly if the person wants to communicate a discrete message. Therefore, the ability to adjust the volume of the speech output makes devices useful for interacting with strangers and speaking before groups of people. Some persons who use AAC prefer a non-SGD, such as a communication board, to convey more personal or confidential messages between the user and a partner. Communication partners should be reminded of a number of dos and don'ts (Table 9-4) when communicating with persons who rely on AAC.

4. *Technology should be usable in all environments and physical positions.* With the advent of integrated systems on mainstream mobile devices, AAC devices have also become more portable (i.e., lighter, sleeker in design, easier to carry), more intelligible, and more responsive to environmental factors (such as bright sunlight). In addition, these devices need to be durable/rugged to withstand physical abuse, including exposure to hostile environments, such as the beach, the playground, and bathrooms. Unless the device is constructed to be sandproof and waterproof, a non-SGD, such as a communication board, may be a more effective option in these environments. Although an AAC user may be able to use direct selection or scanning to operate a communication device, eye gaze may be preferred at certain times (e.g., when fatigued or lying in bed). Multimodal communication should always be encouraged and usually will represent both non–speech-generating and speech-generating options, as well as unaided means of communication, such as gestures or manual signs.

5. *Technology should not restrict the topic or the scope of communication.* Any individual with typical intellectual functioning is capable of constructing an infinite number of highly original and complex messages. Reducing available vocabulary to a set of prestored messages severely restricts the richness of communication. Ideally, a communication device should allow the user access to

TABLE 9-4

Tips When Talking to Persons Who Use AAC

WHAT TO DO	WHAT NOT TO DO
• Take time and be patient • Speak directly to the person • Ask the person to show you yes/no • Ask the person how they communicate • Use the AAC system • Try to elicit stories • Develop topics for interaction • Give choices	• Do not be afraid • Never accept that a person has no AAC • Do not ignore the person • Do not communicate through others (e.g., personal assistant, parents, or caregivers) • Do not guess the AAC user's intended message too quickly • Do not be afraid to ask • Do not assume anything

AAC = augmentative and alternative communication.

the vocabulary they would like to use while also providing options so that the vocabulary can be expanded to express any idea needed in ongoing conversation. Literacy and text-to-speech devices, for example, allow for extensive vocabulary and generation of new ideas. However, this does not always imply the need for speech-generating technology. For example, the use of a non–speech-generating alphabet-based board by an individual with severe dysarthria for the cuing of initial letters of words may assist a listener's comprehension and help the user control rate of speech. A slower rate may also result in increased intelligibility.

6. *Technology should enhance the effectiveness of the AAC user's communication.* One advantage of software-based SGDs is the potential to use computational linguistics to predict communication patterns and enhance communication rate. Because rate is always a major problem for AAC, as discussed earlier in this chapter, any rate increase afforded by word or message prediction is helpful. However, limitations remain because aided communication never approximates rates of normal conversation. Competent AAC users often shift back and forth between prestored messages and typing out novel messages. The AAC user should be able to engage in interactive conversations by sharing control of the interaction, being able to ask questions, expand on topics, and make spontaneous observations. The capacity to express emotion in speech is also desirable, although it remains difficult for text-to-speech technology to add emotion automatically to speech output during message construction. All of this is desirable, of course, with minimal physical and cognitive load.

7. *Technology should allow and foster the AAC user's development (e.g., skills in device usage, motor abilities, and language).* The device should match the current skills levels of the AAC user so it is rewarding to use, but it should also allow for the development of new skills (e.g., literacy) to enhance the effectiveness of communication. Inherent in the development of these skills is also the development of social, educational, and work skills to facilitate improvement in overall quality of life.

8. *Technology should be acceptable and motivating for the user and significant others.* If the device is fun and effective in fostering communication, significant others (e.g., family, friends, and coworkers) will be more likely to participate in communication and to actively encourage the use of the device. Factors, such as the appearance of the device, ease of use and transport, and type and quality of output, are important considerations for the AAC user's and their family's willingness to actively use the device in everyday living. Frequently, AAC users prefer using their own speech, even if not intelligible. A combination of the user's own speech, SGDs, aided communication, and gestures can enhance communication and increase motivation.

9. *Technology should be affordable.* Although the cost of the device (including insurance, maintenance, and upgrade) is an important consideration, it should not be the only one. Cost should be balanced with the features of the device and the individual's needs. Although devices have become less expensive due to widespread use, it still represents a great investment for many families who cannot afford them. It is estimated that only 5% to 15% of people requiring assistive technology in low- and middle-income countries have access to it (Eide & Øderud, 2009). However, this is not only due to the costs of the technology (which may lead to, for example, donations of expensive yet inappropriate technology for these individuals), but also as a result of limited training, professional support, or maintenance required to utilize the technology. Many insurers, schools, or other state agencies seriously question such a financial outlay due to budget constraints. The amounts cited in invoices typically represent only the initial purchase. However, costs will also be incurred for training the AAC user to make effective use of the device and for maintenance costs, such as replacing the battery or electronic components throughout the life of the device. Finally, as the AAC user outgrows the device or as new, more powerful devices come on the market, there will be additional costs for upgrading and/or replacement. The use of non–speech-generating technology options that require the ongoing use of an aide can also represent considerable expense.

10. *Technology should be easily maintained and repaired.* Devices should be designed so the user and caregivers can operate them independently and make simple repairs as needed. The availability of a warranty is an important consideration in selecting a high technology device. Manufacturer's hotlines provide immediate access to information for solving problems in programming, simple maintenance, and repair. When repairs are needed, manufacturers should provide a loan device so the user will have minimal downtime. Non–speech-generating technology options are typically easily modified and easily replaced if necessary and should always be ready as a backup when SGDs need to be repaired.

All the above factors play a significant role in the selection and use of any communication technology. Technology is not to be applied with the expectation that it will be a miraculous solution. It is an important part of AAC, and when properly defined and integrated into the total plan for the AAC user, can increase the overall effectiveness of communication and improve quality of life.

FUTURE PERSPECTIVES

Waller (2019) presents the argument that the real potential for technology to support the needs of persons who use AAC is yet to be harnessed. Authors (Light & Drager, 2007; Light & McNaughton, 2012b, 2014a) have long reflected on the need for technology to support both the development of language and the use of AAC. Instead of users having to expend vital physical and cognitive effort on the operational use of technology, systems can and should be designed to be more usable and easier to support. Designers of AAC technology should also consider ways to support staff in their tasks. For example, in order to keep the vocabulary within VSDs and other graphic-based AAC systems current, updating language content should be simple and include the user. Current graphic-based systems rely on practitioners and families to create, store, and teach users how to access vocabulary. Users are thus restricted to vocabulary prestored by others, running the risk of not providing vocabulary sought by the user.

> John kept on hitting the symbol for star ... after two sleepless nights, his mother recalled an art activity in which John had used glitter ... no one had thought to provide a way for John to talk about glitter!

Although practitioners are encouraged to train users to use **core vocabulary** to extend their communication, the reliance on others to provide access to experiential vocabulary limits the opportunities for users to initiate and engage in novel communication. Can technology support user-directed exploration of vocabulary and sharing experience not already known by the listener? Can technology reduce the complex operational training requirements of systems instead of the load on users and practitioners to do all the work at the moment?

The following three examples illustrate ways in which technology can be designed using aspects of artificial intelligence. As mentioned earlier, persons who use AAC engage in little or no personal storytelling. Creating and articulating stories about oneself is often a real struggle for people who rely on computer-generated synthetic speech. This can be either due to short, prestored utterances or to the tedious preparation of word-for-word text-to-speech output—both impacting negatively on spontaneous social conversation. The "How was school today?" system was designed to enable children who use AAC to talk about their school day by automatically generating utterances (Black et al., 2012). The system uses data-to-text technology to generate narratives from sensor data, such as sensors that track the child's interactions with teaching and other staff, peers, and friends, as well as with objects, such as teaching tools. Sensors were placed on doorways to detect the child's location (e.g., the classroom or hallway), thereby providing additional information to the database. Apart from sensors, modeling was also used as the child's timetable of planned daily activities to provide information about time, activity, interaction, and location. Moreover, observations, interviews, and prototyping were also used to ensure that stakeholders were involved in the design of the system. The system used all the information from the database to generate messages, such as, "I went to the hall. We had music. Mrs. Smith and Jenny were there. I played with the tambourine." Evaluation data showed this system has the potential to support individuals with disabilities to participate better in interactive conversations, as they had more control during the conversation in comparison to their usual interactions where control lay mainly with the speaking partner.

Research in Scotland also demonstrated that computers can provide children who are nonspeaking with opportunities for telling jokes. Instead of relying on practitioner-stored jokes, the System to Augment Non-Speakers' Dialogue Using Puns (STANDUP) project (Manurung et al., 2008) developed a system that provided users with computer-generated puns. Using artificial intelligence, STANDUP generates riddles in a question/answer format by using concepts, like synonyms and homophones, to build vocabulary in a fun-loving way and also to create spontaneous interaction for individuals who use AAC. For example, when asking the question, "What do you call a spicy missile?" the answer "A hot shot!" is produced as the computer finds a synonym for "spicy" (hot) and for "missile" (shot). An evaluation (Waller et al., 2009) with nine children with cerebral palsy revealed that all participants spontaneously used the software without training on the interface. There was some evidence that the children were aware that the jokes had not been prestored by others, and therefore, were more motivated to engage in joke telling.

The ECHOES project (which supports children with autism in learning social interaction skills through intelligent technology; Porayska-Pomsta et al., 2018) demonstrated how a "virtual agent" could interact with children with autism within a language environment. The system was programmed to increase the complexity of interaction to respond to the development of the individual child's skills. Although not a traditional AAC system, ECHOES provides an example of how technology can adapt to the user allowing practitioners to focus on linguistic and social competencies rather than having to spend effort and time on the development of operational and strategic skills required for the user to navigate and retrieve prestored language.

The application of artificial intelligence to AAC technology (Higginbotham et al., 2012) has the potential to deliver systems that allow persons with complex disabilities to develop communication skills and engage in extended communication at a more acceptable rate while reducing the cognitive and physical load needed to operate the technology. Advances in the areas of computer vision and image processing (such as face detection and object recognition to automatically capture vocabulary), natural language processing (such as text prediction, text summarization, and narrative generation to present appropriate language), virtual agents (using intelligent computing to support interaction and language development), and the internet of things (imbuing objects with functionality, such as the use of robots or tangible communication objects) has the potential to transform AAC technology. However, in order to harness this potential, practitioners and family, as well as persons who use AAC, must be empowered to work with designers in order to deliver better communication for all (Waller et al., 2005).

Summary

This chapter began with a historical overview, given the exponential growth of technology over the past 2 decades. Current uses of technology were explored, highlighting benefits for persons with disabilities. The next section focused on feature matching, and after discussing different aspects of communication competency, the matching of technology features with users (and not vice versa) was explained. The features of AAC technology included physical features related to input devices (e.g., automatic speech recognition, BCIs, eye gaze, keyboards, mice, selection strategies and customization options, switches, touch screens), access methods (i.e., direct or indirect), types of displays (i.e., fixed, dynamic, or hybrid), voice (i.e., digitized speech, text-to-speech, and mixed modes), and portability. Next, the discussion focused on language features, and technology was grouped into single-function devices (e.g., attention-getting devices, voice recorders, and voice amplifiers), graphic-based AAC systems (e.g., VSDs, dynamic screens, and semantic compaction), literacy-based AAC systems, and hybrid systems. Acceleration techniques for rate enhancement were highlighted with an emphasis on layout optimization, code expansion, and language prediction. Ten technology mantras were shared before concluding with future perspectives.

Acknowledgments

The authors would like to thank Sarah Wilds, MS, CCC-SLP, Vice President of Product and Service Development at PRC-Saltillo for her help obtaining Minspeak icons. They would also like to thank Olivia Loots for her drawings used in this chapter.

Study Questions

1. How have recent developments in mobile and connected technology advanced the field of AAC, and how has this impacted the lives of persons who use AAC?

2. In the past, AAC technology was organized into a low technology vs. high technology dichotomy. How does this differ from contemporary thinking of AAC technology being viewed from the perspective of non–speech-generating vs. speech-generating?

3. What are the strengths and limitations of the four different types of AAC technology (i.e., single function devices, graphic-based AAC systems, literacy-based AAC systems, and hybrid systems)?

4. Discuss how recent technological developments have extended the type of input devices and systems. How have these advances impacted on access to communication for persons with a wide range of disabilities?

5. How does the content and layout of displays influence the way in which individuals use AAC effectively and efficiently? Consider issues such as context and type of language use, access methods, and communication rate.

6. What is meant by the term "feature matching," and how does this relate to the four communication competencies discussed in this chapter?

10

Applied Technology

Meher H. Banajee, PhD; Janie Cirlot-New, MS;
Cindy Halloran, BS, OTR/L; John Halloran, MS; Lin Sun, MA;
Annette Loring, MA; Amanda Hettenhausen, MA; and Krista Davidson, MS

MYTH

1. Since speech-generating devices (SGDs) have more and higher advanced features than non-SGDs, most augmentative and alternative communication (AAC) users will derive maximal benefit from SGDs.

2. Individuals with severe cognitive impairments lack certain prerequisite skills for SGD use; therefore, they will not be successful users of such technology. Non-SGDs are then AAC systems of choice for such individuals.

3. SGDs provide the AAC user with the most rapid, efficient communication possible. Therefore, it is the preferred approach for most AAC users.

REALITY

1. While SGDs do indeed have numerous desirable features, there is not a one-to-one correspondence between number of features and benefit of use. For many AAC users, a combination of SGDs and non-SGDs, used at situationally appropriate times, will result in maximal communicative benefit. An AAC user who is a student for instance, may require an SGD to support participation in classroom discussions or to generate a hard copy of homework assignments. However, while in the lunch line, a simple, non-SGD, such as a picture menu, may support that same student's effective and efficient communication.

2. Although many SGDs have features (e.g., word prediction or alphabet overlay) that may not be useful to some individuals with severe cognitive impairments, other features (e.g., dynamic screen displays and voice output) may motivate use and facilitate face-to-face communication so significantly that such devices are excellent AAC systems for such individuals. In most instances, non-SGDs and SGDs will combine to offer the most effective multicomponent AAC system.

(continued)

Fuller, D. R., & Lloyd, L. L. *Principles and Practices in*
Augmentative and Alternative Communication (pp. 195-208).
© 2023 Taylor & Francis Group.

REALITY (CONTINUED)

3. In many cases, setting up SGDs may make the communication process *slower* and *less* efficient. For example, using unaided approaches, such as nodding the head, pointing to a picture or word, or using eye gaze to choose a symbol on a display, are much faster and more efficient than waiting for the caregiver to set up an SGD using eye-gaze technology. On the other hand, speech-generating technology can provide an individual a means for communicating more complex ideas where a choice made via binary selection alone may be insufficient. Furthermore, voice output can be less ambiguous than pointing, eye gaze, or head nodding. In the end, selection of technological solutions must always be completed within the context of a full range of communication options and with recognition of benefits and limitations.

INTRODUCTION

The primary goal of an AAC system is independent, expressive communication by individuals who are nonspeaking or who have limited or unintelligible speech. The purpose of an AAC system is not merely to allow someone to participate in activities but for the user to be able to generate novel messages to interactively communicate with others to express wants and needs, transfer information, develop social closeness, and participate fully in education, employment, family, and community life (Light & McNaughton, 2015). AAC may represent existing language or aid in teaching expressive and receptive language. There are no prerequisites to introducing AAC to individuals who are nonspeaking. Individuals can begin at the cause and effect stage, learning to access vocabulary while learning language at the same time. Language and communication develop through the acquisition of single words moving to short phrases and sentences. Therefore, AAC systems should seek to follow a similar pattern, especially for beginning communicators.

Aided AAC systems can be non–speech-generating or speech-generating. Non–speech-generating technology includes, but is not limited to, paper-based communication boards/books, photographs, objects, and writing. Speech-generating technology comprises a wide continuum from simple electronic devices with digitized speech-to-tablet technology with AAC applications and high-level **dedicated** and **integrated augmentative communication devices** created specifically for expressive communication using digitized and synthesized voice output. Simple speech-generating systems have limited vocabulary and features to accommodate access, while more sophisticated technology allows for robust communication and a range of features and access methods. In the past, simple AAC solutions might have been the most often recommended for individuals with augmentative communication needs, as these solutions were more likely to be accessible to most users. Many insurance companies, Medicaid, and Medicare provide assistance with funding so individuals are more likely to have access to sophisticated high-level devices with robust language. It is essential that we help individuals in becoming independent communicators at the highest level achievable. While we should strive to provide access to high-level voice output communication to allow independent communication, non–speech-generating and simple speech-generating technology, as well as unaided communication (e.g., gestures, manual signs), can serve as a backup system when needed.

Regardless of level of technology, expressive/receptive AAC tools are a combination of the hardware or instrument, software, and robustness of the language system. There is some ambiguity about where on the technology continuum some tools would lie, as they may utilize sophisticated electronic devices but have software with limited language and features to adapt to the individual. By the same token, some non–speech-generating technology may provide a gateway to more independently accessed language than an electronic device with few prestored phrases. Both the sophistication of the tool and ability to access language for independent functional communication should be considered.

AAC decision makers must have a depth of knowledge about a wide variety of dedicated and integrated devices and the ability to articulate the differences between devices and how specific features should be considered based on the skills and capabilities of the individual in need of the AAC technology. Technology is rapidly changing, but decision makers must stay abreast of the latest technology and how it will be of benefit to individuals who need AAC.

SPEECH-GENERATING DEVICES

Synthesized/Hybrid Speech Output

The most sophisticated AAC technology is computer-based. These SGDs are an integrated group of components designed to be used to enhance communication (American Speech-Language-Hearing Association [ASHA], n.d.c) by individuals with a variety of disabilities. Individual devices vary in size but all include a symbol set, fixed or dynamic displays, synthesized—or a combination of synthesized—and digitized voice output, operational commands, multiple access methods, and changeable settings to accommodate individual needs. Computer-based AAC technology can be dedicated solely to the purpose of communication or integrated to include access to other functions (e.g., environmental control). The PRC-Saltillo Accent series and Tobii Dynavox Indi and I-110 are examples of sophisticated computer-based AAC devices (Figure 10-1).

Dedicated and Integrated Devices

Computer-based SGDs can be dedicated or integrated. A dedicated SGD has been defined by the Centers for Medicare and Medicaid Services for the purpose of coverage as "… durable medical equipment that provides an individual who has a severe speech impairment with the ability to meet [their] functional, speaking needs … and are used solely by the individual who has a severe speech impairment. Other covered features of the device include the capability to generate email, text, or phone messages to allow the patient to 'speak' or communicate remotely, as well as the capability to download updates to the covered features of the device from the manufacturer or supplier of the device" (2014). An integrated device is one that allows for use as a traditional computer complete with internet access and software or apps that perform tasks unrelated to the production of speech, such as environmental control, word processing, spreadsheets, music, videos, and games. While most insurance companies will not pay for features that are not deemed medically necessary, consumers can opt to pay a nominal fee to allow devices to be "unlocked" and enable internet access along with other computer features.

Hardware

SGDs are a combination of hardware and software. Some devices include all proprietary components (e.g., Accent, I-110) specifically designed to meet the needs of AAC communicators and engineered to be compatible with other assistive technology. A number of features that meet the unique needs of AAC communicators include glare- and break-resistant glass, cases designed to withstand high impact with built-in handles and stands, infrared capabilities for environmental controls, and integrated components to accommodate eye gaze, scanning, or head pointing. Manufacturers of AAC devices categorized as **durable medical equipment** must adhere to accreditation and quality standards. Manufacturers offer technical and funding support and may also provide implementation training.

Speech-generating devices may also be a combination of proprietary and commercially available components, such as a tablet with preloaded AAC software (e.g., ProSlate [Forbes AAC], ViaPro [PRC-Saltillo], Wego [Talk To Me Technologies]). To be considered a fundable dedicated device (at least for Medicaid and Medicare), tablet-based devices must be locked into the AAC software. Figure 10-2 provides examples of combined proprietary/commercially available SGDs.

Consumers also have the option of obtaining commercially available hardware, such as Android or Apple tablets, and downloading their choice of AAC software. Benefits include ready access and lower cost. However, since tablets are used by the general public, they are not considered durable medical equipment for funding purposes. Support for app-based AAC solutions is usually limited to online and email

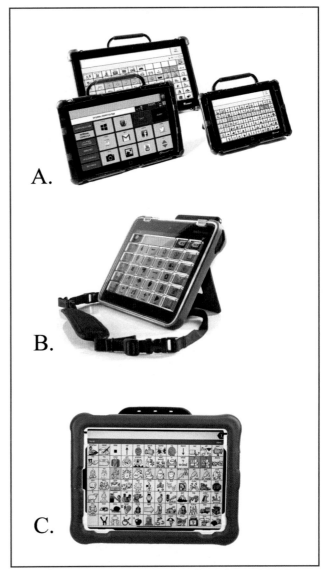

Figure 10-1. Sophisticated computer-based AAC devices. (A) PRC Accent series, including devices with 8-, 10-, and 14-inch screens. (Reproduced with permission from PRC-Saltillo.) (B) Tobii Dynavox I-110. (Reproduced with permission from Tobii Dynavox.) (C) PRC ViaPro. (© Copyright 2020 PRC-Saltillo. All rights reserved.)

support. Because tablets are not constructed for mounting on wheelchairs and heavy use while being transported, they may be unable to withstand excessive and continuous transportation and use from a user with limited motor abilities.

Regardless of the system selected, individuals conducting an AAC assessment should conduct a complete AAC evaluation that includes trials with a variety of AAC solutions. Accessories for different access methods (e.g., eye gaze, head control, switch access) may use Bluetooth connectivity that may not be reliable by working intermittently. In addition, Bluetooth technology may need to be purchased separately from different vendors or companies, which may lead to compatibility issues and limited support.

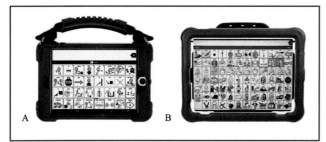

Figure 10-2. Examples of combined proprietary/commercially available SGDs. (A) QuickTalker Freestyle. (Reproduced with permission from AbleNet, Inc.) (B) PRC ViaPro. (© Copyright 2020 PRC-Saltillo. All rights reserved.)

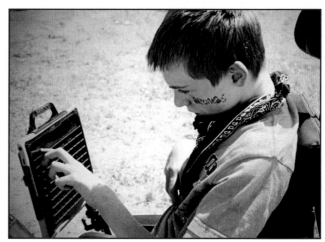

Figure 10-3. NOVA Chat 10 with keyguard to allow for more accurate access to the device's keys. (© 2019 PRC-Saltillo. All rights reserved.)

Device Access and Accessories

To interactively communicate with others, an individual must be able to access the vocabulary and text-to-speech on the communication device. Access can be achieved through direct selection, including access with a finger, mouse, track-ball, joystick, eye gaze, or head pointer. If direct selection is not an option, the user will need to use scanning, which typically involves the use of a switch or interface. The most desired form of access is direct selection, as it is far more efficient and quicker than scanning.

Direct Selection

Direct selection refers to the ability to directly select a symbol, icon, or letter. This can be accomplished through a variety of options. If motor skills are adequate to support its use, direct selection is the preferred means of access because it allows faster, more efficient access to vocabulary and places fewer cognitive-perceptual demands on the user than does scanning (Koester & Levine, 1994; Ratcliff, 1994). The cause and effect aspects of motor movement are easier to learn.

The most common direct selection method is physical touch. For SGDs, the user must either touch to activate capacitive screens or press to activate a mechanical button or resistive screen. Keyguards, clear or dark plastic raised grids with openings to access buttons on a device, can be particularly helpful for those with motoric challenges (Figure 10-3). These raised grids can prevent unintentional access of a capacitive screen while moving the hand to the desired target. Keyguards also improve accuracy by promoting use of an isolated index finger, accentuating the visual target and providing a place for tactile cues for those with visual impairments. By increasing accurate selection, the device user may be able to access smaller buttons and more vocabulary than without a keyguard.

Eye gaze is a method of direct selection that requires refined motor activity. The user gazes at a target on the device and waits a predetermined time, blinks, or accesses a switch and the device is activated. To operate a device using eye gaze, an eye-tracking module is required. Eye trackers work by emitting a near infrared light and reading the reflection of that light in the user's eyes to determine where they are looking on a screen. That location is then activated by blink, dwell, or switch. SGDs may have these modules built into the device hardware or they may be an accessory that is attached externally but integrated via software. While eye-tracking modules are becoming more of a commodity in the general purpose market, through integration of hardware and software, SGDs offer the ability to adapt for positioning challenges, ambient light, eye preferences, and extraneous movement. The activation of smaller targets on a screen requires more precise calibration.

Head pointing can be accomplished through both speech-generating and non–speech-generating means. An example of non–speech-generating head pointing would be the use of a headstick (a device that is secured to the head and has a stick or extension that the user moves with the head) to select symbols on a communication board or other display. Speech-generating head pointing requires sophisticated technology attached to or included with an SGD. The module emits an infrared light. A small, adhesive reflective dot is placed on the individual's forehead, cap, glasses, or other convenient spot in the vicinity of the head. Optical sensors calculate how the infrared light reflects off the dot to detect the head's movement, with the on-screen cursor moving in the same direction as the individual's head movements. Selections are made either by dwelling on a target for a predetermined time (e.g., 0.5 seconds) or by activating a switch. Head pointing can be less tiring than eye gaze and less reliant on positioning.

Scanning

When direct selection is not feasible, scanning can be used to select symbols from a communication display. Scanning is defined as "stepping through" a set of symbols until the desired symbol is available and selected (Church & Glennen, 1992). When scanning is used with speech-generating hardware, the individual will access a switch to control activation and selection. The device is programmed to scan so that a highlighter moves across the display in a specific pattern. When the desired symbol is highlighted, the user accesses a switch with a reliable motor movement. In many SGDs, multiple scanning methods exist, such as step scanning, automatic scanning, and **inverse scanning**. Scan patterns include circular scanning, linear scanning, and row-column scanning. Scanning times can be adjusted based on the motor abilities of the user.

Switches

Numerous types of switches can serve as interfaces between individuals and assistive technology and/or AAC devices based on the motor movements of the user and placement of the switch. The purpose of switch access for someone using a communication device is to access the vocabulary and/or text for interactive communication purposes, not to accomplish another motoric goal (e.g., placement to promote reaching across midline). Switch access should be as easy and efficient as possible for the user with the most reliable and consistent motor movement. The emphasis should be placed on communication. The location may be at any accessible site on the body, including a knee, foot, elbow, hand, head, or cheek. There are various means of activating switches, such as physical touch (button switch), physical proximity, air pressure (e.g., sip and puff), or detection of electrical impulses sent to a muscle (e.g., NeuroNode). The reader is referred back to Chapter 9 for illustrations of various types of switches. Individuals using switches will likely have their SGD mounted to their wheelchair or other positioning aid.

Device Mounts

Individuals with limited mobility often need their device mounted in a stable position for optimal access. Device and switch mounts consist of a plate for attachment of the device or switch hardware with joints for connecting that plate to a device-mounting plate or a stabilizing base. This allows for accurate positioning and stability while accessing the communication device. Types include table, floor, bed, and wheelchair mounts (Figure 10-4).

Software

Software stored within the hardware houses the language system, features, settings, voice synthesizer, etc. Software may be particular to a specific device or downloadable to various platforms (e.g., AAC apps can be downloaded either free or for a price onto a tablet or smartphone).

Language Systems

While some AAC software allows total customization of a language system, most SGDs offer choices of standardized, preprogrammed language systems with the ability to add customizations. Most vocabulary is laid out in a grid system, except for visual scene displays (VSDs). Some AAC software offers limited vocabulary while more linguistically robust systems accommodate various language skill levels within

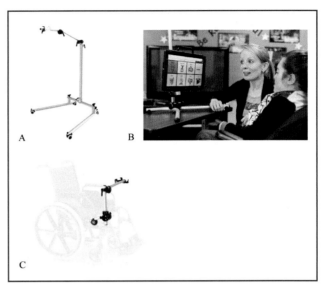

Figure 10-4. Mounts stabilize a device for access for those with limited motor skills. (A) Floor. (B) Table. (C) Wheelchair. (© 2019 PRC-Saltillo. All rights reserved.)

the same representational framework. There are structural differences that should be considered when meeting the individual's needs, accommodating current skills, and providing a pathway for growth or future needs. ASHA states that the goal of AAC is to provide "… the most effective interactive communication possible. Anything less represents a compromise of the individual's human potential" (n.d.c).

A robust language system provides the ability to communicate across environments for a variety of communicative functions and with a variety of communication partners. Components of a robust language system include a wide range of word classes with a large number of core words and the ability to make morphological changes, such as verb tenses, pluralization, and comparative and superlative adjectives, for generation of grammatically correct sentences. The language system should also support motor automaticity with consistent vocabulary arrangement and text-to-speech. The use of a robust language system that can accommodate different skill levels over time alleviates relearning of word location and system navigation as abilities change.

Language can be represented with pictures, symbols, visual scenes, printed words, word prediction, or abbreviation expansion. While most systems rely heavily on one representation strategy, usually multiple strategies are available within the same system. For example, an individual primarily may use symbols to produce words but rely on a keyboard and word prediction when a desired word is not preprogrammed. An individual with a severe motoric disability may rely on strategies that minimize movement and keystrokes, such as abbreviation expansion or word prediction. Language systems based primarily on icons are beneficial to device users who are not literate but may also provide keystroke savings to literate users. Systems relying on the written word or spelling may be quicker to learn for those who are literate.

The method of utterance generation is important to consider. Spontaneous novel utterance generation is possible when AAC users have access to individual words, word combinations, and commonly used phrases to independently create their own utterances in a manner similar to how verbal adults use language and children learn language (Hill, 2001). A phrase or sentence can be stored on a single button to allow access with one touch.

While prestored phrases limit generative speech (as the majority of spoken speech cannot be predicted and most utterances are novel and unique) they can be beneficial to represent frequently used phrases, sentences, and even messages. Examples of prestored phrases include storing a script for calling a doctor or participating in the school play or prestoring a speech. Consideration should also be given to the auditory output created while generating utterances on an SGD. Do utterances sound like connected verbal speech or are categories pronounced while selecting words? For example, does the SGD speak the category "fruit" before it says "apple?"

Robust language systems include thousands of words; therefore, the organization of those words needs to allow for effective and efficient access and accommodate customization of vocabulary within the existing framework. There are multiple vocabulary organization methods, including semantic-, grammatical-, activity-, or environment-based; alphabetic; frequency of use; word prediction; and VSDs. Computer-based technology allows access to multiple changing screens and the navigational requirements will affect rate of communication. The AAC communicator will need to understand how to navigate from screen to screen to find desired vocabulary or rely on motor automaticity.

Levelt's model of language production states that while message generation and monitoring require executive control, speakers do not normally attend to the processes of language encoding and articulation. The speed and complexity of the motor process for verbal speech demands that it be carried out automatically (i.e., without conscious awareness) for the production of fluent speech (Levelt, 1989). When the motor movement to produce a word remains consistent, automaticity can develop, allowing communicators to focus on the content and other aspects of the communicative exchange by reducing the cognitive load of understanding and discriminating icons or understanding the organizational system. Automaticity is possible in systems that always return to a home page once a word is spoken. If the device user must select a navigational button to close a page or produce multiple utterances on the same page of a dynamic system, words will not allow for consistent motor patterns and navigational skills will be required (Halloran & Halloran, 2013).

The number of buttons per screen also affects navigation complexity, as more buttons per screen allows for a greater number of words to be produced with fewer keystrokes. Larger buttons may need to be considered to accommodate access issues, but the tradeoff is either a smaller vocabulary or more navigation, and therefore, greater number of button pushes required to access the same vocabulary.

VSDs are composed of familiar scenes (e.g., a classroom with a desk, chalkboard, teacher, and students) rather than a grid. Hotspots are programmed to produce messages for some portions of the scene, such as, "Ms. Smith is reading a story," or "Tyrone is sitting at the table." For adults, it may be a scene of a familiar living room with the person's spouse looking at photographs. VSDs can represent the environment and interactions of people with each other and with the environment. Some research has indicated success with communication for adults with aphasia using simple VSDs (Seale et al., 2007). There is also research to suggest that young children with developmental disabilities can learn to take more social turns during interactions and learn vocabulary, but there is little research to support the use of VSDs for sophisticated interactive communication (Drager et al., 2009).

Several trademarked language systems are available and most offer different levels to accommodate the individual's skill set. Some language systems are only available on a particular AAC manufacturer's products (e.g., Unity [PRC-Saltillo], TD Snap [Tobii Dynavox]) while some are licensed on multiple companies' products (e.g., WordPower, Gateway).

Unity is designed with a focus on easy access to core words arranged semantically on the screen along with fringe vocabulary arranged categorically. It also has predictable locations for parts of speech. Language Acquisition through Motor Planning (LAMP) Words for Life (PRC-Saltillo) is a variation of Unity that presents one unique and consistent motor pattern per word. WordPower combines core vocabulary, spelling, and next-word prediction. Words outside the base set of core words are arranged alphabetically or categorically. WordPower is available on several device manufacturers' products, including Tobii Dynavox and PRC-Saltillo.

Tobii Dynavox has two proprietary language systems, TD Snap and Communicator 5, that offer a set of core words with added vocabulary stored categorically. Additionally, Communicator 5 offers vocabulary subsets that duplicate non–speech-generating communication options, such as the **Pragmatic Organized Dynamic Display** (PODD). There are also a number of AAC apps with robust language systems.

Features That Support Language/Communication

When learning a robust language system, the ability to only show a subset of vocabulary provides the opportunity to teach targeted words while minimizing distractions. **Vocabulary masking** allows the therapist to accommodate current language ability while keeping the location of words consistent as vocabulary grows, eliminating the need for motor relearning as access to vocabulary is expanded. An efficient masking feature should allow for changes to be made quickly with regard to what words are showing so language can be taught in natural activities. One such software feature is Vocabulary Builder (Figure 10-5).

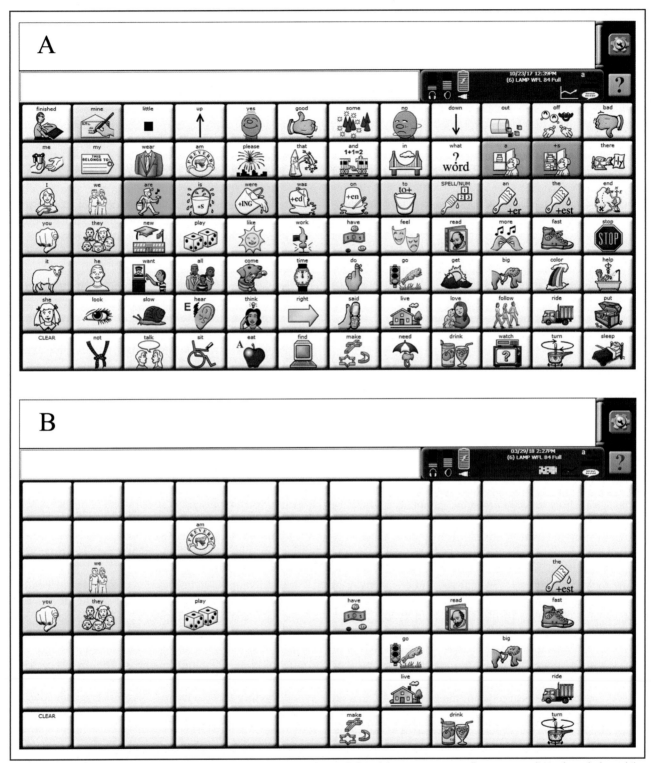

Figure 10-5. The Vocabulary Builder tool in PRC-Saltillo's Unity and LAMP Words for Life language systems allows access to limited vocabulary while keeping the motor pattern to say those words consistently as vocabulary is expanded. (A) Vocabulary Builder off. (B) Vocabulary Builder on with selected words. (Reproduced with permission from PRC-Saltillo.)

One of the challenges of a robust language system is learning where all the words are located. A word search feature allows an individual to look up vocabulary by spelling the word to see the pathway to access that particular word. Some devices also allow the user to see and practice the motor pattern to access the word rather than relying on recall of icon sequences. This feature is useful for beginning users and support team members as the device and vocabulary are being learned.

Language sample analysis is encouraged for collecting baseline data, as well as documenting progress during intervention. It needs to be completed on a regular basis (Heilmann et al., 2010). Cross (2015), Hill (2004), Hill and Romich (2002), and Van Tatenhove (2014b) have advocated for language sample collection and analysis to be part of common practice for the field of AAC. One tool to help with language analysis in AAC is **automated data logging**. Data logging refers to the automatic recording of data that can be analyzed to produce a time-stamped transcript of what has been generated on an AAC device (AAC Institute, 2015). These collected data can then be analyzed to assist in making intervention and management decisions as part of the ongoing assessment process (Lloyd et al., 1997). Automated data logging has been an available feature on some SGDs for over 30 years and has more recently been added to AAC apps.

Automated data log files may look different based on the device manufacturer or app developer. However, most data log files have similar elements, including:

- Timestamp: The time an event occurs
- Output: The words generated by the person using the AAC system
- Language codes: Indicate how the output was formulated (e.g., spelling, word prediction, semantic compaction, from navigating to multiple pages)
- Nonlanguage codes: Include page navigations, key selections, and other actions without output

The length and format of raw data log files makes review burdensome. Additionally, the lack of a universal format for data log files makes analysis more challenging. Traditional language analysis software programs cannot accept data log files without them being manually reformatted and redefined—a time-intensive process. This may pose a challenge for speech-language pathologists with large workloads and high productivity requirements. Examples of software that allow for data log files to be analyzed, either manually or through an automatic process, include Systematic Analysis of Language Transcripts (Miller & Chapman, 1985), ACQUA (HEAD Acoustics; Lesher et al., 2000), and QUAD (Cross, 2010). Additional programs, such as Microsoft Word or Excel, can also be used to reformat and perform simple data analysis.

There are two tools unique to the field of AAC that allow for a more automatic analysis of data log files. These include the Performance Report Tool (PeRT; AAC Institute, 2001) and Realize Language (PRC, 2014). PeRT and Realize Language both have been used to conduct case studies and research. They use different representational methods, making them complimentary.

PeRT was developed by the AAC Institute in 2001 to decrease the amount of time needed to create an AAC performance report from Language Activity Monitor (LAM) data. LAM specifically refers to the data logging feature available on PRC-Saltillo devices. Rather than manual extraction of summary information, PeRT performs automatic analysis on 17 quantitative utterance-based and word-based measures. Appendices include LAM data, utterances, word lists, and a text version of the report (Romich et al., 2003). PeRT is not commonly used in clinical practice.

Another analysis tool is Realize Language. This is a subscription-based web service from PRC-Saltillo that provides an analysis of data log files from several different AAC devices and apps. Data log files can be uploaded manually or via WiFi from devices and apps to the online system. Realize Language allows for data to be analyzed in a variety of ways, including word frequency, parts of speech, performance against target vocabulary, and daily/weekly/monthly device use. It is also possible to search for specific instances of words in order to see them in context. Realize Language utilizes data visualization in that it turns raw log files into charts, calendars, word clouds, tables, and other graphics and reports (Figure 10-6).

Available tools for language use offer a variety of options for clinical application. Regardless of which tools are used, there are certain elements that must be considered, including privacy of the individual, training for all team members, a plan for why and when to collect data, and ongoing analysis and interpretation of the data log files.

Features That Support Programming

To customize vocabulary, speech-generating technology offers libraries of hundreds or thousands of symbols from one or more symbol corpuses. Most speech-generating technology also allows the AAC user or significant others to take and/or import photographs, pictures, or other images. This is helpful when representing specific family members, teachers, pets, a favorite restaurant, or famous person. However, it is important to consider that words used across different settings, people, and activities might generalize better if they are not item- or person-specific.

Speech output can be digitized or synthesized. Digitized speech is prerecorded speech stored in the device to be played back later. Digitized speech is helpful for sounds, such as laughing, whistling, cheering at a sports event, making animal sounds, or while using **voice banked** messages while communicating with family members. Digitized speech does not allow for natural prosody when words and phrases not stored together are combined. Also, the user is limited to saying only what has been preprogrammed rather than being able to produce novel utterances or spell. Memory capacity of a device may limit the length or number of messages stored.

Synthesized speech translates text created by alphabetic letters, words, phrases, pictures, and symbols into a computer-generated simulation of human speech. To produce this type of output, the voice software applies the phonetic rules of the language to translate the text into speech as it is generated, and therefore, is not limited by memory storage. Synthesized speech allows the user to create novel utterances, and speech rate and pitch can be customized for the user. Text-to-speech software offers several voices to match gender and age and is

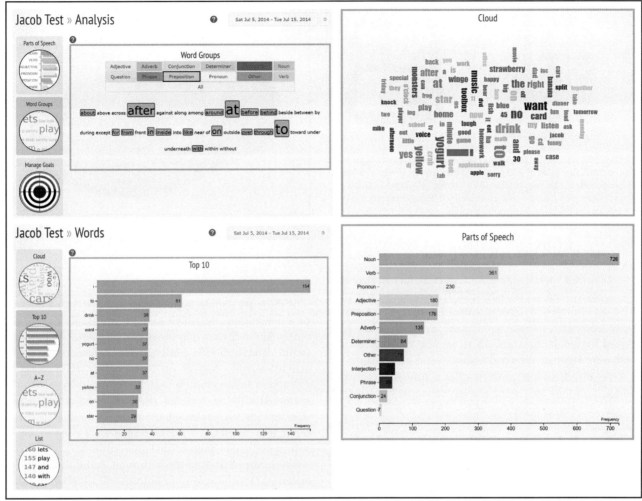

Figure 10-6. Realize Language tracks device use and presents data in charts based on time of use, words used, parts of speech, etc. (Reproduced with permission from PRC-Saltillo.)

available in various languages. Acapela and Ivona voice software are available in a number of SGDs. Additionally, custom and personalized synthesized voices can be created using one's own voice or voices of family members (e.g., My Own Voice by Acapela Group, ModelTalker, or VocaliD).

One of the benefits of computerized AAC technology is that there are many features available to customize the performance of the device to accommodate access challenges for the individual. On the contrary, when consumers are given the ability to access many features, they may make setting changes without understanding the rationale for these settings, making the device less functional. Many posts to social media and calls for assistance to tech support are due to a misapplication of access features. Training and support for speech-generating technology is necessary to guide the clinician through matching accessibility features to a specific individual.

Regardless of access method, computer-based SGDs have the ability to accommodate physical challenges. Dwell (eye gaze, head pointing) or acceptance (touch) time is the length of time that elapses between selecting a key and activation of that key. For example, if dwell or acceptance time is set to 0.5 seconds, a button or key will active one-half second after it was touched. This feature reduces unintentional button activations while moving toward the desired key for the user with extraneous movements, poor finger isolation, or slow saccadic eye movements. Release time, the amount of time that must transpire between a key activation and reactivation, can be adjusted for users who cannot move off a button in a timely manner or who exhibit tremors. This tool can also be used for individuals who tend to engage in self-stimulatory behavior on hearing the same button activated repetitively or who tend to drag their fingers across the surface of a device without lifting them due to physical challenges. Auto repeat determines how fast a key will repeat itself when held down. This time interval can be decreased to benefit an individual who struggles hitting the same key repetitively; on the other hand, the time interval would have to be increased for an individual who cannot move quickly off a key.

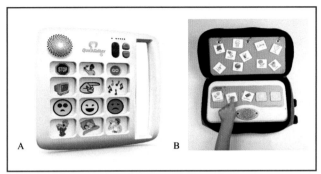

Figure 10-7. Examples of SGDs with digitized speech. (A) QuickTalker 12. (Reproduced with permission from AbleNet, Inc.) (B) Logan Prox Talker. (Reproduced with permission from LoganTech [Proxtalker.com, LLC].)

Digitized Speech-Generating Devices

Digitized speech output AAC devices vary in size, storage capacity, and access methods. They range in complexity from electronic devices with enough storage for hours of recorded speech to battery-operated simple electronics designed for single messages. There are also a couple of apps with only digitized speech available.

Digitized devices tend to offer a limited number of button locations on a static display. Messages can be single words, phrases, or sentences and recorded in a voice similar to the age and gender of the individual who will be utilizing the device and are accessed with software provided by the device manufacturer or with standard picture software, such as Boardmaker. They tend to be considerably less expensive than more sophisticated technology and easier to program. Since button locations are limited, access to a larger number of words or messages than the display will accommodate requires an overlay to be manually changed and/or messages rerecorded. These devices may offer a few features to assist with access, such as switch ports, simple scanning, or various types of feedback when keys are accessed. Voice output usually occurs as each button is activated; however, some devices allow for delayed message playback.

While SGDs with digitized speech may seem easier to operate than higher level technology, language is limited and unplanned real-time conversation is more difficult. Speech output sounds natural at a single button level; however, stringing recorded messages together to create novel utterances is limited, and when recordings are combined, prosody can sound unnatural. Speech output is limited to the words and phrases that have been prestored for the user. When messages change due to the use of overlays, the user must rely more on symbol recognition and discrimination rather than motor planning, thereby increasing the cognitive load to access the device. As the user's need for vocabulary grows, these devices may not meet that need. Some examples of simple SGDs with digitized speech are GoTalkExpress, Prox Talker, Tech Talk 8, and SuperTalker Progressive (Figure 10-7).

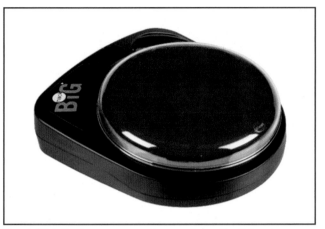

Figure 10-8. Single messages can be recorded on the BIGmack Communicator and played back when the switch is activated. It can also be connected to a toy or appliance. (Reproduced with permission from AbleNet, Inc.)

There are simple, battery-operated SGDs that offer one or a few buttons on which to store words, phrases, or sentences. These devices may be used to develop an understanding of cause and effect, offer a few choices in a predicted activity, or offer easy access to a predictable message. For example, a talking button switch (Figure 10-8) can be programmed with the word "go" and be connected to a battery-operated toy, such as a rabbit that moves upon activation of the button. Similarly, a message such as, "I need to use the bathroom," can be prerecorded on a button SGD mounted to a wheelchair or door of the bathroom. A simple battery-operated SGD with two or four buttons will allow an individual to make choices or answer yes/no questions. Keep in mind that although they provide speech output, these devices do not allow for spontaneous generative communication, as the user has access to only a limited number of message options. The AAC communicator is unable to independently produce utterances other than what was provided.

When the goal is to build or increase functional communication skills, beginning with a few button options that do not promote generative vocabulary offers limited benefit. These devices may also be utilized to make physical access easier for the communicator with motor challenges. However, if motor skills are such that they limit access to just a few buttons, a different access method should be considered.

NON–SPEECH-GENERATING TOOLS AND STRATEGIES

Traditionally, non–speech-generating augmentative communication has been defined as tools to support communication that are nonelectronic, thereby excluding the use of computer technology as an operating system. Non–speech-generating technology has two physical elements: symbols (the means to represent) and displays (the means to transmit). The combinations of symbols and display arrangements that are possible in non–speech-generating applications are almost endless. All types of symbols—object-based, picture-based, representations of manual signs and gestures, alphabet-based, phonemic- or phonics-based, and arbitrary logographs and shapes—can be utilized. If a non–speech-generating display is used as a back up to an SGD, it would be important to utilize the same symbol corpus. A good idea would be to utilize screenshots of overlays from the SGD to construct corresponding overlays for the non–speech-generating display. The amount of language production that is possible depends in part on the display being used, from more complex communication books to manual boards to communication necklaces, strips, and wallets with limited functional or activity-specific vocabulary.

Independent Strategies

A manual **communication board** or book is a static display of symbols, letters, or phrases usually laid out in a grid pattern, printed on paper, and laminated. The individual communicates by pointing to or gazing at symbols on the board. A communication board can be used alone or as a back up to an SGD. Board design should allow for free expression of individual ideas, hence communication boards or books need to include access to core vocabulary, as well as relevant fringe vocabulary, to encourage the combination of concepts and expression of new ideas (see Chapter 12). Therefore, the number of locations (size of the overlay) or concepts should be adjusted to accommodate for a growth in the student's vocabulary and interests. A single board may be used or pages may be bound to provide access to a larger vocabulary, such as core vocabulary boards with flip down strips for fringe vocabulary for a variety of activities and environments. The lack of auditory output may make this modality more difficult to learn for some emergent communicators, as there may not be reliable feedback to their selections. The AAC user's need to transition to a more dynamic electronic display should be assessed on a regular basis to provide more opportunities for expansion and growth. A couple examples of non-SGDs can be found in Figure 10-9.

The **Picture Exchange Communication System** (PECS) was developed in 1985 by Andy Bondy and Lori Frost of Pyramid Educational Consultants in the United States and first used with preschool children diagnosed with autism at the Delaware Autism Program (Bondy & Frost, 1994). Since then, PECS has been used with learners of all ages and varying abilities. PECS is described as a teaching protocol based on B. F. Skinner's book, *Verbal Behavior*, and applied behavior analysis to achieve functional communication. The PECS protocol focuses on teaching the AAC user to approach the communicative partner (via physical vs. verbal prompts, providing errorless learning, immediate reinforcement, and avoiding verbal prompt dependency) through a series of six phases, beginning with the exchange of a single picture

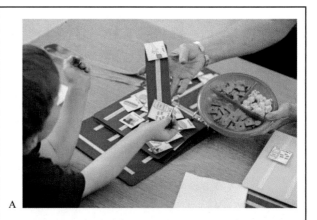

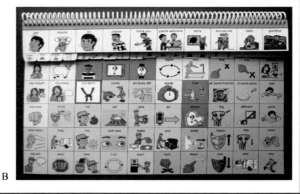

Figure 10-9. Examples of non-SGDs. (A) PECS communication book. (Reproduced with permission from Pyramid Educational Consultants www.pecs.com. All rights reserved.) (B) PIXON communication book. (Reproduced with permission from Semantic Compaction Systems, Inc.)

for a desired item or action. The AAC user is taught in later phases to discriminate pictures, build simple sentences to request, add adjectives and prepositions to sentences, answer questions, and comment. Communication books are used to store picture symbols with hook and loop fastener (e.g., Velcro) and a sentence strip for placing the icons to build sentences. Pyramid Educational Consultants offers an app version to support communicators who might transition to an SGD after Phase 4.

The Pixon Project Kit (Semantic Compaction Systems) was developed in 2009 through a collaborative effort that included speech pathologist Gail Van Tatenhove; other speech language pathologists, educators, and occupational therapists; and linguist Bruce Baker. The Pixon Project Kit is described as an early language development program using non–speech-generating communication boards. Intervention focuses on teaching a small set of high frequency core vocabulary words. Pixon boards can serve as an AAC user's primary mode of communication, as a back up to an SGD, or as a teaching tool to build language skills. The Pixon Project Kit comes with predesigned non–speech-generating communication boards along with templates and symbols to create customized boards.

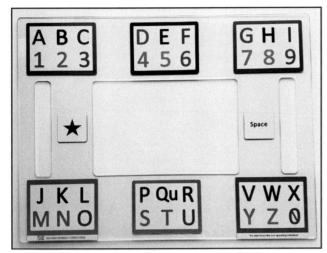

Figure 10-10. An E-TRAN board. In some E-TRANs, the cut-out handles on the left and right may be absent, thereby enlarging the middle and right locations.

Partner-Assisted Strategies

PODD has been developed over the last 15 years by Gayle Porter, a speech pathologist with the Cerebral Palsy Education Centre in Victoria, Australia. PODD is described as being a way of organizing whole word and symbol vocabulary in a communication book that incorporates features to improve the locating of vocabulary. Category and navigational icons have page numbers to indicate which page to turn to next. The communicator selects a symbol on a page. The communication partner voices the selection and turns to the indicated page, so navigational tasks do not inhibit the communication act. Intervention focuses on immersing the AAC user by providing constant modeling of language by all who interact with them. In this way, PODD can not only be used to facilitate more effective communication by the AAC user but also to facilitate the AAC user's understanding of the verbal output of the communication partner (i.e., the communication partner points to PODD symbols as they verbally name the selection made by the AAC user). PODD books can be created and customized to meet individual needs via templates on a purchased CD along with access to symbol software (Porter & Cafiero, 2009). PODD page sets are also available on third-party devices and software.

Partner-assisted scanning can be used with individuals with significant motor impairments. This strategy allows an individual to communicate using non–speech-generating technology. The technique uses a communication board with pictures, symbols, letters, or words. The communication partner points to each picture or row and the AAC user indicates if the partner is pointing to the target item or row in which the target item is located. If the board consists of rows and columns, the partner points to each row in order. If the AAC user indicates "yes" (using a nonverbal means, such as eye blink, thumbs up, or raising eyes), the partner

then begins to point to the item in each column until the user produces some type of signaling response to indicate that the target item (and message) has been encountered. Piché and Reichle (1991) caution that care must be taken in selecting a teachable, salient, socially acceptable, and replicable signaling response.

An E-TRAN (eye transfer) board (Figure 10-10) consists of a non–speech-generating eye-gaze board usually made from a clear material, such as plexiglass, that may contain pictures, symbols, or alphabetic letters depending on the level of the user's language. The E-TRAN is divided into eight group locations—three along the top (left, middle, right), two in the middle (left, right), and three along the bottom (left, middle, right). The center of the board is usually cut out so the communication partners can see each other. In its simplest use, one symbol or picture would be placed in each of the eight group locations. The user would begin by looking at the communication partner through the hole in the center of the board, then gazing at the correct picture or letter, and finally looking back at the partner for confirmation.

When accommodating more than eight options, the user must employ a two-step encoding technique by first glancing at the group location containing the target selection, then glancing at the position on the board that corresponds to the position of their target selection within its group location. To illustrate, refer back to Figure 10-10. (Note that this E-TRAN has the letters of the alphabet, as well as numbers.) To indicate the letter D, the user would first glance to the top middle group location that contains the letter D (the black rectangle), then glance at the communication partner, then move their eyes to the top left group location (the red rectangle), as the letter D is in the top left position within its top middle group location.

Visual Support Strategies

Often non–speech-generating technology is used as a visual strategy to aid receptive language, facilitate learning, support literacy, or provide a means of communication in an isolated activity. These range from the use of visual schedules to assist students in understanding the sequence of activities engaged in during the day, boards used in specific activities, and wall charts to model language (Figure 10-11). While these strategies can be described as communication tools, their range and potential for facilitating interaction between individuals is limited and should not be considered an alternative to an expressive communication system.

A communication necklace, for example, promotes easy access and allows the hands to be free. Similarly, a communication wallet can hold a variety of two-dimensional symbol options. Some AAC users may utilize a wallet because it can be placed in a pocket instead of being worn in full view. Communication boards and symbol vests can be used to provide easy access to activity-specific vocabulary.

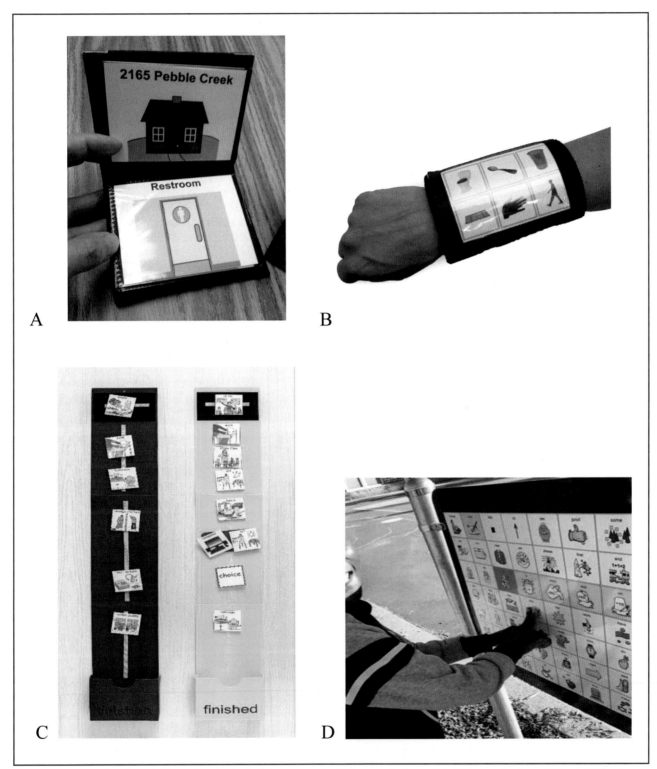

Figure 10-11. Examples of non-SGDs used as visual schedules or prompts. (A) Communication wallet. (B) Communication wristband. (C) Visual schedule. (D) Playground core board.

A **communication wall chart** allows several children in a classroom to make use of the same display. Wall charts can be focused on topic-specific areas (e.g., cooking, playing, or snacking) or can be more generic in nature. **Picture schedule system** and calendar boxes aid in helping the individual understand the steps of a task or sequence of scheduled activities. Symbols, objects, or written lists with check-off boxes are placed in sequential order. Completion of tasks is visually represented by moving the icons or objects to a "finished" area, turning icons over, or putting a check mark by the task.

Symbols can be incorporated throughout the learner's environment to expand exposure to those used in their communication system. Non–speech-generating versions of SGDs can be used for modeling and **aided language stimulation**. Classrooms can use a smart projection board as a more sophisticated wall chart by projecting the language system used by the child on the board to model language in the classroom. Symbols can also be used to label items and locations, as well as supplement written text and support literacy.

Ethical Considerations

Both ASHA and the Council for Exceptional Children provide ethical guidelines for provision of services that include statements concerning the use of evidence-based practice and refraining from practices that can cause harm to a student or client.

Both facilitated communication and rapid prompting method (RPM) have no credible scientific evidence that communication produced via the use of facilitated communication or RPM are the thoughts of the communicator. In addition, use of such techniques can cause harm by reduced opportunities for access to timely, effective, and appropriate interventions and loss of individual communication rights. In August 2018, ASHA's Board of Directors accepted two separate position statements: one on facilitated communication (ASHA, 2018a) and a second one on RPM (ASHA, 2018b). Both position statements are published on ASHA's website along with precautions against using facilitated communication and RPM (ASHA, n.d.a).

Summary

AAC technology covers a broad spectrum from non-SGDs, such as communication boards, to SGDs with limited vocabulary options, to highly configurable computerized SGD technology. Technology for interactive communication has improved significantly over the past 10 years and is more accessible than ever before to those individuals who are nonspeaking and need assistance with interactive communication. Advances in technology ensure an ever-evolving availability of new devices and strategies to assist with communication and provide additional and more efficient means of access for individuals with physical impairments. Chapter 14 will discuss the selection process for technology in more detail.

In this rapidly changing field, proficiencies necessary to make informed clinical judgments include a knowledge of the broad array of current devices, software and their respective features, performance differences, the language production available on a particular device, and how to customize a device to fit an individual's particular needs. It is essential that persons who recommend AAC systems and provide daily support to the individuals using AAC stay informed of the options available to best meet the individual's needs.

Study Questions

1. What differentiates digitized SGDs from computer-based technology with synthesized speech output?

2. Describe three non–speech-generating AAC devices, techniques, or approaches.

3. What is the primary difference between partner-assisted scanning and device-generated scanning using computer-based SGDs?

4. What is meant by text-to-speech synthesizers? Give some examples.

5. Describe at least three encoding systems used for storing and retrieving messages, and comment on their advantages and disadvantages.

6. What is the distinction between "dedicated" and "integrated" communication devices?

7. List at least one ethical concern that needs to be addressed while choosing AAC systems and strategies.

Part IV
AAC Assessment

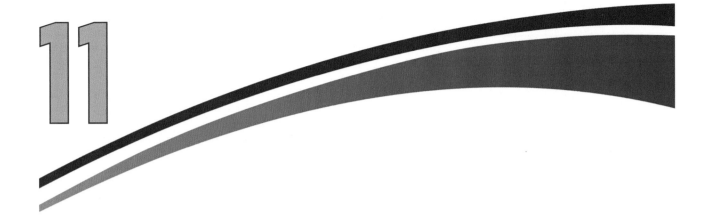

AAC Assessment Process

Elizabeth K. Hanson, PhD; Kristy S. E. Weissling, SLPD;
and Miechelle McKelvey, PhD

MYTH

1. The augmentative and alternative communication (AAC) assessment process may best be accomplished at recognized assessment sites where highly trained specialists and the most current and sophisticated technologies are available.

2. Since AAC assessment is for individuals for whom speech is neither functional nor effective, a person's speech production need not be part of the AAC assessment.

3. For an AAC system to be useful, the communicator must have functional sensory systems to employ it successfully.

(continued)

REALITY

1. It is important to conduct AAC assessments in natural settings where typical routines and daily partners are realistically represented and where the individual with little or no functional speech is most comfortable. AAC *specialists* are not required to perform evaluations or treatment. To the contrary, there is a need for more locally based AAC teams to be developed in schools, hospitals, and clinics, so it is likely that AAC assessments will increasingly be conducted in settings that are most naturalistic to the individual being assessed.

2. The term *augmentative* means to add to or supplement, so the idea of AAC is to use it to add to or supplement natural speech when needed and also to serve as an alternative to speech if speech is no longer useful or if there is no functional speech.

3. It is certainly important to document sensory systems (i.e., vision, hearing, tactile) function during an AAC assessment. However, having deficits in one or more sensory systems does not preclude use of an AAC system. The nature of AAC is to accommodate and adapt to sensory, motor, cognitive/intellectual, and language deficits to make more effective communication possible.

(continued)

Fuller, D. R., & Lloyd, L. L. *Principles and Practices in*
Augmentative and Alternative Communication (pp. 211-230).
© 2023 Taylor & Francis Group.

Myth (continued)

4. "I have no idea how to complete an AAC assessment, so I cannot do one."

5. "I cannot do an AAC evaluation because I do not have access to speech-generating technology at my facility."

6. An AAC assessment is about evaluating a person's ability to use systems that feature microprocessors and speech output.

Reality (continued)

4. Many clinicians already have expertise in dynamic assessment; evaluating the use of gestures, writing, drawing for communication; listing communication modalities observed; and trying different strategies as diagnostic therapy probes. These are all part of AAC assessment! Additional guidance may be sought from a more experienced speech-language pathologist. Continuing education opportunities can add to a clinician's skills to support AAC assessment.

5. AAC assessment is a feature-matching process. You do not need to have a particular device to determine if a client could benefit from a feature. In addition, many states have lending libraries that can be used to acquire equipment for trial use or a short-term assessment. Manufacturers are also sometimes willing to loan equipment or bring equipment to an evaluation to assure the client has the opportunity to work with a particular piece of equipment.

6. AAC is not limited to speech-generating devices (SGDs)! The core of AAC assessment is to evaluate the client's ability to *communicate* using all modalities. This includes gestures, speech, writing, drawing, communication boards, and speech-generating technology. The assessment process identifies communication strengths, current communication skills, and strategies to increase functional communication. This should result in a multimodal AAC system that may or may not include a system with speech output.

AAC Assessment Process and Purpose

AAC assessment is iterative, as the end result leads to intervention, and eventually, continued assessment to address evolving communication needs for the person who uses AAC. This chapter overviews the reiterative assessment process, purpose, and principles. The term "person who uses AAC" is used to refer to the individual with complex communication needs (CCN) who uses or would benefit from an AAC system. "AAC system" refers to the connected aspects of aided and unaided communication, devices that use microprocessors and produce speech, and communication displays, systems, books, and boards that form the individual's entire communication system. This allows for communication using multiple modalities, which is the way all people communicate—not just someone who uses an AAC system. It is assumed that the AAC system consists of multiple parts; it is *never* a single element, such as a display or device. The term "AAC specialist" is used to refer to speech-language pathologists who have a great deal of experience and expertise in AAC assessment and treatment and typically spend 50% or more of their professional time engaged in these activities (Binger et al., 2012). To be an AAC specialist, a person does not need to have specialty certification.

AAC Assessment Principles

The foundation of AAC assessment (and intervention) is the recognition that everyone can communicate and everyone does communicate. There are several principles that reflect a philosophy of service delivery for individuals that use AAC (e.g., Beukelman & Mirenda, 2013; Beukelman & Light, 2020; Blackstone et al., 2015; Brady et al., 2016; National Joint Committee for the Communication Needs of Persons with Severe Disabilities, 2003). Much of the extant literature has focused directly or indirectly on these AAC assessment principles, which have traditionally been built on clinical judgments borrowed primarily from the more general area of speech-language pathology. More recently, some literature has emerged that uses qualitative and quantitative methods to improve assessment practices and decision making (Dietz et al., 2012; Lund et al., 2017, 2021). Brady and colleagues (2016) noted that recent advances in assessment have benefited individuals with CCN; however, there are still individuals for whom communication needs remain unmet. The principles outlined in this section may serve to guide clinicians and advocates of people who use AAC. Additionally, as suggested by Brady and colleagues, a set of principles may be used to advance a research agenda that addresses the theoretical and practical underpinnings of AAC assessment practices.

Records and Tomblin suggested that "[t]here is minimal empirical information available regarding how speech-language pathologists use information from several sources to arrive at a diagnostic decision" (1994, p. 144), and that principles related to assessment decision making are based primarily on an implicit rule system that is passed from one professional generation to another. Records and Tomblin (1994) called for empirical studies of diagnostic decision making in communication sciences and disorders to develop explicit assessment standards. Schlosser and Raghavendra (2004) discussed decision making a decade later saying, "In summary, little is known about how practitioners make decisions in AAC. It could be speculated that most decisions are based on practitioner familiarity, clinical reasoning from experience, practices promoted in continuing education/professional development activities, discussions with colleagues, and some use of research evidence" (p. 2). More recent research (Dietz et al., 2012; Lund et al., 2017, 2021; McKelvey et al., 2018; Quach et al., 2018;

Weissling et al., 2017) evaluated the decision making of clinical and research experts in the field through mixed methods designs. These studies have illuminated trends across several disorder areas (e.g., amyotrophic lateral sclerosis [ALS], aphasia, autism spectrum disorder [ASD], and cerebral palsy), and indicate that decisions occur in three phases in the assessment process: (1) preassessment information gathering (interview), (2) information that may or may not be assessed in an evaluation session based on the individual characteristics of the client (screening), and (3) particular elements of the evaluation session(s) that are specific to the disorder. The evaluation of AAC system features and motor access are central elements that emerged as *always* present in the AAC evaluation trial. This research represents an effort to quantify what historically has been a highly qualitative process. The field of AAC would benefit from further development of theoretically sound, explicit standards for AAC assessment along with refinement of implicit standards specific to AAC. In the interim, the following principles of clinical decision making in AAC assessment provide a foundation.

Principle 1

AAC assessment is based on the premise that everyone can and does communicate. All individuals display behaviors that communicate something, even if unintentional. Individuals with severe communication disabilities often possess some repertoire of both linguistic and non-linguistic speech and gestures. Sometimes these communicative behaviors reveal themselves as unconventional, repetitive, and challenging. For some time now, challenging behaviors have been correlated with the presence of communication difficulties (Carr & Durand, 1985a, 1985b; Neel et al., 1983). Some approaches to communication assessment and intervention view challenging behavior as a way of determining what the communication of the individual may mean. Heath and colleagues (2015) completed a meta-analytic review of 36 articles that used functional communication training with individuals with a disability other than speech alone across ages and developmental disability types. They found that functional communication training worked to decrease challenging behaviors by increasing the communication for participants. The reader can learn more about challenging behaviors in Chapter 20.

Principle 2

AAC assessment must be responsive to people who use AAC and their family and caregivers, all of whom are considered stakeholders in the process. In evidence-based practice, the perspectives of the stakeholders are integrated into the clinical decisions that are made to provide the best possible services (American Speech-Language-Hearing Association [ASHA], n.d.a). These perspectives are crucial, as a lack of input into the development of an AAC system, choice of an SGD, and/or ensuing treatment may result in partial or total abandonment of the system (Parette et al., 2000).

In light of the importance of stakeholder input in the AAC assessment process, it is remarkable that there is little evidence-based guidance for clinicians in appropriate ways to educate and guide those stakeholders in the decision-making process. Siminoff (2013) encourages medical practitioners of all kinds to consider decision making as a social process, as well as an academic- or research-based process.

Principle 3

AAC assessment must involve a team of individuals who have a shared agenda and common goals. This is a long-standing principle and recognizes that successful AAC assessment and treatment involves a team (Yorkston & Karlan, 1986). In a qualitative study of educational teams, Soto and colleagues (2001) identified role boundaries and assigned responsibilities (i.e., who should do what) as themes where disagreements among team members emerged. Teams should be collaborative and team members may find themselves changing existing job roles and responsibilities for the benefit of the person being served (Rainforth & York-Barr, 1997). Rainforth and England (1997) reviewed values and skills needed for teams to achieve inclusion in neighborhood schools, and their findings may be applied more broadly to AAC teams. Specifically, they identified values of equal status, shared goals, shared responsibility, and openness as core values that underlie collaboration. Roles of the team included planning, sharing of observations and impressions, goal development, and problem solving.

Beukelman and colleagues (2008) first identified the roles of various personnel who have a stake in the process of referring a person for AAC assessment, providing the assessment, and supporting the person's communication (i.e., AAC finders, general practice speech-language pathologists, AAC specialists, facilitators, and AAC experts). Binger and colleagues (2012) expanded on the original list, outlining the various personnel involved in AAC assessment. The authors identified the following roles on the team that contribute to AAC assessment:

- AAC finders, who are the people who initially recognize the need for an evaluation and make the initial referral or suggestion
- General practice speech-language pathologists
- AAC clinical specialists
- Facilitators and communication partners (including family members and friends)
- Collaborating professionals (including educators and allied health providers)
- AAC research and policy specialists
- Manufacturers and vendors
- Funding agencies and personnel
- AAC/assistive technology agencies

Beukelman and colleagues (2007) suggest also identifying a communication advocate who is a consistent family member or friend of the communicator and who can serve as a bridge to transfer information about the person's communication needs, supports, and system, which is often lost during life transitions. Beukelman and Light (2020) suggest that members of the team should be selected based on three questions:

1. Who has the expertise needed to successfully complete the evaluation and implement the plan?
2. Who is affected by the decisions of the team?
3. Who is interested in participation on the team?

While the team may not perform the evaluation together in one session, it is imperative that all input is included to support the success of the person who will use AAC.

Principle 4

AAC assessment must include information about typical routines collected in natural settings and multiple environments. One of the aims of assessment is to identify communication needs and develop, enhance, and maintain participation opportunities. At least a portion of the AAC assessment should occur in familiar settings during activity routines that are naturalistically representative, such as at home, school, work, and in the community. A number of observational analyses can be used, along with guided interviews (e.g., Blackstone and Hunt Berg's 2003 *Social Networks Communication Inventory*), to obtain realistic information regarding the typical communication needs of and opportunities for the person who uses AAC. In addition to spoken language routines, routines related to social media usage and written language needs should be considered (Beukelman & Light, 2020; Beukleman & Mirenda, 2013).

Principle 5

AAC assessment must be comprehensive, focusing on functional limitations rather than on the pathologies and impairments. While it is important to understand the individual's pathology and impairment, understanding the functional impact of the communication deficits is more important when determining an appropriate AAC system. Regardless of diagnosis, the AAC system must support improving and sustaining participation in a variety of activities. Certainly, pathology or impairment may inform future decision making in some cases. McKelvey and colleagues (2018) found that in the case of ALS, experts did consider the nature of the disorder in their decision making. To guard against taking a view that is too focused on pathology/impairment, teams should focus on balancing their assessments across the components, including the person who uses AAC, partners, environments, and the AAC system.

Principle 6

AAC assessment must focus on communication strengths and communication limitations. The revised Participation Model (Beukelman & Light, 2020) provides a framework that allows evaluators to identify participation patterns and communication needs by assessing opportunity and access barriers. The framework focuses attention on identifying and modifying barriers that may impede the development and maintenance of maximally effective communication interactions. The revised Participation Model recognizes that strengths and weaknesses are both intrinsic and extrinsic; that is, some strengths and weaknesses lie within the person who uses AAC whereas others are shaped by environments, policies, and practices. All these strengths and limitations require scrutiny if overall AAC service delivery is to be effective and efficient.

Principle 7

Feature matching (Gosnell et al., 2011; Shane & Costello, 1994) is key to a successful AAC evaluation. Ultimately, the AAC system must meet the person's communication needs, rather than trying to make the individual adjust to an existing AAC system simply because it is convenient, available, or less expensive. To do this, assessment teams first determine the current and future communication needs of the individual and then find the AAC systems that have the features to meet those needs. The system should encompass different types of AAC systems, including devices that use microprocessors and produce speech and nonspeaking communication displays. Typically, no one system will meet all communication needs. Therefore, both aided and unaided modes, and both nonspeaking displays and those that produce speech, must be melded together to create a comprehensive communication *system* that meets the needs of the person who uses AAC across partners and environments. Feature matching applies to multimodal communication and is greater than the use of any single technology. Feature matching may also apply to the selection of appropriate symbols (see Chapter 13).

Principle 8

AAC assessment should be efficient. In their development of AAC assessment protocols, Weissling and colleagues (2017) found that experts used preassessment interviews and observations across the disorders studied (e.g., ALS, aphasia, ASD, cerebral palsy). These preassessment interviews are a technique that can assist the clinician in eliminating unnecessary procedures and increase the efficiency of the initial evaluation session. A preassessment phone call or visit is a way of screening for areas where data are sufficient vs. areas where further data need to be collected. Researchers (Lund et al., 2017; McKelvey et al., 2018; Quach et al., 2018) have created protocols that distill assessment methods into three phases:

1. Preassessment information to gather
2. Information to screen for at the time of the evaluation
3. Essential elements of evaluation for each disorder

The protocols were developed across several years and incorporate literature on assessment, information from evaluations completed by experienced AAC providers (i.e., specialists), and information gathered from interviews with such providers. The AAC specialists in the studies were defined as individuals who have particular expertise in AAC and typically spend at least 50% of their workday in AAC-related activities (Binger et al., 2012). Data entered into the protocols are organized to assist the evaluator in synthesizing large amounts of information. Others have proposed assessments and procedures for assessment (e.g., Garrett & Lasker, 2004; Lynch, 2016) in these disorder areas, but these do not usually come in the form of a single protocol for assessment.

Principle 9

AAC assessment is ongoing, often occurring in conjunction with intervention. The revised Participation Model (Beukelman & Light, 2020), as previously discussed, accounts for this process through repeated evaluation of the effectiveness of the AAC system. While the communication needs of people who use AAC typically do not go away, they do change due to maturation, improved function, changes in status/environments, and disease progression. As communication needs change, ongoing assessment is appropriate and essential. It is imperative that the communication supports (including AAC systems) we provide allow access to participation-based experiences that are authentic (Simmons-Mackie et al., 2013).

Some predictable timelines can be anticipated in the lives of people who use AAC. For example, change may be anticipated during transitions to new schools, transitions between grade levels, changes in curriculum, changes in living circumstances, and changes in the individual's medical state. Therefore, ongoing assessment may be needed to minimize the impact of such changes. Other assessments may be initiated because of advances in technology, changes in team members' knowledge of technologies or strategies, changes in the number and types of environments, or changes in the number and types of communication partners. In other words, to promote, maintain, and enhance functional communication, AAC assessment must examine the interrelationship among people who use AAC, partners, environments, and systems on an ongoing basis. Assessment may promote immediate and initial success by addressing the needs of today while continued investigations of the needs of tomorrow are conducted (Beukelman & Light, 2020).

Principle 10

AAC assessment should result in positive change. The service delivery plan should undergo frequent review and, when new information is uncovered, logical modifications should be made. These modifications may involve, for example, adjusting seating and positioning for the person who uses AAC, shaping the use of more effective communication strategies for better social or academic outcomes, or identifying and breaking down various policy and/or attitudinal barriers. Assessing the service delivery plan may also identify a need for new or modified AAC systems, including non–speech-generating displays and microprocessor-based speech output devices and strategies that will be implemented and evaluated in a continuous cycle of evaluation, implementation, and re-evaluation. Accountable service delivery encompasses a balance between assessment and intervention that is so interwoven it seems inseparable.

Scope of AAC Assessment

No one should be left without a way to communicate even when conventional methods, such as speech or writing, are only temporarily disrupted. That means the AAC system that emerges from an assessment may be needed temporarily rather than permanently. For example, the person who is temporarily unable to speak because of postsurgical ventilation needs a way to communicate with health care providers, friends, and family during what is likely a very stressful period. The person recovering from brain injury or stroke may have a positive prognosis for return of speech given time and therapy but needs a system to communicate during what may be a lengthy recovery process. These health-related concerns for communication have been highlighted by professionals advocating for patient-provider communication (Hurtig et al., 2018; Nordness & Beukelman, 2017). Assessment of the needs of these patients falls within the scope of the speech-language pathologist. Preventable health care errors are reduced when patients can communicate effectively in the hospital (Hurtig et al., 2018).

In an educational setting, the young person diagnosed with childhood apraxia of speech may spend years in intense speech therapy and need an AAC system to support immediate communication, support language learning, and to participate academically. It is important clinicians view the assessment process as iterative to address immediate and long-term communication needs for their clients. This chapter provides general guidance for AAC assessment given the range of profiles of persons who can benefit from AAC systems.

It is helpful to consider the person's communication profile in terms of onset, conceptualized here as developmental (i.e., congenital or occurring during the developmental period through about age 21 years; National Institutes of Health, 2010) or acquired (i.e., occurring after the person has achieved some linguistic, cognitive, physical, and emotional milestones). In addition, the evaluator should understand the prognosis of the condition that underlies the need for an AAC assessment and whether it is progressive/degenerative, stable, or improving. Assessment planning will be influenced by the nature of the disorder. More specifically, stable conditions will require plans that account for life transitions (e.g., moving from middle to high school, moving to a new job) and future plans (e.g., a goal to gain employment). In addition, degenerative and improving conditions require the evaluator monitor for changes in motor and vocabulary needs as the client progresses either toward loss or improvement of function. The AAC system will need to be flexible in these cases, such that the individual will have access to it (i.e., a way to interface with the system given changing physical abilities) and the appropriate vocabulary and symbols throughout the duration of the need for AAC. The following sections discuss special considerations for these broad categories of people who may benefit from AAC assessment.

Special Considerations: Developmental Disorders

Progressive/Degenerative

How progressive genetic disorders fit into the categorical framework of developmental vs. acquired could be debated; however, for the purposes of this chapter, degenerative genetic disorders will be considered within the context of developmental disability, as they manifest during the period when developmental milestones are being met. Because they are not diagnosed at birth, their presentation and course do not necessarily parallel developmental disabilities that generally have a stable course.

Several progressive/degenerative conditions manifest during the developmental period and so affect children who use AAC. These include genetic-based seizure disorders (SCN8A), Huntington's disease, muscular dystrophy, neuroimmune mediated disorders (e.g., multiple sclerosis and **opsoclonus-myoclonus syndrome**), and other genetic conditions, such as fragile X syndrome and **leukodystrophies** (rare genetic conditions that are characterized by developmental regression).

Spinal muscular atrophy (SMA) is one example of a progressive condition that results in the need for AAC in children. As a group of conditions, SMA is one of the most common rare genetic diseases in the United States (Spinal Muscular Atrophy Foundation, n.d.). It is categorized by type (I, II, and III) based on age of onset, symptom progression, and severity. Two other forms of SMA, congenital with arthrogryposis and Kennedy's disease, are included in the overall condition description. In general, SMA is a congenital, genetic condition that can appear early in infancy and manifests as deteriorating muscle control causing severe weakness, quadriplegia, and eventual death from respiratory failure. Life expectancy ranges from less than 2 years of age to adolescence, except for the form known as Kennedy's disease, which may develop between ages 15 to 60 years (National Institute of Neurological Disorders and Stroke, n.d.). Children with SMA have intact cognition and develop robust language despite their severe dysarthria, which necessitates the use of AAC. Because of severe fatigue and eventual quadriplegia, children with SMA may be good candidates for speech-generating eye-tracking systems to access their AAC systems (Ball et al., 2018).

Stable

A child born with a condition that remains stable and causes severe dysarthria may not develop the motor control to produce intelligible speech for unfamiliar communication partners. This is sometimes part of the sequela of cerebral palsy (Hustad et al., 2017; Nip, 2017). The child will need to learn language through an AAC system that becomes their expressive mode of communication. Intellectual impairment may be concomitant but is not part of the sequela of cerebral palsy. Further, the child with severe cerebral palsy has a life expectancy of 30 to 70 years (Strauss et al., 2008). Therefore, they will become adults with severe cerebral palsy with personal, educational, and vocational potential and expectations. This scenario illustrates the importance of planning for future communication needs while addressing current communication needs with AAC. Stroke or traumatic brain injury (TBI) in infancy may also result in severe motor impairment that remains relatively stable throughout the lifespan. Such children will have developmental and language learning needs similar to the child born with severe motor impairment.

Improving

Conversely, the prognosis for speech development may be cautiously optimistic for a child born with childhood apraxia of speech. As with other congenital motor speech disorders, this child may learn language through the expressive modalities offered by AAC systems. However, they may attain intelligible speech after several years of frequent and intense speech therapy based on the principles of motor learning.

Similarly, children who sustain brain injury from stroke or other trauma may also improve. Such cases are complex because the child may have reached some developmental milestones prior to the injury. Learning needs and supports may be different for such children due to residual deficits from the brain injury, but their potential for progress must be supported in the near term and future with cyclical evaluations to address advancing communication needs.

Brain injury or stroke in adults may result in speech and/or language disorders with the potential to improve with skilled intervention. They may reach a point in recovery when most communication needs are met through natural speech, relying on AAC as a supplement, and to repair communication breakdowns (Hanson et al., 2013; Hustad & Beukelman, 2000). However, Duffy (2005) suggests that most individuals in this category will likely need persistent AAC systems to supplement natural speech communication, at the very least.

Special Considerations: Acquired Disorders

The previously clear line dividing congenital from acquired disorders is becoming blurry as research explores genetic components in many conditions that are considered acquired. These acquired disorders can be seen in both adults and children, with certain disorders occurring in adults (e.g., ALS, dementia, Parkinson's disease, primary progressive aphasia, and primary progressive apraxia of speech) and others occurring in either adults or children, as addressed above (e.g., brain injury and stroke). For purposes of this discussion, acquired conditions include physical and neurological events that alter the ability of the individual who has already reached milestones in speech and language development.

Progressive/Degenerative

AAC assessment for people with degenerative conditions must address immediate and future communication needs, although not because the condition improves. Rather, the degenerative nature of conditions, such as ALS, multiple sclerosis, multiple systems atrophy, Parkinson's disease, or primary progressive apraxia of speech, requires consideration of changing access needs as the condition worsens. In these cases, the AAC assessment recommendations for immediate communication needs may include systems that are easy to transport and access through physical direct selection (i.e., pointing or physical contact with a display). With disease progression, access needs will become more complex, requiring alternative access methods, such as eye tracking, head tracking, or switch-scanning access. New and emerging access technology is continually evolving to meet those needs (Fager et al., 2019). These access methods are addressed in Chapter 10.

Degenerative conditions in adults may initially present as being a primarily motor impairment in nature but may ensnare language and cognition with progression. Other degenerative conditions initially present with language or cognitive impairment, such as any of the dementias or primary progressive aphasia, a form of frontotemporal dementia. AAC assessment for these conditions will address cognitive-linguistic deficits, such as memory loss and language impairment, that deteriorate over time. In the case of primary progressive aphasia, AAC intervention will address primary language deficits.

Some degenerative processes may occur as the result of disease. One example that falls into this category is **acute flaccid myelitis**, a polio-like condition of unknown etiology but thought to be related to a virus. It primarily affects children. In the case of acute flaccid myelitis, there is a progressive decline in function that may improve over some period of time (Martin et al., 2017). The key factor in AAC assessment for pediatric populations with degenerative conditions is recognition of the communication needs of the child at the time of the evaluation and a plan for adjustments for future communication needs, which may include AAC skills and assistive technology as the disease progresses. Clinicians need to gather information on the disorder and the expected trajectory of change over time. The goals of AAC to meet current needs (today) will need to be balanced with a plan for future needs (tomorrow).

Stable or Improving

Children and adults who acquire stable and/or improving communication disability will also have AAC needs. For example, when conditions, such as TBI and stroke, occur in children, assessment must take into consideration motor, language, and cognitive changes related to development. For those individuals where cognitive, linguistic, and/or motor impairments affect the ability of the person to communicate effectively, AAC assessment should be initiated. The types of deficits the person displays will inform the assessment procedures required. Specifically, evaluators should find AAC and assistive technology solutions that meet current needs but are flexible and can be changed should further recovery require a change or elimination of a strategy.

In this way, stable/improving conditions have different considerations for the future than those of individuals with degenerative or developmental issues. Wherein degenerative diseases require the clinician to consider increased AAC needs over time, improving conditions require the clinician to adjust and reduce AAC intervention when unaided communication emerges. When conditions are stable, there is a continued need for reassessment, which addresses changes in context and age-related factors. As has been previously stated, AAC should be predicated on the communication patterns of same age peers (Beukelman & Light, 2020). Therefore, in the pediatric population, even individuals with unchanged motor or basic cognitive or linguistic skills will go through the same changing participation patterns of developing peers. As such, they will require ongoing assessment and intervention.

AAC Assessment

AAC Assessment Team and Models of Service Delivery

AAC assessment requires the coordinated and unique skills of many individuals to address the CCN of individuals who may benefit from AAC. Collaborative teams are important in service delivery for all individuals with disabilities and particularly in the case of individuals with CCN. Collaborative intervention includes problem solving and goal setting that attends to multiple perspectives (Paul et al., 2006). Successful AAC use is, in part, a reflection of a collaborative AAC team that provides support to the person who uses AAC through training, participation, communication, and dedication of time. Teams that function suboptimally may be a contributing factor to abandonment of AAC strategies (Johnson et al., 2006). Therefore, it is important that the AAC evaluator focuses on team dynamics.

Several factors have been identified as characteristics of successful teams. These characteristics include stakeholders most affected by the use of the AAC system participating as equal members of the team (Beukelman, & Light, 2020; Rainforth & York-Barr, 1997), having adequate time to complete tasks (Johnson et al., 2006), having the ability to provide support through mutual respect and establishment of trust (Parette et al., 2000), and training (Johnson et al., 2006).

Members of the team vary widely and, in addition to the person who uses AAC and the speech-language pathologist, may include family members (e.g., parents, siblings, spouses, children), general classroom teachers, physicians, occupational therapists, physical therapists, special education teachers, vocational counselors, and caregivers. The members of the team vary as much as the individual aspects of the person who will use AAC. The collaborative team approach has been suggested for both children and adults (Beukelman & Nordness, 2015; Rainforth & York-Barr, 1997), and membership in the team is influenced by the age, setting (e.g., medical, school, vocational), and specific characteristics of the individual who may benefit from AAC use. The type of team available is driven by a variety of factors. Policy, practice, and practical factors, such as availability, distance, and personal factors, influence the type of collaborative team used.

Members of clinical teams work together in different ways. The literature identifies **multidisciplinary** teams, in which members work independently and share their results with the team as a whole; **interdisciplinary** teams, in which members work together to evaluate and develop joint treatment goals; and **transdisciplinary** teams, in which professionals share roles during sessions in addition to sharing information. Individuals on transdisciplinary teams may collaborate so closely that their professional roles overlap considerably during evaluation and treatment sessions (Batorawicz & Shepherd, 2011). While the types of teams vary, it is important that the AAC specialist work within the team setting available to create a collaborative and positive team outcome.

Batorawicz and Shepherd (2011) considered clinical teams in their study of the prescription review model of teamwork. The prescription review requires a regular team meeting among members of an AAC clinic to consider evaluation results and recommendations by all clinicians in the group, not just the treating clinicians. They found that family members were included in the evaluation process but not the final team meeting. Despite their finding, the authors support including family members in the prescription review meeting, suggesting that doing so would empower those members and would be educational for all participants in the meeting.

Perhaps the most important part of an AAC assessment report is the recommendations section where the AAC system is specified and the treatment plan is outlined. Therefore, team members must consider the need for someone—one or more team members—to support training and generalization of communication skills beyond treatment sessions. For example, a resource room teacher may be a valuable team member because that is the context at school where new communication skills learned with the AAC system can be transferred and generalized to different communication partners in a different setting. A direct service provider who provides daily support for an adult with an intellectual disability would be a valuable team member during the evaluation and would play an important role in training other caregivers and supporting generalization of skills during treatment. No matter how the service is delivered, the end goal for individuals who use AAC is the application of skills across everyday contexts. Therefore, principles of generalization coupled with individual learning styles and preferences of individuals who use AAC should be combined to determine the best service delivery alternatives.

Adults in medical settings are served in either an individual or group pull-out service delivery model. Home visits and vocational visits may occur, but individuals with acquired disabilities are often seen in settings, such as inpatient hospital units or outpatient clinics/practices. This type of service delivery model is likely driven by reimbursement and system efficiency. That is, it is less expensive and more efficient for clients to come to the therapist than for the therapist to travel to the client.

Milieu models allow services to be provided in the environments where individuals live, work, and play and may improve transfer and generalization of skills by focusing on specific goals in functional contexts. Adults with developmental disabilities may be seen within their vocational setting (e.g., workshop, competitive employment, or supported employment). This model of service delivery may be supported by vocational funding.

Service delivery models for children include direct pull-out methods of individual and group therapy services, as well as models that are more collaborative in nature. The latter may mean individuals other than or including a speech-language pathologist are providing services (Calculator, 2009). Speech-language pathologists have a significant role in the selection of goals and objectives that foster communication and participation in the classroom, training in AAC systems, and monitoring system use (Calculator, 2009). However, other individuals in the child's life will be responsible for implementation, feedback, and recommended adjustments to the AAC system and the training paradigm. A key component of service delivery in schools is inclusion. Calculator (2009) made the case that inclusion cannot be mere placement of the child in a context but rather it must consist of a meaningful context for learning. Beukelman and Light (2020) identified key components of inclusive education, which include being a member of a class with authentic roles and signs of belonging, active participation, and an environment where the person who uses AAC can gain skills that are relevant and important across the curriculum.

Overall, the model of service delivery is influenced by a variety of factors that are not always under the control of the professional. Factors, such as facility policy, local practice patterns, reimbursement, law, and funding, may influence AAC services. In addition, factors, such as distance between the client and clinician, or independent of distance, factors, such as the client's overall health status and endurance, ability to travel and the complexity of arranging transport, and inclement weather, may make in-person evaluation or treatment difficult or impossible. For clients in these circumstances, service delivery by telepractice (tele-AAC services) must be considered as an alternative. ASHA defines telepractice as "the application of telecommunications technology to the delivery of speech-language pathology professional services at a distance by linking clinician to client or clinician to clinician for assessment, intervention, or consultation" (ASHA, n.d.j). Tele-AAC is the application of telepractice to AAC assessment (including evaluation for the purpose of recommending an electronic system with speech output; Anderson et al., 2012). Many funding sources for both speech-language pathology services and for electronic AAC systems with speech output recognize tele-AAC as an equally effective alternative to in-person services and as a form of "face-to-face" service delivery. Those on the assessment team should consider the needs and desires of the people they see and advocate for the best possible models based on person-specific characteristics (e.g., age, attitude, situation).

When considering the long-term goals of the individual using AAC, the evaluation team must hold paramount the goal of insuring the person is able to participate in meaningful activities. With this in mind, the service delivery model should ensure transfer and generalization of skills across contexts (e.g., school, work, home), people (e.g., friends, strangers, family), and situations (e.g., one-on-one interactions, group interactions).

Participation

The Revised Communication Bill of Rights (Brady et al., 2016) for people with disabilities includes the right to participate with others in all environments and situations as full communication partners. Participation may be hindered by barriers to communication, such as policies, practices, and attitudes, that lead to lack of support or access to opportunities for communication. The environment inhabited by the person who uses AAC may not support use of different communication modalities. Caregivers and educators may not have training or experience that would insure support of AAC systems or strategies (Brady et al., 2016; Beukelman & Light, 2020). These must be inventoried as part of the assessment process to identify the contexts, persons, environments, practices, policies, opportunities, and attitudes that are in place to support communication and also those that must be addressed so as not to obstruct successful communication. The idea is that communication is the tool that allows individuals to participate in whatever constitutes their world, be it home life, family, community, work, school, etc. The person who uses AAC is expected to have the same communication needs and expectations for participation as those around them.

Assessment Procedures

Preassessment

AAC assessments are designed to identify and explore the unique strengths and challenges of the individual with CCN. The AAC assessment team begins this complex process by investigating several areas of the individual's life and communication. Conducting a pre-evaluation session interview to systematically gather information prior to a scheduled AAC evaluation will facilitate planning for the actual evaluation session. Team members may choose to contact the person who uses AAC (e.g., using a telephone, digital conferencing, electronic or paper case history information). Although gathering case history information is a standard part of any evaluation, actually speaking with the person being evaluated or their advocate in advance to clarify or expand on this information is encouraged. During this initial direct contact, the interviewer should clarify information about the individual's communication needs and current communication skills. Early identification of communication needs and skills, such as communication partners, environments, favorite topics, current modes of communication (e.g., devices that use microprocessors and produce speech, non–speech-generating communication displays and books), will allow team members to personalize evaluation materials and tasks to maximize efficiency in the evaluation session.

Screening

For the purpose of this section, screening is defined as a process to determine if an area or skill should be included or excluded during the evaluation session. Not all skills and areas identified as appropriate for screening will require in-depth assessment. For example, an individual with ALS who has normal hearing as reported by a recent hearing evaluation will not require in-depth assessment of this area. A child with cerebral palsy whose parents report they suspect vision issues would require more in-depth investigation of visual acuity, visual field, and visual processing.

Assessment

Sensory

Sensory systems (e.g., vision, hearing, touch) have an impact on the use of AAC systems and must be considered in the assessment process. While a specific AAC professional may not be an expert in a sensory system, they should be aware of when to refer, how to screen, and how to engage in basic adaptations based on sensory systems. Specific providers, such as eye care professionals, audiologists, and occupational therapists, may be needed to determine the specific needs and accommodations for an AAC system (including devices that use microprocessors and produce speech, as well as non–speech-generating communication displays and books). However, some basic assessment/screening can be completed by the AAC evaluator.

Vision may be an overlooked area of communication skills during a typical speech/language evaluation, but for a person who would benefit from selecting photographs, line drawings, letters, words, or phrases from a communication display, it is essential to assess visual acuity. This is not to say the person must have vision to benefit from an AAC system. Alternative access methods using tactile or auditory feedback can substitute for seeing a display. However, the clinician needs to understand all sensory strengths and deficits in order to complete a thorough assessment.

Comprehensive explanation of all types of vision assessment is beyond the scope of this chapter. However, vision as it relates to persons with intellectual/developmental disabilities is described here. An ophthalmologist or optometrist can complete a vision evaluation without behavioral tests (e.g., they can use an eye chart with progressively smaller rows of letters that the patient reads with one eye covered). Quantitative assessment of the eye itself for refractive disorders provides a somewhat accurate measure of visual acuity in terms of being far-sighted (hyperopia, not being able to see up close) or near-sighted (myopia, not being able to clearly see things at a distance; Warburg, 2001). Astigmatism is another refractive disorder that distorts both near and far vision (Warburg, 2001). If the person scheduled for an AAC evaluation has not had a vision evaluation, the evaluator may need to advocate for one and be sure the vision health provider knows the person is being evaluated for a communication display that can support text, photographs, and/or line drawings of different sizes.

Individuals who are not literate may be able to learn to respond to an E chart (Azzam & Ronquillo, 2022), which is like a letter chart in that it features progressively smaller letters. However, all the letters are E and are positioned in different directions. To complete the test, the patient needs only to indicate which direction the E is pointing or which direction the "legs" of the E are going (i.e., up, down, left, or right). This test may be useful for adults and children with intellectual/developmental disabilities who may be able to learn the task and respond.

Cortical visual impairment (CVI) is related to brain injury that affects perception and processing of visual images in the brain rather than being a problem with eyesight *per se.* There are many causes. The injury may be the result of brain hemorrhage in premature infants or trauma sustained at any point in development and throughout adulthood (Chang & Borchert, 2020; Philip & Dutton, 2014). Individuals with CVI (sometimes alternatively referred to as cerebral visual impairment) may be able to see but not be able to process what the eyes see. It is common in children with cerebral palsy and in children born with congenital **Zika syndrome** (Philip & Dutton, 2014; Ventura et al., 2017). CVI may not be identified or diagnosed through visual acuity testing (Chang & Borchert, 2020). The condition influences AAC assessment because the individual may have difficulty making sense of a communication display despite intact extraocular anatomy (Blackstone et al., 2021). Wilkinson and Wolf (2021) summarize the design characteristics in an AAC display that may support visual processing for a child with CVI, including movement/animation, high-contrast colors (e.g., yellow on black), simultaneous touch and physical cues, simple displays, and appropriate lighting. Assessment with a qualified vision health provider who is knowledgeable of CVI evaluation is important.

Hearing loss affects approximately 20% of Americans over the age of 12 years as a bilateral or unilateral hearing loss. The prevalence of hearing loss increases with each decade of life (Lin et al., 2011). The overall prevalence of hearing loss supports the need for hearing screenings and evaluations for any person undergoing a speech-language evaluation, and especially for someone with communication impairment who warrants an AAC evaluation. ASHA (n.d.e) provides guidance for hearing screening for adults at 1000, 2000, and 4000 Hz at 25 dB SPL and for children at 1000, 2000, and 4000 Hz at 20 dB SPL. Individuals who do not pass a hearing screening should be referred for a complete hearing evaluation, and the AAC evaluation should not be finalized until the person's auditory acuity and processing are determined.

Some individuals have a difficult time processing tactile information. For example, individuals with ASD or other developmental disabilities may have certain tactile aversions (Baranek et al., 2007). Baranek and colleagues (2007) used the *Sensory Processing Assessment for Young Children* (Baranek, 1999) as a primary outcome measure for a study of hyperresponsiveness in children with ASD and developmental disabilities. They found a relationship between mental age and aversion such that aversion to sensory toys decreased with increasing mental age. Observation and interview can be used to assess sensory sensitivity and preferences of individuals being evaluated for AAC. These factors may influence characteristics of the system and activities completed with the AAC system during evaluation and training. Arthur-Kelly and colleagues (2009) suggest that the successful use of visual supports may be influenced by the sensory preferences of children with ASD. Practically speaking, individuals with a wide range of disabilities show aversion and preferences toward sensory experiences, and for that reason, consideration of tactile responses to stimuli should be considered in AAC assessment.

Language

The assessment of language skills as part of an AAC assessment is completed to assist in decision making regarding a variety of system features and may impact which instructional strategies are initially attempted. For example, vocabulary testing may assist clinicians in selecting vocabulary that is usable by the individual while helping clinicians plan for areas where vocabulary may need to be developed. Information about overall receptive language skills may influence the types of instructional strategies that are attempted and may inform what receptive language skills should be developed through AAC programming. Receptive language skills may also inform semantic and morphosyntactic elements that should be taught or developed. Understanding expressive language skills may help teams make decisions about the types of displays that may support language learning and development. For example, individuals with the ability to combine words and morphemes may benefit from semantic/syntactic grid layouts while beginning communicators with emerging expressive language skills may benefit from activity-based displays. While device trials will be required to inform the final decision-making process in these areas, information regarding basic language skills may give the team members a starting place for device trials.

Expressive language skills are difficult to assess when an individual is unable to speak and has no alternate mode of expression. That is a primary reason for an AAC evaluation, after all. However, rating scales and observation worksheets provided to families, teachers, and caregivers may give insights into the perceived expressive competence of the person being evaluated. The gathering of information for a communication profile helps identify conventional and nonconventional uses of sounds, facial expressions, word approximations, words, sign approximations, signs, etc. that are communicative. Some of this information may be gathered in advance of an evaluation session through interview or case history and/or in-depth observation and interview formats. For example, the online *Communication Matrix* (Rowland, 2013) is a free assessment tool suitable for professionals and nonprofessionals to use to document communicative behaviors in a seven-level matrix ranging from nonintentional behavior to complex language. Additionally, expressive language can be assessed informally through the use of clinician-constructed tasks. Such tasks make use of devices with microprocessors that produce speech, non–speech-generating communication displays or communication books, and appropriate symbols as a means of interacting during a functional communication task (e.g., snack, requesting music, playing a game, directing the completion of a laundry task). Trials with SGDs might include comparing the communication that occurs with a display that is set up for whole-message storage and retrieval vs. a syntactic/semantic display with word-by-word storage and encoding to request, ask questions, and comment. These trials can be set up on apps, SGDs, or non–speech-generating communication displays. The results of such trials provide insight into the individual's ability to encode language to achieve goals during meaningful activities. However, a word of caution is warranted. If the person being evaluated does not understand the symbol system presented on the communication display, that person may not be able to demonstrate their actual expressive language ability.

Receptive language, like expressive language, is difficult to assess if the person being evaluated does not have a conventional way of demonstrating understanding. When individuals cannot participate in standardized tests, adaptation may be required. For example, plates can be enlarged, changes may be made to location (vertical vs. horizontal placement), the field of choices could be reduced, or objects could be used in place of photographic stimuli. While these procedures would invalidate standardization of the test, such adaptations may give the evaluator some practical information about the type of vocabulary, syntax, and morphology the individual understands. Clinician-constructed tasks may include sorting, semantic point-to tasks (e.g., "Point to the one you drink coffee from"), and morphosyntactic point-to tasks (e.g., "Point to the picture of dogs") that can be used to evaluate receptive language skills. Non–speech-generating eye-gaze displays (Figure 11-1) may also be used to evaluate receptive skills. To use an eye-gaze display, the person being evaluated would need to learn how to respond by looking at a location on the display through direct instruction and interaction with the clinician. The assessment should not be undertaken using this response modality unless and until the person uses it effectively to provide reliable responses to questions with known answers. If not, the task may in reality be a test of understanding of the access method rather than receptive language ability.

Clinician-constructed tasks, environmental observation, interviews, and checklists can also be used to estimate the level of receptive language processing. Careful observation has revealed competence in individuals thought to have little receptive language or cognitive functioning. The story of Martin Pistorius (Pistorius, 2013) is a first-hand account of an individual thought not to have receptive language or cognitive skills who actually did. The observational skills of an aromatherapist identified underlying receptive language skills and helped to open the world to Pistorius.

Literacy

The ability to write and spell opens up communication options for those who use AAC. Individuals with literacy skills have more opportunities, are more employable, and are more likely to be viewed as competent communicators. The ability to use the alphabet to code/decode language relates directly to the ability to construct messages using an AAC system. Therefore, literacy skills are essential for individuals who use AAC and must be evaluated. Again, evaluation of literacy skills is not meant to preclude introducing an AAC system, as it may be the means by which a person learns to read, spell messages, and formulate expressive language. However, the evaluator needs to know the individual's literacy level in order to design effective treatment.

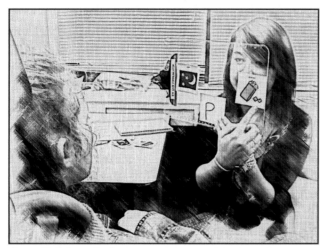

Figure 11-1. Receptive language assessment using eye gaze.

The assessment of literacy in emerging communicators provides a starting point for intervention. The skill may be underdeveloped if the communicator has not had formal instruction in literacy. Therefore, evaluating a person's ability to recognize the letters and sounds in their name, as well as familiar words, is a good place to begin. Another evaluative task is to offer ways for the individual to spell highly familiar, personally relevant words (e.g., family member names and favorite books, games, and toys). Attention to the access method is important here because it would be a tragic mistake to conclude that a person does not know how to spell or recognize print when, in fact, the problem is the way the person is set up to interface with the response system. Also, consider cognitive load when engaging in this type of multifunctional assessment task (e.g., selecting letters to spell or indicating a letter or word in a recognition task). The use of highly familiar, personally relevant words, as mentioned above, may reduce cognitive load and provide an optimal environment for the individual to demonstrate the ability to spell and demonstrate skill during evaluation of access methods.

Literacy assessment in adults may be necessary depending on the underlying condition. For example, individuals with intellectual and/or developmental disabilities have a highly variable range of literacy skills—from being illiterate to reading at a lower grade level—as opposed to an adult with ALS whose literacy skills are intact, and therefore, will not warrant in-depth assessment. In adults with acquired neurological conditions (e.g., aphasia and TBI) it is important to determine if there was a pre-existing difficulty with the individual's ability to read or write. This information can be gathered prior to an evaluation session by interviewing the person to be evaluated or their support person who is knowledgeable and has the authority to answer questions. During the evaluation, the person may be engaged in activities, such as reading directions, filling out a form, and/or reading a newspaper/magazine article, which should all be documented as literacy skills.

Reading ability will impact how information and messages are represented on an AAC display. When assessing a person who has limited experience with print and reading, it helps to begin with offering opportunities and observing if interest in books or written information is apparent. Evaluators can watch for demonstrations of joint attention, page turning, vocalizations in response to a recognized word or letter, or approximations of familiar sight words during literacy activities. Literacy comprehension may include recognition of familiar logos, such as the golden arches for McDonald's, or icons on electronic devices, such as the power and volume buttons. Recognizing such visual images indicates a potential for learning additional literacy skills. The literacy level of an individual will impact how information and messages are represented in AAC systems, and therefore, is an important part of the AAC assessment process. However, literacy is *not* a prerequisite for communicating via AAC.

Cognition

The AAC assessment must include evaluation of cognition; however, specific cognitive skills are not prerequisites for introduction of an AAC system. Levels of cognitive function may be difficult to evaluate, especially with standardized test instruments. Several assessment tools, checklists, developmental scales, and informal tasks may be considered by the AAC assessment team. Using a variety of tasks and tools will lead to a genuine profile of the individual's cognitive strengths and limitations. It is important to note that standardized tests will likely require adaptations to provide useful information. These adaptations will require careful interpretation of assessment data by the assessment team.

An individual with an intellectual disability being evaluated for AAC may display variability in cognitive profile because of experiential deficits (i.e., lack of access to AAC may produce an artificial cognitive deficit that dissipates with AAC access and training). Additionally, the relationship between cognition and language is an intimate one. The act of sentence comprehension requires not only language knowledge and processing but also the simultaneous cognitive processes of reasoning, attention, and memory (Coelho, 2007). Assessing cognition in children or adults with intellectual disabilities is frequently accomplished using informal methods, such as observation during structured tasks, completion of matching activities, and responses to direct questions. Cognitive assessment in adults may be dependent upon the underlying diagnosis. For example, a person diagnosed with ALS may have frontotemporal dementia as part of the sequelae of the condition, which may impact the person's ability to use an AAC system. People with aphasia often have cognitive deficits that impact their ability to navigate an AAC system, switch to a more effective mode of communication, and/or repair communication breakdowns. Such deficits do not preclude a recommendation for AAC but must be considered in developing the AAC system and the training needed to learn to use it.

Speech

Students in speech-language pathology are sometimes surprised to see speech assessment as part of the assessment protocol for a person who will use AAC. The assumption is that people who use AAC do so because they cannot speak. However, one of the terms used to describe the field—*augmentative* and alternative communication—suggests that strategies and systems of AAC may be used to augment or supplement natural speech. In fact, several strategies, such as alphabet or topic supplementation, offer communication partners additional information to decode speech that is somewhat unintelligible (Hanson et al., 2004; Hanson et al., 2013).

Speech assessment should include the person's perspective of communication effectiveness using speech, a measure of intelligibility, a perceptual description of speech (e.g., the perceptual descriptors of speech subsystem performance, such as imprecise consonants, inconsistent voicing, hypernasality, or inadequate respiratory support, provide a helpful description of which subsystems impact speech intelligibility), oral mechanism/cranial nerve assessment, and underlying diagnosis (e.g., mixed spastic-flaccid dysarthria secondary to ALS or childhood apraxia of speech secondary to Down syndrome). Intelligibility measures quantify the percentage of phonemes, words, or sentences that are understandable to an unfamiliar listener. Clinician ratings of speech intelligibility are not acceptable to report, as they are not systematically derived and may vary based on familiarity of the disordered speech to the listener, thus they are neither valid nor reliable (Kent, 1992). There are many published speech intelligibility tests available for children and adults (e.g., *Speech Intelligibility Test* [Yorkston et al., 2007]). In addition, the *Index of Augmented Speech Comprehensibility in Children* (Dowden, 1997) measures speech in terms of the ability of familiar and unfamiliar partners to judge words based on supplemental cues, such as first-letter and topic cues. Results of this nonstandardized test often show that familiar partners (e.g., parents) understand their child's speech better than unfamiliar partners. However, for familiar partners, word intelligibility without additional cues is often much lower than anticipated. This protocol may be created using the word lists with letter and topic cues, published in the appendix of Dowden (1997). Results of this assessment tool are useful in helping family members understand the need for an AAC evaluation even when they feel their child's speech is perfectly intelligible.

Motor Skills

Evaluation of fine and gross motor functioning is a critical part of the AAC assessment process. This process targets positioning and ambulation of the individual as related to the effective use of AAC systems. Included in the assessment are considerations for the individual's use of direct selection or scanning features related to specific AAC systems (Fager et al., 2012; Fager et al., 2011). Although many people who use AAC have motor impairments requiring positional adaptations to maximize communication and other life functions, few specific guidelines are offered to assist the team in motor evaluations (Beukelman & Light, 2020; Schlosser & Raghavendra, 2004; Shane & Costello, 1994).

The AAC team should conduct motor assessment of strength, range of motion, muscle tone, control of voluntary movement, and response to instructions. The goal is not necessarily rehabilitative in that it is not to address deficits of weakness, restricted range, or volitional movement, but rather to identify functional positions that will best support the use of an AAC system and overall attempts to communicate (Brady et al., 2016; also see Chapter 16). Members of the AAC assessment team, specifically physical and occupational therapists, will provide critical information regarding positioning. An appropriate seating position must be established prior to and throughout motor assessment, as proper trunk support contributes to the accurate evaluation of overall motor capabilities (Brady et al., 2016; Rainforth & York-Barr, 1997). The function of the head and neck should be assessed for range of motion, control, and endurance (Brady et al., 2016). Because most individuals require several functional positions across a day's time, the effects of positional changes will require evaluation. For individuals who ambulate independently, maximal ways to transport devices should be sought, whereas in consideration of seating, AAC device mounting and mobility will be key aspects of the motor assessment for individuals who are unable to ambulate independently (Brady et al., 2016).

Identifying the appropriate size, location, and mounting of an augmentative communication device and/or switch mechanism is an additional area of the motor control assessment. If the person who uses AAC is to use direct selection, team members must evaluate the user's range of motion, marking optimal access areas on the display. If the user is being considered for a scanning system accessed via a switch, size and location of the device remain important considerations because auditory- and/or visual-motor coordination and motor control at a reliable switch position will be involved. The person who uses an electronic AAC system with speech output may use multiple access options throughout the day depending on motor control, fatigue level, and external influences, such as lighting and weather. Thus, assessment for access to the system must account for positioning and changing access needs (Beukleman, Fager, et al., 2007).

Communication Needs

Documentation of communication needs includes an inventory of communication partners, environments in which the person currently or potentially may communicate, potential topics of conversation, the support necessary for successful communication (e.g., someone to guide the interaction, create communication opportunities, or engineer the environment for communication success), and the multiple modes of communication that may be used.

Brady and colleagues (2016) summarized current practices to support communication for people with severe disabilities and revised the Communication Bill of Rights, which serves to guide assessment and intervention practices across disciplines for people with severe disabilities. They describe communication assessment as a dynamic and holistic approach that accounts for the person's diagnosis, ability to function in the context of their different environments, and different communication partners. These are all elements that can support or inhibit communication.

Blackstone and Hunt Berg's (2012) Social Networks assessment protocol guides documentation of those elements that contribute to communication strengths and needs. Communication partners are perhaps the most important of the elements documented as they make communication possible. The *communication partner* is usually the other person involved in a conversation. However, the person may fulfill a multitude of roles, including being a relative, friend, voluntary or paid advocate, service provider, or caregiver, to name a few. *Communication environments* are the locations where a person who uses AAC interacts with others, such as at home, work, school, community, restaurants, grocery stores, and other places of business. *Topics of communication* refer to the multitude of possibilities for conversation and interaction, from basic wants and needs to topics germane to social interactions and connections. The concept of communication in *multiple modalities* applies to all people, not just those who use AAC. These include auditory modalities, such as nonspeech vocalizations or sounds, natural speech and synthesized speech from an electronic AAC device and visual modalities, such as body language (including posture and proxemics), facial expressions, gestures, and visual representations, such as text or other communication symbols that represent meaning.

Trials With Speech-Generating Devices

When the focus of evaluation is to determine and recommend an appropriate SGD, multiple devices must be considered and the recommended device must be justified to a funding provider (i.e., health insurance or vocational rehabilitation). The Centers for Medicare and Medicaid Services identify nine categories of SGDs based on type of voice output and duration of available recording time. For example, the first code in the list, E2500, applies to SGDs that provide messages in digitized (i.e., recorded) speech and have up to 8 minutes of recordable time, while near the end of the list, code E2510 applies to SGDs that provide text-to-speech message output using synthesized speech and multiple access methods. ASHA (n.d.g) provides the list of codes, as well as additional resources related to funding, for SGDs (see ASHA, n.d.g, *Medicare Coverage Policy on SGDs*). Selection of technology is discussed in greater detail in Chapter 14 and funding of electronic AAC devices with speech output is detailed in Chapter 17.

Feature Matching

The feature matching approach (Shane & Costello, 1994) is a systematic way of matching the person's communication needs and strengths to an AAC system, as opposed to trying to make the communicator adapt to use a system that may seem to be more convenient. The feature matching approach has withstood the test of time. It can be applied to a wide range of technological applications, including tablet-based technology that uses AAC apps (Gosnell et al., 2011), as well as in the choosing of symbols.

To employ feature matching, the communicator's strengths, abilities, and needs are assessed and identified. Current and future communication needs are considered in order to identify an AAC system that can grow with and adapt to the person's changing skills and new communication needs. Once comprehensive documentation of communication strengths, abilities, and needs is established, available AAC systems are evaluated to find the system that fits or matches the individual's present and future needs. One of the initial decisions is determining the appropriate E25 category on which to focus for an SGD. For this, the feature match approach (detailed later in this section) provides guidance. For example, a person who needs speech output and can spell and compose novel messages but is quadriplegic cannot use a device from the E2500 category because those devices would not have the necessary features. Instead, systems from the E2510 category should be explored because only devices in that category would have the features that meet the person's need for alternative access due to quadriplegia, novel message formulation through text entry, and text-to-speech output.

Once the appropriate category of SGD is identified, devices from that category must be evaluated to determine the best fit for the person. Although each category includes devices with comparable features, there may be characteristics or functions of a specific electronic speech-generating AAC device that provide a better fit for the individual.

Table 11-1 lists assessment areas (addressed earlier in this chapter and expanded upon in later chapters) to consider in a feature matching chart. Table 11-2 lists categories of features that are typically considered when evaluating an AAC system for an individual's use. Features may be presented in rows as they appear in Table 11-2, with columns for the different systems being considered. Gosnell and colleagues (2011) include a "rule out factor" column as the final determinant to easily demonstrate why a particular system is found to be suitable or not. This may be especially useful when writing an evaluation report to obtain funding for an SGD. Table 11-3 shows an example of a feature matching comparison chart with features (including the "rule out factor") specified in rows and three potential SGD choices in columns.

After the team identifies an electronic SGD, any funding agencies require a trial period with it. The client uses the device for a set time—usually 4 weeks—with a plan to use it for communication in multiple settings with a variety of communication partners. This is the time for the assessment team to document communication abilities for different purposes, across multiple environments, and with a variety of communication partners. Goals for trial therapy are not meant to demonstrate mastery of communication skills but rather are a way to show that the person who uses AAC is learning to do so with a variety of communication partners—not just the evaluating speech-language pathologist—in contexts outside the therapy room and for purposes beyond simple requesting. Trial therapy goals must be observable and measurable and should reflect realistic expectations for progress within the time frame of the trial period (e.g., "Tom will answer *wh*-questions, such as "What's your name?" and "Where do you live?" from an unfamiliar communication partner in a public place with gestural support in four of five opportunities during the 30-day trial).

At this point it is important to remember that a complete AAC evaluation will include nonspeaking AAC displays as well as electronic speech-generating systems. However, funding reports for speech-generating systems are typically focused on information related to the category of device that is appropriate for the individual.

Assessment Report and What Comes Next

An AAC assessment is never complete. Rather, it reaches points at which recommendations are implemented, communication skills develop, needs change, and the assessment and recommendations are updated. Report formats follow the information needs of the entity that will receive the report. For example, an evaluation report to obtain funding for a recommended electronic AAC device with speech output will include somewhat different information than an evaluation report designed to identify AAC strategies and non–speech-generating systems to implement in different settings. Some examples of AAC assessment reports for SGD funding are available through the Rehabilitation Engineering Research Center on Communication Enhancement website (http://aac-rerc.psu.edu/index.php/pages/show/id/21) and may be helpful in situations where government or health insurance is pursued. Table 11-4 provides a general outline for an AAC evaluation report. However, one should remember that sections should be modified to meet the purpose of the evaluation and the needs of the person being evaluated.

What comes next, once the assessment reaches a temporary stopping point, is based on the purpose of the assessment. For example, if the purpose is to develop language and learning strategies, then the report with detailed recommendations goes to the team for implementation. If the purpose is to obtain health insurance funding for an electronic SGD,

TABLE 11-1
Assessment Areas to Consider When Developing a Feature Match List
• Academic skills
• Cognitive skills
• Communication needs
• Communication partners
• Environments/settings in which communication occurs
• Language skills
• Literacy skills
• Motor skills
• Perceptual abilities (vision, hearing, touch)
• Supports available from caregivers, peers, educators, family members

then the report goes to the insurance company, often by way of the device's funding department for review and ideally, approval. Regardless, the cyclical process continues, and as it does so, reflects changing abilities, conditions, settings, needs, and partners of the individual.

SUMMARY

The goals of an AAC assessment are to evaluate a person's communication abilities, identify communication strengths (both internal to the person and external, as in partners and supports), identify communication needs, and then design a communication system to address those needs. AAC assessments include much of the same information found in other types of speech-language assessment (e.g., speech, language, literacy, cognitive function). However, the AAC assessment goes beyond standard assessment procedures and includes identification of current communication modalities, communication needs (people, places, and things to be communicated with and about), and the constraints and capabilities of the individual. The evaluation also documents external barriers to communication, such as attitudes, policies, practices, knowledge, and skills that interfere with an individual's ability to participate in all aspects of life through effective communication. These areas of additional assessment are highly individualized. They depend on the person's skills across motor, cognition, language, literacy, social domains, as well as age and life experience.

AAC assessment is dynamic. It involves procedures, such as careful observation of communication in different contexts, interviews of individuals interacting with the person being evaluated, interviews with the individual with CCN to the greatest degree possible, clinician-constructed tasks (e.g., turn-taking, requesting), and, if required for funding, device trials in simulated and functional activities.

Table 11-2

Components of an AAC System Considered in a Feature Matching Assessment

FEATURES	OPTIONS
Display type	Dynamic • Display changes by selecting a hypertext link to a different display Static • Display changes with overlays
Visual representation	Digital photos Grid display Line drawings (e.g., Blissymbols, Picture Communication Symbols, SymbolStix) Text • Variable font Video playback VSD
Visual output	Adjustable color saturation and contrast Printed Visible on display Visible on front-facing display (i.e., facing the communication partner)
Speech/auditory output	Digitized speech (recorded) Synthesized speech (computerized) • Preset • Based on user's voice
Speech/auditory customization	Pitch and rate variation Variable output (e.g., device speaks one letter or word at a time or speaks an entire sentence or message or multiple sentences at a time) Volume control
Feedback (auditory)	Click On/off options Other sound effects Speech (different voice from speech output)
Feedback (visual)	Animation Highlight • Border changes color • Cell changes color On/off options Zoom • Selection area enlarges

(continued)

TABLE 11-2 (CONTINUED)

Components of an AAC System Considered in a Feature Matching Assessment

FEATURES	OPTIONS
Feedback (tactile)	Haptic (i.e., device vibrates with selection) On/off options Variable surfaces (e.g., rough, smooth, small part of object)
Vocabulary	Preprogrammed messages Word-by-word Topic-specific
Rate enhancement	On/off options Settings to increase speaking rate Strategies to decrease keystrokes and/or fatigue • Abbreviation expansion (e.g., HHY = "Hello. How are you?") • Vocabulary prediction (e.g., alphabetical, semantic compaction, syntactic, frequently used, recently used)
Access options	Direct selection • Customized settings • Eye tracking and gaze • Infrared mouse emulation • Touch Scanning • Bluetooth switch capable • Customized scan patterns (e.g., one item at a time, row/column, column/row, group/item) • Customized settings • Hardwire switch capable
Portability (size)	Dimensions (imperial or metric) • Include three dimensions Note: Display size is typically measured diagonally
Portability (weight)	Kilograms, ounces, pounds, etc.
Optional protective case	
VSD = visual scene display.	

TABLE 11-3

Example Feature Matching Chart for a 6-Year-Old Child With Cerebral Palsy

FEATURES	SGD 1	SGD 2	SGD 3
Display type	Dynamic	Dynamic	Static
Visual representations	Colored line drawings Digital photos Digital video Text	Colored line drawings Digital photos Digital video Text	Text
Speech/auditory output	Synthesized Digitized	Synthesized Digitized	Digitized only
Feedback (auditory)	Auditory (speech or sound)	Auditory (speech or sound)	None
Feedback (visual)	Selection highlighted or enlarged	Selection highlighted or enlarged	Can see what is typed on display
Feedback (tactile)	Switch press if switch-scanning access used	Switch press if switch-scanning access used	Key press
Vocabulary	Prelinked customizable displays Preprogrammed core word sets, topic-specific displays	Preprogrammed core word sets, topic-specific displays	Limited preprogramming capability
Rate enhancement	Word prediction (frequency, recency, and alphabetic)	Word prediction (frequency, recency, and alphabetic)	Word prediction (frequency and alphabetic)
Access options	Direct selection: • Touch • Infrared mouse emulation • Eye tracking • Joystick Scanning: • Switch scanning with multiple settings	Direct selection: • Touch • Infrared mouse emulation • Eye tracking • Joystick Scanning: • Switch scanning with multiple settings	
Portability (size)	15″ x 12″ x 3″	17″ x 12″ x 3″	13″ x 6″ x 2″
Portability (weight)	5 lbs	4 lbs	2.5 lbs
Rule-out factor	Smaller and heavier than other viable option		No eye-tracking capability Does not support line drawings, photos, or videos

SGD = speech-generating device.

TABLE 11-4
An AAC Assessment Report Outline

1. Background information
   1.1. Diagnoses
      1.2. Course of condition (e.g., stable, improving, degenerative)
      1.3. Reason for referral/purpose of evaluation
2. Assessment
   2.1. Language (including all modalities)
      2.1.1. Receptive
      2.1.2. Expressive
   2.2. Cognitive/Linguistic
      2.2.1. Memory, attention, executive function
   2.3. Literacy
   2.4. Physical
      2.4.1. Mobility status
      2.4.2. Accessing AAC system
   2.5. Sensory
      2.5.1. Vision
      2.5.2. Hearing
      2.5.3. Tactile
   2.6. Communication needs
      2.6.1. Communication partners
      2.6.2. Communication facilitators
      2.6.3. Communication advocates
      2.6.4. Communication environments
      2.6.5. Opportunities for communication
      2.6.6. Barriers to communication
      2.6.7. Attitudes toward communication
         2.6.7.1. Attitudes of partners, facilitators, and advocates toward AAC
         2.6.7.2. Attitudes of the person toward AAC
   2.7. Feature matching
      2.7.1. Features necessary in an AAC system for effective communication
      2.7.2. AAC systems that have the identified features (and those that do not)
      2.7.3. Demonstrate rule-out factor
      2.7.4. Identify recommended system
3. Summary
   3.1. Communication strengths
   3.2. Communication challenges
   3.3. Findings of evaluation
4. Recommendations
   4.1. Specific components of AAC system
   4.2. Resources (where to obtain recommended materials)
   4.3. Instructions (where to find tutorials and additional training)
   4.4. Timeline for training and follow-up

AAC = augmentative and alternative communication.

Essential elements of the AAC evaluation identify the features necessary in an AAC system to meet the needs of the individual. These AAC systems may include devices that use microprocessors and produce speech but should always include non–speech-generating communication displays and offer multiple modes to use when communicating.

Evaluators must repeat this process as the skills, needs, partners, situations, activities, and settings of the communicator change throughout their life. Initial recommendations must be regularly re-evaluated to ensure that an optimal match between the AAC system and person is achieved. Treatment strategies are essential to AAC system success and are integrated into the assessment cycle. AAC assessment is applied in this way to ensure the person can fully realize their right to communicate all the time, in all places, about all things, and for all purposes that are authentic and meaningful to them.

STUDY QUESTIONS

1. AAC assessment is described as an iterative process. Outline several points in time that a person who uses AAC should be re-evaluated.

2. AAC assessment teams may work under multidisciplinary, interdisciplinary, or transdisciplinary approaches. Describe the similarities and differences among the three approaches.

3. Name and describe the roles of potential members of an AAC evaluation team.

4. Identify several of the key areas of an evaluation for AAC. What types of information are important in each?

5. A preinterview may provide essential assessment information not available through other evaluation procedures. Describe examples of important information that may be learned from a preinterview and how it might inform the assessment process.

6. How might standardized tests be modified when used with a person during an AAC assessment?

7. Both an ecological inventory and use of the Participation Model can be applied easily to observation. Describe the similarities and differences between the two.

8. How does a feature matching procedure inform the AAC assessment process?

9. Why is literacy an important element in an AAC evaluation?

10. Why is speech intelligibility an important element in an AAC evaluation?

12

Vocabulary Selection

Russell T. Cross, DipCST; Karen A. Erickson, PhD;
Lori A. Geist, PhD; and Penny Hatch, PhD

MYTH

1. Standardized vocabulary lists are not helpful when identifying vocabulary for augmentative and alternative communication (AAC).

2. The most important vocabulary selected for AAC users are words that convey basic needs and wants.

3. Core vocabulary is too abstract for some individuals to learn and only should be introduced after they have learned a set of concrete, easy-to-understand nouns.

REALITY

1. Standardized vocabulary lists, especially large-scale corpora, represent one important source from which to select vocabulary for use in AAC.

2. Vocabulary that conveys needs and wants may help some AAC users meet some communication needs but certainly not all. Vocabulary that conveys emotions, ideas, and information is also important.

3. Core vocabulary is not too abstract when it is taught through meaningful interaction and use across contexts. Learning core vocabulary does not require individuals to first learn concrete vocabulary.

INTRODUCTION

One of the most fundamental building blocks of communication is the concept of the "word." It is such a common concept that for most people it is essentially what language is all about—learning words and then stringing them into sentences in order to interact with others. In everyday life, discussion and disagreements about what words mean, where they come from, and how they are used can range from simple conversations over dinner to international legal arguments that dominate the media for weeks. The importance of words in everyday life is so critical that it is easy to forget how much of human discourse depends on how we use vocabulary.

In their spoken form, words are also crucial in establishing and maintaining face-to-face relationships. Everyday events, such as chatting with a friend, asking for help in a

Fuller, D. R., & Lloyd, L. L. *Principles and Practices in*
Augmentative and Alternative Communication (pp. 231-243).
© 2023 Taylor & Francis Group.

store, answering a phone, or even holding down a job, are dependent on individuals being able to express themselves orally in a timely and accurate manner. Inherent in this is the need to have a vocabulary that includes the words necessary to talk about the topic at hand.

For individuals who use AAC, needs for vocabulary are no different from anyone else, and providing that vocabulary along with the means to express it is a primary task for the AAC practitioner. The modes used (e.g., gestures, signing systems, speech-generating devices [SGDs] or manual communication boards) may vary, but vocabulary selection is the process of identifying and representing the words individuals need in order to communicate to their fullest potential. So whether the word "stop" exists in an AAC system as a picture on a board, a sign made with the hands, a spelled word on a piece of paper, or a single or sequence of buttons on an SGD, the availability of the word "stop" itself is what is important from the perspective of vocabulary selection.

Some Words About "Words"

If English speakers are asked to define a "word," they will likely describe it in one of two ways: (1) as an isolated collection of sounds used to refer to a concept or thing, or (2) as a string of letters bounded by spaces or punctuation marks. The former is based on words as spoken phenomena and the latter as written phenomena. The same would go for "dog," "banana," and "thirsty," all of which seem to be easily identifiable as "words." However, what about the words "stops," "stopping," and "stopped?" Are these different words from "stop," or is there some underlying relationship that makes them, in some sense, the same word?

These variations of "stop" are related to **morphology**—the way in which words can change based on how they are used in relation to other words in a sentence. Thus, the word "stop" would appear after the pronouns "I," "we," or "they," but the word becomes "stops" after "he," "she," or "it." Similarly, the word "thirsty" is used when referring to one person ("He is thirsty"), "thirstier" when used between two people ("He is thirstier than Jane"), and "thirstiest" when referring to more than two people ("He is thirstiest of all"). In linguistics, the term **lemma** is used to refer to what might be called the root form of a word, or more commonly, the dictionary entry. As you will see later in this chapter, the distinction between a word and a lemma is important when considering the vocabulary content in an AAC system, especially when it comes to providing an individual with access to systems that support the application of morphological rules during communication.

Vocabulary Characteristics: Core and Fringe

One of the more interesting features of language is that some words are used with extraordinarily more frequency than others. There is also a mathematical relationship, known as Zipf's Law (Zipf, 1936), between the frequency with which a word occurs and its ranking; namely, any word is twice as frequent as the word ranked below it. Thus, the most frequent word "the" is used twice as often as the second most frequent word "of," which in turn is used twice as often as the third most frequent word "and." This holds across languages (Bentz & Kiela, 2014).

This statistical characteristic forms the basis for the notion that all vocabularies contain a relatively small set of words that occur across topics, situations, and demographic groups. These are often referred to as *core* words. In contrast, there are words that will occur only in relation to specific activities, contexts, places, topics, and demographic groups (e.g., Boenisch & Soto, 2015; Witkowski & Baker, 2012). In the field of AAC, these are referred to as **fringe vocabulary**. The distinction between core and fringe words is not based on any judgment of the value of a word but is a manifestation of the statistical properties of word frequencies highlighted by Zipf. It can be helpful to define core and fringe words in the following ways:

> Core words are words that have a higher frequency of use than is statistically expected when compared to a large reference corpus. Core words typically occur across age groups, across different situations, and within many different topic areas.

As an example, the word "want" is found in the vocabulary of toddlers (Banajee et al., 2003; Hadley et al., 2016; Piccin & Waxman, 2007), preschoolers (Bean et al., 2019; Beukelman et al., 1989; Fried-Oken & More, 1992; Marvin et al., 1994; Quick et al., 2019; Trembath et al., 2007), school-aged children (Boenisch & Soto, 2015; Crestani et al., 2010; Wood et al., 2016), and adults (Balandin & Iacono, 1999; Beukelman et al., 1984; Brezina & Gablasova, 2013; Kilgarriff et al., 2014; Stuart et al., 1997). This suggests that including the word "want" in an AAC system is of prime value for any age group.

Fringe vocabulary has different characteristics:

> Fringe words are words that have a lower frequency of use value than is statistically expected when compared to a large reference corpus. Fringe words typical vary across age groups, are found in particular situations, and appear in specific topic areas.

As an example, "teddy" is unlikely to be used with any frequency by individuals from school-age upward, is going to be used most in a play setting, and will be found typically alongside words related to toys and games. Including this word in toddlers' or preschoolers' AAC systems may have value, but the likelihood of it being used much by older individuals is much lower. This is not, of course, to say it will *never* be used, only that when compared to the lexicon of the English language, its expected use in relation to frequency is very low.

There is a third distinction that can be made in relation to word frequencies, and that is the concept of the **keyword**. This is used often in the field of corpus linguistics, a field of study within the general realm of applied linguistics that investigates patterns of use in language by analyzing very large samples of data called "corpora." These corpora are typically of a size that requires sophisticated software search tools in order to make sense of the data. Within corpus linguistics, keywords can be defined as follows:

> Keywords are words that are significantly more frequent in a sample of text than would be expected, given their frequency in a large general reference corpus (Stubbs, 2010).

The essential difference between the keyword and the fringe word is the frequency; a keyword has an unusually high frequency when compared to a large reference set. In the previous example of "teddy" as a fringe word, it could also be classed as a keyword within the environment of play activities or toys. However, keywords can be temporal phenomena and, like bubbles in a glass of soda, they can rise in frequency for a period of time and then suddenly disappear. For example, the words "Santa" and "present" may increase in frequency as Christmas day approaches, but very shortly after, their use can drop back down to almost nothing for a year. The implication of this for vocabulary selection is that deciding where to code or represent such words needs to be carefully evaluated from the perspective of organization and navigation (i.e., where do you put it so that it can be found?). Adding "Santa" to the homepage of an SGD system may make it easy to access in December, but its value from January onward is limited. Left there, it takes up valuable space that could be better occupied by core vocabulary. Knowing that "Santa" is a temporal keyword, it would be better to locate it further inside the system where it can still be accessed with just two or three button presses but would not impede fast access to the more useful, general core words.

Vocabulary Selection Sources

The definitions of core, fringe, and keyword all include the idea of comparisons to a "reference corpus." But what reference corpora are available that can help practitioners in selecting vocabulary for their clients' AAC systems?

Toddlers

A frequently cited source of toddler vocabulary is that of Banajee and colleagues (2003) where the researchers collected naturally occurring language samples from 50 toddlers aged 24 to 36 months. The children were enrolled in five different preschools and the samples were taken over 3 days during play activities and snack time. They found that 23 words accounted for 96% of all the words used by this cohort. Furthermore, they represented a range of different syntactic, semantic, and pragmatic functions:

> Core vocabulary words contained demonstratives (that), verbs (want), pronouns (my), prepositions (on), and articles (the). No nouns were found in this list. Semantic functions included use of agents (I), objects (you), labeling objects (that) and actions (go), possession (my), affirmation (yes), negation (no), location (in), interrogation (what), quantity (some), and termination (finished). Pragmatic functions expressed included initiating interaction by attracting attention (you), maintaining joint attention (this), indicating recurrence (more), and terminating interaction (finished). (Banajee et al., 2003, p. 71)

It is important to note that contrary to naïve expectations, the sample is not dominated by nouns but includes such items as demonstratives, verbs, pronouns, and articles. This does not mean there were no nouns in the sample but that their frequency of use was statistically very small.

This brings up another feature of natural language; although nouns as word tokens constitute the largest part of the English lexicon (Hudson, 1994; Liang & Liu, 2013), the most frequently used words by type are articles, prepositions, conjunctions, and pronouns (Davies, 2008; Francis et al., 1982).

Preschoolers

Beukelman and colleagues (1989) sampled the vocabulary of six preschool children without disabilities with sampling periods ranging from 2 to 7 hours in length. For each subject, sampling ended after 3,000 words (tokens) had been collected, and the number of different words (types) for each ranged from 404 to 468. They found that 45% of the total language sample was represented by the 25 most frequently occurring words, 60% by the top 50, and 85% by 250 words. These figures also serve to reinforce the notion that a core set of high-frequency words can account for a significantly large proportion of the total vocabulary used. Also significant is that the 23 most frequent words in the Banajee and colleagues (2003) study were also found in the top 50 most frequent words in the Beukelman and colleagues (1989) corpus.

These findings were reinforced in a later study (Fallon et al., 2001) in which language samples were recorded from five typically developing children ages 3.9 to 4.9 years of age. Each child wore a small tape recorder that recorded 1 to 2 hours of speech at a time over a 2- to 4-day period. Samples of 1,000 words for each child were transcribed to create a sample of 5,000 total words used. The authors found that the 25 most frequently used words accounted for 44% of the whole sample, and that the 250 most frequently used words accounted for 89% of the sample. Furthermore, the top 25 words were not primarily nouns but a mix of verbs, prepositions, pronouns, adverbs, and even contractions. Nouns were an important element of specific topics but their individual frequencies were relatively low.

Trembath and colleagues (2007) collected spoken samples from six typically developing Australian preschoolers aged between 3 and 5 years. From a total of 18,000 tokens, 1,411 different words were identified and any that occurred with a frequency of at least 0.5 per 1,000 words and were used by at least three (50%) of the participants were labeled as core words. This core of 263 words accounted for almost 80% of the total sample and the authors noted that 34 of the 50 most frequently used words were also featured in the list of the 50 most commonly used words in the Beukelman and colleagues (1989) study.

School-Aged Children

In a study based on longitudinal data collected in the 1970s, Raban (1987) analyzed the spoken vocabulary of 96 5-year-old children based on a corpus of 70,000 word tokens resulting in a vocabulary of 4,174 different word types. The analysis also included frequency scores for words by part-of-speech rather than just the word string itself. For example, the word "look" can be used as either a verb ("Look at that") or a noun ("Take a look at that"), and in the Raban study, these are broken down as noun (17) and verb (443). This can be extremely useful when making a decision about how to teach a word that not only has more than one meaning but potentially represents multiple parts of speech. In the case of "look," teaching it as the verb form would make much more sense from the objective point of view of using the more frequently used form. Current online corpora offer the potential to see these distinctions, and this will be discussed shortly.

Robillard and colleagues (2014) compared the core vocabularies of a group of six monolingual French speakers, 19 bilingual English-French speakers, and 22 French-English speakers. A further 10 were identified as having language impairment, so their data were analyzed separately. Using the same method of identifying core words as Trembath and colleagues (2007; i.e., a word had to be used with a frequency of at least 0.5 per 1,000 words and had to be used by at least 50% of the participants), they found that monolingual and bilingual children essentially use the same core words in French. They also found no significant differences in core frequencies between the groups and when combining them all to create a single corpus. They also found the French core words had the same frequency distribution as their English forms. From this, they concluded that their final list of English/French core words could be used in vocabulary selection for both languages. It is worth noting that studies of vocabulary in non-English languages have tended to support the notion of similar core vocabulary sets in Arabic (Draffan, Wald, et al., 2015), Korean (Shin & Hill, 2016), Zulu (Mngomezulu et al., 2019), and German (Boenisch & Sachse, 2007).

As children develop literacy and begin to use writing as a form of expression and communication, this opens up another source for vocabulary selection studies: written language samples. Not only can such data be used to inform vocabulary selection for an AAC system but similarity in word frequencies between spoken and written language make it possible to provide individuals with two channels through which to express themselves. Zangari and Van Tatenhove (2009) suggest that making high-frequency vocabulary available for both face-to-face and written communication is a priority for intervention with clients using AAC systems.

Clendon and Erickson (2008) collected 2,721 writing samples from 238 students in the United States ($n = 125$) and New Zealand. The students were allowed to write about any topic they wanted and generated between one and 33 writing samples each. A total of 85,759 word tokens were collected, which included 5,724 different words. They found that the top 163 words accounted for 70% of the total words used and the top 39 words accounted for 50% of the total words used. This supported earlier studies of written language (Clendon et al., 2003; McGinnis & Beukelman, 1989) where in the former study, 140 words accounted for 70% of the total sample and 39 words accounted for 50% of the total sample, and in the latter study, 161 words accounted for 70% of the total sample and 46 words accounted for 50% of the total sample.

Clendon and Erickson (2008) also looked at multiword sequences, such as "I like," "I see," and "in the." Although they found some frequency of use variation between the two countries in how some multiword sequences were used, they concluded that "[s]ome multiword sequences may be used with sufficiently high frequency to warrant their storage as whole units in AAC systems" (p. 289). This is a feature of language that is often of interest to linguists working in corpus linguistics and an area of vocabulary selection that will be returned to shortly.

In a follow-up study, Clendon and colleagues (2013) examined the written words and multiword sequences used by 124 typically developing kindergarten and first grade students. They collected 457 samples (11,673 word tokens) and found that 140 words accounted for 70% of the total vocabulary produced (1,590 different words). The article includes the list of those top 140 words with the recommendation that these could form a starting point for developing or implementing an AAC system. The authors were also able to identify the top 10 most frequently occurring two- and three-word sequences, with "I like" being the most frequent two-word phrase and "I went to" as the top three-word phrase, which once again raises the possibility of considering multiword units as part of the vocabulary selection process.

A final example of an available list of core words based on written data is a study by Wood and colleagues (2016) that focused on written samples from 94 first-grade children and 117 fourth-grade children. The entire corpus came from 217 written samples in which there were 27,391 word tokens containing 3,781 different words types. Of these, 191 words made up 70% of the entire written sample and the top 50 words accounted for 51% of the total word count. In reference to parts of speech, 64% of the 50 were nouns, verbs, adjectives, and adverbs with 36% being articles, pronouns, and prepositions. The authors propose that the "… key findings have implications for word selection in designing AAC systems to ensure word selection accommodates not only oral communication but also the demands and opportunities of written language tasks. The overall core vocabulary or word-bank that was identified … may be useful in supporting written personal narrative experiences on a child's AAC system" (p. 206).

The essential takeaway from all these studies is that using core word lists based on data from oral and written sources is a legitimate way of selecting vocabulary for an AAC system.

Adults

One of the earliest studies of vocabulary use in spoken English is that of Berger (1968) where a sample of over 25,000 word tokens were collected over a 2-year period from conversations overheard in restaurants. There were 2,507 different types where 312 accounted for 80% of the total vocabulary used, and the top 100 words accounted for just over 62% of the total used.

Stuart and colleagues (1993) recorded samples of speech used by five retired adults with an aim of looking at variations across topics and commonalities in lexical items. For each individual, a sample of 3,000 word tokens was used, leading to a total sample size of 15,000 lexical items. The researchers found that 100 words represented 63% of the total communication sample and that 200 accounted for just under 78%. The authors noted this would "… indicate that the 250 most frequently occurring words represent the core vocabulary items for this group of elderly women, much the same as previously reported for individuals with a diagnosis of cerebral palsy using Canon communicators, preschool and middle school students" (p. 102).

The reference to the Canon communicators comes from research by Beukelman and colleagues (1984) who collected samples from five adults, who were nonspeaking, using a text-output device. The Canon communicator was a handheld device with a keyboard and a strip printer. A client would spell words out using the keyboard, which would be printed on a strip of paper. The communication partner could then read the text. As the device did not have features, such as word prediction, abbreviated expansion, or other such text-shortening facilities, the client had to be literate in order to use the device, and the data represent a written sample as opposed to a spoken sample. The data were collected for 14 days, at the end of which a core vocabulary of the 500 most frequently occurring words was created from the 34,437 word tokens generated in the total sample. The authors discovered that the 25 most frequent words could be used to cover 35% of the total written sample. Once again, this research supports the critical nature of a core vocabulary.

The difference between core and fringe vocabulary is neatly illustrated by a set of three studies by researchers Susan Balandin and Teresa Iacono. In the first study, Balandin and Iacono (1998b) recorded the meal-time conversations of 34 participants without disabilities across four worksites. A total of 174,877 word tokens were collected of which 7,340 were different. They found that the participants referenced 73 different topics, and further analysis of the 10 most frequently referenced topics revealed 19 topics, five of which (i.e., work, fact-finding, judgments, food, and family life) were used every day.

Having identified topics, they then performed a second study (Balandin & Iacono, 1998a) where they asked 10 professionals (five speech-language pathologists, three rehabilitation counselors, and two teachers) to suggest two topics they thought employees without disabilities might talk about during meal-break conversations for each day of the week and to list five key words for each topic selected. In this instance, the definition of key words was "… words they considered intrinsic to the topic selected" (p. 153). This is close to the keyword definition cited earlier where the words would have a frequency higher than would be expected in a large general corpus. For example, the word "soap opera" appeared in the study as a keyword for the topic of "television," but outside of that topic, it would be seen as having a very low frequency.

In a third article, Balandin and Iacono (1999) used the data from the previous studies and provided a list of 347 core words, where a core word was defined as one that occurred in the sample with a frequency of 0.5 per 1,000. They noted that the vocabulary consisted predominantly of function words, supporting other studies where the most frequently used words are, contrary to what might be expected, not nouns. They said, "This finding was congruent with that of previous vocabulary studies … in that, despite being large, fringe vocabularies account for a smaller proportion of the total words used in conversational samples than to core vocabularies" (p. 105).

Two interesting findings came out of these studies. The first was that the professionals were able to identify the sort of topics that might occur in conversations but were not good at predicting the frequency with which those topics might occur. For example, the topic "gardening" was selected three times yet only accounted for 0.1% of topic use. Similarly, the topics of "television" and "weather" were chosen more than once but used infrequently. The challenge was not in selecting topics but in selecting the frequency with which topics might occur. The second notable observation was that, of the 407 different word types identified as keywords in Balandin and Iacono (1998a), 271 (67%) were used by clients but 136 (33%) were not. In other words, predicting key word vocabulary was more of a challenge than might have been expected. This inaccuracy in predicting key words highlights why including core words in an AAC vocabulary system is so important—they are statistically more predictable. Given the choice between adding "want" or "banana" to a vocabulary set, the probability of a client using the former is much higher than the latter.

Morphology and Vocabulary Selection

As mentioned earlier, there is the lemma or dictionary form of a word and then "word family" variations that come from it. For example, the word "stop" can be imagined as STOP (stop/stops/stopped/stopping) and the word "thirsty" as THIRSTY (thirsty/thirstier/thirstiest/thirstily). By thinking about a word as being part of a cluster or family, it ensures that when vocabulary is being selected, there is some thought given to what forms of the lemma also need to be included and how these forms are represented in the AAC system. The absence of some way to access morphological forms can be a significant impediment to becoming a competent aided communicator (Binger, 2008; Sutton et al., 2000; Sutton et al., 2002).

Being able to understand and use the morphology of a language is essential for conversational proficiency (Hemphill & Tivnan, 2008; Singson et al., 2000) and morphological awareness is thought to be a significant facilitator of vocabulary acquisition (Guo et al., 2011; McBride-Chang et al., 2008; Tong et al., 2011; Wolter & Green, 2013). Studies that investigate the effect of active teaching of morphological awareness suggest that it can improve both spoken and written skills (Apel et al., 2022; Bowers & Kirby, 2010; Good et al., 2015; Goodwin & Ahn, 2010; Goodwin et al., 2012; Levesque et al., 2021), even with children who have significant hearing impairments (Trussell & Easterbrooks, 2017).

Including the morphological variants of words in an SGD can be beneficial to the aided communicator. Binger and colleagues (2011) reported on three children, age 4:09 to 6:03 years, who were all using SGDs that marked the morphological endings for present progressing (+ING), possessive (+'S), regular past tense (+ED), and plural (+S). To access a word ending in one of these morphemes, the client would first select a symbol that represented the root form of the verb and then select the second button to inflect it. As an example, selecting the picture SHOE followed by the +ING button would produce "kicking," whereas SHOE followed by the +ED button would give "kicked." Similarly, adding the +S button to "dog" and "cat" would produce "dogs" and "cats." Using modeling and recasting, specific morphemes were targeted using different ones for different children. In the first instance, all the children learned their target morphemes, but after a break of weeks, they failed on subsequent probes to produce them. After a second intervention phase using contrastive models (i.e., showing one inflected form then another one to illustrate the difference), along with more modeling and recasts, the subjects were eventually able to maintain the morphemes.

In a systematic review of research documenting the effects of language interventions for people with complex communication needs (CCN) that include communication partners modeling the use of AAC, Sennott and colleagues (2016) concluded that "… the 10 studies included in this best-evidence synthesis investigated the impact of aided AAC modeling-based interventions and reported consistently positive and large main effects for pragmatic, semantic, syntactic, and morphological development for young children who are beginning communicators" (p. 110). The evidence provided by all these studies suggests that the vocabulary selection process must also include taking into account all forms of a word to provide a system where the client can have full access to linguistic morphology in order to become a better communicator.

Using Large-Scale General Corpora as Reference Databases

As mentioned, corpus linguistics is a field of study that investigates patterns of use in language by analyzing very large samples of spoken or written language data. Software tools called **concordancers** allow researchers to look at words in context while other tools allow for the analysis of frequency data, which lists all words appearing in a corpus and specifies how many times each one occurs in that set. Concordances and frequency data exemplify, respectively, two forms of analysis—qualitative and quantitative—both of which are critical in research.

The field has grown rapidly since the mid-1980s because of the availability of computer-based methodologies. Prior to that, typical manual analyses of large data samples could take months, even years, but now it is possible to have access to online resources that boast samples in the billions.

One of the most widely used online collections of language corpora is English-Corpora.org (Davies, 2018), which is free to use and provides a selection of analytical tools for examining the different databases. These include the Corpus of Contemporary American English (Davies, 2008; a 560-million word database from 1990 to 2017) the Global Web-Based English corpus (Davies, 2013a; a 1.9-billion word database that includes samples from 20 English-speaking countries collected over the period 2012 to 2013), and the News on the Web corpus (Davies, 2013b; an 8.7-billion word database drawn from online news sources started in 2010 and updated every day).

The application of corpora has been significant in areas, such as lexicography (Hunston, 2002), language learning (Reppen, 2010), and second-language learning (Römer, 2011). More recently, there have been applications in the field of AAC (Cross 2010, 2015; Mühlenbock & Lundälv 2011). Boulton (2010) says that "[c]orpora can provide information on usage in context, especially in the form of concordances, as well as on frequency, distribution, collocation, and so on" (p. 535), which is exactly the sort of data AAC practitioners can use to good advantage when considering how to choose and teach vocabulary.

TABLE 12-1

Relative Frequency Score for Three Word Pairs

WORD	FREQUENCY	WORD	FREQUENCY	WORD	FREQUENCY
tired	4,394	hear	94,421	look	185,176
sleepy	274	listen	30,688	see	277,821

These online corpora have many different uses that include:

- Finding out how native speakers actually speak and write
- Finding the frequency of words, phrases, and collocations
- Looking at language variation and change (e.g., historical, dialects, and genres)
- Gaining insight into culture (e.g., what is said about different concepts over time and in different countries)
- Designing authentic language teaching materials and resources

Here are three simple examples of how the databases can be used in the process of not just selecting vocabulary but also finding out how such vocabulary is used.

1. Using relative frequency scores to determine where to locate words in a system.

    A. When adding words to an AAC system with multiple pages through which to navigate, having the highest frequency words available with the least number of selections is the most efficient way to store vocabulary. Two keystrokes for "coconut" and three for "that" would be inefficient. With some words where you have a choice, checking the relative frequencies can help the decision. Consider the pairs tired/sleepy, hear/listen, and look/see. Which, in each pair, is the more frequently used word, and therefore, the one that needs to be easier to access? Table 12-1 shows the results of a frequency search related to this question.

2. Using part-of-speech search to determine how a multi-meaning word is most frequently used.

    A. A word, such as "light," can have more than one meaning. As an adjective, it means "not heavy"; as a noun, it refers to something you turn on in the dark; as a verb, it means to set fire to something. However, which form of the use of this word is the most common? Using the search feature with the option to show parts of speech, the frequencies of the different meanings of the word are shown (Table 12-2). From the data, teaching the meaning of "light" as the noun first would be more typical than as an adjective or verb.

3. Analyzing multiword phrases.

    A. In some AAC technologies, selecting a pronoun followed by the "to be" verb automatically changes the next set of verbs to their -ing forms. For example, the word "eat" becomes "eating" after selecting "I am" or

TABLE 12-2

Different Meanings of "Light" by Part-of-Speech

PART OF SPEECH	EXAMPLE USE	FREQUENCY
Light (noun)	"Turn on the light."	36,854
Light (adjective)	"I had a light lunch."	8,089
Light (verb)	"Can you light the candle?"	1,203

"he is." But is this always going to work? The verbs "like," "know," and "want" are all core words and appear in almost all AAC word lists. Using the Corpus of Contemporary American English (Davies, 2018), we can see how they vary following the <PRONOUN> + <TO BE> structure in spoken language (Table 12-3). Surprisingly, most of them take the -ed form more frequently than the -ing form, with "known" occurring 22 times more often than "knowing!" What this suggests is that some of our intuitions of how an AAC language system should behave may be different from real-world usage.

An important question to be addressed is whether it is legitimate to use general large-scale corpora in the selection of vocabulary for individuals using AAC systems. Firstly, from all the studies covered in this chapter, it is clear that very large corpora are going to have similar distribution and frequency characteristics to other smaller corpora. The core words that exist in a 450 million–word corpus will have a similar rank ordering to those of a 10,000-word corpus. Therefore, from the perspective of selecting core vocabulary, the words found in very large corpora will be as useful to all individuals with CCN, both children and adults.

Secondly, an overarching aim of vocabulary selection is to provide individuals with the ability to access as large and as regular a vocabulary as those used by speaking individuals. The ultimate target vocabulary for those using AAC is therefore the same as that for anyone else—the lexicon of the language of the community in which they live. If the target is a large, general vocabulary, then the large-scale corpora are precisely that—large, general vocabularies. Of course, there

TABLE 12-3

Frequency of *-ing* or *-ed* Inflection After a Pronoun and "to be" Verb

	FREQUENCY OF USE AFTER		
	"I am …"	*"You are …"*	*"He is …"*
liked	0	3	5
liking	4	11	3
known	7	430	1108
knowing	0	2	68
wanted	1	25	51
wanting	0	55	32

will still be the need to identify keyword vocabulary items for individuals, but online corpora can be helpful tools even in identifying those.

Thirdly, as can be seen in the three previous examples, data analysis with tools such as English-Corpora.org can go much further than simple single-word frequency counts. It is also possible to analyze collocations (which words are found close to each other in discourse) to identify variations between different types of English (e.g., American English vs. Canadian English vs. British English), to chart a word's changing frequency over time, and to create your own corpora and identify keywords.

Finally, general corpora can provide useful information about how and where words are used in the form of concordances. This is an approach already used in teaching English as a second language (Boulton, 2015; Boulton & Vyatkina, 2021; Chujo et al., 2013; Flowerdew, 2009; Yılmaz & Soruç, 2015).

Used intelligently, resources such as English-Corpora. org can enhance the task of vocabulary selection for all demographics and provide analyses that can supplement direct clinical observations and intervention planning.

Vocabulary Selection for Individuals With Severe Intellectual and Developmental Disabilities

Historically, individuals with severe intellectual and developmental disabilities and CCN have not had access to core vocabulary, as they are learning to communicate symbolically. Instead, initial vocabulary considerations for individuals with severe intellectual and developmental disabilities and CCN have focused on fringe vocabulary that represents preferred items or activities (Beukelman et al., 1991; Schlosser & Sigafoos, 2002; Snell et al., 2006) in order to promote requesting (Frost & Bondy, 2002) and functional communication

(Adamson et al., 1992). These items are generally selected through preference assessments (Sigafoos & Reichle, 1992; Snell et al., 2006), which result in a focus on concrete vocabulary allowing communication partners to reinforce successful communication efforts through contingent reinforcement. Vocabulary highlighting preferences also harness the power of attention, increasing the likelihood of joint attention, which is the process assumed to assist learners in mapping words to their referents (Tomasello, 2003). However, the context-specific nature of this fringe vocabulary, an example of the keywords described previously, limits opportunities for teaching and learning while restricting purposes for communication primarily to the communicative function of requesting (Dodd & Gorey, 2013).

An emphasis on preferred items and activities is often accompanied by the prioritization of concrete vocabulary over conceptual vocabulary (Van Tatenhove, 2009). Concrete vocabulary, almost always in the category of fringe vocabulary, as described previously, generally includes object nouns, as well as some action verbs and descriptors. These concrete words are relatively easy to learn because students can physically interact with the objects and perform or observe the actions associated with the words. Learning concrete vocabulary in aided AAC is further supported by the fact that it is possible to represent many of these concrete items, actions, or attributes with highly transparent graphic symbols that visually resemble their referents and are therefore highly guessable (Beukelman & Mirenda, 2013; Schlosser & Sigafoos, 2002).

While this use of concrete, fringe vocabulary may have both cognitive and linguistic developmental advantages, the context-specific nature of concrete vocabulary limits opportunities for teaching, learning, and use while restricting opportunities for combining words (Dodd & Gorey, 2013). For example, consider the graphic symbols for a preferred food (e.g., "cracker") and a preferred activity (e.g., "music"). There are few opportunities to use or see others use these symbols throughout the day, as these symbols can only be used to label or request and cannot be meaningfully combined.

For many individuals with severe intellectual and developmental disabilities and CCN, this focus on context-dependent vocabulary means the vocabulary they are provided routinely changes in order to accommodate particular activities or routines (Deckers et al., 2017; Van Tatenhove, 2009). This context-specific use of vocabulary may also limit access to comprehensive aided AAC systems. For example, Erickson and Geist (2016) reported the results of a large-scale survey completed by teachers of school-aged students with severe intellectual and developmental disabilities ($N = 44{,}787$), many of whom had CCN ($n = 15{,}672$). Fewer than a quarter had access to SGDs with comprehensive vocabulary sets. The majority of students had SGDs or non–speech-generating systems that included nine or fewer messages, and nearly half of the students communicated via symbols presented one or two at a time.

The common approach to selecting and displaying vocabulary related to a specific activity or environment may promote successful use in specific contexts. However, this practice is likely to create barriers to generalized use and communication access, as words available during one activity are often not available in subsequent activities or routines. As individuals with severe intellectual and developmental disabilities and CCN require more intense repetition, stability, and predictability for learning (Kleinert et al., 2009; Nash et al., 2016), continually changing the vocabulary and/or its location to support activity-specific communication may not support optimal word learning and communication development.

Value of Core Vocabulary for Individuals With Severe Intellectual and Developmental Disabilities

As described previously, core words have a high frequency of use across age groups, situations, and topic areas. This leverages the utility of context-independent words to support receptive and expressive communication across contexts, partners, purposes, and functions. It also supports a level of repetition with variety that individuals with severe intellectual and developmental disabilities require to learn in a way that promotes generalization and use (Erickson & Koppenhaver, 2020). Most proponents of core vocabulary acknowledge that it is conceptual and may therefore be more difficult to learn than concrete, fringe vocabulary (e.g., Snodgrass et al., 2013); however, the dramatic increase in opportunities for teaching and learning may counteract this, as core words can be used across contexts, purposes, and partners both in isolation and in combination (Adamson et al., 1992; Deckers et al., 2017).

Creating a Prioritized Core Vocabulary for Individuals With Severe Intellectual and Developmental Disabilities

Using core vocabulary with individuals with severe intellectual and developmental disabilities and CCN requires a process for prioritizing and selecting from the hundreds of words that comprise most core vocabulary lists. To address this need, researchers at the Center for Literacy and Disability Studies in the Department of Health Sciences in the School of Medicine at the University of North Carolina at Chapel Hill followed a process similar to the corpus search suggestions described previously. Instead of using a large corpus, the team compiled the vocabulary lists from four significant core vocabulary studies involving young children (Banajee et al., 2003; Beukelman et al., 1989; Marvin et al.,1994; Trembath et al., 2007). Then, they cataloged the core vocabulary words used in commercially available AAC systems (i.e., various versions of Gateway [Communication

Technology Resources], GoTalk [Attainment Company], TouchChat [PRC-Saltillo Corporation], and Word Power [Dynavox Mayer-Johnson]), by school systems (e.g., Oakland School District in Michigan), and AAC specialists (e.g., Gail Van Tatenhove). This resulted in a list of 394 unique lemmas.

After the list was compiled, a score was created reflecting the number of lists that included each word (the maximum score was 23). This count helped to prioritize the 394 words such that those that occurred regularly across the 23 sources had a higher count than those that occurred only on one or two of the sources. Additionally, the U-score was determined for each word. A U-score reflects the frequency and dispersion of words in written English (Zeno et al., 1995). As such, it provides an indicator of the relative importance of each word in academic contexts. Given the language and literacy abilities of individuals with severe intellectual and developmental disabilities and CCN (Erickson & Geist, 2016), U-scores were determined for written text only at the elementary level.

To further address the needs of school-aged individuals with severe intellectual and developmental disabilities and CCN, the expressive communication demands of college and career readiness standards in use in states across the United States were determined. Specifically, the words in the college and career readiness standards in English language arts and mathematics that are specifically called out as words students need to say were identified. This was accomplished by examining each standard, grade K-12, and highlighting words (e.g., "who," "what," "when," "where") or word classes (e.g., plural nouns, irregular past tense, question words, prepositions) that were explicitly called out.

Many of the specific words called out already appeared in the list of 394 core words. Those that were not already on the list were added. The classes of words called out represent either open- or closed-sets. Open-set categories of words are large, which makes it impossible to identify appropriate individual words (e.g., nouns and verbs). Closed-set categories of words are limited in size, and the specific words that compose this set can be identified (e.g., pronouns or prepositions) or the morphemes that mark them can be identified (e.g., plural -*s* and -*es*). Words that were specified within closed-sets were added to the core vocabulary list. A total of 202 words were added to the list either because they were called out explicitly or were members of a closed set.

The open-set categories, as well as other expressive language demands of college and career readiness standards, were then operationally defined (Table 12-4). Each of the words in the vocabulary list (596 words combining the initial core list and the additional words extracted from the standards) was then coded to indicate which of the 36 open-set word classes or expressive language demands the word could address. For example, each of the adjectives in the list of 596 words was given a score of 1 because it met the open-class category of adjectives. Some adjectives received an additional score of 1 because they were also opposite pairs (e.g., "big" and "little"), which is another expressive language demand of

Table 12-4
Open- and Closed-Set Word Categories

CATEGORIES	DESCRIPTION OF WORDS IN CATEGORY	EXCEPTIONS
Ask questions	*Wh-* question words (e.g., "who," "what," "where," "why," "when," and "how")	Auxiliary verbs and modals excluded because they do not have meaning as single words
Define author/illustrator	Pronouns, verbs, and nouns (e.g., "story," "picture")	The verb "take" excluded because it must be used with an object (e.g., "those" or "pictures") to indicate photographic illustrations
Describe	Adjectives, adverbs, and number words	Adverbs, such as "really," "very," and "too," were excluded
Compare/contrast	Pronouns, nouns (e.g., "dog," "cat"), descriptors, prepositions (e.g., "in," "out"), verbs with a counterpart that is opposite, and the word "not" for broad application	
Opinion	Adjectives, adverbs, verbs	Excluded all pronouns or nouns
Request clarification	Question words, verbs (e.g., "help," "like"), and repetition (e.g., "again," "more")	
Pronouns	Closed set	
Feelings	Emotional states and physical states	Excluded adverbs, such as "so," "very," "really," and "too"
Verbs	Verbs that appear on the top 1,000 verbs in English list (Talk English, n.d.a)	
Nouns	Nouns that appear on the top 1,500 nouns in English list (Talk English, n.d.b)	
Regular plurals	Closed set	
Prepositions	Single-word prepositions (O'Brien, 2020)	"Next" and "because" excluded because they must be combined with other words to be prepositions (e.g., "next to," "because of")
Antonyms	Both words in antonym pairs must be represented in the list	
Possessive pronouns	Closed set	
Conjunctions	Single-word conjunctions	Excluded "either" and "neither" because both must be used with "or"/"nor"
Determiners	Closed set	
Sequences	Prepositions (e.g., "before," "after"), adverbs (e.g., "then," "next"), and numbers (e.g., "first," "fourth"); included numbers 1, 2, 3, etc., and completion words, such as "finished," "done," and "over"	

(continued)

TABLE 12-4 (CONTINUED)

Open- and Closed-Set Word Categories

CATEGORIES	DESCRIPTION OF WORDS IN CATEGORY	EXCEPTIONS
Collective nouns	Closed set	
Irregular plurals	Closed set	
Reflexive pronouns	Closed set	
Irregular past tense	Irregular past-tense verbs that appear on the 50 most common irregular verbs in English list (ESL Lounge, 2020)	
Adverbs	Adverbs that appear on the top 250 adverbs in English list (Talk English, n.d.c)	
Text parts	Included words, such as "chapter," "title," "cover," "paragraph," and parts of a story (e.g., "characters," "plot") or book (e.g., "table") and paper (i.e., "what someone wrote")	Excluded text-type descriptors, such as "fiction," "real," and "pretend"
Time	Prepositions, numbers, adverbs (e.g., "when"), nouns (e.g., "day," "today"), numbers (e.g., "1," "2," "3")	
Cause and effect	Conjunctions, prepositions, adverbs (e.g., "if," "then," "before," "after," "because," "since," "so"), and the specific words "problem," "cause," and "effect"	
Abstract nouns	Closed set	
Future tense	Closed set	
Comparative/superlative	Closed set	
Coordinating/subordinating conjunctions	Closed set	
Measurable attributes	Terms representing dimension, length, long, light, around, high, and measurement (e.g., "inches," "feet")	
Progressive verb tenses	Past, present, and future progressive verb tenses (Note: words are not meaningful as single words given that all progressive tense verbs require word combinations)	Excluded present-perfect progressive, past-perfect progressive, or future-perfect progressive because they must all be combined with "been"
Modal auxiliaries	Closed set	
Correlative conjunctions	Closed set	
Shapes	The names of shapes (e.g., "circle," "square," "triangle")	
Describe angles, shapes, figures, and dimensions	Adjectives, numerals, some prepositions (e.g., "in," "out," "on," "beside")	
Rhyming words	Any pair or more of rhyming words in the entire list	

college and career readiness standards. This scoring provided an important basis upon which the 596 could be weighted for eventual inclusion in vocabulary sets of different sizes.

Weighting the Core Vocabulary Scores

The previously described process resulted in a list of 596 words. Each of the words received a score on the following indices: number of the 23 core vocabulary lists on which the word appeared, U-score, number of closed-sets the word addresses, and number of open-sets and other expressive language demands the word addresses. Summing these raw scores did not adequately reflect the relative importance of each word. For example, the U-scores for words on the list ranged from below 1 to 52,474 as a result of Zipf's Law (Zipf, 1936) and the fact that words, such as "congruent," appear very infrequently in elementary-level written text, and words, such as "the," appear very frequently across all texts. To address this, each of the indices was weighted in order to calculate a composite score of the relative importance of each word included in the total set.

Weighting of AAC Scores. Each word received a score that reflected the total number of the 23 core vocabulary lists on which it appeared. This raw count was multiplied by 10 to make sure the utility of the word in face-to-face communication was given significant weight in determining the relative importance of the word.

Weighting of U-Scores. This measure of frequency and dispersion in written English has a huge range with very few words in the entire corpus of written English having a U-score of 1,000 or more. The weighting system for U-scores was determined based on the U-scores that corresponded with the first 100, 500, and 1,000 most frequent and disperse words. A weighted U-score of 10 was given to words in the 100 most frequent and disperse words in written English. A weighted U-score of 5 was given to words in the 200 to 500 most frequent and disperse words in written English. A weighted U-score of 3 was given to words in the 600 to 1,000 most frequent and disperse words in written English. No words on the list appeared outside of the 1,000 most frequent and disperse list.

Weighting of Open-Class and Category Scores. Category scores were weighted based on the percent of words in the overall list that could be used to address an open class or category. In order to ensure that the selection of words had maximal representation from the range of open classes and categories required by college and career readiness standards, higher weighting was ascribed to the words in classes or categories that had fewer exemplars. For example, in the entire list of 596 words, there are 222 words (37%) in the noun open class but only one that is in the collective noun class. This means that the single collective noun, "school" as in a "school of fish," needs a higher weight than any one of the 222 singular nouns that could be included. As a single word, "school" has a higher weight than the other 221 nouns because it is the only collective noun that students could use to express their understanding of collective nouns.

To account for the percent of the 596 words that address each open class or category, a score of 1 was assigned when 41% or more of the words could be used to meet a college and career readiness standard as called out in an open-class or language category. Scores were multiplied by 2 if 31% to 40% of the words could be used, by 3 if 21% to 30% of the words could be used, by 4 if 11% to 20% of the words could be used, and by 5 if 1% to 10% of the words could be used to meet a college and career readiness standard as called out in an open-class or language category.

Combining the Weighted Scores. Weighted scores for AAC, U-score, and open class or category were summed to create a rank score. The rank scores then served as indicators of the overall importance of each word or its priority as a word to include in supporting the expressive communication of individuals with severe intellectual disabilities and CCN, especially in the context of school.

Narrowing the List for Individuals With Severe Intellectual Disabilities and Complex Communication Needs

The major advantage of core vocabulary as an initial lexicon for individuals with severe intellectual disabilities and complex communication is the utility of the words across communication purposes and contexts. This maximizes opportunities for teaching and learning through ongoing opportunities for repetition with variety. However, this cannot be accomplished with 596 words. Instead, a smaller set of words is required. To address this need, the team at the Center for Literacy and Disabilities set out to identify a small set of words from the prioritized list that was large enough to allow adults to demonstrate use of symbols across every interaction while maximizing repetition. Funded by the U.S. Department of Education, the team selected the words as part of Universal Core vocabulary that is at the center of the implementation model in Project Core (http://project-core.com). The final list of 36 words (Table 12-5) was selected because they met the following criteria:

- They are meaningful as single words
- They can be combined meaningfully
- They are useful across environments, activities, and interactions

The 36 words in the Universal Core vocabulary are only a starting place for students who benefit from a smaller set of symbols to support their initial learning. As students begin using the Universal Core, it is critical to build on those words and move to a robust, comprehensive AAC system. In Project Core, this shift from a focus on maximizing teaching and learning opportunities using the Universal Core to an emphasis on teaching more robust solutions is supported through partnerships with developers and manufactures of SGDs and communication apps (see http://www.project-core.com/app-and-sgd-product-keys/). These supports range from documents that describe where the Universal Core vocabulary is located in various SGDs and apps to specific sets of

TABLE 12-5

The Universal Core Vocabulary in Alphabetic Order

all	can	different	do	finished	get
go	good	he	help	here	I
in	it	like	look	make	more
not	on	open	put	same	she
some	stop	that	turn	up	want
what	when	where	who	why	you

dynamic pages that feature the Universal Core vocabulary with all other vocabulary initially masked and options to unmask as students begin to communicate in increasingly sophisticated ways.

Implementing the Universal Core Vocabulary With Individuals With Severe Intellectual and Developmental Disabilities

Selecting the words to include in an initial vocabulary set is just the first step in teaching flexible symbolic communication to individuals with severe intellectual and developmental disabilities. Identifying the Universal Core vocabulary was just one part of the comprehensive implementation model built by the team at the Center for Literacy and Disability Studies. In addition to providing a robust initial set through the Universal Core vocabulary, the team identified a set of evidence-based practices to support instruction targeting its use. These practices include providing ongoing, personal access to aided AAC (Douglas et al., 2012; Ganz et al., 2012; Holyfield et al., 2017; Romski et al., 2015; Schlosser & Lee, 2000), identifying and attributing meaning to early behaviors (Beukelman & Mirenda, 2013; Cress et al., 2007; Rowland, 2011b; Smith et al., 2016; Yoder et al., 2001), providing aided language input (O'Neill et al., 2018; Sennott et al., 2016) without an expectation for immediate imitation, output, or expression (Smith et al., 2016), and teaching in naturalistic environments and routines (Cowan & Allen, 2007; Pindiprolu, 2012; Romski & Sevcik, 1996; Woods et al., 2004; Yoder et al., 1991). Combining the high-frequency, flexible vocabulary in the Universal Core with these practices is helping individuals with severe intellectual and developmental disabilities move to symbolic communication across purposes, contexts, and partners (Benson-Goldberg et al., 2022; Geist et al., 2021).

SUMMARY

Words play a critical role in everyday life, yet their use is often taken for granted in spoken and written communication. For individuals who use aided AAC, words can never be taken for granted, and the ways words are selected for inclusion in aided AAC systems can have a profound impact on the ease with which individuals can communicate across purposes, partners, and settings. This chapter highlights the importance of frequency of use as a key component of vocabulary selection in AAC and argues for a focus on core, rather than fringe, vocabulary. Specifically, strategies were described that employ large-scale general corpora as reference databases (e.g., Global Web-Based English and News on the Web), and a specific approach to selecting core vocabulary as an initial vocabulary set for individuals with severe intellectual and development disabilities was detailed. Regardless of the modes individuals use in aided AAC (e.g., gestures, signing systems, SGDs, or manual communication boards), vocabulary selection must allow individuals to effectively communicate to their fullest potential. While fringe vocabulary is important, especially when the words are keywords in specific contexts, it cannot match the flexibility and utility of core vocabulary in addressing the communication needs of AAC users.

STUDY QUESTIONS

1. Discuss the role of words in everyday communication across modalities.

2. Describe the difference between core, fringe, and keyword vocabulary in the context of AAC.

3. Discuss large-scale reference corpora and how they can be useful in vocabulary selection.

4. Describe two or more vocabulary selection sources.

5. Explain the role of morphology in communication and the ways AAC users can access morphology to support their communication.

6. Discuss the pros and cons of using core vocabulary as an initial vocabulary set with individuals with intellectual and developmental disabilities.

13

The Process of Symbol Selection

Donna R. Brooks, PhD
and Donald R. Fuller, PhD

MYTH

1. If clinicians/educators have the most common aided and unaided symbols at their disposal, the communication needs of all augmentative and alternative communication (AAC) users will be met.

2. Symbol selection is a simple process. Just determine the AAC user's vocabulary needs, then find an aided or unaided symbol to match each vocabulary word.

3. It is best to choose all symbols from the same aided or unaided symbol corpus. Similarly, it is best to choose symbols from only the aided or unaided domain for any given individual (i.e., aided and unaided symbols should not be combined in the same AAC system).

REALITY

1. Not all AAC symbols are created equal. Clinicians/educators should know and have at their disposal all possible aided and unaided AAC symbols. There are wide differences in the manner in which concepts are depicted by symbols and in their value for different individuals in different environments. If clinicians/educators have only a small number of symbols from which to choose, there is a great chance that the best symbols will not be chosen.

2. Symbol selection, if conducted properly, requires clinicians/educators to consider many characteristics of the user and potential symbols. The symbols must then be closely matched to their referents and grouped in a way that facilitates acquisition and retention.

3. Whether clinicians/educators choose all symbols from within the same aided or unaided corpus is dependent upon the intended use of the AAC system. In some cases, it will be more appropriate to choose symbols from a variety of aided and/or unaided corpuses. A truly effective AAC system most likely will contain both aided and unaided symbols.

Fuller, D. R., & Lloyd, L. L. *Principles and Practices in Augmentative and Alternative Communication* (pp. 245-257).
© 2023 Taylor & Francis Group.

TABLE 13-1
AAC Symbol Selection Considerations

CATEGORY	CONSIDERATIONS
User	Abilities and limitations
	Preference
	Experiential and cultural background
Acceptability	Cosmesis or aesthetic quality
	Perceived difficulty or complexity
	Previous intervention outcomes
	Correspondence to the language of the general community
Use	Accessibility
	Display permanence and reproducibility
	Durability and portability
Vocabulary	Initial vocabulary size
	Expansion capability
Intelligibility	Intelligibility of synthetic speech
	Symbol iconicity
Linguistic	Degree of inherent linguistic structure
	Correspondence to oral and written language
	Development of literacy
Interaction	Assertiveness
	Active participation
	Face-to-face and text interactions
	Projectability
	Facilitation of independence
Efficiency	Overall corpus efficiency
	Rate of communication
Audience	Potential communication partners
Teaching and learning	Adaptability to the educational environment
	Ease of teaching and learning

PHASE I: GENERAL AAC SYMBOL SELECTION CONSIDERATIONS

A primary principle all service providers should know is all symbols are not created equal. What may be an excellent selection of symbols for one individual in one situation may be a poor selection for another individual in the same situation. Alternatively, what may be an excellent selection of symbols for one individual in one situation may be a poor selection for the same individual in a different situation. Therefore,

the practitioner's selection of symbols should always focus on the individual user and that user's unique situation. Armed with the knowledge of available symbols, clinicians and educators turn their attention to the selection process.

Over the years, several guiding principles have been suggested to assist service providers in selecting AAC symbols for potential users. These guiding principles have come primarily from practicing clinicians and service providers with a smaller number of principles coming from empirical research. Collectively, these principles have been referred to as selection considerations, and they govern the choice of assistive technology and symbols.

Variables to Consider

Several symbol selection considerations have been presented over the past few decades (Goodenough-Trepagnier, 1981; Jones & Cregan, 1986; Kiernan et al., 1982; Lloyd & Karlan, 1983, 1984; Musselwhite, 1982; Musselwhite & St. Louis, 1988; Nietupski & Hamre-Nietupski, 1979; Shin & Park, 2022; Silverman, 1995; Vanderheiden & Harris-Vanderheiden, 1976; Vanderheiden & Lloyd, 1986; Yoder, 1980). Some of these considerations have focused on the characteristics of potential AAC users, whereas others have dealt with the characteristics of symbols, and yet, other considerations are relevant to clinical and/or educational environments. A discussion of symbol selection considerations can be aided by grouping them into ten major categories:

1. User
2. Acceptability
3. Use
4. Vocabulary
5. Intelligibility
6. Linguistic
7. Interaction
8. Efficiency
9. Audience
10. Teaching and learning

These categories and their pertinent selection considerations are listed in Table 13-1.

In the following sections, different symbol selection considerations are defined and discussed followed by suggestions for rating symbols with a few aided and unaided symbol types used for comparison. The second major section of this chapter discusses phase II of the symbol selection process: selecting specific symbols and teaching considerations.

User Considerations

User considerations pertain to the individual who will be using symbols as a means of communicating messages. These characteristics may be the most important ones of all and include the individual's abilities and limitations, preferences, and experiential and cultural background.

Abilities and Limitations

Service providers must consider variables relative to the cognitive, physical, and sensory abilities of the potential AAC user. Type and severity of impairment(s) are two important variables to consider in selecting AAC symbols. The demands different symbols place on an individual's auditory, cognitive, memory, motor, receptive language, tactile, and visual skills vary widely and must be matched with individual abilities.

A potential AAC user's abilities and limitations must be thoroughly assessed. Service providers must be careful not to overgeneralize the limitations of a condition and rule out specific symbols prematurely because it first appears that they may not be the best choice. For example, Blischak and Lloyd (1996) described a young woman with hearing impairment who, despite sensory and physical impairments, developed some competency using manual signs as part of her multimodal communication system.

Bates and Macleod (2017) discussed assessing the use of AAC with children with movement disorders. They noted vision as one factor to consider. In evaluating an individual's visual abilities and limitations, the clinician or educator should consider the following:

- Does the potential AAC user detect, see, and look at visual materials?
- Can the user deliberately fix and shift their gaze on the materials they are shown?

Fatigue was another area of concern for Bates and Macleod (2017), which gets to how cognitively and/or physically demanding symbols may be to the user. Additionally, a more recent study by Shin and Park (2022) indicated that the working memory of the user had a significant effect on graphic symbol selection. While the focus of the Bates and Macleod (2017) study was on assessment, it is equally important to consider a potential AAC user's abilities and limitations in the context of symbol selection, as these will likely assist the clinician/service provider in determining which symbol sets and/or systems are the most appropriate and effective for their clients or patients.

Preference

Service providers must also consider the potential AAC user's preferences for expressive modality and symbols to the extent possible. No matter how effective service providers think a set of symbols may be or their potential benefit in meeting the user's needs, if the AAC user does not like or want the symbols, they may be of little use.

Experiential and Cultural Background

Service providers must also get to know potential users well enough to learn about their experiential and cultural background so appropriate symbols can be selected (Fannin, 2016). For example, a symbol depicting a cow being milked may be an inappropriate symbol for "milk" if the user's only reference to milk is a carton or glass of white liquid.

Cultural background is also important. DeKlerk and colleagues (2014) found that children from different language groups in South Africa may not perceive graphic symbols the same way. Nigam and Karlan (1994) conducted a cross-cultural validation study of Picture Communication Symbols (PCS) with Asian-Indian individuals. Their findings indicated that not all PCS were appropriate for referents in the culture studied. This would seem to indicate culturally relevant depictions of vocabulary are needed to increase communicative success. Soto and Yu (2014) noted irrelevant vocabulary and culturally inappropriate symbols and messages may be barriers to family buy-in. To address this problem, Mindel and John (2018) suggest setting up AAC systems to facilitate code-switching between different environments (e.g., the AAC user's school and home). Essentially, increased use in one environment will usually generalize to increased use in the other. While service providers must understand the culture of potential users to select the most appropriate symbols for them, there continues to be a need for more research to support vocabulary selection frameworks for culturally and linguistically diverse populations (Mindel & John, 2018).

Acceptability Considerations

Service providers need to assess the acceptability of the symbols to the potential user, individuals close to the user (e.g., caregivers, peers), and other communication partners in the general community. Spoken language is commonly accepted and rewarded in the general community, and therefore, is the standard by which other symbols are compared. Individuals who do not have functional speech to communicate rely on AAC systems that may or may not be accepted when compared to the benchmark of spoken communication. In the following sections, acceptability will be discussed in relation to cosmesis or aesthetic quality, perceived difficulty or complexity, previous intervention outcomes, and correspondence to the language of the general community.

Cosmesis or Aesthetic Quality

Cosmesis or the aesthetic quality of an AAC system is usually in reference to the aid or device being used to transmit messages (e.g., a communication board, E-TRAN board, or speech-generating device [SGD]) than to symbols themselves. However, symbols do have some degree of aesthetic appeal. Some symbols may be more visually or psychologically appealing than others due to such factors as design, use of color, amount of detail, and figure-ground differential. What is aesthetically appealing to one individual may not be to another. Therefore, it is important that the symbols chosen are aesthetically appealing to the user. Less important—but important nonetheless—is that the symbols chosen are also aesthetically appealing to communication partners. It is important that service providers remember that cosmesis or aesthetic quality of symbols is in the eye of the beholder.

Perceived Difficulty or Complexity

Variables other than cosmesis may also influence acceptability. One is the perceived difficulty or complexity of symbols. For example, McNaughton and Kates (1980) found that acceptability of Blissymbols is generally low because many people who are introduced to the system perceive it initially as being complicated. However, once the system is understood, it may become more acceptable.

Previous Intervention Outcomes

Another variable that may influence acceptability is the experience of the AAC user and/or caregivers with prior intervention outcomes. Previously failed attempts at using AAC may adversely affect acceptability of a newly introduced symbol corpus. In an anecdotal report, Reuss (1991) noted that the parents of her student with physical disabilities viewed the introduction of Blissymbols as just another approach that would probably be unsuccessful in improving their daughter's life. Although Blissymbols (or any other symbol corpus, for that matter) may have been an excellent choice for this child, due to past failed intervention attempts, her parents' perceptions may have been adversely affected. Therefore, it is important that clinicians, educators, and other practitioners are cognizant of previous intervention attempts so they can work to alleviate any negative beliefs or perceptions on the part of the potential AAC user or significant others in their life.

Correspondence to the Language of the General Community

Finally, acceptability may be influenced by the degree of connection to the community language. As more and more AAC users move to less restrictive environments, the acceptability of symbols by general education classroom teachers, employers, and the community at large becomes increasingly important. Symbols that more closely match the community language (e.g., traditional orthography–based systems, synthetic speech) or symbols that can be readily adapted to the community language (e.g., Blissymbols, manually coded English [MCE]) may be more acceptable than symbols that are not as closely matched to the community language (e.g., objects, photographs and pictures, American Indian Hand Talk). Although graphic symbols typically are accompanied by their meanings spelled out in traditional orthography, accessible vocabulary may not be sufficiently robust to allow the individual to generate messages as grammatically complete as the language used in the general community. For persons who rely on AAC and are literate, this shortcoming may in some way affect their perception of the symbols used with their AAC system.

Use Considerations

"Use" refers to the characteristics of symbols that affect how effectively and efficiently they are used by the individual with complex communication needs (CCN). These include such considerations as accessibility, display permanence and reproducibility, and durability and portability.

Accessibility

Accessibility refers to how easy it is to access symbols for message transmission. This characteristic may not be as directly relevant to symbols as to the aids or devices that are used to transmit messages. In general, aided symbols tend to be less readily accessible than unaided symbols because the user of aided symbols must access them through a device or display that is external to the user's body. Unaided symbols, on the other hand, require only parts of the user's body for message transmission. With unaided symbols, the ability to access symbols is governed to a large extent by the individual's motor skills. Motor skills are also necessary to access aided symbols on a display, and the display must be with the AAC user at all times.

Display Permanence and Reproducibility

Display permanence and reproducibility are more specifically related to AAC symbols. Display permanence refers to whether a symbol is visually permanent and enduring vs. dynamic and temporary. Reproducibility is defined as the ease with which a symbol can be copied or drawn in the immediate clinical or educational environment. These two variables are related to each other in that permanent and enduring symbols generally are easier to reproduce. Most aided symbol corpuses are graphic, and therefore, permanent. Symbols with greater display permanence place fewer demands on a user's recall memory. On the other hand, unaided symbols are predominantly dynamic, and therefore, are nonpermanent and more difficult to reproduce. They also tend to place a greater demand on recall memory.

Durability and Portability

Durability and portability are more relevant to the AAC displays or devices but apply to symbols as well. Because aided symbols are used with communication aids, their durability and portability are affected by the devices that house them. Aided symbols, such as objects, have the risk of being misplaced or lost and even graphic symbols displayed in calendar boxes or communication vests can be lost, torn, or otherwise damaged. By contrast, since they are produced using body parts, unaided symbols are easily portable and are as durable as the individual's body.

Vocabulary Considerations

Vocabulary variables include the initial size of a corpus of symbols, but more importantly, the ability (or lack thereof) to expand vocabulary beyond the initial corpus. The former is applicable to all persons who must rely on AAC symbols to communicate while the latter pertains more specifically to persons with CCN who are literate, and therefore, possess the ability to use the full depth and breadth of language.

Initial Vocabulary Size

Aided and unaided symbol sets and systems discussed in Chapters 7 and 8 differ considerably in the numbers of symbols that comprise their initial vocabulary. Initial vocabulary size ranges from small symbol sets having only a few symbols to sophisticated corpuses having literally thousands of symbols. Obviously, symbol corpuses having a larger initial vocabulary from which to choose are preferred for persons who have the potential to communicate abstract, as well as concrete, ideas. Larger vocabularies represent a wide range of concepts, from objects to feelings to action words, and in some cases, function words (e.g., articles, conjunctions, prepositions). Symbol systems tend to have a larger initial vocabulary size than symbol sets, although this is not always the case. For example, PCS is classified as a pre-linguistic symbol set, yet it consists of 37,000 symbols representing over 40 different languages.

Expansion Capability

What separates symbol sets from symbol systems is not the size of the initial vocabulary but the fact that symbol systems have an internal logic (i.e., generative rules) that allow for expansion capability. A symbol collection or set, by comparison, does not have logic or rules for expansion beyond the original corpus. Across the domains of aided and unaided symbols, one can see varying degrees of logic and expansion capability. The reader is referred to Figure 3-5 in Chapter 3. Systems with expansion capability allow the clinician or educator to create symbols beyond the initial corpus, thereby increasing vocabulary size. An increase in vocabulary size tends to result in good to excellent representational range (i.e., representation of abstract, as well as concrete, ideas and most, to all, parts of speech). With symbol corpuses having excellent expansion capability, the end user is able to utilize the full power of language.

At least for aided symbols, in many cases, AAC users' available vocabulary is not limited exclusively by the number of symbols at their disposal but rather by limitations imposed upon them by their communication display. In such cases, symbols that represent concentrated message pools (i.e., those having a high frequency of use) should be displayed first, with symbols that represent special messages being added as needed (Goossens' et al., 1992). Quick and colleagues (2019) add to this belief by showing there is a common set of words frequently used by mothers in the daily interactions with infants and toddlers, and these same words make up a large proportion of the words frequently used by young children.

Intelligibility Considerations

Intelligibility is a term that is synonymous with iconicity, although it does not pertain exclusively to symbols and referents. When used synonymously with iconicity, intelligibility is the visual relationship symbols have to their referents (i.e., the things or ideas being represented by symbols). A second definition of intelligibility is the degree to which an individual can understand synthesized speech. Synthesized speech that is easily comprehended is said to be intelligible; poor synthetic speech quality is likely to be judged as unintelligible.

Intelligibility of Synthetic Speech

Intelligibility is discussed briefly here in relation to synthesized speech as words, phrases, sentences, and in some cases, lengthy messages may be produced via SGDs. These lower-end and typically lower-cost SGDs produce synthesized speech using text-to-speech input. The SGD user types a message and the typed letters pass through an algorithm that converts them into speech sounds. Truly synthesized speech tends to sound robotic, as it does not possess the capability of regulating pitch or prosody. Several comparative intelligibility studies were conducted in the earlier years of the field, as at that time, synthesized speech was more commonly used in SGDs than it is today. Synthetic speech output today may be digitized (i.e., digitally recorded), synthesized (i.e., using text-to-speech), or a combination of both (i.e., hybrid speech output) and is being continuously improved to the point that some synthetic speech output—digital and hybrid speech output, especially—is near-natural in terms of quality and intelligibility.

Symbol Iconicity

When used to describe symbols, intelligibility refers to the ease with which symbols are understood by AAC users and their communication partners. In the case of symbols, a more commonly used term for intelligibility is iconicity, which refers to the degree to which an individual perceives the relationship between a symbol and its referent (Bellugi & Klima, 1976; Brown, 1977, 1978). Symbol iconicity includes **transparency** and **translucency**, while the absence of iconicity is referred to as **opaqueness**. Transparent symbols are those in which the observer easily can see the relationship between symbols and their referents in the absence of the referent. In other words, for transparent symbols, referents are guessable. For example, most individuals would guess that Symbol 1 in Figure 13-1 represents "house," and indeed it does. On the other hand, some symbols are arbitrarily

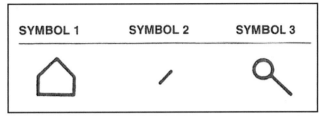

| SYMBOL 1 | SYMBOL 2 | SYMBOL 3 |

Figure 13-1. Illustrations of iconicity and opaqueness using Blissymbols as an example.

assigned to referents so that the relationship between the symbol and its referent is generally not understood even when the symbol and referent appear together. These symbols are classified as opaque. Symbol 2 in Figure 13-1 is an example of an opaque symbol that represents the article "the." Most symbols are neither transparent nor opaque and are classified as translucent. Translucent symbols may not be readily guessable like transparent symbols, but the relationship between symbols and referents is generally understood once the two appear together. Symbol 3 in Figure 13-1 is an example of a translucent symbol. Some individuals may guess that this symbol represents "lollipop," some may think it represents "tennis racket," and others may believe it represents "balloon." This symbol is not readily guessable. However, once its true meaning ("spoon") is provided, most people can understand the relationship. Intelligibility—as defined as symbol iconicity—is relevant to all aided and unaided symbols, including speech. For example, natural speech is by and large opaque. For the most part, the acoustic signal produced when a person says a word bears little relationship to the referent symbolized by that word. For example, the combination of the letters C, A, and T to form the word "cat," and the combination of speech sounds /k/, /æ/, and /t/ to produce the acoustic symbol /kæt/ bear little resemblance to the pet with pointed ears and whiskers. However, a small number of English words do sound like their referents (e.g., "cuckoo," "buzz," "hiss"). These onomatopoetic words are iconic. Other aided and unaided symbol sets and systems have varying proportions of iconic and opaque symbols.

Symbol intelligibility or iconicity applies to both AAC users and their communication partners (e.g., caregivers, peers, and the general community). Of all the symbol selection considerations discussed in this chapter, iconicity has received the most empirical attention. Fristoe and Lloyd (1979a) postulated what is commonly referred to as the iconicity hypothesis, which states that the visual representation (i.e., iconicity) afforded by some AAC symbols may facilitate the learning and memory of symbol-to-referent associations. In other words, "[i]conic symbols having a strong resemblance to their referents would be easier to learn and remember than those symbols having a weak visual relationship" (Fuller & Stratton, 1991, p. 52). Subsequently, a vast body of research predominantly has supported the iconicity hypothesis for graphic symbols (Clark, 1984; Fuller, 1988; Goossens', 1984; Hern et al., 1994; Luftig & Bersani, 1985; Mizuko, 1987; Nail-Chiwetalu, 1992; Yovetich & Paivio, 1980) and

for unaided symbols (Brown, 1977, 1978; Doherty, 1986; Goossens', 1984; Griffith, 1979; Griffith & Robinson, 1980; Konstantareas et al., 1978; Luftig & Lloyd, 1981; Mandel, 1977; Polzer et al., 1979; Snyder-McLean, 1978). This finding is consistent for children and adults having typical cognitive and physical abilities, as well as for individuals with autism and cognitive impairments (except in persons with cognitive impairments, the iconicity hypothesis is supported only when comprehension tasks instead of production tasks are considered). Nevertheless, with all other factors being equal, iconic symbols should be used, especially by individuals with cognitive impairments (Mirenda & Locke, 1989; Mizuko & Reichle, 1989). However, iconicity is in the eye of the beholder. What may be a strong visual relationship between symbol and referent for one individual may not be strong for another. Consequently, for iconicity to be used to its greatest advantage, it must be in relation to the individual who uses AAC and their communication partners, not the clinician, educator, or other practitioner.

Linguistic Considerations

Linguistic variables include the degree of inherent linguistic structure of an AAC symbol corpus, the level of correspondence to the spoken and written language of the community at large, and how well the symbols provide for the development of literacy. All these variables are related to a large degree. For example, if a symbol corpus has a strong degree of inherent linguistic structure and corresponds well to the spoken and written language of the community, it most likely will facilitate the development of literacy.

Degree of Inherent Linguistic Structure

Some aided and unaided symbol corpuses have their own unique linguistic structure; although, their structure may not be used as part of an AAC system. For example, Blissymbolics has its own syntactic structure that is not the same as the linguistic structure of English. American Sign Language (ASL; and all sign languages, for that matter) also has its own unique linguistic structure. Typically, when these symbols are used as part of an AAC system, they are simply borrowed and placed in English syntactical order. For ASL, adaptations of this nature have resulted in a number of pedagogical sign systems, such as Seeing Essential English, Signing Exact English, and Signed English. Although systems with their own unique linguistic structure may not correspond well to the spoken and written language of the larger community, they are still useful and effective in other environments.

Correspondence to Oral and Written Language

As a whole, symbols that are an analog of the community language correspond well with the spoken and written language of that community and assist in the development of literacy. Traditional orthography, fingerspelling, Morse code, and Braille are representations of the English language because they use letters or codes for letters that can be combined into English words. On the other hand, objects, simple pictures, pointing, yes/no gestures, and other simple gestures (when used as the primary means of communication) have virtually no linguistic structure, and therefore, do not have correspondence to the spoken and written language of the general community due to their limited nature.

Development of Literacy. Approximation to the spoken and/or written language of the community can be achieved through symbols representing function words or through other strategies. For example, the use of Blissymbolics has been suggested as a means to facilitate the development of literacy because some of the processes involved in the reading of written language are similar to those used in the linguistic processing of Blissymbols. Schulte-Sasse (1991) hypothesized that users of Blissymbolics may have the potential to develop a level of visual perception that is a crucial skill in the reading process. Because of the parallels between Blissymbols and written language, the use of Blissymbolics may further facilitate the development of the following skills: (a) understanding of pictographs and word pictures, (b) providing insight into the utility of language, (c) differentiating between word and object, (d) formulating of concepts and word finding, (e) utilizing segmentation in reading (e.g., semantic elements in Blissymbolics may facilitate segmentation), and (f) understanding grammatical rules that govern sentence structure. Any aided or unaided symbol system that has a large proportion of function words or that approximates the skills necessary for literacy easily may be adapted to the community language, and therefore, may benefit the development of literacy.

Interaction Considerations

Interaction variables describe the ease with which a user can communicate with others. Although the considerations included in this category may relate more to the transmission technique being used, they pertain, at least to some degree, to AAC symbols as well. These variables include assertiveness, opportunity for active participation, face-to-face and text interactions, projectability, and facilitation of independence.

Assertiveness

Assertiveness refers to the ability of the user to interrupt a communication partner, to protest about something, or to ward off interruptions from others. Although some may consider these behaviors rude, many able-bodied individuals use them in the course of typical conversations. The AAC user should be afforded the opportunity to engage in these behaviors as well by being given access to symbols conducive to these behaviors.

Opportunity for Active Participation

Opportunity for active participation refers to both AAC users and their communication partners. As a general rule, aided symbols allow for active participation because the aid or device displaying the symbols becomes the focal point of the conversation. Both user and communication partner must attend to the symbols on the aid or device for effective exchanges to take place. Ideally, conversational input from the communication partner should also occur via the user's aided symbols. This has been referred to as **augmented input** (Romski & Sevcik, 1988). When several AAC users have the opportunity to communicate with each other, interaction is promoted through use of the same symbols (Mizuko & Reichle, 1989).

Face-to-Face and Text Interactions

Face-to-face interaction is adversely affected by aided symbols as a whole because the AAC user and communication partner must attend to an aid or device during message transmission. Unaided symbols, on the other hand, allow for better face-to-face interaction between AAC users and their communication partners. There is increased recognition that communication goes well beyond face-to-face interactions (Light & McNaughton, 2012b). Communication can also occur via email, text messages, and real-time text interactions via cellphones and the internet. It is important that clinicians and educators provide opportunities for AAC users to access these communication options, as they become an essential part of daily life.

Projectabilty

Projectability is defined as the ability to communicate effectively over a distance. With the exception of synthetic speech, aided symbols tend to rate poorly on this consideration. Typically, the communication partner must be within at least 3 feet of the AAC user for effective communication to take place. Conversely, many unaided symbols can be projected over fairly long distances. This is especially true of unaided symbols that use a fairly large **sign space** (e.g., American Indian Hand Talk, some manual signs, and pantomime). Unaided symbols that have a more restricted production space (e.g., fingerspelling, hand-cued speech) are not as easily projectable.

Facilitation of Independence

Facilitation of independence only partially depends on the specific symbols being used. It is more related to the type of aid or device that houses aided symbols, the method of access, and the motor abilities of the potential user. Generally speaking, aided or unaided symbols that are idiosyncratic or arbitrary may require an assistant or aide to decipher the user's messages. This in turn inhibits independence and may lead to the abandonment of an AAC system.

Efficiency Considerations

The efficiency of AAC symbols in communicating a message is determined by overall symbol corpus efficacy and rate of communication. Efficiency considerations are related to some degree to the vocabulary and linguistic considerations discussed earlier in this chapter.

Overall Symbol Corpus Efficiency

Overall symbol corpus efficiency is evaluated by the relationship between symbols and the messages they convey. Blissymbols, PICSYMS, Sigsymbols, manual signs from ASL, and pedagogical sign systems tend to have high overall efficiency. These transitionary and linguistic symbol systems tend to have a one-to-one relationship between symbols and concepts (i.e., a single symbol represents a concept or word). Aided and unaided symbol systems that have a less than one-to-one relationship are less efficient. For example, all systems based on traditional orthography (e.g., Braille, fingerspelling, Morse code) require the user to combine alphabetic letters or other representations of alphabetic letters to form words. If words must be spelled individually, then the user must engage in many activations to produce single words, thus reducing efficiency. For example, fingerspelling of Y-E-S-T-E-R-D-A-Y involves the production of nine symbols to convey that single concept.

Rate of Communication

Rate of communication refers to the speed of message transmission. Because natural speech is the standard by which all other symbols are compared, having a rate of communication that approximates that of spoken communication is desirable. Examples of AAC symbols that can accomplish this are ASL, MCE, Tadoma, and hand-cued speech. However, a high degree of proficiency is required to approximate the rate of natural speech. Although producing manual signs takes more time than producing the acoustic symbols of natural speech, ASL has much less redundancy than spoken English. In some cases, expression in ASL can convey the same amount of information more quickly than a spoken phrase. The net effect is that identical messages in ASL and natural speech tend to be transmitted at a comparable rate. Proficient users of MCE, Tadoma, and hand-cued speech (which make natural speech more visual and/or tactile) also can communicate at a rate that approaches natural speech. Digitized and synthesized speech are capable of approximating the rate of natural speech, but a user may only be able to produce about two to five words per minute due to motor impairment.

Aided symbols are typically more slowly transmitted than unaided symbols because a selection technique must be used (e.g., direct selection, scanning). When feasible, it may be advantageous to use the same symbol type across non–speech-generating and speech-generating applications. AAC users should have access to the most flexible and efficient symbol types that meet their needs (Silverman, 1995). Additionally, the findings of Perrin and colleagues (2017) suggest symbol location within an AAC device and individual cognitive abilities influence the speed and accuracy of retrieving symbols.

Audience Considerations

Audience refers to the number of potential communication partners who are available to a person using AAC. Symbols that are equivalent to or closely approximate the community language allow for a large number of potential communication partners. As a whole, aided symbols provide for a relatively large potential audience because the gloss (i.e., the written word depicted by a symbol) is typically displayed with the symbol. Most aided symbols also tend to be relatively iconic, so that even if potential partners cannot read, they still may be able to understand symbols' meanings. On the other hand, unaided symbols are generally limiting because most have to be learned by communication partners. Potential audience is affected by the knowledge members of the community have of different symbol corpuses. A person who uses ASL or manual signs from ASL may have a relatively small potential audience within the community at large but a relatively large potential audience within the Deaf community.

Teaching and Learning Considerations

Teaching and learning considerations relate to whether the symbols are adaptable to the educational setting, as well as their ease of teaching and learning. These considerations may be dependent on many of the other categories of considerations, such as audience, efficiency, intelligibility, interaction, linguistic, use, and user.

Adaptability to the Educational Environment

Adaptability to the educational environment depends on several factors:

- The degree to which symbols approximate the language being used in the educational setting
- The capability of the user to convey abstract, as well as concrete, ideas through the use of symbols
- The degree to which symbols facilitate user independence
- The ease with which symbols can be reproduced or generated

Symbols that are analogs of the English alphabet may be the most easily adaptable to the educational setting. These include Braille, digitized and synthesized speech, expanded rebus symbols (to a certain extent), and Morse code. Other symbol sets and systems that may be readily adapted to the community language (e.g., Blissymbols, hand-cued speech, pedagogical sign systems, PICSYMS, Sigsymbols) may also be adaptable to the educational setting. Symbols that are easily reproducible on the spot (e.g., Cyberglyphs, PICSYMS,

Sigsymbols) also have an advantage over those that are not. More powerful aided and unaided symbol systems will also allow the individual to express a wide range of ideas, thereby enhancing independence. Independence is also enhanced when symbols are easily understood and do not require an aide or interpreter.

Ease of Learning and Teaching

Ease of learning and teaching are interdependent variables (Hooper & Lloyd, 1986; Hurlbut et al., 1982; Raghavendra & Fristoe, 1990; Schlosser & Lloyd, 1993; Schlosser et al., 1991). By having strong visual relationships to their referents, iconic symbols are easier to acquire and retain. One could then argue that iconic symbols should be taught first. However, the manner in which symbols are taught may be just as important (Hooper & Lloyd, 1986; Hurlbut et al., 1982; McNaughton & Warrick, 1984; Quist & Lloyd, 1990; Raghavendra & Fristoe, 1990; Schlosser, 1995; Schlosser & Lloyd, 1993; Schlosser et al., 1991). Light and McNaughton (2012a) called for greater focus on research to investigate the most appropriate symbols for young children, not simply to determine whether children can learn AAC symbols but what types of symbols are most readily acquired. Caron and colleagues (2020) concluded the effects of software features, such as dynamic text and speech output upon selection of a graphic symbol within a display grid, were positive. Carter and Hartley (2021) demonstrated children with autism spectrum disorder benefitted from greater iconicity when learning words from color pictures. However, at present, there is not a solid research base from which to draw conclusions regarding the manner and ease of teaching, but one can deduce that at least some of the considerations related to learning apply equally to pedagogical strategies and ease of teaching.

Several cross-symbol set and system comparisons have been made regarding the ease of learning of various aided symbols. In order of most to least difficult to learn, the general trend appears to be traditional orthography, Blissymbols, rebus symbols, Pictograms, PICSYMS, and PCS (Briggs, 1983; Burroughs et al., 1990; Clark, 1977, 1981; Clark et al., 1974; Ecklund & Reichle, 1987; Goossens', 1984; Hughes, 1979; Hurlbut et al., 1982; Kuntz, 1975; Leonhart & Maharaj, 1979; Mizuko, 1987; Romski et al., 1985; Woodcock, 1968). However, this observation should be viewed with caution because it is based on studies that predominantly explored short-term learning and recall of aided symbols. Retention and generalization of symbols were not addressed. Studies related to the ease of learning of unaided symbols have not been conducted.

Comparing Aided and Unaided AAC Symbols

Symbol selection requires that clinicians and educators know about available aided and unaided symbols. Through the use of the selection considerations just described, clinicians, educators, and other service providers can evaluate systematically a wide range of aided and unaided symbols to determine which ones are most suitable for inclusion in AAC systems for specific users. General comparisons can be made between and among symbol types with more in-depth analysis being conducted according to characteristics of the user.

Natural Speech Is the Gold Standard

Natural speech is the standard by which all other symbols are compared. However, shortcomings of natural speech are its lack of display permanence, reproducibility, and iconicity. Synthetic speech closely approximates natural speech, except that accessibility, durability, and portability are not rated as highly as natural speech. These variables depend to a large extent on the SGD that houses synthetic speech, and more specifically, the means by which symbols are accessed on an SGD. As a general rule, unaided symbols have greater capacity for more closely approximating the rate of natural speech than aided symbols.

Use of Feature Matching to Make Judgments

In determining the best symbols to use for a given client or patient, clinicians and service providers can use a rating system based on research, clinical judgment, and intuition (an example of a feature matching approach). For example, a simple three-point rating scale (e.g., poor, fair, good) or a more elaborate five-point scale can be used to describe the degree to which each symbol type meets the selection considerations discussed in this chapter. User and acceptability considerations that relate more to users' abilities and personal preferences than to symbol characteristics are critical considerations for making in-depth analyses and judgments regarding which symbols to choose for specific AAC users. Ratings of the other selection considerations are helpful in making general comparisons.

To support this concept, Groba and colleagues (2021) conducted a study that resulted in a guide with suggestions to support an AAC design that emerges from the user's perspective and facilitates the understanding of the user's daily life. Rating symbols allows clinicians, educators, and other practitioners to make gross judgments about particular AAC symbols based on how they compare with one another and how closely they compare with the gold standard of natural speech. Effective judgments can be made only when the user is placed in the center of the decision-making process. By taking user characteristics and acceptability variables into consideration, clinicians and educators will be able to refine their general judgments concerning symbols, thus focusing on the type of symbols that would be most appropriate. Once a decision has been made as to which symbols (aided and/or unaided) are best for inclusion in an AAC system, clinicians and educators are ready to enter phase II of the symbol selection process.

Phase II: Selecting Specific Symbols and Teaching Considerations

One of the first decisions to be made with an individual who is being provided symbols for the first time relates to the purpose of AAC, because the purpose to some extent governs the symbols used. Will AAC serve only as a means of here and now communication, or should it also provide powerful language that can serve as a bridge to literacy? Should the AAC symbols include an eclectic blend from several symbol corpuses (e.g., will manual signs be used in conjunction with graphic symbols)? If the purpose is to provide a means of immediate communication without regard to language or literacy, a more eclectic approach to symbol selection may be desirable. That is, it is often advantageous to select symbols from a variety of aided and/or unaided sets and systems. However, if the user has the capability to learn language and/or develop literacy, symbols from a single transitionary or linguistic symbol system may be preferred for consistency and for the capacity to generate sentences. Selecting symbols from specific aided and unaided corpuses (e.g., exclusively Sigsymbols or Signed English) may be more appropriate than selecting symbols from several differing symbol corpuses. If the user is already using symbols in the school and/or other environments, the symbols should be retained whenever possible. If the goal is to update or expand vocabulary, the decision becomes whether to continue using symbols from the AAC user's established corpus or to select symbols from other sets and/or systems. Once again, knowing the purpose for AAC can guide clinicians, educators, and service providers in determining which symbols may be most appropriate.

Choosing Symbols to Represent Vocabulary

The remainder of this chapter describes a process by which symbols can be selected for specific vocabulary and how they can be arranged to maximize the possibility for immediately successful communication. This section assumes AAC will serve only as a means of communication without regard to language learning or literacy. This assumption allows the clinician or service provider to use symbols drawn from several symbol corpuses. The following exercise illustrates the appropriateness of taking an eclectic approach by choosing symbols from more than one collection, set, and/or system when the goal of intervention is to provide a means of communication for an individual without regard to language and literacy.

Refer back to Chapter 7 and note how a number of different concepts are depicted in various aided symbol corpuses by studying the following figures:

- Figure 7-2: Microsoft ClipArt
- Figure 7-4: Emojis
- Figure 7-11: Imagine symbols
- Figure 7-13: Mulberry Symbols
- Figure 7-15: ParticiPic symbols
- Figure 7-16: Pics for Picture Exchange Communication System symbols
- Figure 7-17: Pictograms
- Figure 7-19: SymbolStix symbols
- Figure 7-20: Talking Mats symbols
- Figure 7-21: Makaton graphic symbols
- Figure 7-22: PCS (Classic symbols)
- Figure 7-23: PCS (ThinLine symbols)
- Figure 7-24: PCS (High Contrast symbols)
- Figure 7-26: Widgit Symbols

Pay particular attention to how each of these corpuses depicts the concepts "mother" (which appears in all listed corpuses), "angry" (in all listed corpuses, except Widgit Symbols), "yes" (in all listed corpuses, except Pics for Picture Exchange Communication System symbols), and "want" (in all listed corpuses, except Imagine and Talking Mats symbols). It is the authors' intent to drive home two points about symbol selection. The first point can be realized by the reader alone. The second point requires a number of classmates or colleagues—at least one but even more will drive the point home even more effectively.

The first point is that for any given individual (*you*, for example), chances are good that the same symbol corpus was not selected for all four concepts: "mother," "angry," "yes," and "want." Instead, symbols were probably chosen from two or more of the available corpuses. Indeed, for some individuals, the choice of symbol to represent each of the four concepts came from a different corpus! The lesson here is *no single symbol corpus possesses the best representation of all concepts.* This is equally true for unaided symbols as for aided symbols.

To drive home the second point, find at least one—and better yet, a few—classmates or colleagues and have them join you in the exercise described before. If a number of people were asked to perform the same task previously described, it is doubtful the entire group would agree which symbols best depict the various concepts. Not only would each person in the group likely choose representations of "mother," "angry," "yes," and "want" from different symbol corpuses, but for each of these four concepts, there likely would be considerable variability as to which symbols were chosen for each concept. Each individual likely used their own criteria (e.g., aesthetic appeal, iconicity, or personal preference) in deciding which symbol to choose for each of the four concepts. This is also just as true for unaided symbols as aided symbols.

This is a compelling reason clinicians, educators, and service providers must know the symbol corpuses that are available, have access to all possible symbols, and work with the AAC user to the extent possible when choosing symbols. *When at all possible, AAC users should be at the center of the symbol selection process, as it is their judgment—not the professional's—that should determine which symbols will represent the various concepts being depicted in their AAC system.*

Other Variables Pertinent to the AAC User

Conceptual Development

Keeping in mind that the individual with CCN is at the center of symbol selection, there are other considerations that relate directly to the AAC user. One of the earliest determinations that must be made when selecting aided symbols is the conceptual development of the user. Graphic (and therefore, visual) symbolic representation consists of several levels of conceptual development. From simplest to most complex, these are:

- Level 1: Identical object-to-object associations (i.e., an object is used to represent itself)
- Level 2: Nonidentical object-to-object associations (i.e., a nonidentical object, such as a miniature, is used to represent the real object)
- Level 3: Picture-to-object associations (i.e., the individual must understand that a two-dimensional picture is being used to represent the corresponding three-dimensional real object)
- Level 4: Part-to-whole associations (i.e., the individual must recognize a concept although only part of it is being depicted)
- Level 5: Ideographic symbol-to-picture or -object associations (i.e., the symbols become less realistic and more schematic)
- Level 6: Abstract symbol-to-picture or -object associations (i.e., the relationship between symbol and referent is arbitrarily assigned, and therefore, must be learned)

Choosing appropriate symbols will be determined to some extent by the AAC user's level of conceptual development. As an example, selecting traditional orthography or fingerspelling (which requires abstract symbol-to-picture or -object associations at Level 6) would be inappropriate if the AAC user is functioning at conceptual Level 1 or 2. The work of Thistle and Wilkinson (2015) further supports this concept. When asked what factors influenced their selection of symbol type, a majority of respondents in their study indicated that the user's cognitive level should be considered. Ogletree and colleagues (2018) cited work where children were asked to identify select PCS symbols and then draw their representation of the symbols. The children drew contextually based pictures. It was concluded that children's representations of some symbols may differ significantly from adults and more complex concepts may be difficult to represent for young children. Since no single aided or unaided

symbol set or system has all the best symbols, a determination of conceptual development should occur during a thorough AAC assessment.

Functionality

Functionality is an important consideration in selecting symbols. Individuals must have certain physical abilities to use certain symbols. Symbols should be as functional as possible for the AAC user. Selecting traditional orthography for an individual who is blind, for example, would not be a functional choice. Braille, on the other hand, may be. Roche and colleagues (2014) reviewed the use of tangible symbols as an option for individuals with developmental disabilities who were blind or had significant visual impairments. The symbols consisted of three-dimensional whole or partial objects and were taught primarily as requests for preferred objects or activities. Although Roche and colleagues (2014) concluded tangible symbols appeared to yield promising results, communication was limited to requesting. Additional research is warranted on how functionality may interact with symbol selection and communication acts.

Variables Pertinent to Symbols

The selection of symbols to represent vocabulary not only includes variables related to the AAC user but to the symbols themselves. One variable—visual complexity—applies to aided symbols (this variable also applies to unaided symbols, but in this case, the variable refers to complexity of production). Another variable—iconicity—applies to both aided and unaided symbols. Finally, several variables pertain to just unaided symbols.

Aided Symbols

Visual Complexity. For aided symbols, visual complexity is also a variable to consider (Fuller, 1988, 1997; Fuller & Lloyd, 1987; Hern et al., 1994; Luftig & Bersani, 1985; Nail-Chiwetalu, 1992). Visual complexity has been defined in two ways: (1) the number of semantic elements needed to create a composite symbol (Luftig & Bersani, 1985) and (2) the number of strokes required to create a symbol (Fuller & Lloyd, 1987).

To date, empirical research on visual complexity has yielded mixed results. For example, Fuller (1997) found that for typically developing children, visual complexity (defined by the number of strokes) had a facilitative effect on learning of Blissymbols when they possessed a low degree of translucency but had no effect at all on adults without impairments. Hern and colleagues (1994) studied institutionalized persons with severe cognitive impairments and found visual complexity had a facilitative effect only on learning of highly iconic Blissymbols. Such mixed results suggest complexity has not yet been defined consistently. Until visual complexity is more thoroughly investigated, clinicians, educators, and service providers must rely on the AAC user's perception and their own professional intuition in determining what constitutes visual complexity for aided symbols.

Aided and Unaided Symbols

Iconicity. As was discussed earlier in this chapter, iconicity should be considered a factor in symbol selection for both aided and unaided symbols (Doherty, 1985; Fristoe & Lloyd, 1979a; Fuller, 1988, 1997; Fuller & Lloyd, 1987; Hern et al., 1994; Lloyd & Fuller, 1990; Luftig & Bersani, 1985; Luftig & Lloyd, 1981; Nail-Chiwetalu, 1992). Research has shown that iconicity is a powerful variable in the acquisition and retention of both aided and unaided symbols. Selecting symbols that are more representative of their referents maximizes the possibility for immediate success.

For aided symbols, it may be possible to improve the iconicity of some symbols through the utilization of animation and environmental sounds. Fujisawa and colleagues (2011) and Schlosser and colleagues (2014) found that animation improved the iconicity of aided symbols while Harmon and colleagues (2014) concluded animation plus the addition of environmental sounds helped typically developing children learn symbols more readily. While determining iconicity for a specific user can be difficult, it is somewhat generalizable to a number of different populations. One should always keep in mind that iconicity should be determined in reference to the AAC user.

Unaided Symbols

For unaided symbols, several variables should be considered during the selection process to facilitate successful acquisition. These include:

- Touch vs. nontouch (manual signs in which the hands touch each other or the body are easier to produce and learn than those that do not)
- Symmetrical vs. asymmetrical (manual signs in which handshapes and/or movements are identical for both hands are easier to produce and learn)
- One-handed vs. two-handed (manual signs requiring only one hand during production are easier to learn)
- Complexity of handshape and/or movement (some handshapes and movements are simpler than others, and therefore, easier to produce and learn)
- Visible vs. invisible (manual signs that are more readily seen, as they are not obscured by another aspect of the same sign, are easier to learn)
- One movement vs. two or more movements (manual signs utilizing simple, single movements are simpler to produce and learn)

When choosing unaided symbols, clinicians, educators, and service providers should select manual signs and gestures that match the user's cognitive and physical abilities.

Creating a Teaching Environment for Success

Once symbols have been chosen for a user's vocabulary, clinicians, educators, and service providers should set up the teaching environment to heighten opportunity for success. One strategy that has been successful in increasing opportunity for productive use of aided AAC in the educational setting is implementation of peer network interventions. Research has shown that the use of peer networks in AAC modeling results in increasing students' use of communication within interactions with peers (Biggs et al., 2018; Kamps et al., 2014; Kamps et al., 2015). Increases in peer interaction are likely to facilitate independence and increase student use of AAC in the educational setting and beyond.

Another strategy clinicians, educators, and other practitioners may want to consider is grouping vocabulary so the easiest symbols are taught first. Consider an AAC user who has a relatively large vocabulary of 200 symbols. Teaching all these symbols at once would be difficult, if not impossible. Therefore, clinicians may want to group symbols in sets to facilitate teaching and learning. For example, for the individual just described, symbols could be taught in several sets of 10 to 20. Symbols assigned to the first few sets should be those that are highly preferred by the user, transparent or highly translucent, easy to produce (for unaided symbols), as dissimilar as possible to reduce visual discrimination issues, and likely to have immediate communicative impact.

Minimal pairs exist in many aided and unaided symbol corpuses. For example, the Blissymbols for "happy" and "sad" are identical, except for the orientation of the arrow: both utilize a heart element; an up arrow is to the right of the heart for "happy" and a down arrow is to the right of the heart for "sad." Similarly, many manual signs have identical handshapes, locations, and/or movements. This is referred to as **topographical similarity** and is equivalent to minimal pairs for aided symbols. Minimal pairs should be avoided when teaching initial sets of aided and unaided symbols. Immediate success in communication is virtually assured if clinicians and educators begin the teaching process with symbols that are highly motivating to the AAC user, functional, highly iconic, easy to produce, and visually distinct.

SUMMARY

Symbol selection is a process that requires considerable thought and planning on the part of clinicians, educators, and other service providers. With the large number of aided and unaided symbols available, one must make a systematic attempt to determine which symbols are most appropriate for a specific AAC user. In other words, individual symbols (drawn from several different symbol corpuses) or complete sets or systems that best match the user's purposes, abilities, and needs and facilitate communication with a wide range of partners across several environments, should be determined in a thoughtful and systematic manner. The first phase in this process is to evaluate all possible symbols to determine which are most appropriate. By using the selection considerations discussed in this chapter, clinicians, educators, and other service providers should be able to eliminate inappropriate symbols or even complete symbol corpuses, thus reducing the number of potential choices to a more manageable number. Once this is accomplished, professional service providers are ready to enter phase II of the selection process—matching complete symbol corpuses, or individual symbols drawn from a number of symbol corpuses, with their referents in a manner that maximizes the potential for successful communication.

STUDY QUESTIONS

1. Describe the two phases of AAC symbol selection.

2. Name and briefly discuss two user variables. How do they relate to the process of symbol selection?

3. Briefly describe how vocabulary variables are interrelated.

4. Of all the symbol selection considerations, which one has received the greatest empirical attention? What do the research findings suggest?

5. Take one aided and one unaided symbol corpus. Compare them in terms of all appropriate symbol selection considerations.

6. What is the guiding principle behind the process of matching symbols to referents?

7. Briefly discuss conceptual development. What is its importance in the symbol-referent matching process?

8. What are some inherent characteristics of unaided symbols that can be manipulated to maximize the possibility of immediate communication success? What are a couple of these characteristics for aided symbols?

14

Technology Selection

Amanda Hettenhausen, MA; Krista Davidson, MS; and Lyle L. Lloyd, PhD

MYTH

1. People who use or could benefit from augmentative and alternative communication (AAC) and their family members often lack knowledge about the features of various AAC systems. Therefore, the responsibility for selecting technology should fall primarily to professional members of the AAC service delivery team.

2. People who use AAC want the latest, most advanced, or most expensive AAC technology available.

3. The end goal of technology selection is acquiring the AAC system.

REALITY

1. Even though people who use or could benefit from AAC and their family members may have minimal knowledge about AAC systems and devices, they are major stakeholders in selecting the AAC system. It is the responsibility of the professional members of the AAC team, who have systems and device expertise, to educate people who use AAC and their family members about systems with appropriate features so that informed decision-making is possible (Lloyd & Belfiore, 1994). Technology selection should be the joint endeavor of the entire AAC team (Musselwhite & St. Louis, 1988; Parette et al., 1993).

2. People who use AAC, like most other individuals, want a system that provides the most reliable and efficient means of communicating. The value of an AAC system is much more than its cost or newness.

3. Although a team may face many challenges in the acquisition of appropriate AAC technology, acquiring the device is just the beginning rather than the end goal in AAC intervention. AAC technology is part of an approach, not solely a solution to a problem.

INTRODUCTION

The purpose of **technology selection** is to match the strengths and needs of people who use or could benefit from AAC to the features of the technology (Costello & Shane, 1994; Demasco, 1994; Light & McNaughton, 2013; McNairn & Smith, 1996). Due to the rapidly evolving nature of technology, the number of AAC options continues to grow. AAC solutions are available on mobile technology, dedicated

Fuller, D. R., & Lloyd, L. L. *Principles and Practices in Augmentative and Alternative Communication* (pp. 259-266). © 2023 Taylor & Francis Group.

TABLE 14-1

Steps Involved in Selecting an AAC System

1. Assess the person who could benefit from AAC, including consideration of communication partners and environments.
2. Assess person's communication needs and the symbols to represent the vocabulary/messages.
3. Determine relevant features needed based on the assessment.
4. Identify AAC systems that have the desired features.
5. Carefully consider AAC systems that will enable the person to meet all communication needs.
6. Conduct trial(s) with selected AAC system(s), to reinforce the preliminary decision regarding goodness of fit and/or satisfy funding requirements.
7. Select the most appropriate AAC system.
8. Assist in procuring AAC system.
9. Provide further training in its effective use.

AAC = augmentative and alternative communication.

devices, and other computer platforms. The availability and awareness of mainstream systems (e.g., mobile technology) continues to move the industry to provide more portable, affordable, and personalized solutions. Additionally, it has empowered consumers and increased the acceptance and use of AAC to those who may not have previously considered it (Caron, 2015; Caron et al., 2014; McNaughton & Light, 2013).

As these options continue to expand, two complications may occur. First, selecting the right AAC solutions may become more difficult or overwhelming, as technology changes rapidly and continuously. Second, the technology selection process may be shortened or bypassed altogether. Scherz and colleagues (2010) found that mobile technologies and AAC apps are often purchased without an assessment or stakeholder input. Despite the influx of and access to new technologies, it is important that teams continue to collaborate using established selection procedures in order to select the most appropriate technology to meet current and future communication needs (Beukelman & Mirenda, 1992; Fried-Oken, 1992; Leighton, 2015; Light & McNaughton, 2013). Decisions related to technology selection should include feature matching, which is the term for the process of matching the features of technologies to the strengths and needs of the person who uses or could benefit from AAC (Light & McNaughton, 2013).

As indicated in Chapter 11, the assessment process involves consideration of the person who uses or could benefit from AAC, the communication partners, the environments, and the AAC system. Table 14-1 provides a list of the steps involved in selecting an AAC system. Steps 1 through 2 are

discussed in Chapters 11, 12, and 13. Step 8 is discussed in Chapter 17, and Step 9 is covered across the chapters related to intervention. This chapter will focus on Steps 3 through 7. This chapter discusses the roles and responsibilities of the AAC service delivery team in selecting technology, technology selection variables to be considered, the process of feature matching, and the purpose and process of evaluating **trial** use during the selection process.

ROLES AND RESPONSIBILITIES IN SELECTING TECHNOLOGY

The importance of a team approach in AAC cannot be understated. As with other parts of the AAC assessment process, all team members should continue to collaborate to select the most appropriate AAC technology for an individual. For a complete description of possible team members and their roles, see Chapter 11. The makeup of each team will vary, and the roles that each person serves during the technology selection process will depend on their experience, knowledge, and skills. The team must be consumer-responsive and, as such, always include the individual who uses AAC, as well as their family to whatever extent possible. Abandonment of the AAC system is less likely when the family is involved in the technology selection process (Fishman, 2011; Mitchell & Alvares, 2015).

In addition to a team approach, it is essential that at least one or more of the team members possess expertise related to AAC technology. This could be any member of the team but is often a speech-language pathologist, assistive technology specialist, occupational therapist, or other related professional. Expertise implies a strong knowledge base of the technology (see Chapter 10) and current best practice, as well as experience using the various technologies. Familiarity with selecting apps, one or two speech-generating devices (SGDs), or specific computer software is insufficient. Unfortunately, given the readily available nature of technology, teams often make decisions based on familiarity and/or immediate access or availability of technology instead of what is the best fit for the individual. In the event that a team does not have someone who demonstrates expertise in AAC technology, the responsibility shifts to educating oneself and accessing resources. Resources may include but are not limited to, experienced colleagues, AAC companies and local representatives, books, feature comparison charts, research articles, university courses, independent studies, conferences, and webinars.

A number of responsibilities will continue well beyond the initial process of the technology selection, as assessment is an ongoing process (Fishman, 2011). The following list offers a number of these roles and responsibilities to be shared by the service delivery team (Golinker, 1992; Parette et al., 1993; Uslan, 1992, Yaida & Reuben, 1992):

- Establish, conduct, and monitor trial use with selected AAC system(s) to reinforce the preliminary decision regarding goodness of fit and/or satisfy funding requirements.
- Train the person who uses or could benefit from AAC and their communication partners in the use of the AAC system
- Conduct administrative activities related to acquisition and use of the AAC system
- Modify the environment to support the use of the AAC system
- Evaluate the continued suitability of the selected AAC system
- Assist in the development, modification, maintenance, and/or upgrade of the AAC system

Technology Selection Variables

Technology selection is a challenging process for two primary reasons. First, it is difficult to navigate the ever-growing maze of mass-market applications and advancements in technology (Gosnell et al., 2011). Second, decisions are complex because they are shaped by multiple interrelated user, partner, environmental, and AAC system variables that influence the appropriateness of one group or piece of technology over another (Beukelman et al., 1985; Fried-Oken, 1992).

In general, AAC technology selection is based on determining systems that provide the desired vocabulary and language organization, support access needs, have the necessary symbols and output(s), can be supported and maintained, develop social networks, and meet other individual needs or considerations. Selection of technology should be equally influenced by the person who uses AAC and their preferences, which may include factors related to availability, cost, familiarity, and social acceptability (Caron, 2015; Meder & Wegner, 2015). Technology selection is a delicate balance. Both client preference and clinical expertise must be integrated into the selection process because, in the end, the best AAC system is the one that will be used and supported (Light & McNaughton, 2013).

As part of their work on a symbol taxonomy, Fuller and colleagues (1991) determined that nearly 50 discrete AAC selection variables exist in the AAC literature. These variables were grouped into three areas of (1) functionality/ability to meet needs, (2) availability/usability, and (3) acceptability/compatibility (Vanderheiden and Lloyd, 1986). Several others (e.g., Cress & French, 1994; Cress & Goltz, 1989; Demasco, 1994; Goodenough-Trepagnier, 1994; Koester & Levine, 1994; Light, 1989; Light & Lindsay, 1991) have suggested design goals or variables to be considered in selecting AAC technology. Systems that (1) support learnability, (2) promote consistency, (3) provide immediate utility, (4) promote spontaneity, (5) minimize motor demands, (6) minimize

cognitive/memory demands, (7) minimize attention shifting, and (8) support updates/upgrades should receive high consideration when selecting devices for trial use. Each of these eight variables is briefly discussed below relative to the abilities and needs of the person who uses AAC.

Learnability

Learnability relates to the ability to use and understand an AAC system. As technology is considered and selected, the ease of learning for the person using the system, the family, and the team members must be considered. A highly learnable system is said to be intuitive, and the intuitive nature of a system varies across individuals. Most AAC systems require some level of learning, and one cannot underestimate the value of a knowledgeable support network to assist in this learning process. If a system is considered difficult to use by either the person using the device or relevant stakeholders, it may lead to abandonment (Johnson et al., 2006). Therefore, the ability to learn an AAC system, given support and time, is an important consideration in the technology selection process.

Consistency

Another key consideration is the consistency of the AAC system based on past experiences and future needs. The team should ensure that the technology is compatible, or consistent, with other products with which the person who uses AAC is familiar or has mastered. For example, if a person is already familiar with technology on the iOS platform, they may prefer AAC solutions on this same platform. Additionally, if an individual has had experience with standard keyboards, considering systems that have QWERTY arrangements seems appropriate. Similarly, some individuals may begin their AAC journey with a manual communication board. When transitioning to speech-generating technology, it is imperative to consider the symbol set and layout they have already been using (Halloran & Halloran, 2013). Increased consistency helps to decrease cognitive load.

Initial Utility

Although achieving instant benefits along the continuum of technology is often difficult (Goodenough-Trepagnier, 1994), some immediate, positive change in communication will help maintain enthusiasm for further use and learning. Teams should consider the use of technology features that support some initial utility of the AAC system (e.g., temporarily minimizing the number of words/icons on the screen, looking up where words are located within the vocabulary). Extrinsic factors, such as providing prompts or structuring interactions around highly motivating and meaningful communication, will also support initial success and utility of the technology. Teams generally agree that the use of technology should lead to some immediate improvement in communication; however, becoming a competent communicator is a process, and the time required is unique to each person (Light, 1989).

Spontaneity

The production of speech via AAC is typically 15 to 25 times slower than the production of natural speech (Beukelman & Light, 2020). For many people who use AAC, communication rate and spontaneity are important factors in judging technology success. They are directly related to effectiveness in communication interaction, especially in educational and employment settings when communication rates are even greater (McNaughton & Bryen, 2007; Vanderheiden & Kelso, 1987). Advancements in technology provide tools to support rate enhancement and more natural interaction. For example, word prediction and abbreviation expansion are two available features that may enhance the communication rate for some people who use AAC. Other features that may promote increased rate and/or spontaneity include prestored phrases, logical next words, recents list, encoding, and consistent location of vocabulary for efficient access (American Speech–Language–Hearing Association, 2017). During the selection process, it is important to consider which features may help increase rate and spontaneity for the individual.

Motor Demands

The motor skills required to use technology are relevant because they may increase cognitive and physical demands for individuals using AAC (Goodenough-Trepagnier, 1994). Therefore, goodness of fit has been achieved when a device minimally taxes the motor system to whatever extent possible. As a person uses an AAC system, they often develop a motor plan for the features of their system (Dukhovny & Thistle, 2017). A motor plan facilitates efficient and effective use, which allows for increased automaticity and decreased cognitive load. One approach, **Language Acquisition through Motor Planning**, capitalizes on this strategy (Naguib Bedwani et al., 2015). See Chapter 10 for additional information about this method.

The challenge of selecting technology is compounded for those with significant physical disabilities. There is often an incongruity between the identified need for a robust vocabulary in the system and the ability to determine an appropriate access method for the person to learn the system (Kay, 2014). If an alternate access method (e.g., eye gaze, switch scanning) is necessary, motor demands may become the primary determining factor in selecting AAC technology. However, it is important that information regarding motor demands is considered jointly with communication and language. A period of use with any device is recommended prior to procurement because consistency, speed, and economy of motor activity typically improve with device use and practice (Koester & Levine, 1994; Treviranus, 1994).

Cognitive/Memory Demands

Cognitive and memory demands are inherent in learning anything new, including an AAC system. Similar to motor demands, the aim should be to select technology and use strategies that work to decrease cognitive load (Cress & French, 1994; Cress & Goltz, 1989; Demasco, 1994; Koester & Levine, 1994; Light, 1989; Light & Lindsay, 1991). Multiple interrelated elements of a device (e.g., access mode, symbols, symbol arrangement, navigation, output) are noted to concomitantly influence cognitive load. For example, the task of symbol selection is complex, and individuals must use memory functions for object, spatial, and temporal processing (Wagner et al., 2012). As technology advances, features continue to be added to AAC. It is necessary to consider whether these features are beneficial for the person using AAC or if they increase cognitive complexity. For example, when certain features (e.g., word prediction) are available in a device but are not readily visible, the cognitive load required to recall and access them may be too great that the person using AAC avoids their use (Demasco, 1994; Thistle & Wilkinson, 2013). When so much mental energy is invested in achieving the means to an end (e.g., message construction), then too little may be left to achieve the end itself (e.g., functional communication; Treviranus, 1994). As with motor demands, cognitive demands may only be truly assessed after the individual has had repeated use of the technology with sufficient opportunities to increase familiarity (Goodenough-Trepagnier, 1994; Wagner & Shaffer, 2015).

Attention

The addition of an external AAC system compounds the attention demands during a communication exchange. The person who uses AAC must not only attend to the communication partner, subject matter, and possibly additional stimuli (e.g., TV show, book, toy) but also to the AAC display (Thistle & Wilkinson, 2012). Technology should be chosen to minimize monitoring of auditory or visual features so that energies can be conserved for the actual process of communication. Although everyone expends some energy monitoring the sensory demands of the communication process, speaking individuals do so using minimal mental energy (Demasco, 1994). The team must determine the individual's visual scanning capacity, their ability to focus on a relevant target, and the ability to attend to multiple tasks (Wilkinson & Hennig, 2009). Special attention to symbols, organization, array, color, and layout is again required to account for attention demands (Thistle & Wilkinson, 2012). For a review of cognitive, attentional, and motivational demands in AAC, see Wilkinson and Hennig (2009).

Updates/Upgrades

The goal of the AAC service delivery team is to select technology that can grow and evolve, not only with the person who uses AAC but also with the advances of technology. Advancements in AAC technology will continue as manufacturers and developers provide updates/upgrades to benefit those who use AAC. The team should attempt to predict skill acquisition and device modifications in order to achieve current and projected goodness of fit. Adding new vocabulary, changing symbol types, or rearranging an existing display may all disrupt the current skills or abilities of the person using AAC; therefore, teams must engage in forward thinking in anticipation of the effects of possible updates/upgrades. Software updates may add new features and/or resolve existing bugs. It is important to consider the cost-benefit analysis of updates/upgrades and new learning (Smith-Lewis, 1994; Treviranus, 1994). Most technology allows for updates to be completed quickly and easily without removing it from the person who uses AAC. For example, both mobile and dedicated solutions take advantage of wireless connection capabilities and/or a USB transfer to complete software updates.

There may be times when it is appropriate and/or necessary to upgrade the AAC system. For example, the communication and/or medical needs of the individual may change and require different access methods, strategies, features, or supports (Fishman, 2011). An upgrade may also be mandated due to outdated technology. For example, older tablets no longer support software updates of many AAC applications. If a new feature is released that is determined by the team to be necessary to support the person using AAC, then a technology upgrade may be appropriate. The decision to upgrade the system will typically involve a discussion regarding funding and access to the new technology. Funding sources, such as Medicare and private insurance, may require 5 years before a new device will be considered. There are exceptions in which a new device may be funded sooner; however, the medical necessity for the new device must always be well documented.

Decisions to update and/or upgrade technology are part of the ongoing technology selection process. Not only is it imperative to decide which technology to update, but it is also important to consider when to introduce the new technology. For example, the person using AAC may prefer to switch to the updated technology all at once, or it may be more appropriate to provide a gradual transition. It is essential that the team continue to collaborate through the technology selection process in order to choose the best fit to meet the needs and preferences of the person who uses AAC and their family.

FEATURE MATCHING

After considering user, partner, environmental, and device variables, the team begins the feature matching process (Steps 3 and 4 in Table 14-1). Feature matching is a predictive means for pairing the current and future capabilities and needs of the person who may benefit from AAC with the relevant features of the AAC system (e.g., language system, hardware, mode of access, symbols, feedback methods; Light & McNaughton, 2013). It may help to group features according to three domains of consideration: sensory-motor, cognitive-communication, and environmental. For example, features in the sensory-motor domain would relate to the individual's physical, sensory, and motor needs and abilities. This would include access features and auditory, visual, and tactile feedback (Helling & Minga, 2014). Due to the evolving nature of technology, the list of features is constantly changing and expanding. AAC teams can locate common feature-matching lists in AAC evaluation resources and articles. Examples may include the Georgia Project for Assistive Technology, the Dynamic AAC Evaluation Protocol (Clarke, 2016), Gail Van Tatenhove's assessment tools (Van Tatenhove, 2020), and the clinical framework for selecting apps, suggested by Gosnell and colleagues (2011).

Although there are feature matching tools available, a team can also create one based on the person using AAC. Table 14-2 is one such example of a feature matching worksheet for Ian. The left column lists 15 features that have been determined to meet his needs. Three options appear across the top that have been identified as having most of these features. Notations in the individual cells indicate availability of the features that enable the team to determine the most appropriate options for trial. Ian, a 5 year old with above average cognitive abilities and severe physical impairments, was enrolled in an inclusive kindergarten classroom at his local elementary school. He required an AAC system that could accommodate both traditional orthography and other graphic symbols he could access with his right index finger. Because of the tendency to drag his hand and his fluctuating range of motion, Ian needed a keyboard with specific cell sizes and a keyguard. He demonstrated poor visual acuity and required auditory feedback for cell activations. Other specific features he needed included a computer interface so he could email his written work, adjustable activation delays so the length of time a cell must be activated could be adjusted based upon his fatigue level, and a no-repeat function so if his hand or finger rested on a key it would only produce a single character or command. Three systems were identified by the team to be procured for assessment. Of the three options considered during the assessment, the team decided to pursue a longer trial with Option A, to verify the team's preliminary decision of goodness of fit. Option A had all available features, and during the assessment, Ian demonstrated initial utility. The family also indicated it had a high degree of learnability of that option for

TABLE 14-2

Sample Feature Matching Worksheet

NAME: Ian		DATE: 11/3/22	
NEEDS/ FEATURES	**OPTION A**	**OPTION B**	**OPTION C**
Direct selection	✓	✓	✓
Auditory activation feedback	✓	✓	✓
Flexible grid size	✓	✓	
Voice output: Digitized and synthesized	✓	✓	✓
Text-to-speech	✓	✓	✓
Mounting capability	✓	✓	✓
Durability/ warranty	✓	✓	
Keyguard	✓	✓	✓
Technical support	✓	✓	
Computer interface	✓	✓	✓
Symbol type: PCS	✓	✓	
Symbol sequencing potential	✓	✓	✓
Adjustable activation delay	✓	✓	✓
No-repeat function	✓	✓	
Portability	✓		✓
Customizable for diversity and inclusion	✓		✓

PCS = Picture Communication Symbols.

The advent of the portable tablet and the rapidly changing world of communication applications have revolutionized the AAC world. One of these changes is increased accessibility to technology, which may result in teams abandoning the feature matching process in order to fit someone to an available tablet or app. Selecting the most appropriate AAC system (including hardware, software, and intervention strategies) is still the result of a methodical process by which a person's strengths, abilities, and needs (current and future) are matched to available tools and strategies (Gosnell et al., 2011). Comparison tools for examining and selecting AAC apps are constantly being produced and updated. Gosnell and colleagues (2011) suggest app features be analyzed according to 11 categories for comparison, including customization of these settings:

1. Access
2. Display
3. Feedback features
4. Output
5. Support
6. Speech settings
7. Purpose of use
8. Rate enhancement
9. Representation
10. Required motor competencies
11. Miscellaneous

Any feature matching tool used in the comparison of apps (or other AAC systems, for that matter) must be dynamic, as new solutions continue to develop and change.

No one item of AAC technology is likely to have all the features desired to meet an individual's current and projected communication needs. Rather, several types of AAC will have some of the desired features. Consider Imani, a young woman with autism spectrum disorder whose AAC team is now assisting her with technology selection. The team's consensus is that Imani will be successful in pairing a non–speech-generating communication board with her existing unaided gesturing and limited natural speech to achieve functional communication in brief interactions with familiar communication partners. However, the team has agreed that Imani will require an SGD with a QWERTY keyboard and internet access as a viable communication and employment tool for use at her workstation in a telecommunications office. The team also considered features that would support Imani's uniqueness. They included symbols that were representative of her skin tone on the non–speech-generating board and explored the voice options on the SGD to ensure she had a synthesized voice that reflected her dialect. Once Imani's needs have been identified, several potentially useful communication devices are selected, and two to three of these systems are recommended for further assessment. After considering the selected devices, Imani, assisted by her AAC team and family, selects the one that best fits her communication, diversity, social, and work needs, and eventually pursues purchase via insurance.

both them and their son. During the 3-week trial period, non–speech-generating displays were developed to support communication across all environments (e.g., in the bathtub, riding the bus). These displays were also used to maintain continuity of communication when the trial device was returned to the loan program at the end of the trial period.

Many people who use AAC, like Imani, achieve maximal benefit when both non–speech-generating and speech-generating technology systems meld with one another and with various unaided communication options to yield multimodal communication (Iacono et al., 1993; Murphy et al., 1995). A thorough overview of the basic components of the technology continuum is provided in Chapter 10.

CONDUCTING TRIALS WITH AAC SYSTEMS

Despite the excitement and potential benefits surrounding AAC, simply having access to the technology does not always guarantee its success (Caron, 2015; Caron et al., 2014; Gosnell et al., 2011; Shane et al., 2012). As listed in Table 14-1, once the team has identified AAC systems that have the desired features, the next step is careful consideration of those systems to select the best fit to meet the needs and expectations of the person who uses or could benefit from AAC. It is important to ensure the selected technology provides the individual with the most effective communication and social interaction possible, considering both current and future needs (American Speech-Language-Hearing Association, 2004b).

Prior to acquiring the technology, the team may decide to conduct a trial(s) with the selected AAC system. A trial is a systematic examination of the performance, quality, or goodness of fit. It can aid in determination or reinforce the preliminary decision regarding which features and/or system is most appropriate. Additionally, a trial may fulfill possible funding agency requirements, provide insight into use across environments and communication partners, and allow for additional data collection (Zangari, 2016b). A trial is not intended as a test of performance or independence. For this reason, a successful trial would show whether the AAC system provided an opportunity for meaningful improvement in current communication performance and demonstrate potential for improvement in future communication performance (J. Riley, personal communication, March 18, 2016).

Trials are available through a variety of different sources, including assistive technology lending libraries, trial versions of communication apps, and AAC manufacturers. The length of a trial may vary between a single session, a few weeks, or several months. This will depend on a variety of factors, including the needs of the individual, familiarity with the AAC system, expertise of the individuals on the team, availability of AAC system(s), and/or funding source requirements. In some cases, a particular device may more immediately show a strong potential for being effective and efficient, whereas in other cases, the device's potential will take longer to determine. The environment in which the trial occurs may also vary, depending on these same factors. In some cases, a particular device may only be available in the clinic or school setting. Multiple trials across AAC systems may not be possible or may be unduly burdensome, especially when there is no perceived functional value (E. Davis-McFarland, personal communication, September 14, 2018).

A systematic approach to a trial will help maximize success. Zangari (2016a) proposed the following as important considerations:

- Determine goals for the trial. This will help drive many decisions, including where, with whom, and for how long to trial the AAC option(s).
- Establish a plan for training. Stakeholders must be able to support the use of the AAC system during the trial. The technology may influence the training resources available. Examples include in-person support from AAC representatives, free online trainings, or self-guided learning (Higdon & Hill, 2015).
- Customize the technology. The technology should reflect the needs, preferences, and diversity of the person using AAC and their family. This may include personalization to the vocabulary, symbols, voice output and dialect, and/or access settings.
- Engage in team conversations. Stakeholders should discuss what works and what does not. The preferences of the person using AAC and their family should be highly valued.
- Consider environmental factors. Whenever possible, complete the trial across the natural environments of the individual. If this is not possible, complete careful consideration of the individual's social network and environments (Blackstone & Hunt-Berg, 2012) or consider the use of videotaping or telepractice (Mitchell & Alvarez, 2015).
- Collect data. Both qualitative and quantitative data should be gathered.

The next step is to determine whether the selected AAC system improved the current communication performance and demonstrated potential for improvement in future communication performance. Teams may find it difficult to find functional outcome measures valid and reliable tools that evaluate the effectiveness of a treatment or assessment that capture the often subtle but critical changes that document progress for people who use AAC (Hanson, 2007). Several tools have been developed; however, they are not one size fits all. The team must use the tool that is most appropriate to document progress for the individual using AAC. Documenting progress is an integral part of the ongoing assessment, technology selection, and intervention process. Table 14-3 includes examples of available checklists, frameworks, and profiles. Positive functional outcomes measures would likely result in a decision to procure the AAC system. Although multifaceted and sometimes challenging, trials can serve as an integral part of the technology selection process.

Table 14-3
Assessment Tools to Document Progress

Augmentative and Alternative Communication Profile: A Continuum of Learning	Kovach, 2009
Checklist of Communicative Competencies, Revised	Bloomberg et al., 2009
Functional Communication Profile, Revised	Kleiman, 2003
Goal Attainment Scale	Kiresuk & Sherman, 1968; Hanson, 2007
Social Networks: A Communication Inventory for Individuals with Complex Communication Needs and Their Partners	Blackstone & Hunt-Berg, 2012
The Test of Aided-Communication Symbol Performance	Bruno, 2017
Communication Matrix	Rowland, 2011a

Table 14-4
Suggestions to Ensure Goodness of Fit in Technology Selection

1. Select technology with team input, especially including the input of the person who uses AAC.
2. Complete a thorough assessment, using a trial when needed to verify suitability or collect data for funding purposes.
3. Understand acquiring the technology is the beginning not the goal in AAC intervention.
4. Consider both aided and unaided communication.
5. Consider time and funding for communication-partner training.
6. Consider long-term communication needs in different contexts.
7. Consider the importance of environmental support.
8. Continue intervention while waiting for recommended technology to be trialed and/or obtained.
9. Maximize resources to make an informed decision.
10. Follow up on funding denials.

AAC = augmentative and alternative communication.

SUMMARY

This chapter has outlined steps in selecting appropriate AAC technology using a transdisciplinary team and a model that considers the person who could benefit from AAC, the partners, the environments, and the total AAC system. The goal of technology selection is to match the strengths and needs of the person who could benefit from AAC to the features of the AAC technology. Blischak (1993) identified suggestions to avoid common AAC selection pitfalls. These continue to be true today and are presented in Table 14-4 to help ensure successful technology selection.

The future of AAC should not be driven by advances in technology but rather by how well we can take advantage of those advancements to enhance communicative opportunities for individuals who use AAC (Cook, 2011). The vast number of features across the technology continuum and the interrelationships of variables influencing the feature matching process (e.g., environmental factors) might seem to suggest that achieving any goodness of fit is overwhelming, if not virtually impossible. Teams that are most successful in technology selection are those that systematically proceed through the process. The process begins by identifying the current and projected communication needs of the individual who uses AAC, which forms the basis for determining the various technology features needed. The team must then identify the technology—either expressive non–speech-generating or speech-generating—that offers the maximal number of desirable features.

Some of the most challenging issues of AAC service provision relate to selecting technology that will provide people who use AAC with maximal communication support with numerous communication partners across a variety of functional environments. Consequently, technology selection will continue to be integral to the assessment process, as the cost and benefit of technology use are further investigated and mobile technology continues to evolve. Despite the growing number of variables, the benchmark of successful technology selection is when a person uses their AAC system to meet multiple daily communication needs and bring about positive life changes.

STUDY QUESTIONS

1. What are the major roles and responsibilities of AAC service delivery team members as they relate to selecting technology?
2. What are six important considerations when formulating the trial period?
3. Describe feature matching and identify at least one available tool to assist in this process.
4. Define functional outcome measures.

Part V
AAC Intervention

15

Intervention Principles

Erin Colone Peabody, MA; Erna Alant, PhD; and Lin Sun, MA

<table>
<tr><td>

MYTH

1. There are certain prerequisite skills that an individual needs to exhibit before using any augmentative and alternative communication (AAC) strategy (e.g., make eye contact, pay attention, show object permanence, imitate motor skills).

2. The use of AAC strategies impedes the development of speech. Thus, it is best to wait and see if speech develops before working on AAC.

3. The main task of AAC intervention is to provide the AAC user with strategies and techniques for the transmission of messages and information.

4. AAC intervention is focused on the use of AAC devices to supplement existing communication.

</td><td>

REALITY

1. There is no evidence that one must exhibit these skills prior to using AAC strategies. The range of AAC strategies available accommodates a diversity of skill levels and allows for all to develop skills while using AAC strategies.

2. There is no evidence that AAC intervention inhibits the development of oral language skills. The focus of AAC is effective communication, which includes speech. Since AAC does not deter speech development, there is no rationale for delaying AAC intervention until an individual has failed to develop or regain speech.

3. Although the ability to send and receive messages are necessary, it is not sufficient for effective social interaction. AAC intervention also needs to address the individual's motivation to communicate and the social environment (e.g., communication partners) of the person who uses AAC.

(continued)

</td></tr>
</table>

Fuller, D. R., & Lloyd, L. L. *Principles and Practices in Augmentative and Alternative Communication* (pp. 269-278).

REALITY (CONTINUED)

4. Although the use of AAC devices can play an important role in facilitating communication with others, technology is not magic. Infusing the use of AAC devices into the everyday interactions of an individual requires significant training and support not only of the individual but also of those in the individual's environment. Therefore, a team approach is critical and can include professionals from a variety of disciplines, as well as parents, siblings, and peers.

A CHANGING LANDSCAPE IN AAC INTERVENTION

The past decades have seen dramatic changes in the technology used by people who have severe communication problems. Technological innovations related to dedicated communication systems and the provision of broader access (e.g., eye gaze and switches) to these systems have been significant. In addition, recent developments of mobile devices and tablets have changed the AAC technology landscape to become more mainstream as an increasing number of communication and AAC applications are available for mobile technology. This change in particular has impacted service delivery in AAC intervention as it encouraged a move from an expert-based to a consumer-driven model of intervention (Herschberger, 2011). For example, it is not uncommon for a child in need of AAC services to arrive at the therapist's door with a communication app downloaded on a mobile device as parents, caregivers, or educators become more empowered to search and acquire technological solutions on their own with the use of the internet.

However, significant change is not only noticeable in the technologies available for communication but also in relation to the clients we serve. For example, Huer (1999) stated that while the majority of services at that time were offered to persons who are of European American ethnicity, projected estimates indicated that an increasing number of families within other ethnic groups would become eligible for services. This prediction has become a reality in most school districts as speech-language pathologists grapple with students from different ethnic backgrounds who need AAC (Dukhovny & Kelly, 2015; Pickl, 2011; Soto & Yu, 2014). Apart from accommodating different cultural factors in intervention, bilingualism and its role in AAC intervention has also become more prominent, as students who use AAC from different linguistic backgrounds have to be accommodated within mainstream education (DeKlerk et al., 2014). In addition to an increase in cultural and linguistic diversity over the past decade, the field of AAC has also seen a change in the types of disabilities we serve.

Although the majority of AAC clients during past decades included adults and students with physical disabilities (e.g., cerebral palsy and acquired disorders), this population has changed quite dramatically. According to the Centers for Disease Control and Prevention, the overall prevalence of autism spectrum disorder diagnosis in 2014 was 23.0 per 1,000 children aged 8 years (i.e., 1 in 44; Baio et al., 2018; U.S. Department of Health & Human Services, 2022). Of the individuals with this diagnosis, it is reported that approximately 25% present as minimally verbal (Rose et al., 2016). AAC services for these individuals require not only an emphasis on the development of interpersonal communication skills but also on increasing the students' linguistic abilities to facilitate learning. Consequently, intervention for these students entails not only a focus on interpersonal communication abilities (i.e., basic interaction communicative skills) but also on facilitating curriculum-based learning in the classroom (i.e., cognitive academic language proficiency).

An increase in the older adult population also has necessitated more services for people with Alzheimer's and dementia (Crema, 2009). Beukelman and colleagues (2008) differentiated between intervention focused on restoration and intervention focused on compensation. They stated that although more attention has been paid to adult-acquired problems to facilitate restoration of abilities, relatively little attention has been paid to those chronic adult disabilities that require a focus on compensatory strategies for interaction. Although there has been some interest in the use of AAC in people with dementia (e.g. Alant, 2017b; Alant et al., 2015; Beukelman et al., 2007; Bourgeois et al., 2001; Murphy & Oliver, 2013), this area still requires further investigation to strengthen intervention efforts.

BROADER FRAMEWORK AND PURPOSE OF AAC INTERVENTION

The complexity and increasing diversity of the population we work with necessitate ongoing reflection on the goal of AAC intervention to ensure that intervention efforts are not only oriented to facilitate predefined outcomes, but also include goals to facilitate *authentic* interactions relevant to the individual and their family. For this chapter, we would like to focus on two different purposes of communication that typically require diverse interactional skills: skills related to authentic *social interaction* that focus on face-to-face interaction (e.g., more symmetrical relationships typically found in interactions with friends with an emphasis on basic interactive communicative skills) and *task-oriented interactions* that are goal-focused and strive to achieve predefined outcomes typical of more formal learning contexts. These learning contexts tend to be more asymmetrical in nature with an emphasis on cognitive academic language proficiency.

The importance of this differentiation is two-fold. First, it highlights the underlying purpose and different outcomes of intervention. Direct training and teaching goals mostly target specific language or interactional skills. These efforts, although well-intended, often do not impact interactions between the client and their communication partners, and therefore, have limited impact on daily live interactions. Intervention goals related to "what the school requires" or "what the parents or family want" or "what the next developmental stage requires" do not necessarily translate to meaningful engagement between the client and those in their environment. Although learning new skills is important, the context within which it is acquired is vital for sustained use. Participation of the individual who uses AAC in intervention activities should transcend the mere exchange of messages; for example, responses to specific instructions. Intervention goals need to facilitate the individual's interest and curiosity in communicating with others across environments to encourage dialogue beyond the formal teaching context.

The second reason for this differentiation is to stress the importance of moving intervention goals beyond the mere formal teaching of skills. Interventionists need to move beyond direct, structured intervention to engage with the individual who uses AAC in a meaning-making process. Although generalization of skills has been a concern over many years in the field of AAC (e.g., Kent-Walsh & McNaughton, 2005; Schlosser & Lee, 2000), the focus here is on ensuring that the individual is able to engage in meaning-making with another. This requires that some time during sessions be allocated to engaging with the client for the sake of getting to know each other better without any specific teaching outcomes in mind. Openness in interacting with the individual who uses AAC and being present to engage with another is core to effective communication intervention. AAC intervention is not just about *doing with* but also *being with* the individual who uses AAC (Alant, 2017a). AAC clients need to experience meaning-making in interaction with their family, teachers, and therapists to provide a basis for meaningful engagement with others.

Meaning-Making, Relational-Oriented Interaction, and Social Closeness

Social interactions are about making contact with others and form the basis for building friendships. These interactions are usually more informal and focus on dialogue, mutual understanding, emotional resonance, and expression. Alant (2017a) described communication as a meaning-making process whereby both communication partners engage in a creative exchange of messages that culminate in the development of *new nuanced meaning* (Alant, 2017a) between them. New nuanced meaning refers to the unique associations that develop between people in an interaction as they interpret and influence each other's messages. These unique associations form the glue that facilitates the development of friendships and long-term interactions. A lack in the ability to pay attention to and show interest in others commonly leads to routinized interactions that are very limited in intersubjective meaning-making, as discussed above. To further describe this process of meaning-making, Table 15-1 explains the different levels of meaning-making in interaction by highlighting the two components of participation and engagement that form an integral part of the meaning-making process.

From Table 15-1, it is evident that meaning-based interaction is defined in terms of a creative interaction between the individual's ability to *engage* in interaction with another (i.e., interest in, attention to, and understanding of the other), as well as the ability to *participate* in exchanges with another (i.e., ability to express oneself and exchange messages in interaction). Meaning-making here is not only related to a cognitive process of exchanging and understanding messages but also includes the ability to *be with another* (i.e., the ability to emotionally resonate with another).

Therefore, the development of friendships and social closeness is of primary importance in this type of interaction (Alant, 2017a). The process of meaning-making is aimed at getting to know the other and creating new nuanced meaning together rather than achieving a specific goal as an outcome of the interaction.

Task- or Goal-Oriented Communication

Task- or goal-oriented communication is focused on predefined outcomes; for example, using a structured approach to teach a student specific language structures. Although there is an exchange of messages that could include the use of positive reinforcement strategies (e.g., teaching practices that utilize principles from applied behavior analysis) to facilitate learning, this process endeavors to teach specific language structures and concepts. Consequently, this type of interaction is more asymmetrical, as the therapist or teacher is supporting the client or directing learning in a more overt way (Alant, 2017a). Interactions are highly structured and require the teacher or interventionist to follow a specific script to facilitate learning. This teaching style places greater value on teaching *skills* vs. emphasizing the teacher's or interventionist's role in promoting attention and sensitivity to the other. Positive reinforcement for target behaviors (i.e., molding of behavior) together with the use of drill and practice focus almost exclusively on modifying behaviors or responses to comply with expectations. Although relevant to learning and increasing skills of the client, these learning situations generally provide little if any opportunity for meaning-making between communication partners.

TABLE 15-1

Different Levels of Meaning in Interaction With Communication Partners

LEVEL OF MEANING IN COMMUNICATION	DESCRIPTION OF COMMUNICATION	PARTICIPATION	ENGAGEMENT
Level 1: Formalistic meaning	Structured meaning, use of predetermined utterances, highly predictable	Routinized, short, superficial, fleeting contact Social greetings, "small talk"	Minimal
Level 2: Literal meaning	Here-and-now–focused exchanges primarily for the purpose of exchanging information; often focused on preprogrammed utterances	Few exchanges, with limited opportunity for development of meaning between partners	Short periods of involvement
Level 3: Extended meaning	More extensive discourse, topic development, coherence exchanges dialogue characterized by sensitivity to context and adjustment to uniqueness of the interaction partners; semantic connectedness	Longer exchanges Adjustment to the communication partner (e.g., vocabulary, topic adherence) Ability to understand the perspective of the other Manifestation of multiple meanings of words and phrases as partners adjust to interaction with each other	More extensive involvement in interaction
Level 4: Versatile meaning	Intuitive use of language and ability to infer meaning with ease; dynamic flow between levels of communication	Dynamic expression and use of communication modes in interaction Skill in adjusting to partner communication needs on different levels Ease in moving from seemingly superficial exchanges to more serious exchanges	Extensive involvement, which allows for dynamic levels of meaning in interaction

Reproduced with permission from Alant, E. (2017a). *Augmentative and alternative communication: Engagement and participation.* Plural Publishing.

Long-Term Sustainability of AAC Intervention: Building Communicative Competence

From the description above, it is evident that one needs both relational- and task-driven goals to increase the long-term impact of intervention efforts. While children participate in formal learning situations at school, adults typically participate in a variety of functional routines of daily living, employment activities, and tasks that require attention and high-level skills without necessarily interacting with others. Although these goal-driven activities are essential in life, it is the balance between task- and relational-oriented communication situations that is important in facilitating the development of friendships and social closeness between people. Being part of a structured training program does not guarantee that a student who uses AAC has opportunities to develop skills necessary for meaning-making and interacting with others. However, the creative synthesis between relational- and task-/goal-driven contexts provides an opportunity for enhancing communicative competence of users of AAC and their communication partners. By focusing on the overlap between relational- and task-driven contexts, communication partners learn not only to do activities with the other but also to develop the skill of interacting with each other about what they are doing (see Figure 15-1 for a visual presentation of the overlap).

When viewing AAC intervention and its progress over the past decade, it becomes evident that technological development has necessitated an emphasis on the use of devices to enhance participation of users of AAC in daily life (e.g., Anderberg & Jönsson, 2005; Cohen & Light, 2000; McNaughton & Bryen, 2007; Raghavendra et al., 2012; Thirumanickam et al., 2011). Although necessary, this focus on technology and its use has proliferated interventions focused on goal-driven outcomes to enhance communicaton competence by, for example, attending to operational, linguistic, and social and strategic competence (Light, 1989). Our relative inability to document variables that relate to engagement and interpersonal sensitivity in interaction has contributed to a lesser emphasis on these components as part of meaning-making between users of AAC and their communication partners.

Although restricted levels of meaning-making is not the only factor contributing to research documenting loneliness and social isolation of people who use AAC, our preoccupation with teaching skills and strategies are not necessarily helpful in promoting friendships and social closeness between users and their communication partners (Alant, 2017a; Klein, 2016).

IMPLICATIONS FOR AAC INTERVENTION

One of the challenges in AAC intervention deals with how to integrate the use of AAC strategies into the daily lives of individuals who use AAC and their families. A large part of this challenge relates to the art and skill required to understand the interactional context (e.g., communication partners; personal, social, and cultural contexts) by not only cognitively analyzing communication partners' behavior but also paying attention to how communication partners engage and emotionally resonate with each other (Alant, 2017a). Communication is, after all, not merely about exchanging messages. It is about the ability to see another, to have shared moments while using language, and to make adjustments to one's own way of expression in an effort to enhance meaning-making with the other.

Therefore, intervention goals need to address ways to infuse skills within natural interactions by enhancing the interpersonal sensitivity of communication partners and users of AAC. In this intervention framework, a focus on relational- and task-driven goals needs to include a dimension focused on the meaning-making component (see the overlap in Figure 15-1). Perhaps one of the best examples of how meaning-making occurs early in life is to look at early language development in typically developing toddlers' interactions.

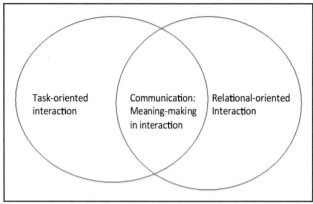

Figure 15-1. Relational- and task-oriented contexts and meaning-making.

Learning to Communicate and Communicating to Learn

From the moment an infant enters the world, the young child engages in developing relationships with others. By the time babies grow into toddlers, they have been exposed to approximately 4,380 hours of oral language, which is an average of 8 hours of spoken language per day (Korsten, 2011). Much of this language exposure is embedded in social interactions with parents, caregivers, and family members.

Take a typical interaction between a toddler and parent for example. A 24-month-old boy hears a plane flying in the sky. He looks up and points to the sky. Almost simultaneously, the toddler, still with an outstretched arm pointing to the moving object, looks at his parent and speaks, "Mama, Mama" with rising intonation. The parent looks at her child and smiles. The parent then looks up at the object zooming in the sky. The parent returns her gaze to meet that of the toddler and says, "Plane. That's a plane. It's up in the sky. It takes people on trips." This is a layered interaction between parent and child. There is initiation of an interaction ("Mama, Mama"), joint attention to a shared experience (mother looking at the object the child is pointing to in the sky), the labeling of an unknown object and sound ("plane"), a model of how to place this new label into a rule-governed linguistic structure ("That's a plane"), and an introduction of how this label fits into the world ("It's up in the sky. It takes people on trips.").

Although the verbal exchange between parent and child is evident, much of this interaction revolved around communication partners portraying mutual interest in and attention to the other. The mother communicates to the child that his utterances were meaningful and worthy of her attention. She then continues to affirm and expand on the child's utterance. This is moving beyond a moment of sharing to develop meaning in interaction (see Level 2 in Table 15-1).

Typically developing language learners appear to learn language and how to communicate with ease across all environments. Most of what is learned has not been formally taught but rather acquired in the natural environment, as parents, siblings, and others in the child's environment model language use and interaction skills. As children begin to develop their verbal language, parents begin to expand upon the communicative messages by lengthening the child's utterance or recasting what the child has said in a different way. Typical language learners develop language in a systematic and progressive manner. The child first develops an understanding of words, then around 1 year of age, they start to speak in single words. As their receptive and expressive vocabularies increase, they start to combine these words. As the combination of words increases in length, the addition of morphological markers appear. Roger Brown (Brown, 1973) formulated the stages of language development of children starting at 15 months through 52 months and up. At Stage V, children have a mean length of utterance ranging from 3.7 to 4.5 and use more complex morphological markers, such as third-person irregular, uncontractible auxiliary, and contractible auxiliary. Van Tatenhove (2009) stated that when children enter kindergarten, they have already learned and become masters of language and communication. They have "learned to talk"; now it is time for them to "talk to learn."

In addition to charting the way in which toddlers learn to verbally express, we also need to pay attention to how they are able to develop social closeness and increase their ability to develop meaning interaction with others. For example, take the conversation between Henry, an almost 4-year-old, and his mother talking about his upcoming birthday while she is getting ready for work. "Mommy?" His mother looks up from applying her makeup, "Yes, Henry." Henry responds, "I want Paw Patrol." His mother continues to look at him and asks a follow-up question to better understand her son's request. She asks, "You want Paw Patrol presents for your birthday?" He exclaims, "Yes! I like Paw Patrol the best. So, you can get me Paw Patrol." His mother smiles and responds, "Okay Henry, I will get you something from Paw Patrol." Henry looks at her with concern. "No Mommy, I want someone else to get me Paw Patrol. I already have a toy that I want you to get, silly," he says as he smiles at her. His mother chuckles and pats his floppy blonde hair. "Oh, you want someone else [emphasizing "someone else" by saying the words louder and extending them out] to get Paw Patrol for you." He nods and says, "Remember, Mommy. I told you to get Mickey Mouse. I like the Clubhouse."

The short exchange between Henry and his mother shows the quick succession of communication acts and behavior contributing to meaning-making between them. First, Henry attracts his mother's attention by saying "Mommy" and then he proceeds to tell her what he wants. Then, he realizes that she got the message wrong in that if she gives him the Paw Patrol toy, he will lose out on another gift he wants, one they have decided on before (Mickey Mouse Clubhouse).

On the surface, this interaction seems quite simple; however, it demonstrates a meaning-making level of 3 to 4 between the two communication partners. The meaning developed in this interaction is conveyed not only by the verbal interaction, but also eye gaze, gestures (mother touching his hair), tone of voice, and facial expression (Henry's expression of concern). These rich interaction experiences typical children are exposed to in their home provide a solid basis for the children's attention to and interest in meaning-making with others.

A Different Path

Children who have little or no ability to speak have different experiences during their early years. While most children enter kindergarten with a sizable vocabulary and are able to combine words into sentences with ease, children with limited speech are often still in the process of learning how to use concepts and words and how to embed these into the utterances. In some cases, these children have a good understanding of language but no effective expressive modality to facilitate interactions with others.

Van Tatenhove (2016) asked the question, "How should a normal language acquisition model be used when working with children who use AAC systems?" In her paper, *Normal Language Acquisition and Children using AAC Systems*, she suggested that interventionists use typical language acquisition as a *guide* to AAC intervention rather than as an *evaluation* of the child's language abilities. However, she cautioned that AAC users cannot be evaluated fairly against their peers who developed language typically and listed a few reasons why this type of approach is unfair:

- An introduction to AAC systems after the age of 3 years places an unfair comparison to typical milestones due to different language experiences
- Normal language development models focus heavily on expressive language, which puts the AAC user at a disadvantage because of the often late introduction to an AAC system vs. assessing receptive language skills, which is often an area of strength
- Access to preselected vocabulary may be heavily noun-based and typically has little to no access to morphological markers
- Limited access to modeling of language on the AAC system

These reasons highlight the constraints in natural-occurring meaning-making interactions between young children who use AAC and their communication partners. Early meaning-making experiences for children who use AAC are often not only different but limited by the types of messages they can use to engage in interaction with others. Similarly, communication partners are often uncertain about how to interact with users of AAC. For example, it is well reported that parents are more leading in their interactions with children who use AAC (e.g., Light et al., 1994). At times, the tendency is also to focus on the communication board or device to find something to communicate rather than focus on the interaction with the child. Early interactions between caregivers and typical children provide interventionists with a guide to AAC intervention, as it highlights meaning-making during exchanges in a natural context.

The Importance of Meaning: Semantics as a Starting Point

Perhaps one of the most important early AAC intervention principles relates to forefronting meaning-making in interactions between a young child who uses AAC and their communication partners. When developing vocabulary to teach and facilitate language development, interventionists need to keep in mind that the ultimate goal is for users to be effective communicators able to develop meaningful social relationships. An interventionist's and parent's instinct might be to start with teaching nouns (or the labels of preferred items) or often the immediate goal is to decrease maladaptive behaviors that stem from the individual's frustration due to an inability to express themselves or get access to preferred items due to an ineffective communication system. In the immediate term, providing a child with a communication system (e.g., depicting nouns/objects of choice) could help to decrease maladaptive behaviors (Mirenda & Brown, 2007); however, this type of needs-based vocabulary has limited long-term impact on developing relationships with others. Similarly, focusing on nouns will allow for the user of AAC to meet basic wants and needs, but how do these interactions resemble naturalistic interactions between parents and their children? While the child might have access to some vocabulary, the interaction pattern imposed by the type of vocabulary on the device or board can be restrictive in facilitating natural interaction patterns between the user of AAC and their communication partners. Early AAC intervention goals, although immediately useful, could therefore stifle the AAC user's ability to meet the overall goal of being an effective communicator in interaction with others (Alant, 2017a). Therefore, access to and the selection of an AAC users' vocabulary is critical. Again, think about a typically developing language learner. The vocabulary that they are exposed to includes not only nouns but verbs, attributes, prepositions, etc. These individual words are used to communicate a variety of functions that go well beyond requesting. Studies conducted by Banajee and colleagues (2003) and Stuart and colleagues (1997) found that individuals across the lifespan use a similar core set of words. The English language has more than 100,000 words, and an educated adult uses as many as 15,000 words. However, 80% of words used in spoken daily interactions consists of only about 350 words. These words, referred to as core vocabulary (Cross et al., 1997), can include

words like "I," "no," "yes," "my," "the," "want," it," go," "mine," "what," "here," "more," "out," etc. and show notable consistency across environments, activities, and social interactions of typical communicators across the lifespan (Balandin & Iacono, 1998a; Banajee et al., 2003; Beukleman et al., 1989). Therefore, this is the vocabulary that interventionists should be aware of in promoting communication of clients who use AAC. Core vocabulary provides a strong foundation for the development of flexible and dynamic interactions between the user of AAC and communication partners, as it provides a framework for the learning of multiple meanings of words and concepts. Therefore, an understanding of and access to core vocabulary allows the AAC user to move beyond the limited social interactions of requesting or scripted conversations. Core vocabulary lends itself to allowing the user of AAC and their communication partner to engage in dynamic interactions that facilitate meaning-making in a variety of contexts.

Moving Beyond Requesting and Communicating in Single Words

Although the different language functions typically used by speaking individuals in everyday interactions are commonly acknowledged by interventionists, it can be challenging to assist users of AAC to use a variety of language functions. While the user of AAC might have the appropriate vocabulary, they still need to know which of these are appropriate for use in which context. Van Tatenhove (2016) described this situation as similar to doing a specific task or job. If you need to do something (e.g., use a specific language function), you need to identify the correct tools (i.e., words) to complete the task. For example, the AAC user needs to be able to communicate a wide variety of communicative messages. These messages range from requests, to comments, to asking questions, to protesting, to greeting, etc. If the user wants to communicate a rejection message, they should include words like "no," "stop," or "finish." Van Tatenhove (2016) stated that a well-selected AAC core vocabulary will fulfill most of the functions of language and ensures that the child using an AAC system has the opportunity to learn how to communicate for a variety of reasons, experiencing the power of language to meet a range of their communication needs (Beukelman & Light, 2020; van Tilborg & Deckers, 2016).

As young children use different types of messages and language functions, they not only combine words into sentences but also develop the ability to use morphological markers in interactions. Therefore, they learn morphological and syntactical rules that govern language. These features should also be available to the AAC user. However, getting AAC users to move beyond using single words can be quite challenging (Beukelman & Light, 2020; Loncke, 2014).

Aided Language Stimulation: Use of Modeling And Recasting

Aided language stimulation is an umbrella term for strategies (Elder & Goossens', 1994; Goossens' et al., 1992; Romski & Sevcik, 1996) focused on combining the spoken language of the communication partner with modeling of the use of the AAC system (i.e., the full range of technology). This is done by pointing to (or activating) the targeted vocabulary to ensure that the user receives the message by using multimodal input. Researchers have demonstrated the usefulness of aided language stimulation in teaching language skills. For example, Drager and Light (2006) found that modeling and responding to the child's communicative attempts not only led to increased understanding of concepts but also to increased rates of turn taking in play, increased expressive vocabularies, and ultimately, morphological development. Bruno and Trembath (2006) also stated that this method improves the complexity and length of utterances.

However, like the use of all strategies, the challenge is how to use aided language stimulation strategies to facilitate meaning-making in interactions with others. Although evidence suggests that aided language stimulation can be effective in facilitating predetermined language outcomes (e.g., task-oriented activities), there is little evidence of its impact in promoting meaning-making and social closeness with others. Conversational recasting and modeling (Cleave & Fey, 1997; Loncke, 2014) are two strategies that communication partners may use to provide aided language stimulation.

Conversational recasting is defined as a response (to an individual's utterance) that maintains the core idea, but expands on it by modeling a corrected or expanded version of the original utterance (Baker & Nelson, 1984; Cleave & Fey, 1997). For example, in response to a parent asking their child what happened at school during the day, the child says, using their AAC system, "play Sarah." The parent acknowledges the message and provides an example of an expanded, syntactically correct form by orally saying, "You played with Sarah," while activating "you play Sarah" on the device or communication board. Then, the parent might model orally and select the symbols, "How fun!"

In this example, the caregiver is providing a correct and expanded utterance. In addition, the caregiver demonstrated interest in the child and showed the child that the communicative message was understood. They then proceeded to make a comment ("How fun"). Although the interaction lasted a couple of exchanges, the level of meaning in interaction will depend on the level of mutual interest between parent and child. The more scripted the interaction routine is, the less potential it has for expanding meaning-making between communication partners.

The second strategy is modeling. The use of this strategy focuses on providing the correct model of language in different contexts. This may be used in the context of a language lesson (goal-driven, task-oriented) or in a communicative interaction between the AAC user and a communication partner (more relation-oriented). For example, when reading the book, *One Fish, Two Fish, Red Fish, Blue Fish* by Dr. Seuss, the teacher would orally read the phrase, "This one has a little star." This is paired with the teacher selecting the symbol "this" then pointing to the fish, followed by selecting the symbol of "little," then pointing to the star. The AAC user benefits from seeing a model of how the AAC system can be immersed in the book-reading context. Specific language targets and communication functions are taught all the while providing a framework for these targets within syntactical structures with morphological markers applied.

Typical language learners benefit from these teaching strategies because they are constantly and continuously used across all environments and with all communication partners. AAC users need the same accessibility to these strategies to maximize their understanding and use of language with an AAC system. In order for this to be achieved, the AAC system must be available for use throughout the day and across environments and activities.

Finally, there is a cautionary note that modeling expression and recasting another's utterances do not necessarily facilitate meaning-making in interactions with others. Although these strategies can certainly assist in expanding exchanges with others, meaning-making requires an awareness of and sensitivity to the other individual in interaction (Alant, 2017a). Interventionists need to be upfront in differentiating between task-/outcomes-oriented (e.g., an increase in utterances and language ability) and relational-oriented (i.e., ability to emotionally resonate) interactions to ensure a realistic assessment of the individual's ability to engage with others in interactions.

SUSTAINABILITY OF INTERVENTION: ENHANCING RELATIONSHIP DEVELOPMENT AND FRIENDSHIPS

Choosing and purchasing an AAC system for a client, albeit a challenging process including assessment and securing funding, is the easy part. Once a device is acquired, interventionists need to be thoughtful about how this device will be weaved into the everyday experiences of their client and how to train and empower the client's everyday communication partners to provide access and facilitate the use of the device. If we view the frequency with which typical communicators interact with those around them, it reminds us of the importance of access to an AAC device for all users across contexts and communication partners. Therefore, it is crucial that the AAC system be embedded into the natural environment and others are trained to act as teachers and communication partners. Embedding a system in the natural environment implies not only availability of the AAC system to increase the frequency of interactions but also the relevance of the exchanges in facilitating meaning-making with others.

Factors to Consider in Facilitating Sustainability in Intervention

Teaching and Interacting

Kent-Walsh and McNaughton (2005) stated that an individual's communication skills influence the communication interaction between individuals. Therefore, the quality of an interaction between an AAC user and a communication partner is greatly dependent upon the interaction skills of the communication partner. Many of the communication partners who interact with the user and the device have no formal or even informal training on how to use or teach the system. Without instruction or opportunities to see modeling of how to interact using AAC strategies, communication partners have great difficulty engaging in successful communicative interactions with users of AAC (Kent-Walsh & McNaughton, 2005). Therefore, the goal is to expose communication partners to experiences of what meaning-making could look like in interaction with users of AAC. Teaching AAC strategies to communication partners can be useful; however, they can also impose a level of artificiality in the interaction. What could have been a relaxed and natural process of being together can often be transformed into a teaching or a work interaction. Clearly this type of experience does not provide a good basis for sustained use of AAC systems in interaction. The gains derived from being together and developing meaning in interaction are vital in promoting consistent use of AAC systems in interactions. Therefore, the art is to infuse the use of the device within the natural context in small steps to minimize it becoming a significant distraction in interactions.

A clear and well thought-out training plan should be put in place that supports the learning of the basics, such as how to navigate the system. Communication partners need to understand that core vocabulary is a vital part of creating meaningful interactions with users of AAC (Van Tatenhove, 2016). Aided language stimulation and the use of strategies, like recasting and modeling, can be effective, as communication partners can learn to infuse these in social interactions across all activities and environments of the day. This infusion requires patience and incremental steps to ensure the use of these strategies do not overpower the meaning-making process between the user of AAC and their communication partners (Alant, 2017a).

Understanding the Communication Partner

It is important to understand each individual communication partner's beliefs regarding the user as a communicator, the actual system as a communication tool, and their role as a communication partner. Understanding those beliefs will allow the interventionist to tailor training and support to meet the individual's needs. If a communication partner believes they are able to communicate well enough with the client without the system, then intervention needs to focus on assisting the communication partner to understand and *experience* the contribution that AAC strategies can have in extending their interaction with the user of AAC. Feelings of being overwhelmed by technology generally is counterproductive in exploring ways to integrate the use of AAC strategies into daily life. McNaughton and colleagues (2008) conducted an online focus group discussion to better understand parents' perspectives on learning and engaging with AAC systems. This study emphasized the need to consider the comfort level of the communication partner with technology and how that individual will learn the system.

Experiencing Meaning-Making

Persuading communication partners to interact with users by using AAC strategies often infuses a dimension of artificiality into the interaction. It is important for communication partners to be able to identify these contrived events of limited meaning-making to allow them to develop the sensitivity to realize the difference between using an AAC strategy and infusing it into meaning-making interactions. Interventionists need to help tear barriers down by encouraging problem solving that yield solutions or alternatives. Creating a sense of ownership will empower communication partners to be active participants in the process. For example, when asked how it was going with using the AAC system outside of therapy, the communication partner stated that the system is not being used when they and the AAC user go out for walks in the park because they are concerned that the device may be dropped and break. The interventionist acknowledged the concern and then provided them with information about how the mount attached to the client's wheelchair was designed to allow access to the AAC system when in the wheelchair. The interventionist could provide examples of ways that aided stimulation may be used in this environment, as well as by using manual signs. They also could explain that the AAC system is not a show piece and should be enriching their interactions with each other. Similarly, AAC systems of students are often not used in schools. The devices are in classrooms but hidden away in backpacks, on counters or shelves in homes, or even on the desk in front of an AAC user without any activation or selection. Some users will figure it out independently, but in most cases, the AAC user will require assistance to get to know the device and how it can be used to facilitate interactions with others. The clearly defined role of communication partners in supporting the infusion of the AAC system into interactions with the client is critical. They do need to understand the importance of bridging the gap between using the device as a teaching tool and using the device in developing relationships and friendships with others (Alant et al., 2013). An AAC system is only as effective as a communication tool as the AAC user and the communication partners allow it to be.

Core Vocabulary and Small Steps

Many interventionists are good at teaching task-oriented goals, as these represent a clear plan with specific goals that are easily met. These types of goals are necessary for language development and learning how to effectively use an AAC system to communicate. Social skills can even be taught in this manner; for example, greetings can be worked on with peers and staff in a school environment. Working in this manner does not guarantee the development of social closeness or the development of friendships. The benefit of using a core vocabulary approach with communication partners is that it can be less overwhelming for communication partners. Core vocabulary provides the user with words that can be easily sequenced together to create messages that express ideas, thoughts, questions, or even humor during an "in the moment" conversation that was not planned or pre-programmed. This allows for a shared moment between people that is authentic and dynamic. Shared moments, common bonds, and interest in one another is what leads to the development of a friendship. This cannot happen without the ability to use one's language to share and gather information to create a connection. AAC users need to be able to communicate more than just requests. Core vocabulary can allow for this to happen. Like any other strategy, the use of core vocabulary is as effective in promoting authentic interactions as the ability of the communication partner in infusing rather than imposing the use of the system in interactions with the user (see Chapter 12).

SUMMARY

The landscape in AAC intervention has experienced dramatic changes in recent years. Technological innovations (e.g., eye gaze and head pointing) along with increased availability of communication applications on mobile devices has allowed for a wider range of individuals to communicate using AAC. Due to the complexity and increasing diversity of users of AAC, it is critical that interventionists plan for goals that not only address cognitive academic language proficiency, but also basic interaction communicative skills.

Additionally, interventionists must keep in mind the potential barriers that may impact the user of AAC from fully meeting their communicative potential. Interventionists must consider which vocabulary and teaching strategies, such as core vocabulary and aided language stimulation respectively, will allow for not only the development of language and the ability to communicate a variety of message types but also generalization of use. Consideration of the communication partners' needs must be realized and planned for accordingly in order to ensure positive outcomes.

The ultimate goal of AAC intervention is to help users of AAC develop friendships and social closeness with their communication partners. This is not a guaranteed outcome of intervention. This requires that the device be weaved into the day-to-day framework. This will ensure access to the device and increase the frequency of interactions. However, the device must be viewed as more than a means to participate and to gain access to wants and needs. It is critical that it be viewed as the communicator's voice and the means for developing relationships. Finally, it requires that the interventionist and communication partners are sensitive and have a deeper awareness of the user of AAC as an individual in order to create an authentic interaction, which ultimately facilitates the goal of developing meaningful relationships.

STUDY QUESTIONS

1. How has the changing landscape of AAC impacted assessment and intervention?
2. Describe the differences between a task-oriented interaction and authentic interaction.
3. Discuss the diference between "imposing" and "infusing" the use of AAC strategies into an individual's life.
4. Provide an example of how a clinician could use aided language stimulation to enhance meaningful interaction with a young child.
5. Explain how the communication partner impacts the effectiveness of AAC intervention.
6. What is the ultimate goal of intervention for AAC users?

16

Seating, Positioning, and Communication

Shirley Wells, DrPH; Jack Ruelas, OTR;
John Luna, OTD; and Sayda E. Ruelas, MPT

<table>
<tr>
<td>

MYTH

1. If an occupational therapist, physical therapist, or other specialist has prescribed positioning, then other team members should not question it.

2. A person should remain in one position no longer than 2 hours.

3. Sidelyers and prone positioners encourage development of head control, shoulder stability, and hand function by helping people with disabilities to approximate the positions of developing infants.

</td>
<td>

REALITY

1. All team members, including the person being positioned, have a role in deciding upon positioning and ensuring that it is optimal.

2. It is important to individually determine how long each person can sit comfortably and safely. Some people need to have their positions changed more often than every 2 hours and others can sit in a well-designed seat for much longer than 2 hours.

3. Current intervention theories no longer support these presumed development effects of sidelyers and prone positioners, especially beyond infancy and for people with severe disabilities.

</td>
</tr>
</table>

SEATING AND POSITIONING

Approaching Seating and Positioning

Many children and adults with disabilities may not be able to use speech as their primary mode of communication and may therefore require augmentative and alternative communication (AAC; Treviranus & Roberts, 2003). Those with complex physical and communication needs rely on assistive technology and AAC to participate wholly in daily life. However, some will frequently have problems with their posture, controlling their extremities, and seating. They often require adaptive seating and positioning systems to provide greater body stability, trunk/head support, improved posture, and reduced pressure on the skin surface (Assistive Technology Guide, 2016). Seating and positioning may also influence other aspects of a person's communication, such

Fuller, D. R., & Lloyd, L. L. *Principles and Practices in*
Augmentative and Alternative Communication (pp. 279-292).
© 2023 Taylor & Francis Group.

as cognitive performance, hearing, vision, attention, arousal, and opportunities for interaction (Costigan & Light, 2010b; Falkman et al., 2002). For verbal communication, we need appropriate head and trunk control for physiological function, vocalization, endurance, and self-esteem. Thus, optimizing motor skills and seating position for access to AAC is imperative.

Individuals with disabilities with spinal cord injury, traumatic brain injury, cerebral vascular accidents, cerebral palsy, multiple traumas, spina bifida, musculoskeletal problems, cardiac diseases, and metabolic disorders are most commonly identified with seating, positioning, and mobility problems. Each of the sections of this chapter contains background information, current information, and questions to guide clinicians through the decision-making process, as well as a continuum for positioning, seating, and mobility.

Interprofessional Practice

Wheelchair seating and mobility is a technical and specialized area of rehabilitation. The unique characteristics of the individual and current technology must be considered when choosing the best AAC. A complete understanding of the individual's health condition and associated impairments will direct the provider in assessing optimal positioning, mobility, and AAC for the individual with a disability. Due to this complicated intervention process, an interprofessional team approach to assessment and intervention is ideal. Successful AAC services require a collaborative team approach, involving the individual who requires AAC, their families, and members from various professional disciplines.

The members of the team depend on the complexity of the impairments of the individual being evaluated, availability, and funding. The team may be composed of any of the following:

- *Physician:* The physician is required to assess the client's medical status as it relates to seating, positioning, and mobility issues. The physician provides the certificate of medical necessity, which is needed for payment of technology.
- *Occupational therapist:* The role of an occupational therapist involves the evaluation of body movement and physical capabilities, including fine motor and gross motor skills, touch and sensory perception, posture and positioning, and analysis of the environment, user needs, and access methods when considering the provision of assistive technology.
- *Physical therapist:* Working as part of the team, physical therapists may work closely with occupational therapists to evaluate seating, positioning, and mobility and to examine a person's posture and movement to find the best position or adaptation for the provision of assistive technology for optimal access.

- *Speech-language pathologist:* The role of a speech-language pathologist is to evaluate disabilities affecting speech and language, including swallowing disorders. The evaluation will involve assessing the person's communication abilities and needs to identify proper AAC options with appropriate vocabulary with the seating, positioning, and mobility recommendations.
- *Rehabilitation engineer:* Engineers usually work as part of a multidisciplinary team and may be involved from the initial client assessment or at any stage from assessment to equipment delivery and client support.
- *Seating-and-mobility specialist:* This discipline is earned by certification through the Rehabilitation Engineering and Assistive Technology Society of North America that may be held by physical therapists and occupational therapists who demonstrate advanced seating and mobility skills.
- *Assistive technology professional:* This discipline is earned by certification earned through the Rehabilitation Engineering and Assistive Technology Society of North America that may be held by physical therapists and occupational therapists. This individual specializes in matching the AAC user's strengths and limitations to the procurement of assistive technology.
- *Rehabilitation technology specialists:* These are earned credentials of durable medical equipment providers. The assistive technology professional is a required certification for a rehab technology specialist who is evaluating a client for a rehab-level power wheelchair funded by Medicare. The vendor should have extensive knowledge of commercially available equipment, as well as the ability to acquire equipment for trial or extensive evaluation before equipment purchase. The vendor may assist the team in funding procurement, fitting, training, and ongoing service of the technology provided.
- *Education and teaching professionals:* Education professionals have important roles during an assessment within the educational setting. Assessments require a good understanding of a student's characteristics and capabilities of education and technology in accessing the curriculum and academic performance. The education professional should also have the knowledge, skills, and competencies to support students with the use of assistive technology in an educational environment.

Although occupational therapists and physical therapists may be the leading "positioning" players, the creation of a team that possesses the knowledge, skill, and abilities needed to service the client are essential tools for any AAC team. The team will permit the solving of straightforward problems and encourage the seeking out of expert input as complex issues arise. Not every occupational or physical therapist specializes in seating, positioning, mobility, or AAC. Thus, it is essential for clinicians to become familiar with resources that are available and the capabilities of local service providers.

A family-/client-centered approach is a critical element for selecting the most appropriate AAC. The end-user must be satisfied with the product to ensure its use. Outcome measures may be used to ensure that identified goals are being met and recommended equipment continues to meet the client's needs in the future. Optimally, the client and family should see and try different equipment options in natural environments to effectively assess how equipment can be used and can identify barriers that impact their daily function. The opportunity for a group of well-qualified personnel with an understanding of basic principles of seating, positioning, and AAC to demonstrate and recommend appropriate equipment is a crucial component to maximize a client's independence and productivity.

CLIENT ASSESSMENT

People who use AAC have many different medical diagnoses, most of which result from congenital or acquired central nervous system (CNS) pathology. Brain damage or malformation can contribute to neuromotor, musculoskeletal, and sensory impairments. Impairments at this level impact body function, such as motor control, and affect both oral communication and communication through AAC devices. Because of the complexity of the CNS, the type and severity of motor problems depend on the location and the extent of the brain damage or malformation. For this reason, even people who have the same diagnosis, such as cerebral palsy, traumatic brain injury, or stroke, may have variations in the presentation of their muscle tone, motor abilities, and sensory functions. These factors are important when considering seating and AAC device implementation to maximize function and promote participation for the user with their environment, be it at home, school, work, community, or elsewhere.

Factors for Consideration

Neuromotor

The **neuromotor system** pertains to both the nerves and muscles or to nerve impulses transmitted to muscles to create movement (Mosby, 2017). An abnormality of—or damage to—the brain, spinal cord, or nervous system that sends impulses to the muscles of the body can create a neuromotor impairment. These impairments may be acquired at or before birth and often result in complex motor problems that can affect several body systems. Motor problems can include limited limb movement, loss of urinary control, and loss of proper alignment of the spine. The two most common types of neuromotor impairments are cerebral palsy and spina bifida (Ohio Department of Education, 2017). These motor problems can impact not only oral communication for

speech production but also the ability to engage in written communication. Individuals with a high spinal cord injury, for example, can usually speak but are unable to use their hands, so they may require adaptations to written communication. Speech production can be affected by cranial nerve damage (Ziegler & Ackermann, 2013). Many of these associated problems can be modified or controlled through proper seating positioning.

Common Neuromotor Problems

Abnormal Muscle Tone

Abnormal muscle tone is a neuromotor issue commonly seen by therapists. Tone can be increased or decreased depending on the type, location, and severity of the neuromotor damage. **Muscle tone** refers to the state of tension within muscles. Muscles are always in a slight state of contraction; without this tension, we would not be able to maintain and control upright posture and resist the force of gravity. Abnormal muscle tone presents in many different forms (Gutman, 2017):

- Hypotonia (low tone; e.g., floppy baby syndrome)
- Hypertonia (high tone; e.g., stroke and traumatic brain injury)
- Rigidity (e.g., Parkinson's disease)
- Dystonia (e.g., cerebral palsy)
- Spasticity (e.g., stroke and traumatic brain injury)

The wheelchair can be used to inhibit abnormally increased tone and improve function via improved postural alignment, especially of the pelvis. Position, emotions, arousal, and health are some of the factors that can cause variation in a person's muscle tone. In patients with hypotonicity or low tone, the wheelchair seating system can provide support for the trunk and extremities to prevent collapse and to avoid unwanted pressure on bony landmarks. These are common strategies used when treating individuals with neuromotor dysfunction. Seating equipment and a properly prescribed wheelchair can serve to provide proximal stability and promote distal mobility and function.

Postural Stability

Postural stability is an automatic function, whereas postural orientation is a conscious decision. It involves the control of the body's position in space to obtain stability and orientation. Stability (or balance) maintains or regains the position of the body over the base of support (BOS; center of body mass [COM]) to prevent falling during static or dynamic activities. Orientation aligns the body parts about one another, so they are appropriate for the task being accomplished (Shumway-Cook & Woollacott, 2017). Functional goals of postural control include:

- Postural orientation: This is the active alignment of the trunk and head with respect to gravity, support surfaces, visual surrounding and internal references, and postural equilibrium.
- Coordination of movement: These entail strategies to stabilize COM during both self-initiated and externally triggered disturbances of stability.
- Proximal stability: Stability involves movement of COM relative to BOS.

The purposes of these body control systems are to maintain equilibrium and orientation in sitting and standing (Gaebler-Spira & Girolami, 2013).

When people have deficits that interfere with normal control of posture, they lack both the necessary stability and alignment for optimal function. Postural control is crucial because it provides a basis of support that allows the arms and legs to move smoothly. An individual who has difficulty sitting with good posture will struggle to write or do any table-top activities that require fine motor precision, such as operating an AAC device, as they will need to put all their attention into making sure they will not fall off the chair. The relation between postural control and fine motor skills is the primary focus of therapy. Clinicians should consider postural control and fine motor skills as two interdependent systems when choosing seating systems and AAC devices (Wang et al., 2011).

Motor

Motor performance problems can be both related to and independent of other neuromuscular problems. People with neuromotor conditions often have difficulty with several components of motor performance, such as abnormal timing and force of muscle activation; difficulty with initiation, sustained holding of contraction, and/or termination of movement; decreased speed of movement; and use of abnormal compensatory patterns of movement as a person attempts to accomplish motor goals (Sakurada et al., 2017). People with severe neuromotor problems often have few movement options available to them, so they must approach different tasks with stereotypic movement (repetitive, non-functional movement) or paucity of movement.

Neuromotor Problems' Impact on AAC

Neuromotor problems must be considered when selecting AAC devices. From the proportional joystick to specialty devices, such as switches, head arrays, or a sip-and-puff system, the selection of access methods is dependent upon muscle tone, postural stability, and motor performance of the individual. Problems in these areas can be related to and independent of the selection and use of AAC devices. Because of muscle weakness, spasticity, tonicity, patterned movements, or limited range of motion, individuals with physical disabilities may not be able to press a key or switch or make

reliable and interpretable movements (Higginbotham et al., 2007; Lange, 2018). Muscle tone affects eye musculature, impacting ocular-motor control. Good posturing improves eye gaze, hand and arm function, and head position. With the trunk and head supported at midline, the individual with a disability can direct their gaze more functionally. A proper seating system can inhibit abnormal muscle tone and movements. Thus, the evaluation of the individual's body contours, range of motion, and orientation in space can ensure implementation of a seating system that best positions and supports the person for comfort and AAC function.

Musculoskeletal

The musculoskeletal system provides form, support, stability, and movement of the body. This system consists of muscles, tendons, ligaments, bones, joints, and associated tissues that move the body and maintain its form. The integrated action of joints, bones, and skeletal muscles produces movements, such as walking and running, as well as subtle movements that result in facial expressions, eye movements, and respiration (National Library of Medicine, n.d.). Musculoskeletal disorders are injuries and disorders that affect the human body's movement or musculoskeletal system (i.e., muscles, tendons, ligaments, nerves, discs, blood vessels).

Common Musculoskeletal Problems

Joint Contractures and Skeletal Deformities

Joint contractures and skeletal deformities can be present at birth, but they usually develop over time, secondary to neuromuscular impairments. When a joint is contracted, it cannot be moved passively through its full range of motion. Other common skeletal deformities include scoliosis (sideways bending of the spine, which is usually combined with rotation of the vertebrae), kyphosis (forward bending of the spine), and hip dislocation (the hip joint separates, with the ball on the top of the femur coming out of the socket in the pelvis).

The primary causes of contractures and other deformities are position and muscle imbalance. Positional deformities occur when muscles and other soft tissue around a joint become tight due to lack of joint movement. A person who sits all day, for example, and whose hips and knees are not in extension for a sufficiently long period will likely develop hip and knee flexion contractures. Although there is little evidence to indicate how long is enough, research suggests that joints must be at their maximum range for at least 6 to 7 hours each day (Institute of Medicine and National Research Council, 2001; LeBlanc & LeBlanc, 2010). Thus, the value of periodic passive range-of-motion exercises to prevent contractures is questionable, and contracture prevention through selective positioning to provide a prolonged stretch is more likely to be of benefit. Achieving and maintaining pelvic alignment is also key to optimal positioning. The pelvis should be positioned in a level and anterior position. A level pelvis allows for symmetrical weight-bearing and equal pressure distribution and improves alignment above and below the pelvis. Seating considerations of the pelvis are key to achieving proximal stability, which is necessary for distal mobility and control of the upper extremities for AAC use.

Muscle Imbalance

Muscle imbalance can also contribute to joint contractures and is usually compounded by position. For example, if the muscles (adductor muscles) pull the thighs together (inward and internally rotated), an abduction contracture will result if the individual is allowed to remain in this position. This contracture creates an imbalance with the thigh muscles (abductors) that pull the leg outward and externally rotate. One way to prevent this and other contractures caused by muscle imbalance is through positioning that maintains the body in alignment opposite the pull of the more active muscles. It must be determined if optimal alignment can first be achieved passively on a flat surface in a supine position and then in the seated position. Sometimes it is better to accommodate range of motion limitations rather than overcorrect alignment, as this may become uncomfortable for the patient and end up causing rotational forces above and below the pelvis. The pelvis is the key to optimal alignment in a wheelchair (O'Sullivan et al., 2014).

While the pelvis is the BOS for distal upper extremity movements and sensory systems (e.g., visual, proprioceptive, tactile, and vestibular) function, it provides the input to the CNS to generate efficient motor responses to access AAC devices. Considering sensory, neuromotor, and musculoskeletal factors can assure an optimal match when selecting seating to optimize a client's functional mobility.

Musculoskeletal Problems' Impact on AAC

Musculoskeletal problems related to arm and hand movements for control, ocular scanning, and duration and comfort of usage can impact many aspects of the selection of an AAC system. Muscle imbalance and joint contractures affect some limbs more than others. Because of this difficulty in moving, joints stay in one position for a long time. The limitations of musculoskeletal problems can lead to physical issues, such as pain, limited mobility, and an unbalanced appearance. These problems lead to an increased risk of injury due to a lack of stability. This instability can lead to an increased risk of damage to joints, muscles, bones, tendons, ligaments, and the surrounding connective tissue. A misplaced muscle or weak muscle of the eye can result in difficulties in fixating, shifting and focusing, and scanning and tracking a moving target, as well as result in fatigue and reduced acuity.

Upper and lower extremity physical functioning influences AAC aids and systems. For example, if the upper extremities are not functional for access but the individual has sufficient control of their head or other body part, an optical pointer, head mouse, or microswitch with scanning may be selected to access an AAC device. Individuals using a wheelchair may require a wheelchair mounting system to transport the AAC device. To improve outcomes, physical and occupational therapists work together to create a postural support system for a patient with neuromuscular problems in need of a mobility system. Occupational therapists work with speech-language pathologists to create a communication system for individuals and their families.

Vision

Many AAC systems rely on a dynamic visual interface for use (e.g., graphic symbols, communication boards and books, manual signs, computer displays, gestures and body language). Vision can contribute to, or detract from, the success of AAC interventions (Blackstone, 2005). Thus, accounting for the function of the integrity of the visual field during the wheelchair seating and alignment evaluation can ensure a good match between technology and the client's abilities for optimal participation. When assessing the visual system, it is essential to assess the client's visual field and visual scanning abilities.

Common Visual Problems

Visual Field

There are numerous ways to assess **visual field** integrity during a wheelchair assessment. First, observe for asymmetries during a period of general observation. Posture associated with a visual impairment includes the client's preference for their head shifting away from midline or bringing their head either above or below the horizon in order to compensate for a visual field deficit. The person constantly will be shifting positions to see. A more formal method of assessment of visual conformation involves occluding the vision of one eye while checking for visual field integrity in the vertical and horizontal planes and each of the four quadrants (superior, inferior, right, and left) of the uncovered eye. The process is then repeated on the opposite side (Blaikie, 2014; Gutman & Schonfeld, 2009). The client's inability to see visual stimuli or delay identifying the stimuli in a specific quadrant could be indicative of a visual field cut. These findings should be noted and retained as consideration for both wheelchair and AAC device selection. If a visual field deficit is detected that had not been previously diagnosed, make sure to share these findings with the rehabilitation team (which should include the client and a primary medical physician and/or an optometrist).

Visual Tracking

It is critical to assess **visual pursuit/tracking** when performing a wheelchair assessment, not only to increase participation through improved communication via an AAC device but also to assure safe community mobility. Visual tracking is a product of oculomotor control, or the ability of the eyes to coordinate their movement in unison to process visual information. It is the ability to lock onto and maintain fixation on a moving target across all visual fields (Gutman, 2017). When screening for the integrity of oculomotor control, the client's head is held in a midline position. Present an object at midline and slowly move the object across all fields making the shape of an H and diagonally making the shape of an X. The client can also be observed tracking the movement of people within the room. An impairment is indicated if the client is unable to track objects across the visual fields, coordinate movement of both eyes simultaneously, or isolate the head from eye movement (Gutman, 2017).

An additional function of ocular motor control includes convergence and saccadic movements. The inability of both eyes to move inward during a task, such as reading, is indicative of convergence insufficiency. The client may complain of losing their place when reading or writing and difficulty performing tasks up close. Convergence/divergence deficits are indicated if one or both eyes fail to move inward and symmetrically toward and away from the nose. Saccadic vision is quick, precise eye movements during visual scanning or visual search. Saccadic eye movement is used to read and to look for a person in a crowded room. Screening is the same visual pursuit, except for the examiner request: The client shifts their gaze as quickly as possible between two static point positions on contralateral sides of the body. Overshooting or undershooting between targets demonstrates a visual impairment (Gutman, 2017; Mucha et al., 2014).

Findings from the ocular motor screening should be noted in the client's wheelchair assessment for further consideration. Additional consideration should be made in the selection and placement of AAC devices if the client has additional visual acuity or visual perception deficits noted when completing the visual screening.

Visual Impairments' Impact on AAC

The range of visual impairments may be caused by diseases or problems of the eye, the visual pathway, or the brain. Terms such as visual impairment, blindness, legal blindness, and low vision are used to describe different degrees of visual impairment. Common diagnoses associated with visual impairment include age-related macular degeneration, retinopathy, glaucoma, cataracts, and refractive error. Visual impairments can also coexist or occur secondary to another diagnosis, such as cerebral vascular accident, diabetes, and cerebral palsy. Visual field disturbances can impair the use of a wheelchair for community mobility, prescribed AAC device, and the client's ability to participate in their environment. Visual acuity loss, such as myopia, hyperopia, and astigmatism, may impact the positioning of an AAC device. Visual field deficit or loss may affect the arrangement and placement of a static display or locus of production of unaided symbols. Point of fixation and head control and oculomotor problems may impact spacing of items on a display, the location of a device, and visual scanning.

It is essential to correlate impairment with the appropriate modification to reduce or eliminate barriers to AAC access while preserving function. For example, mounting an AAC device to a wheelchair on the right would be appropriate for a client who has a left visual field cut. It is vital that the client preserves optimal sight lines to use their wheelchair safely for community mobility. Matching access with a function to eliminate barriers to participation should be a primary goal. The utilization of all available services can help address these issues not only from a compensatory (AAC and wheelchair implementation) but also from a rehabilitative approach to achieve optimal participation. Making basic accommodations can make a huge difference in supporting the communication efforts of people with visual impairments (Blackstone, 2005).

Sensory Systems

The **sensory system** is vital to achieving functional motor performance, providing safety, and protecting the body. The body receives impressions of warmth, softness, pressure, and pain through the sensory system, as well as the sense of equilibrium; that is, knowing whether the body is moving and sensing the body's posture and position. By detecting environmental changes, the sensory system provides individuals with protection and with mechanisms for experiencing the world. The sensory system consists of sensory receptors, neural pathways, and parts of the brain involved in sensory perception. The sensory systems include those for vision, hearing, somatic sensation (touch), taste, and olfaction (smell).

Common Sensory Problems

Vestibular

The **vestibular system** is responsible for detecting the effects of gravity, movements of the head, and the development of balance (Ayers, 2005). Sensory information about motion, equilibrium, and spatial orientation is provided by the vestibular apparatus, which in each ear includes the utricle, saccule, and three semicircular canals. The vestibular system is responsible for processing movement, changes in head position, and direction and speed of movement. When the vestibular system is activated, the brain is both calmed and aroused.

Movement can calm, arouse, work muscles, and provide comfort by varying our position. An agitated client may become calm when the vestibular system is activated, and a client who is not alert may become alert. From a sensory standpoint, movement provides vestibular input. Static seating does not move with the client. The client may be able to move within and separate from the wheelchair seating system, but the more restrictive the seating system is, the less the client will be able to move in it.

Consideration of the vestibular system includes accessing the overall position of the client about their vertical position. Positioning a client in a more reclined position may reduce the effects of gravity to the benefit of the integumentary system; however, this position may also elicit undesired reflexes or an increase in muscle tone. Since it is difficult to impose normal movement over abnormal tone, the client's ability to access their AAC device via direct or indirect selection may be impaired. Suspected sensory impairments should be relayed to other members of the rehabilitation team, such as the occupational therapist, for more formal assessment and intervention.

Proprioception

While the vestibular system is responsible for detecting movement, the **proprioceptive system** is responsible for generating a sense of body awareness. Proprioception, also referred to as kinesthesia, is synonymous with body position and movement (Ayers, 2005). The proprioceptive system through nerve receptors in the joints and muscles is the sensory component of the sensory-motor loop, which coordinates movement (Witchalls et al., 2012). Proprioception helps to maintain balance during static and transitional movements, motor control, and all aspects of activities of daily living (Gutman & Schonfeld, 2009).

Assessing proprioception consists of active/passive movement detection and discrimination (Hillier et al., 2015). Evaluating proprioceptive function begins with a general observation regarding the client's quality of movement when engaged in functional reaching activities. With the client's eyes occluded, primary screening involves moving each joint through the planes of motion while holding at the last position. Ask the client where the extremity is or if they can replicate the motion with the other extremity. Additional screening includes monitoring the accuracy of movement when the patient is asked to bring their finger to their nose with vision occluded (Gutman & Schonfeld, 2009). Impairments in the proprioceptive system can affect the client's body awareness and upper extremity coordination.

Given the pivotal role of proprioception in movements, individuals diagnosed with cerebral palsy (Wingert et al., 2009) and other disorders affecting the CNS (e.g., cerebral vascular accident) may experience proprioception or kinesthetic impairments. Impaired sensory-motor function (with underlying proprioceptive system dysfunction) can limit available control for AAC technology. It is essential to assess the client's ability to activate a desired switch, as well as the

level necessary to activate a switch. These can impact both the type and location of the switch. General strategies for seating to reduce the effect of proprioception impairments should center around providing a stable BOS (proximal stability) and to support distal manipulation of items.

Tactile

For a wheelchair evaluation, it is important to consider the sensory aspect of touch and the role it plays in protecting the integrity of the skin through registering heat, cold, pain, and pressure. Functionally, the ability to localize touch allows the client to feel clothing on their body, identify and remove an annoying fly on the arm, and find a pressure spot on the surface of a shoe. **Tactile** assessment (Gutman & Schonfeld, 2009) includes:

- Tactile localization
- Two-point discrimination (ability to determine whether one has been touched by one or two points)
- Stereognosis
- Vibration
- Simultaneous stimulation

Screening results should be documented through the **dermatome** areas and functionality. Stimuli should be presented randomly. Impairments in touch-processing play a crucial role in recognizing noxious stimuli or discomfort, which can pose a potential risk to skin integrity and/or injury, difficulty in fine motor tasks, identifying objects when vision is occluded, and bilateral coordination and manipulation. The most common impairment is excessive sensitivity to light touch. Hypersensitivity to light touch is often accompanied by lack of normal sensitivity to heat, cold, and pain. It is crucial for survival that these receptors work efficiently, and that their input is organized and processed quickly so appropriate action can be taken. Thus, sensory evaluation is imperative for wheelchair and AAC usage. It will allow the team to assess the extent of the sensory loss, determine functional impairment and limitations, and guide decision making for optimal AAC technology.

Sensory Impairments' Impact on AAC

Intact sensory receptions are required for communication. Each person's sensory system has preferences related to positioning, movement, touch, taste, and smell. Motor control and proprioceptive input are needed, for example, to position the hand and move it over an AAC device particularly for extensive time periods. Vestibular input is needed for spatial orientation and head control for visual scanning. When visual representation is inaccessible, auditory and tactile stimulation are often the preferred modes of language representation. Sensory receptors are mostly concentrated in the hands and upper extremities but can be limited by abnormal muscle tone and poor manual manipulation skills. Active touch is our sense of touch that enables us to modify and manipulate the world around us.

Individuals with sensory dysfunction do not have adequate sensory processing skills to receive, organize, interpret, and respond to sensory information efficiently. This dysfunction negatively affects their attention, behavior, and movement. An AAC system that simplifies the sensory processing and motor planning involved in communicating allows individuals to participate in everyday activities.

Summary

The functional use of AAC in the context of wheelchair seating and mobility occurs as the result of the dynamic interaction of all the sensory systems. Therapeutic seating can provide support for trunk and extremities, reflex inhibition, and control for abnormal movement, thus allowing the client to focus on the voluntary motor control needed to operate communication equipment and participate in functional activities (Costigan & Light, 2010b; McNamara & Casey, 2007). Therapists must employ clinical rationale in the context of the most current evidence to ascertain not only the immediate needs of the client but also the needs of the client for the next 3 to 5 years and beyond. Assessment and intervention for our clients must occur in the context of the clinical, home, and community environments.

WHEELCHAIR ASSESSMENT AND SEATING POSITION

Evaluating for and choosing wheeled mobility and seating can be a daunting task. However, if a therapist can understand the reasons for specific functions, then the therapist is better able to choose or recommend specific equipment for mobility and AAC access. Both manual and power wheelchairs provide the same functions even though they are powered differently. Another concern is the effect of the seated position on access and use of AAC. What follows will be a discussion of the basic functions and positioning that are available throughout the gamut of mobility options and the types of seating and mobility equipment.

Basic Functions of Wheelchairs

The **wheelchair** is one of the most commonly used assistive devices for enhancing personal mobility and communication (a precondition for enjoying human rights and living in dignity) and assists people with disabilities to become more productive members of their communities. For many people, an appropriate, well-designed, and well-fitted wheelchair can be the first step toward inclusion and participation in society (World Health Organization, 2008). Thus, the essential functions of a wheelchair are to provide appropriate seating and independent mobility to assist an individual in completing activities of daily living and instrumental activities of daily living. These activities can range from independent mobility around the home to providing independence in pressure relief and repositioning several times a day. The goals of the seating system include postural support, stability, and pressure distribution. The goals of the mobility system include providing optimal mobility and function.

Wheelchairs are used by people for whom walking is difficult or impossible due to illness, injury, or disability. A basic manual wheelchair incorporates a seat, footrests, and four wheels: two caster wheels at the front and two large wheels at the back. The two larger wheels in the back usually have hand-rims. The device is propelled either manually (by turning the wheels by the hand) or via various automated systems. Many different types of wheelchairs are used for various reasons. It is essential to understand the limitations and safe operation of whatever wheelchair is chosen (Disabled World, 2017).

Types of Wheelchairs

There are many types of wheelchairs, including manual, power, sports, and recreational chairs, for all ages and sizes. There are standard (folding) wheelchairs that fit most general needs, and then there are custom-built (i.e., rigid) wheelchairs. Wheelchairs are categorized by weight, frame, usage, or propulsion. According to Chairdex (n.d.), Disabled World (2017), and Wilson and Kishner (2016), they include:

- Manual wheelchairs that are propelled by the user or moved by an attendant. A manual wheelchair is easy to maintain, is lightweight, and is the least expensive to buy. Manual wheelchairs are best used by people with good muscular strength and coordination in their arms and shoulders. Specialized manual wheelchairs include lightweight, ultralightweight, bariatric, pediatric, and dynamic frames.
- Electric wheelchairs that are propelled by a motor and battery. They are operated with a joystick or push buttons. Some electric wheelchairs use advanced technology. Electric wheelchairs need sturdy frames to support the motor and battery, so they are very heavy and quite expensive. The average cost of an electric wheelchair is $7,000 but can cost anywhere from $3,000 to $30,000. Electric-powered wheelchairs are ideal for anyone who does not possess the strength or ability to cope with a manual chair (many people own and use both manual and electric chairs).
- Wheelbase or scooters, which are wheelbase chairs with four small wheels extending from a low platform. The type of chair mounted on this platform varies according to the disability and needs of the user. The chair can swivel and allow the user to mount and dismount from either side; however, the user must maintain a rigid posture when driving the scooter. This means that wheelbase chairs are rarely suitable for people with severe disabilities.

- Sports wheelchairs that are designed for playing sports. They are ultralightweight yet very stable. They are often used for tennis, wheelchair basketball, and marathons. Depending on the sport, chairs vary in design.

- Standing wheelchairs that support the user in a standing position. They can be used as both a wheelchair and a standing frame, allowing the user to sit or stand in the wheelchair. Movement from sitting to standing is accomplished with a hydraulic pump or electric-powered assist.

- Stair-climbing wheelchairs that have been designed with the ability to climb flights of stairs. These sometimes include battery-operated supports at the back that act as stabilizers as the chair climbs and independent stair-climbing wheelbases onto which the wheelchair is fastened. Most stair-climbing chairs still require a separate human attendant to operate. Alternatively, the wheelchair user must be able to grasp a suitable handrail.

- Pediatric wheelchairs that are both in manual and electric form. They are just smaller-scale versions of the larger adult wheelchairs. These are usually adjustable to accommodate a child as they increase in weight and bulk with age.

- Beach wheelchairs that are recognizable because of the large wheels that enable it to ride smoothly over sand without sinking. This chair also allows users to enter the water.

Recent technological advances are slowly improving wheelchairs. These advances are enabling the chair to balance and run on only two of its four wheels on some surfaces, thus raising the user to a height comparable to a standing person. Four-wheel-drive chairs are becoming more available and advanced. Different wheelchairs come with different capabilities and different prices as well. Wheelchairs today come in festive colors and seat prints. They can also be further customized to make them unique to the user. As there is such a wide range of prices for wheelchairs, the provider should be cognizant of cost and ensure that the person who will be using the chair gets the best chair available for the money invested.

Wheelchair Functions and Features

Wheelchair seat size (width and depth), seat-to-floor height, footrests/leg rests, front caster outriggers, adjustable backrests, controls, and other features can be customized for, or added to, many basic models. Some wheelchair users, often those with specialized needs, may have custom-built chairs.

Tilt, Recline, and Elevating Leg Rests

Tilt, recline, and elevating leg rests are the most common medically necessary positioning features available on almost any manual or power wheelchair. These three functions can facilitate a client's basic functions, such as postural alignment, improved circulation, pressure relief, change in the visual field, improvement of physiological processes, and regulation of spasticity and edema (Dicianno et al., 2015). The ability to manipulate these features allows for either the client or caregivers to manage seating positions to enhance quality of life.

Tilt refers to the ability to rotate a specific seating system around a fixed axis (Cook & Polgar, 2015; Figures 16-1A and 16-1B). Tilt allows for changes in the seat angle as it relates to the ground while retaining a constant seat-to-back angle (hip angle). Virtually the whole of the chair moves as a unit on a pivot. Think of a child who leans their seat back in the classroom (Figure 16-1C).

Tilt allows a client or their caregivers to manage pressure relief on bilateral lower extremities and crucial points, such as under the hips on the ischial tuberosities. As the client is tilted backward, the pressure is redistributed from the lower extremities to a larger surface area, including the client's back (Figure 16-2).

The most commonly used systems tilt the client posteriorly. Some powered wheelchairs have the option to tilt anteriorly. The purpose of anterior tilt is to assist those clients who retain the ability to complete a transfer independently. The anterior tilt also affords the client an increase in forward reaching. Manual specifications allow for up to 10 degrees of anterior tilt while power options can range from 10 degrees to 30 degrees of anterior tilt.

Recline refers to the change in position of the seat-to-back angle. This back angle can range from the typical 90 degrees to nearly horizontal. A benefit of recline is the ability of the client to change the angle from an upright sitting position to relieve back pressure when fatigued. Recline is useful for individuals with limitations in hip flexion that require the hip angle to be greater than 90 degrees. Recline may also facilitate bowel and bladder function, alleviate orthostatic hypotension, and reduce edema and increase circulation of bilateral lower extremities when combined with elevating leg rests (Cook & Polgar, 2015). Recline is beneficial in work or social situations where changes in the seat-to-floor angle would prevent the client from being able to remain under a table or desk or to continue working or engaging in social situations.

There are two main areas of concern when considering tilt and recline for a specific client: shear and seating system. **Shear** occurs when opposing forces occur parallel to each other (Figure 16-3). The use of a recline system increases the shear that the client experiences between their back and the seat back surface (Figure 16-4). Shear force can lead to tears in the skin, which can lead to pressure ulcers. Most recline systems on the market are considered low-shear systems; however, they are unable to eliminate shear. Custom-molded seating systems provide significant support for a client who needs to maintain corrected body alignment. However, these systems are static and do not allow for dynamic movement of the client. Because of the inherent shear found in recline

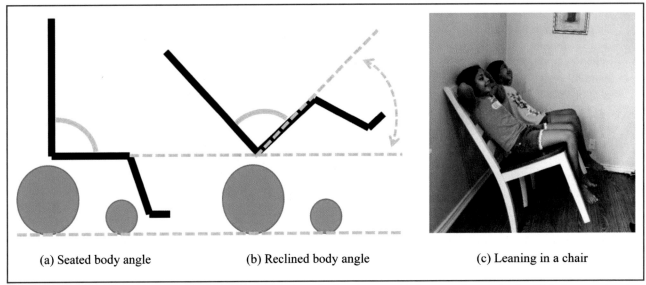

(a) Seated body angle   (b) Reclined body angle   (c) Leaning in a chair

Figure 16-1. Wheelchair tilting. (A) Normal wheelchair position with seat back and seat at a 90-degree angle to each other. (B) Both seat and seat back tilt backward, maintaining the 90-degree angle. (C) An everyday example of children tilting their seats back.

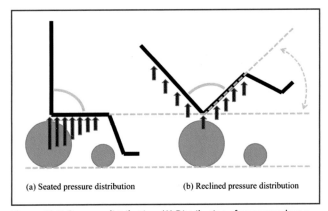

(a) Seated pressure distribution   (b) Reclined pressure distribution

Figure 16-2. Pressure distribution. (A) Distribution of pressure when a wheelchair is in its normal position. (B) Redistribution of pressure when seat back and seat tilt backward, maintaining the 90-degree angle.

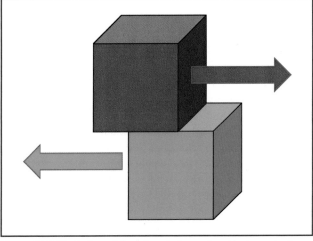

Figure 16-3. Illustration of shear force between two blocks contacting each other as they move in opposite directions.

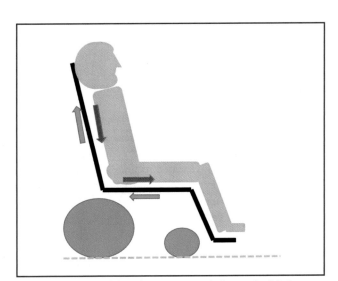

Figure 16-4. Potential shear forces generated when a wheelchair seat back is tilted backward, changing the angle between it and the seat.

systems, a custom-molded back would not maintain its alignment on the client's body when moved from the normal position. This would magnify shear and pressure on specific points of contact on the client's body.

Another point to assess is the shifting of the COM when the chair has a tilt function. The COM of the client and seat must not move outside the BOS of the wheelchair base. A simple tilt system will move the COM posteriorly to the COM of the base (Figure 16-5). If the COM is moved too far, the base can become unstable and can tilt over, leading to client injury. A tilt in space system is available and has additional mechanisms to keep the COM of the client and seating centered on the base (Figure 16-6). However, this will add additional weight to the wheelchair system.

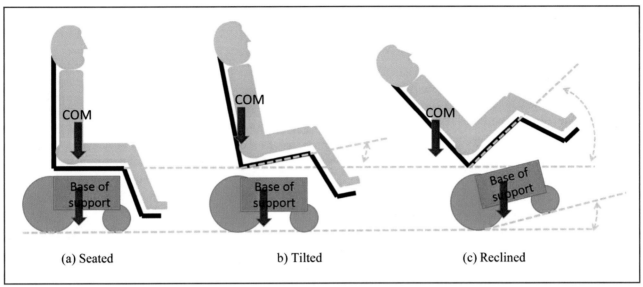

Figure 16-5. Changes in COM and BOS depending on wheelchair position. (A) Normal seating. (B) Seat back and seat both titled backward at a relatively small degree. (C) Seat back and seat both titled backward at a greater degree. Note in (C) the seat is positioned over the back wheels; if the seat is tilted back too far, COM and BOS are so far out of alignment that the wheelchair is in danger of tipping backward.

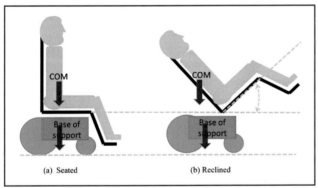

Figure 16-6. Alignment of COM and BOS in client seating. (A) Normal seating position. (B) Both seat back and seat tilted backward. Note the seat is positioned forward, toward the front wheels, to allow for BOS and COM to align. This will prevent the wheelchair from tipping over.

Elevating leg rests allow a client to change the leg and footrest angle relative to the seat to flex or extend the lower extremity at the knee (Dicianno et al., 2015). Edema can be effectively managed with the use of elevating leg rests in combination with tilt, when the legs are elevated above the heart. Elevating leg rests can be either manual or powered.

Seat Elevator

A **seat elevator** will lower and raise the seat height relative to the ground, usually through use of an electromechanical system. This change in elevation does not affect the seat or back angles. Seat elevators have several medical benefits, including assisting with safe transfers, increasing reach, and increasing psychological benefits (Arva, Schmeler, et al., 2009).

A client can more easily complete a transfer if the transfer occurs across level surfaces or with the assistance of gravity in a downhill direction. With the use of a seat elevator, the client can control in which direction the transfer will happen (Arva, Schmeler, et al., 2009). The use of the seat elevator allows for a client, especially one with limited upper extremity reaching abilities, to engage in reaching for objects and surfaces encountered in their home, work, school, or community. This in turn allows them to complete mobility-related activities of daily living. Also, reaching from a seated position limits the client's vertical reach even if their upper extremities are not affected. Seat elevators reduce upper extremity fatigue and pain from continually reaching overhead (Arva, Schmeler, et al., 2009).

By raising the seat height, a client can communicate with their peers at eye level, thereby affecting the client's self-confidence. If the client can control the height of their chair, they are better able to engage socially at a level that is "normal." Seat height will help prevent fatigue from the client having to look up at their peers or their environment the majority of the time. The client is better able to position themselves to engage in conversations more effectively or to navigate their environment safely in a crowd (Arva, Schmeler, et al., 2009).

Standing Function

The standing function for wheelchairs is not a standard function found on most wheelchairs. The majority of standing functions are found on power wheelchairs. Individuals who use wheelchairs on a frequent basis can suffer secondary complications due to long-term sitting (Arva, Paleg, et al., 2009). Standers that are mechanically or electromechanically integrated into wheelchair bases allow the client to independently manage frequent and random standing to alleviate the adverse effects of constant sitting.

Being in a standing position provides a wide array of medical benefits, such as improving functional reach, maintaining vital organ capacity, maintaining bone density, improving circulation, improving passive range of motion, and reducing the occurrences of urinary tract infections, pressure sores, and skeletal deformities (Arva, Paleg, et al., 2009). Functional reach in the vertical direction is greatly enhanced with a standing feature. While in standing mode, the wheelchair facilitates movement in the client's environment by allowing them to access everyday items like light switches and countertops. The standing feature can assist with managing contractures of the lower extremities by allowing the caregiver or client to perform range of motion exercises for the legs. The ability to stand also changes the alignment of the pelvis and spine, allowing for an increased capacity of vital organs. With movement in standing, gravity can assist with vital organ function. Users of wheelchairs with the standing feature present with better functioning of the respiratory and gastrointestinal system, including better voiding of both the bowel and bladder (Arva, Paleg, et al., 2009).

Seating

A significant goal of seating is to provide a stable BOS to promote general and autonomic nervous system function (Jones & Gray, 2005). Biomechanical fundamentals, medical essentials, and requirements of occupational and physical therapists have to be considered, as well as the needs and desires of the client. The optimum outcome is a comfortable seating device that improves function and helps the client increase their participation in social life. Functioning seating includes an upright position of the trunk with a balanced head position and the pelvis positioned in three dimensions with bilaterally flexed and slightly abducted hips. Sitting should be comfortable for several hours (Strobl, 2013).

The **seating system** is composed of the primary support surface (seats and backs) and secondary supports (lateral trunk supports, head supports, and pelvic-positioning belts). Support surfaces may be planar, generically contoured, or custom-molded to an individual (Cook & Polgar, 2015; Wilson & Kishner, 2016). Planar seating is plane seating that provides the most minimal contact with the client's body. This minimal contact allows for clients to move around in the seating system freely (Cook & Polgar, 2015). Custom-molded or custom-contoured seating is used with clients who require significant physical support to maintain their seating positions. This type of seating system enhances postural alignment, decreases abnormal posturing, provides pressure relief, and ergonomically supports the individual. This seating is needed when the client presents with significant skeletal deformities, such as scoliosis, pelvic obliquities, and hip deformities due to moderate to severe CNS dysfunction or neurological disease. Custom molded seating is very specific for each client and for that moment in time when the mold was created. Special considerations need to be made that track growth or continued skeletal deformations (Costigan & Light, 2010b; Strobl, 2013; Wilson & Kishner, 2016).

Summary

Prescribing seating for individuals who use wheelchairs often entails consideration of posture, comfort, function, and pressure management. According to Costigan and Light (2010b), "[a] seated position that ensured a neutral pelvic position, appropriate weight-bearing surface, and vertical alignment of the upper extremity is successful in improving access to a computer-based AAC device" (p. 603). The use of wheelchair functions that include tilt-in-space, backrest recline, and seat elevation enhance comfort and sitting tolerance (Ding et al., 2008). These seating functions provide a wide array of benefits to those clients who need them. However, each seating function adds additional hardware, and therefore, weight to the seating system. When considering AAC devices, the therapist needs to consider the type of wheelchair the client has, as well as what seating functions the client uses.

POSITION FOR COMMUNICATION

Motor access to an AAC device or display can be considered after a person is positioned well. The configuration of the wheelchair is specific to the manufacturer. The controls the client uses are based on their functional abilities. Determining the most effective method for a person to operate a device is an art rather than a science that takes time and trial and error, particularly when a person has severe motor control problems. Two fundamental questions need to be answered when deciding how a person will control a device: Which body part will be used? Is direct selection or scanning (typically via the use of switches) likely to be most effective?

The motor aspects of communication should be as effortless as possible. The hands are the preferred site for access because of the fine motor control that may be possible. Many people also prefer to use their hands, and hand use tends to be more socially acceptable. The head also may be the control site of choice. The head can be used either to directly select symbols with a pointer or through eye gaze, or to activate a switch if direct selection is not possible. Many people with severe disabilities have better control of their eyes than other body sites so that eye-gaze techniques can be developed. Controls can be as simple as a joystick mounted to the armrest or as technologically advanced as a head array (Figure 16-7).

The concern with assistive technology is that the hardware must be mounted onto a location that will ensure the client has access to their communication device regardless of the position the client wishes to be in. The armrest is a typical mounting location for controllers and other devices. The armrest may either be attached to the base of the wheelchair or the seat back. If the armrest is mounted to the base of the chair and the client reclines, the client may lose contact with the controller. The torso and arms are moved posteriorly and away from the controls when the seat is reclined. If the

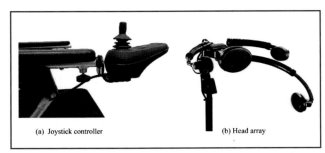

Figure 16-7. Types of controls for AAC. (A) A simple arm-mounted joystick controller. (B) A more sophisticated and complex head array controller.

armrest is mounted to the seat back, the armrest and controls will move backward with the client. The client will not lose contact with their controls.

Should there be AAC devices that incorporate controls via eye gaze? The location of the device within their field of vision is essential. Care must be taken to mount the AAC hardware to a location that allows the client to access both their seat functions and communication devices a majority of the time. When mounting AAC devices for access by the lower extremities, consideration must be given to the movement of the elevating footrests. Most wheelchair systems extend the foot platforms to allow for full extension of the knees. Some people can use more than one site, which can improve the efficiency of AAC use or may permit one site to be used for AAC and another to control other assistive technology, such as a power wheelchair (Cook & Polgar, 2015).

Assessment Considerations for AAC

With direct selection, the person chooses from among an array of symbols by pointing with a hand, finger, eye, or other body part. There are six elements of motor control to determine whether a person can use direct selection. These elements are:

1. Fine motor control: The degree of control needed to accurately select small targets that are close together, such as keys on a computer keyboard.

2. Range of motion: The distance that a person can move a body part in conjunction with their trunk, shoulder, and elbow movement. Providers must determine not only the range of motion of the specific body site that will operate a device but also other potential body parts that may be responsible for positioning the primary body site so it can do its work.

3. Strength: Strength is needed to press keys or to raise an arm against gravity to reach a display. Sometimes people with motor control problems move too forcefully, so a device that is not sturdy enough can break.

4. Endurance: If the movement required to operate a device is too tiring, the person will not be able to communicate at will. Sometimes endurance will increase as the person gains strength.

5. Versatility: The most versatile body part is a finger, and more than one usable finger increases versatility. One or more fingers can press keys, point to symbols, operate a joystick, or press a switch.

6. Speed: Speed can be affected by the location and the type of display, as well as the body part being used.

Evaluations of range, strength, endurance, versatility, and speed are generally more useful for determining which body part will operate an AAC device and the features of the device. These elements can often be accommodated by the size, location, and type of communication display. Versatility usually comes into play when deciding which body part will give the most options. Potentially, any movement can be used to activate a switch, including eyebrow elevation, eye blinks, sipping and puffing of air, as well as the more common methods of pushing, tapping, or squeezing or deforming through movements of the head, hand, or foot. Gaining knowledge of the person's voluntary movement during other activities is usually the best place to start. Seating, other types of positioning, and motor control are critical components of the successful implementation of AAC. Wheelchairs are essential bases for the attachment of AAC devices from which a client can communicate and control their environment remotely.

CASE EXAMPLE

Ramon

Ramon is a 16-year-old with spastic quadriplegic-type cerebral palsy and a seizure disorder. Secondary to the cerebral palsy, he has a dislocated hip, thoracic kyphosis, and severe flexion contractures of his elbows, knees, and hips.

Ramon's wheelchair had a planar seat and back. Because of his kyphosis, Ramon leaned far forward in the chair, which required an H-strap to hold him upright, a thick cushion behind his head, and a strap around his forehead to keep his head up. Because positioning was difficult and Ramon was uncomfortable in his chair, he spent much of his day at school lying on his side on a wedge or in a beanbag chair.

- What are some of the body functions/structures that should be considered when selecting his new wheelchair?

- What are the roles of the members of the interdisciplinary team?

- As a speech practitioner, how can you coordinate these services for your client with other members of the interprofessional team?

A primary educational goal for Ramon has been to improve his basic non-linguistic social-communicative interaction. At the beginning of the last school year, Ramon received a new wheelchair that was designed to accommodate his severe trunk and limb deformities. The most critical feature of the chair is a custom-contoured chair back designed to accommodate his kyphosis while maintaining his head in an upright position. The chair also has a custom-contoured seat to level his pelvis and accommodate his dislocated hip, and footrests are placed slightly under the seat to accommodate his knee flexion contractures. Because Ramon lacks postural control, a chest restraint and posterior head support are still needed, but he no longer leans heavily into the chest panel and straps, and he can hold his head up without the anterior strap.

- How will Ramon's new wheelchair impact his participation in his educational environment?
- How will the wheelchair impact his body positions?
- How can the new wheelchair facilitate the AAC implementation?

In his new chair, Ramon has been able to sit comfortably for several hours at a time, his eating has improved, and he has learned to press a switch. As a result of his increased comfort, Ramon is learning necessary dyadic interaction skills that have never been possible for him before.

Summary

A well-seated position is the best position for communication. It can offer opportunities for interaction, promote motor control, and provide mobility to "where the action is." Seating position is efficacious in improving the accuracy of target selection from a computer-based AAC device. Improved balance and stability can enable a greater range of motion of upper extremity movement. Having the appropriate weight-bearing surfaces and supported vertical alignment of the upper body improves control of motion, increases the functional distance of reach, and facilitates the accurate selection of targets. It is recognized that appropriate positioning for children and adults with physical disabilities is vital to facilitate engagement in functional activity and enable participation with the environment.

Proper positioning can improve upper extremity function, postural alignment, and prevent the development of deformity. Children and adults who lack postural control and are unable to maintain appropriate posture will therefore require external support from seating systems. The goal then is to provide adaptive seating to create a functional seated position to maintain health and function as part of a postural management approach. A well-seated position requires attention to specific guidelines. Members of the AAC team require basic knowledge of seating to address not only simple issues for people with mild motor impairments but also for those with severe motor impairments. Vigilance in ensuring a functional seated position for physical access to AAC across and within all communicative exchanges—through regular seating analysis and modifications—may be a critical step toward functional communication.

Study Questions

1. Describe the role and function of each potential interprofessional team member who may be involved in seating and positioning assessment and intervention for AAC.

2. When considering a client who has severe physical and/or sensory impairments, what factors should be assessed and considered when choosing an AAC device?

3. Identify the purpose and types of wheelchairs.

4. What wheelchair components may be customized or added to a basic wheelchair to optimize proper positioning?

5. What is the relationship between seating positions, communication, and AAC devices?

6. Name and describe the six elements of motor control that determine whether a person can directly access an AAC device or may have to rely on indirect access, such as switches.

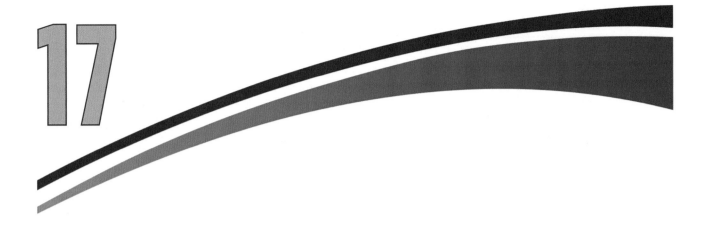

Speech-Generating Device Funding

Lewis Golinker, Esq

Editor's Note: This chapter was written by an attorney who is an expert in disability law. As the system of referencing differs considerably between the legal profession and the social/behavioral sciences, the referencing for this chapter shall be in accordance with the conventions used in the author's profession. Superscripted numerals throughout the text refer to endnotes that appear at the end of this chapter. Documents referenced in this chapter will be provided by the United States Society for Augmentative and Alternative Communication upon request.

<table>
<tr><td>

Myth

1. With the introduction of tablet computers and speech-generating device (SGD) apps, funding of speech-generating technology is no longer necessary.

2. Funding of speech-generating technology is so difficult that one may as well not even bother trying to procure funding.

3. Medicare and Medicaid do not fund SGDs.

4. The identification of medical need for an SGD is the responsibility of a client's doctor.

5. Funding for speech-generating technology is only available for children.

6. School-aged children with SGD needs will have an educational but not a medical need for speech-generating technology, and the public school rather than health benefits sources should pay for that technology.

</td><td>

Reality

1. There is no basis to assume that all clients will be able to afford SGDs using their own resources, regardless of the device used as SGD hardware. "Low cost" is a subjective phrase: What is low to some will not be low to others. There is also no basis to assume that all clients require SGDs based on off-the-shelf tablet computers and SGD apps. The speech-language pathologist's role is to identify SGD need and to recommend the most appropriate device that will enable clients to meet all their daily communication needs. While off-the-shelf tablets and apps will be effective for some clients, other clients will require other devices, some with much higher prices. The reality is that some—perhaps most—clients still require funding assistance to acquire their SGDs.

2. The process of funding is not as difficult as it may at first appear. Various funding sources have clear guidelines and requirements for funding of SGDs. It is the responsibility of the speech-language pathologist to become well versed as to the guidelines and requirements of funding sources.

(continued)

</td></tr>
</table>

Fuller, D. R., & Lloyd, L. L. *Principles and Practices in Augmentative and Alternative Communication* (pp. 293-349).

REALITY (CONTINUED)

3. This may have been true several decades ago, but both government-funded programs will fund speech-generating technology, as long as their requirements and regulations are met.

4. Augmentative and alternative communication (AAC) is within the scope of speech-language pathology as a form of speech-language pathology treatment. The purpose of all speech-language pathology treatment, including all AAC interventions that include SGDs, is to enable clients to meet all their daily communication needs. Speech-language pathologists are specially trained to identify speech and language impairments and to plan and implement treatment. For all these reasons, it is the speech-language pathologist, not the client's physician, who is responsible for identification of SGD need and for the recommendation of the most appropriate SGD to meet that need. Speech-language pathologists are the professionals primarily responsible for supporting client access to health benefits source funding to acquire needed SGDs.

5. Funding is available not only for children but for adults as well. Programs such as Medicare, Vocational Rehabilitation, the Veteran's Administration, private insurance, and Medicaid will fund speech-generating technology for adults.

6. That speech-generating technology is needed is based on the existence of a speech or language impairment that interferes with the client's ability to meet *all* daily communication needs. The speech-generating technology is a form of speech-language pathology *treatment*. The purpose of or medical need for any speech-language pathology treatment is to enable the client to produce understandable speech regardless of the content of the speech, the location of the speech, the relationship between the client and a communication partner, or when the speech occurs. For a client enrolled in school, speech-generating technology will be used in school because that is where the client will be. It does not change the *medical* need for the device to an educational need. This conclusion is equally true for students who require a ventilator to assist with breathing or a wheelchair to assist with mobility. Their needs are medical regardless where they come or go with and use these devices.

INTRODUCTION

Having a disability is not cheap. Many people with disabilities have multiple needs, some or all of them may be beyond their personal financial resources. Faced with the prospect of doing without or having to settle for an unequal substitute offering fewer benefits, people with disabilities will look for any and all possible sources of funding assistance to secure what they need. People with complex communication needs (CCN) are no exception.

For people with CCN, SGDs[1] are important tools to enable them to meet daily communication needs. However, since their introduction in the mid-1970s, SGDs have been too costly for most people to purchase directly. Instead, SGD access has required funding assistance from third-party sources. They include both public and private health benefits sources (Medicare, Medicaid in all states, Tricare, the Veterans Administration, commercial insurance, and employer-sponsored health benefit plans), public schools, telecommunications equipment distribution programs, and vocational rehabilitation programs. Today, funding assistance for SGDs is provided by all these sources. For this reason, access to SGD funding has become largely a matter of procedure and routine for the overwhelming majority of clients. Today, active efforts to persuade funding sources to accept SGDs as covered benefits will be needed only in exceptional circumstances. These funding opportunities exist because of ongoing advocacy by individuals with CCN and their families, speech-language pathologists, SGD manufacturers, organizations (including the United States Society for Augmentative and Alternative Communication [USSAAC] and the American-Speech-Language-Hearing Association [ASHA]), and advocates.

Even where SGD coverage and funding is accepted, the procedure and routine to gain access to an SGD is unlike a system that operates largely automatically and in the background, such as a building's heating, ventilation, and air conditioning. Access to those systems may require no more than the flip of a switch. By contrast, access to SGD funding requires far more. The SGD funding process requires of speech-language pathologists an evaluation, reporting, advocacy, and training. Clients and their families, SGD manufacturers, and often advocates have additional roles and responsibilities. Perhaps a closer analogy is to a wood stove: the tasks required to access SGD funding are comparable to felling the tree, chopping logs, feeding wood into the stove, removing the ash, and cleaning the flue.

Because SGD funding is not automatic or guaranteed, knowledge of the key principles, questions, and answers related to SGD funding is essential, both to ensure the funding process works as it should and to repair the process when for one reason or another, it does not.

A Speech-Generating Device Funding Discussion Is Still Necessary

Despite wide acceptance of SGDs by sources of funding, there are at least four reasons discussion of SGD funding remains a highly relevant topic. First, some funding sources still refuse to acknowledge SGDs as program benefits. Second, some sources "forget" that SGDs are covered benefits and deny SGD funding requests. Discussion of funding principles is necessary so speech-language pathologists and others know the appropriate strategy and have the necessary information to remove these barriers and to ensure SGD access. Third, the introduction of relatively low-cost, off-the-shelf tablet computers as SGD hardware does not make SGD funding an anachronism. Although some available SGD models, for some clients, have become affordable and can be acquired without the need for funding program assistance, the discussion of and need for SGD funding remains as important today as ever. These SGD models are appropriate for only *some* clients, and when recommended, they are affordable for direct purchase by only *some* clients. Many—perhaps most—clients who receive SGD recommendations, including for these models, still require funding support. Fourth, a speech-language pathology evaluation remains the recommended procedure to identify SGD need and the most appropriate device, mounts, and access aids. Speech-language pathologists are also responsible for writing the treatment plan for clients to develop communicative competence. All these speech-language pathology tasks have been shaped by the SGD funding process. A review of this process will inform speech-language pathology clinical practice whether funding is needed or not.

Scope of This Chapter

This chapter will discuss SGD funding by health benefits sources in the United States. They are the largest sources of SGD funding, they provide benefits to the largest number of people, their benefits are available without regard to client age (i.e., eligibility runs from birth to death), they do not focus on client activity (e.g., enrollment in school, interest in or pursuit of vocational goals), and they have primary funding responsibilities (i.e., a duty to pay first) when clients are also eligible for special education or vocational rehabilitation funding.[2]

ORIGINS AND EVOLUTION OF SPEECH-GENERATING DEVICE FUNDING

Introduction

SGDs were introduced for client use in the mid-to-late 1970s. From the outset, SGDs were too expensive for many if not most clients and their families to purchase with their own funds. As a result, from the very beginning of SGD availability, funding assistance from third parties was recognized as necessary for client access to these devices.

Possible Sources of Speech-Generating Device Funding

All the public sources of health benefits (e.g., Medicare, Medicaid, Tricare, Veterans Administration, special education, telecommunications equipment distribution funds, and vocational rehabilitation) and private sources (e.g., private health insurance and employer-sponsored health benefits plans) now recognized as SGD funding sources predated the introduction of SGDs. However, *none* of the laws creating publicly funded health programs, special education, and vocational rehabilitation programs identified SGDs as a covered benefit. Review of health insurance policies and health plans led to the same conclusion: In general, there was no mention of SGDs. For this reason, if these programs were to be SGD funding sources, they would have to be persuaded that SGDs "fit."

Key Elements of Speech-Generating Device Funding Sources

All SGD funding sources share three characteristics: (1) devices and equipment are among their covered benefits categories, (2) the scope of device and equipment coverage is sufficient to include SGDs, and (3) the benefits provided by SGDs further the goals or purposes of the program, that is, SGDs address clients' health, education, and vocational needs.

Sources of Health Benefits

The largest sources of health care or funding assistance to access health care in the United States are Medicare, Medicaid, Tricare, the Department of Veterans Affairs, commercial health insurance, and employer-sponsored health plans. These sources rely on thousands of administrative units to make decisions regarding who is eligible, what is covered, and whether access to covered benefits will be provided. They include Medicare and Tricare regional contractors, Veterans Affairs hospitals, Medicaid programs in every state, and countless health insurance policies and health plans.

Notwithstanding the large number of decision-making units, generalizations about whether each will be an SGD funding source are possible. All health benefits sources apply a common template that governs their obligations. It asks four questions:

1. Is the client eligible—a beneficiary, participant, or recipient—of the program, policy, or plan?
2. Is the intervention (health care service or medical device) being sought covered (i.e., does it fit within the scope of benefits covered by the program, policy, or plan)?
3. Is the intervention medically necessary for the client?
4. Is the request unaffected by any program, policy, or plan exclusions or limitations?

When all four questions are answered with yes, health benefits sources are obligated to provide the requested service or device.[3]

Another common characteristic of health benefits sources is their use of identical or substantively similar vocabulary to describe their covered benefits, medical need standards, and exclusions and limitations. Discovery of these overlaps simplified the task of establishing whether SGDs are covered health benefits. They supported a "domino" or "snowball" effect: The facts and principles that persuaded one source to accept SGDs as benefits were then presented to other sources, and their persuasive force grew as more sources reached the same conclusion.

Program Eligibility

In the United States, no single source of health benefits serves everyone. Instead, there are multiple sources, each with distinct eligibility criteria. It is also true that individuals may be eligible for more than one source, that is, have "dual eligibility." Insurance-insurance, insurance-Medicaid, and Medicare-Medicaid are common forms of dual eligibility. In general, clients' dual eligibility may increase the number of tasks speech-language pathologists must complete when conducting an evaluation and increase the reporting required to support an SGD recommendation, but it should not interfere with SGD access. Clients and speech-language pathologists should not be concerned that with dual eligibility the client is enrolled in one program too many to gain SGD access.

Speech-language pathologists must identify all the funding sources to which a client may be eligible; however, it is not the speech-language pathologist's responsibility to pursue eligibility for clients. Instead, clients will present some form of identification (e.g., a card) that identifies them as eligible for one or more health benefits sources.

It is also possible that a client will not have any source of health benefits funding assistance. For these clients, assistance may be sought from educational, vocational rehabilitation, or telecommunications equipment distribution programs, as well as sources of long-term device loan or from charitable sources.

A Word About Charities

A wide range of charities may provide SGD funding on a voluntary basis. They are not discussed in this chapter because they have no legal obligations to respond to SGD funding requests. Also, those who seek help have no enforceable rights if requests are not answered in a timely manner or are denied. For these reasons, charities may be of help to some people, for some things, some of the time. Because they *might* be of help, speech-language pathologists and clients and their families should investigate them as possibly available funding sources or as sources of no- or low-cost equipment loans, but charities are not and should not be thought of as substitutes for the funding sources discussed in this chapter.

Devices and Equipment Are Covered Benefits

Once eligibility is identified, the next question asked is whether the benefits of these sources include (i.e., *cover*) devices or equipment *of any kind*? For all of them, the answer is yes. The most common benefits categories in which devices and equipment are covered are durable medical equipment (DME) and **prosthetic devices**.

Medicaid programs are an exception. They offer a prosthetic devices benefits category,[4] but they have no DME benefits category and also use slightly different vocabulary. Instead of "durable medical equipment," Medicaid programs cover "medical equipment" items. Instead of a stand-alone benefits category, "medical equipment" is a component of home health care services;[5] occupational therapy, physical therapy, and speech-language pathology services;[6] rehabilitative (including habilitative) services;[7] nursing facility services;[8] and intermediate care facility services for individuals with developmental disabilities.[9]

Health insurance policies subject to the Patient Protection and Affordable Care Act (ACA) also use distinct vocabulary. The ACA requires insurance policies to offer "habilitative and rehabilitative services and devices,"[10] which include the devices and equipment other sources recognize as DME or prosthetic devices.

Device and Equipment Coverage Includes Speech-Generating Devices

That all sources of health benefits cover devices and equipment items, whether as DME, prosthetic devices, or under another category label, was a necessary but not sufficient basis to establish SGDs are covered benefits. Still necessary was a determination that these sources will accept SGDs as being among the *types* of devices and equipment that are covered.

Establishing Speech-Generating Devices Fit as Durable Medical Equipment or Medical Equipment

DME or medical equipment is the most common benefits category health benefits sources use to classify or cover SGDs. Medicare, almost all Medicaid programs, and most insurers acknowledge SGDs fit within this benefit. To reach this conclusion, these sources had to accept that SGDs match the physical and functional characteristics stated in the sources' DME definitions. This task was made significantly easier because most health benefits sources copy and use the Medicare DME definition and other coverage guidance either in whole or substantial part.[11] The Medicare statute (law) states a DME "definition" consisting of a list of specific equipment:

> The term 'durable medical equipment' includes iron lungs, oxygen tents, hospital beds, and wheelchairs … used in the patient's home … Blood-testing strips and blood glucose monitors for individuals with diabetes …[12]

This statement of coverage is supplemented by a definition of DME in Medicare regulations. It identifies several required device characteristics:

> Durable medical equipment means equipment … that:
> 1. Can withstand repeated use;
> 2. Is primarily and customarily used to serve a medical purpose;
> 3. Generally is not useful to an individual in the absence of an illness or injury; and
> 4. Is appropriate for use in the home.[13]

SGDs fit this DME definition because they possess all the characteristics required of covered DME items.

Speech-Generating Devices Can Withstand Repeated Use

According to Medicare, an item that is *durable* is one that can "withstand repeated use."[14] Some insurers and health plans use different vocabulary to describe this characteristic of DME items: They state that items of DME are "not consumable or disposable." These phrases are synonymous. All SGDs are durable and are not consumable or disposable.

The common meaning of durable is something that is "long-lasting" and "able to exist for a long time without significant deterioration." Medicare has clarified "long-lasting" and "long time" to mean a "minimum lifetime requirement" of 3 years.[15] Although this minimum lifetime requirement provision does not apply to SGDs, they historically have had useful lives longer than 3 years. SGD manufacturers report their devices—both historic and current models—are intended for everyday use for periods of at least 5 years.

SGDs are also not disposable. A disposable item is the polar opposite of one that is *durable*. A standard dictionary definition for "disposable" is something designed to be used once and then thrown away. As just reported, SGDs are designed to be used every day for several years. Also, as a practical matter, the cost of SGDs presents a strong rebuttal to any suggestion that they are disposable. That SGDs may cost several thousand dollars and necessary mounts and accessories may add several thousand dollars more makes clear beyond question that they are *not* intended to be used once and thrown away.

Likewise, SGDs are not "consumable," that is, something that is used up or destroyed. An SGD is not "consumed" in any way, as clients select or construct messages for the device to speak. SGDs do run on batteries, but these are rechargeable and are designed to enable use day after day for years. A Medicare administrative law judge concluded SGDs are durable *because* they ran on rechargeable batteries.[16] Other similar items that rely on components that are rechargeable or refillable are recognized as DME. These items include oxygen tanks, which are emptied through use, and portable ventilators and power wheelchairs, which, like SGDs, run on rechargeable batteries. They are not "destroyed" through use. None of these equipment items is "consumable." Not surprisingly, funding sources have not challenged SGD coverage on the basis that they are not durable or are consumable or disposable.

Speech-Generating Devices Primarily and Customarily Are Used to Serve a Medical Purpose

The second required characteristic of an item of DME is that it "is primarily and customarily used to serve a medical purpose." This DME characteristic has been the basis most frequently cited to deny SGD coverage.

As with the "durability" element, some benefits programs use synonyms for the phrase "medical purpose," such as "treatment" or "therapeutic" purpose. All three share a common meaning. The words "medical" and "therapeutic" both include "treatment" as part of their definition.[17] One court noted:

> We, however, must give the word 'medical' its ordinary sense, as referring more usually and broadly to the treatment, cure, or alleviation of any health condition, including [disability].[18]

Simply stated, an equipment item will serve a "medical purpose" if it can be established as treatment for an illness, injury, or condition.

There are many different *goals*, *purposes*, or *types* of treatment, including amelioration, correction, cure, habilitation, palliation, prevention, and rehabilitation.[19] SGDs can be described as serving several of these purposes, including amelioration,[20] habilitation,[21] and rehabilitation.[22] SGDs *ameliorate* by reducing the functional communication impacts of complex and severe communication impairment whether developmental or acquired. For example, clients may be able to say more to more people about more topics in more settings than they are able to express without the device. By expressing themselves more effectively, they will experience fewer communication breakdowns and will have an easier and less frustrating way to recover when communication breakdowns occur. These effects also describe SGDs' *habilitative* purpose. SGDs provide a more effective means of expression and a means to develop language for clients with conditions, such as autism and cerebral palsy, who have not developed functional speech. Likewise, these effects describe SGDs' *rehabilitative* purpose. SGDs provide an alternative or supplemental means of expression for clients who have lost their ability to functionally communicate due to acquired impairments, such as amyotrophic lateral sclerosis (ALS), traumatic brain injury, or stroke.

All SGDs are recommended, prescribed, and used to implement a program of speech-language pathology treatment for complex and severe communication impairment. The generally accepted principle—supported by ASHA guidance, professional literature, position statements of the nation's leading medical professional associations, the decisions of other government agencies, and adopted as the coverage standard by health benefits sources—is that AAC interventions, including SGDs, are medically necessary and appropriate treatment when a speech-language pathologist determines an individual cannot meet all daily communication needs using natural communication methods, such as oral speech or writing.[23]

Since 1981, ASHA has formally recognized AAC interventions, including use of SGDs, as a speech-language pathology treatment method and is therefore within the scope of practice of speech-language pathologists.[24] This position has been renewed and updated, and it remains ASHA's current and official position.[25] In short, SGDs are one form of

AAC treatment, which is a form of speech-language pathology treatment. There is also more than 40 years of professional literature and practice related to AAC interventions, including SGDs, as treatment for severe expressive communication disabilities and to prevent the adverse effects associated with an inability to speak or otherwise expressively communicate.[26]

Position statements of the nation's leading professional medical associations also confirm the treatment role of SGDs for a range of severe communication impairments. In 2000, the American Medical Association (AMA), American Academy of Neurology (AAN), and American Academy of Physical Medicine and Rehabilitation wrote to Medicare to support SGD coverage by that program. The AAN stated the following as the basis for its support:

> In general, the [AAN] supports a policy that includes [AAC] devices to be covered … when incorporated into a speech-language pathology treatment plan. The treatment plan which authorizes this coverage should … conclude the individual is unable to meet communication needs arising in the course of daily activities using natural communication methods … [T]he AAN believes that [AAC] devices are a form of [DME] which can be of great help to selected individuals with neurological disorders unable to communicate during the course of daily activities. They can be a successful form of treatment as part of a speech-language therapy plan in carefully selected and evaluated individuals.[27]

AMA stated:

> The AMA agrees with the [AAN] that these devices are medically necessary for severely speech-impaired patients to meet the communication needs arising in the course of their daily activities …[28]

The American Academy of Physical Medicine and Rehabilitation stated:

> The Academy strongly believes that [AAC] devices are medically necessary aids for communication … The Academy lends its full support for Medicare coverage of these devices for patients with severe communication impairments, such as dysarthria, apraxia, and aphasia, regardless of the motor or neurological condition that gives rise to the communication impairment … They are necessary to meet the communication needs arising in daily activities.[29]

Several years later, the American Academy of Pediatrics stated:

> Many children and youth with special health care needs can improve day-to-day functioning with the aid of assistive technology, including alternative and augmentative technology.[30]

The general acceptance that SGDs serve a medical, therapeutic, or treatment purpose or role also extends to other federal agencies. For example, the U.S. Food and Drug Administration (FDA) is a regulatory, not a funding agency. The FDA is the federal agency responsible for classification of medical devices. It concluded that SGDs serve a medical purpose *in 1983*. At that time, the FDA created a classification called "powered communication systems," which it defined as:

> An AC- or battery-powered device **intended for medical purposes** that is used to transmit or receive information. It is used by persons unable to use normal communication methods because of physical impairment …[31]

Additional reinforcement for the conclusion that SGDs serve a medical purpose is supplied by Medicare and Medicaid. Congress expressly prohibits Medicare from providing reimbursement for any item or service that is "not reasonable and necessary for the diagnosis *or treatment* of illness or injury or to improve the functioning of a malformed body member."[32] Medicare guidance expressly states the concept of "reasonable and necessary" limits coverage only to "services or supplies that are needed for the diagnosis or *treatment* of your medical condition and meet accepted standards of *medical* practice."[33] Medicaid programs are required to make determinations about coverage of items or services consistent with accepted standards of *medical* practice.[34] Both programs cover SGDs as DME.

That health benefits sources cover *speech-language pathology* services provides another way to establish the *medical purpose* served by SGDs. All publicly funded health benefits programs and almost all health insurers and health benefits plans cover speech-language pathology services. They may be identified as a specific benefit category or as a benefit within home health care services or rehabilitative therapy services.

The goal of all speech-language pathology treatment is the same: to enable clients to overcome or ameliorate the communication limitations that preclude or interfere with their meaningful participation in daily activities.[35] Meaningful participation means effective and efficient communication of messages in any form the clients choose.[36] AAC interventions, including use of SGDs, serve the same purposes and have the same goals as all other forms of speech-language pathology services. In other words, *because* speech-language pathology services are included as covered benefits and *because* they are recognized as serving a *medical purpose*, SGDs also must be recognized as serving a *medical purpose* because SGDs are recommended and used to achieve the same goals.

The truth of this assertion is demonstrated most directly by the example of ALS. One of the first texts written about AAC interventions recognized the value of an SGD for clients with this condition:

> [A] person with [ALS], for example, who becomes incapable of speaking and writing, can be provided with augmentative techniques that allow full access to expression of ideas, wants, and needs.[37]

Before AAC interventions and SGDs are considered or recommended, clients with ALS will experience speech impairment of ever-increasing severity. As the speech function deteriorates, a range of speech-language pathology services will be provided to maintain clients' ability to communicate functionally. However, when their speech intelligibility deteriorates to 80% or speaking rate slows to less than 125 words per minute, it is generally accepted that the threshold for consideration of AAC interventions, including use of SGDs, has been passed.[38]

For clients with ALS, the appropriateness and effectiveness of SGD use is beyond question. It is accepted that "the loss of communication in ALS [as compared to the loss of speech ability] is not inevitable and that [AAC] strategies can preserve this critical function even in the face of profound motor deterioration."[39] For more than 20 years, SGD use has been declared *the standard of care* to maintain functional communication for clients with ALS.[40] No rational basis exists to conclude that speech-language pathology services for clients with ALS serve a *medical purpose* when their goal is to maintain the clients' ability to report about their needs, wants, thoughts, or feelings using speech, but recommendation and use of an SGD to enable the same messages to be reported (when clients can no longer communicate effectively by speaking) does not.

Other conditions, such as head and neck cancers, which may result in a sequence of surgeries, including a tracheotomy and/or a glossectomy, illustrate how a single client can progress through different types of speech-language pathology services directed to speech and also different types of devices to aid speech production, including the artificial larynx, tracheaesophageal voice prosthesis, and SGDs. In this example, as with ALS, although a range of speech-language pathology treatment methodologies are provided, the treatment goals and *medical purpose* of all treatments remain the same.

A characteristic common to ALS and cancer is that they are progressive. Many other conditions that impair speech are described as stable. These conditions also have a broad continuum of severity for which different speech-language pathology treatment methodologies will be employed. It is the speech-language pathologist's responsibility as part of the speech-language pathology evaluation to determine the most appropriate intervention for each client. That, for some clients, the treatent recommended may be directed to speaking, and for others, it may be directed to use of an SGD may reflect no more than the difference in the complexity or severity of the *same* speech impairment. For either one, there is no difference in the *medical purpose* of the treatment recommended or provided.

In general, the following rhetorical question helped establish that SGDs serve a *medical purpose*:

> If there was a form of surgery or a pill that will improve the client's functioning to the same level that can be achieved with the recommended device, will providing that drug or performing that surgery be recognized as serving a medical purpose?

When intended to improve function, surgery and use of medication are generally presumed to be *medical* interventions serving *medical* purposes. That no surgery or pill may exist to achieve a particular outcome for a client's communication needs, but instead, an item of DME must be used to serve the same purpose and achieve the same goal should make clear the equipment item will serve a *medical* purpose.

In individual funding requests, speech-language pathologists helped to persuade funding sources that SGDs, mounts, and access aids serve a medical purpose by reporting that the recommended equipment was *the most appropriate form of treatment available to enable the client to meet daily functional communication needs.*

That SGD use is a form of speech-language pathology treatment, and therefore, serves a medical purpose, satisfies part of this element of the DME definition. In addition, this treatment role must be established as the "primary and customary purpose" of the SGD use. This requirement is met because for many clients, the *only* purpose the SGD will serve is speech generation. This SGD characteristic is described in greater detail in the next section.

Speech-Generating Devices Are Not Generally Useful to an Individual in the Absence of an Illness or Injury

The third element of the DME definition states that the item "generally is not useful to a person in the absence of an illness or injury." For something to be "useful," it must fill a need. It must be likely the individual *will* use the item to accomplish a functional goal. "Will use" is the key phrase; this criterion does not ask whether an individual *can use* the item. The latter standard is unworkable as a practical matter: Almost everyone *can* use a wheelchair for mobility; almost anyone *can* use an SGD to speak. But, when mobility or speech is not impaired by illness, injury, or disability, no one will want or need to use a wheelchair or a communication device. Walking or speaking are far more efficient, and in many cases, more effective means to accomplish these goals.

SGDs satisfy this requirement because they are used *only* by clients who, due to complex or severe communication impairment, are unable to meet all daily communication needs using speech or other natural communication methods, such as writing, gesture, or manual sign. Only clients with severe communication impairment will be evaluated for, recommended, want, use, or benefit from an SGD. Those able to speak effectively will not want, need, or use an SGD because speech is far faster and more flexible than any other method of expression[41] and speaking, in contrast to an SGD, is accomplished for free. No one will spend thousands of dollars for equipment items that will accomplish the same goals. In other words, if no one will buy or seek funding for an SGD when the same goal can be accomplished without charge, then SGDs will *not* "generally be useful" to anyone without specific need for them.

These explanations were sufficient to establish that purpose-built SGDs met this requirement of the DME definition. These SGDs were designed and manufactured for the specific purpose of speech generation and were intended to be used exclusively by clients with CCN. Also, they were marketed exclusively to clients and their families, diagnosis- or disability-focused organizations, and to professionals, such as speech-language pathologists, occupational therapists, and special educators who served clients with speech impairment. This focus established that only someone who truly *needed* an SGD would have any interest in them.

Ancillary Features. Among even the first generation of SGDs were those that offered clients ancillary features—additional, extra, supplemental to[42]—their primary speech-generating capabilities. That these features were incorporated in SGDs is easy to understand. Years before smartphones and touchscreens for computers, engineers designing SGDs recognized the tension between the physical space within clients' effective reach and control and the many things they might want to do within that space. Creating messages is one, but others included noting the time, controlling the environment,[43] using the phone, and taking notes. Clients might try to use single-purpose devices for each function, but there would be nowhere to put them. Only by offering devices with multiple capabilities could the small space available be used efficiently. The result was the creation of SGDs that included a clock and alarm; environmental control capabilities for lights, shades, and doors; phone and TV control capabilities; and calculators and files for storing notes or lists.

Ancillary features generally have not been relevant for funding purposes. By definition, ancillary features will not be the "primary and customary" use of the device, so they do not affect that element of the DME definition. They are also not relevant in regard to the "generally not useful" criterion. As already mentioned, to be useful, the item must fill a need, and the item must meet that need better or as well as other alternatives at less cost. SGD ancillary features do not cause SGDs to pass that test. No one will express interest in an SGD whose size, shape, weight, performance, quality, and cost compares adversely to a watch, clock, calculator, or TV or other appliance remote control. A comparison: Perhaps all microwave ovens include a clock feature, but no one will buy a microwave oven just because it will tell the time.

There was one notable instance when SGD ancillary features were the focus of attention in regard to SGD funding. In February 2014, Medicare issued a coverage reminder related to SGD coverage. Without explanation, this reminder stated:

> [Medicare] does not extend [SGD] coverage to the broader range of [AAC] devices that have capabilities exceeding the sole function(s) of speech-generating, such as (not all-inclusive); wireless and cellular communication capabilities; environmental control capability, non–speech-generating software (e.g., games, word processing, email).

This guideline effectively barred SGDs from offering *any* ancillary (i.e., non–speech-generating related) features and it represented a dramatic, unwelcome change in Medicare SGD coverage policy. In 1999 to 2000, when Medicare staff were reviewing whether to cover SGDs, they reviewed product literature and were given demonstrations of then-current devices. The product literature from that period openly reported that some SGD models from the largest SGD manufacturers offered environmental control and other ancillary features. Medicare staff offered no concern or objection, and all these devices were approved for Medicare coverage as DME.

In late 2014, Medicare staff began a reconsideration of its SGD coverage policy. Updated guidance issued at the conclusion of that review rejected the assertions made in the coverage reminder, and once again, ancillary features offered by SGDs were not relevant for coverage purposes.[44]

"Off-the-Shelf" Computer-Based Speech-Generating Devices. Throughout the history of SGD availability, some device models relied on off-the-shelf computer hardware. SGDs manufactured by Words+ Inc., one of the earliest SGD manufacturers, were one example. Words+ Inc. produced SGDs that used industrial- or military-grade laptop computers—devices with cases and components designed and built to withstand rough handling. One of its SGD models was called the Toughbook. Another SGD manufacturer, Enkidu, introduced SGDs that were based on small handheld computers, then called personal digital assistants (PDAs).

While these devices functioned as SGDs, they also had general computer functionality. Obviously, devices able to perform general computer functions will not satisfy the criterion of "generally is not useful to an individual in the absence of illness or injury." However, the reaction of most funding sources had been to ignore the distinction among SGDs based on their hardware; funding sources that adopted SGD coverage did so for all models. A few took note that some SGDs were computer-based but did so only to create an exception that allowed them to be covered. For example, Indiana Medicaid stated:

> If authorization is requested for a computer or computerized device, the intended use of the computer or computerized device must be compensation for loss or impairment of communication function.[45]

Other programs responded by including computers or computerized devices in their description of covered SGDs, that is, SGDs include "methods that use communication boards, charts, and mechanical or electronic aids, or computerized devices."[46]

This *laissez faire* attitude toward computer-based SGDs continued until 2000 when Medicare issued an updated National Coverage Determination (NCD) for SGDs. Medicare announced that effective January 1, 2001, SGDs will be covered as items of DME. However, Medicare rejected coverage for:

… devices that are not dedicated speech devices, but are devices that are capable of running software for purposes other than for speech generation, *e.g.*, devices that can also run a word processing package, an accounting program, or perform other non-medical functions; laptop computers, desktop computers, PDAs, which may be programmed to perform the same function as a[n] [SGD], … and a device that is useful to someone without severe speech impairment is not considered a[n] [SGD] for Medicare coverage purposes.[47]

This NCD introduced the concept of a "dedicated" SGD and adopted three qualifying criteria. Off-the-shelf laptop computers and PDAs did not meet any of them.

Several proposed responses to this guidance were discussed and quickly abandoned. Asking Medicare to reconsider this requirement was rejected as unlikely to succeed. Designing new cases for computer-based SGDs was rejected as too costly and too time-consuming. Court action to challenge Medicare's "dedicated device" requirement was rejected as too time-consuming, too costly, and as impossible to predict its chances for success.

Instead, review of the computer and PDA operating software identified changes that would make these devices *functionally* dedicated, that is, functionally indistinguishable from SGDs that were purpose-built. Software changes could lock out general computer features but leave access to those that supported speech generation. Prototypes of several dedicated computer-based devices were presented to Medicare managers, who accepted them for coverage. They acknowledged their interest was on SGD functionality. They reported no interest in whether SGDs rely on hardware that is specially designed and manufactured for use as an SGD or on an off-the-shelf computer.

On May 4, 2001, Medicare issued an "interpretive clarification" to the NCD that stated:

Computer-based and PDA-based AAC devices/[SGDs] are covered when they have been modified to run only AAC software.[48]

Medicare's approval of these changes allowed all SGDs to satisfy the "generally not useful" DME criterion. Regardless of their hardware, their only use was for speech generation, and thus, only a person who *needed* an SGD to treat complex and severe communication impairment would want or use one. Beyond Medicare, other health benefits sources either continued their pre-existing acceptance of computer-based SGDs or adopted the coverage framework stated in Medicare's NCD and interpretive clarification.

Since 2001, SGD manufacture has evolved. It has become far more economical to rely on off-the-shelf as compared to custom-made subsystems and on complete off-the-shelf computer products. The trend has been for increasing numbers of SGD models to be based on off-the-shelf computer products. Because all these SGDs can be modified in compliance with Medicare's "dedicated" device requirement, they continue to meet the "generally not useful" DME criterion.

Medicare's reconsideration of its SGD guidance, completed in 2015, reinforces that any type of computer or similar device will be acceptable when it has been modified as follows:

As long as the [SGD] is limited to use by a patient with a severe speech impairment and is primarily used for the purpose of generating speech, it is not necessary for a[n] [SGD] to be dedicated only to speech generation to be considered DME.[49]

In the revised Local Coverage Article for SGDs issued at the conclusion of the reconsideration process, Medicare acknowledged that desktop, laptop, tablet, or other forms of computers, smartphones, and any similar devices will be acceptable for use as SGD hardware "if it is designed by the manufacturer to function as an SGD at the time of initial issue."[50]

In sum, there is no basis for health benefits sources to object to any SGD as long as it has been modified to meet the Medicare SGD coverage requirements. For this reason as well, it is recommended that for a client with health benefits from any source, speech-language pathologists always recommend the Medicare-compliant model of SGD if one is available.

Tablet Computers as Speech-Generating Devices. All SGDs that produce synthesized speech output always have been computers based on their component parts. All rely on operating systems, software, memory, microprocessors, methods to input information, and means of information output. Most have also been *tablet* computers, a term that has never been defined for discussion related to AAC. As used here, tablet computers are computers that rely on a touch-screen as the primary method to input information and do not have an attached keyboard (in contrast to a laptop computer) or include an accessory keyboard as a standard hardware component (in contrast to on-screen, software-generated keyboard emulators). Use of tablet computers as SGDs is anything but new. Approximately 20 years ago, Enkidu, and subsequently Dynavox, marketed a family of SGDs called the Tablet with several models that had different screen/display sizes. As just discussed, off-the-shelf devices—laptop computers and PDAs—have also been used as SGD hardware. All these devices have been scrutinized for DME coverage and all have been found acceptable.

Because off-the-shelf laptop and tablet computer-based SGDs have long histories of acceptance as DME, the introduction in 2011 of Apple iPad tablet computers and other similar models that rely on different operating systems (e.g., Android, Windows) and their use as SGDs present no new issues from the standpoint of SGD coverage for funding purposes. None of these devices alone nor all of them as a group represent a new or different type or class of SGDs, notwithstanding the popular reference to these devices as mobile technology. Mobile also describes nothing new. SGDs specifically designed to be mobile—to be carried comfortably by individuals who are ambulatory (as compared to devices mounted to a wheelchair)—have been available since the early to mid-1990s.[51] All these devices can be modified to meet the requirements of "dedication" or otherwise can be limited to speech-generating functions, which is the key factor that will enable these devices to satisfy the "generally not useful" criterion of the DME definition.

That several named or branded SGD models based on these off-the-shelf tablet computers are available from SGD manufacturers is further evidence of the ordinariness of these SGDs for funding purposes. Other sources offer no-name **T+A+C** (Tablet + App + Case) SGDs based on speech-language pathologist recommendation and physician prescription.[52] As long as these devices meet the functionality limitations that will transform them into SGDs, their coverage for funding purposes should not be controversial.[53] Indeed, several funding programs, including Medicare, acknowledge in their SGD coverage guidelines that these devices will be accepted as SGDs for funding purposes.[54]

Speech-Generating Devices Are Appropriate for Use in the Home

The final criterion of the DME definition is that the item "is appropriate for use in the home." Another phrasing of this element is that the item has been "*designed* for outpatient use." All SGDs meet this criterion. SGDs have been designed and are intended to come and go with clients whenever and wherever they want to speak. SGDs are best described for use that is intended to be setting-independent. Nothing about them can characterize them as institutional equipment (the opposite of equipment designed for outpatient use).[55] That Medicare covers SGDs as DME reinforces the conclusion that SGDs satisfy this criterion. Medicare does not provide DME to residents in institutional settings, such as hospitals or nursing facilities.[56] Data from SGD manufacturers and vendors also support the conclusion that SGDs are not designed or intended for institutional use. They can relate the history of their sales to establish their SGDs are sold and are used by individuals residing at home and were not designed or intended primarily for use by residents of institutions.

Likewise, SGDs are not items that are intended or appropriate for use only in therapy sessions or settings. They are intended and appropriate for use in all settings throughout the day, including use at home. This criterion has never been cited as a basis for denial of SGD coverage or funding.

Speech-Generating Devices Have Much in Common With Equipment Identified as Examples of Covered Durable Medical Equipment

Medicare and some other health benefits programs supplement their DME definitions based on physical or functional characteristics with examples of specific items that are covered as DME.[57] These examples provided additional opportunities to establish SGDs are DME. Reduced to its essence, funding sources were told *because* "A" is identified as the type of device that is covered and *because* SGDs are just

like "A"; *therefore*, SGDs also should be covered. For example, wheelchairs very often are identified as an example of a covered DME item. Although they address different functional impairments, SGDs and wheelchairs have much in common. They both provide the same *type of treatment*: They are *ameliorative*, that is, they lessen the functional effects of impairments but do not address the underlying cause of the impairment.[58] They are also *habilitative* or *rehabilitative*, enabling individuals to meet daily mobility needs when they are not otherwise able to do so due to disability, just as SGDs enable individuals to meet daily communication needs when they are otherwise unable to do so due to disability.

SGDs and wheelchairs also serve the same medical, or functional, purpose.[59] Specifically, they both are tools that serve as a functional complement or substitute of mal- or nonfunctioning body parts that make it impossible to perform a motor task, such as ambulation or speech. Both devices permit an individual to accomplish a specific functional intent, for example, to move from place to place or to speak, by bypassing body parts that are necessary for the normal accomplishment of those intents but are not working due to disability. For mobility, the brain generates an intent to move from point A to point B; it then generates motor instructions for the muscles of the legs to accomplish that intent, and it sends those instructions along the nerves to the muscles to implement that intent. If due to disability, those instructions cannot be carried out in the normal fashion, the brain can bypass the nonfunctioning body parts and redirect the instructions to the arms and hands, which can propel a manual wheelchair or control a power wheelchair through a joystick. Thus, by bypassing the nonfunctional body parts *and* with the aid of an item of DME, the original intent can be accomplished.

The same bypass exists for SGDs. Ordinarily, speech is the outcome of a series of linked physiological steps. The "communication chain" is a more than 100-year-old metaphor for how the body produces expressive communication (and extends to the steps related to hearing and receptive communication).[60] It states that expressive communication results from a series of five linked steps that must work properly to be successful. These steps include:

1. The brain generates a thought.
2. It is then linguistically encoded into speech.
3. Motor instructions are generated for the speech organs.
4. The nerves then carry those instructions to the speech organs.
5. The speech organs execute the motor instructions.

Figure 17-1 illustrates the communication chain.

Disability can affect any of these "links" or steps in the communication chain. ALS, for example, directly interferes with the fourth link of the chain. It causes the loss of the motor neurons to carry instructions from the brain to the speech organs. Because those body parts are no longer receiving motor instructions, they cease to function and atrophy, making them unable to operate.

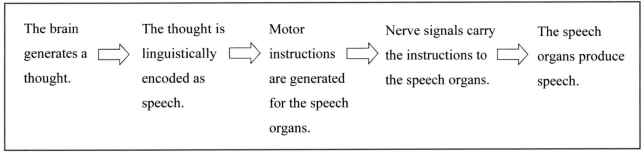

Figure 17-1. The sequential links in the communication chain.

When there is a break in the communication chain, items of DME, such as an SGD, are available to provide a bypass around the nonfunctioning body parts and enable the person to perform the speech task. For example, a person with ALS who still has the use of their hands will bypass the nonfunctioning motor neurons to the speech organs and instead redirect the motor instructions for speech to the hands, which will direct an SGD to create and speak a message.

Peggy Locke, former president of the Communication Aid Manufacturers Association, explained this functional equivalence in a letter to Medicare staff in 1999 as they reviewed Medicare SGD coverage:

> [SGDs] allow their users to achieve [their communication] goals by providing a functional substitute for body organs and structures that are necessary for the production of speech but which are nonfunctioning or malfunctioning due to illness, injury, disease, or condition. Another way to describe the purpose of [SGDs] is as a functional bypass of these non- or malfunctioning body structures, *i.e.*, they allow the [SGD] user to express a thought (message) as speech, by bypassing the nerves, muscles, and organs of speech which, due to impairment, make natural speech ineffective. The [SGD] is the bypass. Viewed in this way, [SGDs] provide the same benefits and serve the same functional purposes as power wheelchairs ... [61]

Several funding sources specifically recognized these functional similarities between SGDs and wheelchairs as the basis to accept SGDs as covered DME items.[62]

Health Benefits Sources' Objections to Speech-Generating Device Coverage as Durable Medical Equipment

When first asked to accept SGDs as DME, not all funding programs were persuaded to do so. Some of the most frequently cited objections are reviewed here.

"Discretion" to Not Cover Speech-Generating Devices. Several state Medicaid programs refused to accept SGDs as DME by claiming they had the discretion to select what health care they wished to cover and what they did not wish to cover. Although state Medicaid programs do have *some* discretion to determine the extent of medical services they

offer, it is not as broad as Medicaid programs claimed. When challenged, this claim was never upheld to cause the exclusion of SGDs.

For example, the Iowa Medicaid program refused SGD coverage because it claimed the right not to provide any equipment as an adjunct to its coverage of speech-language pathology services. A reviewing court rejected this claim of discretion, noting that the federal Medicaid regulations for speech-language pathology services stated the scope of the service "includes any necessary supplies and equipment."[63] State Medicaid programs are obligated to follow the federal statute and regulations.[64] They cannot choose parts of regulations they will comply with and ignore others. The court stated, "Iowa cannot arbitrarily exclude electronic speech devices from coverage under its Medicaid program."[65]

Utah Medicaid tried a somewhat different approach. Iowa attempted to not cover SGDs as a specific form of care within the scope of a *covered* benefit category. By contrast, Utah claimed the right to declare that SGDs will be considered *only* as a benefit of a category that was *not* covered. Utah Medicaid declared that for adults, SGDs were equipment *exclusively* under the speech-language pathology benefit. Because speech-language pathology services is an optional Medicaid benefit category for adults and Utah elected not to provide this benefit, it claimed SGDs were not covered for adults. This claim of discretion was rejected by a reviewing court. SGDs, like many other types of care, can fit and can be covered under several Medicaid benefits categories. There was no reasonable basis to declare that SGDs *had* to be considered under only one benefit category, in particular one that was not covered when SGDs easily fit within one or more that *were* covered.[66]

Other Medicaid claims of "broad discretion" to not cover other services and devices have also been rejected. Courts ruled that coverage of a medical service or device that otherwise fits within the one or more covered benefits categories may not be refused simply because the service or device is disfavored.[67] Instead, coverage decisions must have a reasonable basis. To be reasonable, it must be related to the goals of the program as a whole, that is, there must be some *medical* basis for a coverage exclusion.[68] When no medical basis exists, refusal to cover an item or service is arbitrary and is prohibited. For DME items in particular, federal Medicaid authorities have stated that equipment items that satisfy the definition of DME must be covered. Interpreting a Medicaid regulation that requires covered benefits to be offered in sufficient amount, duration, and scope to reasonably achieve their purpose, federal Medicaid administrators stated, "[B]ecause of the unique nature of medical supplies, equipment, and appliances, scope [of coverage] limitations within the applicable federal and state definitions *are not consistent with sufficiency of the benefit.*"[69]

Exclusive Coverage Lists of Durable Medical Equipment. Another Medicaid program rationale to refuse coverage for SGDs and other equipment items was to add an *exclusive* list of covered items to its descriptive DME definition. Items on the list were covered; items not on the list, even if they met the requirements of the descriptive definition of DME, were not. Medicaid staff responsible for review of benefits requests were required to apply the list when making decisions. This approach had several practical flaws: No claim was made that all possible equipment items had been considered. Thus, omission from the list might be based on no more than the device had never been reviewed. There were also no specific criteria for what justifies inclusion on the list, and no procedure had been identified for new or overlooked items to be considered for coverage.

From a legal standpoint, Medicaid program coverage must be based on reasonable standards consistent with the objectives of the program, that is, standards must be related to the goals of the program, hence they had to have some *medical* basis.[70] Creating a list of covered items, calling it exclusive, and requiring decision makers to apply it satisfies none of those obligations. When challenged, Federal Medicaid authorities rejected this approach, first in what is known as the DeSario Letter. Instead of exclusive lists of covered DME, state Medicaid programs were allowed to:

> Develop a list of preapproved items of ME [medical equipment] as an administrative convenience because such a list eliminates the need to administer an extensive application process for each ME request submitted. An ME policy that provides no reasonable and meaningful procedure for requesting items that do not appear on a State's preapproved list, is inconsistent with [the Medicaid Act]. … [There also must be a process] for seeking modifications or exceptions [and this process] must be made available to all beneficiaries and may not be limited to subclasses of the population (*e.g.*, beneficiaries under the age of 21).[71]

The U.S. Supreme Court subsequently relied on the DeSario Letter to set aside a court decision that had upheld the use of an exclusive list.[72]

Several years later, a court carved out an exception to the DeSario Letter, allowing Texas Medicaid to create a list of "never covered" items and allowed the placement of items on such a list to escape judicial review.[73] This exception subsequently was rejected by Federal Medicaid authorities. "States should not be implementing policies that unreasonably restrict access to specific items of medical equipment."[74] Federal Medicaid regulations applicable to DME were amended to address both of these circumstances:

> States can have a list of preapproved medical equipment, supplies, and appliances for administrative ease but States are prohibited from having absolute exclusions of coverage on medical equipment, supplies, or appliances. States must have processes and criteria for requesting medical equipment that is made available to individuals to request items not on the State's list. The procedure must use reasonable and specific criteria to assess items for coverage.[75]

Those regulations also state equipment items that satisfy the definition of DME must be covered.[76]

Speech-Generating Device Coverage Criteria Based on Client Age. Another discretion-based rationale advanced by several Medicaid programs was that they were permitted to reject SGD coverage as DME on the basis of client age, specifically to reject SGD coverage for adults (recipients ages 21 years and older). Medicaid program discretion was again cited as the basis. This rationale has been rejected each time it has been raised.

Reviewing courts noted client diagnoses and need for an SGD were not related to age. For example, clients who obtained an SGD as children would continue to need the device independent of the arrival and passage of their 21st birthday. They also noted that all the relevant standards for access to Medicaid benefits were the same for recipients of all ages. DME was a covered benefit, the DME definition was the same, and the medical need definition was still the same. The first court to review this claim concluded:

> The … selection of age as the sole criterion for denying benefits is wholly unrelated to the medical decision at hand [*i.e.*, does the client need the SGD] and cannot meet the fundamental legal concept of reasonableness.[77]

All other attempts by Medicaid programs to impose an age-based coverage limitation for SGDs were also rejected.[78]

Speech-Generating Devices Serve "Educational" Not "Medical" Purposes. Another attempt to reject SGD coverage was based on the DME criterion that a device "is primarily and customarily used to serve a *medical* purpose." Health benefits sources claimed that for clients who are of school age (i.e., 3 through 21 years), the purpose of the SGD is "educational." They offered multiple justifications for this conclusion by pointing to the location where the device is used, to the content of speech, and to where the speech-language pathologist who conducted the evaluation worked. Basically, Medicaid programs asserted: *Because* the device will be used in school, its use must *therefore* be for an educational purpose.

None of these explanations withstood even the most superficial scrutiny. Even if all that funding sources claimed was true, SGD use in school will not be the "primary and customary" use of the SGD. Clients who require SGDs need them to communicate effectively when they are in school and when they are not in school. They will need the device before school begins, after it ends, on weekends and holidays, and during vacations when school is not in session. The National Joint Committee noted:

> [A] special education student's communication needs do not depend on school attendance but exist through the course of the student's day and year. In fact, time in school represents less than 20% of a typical student's waking hours during the course of a year.[79]

Thus, the alleged "educational" purpose of the device cannot be its "primary and customary use."

Equally baseless was the assumption that all speech—and by extension, all activity—on school grounds or during the school day serves an "educational" purpose. Throughout the school day, many activities serve a wide variety of purposes, including both educational and medical purposes. For example, consider a student who requires a ventilator to assist with breathing. Obviously, the student must breathe in school; indeed, the ventilator can be viewed as a prerequisite to school attendance. Nonetheless, it is baseless to claim that the breathing assistance it provides serves any real *educational* purpose. It is a medical device that is essential for life. It is also essential for school attendance, but the latter is hardly its purpose.

Another easy example is a student who falls on the playground and is bleeding. That student has a *medical* not educational need to go to the school nurse's office. The nurse serves a *medical* not an educational purpose when the injury is cleaned and bandaged. Likewise, a student unable to speak, write, or sign effectively due to disability requires an SGD to overcome the effects of that disability. That need is *medical*, regardless of what message the student communicates. Whether a message is about a personal care need or sports or a class assignment, the *need for* or *purpose for* the SGD remains the same: It is treatment for the student's communication impairment.

SGDs, along with ventilators, wheelchairs, standing devices, administration of medications, and other health-based services all serve *medical* purposes. That any of these devices may be essential for school attendance, are provided during the school day, or are used at school reflects no more than where students spend the day.

There is a legal as well as a common sense basis for rejecting this objection. Medicaid programs are expressly prohibited from rejecting requests for otherwise covered services on the basis that they are educational and not medical because they may be needed at school. The Individuals with Disabilities Education Act requires schools to provide a "free appropriate public education" to students with disabilities, which includes "related services."[80] Related services include audiology, nursing, occupational therapy, physical therapy, psychological counseling, and speech-language pathology services,[81] all of which are also Medicaid health or medical services. The Individuals with Disabilities Education Act also states that "assistive technology devices" are a related service,[82] a category that overlaps significantly with the Medicaid DME benefit and includes SGDs. That these services fit within the scope of these two programs does not empower either to refuse to provide or pay for them by claiming the other is responsible. The Medicaid statute expressly prohibits this[83] and this prohibition was applied to reject a Medicaid program's denial of an SGD because the recipient was of school age, and therefore, the school was required to provide the device.[84] When schools attempted to apply the same claim of *them, not me*, that is, that occupational and physical therapy services were medical not educational, they were expressly prohibited from refusing to provide these or other health-based related services.[85]

Establishing Speech-Generating Devices' Fit as Prosthetic Devices

The majority of health benefits sources cover SGDs as DME, but Veterans Affairs and Tricare (both with express support from Congress),[86] and some insurers, health plans, and Medicaid programs, cover them as prosthetic devices.

SGDs are accepted as prosthetic devices by these sources for the same reason they are accepted as DME by others: They "fit" within the scope of their prosthetic device benefits categories. Specifically, they match the physical and functional criteria stated in their prosthetic device definitions.[87]

As with DME, the Medicare prosthetic device guidelines are copied in full or significant part by most other sources. Medicare defines prosthetic devices as, "Prosthetic and orthotic devices means devices that replace all or part of an internal body organ …"[88] This definition is supplemented by additional guidance that states:

> Prosthetic devices (other than dental) are covered under Part B as a medical or other health service … and are devices that replace all or part of an internal body organ or replace all or part of the function of a permanently inoperative or malfunctioning internal body organ …[89]

The broader *function-based* definition supports Medicare coverage of devices, such as cardiac pacemakers, as prosthetic devices. Pacemakers do not replace all or part of the heart or brain. Instead, they provide electronic pulses to regulate and support heart function. Devices of this type are covered because Medicare acknowledges that *functional* substitution or restoration rather than *actual* substitution or replacement of the body part itself is a characteristic of prosthetic devices. This reasoning also supports Medicare coverage of cochlear implants as prosthetic devices. They do not replace the inner ear; rather, they substitute for and enhance its function.

SGDs also satisfy these criteria. They provide a functional substitute for malfunctioning or permanently inoperative body organs and other body structures needed to produce speech. This includes the nerve pathways and muscles that control the larynx, vocal folds, tongue, teeth, and lips, all of which must function properly and in coordinated fashion to produce intelligible speech. In this regard, SGDs cannot be distinguished from the artificial larynx (electronic speech aid)[90] and tracheoesophageal voice prosthesis[91] for individuals who have had a tracheostomy or have a nonfunctioning larynx due to prolonged intubation or other cause. These two devices are very useful for comparison to SGDs. They are commonly covered prosthetic devices that address impairment to the speech function, as do SGDs. But neither of these devices *replace* the larynx or vocal folds. To the contrary, they provide a substitute that enables an exhaled column of air to be converted to speech if the larynx has been removed or the vocal folds are not functioning.

The functional equivalence among these speech aids and SGDs has been most important to respond to United Healthcare, one of the nation's largest insurers, which also serves as claims and appeals fiduciary for many health plans. It often includes an exclusion for "devices and computers to assist communication and speech," which appears to target SGDs.[92] However, quite often added to this exclusion is an exception for "speech aid devices [or speech aid prosthetics] and tracheoesophageal voice prostheses." An exception to an exclusion in a health insurance policy or health plan is a statement of coverage. In other words, some speech devices are excluded, and others are covered.

SGDs fit in the latter category. Because SGDs have been shown persuasively to be "speech aid devices," several have been approved under this exception. These favorable decisions were supported by Medicare, which defines SGDs as "speech aid devices." In 2015, as part of the update of its SGD coverage guidelines, Medicare specifically recognized the importance of this characterization of SGDs to support funding by other funding sources:

> *Comment:* One commenter recommended that the phrase 'speech aids' be included in the definition of SGD: '[SGD] are speech aids considered to fall within the DME benefit category ...' The commenter believed that the addition of this phrase may be beneficial to individuals with insurance other than Medicare.
>
> *Response:* We agree with this comment and will add the phrase 'speech aids' in the definition of SGD.[93]

The Tricare program also covers SGDs as prosthetic devices and calls them "speech aids."[94] Anthem Blue Cross Blue Shield (BCBS), another of the nation's largest health insurers, is one of several that state SGDs are speech aids.[95]

That SGDs fall within the exception for "speech aids" is also based on a comparison of SGDs to "tracheaesophageal voice prostheses." As already noted, these devices, like SGDs, substitute for the function of impaired or nonworking speech organs. They operate in different ways but they both provide the same benefit.

Establishing Speech-Generating Devices Are "Medically Necessary"

The foregoing discussion reviewed how SGDs are established as covered benefits. The next step is to establish that they provide the benefits that fall within the goals and purposes of health benefits programs, that is, that they are *medically necessary*.

All health benefits programs require proof of medical necessity to gain access to or funding for any covered benefit. The following is an example of a medical need definition:

> Where prior approval of medical, dental, and remedial care, services, or supplies is required under the MA [medical assistance—Medicaid] program, such prior approval will be granted when the medical, dental, and remedial care, services, or supplies are shown to be medically necessary to prevent, diagnose, correct, or cure a condition of the recipient which: (1) causes acute suffering; (2) endangers life; (3) results in illness or infirmity; (4) interferes with the capacity for normal activity; or (5) threatens to cause a significant handicap.
>
> *Necessary to prevent, diagnose, correct, or cure a condition* means that requested medical, dental, and remedial care, services, or supplies would: meet the recipient's medical needs; reduce the recipient's physical or mental disability; restore the recipient to [their] best possible functional level; or improve the recipient's capacity for normal activity. Necessity to prevent, diagnose, correct, or cure a condition must be determined in light of the recipient's specific circumstances and the recipient's functional capacity to use or make use of the requested care, services, or supplies and appropriate alternatives.[96]

The preceding text is just an example. Health benefits sources have no uniform definition of medical necessity. Instead of common vocabulary, four principles are common to all medical need definitions. Medical need is established by evidence of:

- An identified illness, injury, or condition
- That causes or will cause identifiable adverse effects on client health status or functional abilities
- For which the care, device, or service being recommended is recognized as an effective form of treatment that will meaningfully address the condition (e.g., prevent, cure, or correct it) or will meaningfully address its effects (will ameliorate it, will prevent adverse effects, eliminate or lessen the severity of the effects, or slow or stop their progression)
- As compared to other forms of treatment that will provide the same benefits, the one being recommended is the least costly of these equally effective alternatives

For more than 40 years, both speech-language pathologists in their evaluation of clients and SGDs as a class of DME items have satisfied all these principles.

That SGDs are an effective form of treatment already has been discussed. The same facts established both this principle and that SGDs "serve a medical purpose," which led to their acceptance as DME. That discussion explained that SGDs are a long-accepted form of AAC intervention, which is a long-accepted speech-language pathology treatment methodology. SGD use has been accepted as effective treatment for individuals with complex and severe speech impairments.

Still to be addressed is the question, *Is this SGD medically necessary for this client?* This is the critical SGD funding question. It must be answered for every client, for every SGD request. Primary responsibility to answer it lies with speech-language pathologists.[97]

The speech-language pathology evaluation and report establish clients' medical need for specific SGDs, mounts, and access aids. To guide speech-language pathologists through the evaluation and report-writing process, almost all health benefits sources have SGD coverage criteria. These criteria outline the scope of the speech-language pathology evaluation, identify the topics to be addressed in the speech-language pathology report, and often state an eligibility standard for SGD approval. Once again, Medicare serves as a model. Its guidance outlining the required speech-language pathology evaluation and report to support SGD funding has been copied in whole or part by many other sources.[98] Medicare's guidance states:

A[n] [SGD] (E2500-E2511) is covered when all of the following criteria (1 through 7) are met:

1. Prior to the delivery of the SGD, the beneficiary has had a formal evaluation of their cognitive and communication abilities by a speech-language pathologist. The formal, written evaluation must include, at a minimum, the following elements:

    a. Current communication impairment, including the type, severity, language skills, cognitive ability, and anticipated course of the impairment

    b. An assessment of whether the individual's daily communication needs could be met using other natural modes of communication

    c. A description of the functional communication goals expected to be achieved and treatment options

    d. Rationale for selection of a specific device and any accessories

    e. Demonstration that the beneficiary possesses a treatment plan that includes a training schedule for the selected device

    f. The cognitive and physical abilities to effectively use the selected device and any accessories to communicate

    g. For a subsequent upgrade to a previously issued SGD, information regarding the functional benefit to the beneficiary of the upgrade compared to the initially provided SGD

2. The beneficiary's medical condition is one resulting in a severe expressive speech impairment

3. The beneficiary's speaking needs cannot be met using natural communication methods

4. Other forms of treatment have been considered and ruled out

5. The beneficiary's speech impairment will benefit from the device ordered

6. A copy of the [speech-language pathologist]'s written evaluation and recommendation have been forwarded to the beneficiary's treating physician prior to ordering the device

7. The [speech-language pathologist] performing the beneficiary evaluation may not be an employee of or have a financial relationship with the supplier of the SGD

If one or more of the SGD coverage criteria 1 through 7 is not met, the SGD will be denied as not reasonable and necessary.[99]

Identify Clients' Illnesses, Injuries, or Conditions

Clients with CCN will have health conditions that adversely affect their body structures, their activities (e.g., expressive and receptive communication), and their participation, that is, their ability to meet all daily communication needs.[100] These health conditions can affect clients' speech, language, cognitive, physical, and sensory functioning. They include congenital or developmental conditions (e.g., autism, cerebral palsy, Down syndrome, and intellectual disability) and acquired conditions (e.g., ALS, head or neck cancer, stroke, and traumatic brain injury). They also include conditions that directly impact speech and language, such as aphasia, aphonia, apraxia, and dysarthria. These conditions are all associated with a need for AAC intervention, including SGD use. Speech-language pathology reports must identify all conditions relevant to clients' ability to meet daily communication needs (refer back to Medicare SGD Coverage Guideline items 1a and 2).

The *Formal Request*, submitted to Medicare staff in late 1999 to aid their reconsideration of Medicare SGD coverage, discussed the conditions associated with SGD need based on a review of the professional literature current to that date.[101] The AMA and the American Academies of Neurology, Physical Medicine and Rehabilitation, and Pediatrics all subsequently acknowledged SGDs are medically necessary for treatment of severe communication impairment, including serving as the "standard of care" to address adverse effects on expressive communication associated with ALS.[102] Neither the *Formal Request* nor medical society input proposed any limitations on SGD access on the basis of condition. Medicare's SGD guidance is consistent with this input. It supports SGD coverage without condition-based limitation or exclusion. Other health benefits sources also do not limit SGD coverage by condition.

In addition to the identification of all relevant impairments, speech-language pathologists must assess and report their severity and anticipated course and related factors that may affect speech, such as clients' language skills and cognitive ability (refer back to Medicare SGD Coverage Guideline, item 1a). Clients' conditions that affect physical and sensory functioning, as well as their severity and course, must also be evaluated and reported. In general, this section of the speech-language pathology evaluation and report will establish clients' baseline functioning, that is, clients' abilities and limitations without consideration of past or current AAC interventions.

Although not mentioned specifically in the Medicare template, speech-language pathologists should always gather and report facts about clients' receptive language abilities. These facts are important because the existence of a gap between clients' receptive and expressive communication skills (a disparity between what one is able to understand and what one is able to express) is a long-recognized justification for pursuing AAC assessment and recommendation of AAC interventions, including SGDs. One of the first textbooks on AAC interventions reported that this functional communication gap justified AAC assessment and recommendation:

> Individuals with severe expressive communication disorders typically exhibit a notable discrepancy between their level of comprehension and their ability to speak and/or write. [An article in press reports] "communication augmentation should be considered in addition to more traditional speech and language therapy if an individual experiences or is at some risk for experiencing 'communicative dissonance,' a dissociation between communication needs and capabilities." Communicative dissonance … occurs when intelligible speech fails to develop, when the ability to speak is lost, or when physical or cognitive disabilities preclude the use of written language … The degree of communicative dissonance experienced depends on the disparity between an individual's communication needs and capabilities. Thus, a major goal of augmentative communication interventions is to employ compensatory interventions that will result in enhanced expressive capabilities and a reduced level of discrepancy. The greater the communicative dissonance, the greater the potential contribution of augmentative interventions.[103]

It is noteworthy that no limitations are imposed on speech-language pathology discretion regarding *how* these data are gathered. It is not common that health benefits programs' SGD coverage guidelines will direct speech-language pathologists to conduct specific procedures or perform specific tests.[104]

Describe the Conditions' Adverse Effects on Health Status or Functional Abilities

Speech-language pathologists' next evaluation and reporting task is to identify and describe all the adverse effects of the clients' conditions and all past and current speech-language pathology treatment efforts and their effects. The context for this task is whether clients are able to meet all their daily communication needs. To begin, speech-language pathologists must identify and explain clients' current and reasonably foreseeable future daily communication needs. One tool to help accomplish this task is Social Networks (Augmentative Communication, Inc), a template to aid identification of all typical communication partners and important facts related to each partner. This tool directs attention to the existence and nature of the relationship between the client and each partner, which often affects the frequency, location, content, and other factors that may affect the effectiveness and efficiency of their communication.[105] It allows speech-language pathologists to assess whether clients are able to communicate effectively with each current or potential communication partner and whether there are special factors that must be considered for effective communication with each partner.

Clients' functional goals complement their daily communication needs (refer back to Medicare SGD Coverage Guideline, item 1c). Clients' communication goals should address the four "any's:" the ability to engage in effective and efficient communication with *any*one, about *any*thing, *any*where, and at *any* time. Beukelman and Mirenda stated the "purpose of AAC intervention is to facilitate meaningful participation in daily life activities."[106] The National Joint Commission defined "meaningful participation" as the effective and efficient communication of messages in any form the beneficiary chooses.[107]

Once clients' daily communication needs and functional communication goals have been identified, the focus shifts to what speech-language pathology treatment, if any, was or is now being directed to help clients meet those needs and achieve those goals. A note about prior or current treatment: Although it is very common clients have received or are receiving some form of treatment before being evaluated for an SGD, it is not required. There is no sequence of alternative treatments clients must satisfy (i.e., no alternative treatment prerequisites) before an SGD evaluation can be conducted, before an SGD can be identified as the most appropriate treatment, or before access to specific types of SGDs will be provided.[108] Among the first clients identified as having AAC and SGD need were individuals warehoused in long-term care facilities who were believed by staff to be beyond help, and as a consequence, received no treatment. For example, a woman who had this experience following a stroke later (with the use of an SGD) wrote:

Now I am horrified … I know I have a throat and should be able to scream for someone to take me away. I realize there is no power in my legs, arms, hands, voice, body. I realize that I am paralyzed.

She [a nurse] doesn't speak to me or look me in the face to see if I'm alive, and I suddenly realize that I'm not going to get better. I'm just going to get worse. The nurse … is waiting for me to die.

She [the nurse] stops singing and calls another nurse into the room … "This one doesn't got a brain. Can't do nothin' but cry, so don't mind her."

This continued for *6 years* until she was finally approached as an intelligent person and examined by a speech-language pathologist who was skilled in AAC assessment and treatment. The woman later described this initial encounter with the speech-language pathologist:

This is no dream: I'm actually being spoken *to* … For the first time in 6 years I feel whole … I raise my eyes for *yes*, hardly able to believe that someone is asking permission before she does something to me.[109]

As this client's experience illustrates, the need to provide AAC treatment and use of an SGD may be a first response. It may be obvious in the evaluation that other forms of speech-language pathology treatment will not be appropriate. Regardless what treatment has been or is being provided, clients must be evaluated and recommended the most appropriate treatment based on how they are at the time of the evaluation with consideration also given to reasonably foreseeable changes in their current condition. This observation and response is the same for clients with cardiac impairments as for clients with speech impairments. Change of diet and lifestyle may be part of the overall treatment protocol for individuals with mild cardiac impairment, but they are not appropriate for clients who present far more severe impairment and for whom the immediate need is for an angioplasty, stent, or cardiac artery bypass. Analogies beyond medical care present the same absence of mandatory sequencing or prerequisites. Speech-language pathologists encounter clients just as do clothing stores: The latter may stock all sizes, but their task is to provide clients only with items that are appropriate to their current needs.

For clients who have received or are currently receiving some form of treatment, all treatment must be described, including services for speech and language development, speech production, writing, signing, use of non–speech-generating communication aids, use of SGDs, and use of alternative access methods. What was or is being provided, for how long, what effect it had, and if discontinued, the reason why must all be explained. Among possible explanations for services that were tried and discontinued are that they limited what the client could say; for example, the treatment did not provide access to all of the client's language. Alternately, it limited who the client could communicate with or where the communication could occur, such as the treatment required something (e.g., a specific skill or action) that could only be performed by specially trained communication partners, leaving clients unable to communicate with others when those partners were not present to interpret or translate clients' communicative actions into messages. Other reasons a form of treatment may have been abandoned are that its operational demands resulted in ineffective or inefficient expression or required unnecessarily burdensome effort. Message creation may have been too slow to permit effective communication or required effort that was very fatiguing. The discontinued intervention may have led to communication breakdowns but did not support efficient recovery from them. In each of these examples, a form of treatment might have been abandoned because it did not allow the client to communicate effectively and efficiently with all typical communication partners.

Having identified clients' daily communication needs, functional communication goals, and all treatment efforts that have been or are being offered to help clients meet those needs, two speech-language pathology judgments must be made. First, are clients able to meet daily communication needs using *natural* communication methods, that is, will speech-language pathology services directed to speech, writing, or sign be sufficient for clients to meet their daily communication needs (refer back to Medicare SGD Coverage Guideline, item 1b)? Second, do past or current AAC interventions enable clients to meet all their daily communication needs (refer back to Medicare SGD evaluation template, item 4)? If the answer to the first is yes, then clients will not have a medical need for AAC intervention. If the answer to the second is yes, then clients' needs will be met by the AAC intervention just described. Only if the answer to both questions is no will the evaluation continue to consider new or different AAC interventions, SGDs, mounts, and access methods to help clients meet their daily communication needs.

Speech-Generating Devices Considered

Once it has been determined that clients are unable to meet all their daily communication needs using speech or other natural communication methods, speech-language pathologists' next steps are to identify the treatment methodologies that will change the *status quo*, that is, will improve clients' communication functioning and reduce or eliminate clients' unmet communication needs. This task may lead to identification and recommendation of multiple solutions, each addressing some of the clients' unmet needs. One of those solutions may be an SGD, and for funding purposes, the SGD will be the focus of attention. However, it is neither expected nor required that an SGD will be the only method clients will use for expression.

A health benefits program once stated: If clients are functional communicators in all customary environments, then the SGD would be the *only necessary means of expressing themselves*. This assertion has no basis in fact or professional practice. Clients are unlikely to ever have only a single means of expression. Clients with an SGD need will want to add this tool to their other means of expression, so together they will be able to meet all their daily communication needs. One of the pillars of communicative competence is strategic competence, the repertoire of skills clients must learn to ensure messages are communicated efficiently and effectively.[110] This includes learning when it will be most effective and most efficient for each client to use an SGD or to rely instead on other available communication strategies or tools, which may include voice, vocalizations, gesture, manual sign, body movement, or eye gaze. The program subsequently abandoned this assertion.[111]

In addition, there is no expectation or requirement that speech-language pathologists speculate about the frequency of expected use of different communication methods. For example, one Medicaid program stated in proposed guidance that "an SGD is intended to be *the primary source* of communication." Like the claim that an SGD be the only communication method, this assertion has no basis in fact or professional practice. **How** speech-language pathologists can reach such a conclusion (or on what objective data it can be based) was never explained: It asks about how frequently the device will be used in relation to other forms of communication **before** the device is provided. It also does not set a time parameter for when this measure is to be taken. It is reasonable to expect clients' use of the SGD will change based on their communication partner: Familiar partners may understand more of clients' speech, vocalizations, and gestures, thereby reducing the need to rely on the SGD. By contrast, less familiar partners and others, such as children, may be less able to extract meaning from those efforts. Thus, clients' primary means of expression may vary throughout the day or among the days of the week. Clients' use of their SGDs may also change over time, as their operational skills and strategic competence develop and improve, a process that will continue for years.

> The attainment of communicative competence by individuals who use AAC is a complex process that requires significant time and effort. Communicative competence is not attained in days or weeks; rather, the growth toward communicative competence takes place during many years of learning and practice.[112]

> Communicative competence needs to be learned. Becoming a competent communicator is a step-by-step incremental process. It requires a long-term investment. It is the culmination of years of learning—the outcome of commitment, appropriate instruction, and hard work.[113]

This variability of SGD use illustrates the difference between facts that can be measured (i.e., what a funding source *may claim* are important) and the facts *that are* important to SGD assessment, recommendation, and funding requests. The program subsequently deleted this sentence when it published final guidelines.

Instead of searching for clients' sole or primary means of expression, speech-language pathologists consider specific SGD models in order to identify the device, mount, and access aid that will be the "most appropriate form of treatment to enable clients to meet all their daily communication needs" (i.e., will provide the maximum reduction of their unmet communication needs).[114] This search process is known as *feature matching*, matching clients' abilities and needs with device characteristics. Feature matching is a process of comparison, elimination, and selection. SGDs, mounts, and access aids that do not match clients' abilities and needs at all or not as well as others will be ruled out. The equipment that best meets clients' needs will be recommended. By contrast, feature matching does not require clients to need or intend to use all or any specific percentage of an SGD's features. Once it is determined that a device has the features that will match client needs, what else the device may be able to do is beside the point.

Health benefits sources generally do not impose strict protocols for how speech-language pathologists consider alternatives, such as which types of SGDs they must consider. Some programs require consideration of a minimum number of SGD alternatives (e.g., three SGDs from different codes [i.e., device types] or different SGD manufacturers), but specific demands are not common. Even if not specifically required, speech-language pathologists should consider multiple AAC and SGD alternatives starting with those that are least costly. This approach is sensible because all funding sources require speech-language pathologists to select the least costly, equally effective alternative. Following this course will lead to consideration of non–speech-generating solutions first, then SGDs that produce digitized speech, and then those that produce synthesized speech. Client access needs (i.e., how clients will operate the device) must be a matter of concern throughout.

Programs cannot require that every SGD model be considered. Such a demand would be impractical due to the large number of SGD models and unnecessary because of the functional similarities of SGDs with the same "code." A system of coding known by its acronym HCPCS was created to aid both coverage and payment of medical equipment items.[115] SGDs have been grouped into six codes on the basis of shared functional characteristics. Four codes are for SGDs that produce digitized speech output. The other two codes are for SGDs that produce synthesized speech output. Figure 17-2 provides the definition of the six SGD codes. There are also codes for SGD software (E2511), for SGD mounts (E2512), and for SGD accessories (E2599).

Because of the similarities of devices within these codes, speech-language pathologists are often able to perform their initial feature matching tasks at the code- or device-type level. They can identify clear mis- or nonmatches between clients' abilities and needs and device features, and as a result, conclude that all similar SGD models in the same code

HCPCS Code	Code Description
E2500	SGD, digitized speech, using prerecorded messages, less than or equal to 8 minutes of recording time
E2502	SGD, digitized speech, using prerecorded messages, with greater than 8 but less than or equal to 20 minutes of recording time
E2504	SGD, digitized speech, using prerecorded messages, with greater than 20 but less than 40 minutes of recording time
E2506	SGD, digitized speech, using prerecorded messages, with greater than 40 minutes of recording time
E2508	SGD, synthesized speech, requiring message formulation by spelling and access by physical contact with the device
E2510	SGD, synthesized speech, permitting multiple methods of message formulation and multiple methods of device access

Figure 17-2. SGD code definitions.

can be ruled out as not appropriate. Health benefits sources do not prohibit or object to this procedure, which enables speech-language pathologists to narrow SGD choices that will be subject to closer scrutiny.

Stated next are some facts speech-language pathologists may use to consider whether it is appropriate to rule out all devices within SGD codes. The material that follows is not intended as a complete outline of how speech-language pathologists should assess SGD alternatives. Readers are directed to Chapters 11 through 14 for a more complete discussion of speech-language pathology tasks leading to an SGD recommendation.

Non–Speech-Generating Solutions (E1902). Rather than looking to identify the single or primary means of expression to enable clients to meet all daily communication needs, speech-language pathologists look for as many forms of treatment as may be needed to achieve that goal. For all or almost all clients, non–speech-generating solutions, such as communication boards, books, and cards,[116] and nonaided solutions, such as clients' limited speech ability, vocalizations, manual signs, gestures, facial expressions, and eye gaze, will be part of the solution. Some or all will be appropriate and necessary but not sufficient by themselves to enable clients to meet all their daily communication needs.

These strategies and tools will likely be appropriate for only some communication partners, messages, and settings. However, communication is also likely to occur in settings where partners will not be in a position to observe clients' messaging, with partners who will not recognize clients' pointing or eye gaze as communication, and with partners who will not understand what clients are trying to communicate, that is, they will not be able to interpret or translate the message. For clients who must rely on eye gaze, communication will occur with partners who have no duty to hold or change the boards.[117] Consider a child in school. Their

peers may not be able to see what the child is pointing to on a board based on where they are seated in the classroom. They may not be literate to be able to read messages on a letter or word-based board. They may not know what the symbols represent on a picture- or symbol-based board. A child could not expect cafeteria staff, separated by a serving counter, to see selections made on a letter, word, picture, or symbol board or to pick up and use eye-gaze boards to let the student make food choices.

Vocabulary size is another limiting factor for non–speech-generating aids. As a client's vocabulary increases, more words, messages, or picture symbols must be displayed, leading to more pages or cards that must be managed. Sorting through the cards or pages becomes a barrier to independent, easily accessible expression. Navigating through multiple pages of language or cards slows down and may completely stop the communication process. A common observation in speech-language pathologists' reports is that: "The focus inevitably shifts to managing the communication system at the cost of the client independently communicating desired messages." One of the developers of the Picture Exchange Communication System (PECS) estimated that at 80 to 120 cards "changing to an electronic system that can accommodate more symbols would be appropriate."[118]

In all these circumstances, non–speech-generating solutions will not be appropriate to address all of clients' unmet communication needs. Thus, the search must continue to identify other treatment methods. For these reasons and others, a voice is required. In general, speech output will be necessary because speech is the common denominator. It is the method of expression able to be understood by the greatest number of potential communication partners in the widest variety of settings, and to be effective, speech requires no special skills, training, actions, or positioning on the part of the communication partners.

Speech-Generating Devices: Digitized Speech Output Devices (E2500, E2502; E2504, E2506). There are many digitized speech output SGD models ("digitized speech SGDs"), but characteristics they share make these devices inappropriate—as a class or device type—for many clients.

Digitized Speech Output Speech-Generating Devices Do Not Support Eye-Gaze Access. Clients who require use of an eye-gaze accessory to operate an SGD must be recommended for a synthesized speech output device. The entire category of digitized speech output devices can be ruled out because none supports eye-gaze access. The clients' access needs cannot be met by these devices.

Digitized Speech Output Speech-Generating Devices Do Not Support Word or Message Creation by Spelling. A second basis to rule out all digitized speech output SGDs is clients' use of or planned training to use letter-by-letter spelling to create words and messages. No digitized speech output SGD will support this method of message formulation. As a group, digitized speech SGDs do not have text-to-speech capability. Clients able to spell or who are or will be learning to spell have communication abilities that exceed the capabilities of these devices.

However, a distinction is required between the ability to spell that supports ruling out all digitized speech output SGDs and the ability to combine or sequence symbols to form novel messages, which does not. Speech-language pathologists often inappropriately equate these abilities. It is correct that almost all digitized speech output SGDs will not support combining or sequencing symbols to create messages, but a few do have this capability. For this reason, speech-language pathologists must be more specific: The ability to combine or sequence symbols should be identified as part of a decision to rule out all digitized speech SGDs that will not support this method of message formulation. But, other reasons must be identified to rule out the remaining digitized speech output SGD choices.

Digitized Speech Output Speech-Generating Devices Do Not Offer Access to All of Clients' Vocabulary. The goal of all speech-language pathology services, including SGD use, is to enable clients to produce whatever they want to say, whenever, wherever, and to whomever they want to speak. SGDs that provide access to only some of the clients' messages are not appropriate. Digitized speech output SGDs have two characteristics that may interfere with clients' access to all their vocabulary.

One is that almost all digitized speech SGDs have a fixed upper limit of the number of words or messages each can produce. If clients' functional vocabulary exceeds the message total available on any digitized speech SGDs, those devices are not appropriate. When considering clients' functional vocabulary, speech-language pathologists must estimate both clients' current vocabulary and its reasonably foreseeable growth over time.

Static (or fixed) displays are the second characteristic of digitized speech output SGDs that may interfere with clients' access to all their vocabulary, and thus, render digitized speech output SGDs inappropriate. A static display "refers to any AAC display in which the symbols and representations are fixed in a particular location."[119]

Digitized speech output SGDs have static displays with a wide range of messaging capability: from 1 to 128 message options. Some digitized speech output SGDs will also provide access to more messages than can fit on a single display "page." They accomplish this by offering multiple "levels," each of which will offer an additional page of messages (i.e., a multiple of the number of messages on their displays). For example, an SGD with a 12-message display with 8 levels will have a total messaging capacity of 96 messages (12 per page times 8 pages equals 96 messages), and a 32-message device with 8 levels will have a total messaging capacity of 256 messages (32 per page times 8 pages equals 256 messages).

The availability of multiple levels may result in the total number of messages some digitized speech output SGDs can produce being greater than clients' estimated current and reasonably foreseeable future vocabulary. However, that comparison may not be appropriate. Rather than just considering the total number of messages that can be produced, speech-language pathologists must consider the number of messages clients will be able to access on SGDs with static displays. That total may be significantly smaller than the total number of messages the device can produce and smaller than clients' vocabulary.

Clients Cannot Change Paper Overlay Pages Independently. The total message capacity of digitized speech output SGDs with multiple levels may be beside the point because clients may not be able to access more than the first display page. To change the pages on a multiple-level digitized speech output SGD, a seven-step procedure must be completed:

1. The additional page(s) must be removed from a storage carrier.

2. The additional page(s) must be searched to locate the word or message the client wishes to say.

3. The existing display page must be removed from the device.

4. The new display page must be inserted in its place.

5. A selection knob on the device must be changed to correspond to the new page.

6. The client must select the new word or message for the device to speak it.

7. The removed display page must be inserted in a carrier for storage and transport.

These operational demands make multilevel digitized speech output SGDs inappropriate for clients unable to perform these tasks independently whether due to cognitive, sensory, physical, or other causes.[120] As one decision-maker reported:

The … speech-language pathologist reported that the Appellant's physical inability to insert, remove, store, and retrieve the paper overlays that must be changed to access stored messages ruled out the static display SGD. [The Appellant's attorney reported] that if the Appellant relies on 4-button displays but cannot change the overlays, then the static display SGD will offer him only 4 messages in total despite its ability to store 190+ messages. What else the device might be able to offer [literally] will be beyond his reach.[121]

Clients must be able to perform page changes independently—on their own—because no one is responsible to provide this assistance. That, *in some circumstances*, a communication partner may be likely to provide this assistance is not responsive. The required goal is to identify a device that will provide access to all of a client's vocabulary, not to some of it, and to enable communication with any communication partner, not just some of them. Moreover, no funding source will provide a communication assistant with specific responsibility to change static display pages. One funding source representative bluntly stated in response to a question about providing a communication assistant, "We don't hire anybody for anything."[122] One reason why a communication assistant will not be provided is cost. Considering the number of hours an assistant will be required per day, every day, multiplied by that person's hourly wage, an assistant's costs will exceed that of any SGD within just a few months. And those costs will continue to increase as long as the client must rely on this type of SGD. The support needed to make such an SGD an appropriate choice disqualifies it from further consideration because it is not the least costly, equally effective alternative.

Even if a client could change static display pages independently, the maximum number of messages a digitized speech output SGD can produce still may not be the appropriate comparison because clients may not be able to access the maximum number of cells on a display page. They may require fewer or larger targets to accommodate physical, sensory, or cognitive limitations. For example, instead of 12 cells per display page, the client may be able to access only 4. Even if the client could access multiple pages, the maximum number of messages the client could access will be cut by two-thirds. That total may not be sufficient to enable clients to access all their current and reasonably foreseeable future vocabulary.

As just explained, speech-language pathologists must ensure there is a match between the messaging capacity of digitized speech output SGDs and clients' current and reasonably foreseeable future messaging abilities. This match may not exist for any SGD of this type.

Digitized Speech Output Speech-Generating Devices Do Not Provide Appropriate Access. Already discussed is that no digitized speech output SGDs will support access by eye tracking. It also is true that some digitized speech output devices will provide for access only by physical contact direct selection; they will not accept switches to support indirect access by scanning. For clients who require switch access, this subgroup of digitized speech SGDs will be inappropriate. Also, even for digitized speech SGDs that will support switch access, independent page changes must still be considered.

Another switch access issue arises for clients who may be able to use multiple switches for direct selection. This opportunity exists only for a few digitized speech SGDs that are able to assign switches to specific locations on a device display.[123] To be appropriate, there must be a match between the number of switches the client can effectively and efficiently control and the number of switches the SGD can support. If the client can access more cells on a display with switches than the device can support, then this small group of digitized speech SGDs is not appropriate. Here too, clients' abilities to change pages independently must also be considered.

Speech-Generating Devices: Synthetic Speech Output Devices That Require Physical Contact Direct Selection and Message Formulation by Spelling (E2508). Another category of SGDs operates as "talking typewriters" or "talking keyboards." These devices require physical contact direct selection, either with a finger, stylus, or head pointer, and message formulation by letter-by-letter spelling. The highly specific operating requirements of these SGDs cause them to be inappropriate for clients for whom any form of alternative access is necessary or who will be most effective or efficient creating messages by any means other than just spelling. These devices are rarely recommended.

Speech-Generating Devices: Synthesized Speech Output Devices That Offer Multiple Methods of Message Formulation and Multiple Methods of Access (E2510). SGDs within the E2510 code are the most frequently recommended SGDs. This may be because they have the greatest flexibility regarding their operation. These SGDs produce synthesized speech and have no limits on the number of messages they can produce or on the length of any single message.[124] These SGDs also permit multiple methods of message formulation and multiple methods of access. They are sometimes described as "touchscreen SGDs." As a group, these SGDs have dynamic displays that allow the pages to be changed electronically. Clients will accomplish this task by the same method they use to access the device.

The SGDs in this code will be recommended when clients are unable to meet all their daily communication needs using speech or other natural methods of communication, or through use of non–speech-generating aids, or use of other types of SGDs. It is speech-language pathologists' responsibility to explain the basis for their professional judgment that an E2510 SGD is most appropriate.

Historically, the point of greatest disagreement related to SGD funding was clients' need for an E2510 device as compared to a digitized speech output device. While this distinction remains important, the primary focus of funding source review (and dispute) may be shifting to speech-language pathologists' judgments among devices *within* the E2510 code. The shift of attention may be based on the E2510 code's range of device choices and prices. Speech-language pathologists must recommend the least costly, equally effective alternative device and access method. However, because all E2510 SGDs share some characteristics, funding sources may assert that they are interchangeable, and therefore, can be distinguished just on the basis of their price. For example, one Medicaid program stated without producing any evidence that "low-cost generic tablet SGDs have the same functionality and quality as those from an SGD manufacturer and can meet any recipient's needs." The program subsequently withdrew that assertion, but it can serve as a possible preview of SGD funding source denial excuses in the future.

To pre-empt such claims or in response to them, speech-language pathologists must explain why "one size does not fit all" and that cost is not the only fact required to distinguish E2510 SGD or access aids. To meet this burden, speech-language pathologists must provide specific reasons why one model or access aid was judged to be most appropriate while others in the same code were ruled out as not appropriate at all or not as appropriate as the one recommended. Differences in capabilities, features, and performances among various SGD models and access aids must be identified. However, pointing to differences is not sufficient: The differences must be meaningful to the client whose needs are being assessed. They must relate to clients' ability to use or benefit from the device or access method.

Speech-language pathologists should identify and discuss the differences among device choices in regard to SGD hardware, SGD software, access methods, and support, training, and other services offered by the device manufacturer or supplier. Objective differences, as well as subjective differences, should be considered and reported: any factors that are clinically significant (i.e., that will influence speech-language pathologists' clinical judgment as to which SGD, software, and access method is most appropriate). Among the factors to be considered will include:

- Differences in device and access aid features
- Differences in clients' ability to use and benefit from device and access aid features (easier to understand, easier to use, faster, more accurate, less fatiguing, easier to correct errors, sufficient speech output volume, weather resistance, glare resistance, ability to accommodate greater head movement)
- Differences in the amount, duration, and scope of the support, training, and other services offered by the device manufacturer or supplier[125]
- Clients' and primary communication partners' preferences

Clients' needs for SGD manufacturer or supplier services, supports, and training will vary, as will all other factors considered in the assessment, and it will be speech-language pathologists' responsibility to assess whether all the post-SGD delivery services clients will need will be available. Among the services that should be considered include:

- Whether in-person assistance will be provided for set-up following delivery; initial programming; initial orientation and training for clients, clients' families, or other frequent communication partners; or clients' services providers, such as school staff
- Whether a library of page sets exists to make access to additional vocabulary easier and reduce the need for programming
- Whether software support and technical assistance will be provided, and if so, how much and by whom
- Whether troubleshooting assistance will be provided, and if so, how will it be available (e.g., in-person, by phone, email, or electronically)
- Whether training related to SGD hardware, software, and access methods is provided and whether a library of website resources exists related to programming, training, and troubleshooting[126]
- Whether customer and technical support will be provided, and if so, how will it be available (e.g., by phone or email)
- What is the duration and scope of warranties (what is covered [unlimited or limited], all equipment, number of years)
- Repair services
- Device loan opportunities during repair
- SGD and access method manufacturer or supplier reputation

The reputation of the SGD manufacturer or supplier is important to consider because some clients' ability to use and benefit from an SGD may depend greatly on the certainty of strong support for years. However, not all SGD suppliers have such a reputation, and none can guarantee what will happen in the future. Speech-language pathologists and clients must consider SGD sources' reputation, including how long have they been part of the AAC community, are they a product developer or manufacturer or just an assembler of SGDs from generic tablets and downloadable software, and are SGDs their primary business. Speech-language pathologists and clients must become as educated as possible about the amount, duration, scope, and reliability of the support, training, and other services from SGD manufacturers and suppliers that clients will rely on.

This is not an exclusive list. Historically, with the exception of device warranties, these services have been provided by SGD manufacturers without charge, without limit, for the life of the device.

Access Methods

Throughout speech-language pathologists' consideration of SGD alternatives, additional careful consideration must be directed to clients' impairments (e.g., physical, sensory) that will affect their ability to access (i.e., operate) SGDs. As noted above, some SGD models may not be appropriate because they cannot accommodate clients' access needs.

Access methods are discussed in greater detail in Chapters 14 and 16, but a short discussion of these methods is necessary here within the context of funding. In general, direct selection is a faster and less burdensome method of SGD access than indirect selection alternatives.[127] Direct selection methods include physical contact with the SGD, most often with a finger or by use of a stylus or head pointer. There are also electronic aids that support direct selection, including the head mouse and eye-tracking accessories. Also noted above is a very limited capability for switches to be used as direct selection aids.

Indirect selection relies on scanning with access provided by switches. Consideration of switches requires speech-language pathologists to assess clients' motor planning, as well as cognitive, motor, and visual abilities. Clients must be able to effectively and efficiently control scanning so that cells on the display will be selected at the correct time and in the correct sequence. Clients must also be able to effectively and efficiently activate and release switches.

Health benefits sources generally provide no guidance to speech-language pathologists regarding how clients' need for alternative access is to be assessed (e.g., demonstrate use of actual switches as compared to models or facsimiles), the numbers or types of switches or the number of locations that must be considered, or the performance data that must be reported to justify ruling out particular access methods. However, just as there is no required sequence or prerequisites regarding which SGDs can be recommended, none is applicable to alternative access. Speech-language pathologists must recommend the SGD model *and the access method* that is most appropriate to meet clients' current and reasonably foreseeable future needs. Clients do not have to use specific types of alternative access tools for some period of time then *prove* each is not appropriate because it will not support effective or efficient communication.

Among alternative access methods, recommendations for eye-gaze accessories will receive the most scrutiny, most likely due to their high cost. However, SGD coverage guidelines generally include no eye-gaze assessment and selection criteria. In the absence of specific instructions to the contrary, speech-language pathologists should approach eye gaze the same way they approach consideration of SGDs and any other form of alternative access. They must identify the most appropriate tools that will enable clients to communicate effectively and efficiently. Speech-language pathologists must also recognize that all eye-tracking accessories are not functionally equivalent and may have different performance characteristics, such as their ability to accommodate clients' head movements. All objective and subjective clinically significant differences between eye-tracking accessories must be identified and explained.

As to access, speech-language pathologists must identify the method that will provide clients greater speed and greater accuracy in making selections on the display and the method that will be least visually, cognitively, and physically demanding. They should not consider eye gaze as a "last resort only" alternative (i.e., eye gaze will be appropriate only if no other access method can be used at all). For eye gaze, as for all other access tools that are considered, that it *can be used* is a necessary but not a sufficient fact to establish that it is "most appropriate."

Speech-Generating Device Software and Apps

When Medicare was updating its SGD coverage guidance between 1999 to 2000, staff were informed that some clients already owned desktop or laptop computers and would be willing to use these devices as their SGDs. To accomplish this goal, AAC software had to be acquired and loaded onto the computer. Medicare staff was told that acceptance of AAC software as a benefit would be equally effective for these clients and far less costly to the program. If not covered, Medicare would have been asked to pay for a new device, including AAC software, instead of just the software alone.

Medicare staff agreed and its 2001 guidance included "software that allows a laptop computer, desktop computer, or PDA to function as an SGD." Medicare created an HCPCS code for AAC software: E 2511. AAC software coverage was retained when Medicare updated this guidance in 2015, but it was restated as "software that allows a computer or other electronic device to function as an SGD."[128] Medicare acknowledges that AAC software can be installed on a desktop, laptop, tablet, smartphone, and other handheld computers.[129] Medicare guidance states no limitations on the software that will qualify for funding as AAC software. Because it also acknowledges software can be added to a wide range of devices, including tablet computers and smartphones, it is reasonable to expect that AAC software, commonly called apps, will be covered by Medicare. While this guidance and the conclusion about its scope applies only to Medicare, other health benefits programs have followed Medicare's policy and practice. Speech-language pathologists should review funding source SGD coverage criteria to determine whether reference is made to SGD software and apps as covered benefits.

Because a software-only option may be available and will be less costly than an SGD, speech-language pathologists who recommend an SGD must consider this option in their assessments. However, in almost all circumstances, the benefits of a software-only solution will be too few and this option will be ruled out as inappropriate.

Many possible reasons will support this conclusion. There must be a device available for exclusive use by the client. Some clients' families do not have a tablet or laptop computer that can be used as an SGD. The possibility a device will have to be shared with other family members who want to access its non-SGD features should disqualify that device for this purpose. Even if a device is available for clients' exclusive use, speech-language pathologists must consider the services and support that may or may not be available when only an app or software is purchased. SGD manufacturers may limit training and other support services to clients who acquire their SGD as well as their software. If so, clients who purchase software alone may have to search for training and support from other sources (and may have to find funding for this assistance or pay privately for it). App developers and tablet sources must also be queried about whether they will provide support and training services, and if so, what amount, duration, and scope of those services will be provided. Speech-language pathologists must also consider whether the funding source's SGD coverage criteria rule out repair or replacement of devices that are not purchased by the funding source or do not meet the funding source's coverage criteria. When all relevant factors are considered, it is not easy to identify a circumstance in which a software-only option will ever be in a client's interest to accept.

Trial Periods

From the perspective of funding, any task that interferes with the process leading to "yes" is unwelcome. At first glance, that reasoning will cast SGD trial periods in a negative light, especially those mandated by funding source SGD coverage guidelines. From the outset, mandated SGD trials are inconsistent with ASHA guidance. About 40 years ago, ASHA determined that SGD trials should be pursued when speech-language pathologists consider them necessary to aid decision making, that is, the judgment about whether a trial is needed is a matter of speech-language pathologists' discretion.[130]

Additional negatives are that trials require time and effort for speech-language pathologists to arrange, coordinate, and complete. Also, most often, trials are performed *after* speech-language pathologists have exercised professional judgment to identify the most appropriate SGD and access method to help clients meet all their daily communication needs. Trial outcomes almost never lead speech-language pathologists to change their recommendation: Almost all SGD and access method trials lead to purchase requests for the same equipment items.

Based on these facts, it is reasonable to question whether mandated trials are necessary for or otherwise aid speech-language pathologists' decision making. Nonetheless, many (but not all) SGD funding sources state in their SGD coverage guidelines that SGD and access method trials are required. Thus, although SGD trials are presumptively more burden than benefit, they are part of the SGD assessment, and speech-language pathologists must design, oversee, and then report about them.

If SGD trial periods create more work for speech-language pathologists, do not aid clinical decision making, and delay SGD access by clients, do they confer *any* benefits? The answer is yes. Trials may be perceived as lemons, but they can be made into a very sweet lemonade. Trials will provide an opportunity to reinforce speech-language pathologists' predictive professional judgment with evidence (i.e., data) based on actual device use and benefit. This try-before-you-buy opportunity is not available for many other types of health care.

When trials are required, funding source SGD guidelines will identify the equipment subject to trial. Almost always it will be the device and access method being recommended for purchase. Speech-language pathologists will not have to conduct a trial before ruling out equipment that is not appropriate at all or not as appropriate as other items. Thus, one trial—not multiple trials—is all that will be required. ASHA has stated that a requirement for multiple trials violates speech-language pathology professional practice.[131]

SGD guidelines will sometimes state the required trial duration. Most common is a 30-day trial; less common is a 90-day trial. Thirty days also is often the maximum amount of time that SGD manufacturers and suppliers (who are the primary sources of trial devices) will offer equipment for trial use. This time period is based on their *business* necessity and not on clients' *medical* necessity, even though the latter is the ostensible purpose for SGD trials.

Some trials are for shorter or longer periods. Trials that are longer generally involve SGDs that have been obtained from sources other than the device manufacturer or supplier, such as a device owned by the evaluating speech-language pathologist, the client's school, or a clinic. SGDs may also be borrowed from other similar sources, such as from a neighboring school district or assistive technology loan closets. SGD guidelines may state that SGD rental is available for trial purposes, but these funds are pursued rarely, if ever. The procedure to access these funds will create even more delay for speech-language pathologists and clients and will create administrative costs to the SGD manufacturer or supplier. Also, the funding source payment for trial equipment rental will not be income to SGD manufacturers and suppliers. As noted above, almost all trials lead to purchase requests for the same SGD model and health benefits programs will offset rental payments from the chosen device's purchase price. Thus, the rental payment offer provides no tangible benefit. For this reason, SGD manufacturers typically provide trial devices on a loan basis. When clients also require mounts and access aids, it is expected that these too will be part of the trial. These additional equipment items typically come from the same sources as the trial SGDs.

Beyond these few particulars, SGD funding sources generally grant speech-language pathologists broad discretion regarding the design and implementation of SGD trials. To enable trials to reach their potential as valuable documentation aids that support speech-language pathologists' clinical judgment, USSAAC and International Society for Augmentative and Alternative Communication have identified the clinical purposes or goals of trials:

> The key facts to be explored in a device trial are whether the client demonstrates interest in using the SGD for the purpose of expressive communication; whether the client demonstrates basic understanding of the device, software, or accessory operation and is able to use them to produce speech; and whether the client has benefited from the opportunity to produce speech, as compared to the client's current means of expression.[132]

For example, trials can provide actual data that clients expressed interest or motivation to use the device (e.g., as demonstrated by the client's positive reaction to having access to the device or by the client's negative reaction to having the device withdrawn at the end of the trial period). Trials can document that clients demonstrated an understanding of the device's basic operational requirements (e.g., the meaning of picture symbols, categorization of words and messages, sequencing, page navigation, waking devices or turning them on or off, adjusting device volume) and that clients demonstrated an ability to use the device to produce functional communication (e.g., report of successful access and actual functional use of the device for communication with others during the trial). Finally, trials can document how clients benefitted from use of the device (e.g., communicated more effectively and efficiently with more partners, about more topics, more frequently, in more settings, as compared to current communication methods that do not include the trialed device and access method; increased access to vocabulary).

Although not typically required by SGD coverage guidelines, speech-language pathologists should write a plan for the design and implementation of the trial. A plan can serve as a checklist to ensure the trial and post-trial report will be complete. It should identify all the people who will be involved and their roles: who will acquire and set up the equipment, who will provide instruction, support, and reinforcement to clients and communication partners, who will record data about clients' trial experiences, and who will prepare the trial report. There is no requirement that the evaluating speech-language pathologist fill any of these roles; depending on when and where the trial will occur, it may not be possible for the evaluating speech-language pathologist to do so. It is also necessary for the plan to address the trial location(s) and describe the amount, duration, and scope of instruction and support services to be provided to each person so that all tasks will be performed accurately, efficiently, and effectively.[133]

Because there are so many variables, each trial will be unique. For example, for some clients, access to the device, necessary instruction and support services, and opportunity to practice may be extensive and may be provided throughout the day and in multiple locations every day for the duration of the trial. In other SGD trials, these opportunities may be limited to specific times, personnel, and settings. These parameters should be stated in the speech-language pathology plan and again in the trial report.

The trial plan should also identify the trial goals. Just as each client and the parameters for device use and support during trials will be unique, so too will be their goals. Substantively, at least some trial goals must be objectively measurable. Additional goals that are subjectively measurable will be acceptable, but these should not be the only goals stated or reported. Of greatest importance, speech-language pathologists must ensure that the goals stated are *reasonably achievable*.

In general, speech-language pathologists have complete discretion regarding the number and focus of goals that will be stated and pursued. However, SGD coverage criteria that will apply to clients' funding requests must be considered in setting trial goals. This guidance may state specific topics that must be addressed and reported, and if so, these must be incorporated into the trial goals. For example, one funding source requires that during the trial, clients demonstrate functional communication with multiple people in multiple settings on multiple occasions.[134] For clients who will seek funding from this source, speech-language pathologists must ensure these opportunities are part of the trial design and implementation and are discussed in the trial report.

When developing trial goals, it is important that speech-language pathologists maintain their focus on the overall trial purpose. As previously stated, trials are *documentation* aids. Therefore, they should be designed to provide actual use and benefit data that confirm or reinforce the facts that led speech-language pathologists to conclude the equipment being trialed is most appropriate to help clients meet all daily communication needs. In other words, by the start of the trial, speech-language pathologists will already have compared clients' communicative functioning with current strategies and tools and with several possible alternatives and will have reached a preliminary conclusion about specific equipment that is believed to be most appropriate. The trial will now provide an extended use opportunity to gather data to support that judgment. Because only one trial will be conducted, trials are only a comparison between the trialed equipment and the strategies and tools clients used before the SGD assessment; trials are not comparisons between or competitions with the equipment choices that were ruled out as not appropriate or not as appropriate.

For trials to provide their greatest value, their goals need not and should not require clients to demonstrate new skills or perform new tasks. While it is appropriate to report if there is improvement in clients' performance of tasks during the trial (e.g., reduced need for assistance in navigation or creating messages), an expectation of improvement should not be built into trial goals. Not demanding improvement or introduction of new skills during trials is easy to justify: trials are of very limited duration and clients may just require more time to improve or learn the new skill. Also, a 30-day trial does not mean the client had access to the device and necessary supports all day, for 30 days. To the contrary, access to the device and to instructional and support services necessary to improve existing skills or learn new ones may have been limited by many factors unrelated to clients' actual or potential abilities (e.g., illness to the client or instructional or support staff, inclement weather, or device malfunction). That clients did not demonstrate improved performance of existing abilities or new abilities by the trial's end may say more about the trial's design and duration than about the client's actual or potential abilities.

Equally true, speech-language pathologists must be alert to SGD funding guidelines that may require clients to demonstrate specific abilities or skills during or following a trial, such as independence in device use, the ability to create novel messages or messages of specific lengths, or the ability to independently navigate between pages. Or, guidelines that demand clients achieve post-trial performance standards, such as "competence," "proficiency," or "mastery." All these examples are inappropriate. Consider "mastery" for example. It is defined as comprehensive knowledge or skill in a subject or accomplishment,[135] possession of consummate skill or full command of a subject of study,[136] and as expert skill or knowledge.[137] These phrases do not describe clients' skills at the conclusion of an SGD trial period.[138]

Demands or expectations such as these are not appropriate as SGD eligibility criteria: Demonstrating any of these abilities or achieving any of these levels of performance has no relationship to whether clients require SGDs to meet all daily communication needs or which SGD model and access aid is most appropriate to achieve that goal. Also, demanding that all clients must meet a specific performance standard is not appropriate because of the enormous variability of clients' pre-existing skills and impairments. For some clients, the trial will be their first opportunity to use the device. It is a truism that "[t]hose who rely on AAC strategies [including SGDs] begin as AAC novices and evolve into competence …" over time.[139] And more than just time is likely to be required. Clients will also require instruction, support, and opportunity to practice to learn and to improve their abilities. Competence, for example, is a level of performance that is achieved over a period of years; it is not a reasonably achievable post–30-day trial period level of performance.[140] Demanding clients reach such performance standards with use of alternative access methods, such as eye gaze, is especially unreasonable.[141] SGD eligibility standards incorporating requirements such as these are inconsistent with Medicaid programs' duty to develop and implement "reasonable standards" governing eligibility for covered services,[142] and they are also inconsistent with Medicaid programs' responsibility to ensure eligibility standards are consistent with professional practice standards.[143] Medicare applies a similar standard.[144]

In addition to not being reasonably achievable standards for SGD trial outcomes or for SGD eligibility, standards that require demonstration of some amount of improvement or achievement of a specific or general performance goal are not consistent with medical need standards. As previously mentioned, treatments that are medically necessary will reduce deterioration, restore functioning,[145] or ameliorate impairments.[146] Clients whose trial experiences showed improvement over their existing expressive communication strategies and tools and who show promise for ongoing improvement over time, will have demonstrated the functional requirements of medical need, even if they did not reach a specific performance demand stated in a funding source's SGD coverage guidelines. Use of those standards may cause

SGD purchase requests to be denied simply because after a trial period the clients did not improve high enough or did not do so fast enough. Such an SGD eligibility standard is not appropriate.

Demands that clients achieve specific post-trial performance goals also ignore almost all clients' eligibility for additional speech-language pathology training services after the SGD is delivered. For Medicaid recipients who are children, in all states, there is an entitlement to ongoing speech-language pathology services until age 21 years.[147] For adults, in almost all states, speech-language pathology services are also covered, meaning speech-language pathology services will be available throughout clients' lifetimes to the extent they continue to be needed. Medicare,[148] Tricare,[149] and Veterans Affairs[150] also cover speech-language pathology. For clients with insurance and health benefits plans, speech-language pathology services are common benefits. The availability of these ongoing speech-language pathology services raises the practical question: What's the rush? Stated another way, demands that clients demonstrate specific skills or reach specific performance levels following an SGD trial are arbitrary and lack a factual, professional practice, or even a practical, common-sense basis.[151]

Treatment Plans

Treatment plans are an almost universally required component of speech-language pathology reports (refer back to Medicare SGD Coverage Guideline, item 1e). They are often the last section of speech-language pathology assessment reports, but their placement does not reflect their importance.

Asserting treatment plans are important regarding SGD funding requests may seem counterintuitive: They describe future events to occur after funding approval is issued and the device is delivered. Also, no funding source has the authority to force clients to return devices because some use-related goal has not been met. So, what difference can a plan for future services delivery and goals development make to SGD funding requests?

Treatment plans serve two purposes. They are a valuable opportunity to further educate and persuade funding sources that they should invest in recommended SGDs, mounts, and access aids. Funding sources know they are being asked to approve equipment items, often *expensive* items that clients may have had only a limited opportunity to use. Treatment plans enable speech-language pathologists to allay funding source concerns about whether devices will be used and will provide predicted benefits or will be abandoned. They do so by explaining how the approval of SGD purchase requests is not an end in itself but one step along a path. As Dave Beukelman wrote:

> [s]peech generating technology is not magic. A piano alone doesn't make a pianist, nor does a basketball make an athlete. Likewise, AAC technology alone doesn't make one a competent, proficient communicator. Those who rely on AAC begin as

AAC novices and evolve in competence … with appropriate support, instruction, practice, and encouragement.[152]

Treatment plans show that speech-language pathologists have thought about clients' futures and have developed *a plan* to guide them from their starting points as "novices" to become "competent, proficient communicators." Or, if the client's condition is progressive, such as ALS, the treatment plan will describe the services intended to enable clients to continue to communicate effectively until the end of their lives. The plans explain that clients and their devices will be part of a services environment that will provide orientation, instruction, training, and skills development over time.

The second purpose they serve is to enable speech-language pathologists to cross-reference and reinforce their judgments that one SGD is most appropriate (is best able to meet clients' skill- and competency-development needs) while others are not appropriate at all (do not have features, performances, or services that match clients' needs) or not as appropriate as the recommended device (do not have needed features, performances, or services in the same amount, duration, or scope). An example: To report in a treatment plan that the client will receive services directed to a goal of spelling and literacy enables speech-language pathologists to add that these services support the decision to rule out *all*—the entire category of—digitized speech output devices because none of them will support spelling as method of message assembly.

The design of treatment plans raises the same who, what, where, and when questions that speech-language pathologists must consider in their design of SGD trials. As with trials, treatment plans must identify objective goals related to the development of client abilities and skills and to describe the instruction, services, and supports clients will need and receive to achieve those goals.

One significant difference between trial goals and treatment plan goals is that the former are directed to clients' *current* abilities and skills: Neither the improvement of existing skills nor the development of new skills are appropriate or necessary for *trial* goals. By contrast, treatment plan goals will identify skills improvement and development that will help clients proceed toward communicative competence.

The services to support achievement of treatment plan goals can come from many sources. Clients may have access to ongoing speech-language pathology services from their health benefits sources and/or from their public schools. In addition, clients may be identified as needing and receiving a variety of services and supports from the source of their SGD. However, all SGD manufacturers and suppliers do not offer the same amount, duration, and scope of services and supports. These differences may be cited among the reasons that the SGD being recommended is the most appropriate choice.

The services from SGD manufacturers and suppliers that may be needed and may be of benefit to achieve treatment plan goals may include:

- In-person field staff who provide set-up assistance for the SGD, mount, and access aid; orientation and programming assistance; training for family, caregivers, school personnel, and clients' other frequent communication partners; and trouble-shooting assistance
- Additional training in group sessions, in person or online
- Libraries of prior training sessions available for review as needed
- A library of page-sets that will aid clients' access to vocabulary if access to programming assistance is not readily available
- Live technical assistance and a variety of support services throughout the week, by telephone, text, or online communication
- One-stop assistance for any component of an SGD system as opposed to having to find support from the manufacturer or supplier of hardware, software, and access aids

When needed or of potential benefit, any or all of these services should be referenced in the treatment plan as tools to help clients achieve their treatment plan goals.

In addition, speech-language pathologists must ensure that the stated amount, duration, and scope of these services will support the conclusion that the goal is reasonably achievable. For example: A goal stating that by a specific date a school-age client will independently perform some form of functional communication must identify sufficient speech-language pathology services to reasonably achieve that goal in the stated time period.

How Long? A second significant distinction between SGD trials and treatment plans is their duration. The length of SGD trials most often is set at 1 month by the SGD manufacturers and suppliers. By contrast, treatment plans describe actions to occur after clients receive their devices. Also, the services and supports described in treatment plans can extend for a much longer duration. Health benefits source services, such as Medicaid speech-language pathology services, may be available for the client's lifetime. For clients of school age, public school–related services, including speech-language pathology services, may be available for many years (up to age 21 years).[153] Services and supports available from some SGD manufacturers and suppliers may be available for the life of the device; others may extend for 5 years.

However, speech-language pathologists have no special skills related to predicting the future. Thus, for treatment plan goals to be credible, the planning horizon must be relatively short. In general, the longer the duration of the plan (i.e., the longer clients will need to achieve a goal), the less credible will be the goal. As time passes, both clients and service providers will be subject to increasing numbers of variables that will be impossible to predict or control.

On this point, funding source SGD coverage criteria may be flawed. While it is important that funding sources recognize a need for the assessment to consider the reasonably foreseeable future, some set specific planning horizons that are too far into the future to be considered reasonable. For example, some SGD coverage criteria direct speech-language pathologists to plan for clients' abilities 2 years after device delivery. That is far too long. How clients will use their SGDs 2 years after delivery will be no more than a guess—speculation.

In a circumstance such as this, speech-language pathologists should divide goals into two categories: those for which it is reasonable to predict clients' ability to perform specific tasks within a specific time, which may be 6 to 9 months after SGD delivery, and those goals that will require longer to achieve. For the former, the treatment plan should describe the specific services clients will require to achieve these goals within the stated time period. For the second group of goals, speech-language pathologists should write goals to reflect progress along a pathway (i.e., "the client *will begin to develop* [some new skill that will require a long time to achieve]" or "the client *will continue to develop or improve* [an existing skill for which improvement over a long time period will be required]").

Just as each client presents unique abilities, skills, and unmet communication needs, each treatment plan will be unique as well. In regard to specific goals, speech-language pathologists will have complete discretion regarding their content. As with trial goals, at least some treatment goals must be described in objectively measurable terms. Most common is a ratio of success per total attempts, stated as a percentage. Speech-language pathologists have total discretion to define success. Speech-language pathologists can also add goals that are subjective, but they cannot be the only goals. Finally, speech-language pathologists should be careful not to exaggerate improvement. Predictions of "significant" or "substantial" progress are not necessary or appropriate.

Least Costly, Equally Effective Alternatives

The key outcomes of the speech-language pathology evaluation are the determination whether clients are able to meet all their daily communication needs, and for those who cannot, the identification of the most appropriate form of treatment that will enable clients to do so. The evaluation process includes consideration of clients' current communication functioning, current unmet communication needs, and identification of the treatment method, such as an SGD and access aid, that will provide the most benefit (i.e., that will provide the maximum "reduction" of the communication impairment, will "restore" clients to their best possible functional level, or will provide maximum "improvement" of clients' communication functioning as compared to current communication methods and as compared to other possible alternatives[154]).

As part of the assessment and decision-making process, speech-language pathologists must compare the benefits that will be provided by the various options and make judgments that rule out those that are not appropriate at all or not as appropriate as the one ultimately recommended. With so many client- and tool-based variables to be considered in the evaluation, it is reasonable to expect that a single choice will emerge as most appropriate for each client. On the other hand, it is possible that as this process nears its conclusion, two or more options appear able to provide all the same benefits, that is, will be equally effective for the client. If so, then all health benefits sources require speech-language pathologists to recommend the least costly SGD, mount, or access aid among them.

Quantifying benefits—identifying which factors are clinically significant—is a matter of speech-language pathology professional judgment and will be client-specific. All the facts previously discussed in the Speech-Generating Devices Considered, Access Methods, and Speech-Generating Device Software and Apps sections will lead to the answer of whether equally effective alternatives exist or not. For all clients, speech-language pathologists must explain carefully and in detail how they decided to rule out alternatives and must explain their rationale for selecting the SGD, mount, and access aid being recommended as most appropriate.

It is essential to remember that funding sources may try to claim that SGDs, software, mounts, and access aids are functionally equivalent and interchangeable, and therefore, are able to be considered solely on the basis of their cost. It is speech-language pathologists' duty to demonstrate why that conclusion is not justified by the facts presented by the clients they evaluate and for whom they are recommending treatment. Although the phrase *least costly,* equally effective alternative begins with reference to cost, in practice, cost is considered last. The "least costly alternative" is *not* the standard. Cost must be compared *only* for alternatives that are equally effective.

Speech-Language Pathology Independence

Speech-language pathologists have been assigned the responsibility to identify medical need and to recommend the most appropriate treatment to address those needs. As previously stated, this responsibility is assigned to physicians for almost all other types of health care benefits. Speech-language pathologists have been given these roles because of their education and experience and also because their decisions are exclusively the product of their professional judgment. Many health benefits sources require speech-language pathologists to certify that they have no financial interest in the recommendations they make. They must not work for the manufacturers or suppliers of SGDs and must not derive financial gain from their treatment recommendations (refer back to Medicare SGD Coverage Guideline, item 7).

Speech-Generating Device–Specific Medical Need Standards

The overarching goal of speech-language pathologists' reports that support SGD recommendations is to establish that devices, software, mounts, and access aids are medically necessary, consistent with professional standards of practice.

It is generally accepted by speech-language pathologists as a matter of professional practice that "AAC is needed by individuals with such complex communication limitations that they are unable to meet their daily communication needs through natural speech (and/or language)."[155]

If funding assistance is required, speech-language pathology reports must also be consistent with the medical need and other eligibility standards of health benefits funding sources. It is common that speech-language pathologists will encounter SGD-specific medical need standards. These may require clients to establish or demonstrate that:

- They have the cognitive, physical, and sensory ability or willingness to use the SGD and accessories effectively
- They will benefit from use of the device
- They have the ability to learn to use the device
- They show potential abilities to use the device

Or, the standards may be more specific:

- The recommended device can be used to communicate with multiple individuals in multiple settings within the trial location while conveying varying message types without being fully dependent on prompting or assistance in producing the communication
- The member has demonstrated the ability to use the recommended device and accessories or software for functional communication as evidenced by a data-driven device trial showing that skills can be demonstrated repeatedly over time, beyond a single instance or evaluation session[156]

Speech-language pathologists must search for key terms and phrases such as those in funding sources' medical need definitions and SGD coverage guidelines. Where they exist, these phrases (and the actions they may require) must be incorporated into speech-language pathology reports. Doing this will show reviewers that the speech-language pathologist is aware of the requirements for SGD approval and hopefully will reinforce that the report satisfies all requirements.

The phrases referenced here focus on demonstrated or potential "use" of the device, but they impose no limitations regarding how or where it can be used, with whom, or what messages will be produced. However, speech-language pathologists must remain alert to phrases in funding source guidance that impose limitations that may not be consistent with generally accepted standards of practice. Several are discussed here.

Health Benefits Sources' Objections to Speech-Generating Device Medical Need

Some health benefits sources have claimed SGDs are not medically necessary because they serve as treatment for the effects rather than the causes of conditions. On its face, this objection is factually correct. SGDs do treat the effects of conditions, not their causes. Nonetheless, this objection is baseless as a medical need objection.

Medical care directed to reduce the adverse effects of conditions is common. The Medicaid Act's Early and Periodic Screening, Diagnostic and Treatment benefit, applicable to all recipients younger than age 21 years, mandates that treatment be provided for causes and for effects. It states that care is medically necessary and must be provided when it will correct or ameliorate a mental or physical health condition. Amelioration is treatment directed to lessening the effects of conditions.[157]

Even without a statutory mandate, no health benefits sources limit the meaning of "treatment" or of medical necessity to exclude effects-directed care. For this reason, even though the Medicaid Early and Periodic Screening, Diagnostic and Treatment benefit does not apply to individuals age 21 years and older, treatment that will ameliorate conditions must be viewed as medically necessary independent of age.[158]

Also true is that SGDs are not unique as an effects-directed form of treatment. A Medicare decision illustrates this broader principle. It notes that many other forms or types of medical care are directed to the effects of conditions, not their cause:

> With regard to common sense, many commonly recognized items that Medicare approves as [DME] do not cure an illness but rather treat the effects of an illness. A wheelchair is an obvious example.[159]

Clients with mobility impairments still have a spinal cord injury or cerebral palsy when they use a wheelchair to meet daily mobility needs. Every objective measure of the severity of these conditions will remain the same, regardless of whether a wheelchair is provided. What changes (i.e., are reduced) are the adverse effects of these conditions on clients' mobility. Many other DME items and prosthetic devices, including SGDs, treat only the effects of conditions.

Treatments for the effects rather than the causes of conditions are not limited to medical devices. For example, clients with severe cardiac impairment may require angioplasty and insertion of a stent or cardiac bypass surgery. These procedures will be treating the effects of plaque build-up in coronary arteries, not the cause. Clients who require surgery to prevent blood vessel rupture from an aneurism will receive treatment specifically to prevent the effects of that condition, not its cause.

That treatment will be directed to the effects of conditions may be a matter of necessity. For some conditions, such as ALS, there is no current effective treatment to prevent or reverse the process of motor neuron deterioration. For spinal cord injury, there is no current effective treatment to restore the nerve pathways. Only treatment directed to the effects of these conditions offer benefit. For other conditions known as idiopathic, treatment is directed to effects because their cause is unknown.

***Med-Speak*: Speech-Generating Devices Must Allow Clients to Communicate Only Medical Needs.** Health benefits sources have objected to SGD funding requests by saying that the purpose of an SGD is to enable clients to produce "medically necessary communication" or "to communicate medical needs" or that SGDs are medically necessary for clients unable to "communicate their basic needs through oral speech or manual sign language." These objections are commonly called med-speak because they focus on communication of medical-related words, phrases, and messages to physicians and other care providers. In essence, they are saying that the basis for SGD medical need is the content of the messages to be produced and the nature of the relationship between clients and their communication partners. Med-speak objections fail because they are not consistent with speech-language pathology assessment or treatment, with how SGDs and other speech aids (e.g., the artificial larynx) operate, or with the general principles of medical necessity.

The focus of speech-language pathology assessment is whether clients are able to meet all daily communication needs. Assessments will explore whether clients are able to communicate with any communication partner, in any setting, about any topic, and at any time. For many clients, daily communication needs will include communication with caregivers about health-related topics. But communication with these specific partners or about these specific topics has no special status. *All* daily communication needs must be assessed, and the recommended treatment must enable clients to meet *all* daily communication needs. These principles apply to all forms of speech-language pathology treatment (i.e., oral speech, use of a speech aid, such as an artificial larynx, or use of an SGD). None focuses on improving clients' ability to say specific words, phrases, or messages or to communicate more effectively exclusively with physicians or other care providers.

Med-speak objections are also completely inconsistent with the way SGDs—and the artificial larynx—operate. For example, a funding source once stated that SGDs must be intended to be used "100 percent of the time to express pain, hunger, or medical symptoms."[160] Upon review, this claim represented a complete exclusion of SGDs, not a limitation based on medical need. No SGD from a single message switch to an E2510 SGD can satisfy such a medical need description. None has any restriction on the content of speech it can produce. Digitized speech output SGDs have upper limits on the number but not the content of messages they can produce. An artificial larynx causes a column of exhaled air to vibrate, supporting the production of any words clients wish to say.[161]

Moreover, while it is easy to say an SGD should provide access to "medically necessary" communication, there is no list of letters, words, or phrases that are inherently medical or nonmedical. Words achieve their meaning from their context, along with their order in a phrase or message.

Yet another reason med-speak objections fail is that they are inconsistent with the general goals of medically necessary treatment (i.e., to improve clients' ability to engage in or perform normal activity). For clients with expressive communication impairments, normal activity is effective speech: able to be understood by all communication partners. Med-speak objections ignore this goal. Instead, they focus exclusively on clients' ability to report information about and to obtain care for other impairments. Yes, SGDs can and will enable clients to obtain access to that care more effectively and efficiently, but those needs and benefits are not why SGDs are medically necessary. Clients' need for an SGD is not greater when they have a headache than when they do not. A decision maker accurately concluded:

> 'Medical need' for a[n] [SGD] is not merely that need that results from or relates to, the communication of symptoms or complaints of illness, or to the necessary treatment thereof … Rather, … [t]he provision of a[n] [SGD] is intended to correct the inability to speak, and is thus necessary to meet [their] medical need.[162]

Nonetheless, almost 20 years later, the same funding source again relied on med-speak, and again it was rejected:

> The agency's contention that the Appellant's need for enhanced communication skills in employment and social settings is not medical in nature misses the mark since the communication skills themselves are medical in nature irrespective of the environment [in which] the Appellant is being asked to communicate. Accordingly, the evidence … supports the Appellant's medical need for an augmentative communication device at the present time.[163]

Comparison can also be made to other types of treatment and other DME items, such as services related to mobility impairment. Services include physical therapy treatment to improve balance, gait, endurance, and wheelchairs and other mobility assist devices. These services are provided to enable clients to meet all daily mobility needs. No funding source has been identified that limits these services to clients unable to walk or otherwise get to a doctor's office or pharmacy, the equivalent of med-speak in the mobility context. Services are provided to aid independent living, not to provide access to specific locations.

Speech-language pathologists should respond to attempts to limit SGD medical need through med-speak by stating the generally accepted professional standard for AAC and SGD need, that clients are unable to meet all their daily communication needs using speech or other natural communication methods. An assertion that clients are only able to access medically necessary treatment to enable them to meet only some of their daily communication needs is not appropriate.

If funding source guidance or a decision refers to "basic needs" or "basic communication needs" in the context of SGD medical need, speech-language pathologists should look carefully as to whether there is any further description of "basic." It is possible there will be none, which grants speech-language pathologists broad discretion to explain that clients' basic needs are the same for all speech-language pathology services—the ability to meet all daily communication needs.[164] Alternately, the funding source may define this phrase in a helpful way, for example, to include "a consumer's ability to communicate needs and wants, transfer information, achieve social closeness, and demonstrate social etiquette."[165] This definition of "basic communication needs" mirrors the generally accepted broad purposes of communication.[166]

There Is No Claim That Necessary Care Has Not Been Provided. Some health benefits programs objected to SGD funding requests for children who require continuous parental supervision and for clients who live in facilities or who have extensive direct care support. The basis for these denials was that another person—a parent or other caregiver—was present to meet the clients' medical needs, the SGD funding request did not identify any medical needs that had not been addressed, and there had been no complaints directed to oversight authority that necessary care was being withheld.

This objection is another version of med-speak; it presumes that only direct care–related messages are medically necessary *and* that only direct caregivers must be considered as communication partners. In addition, this objection presents a "Catch-22" circumstance: There will never be unmet medical needs because once needs are identified, they will be addressed. This logic is flawed because:

> [f]or a person lacking the ability to communicate, [a parent, other caregiver] or [facility] staff is unlikely to have the ESP [extra-sensory perception] necessary to intuit what the person may need or want.[167]

Once recognized, needed care will be provided; it will not be denied intentionally. But whether care is needed, is provided in the amount, duration, and scope responsive to clients' needs, and is fully effective can only be answered by clients.

Moreover, the goal of AAC interventions, including SGDs, is to enable clients to express themselves, not to have someone speak for them:

> Preferred practice for AAC system design is to … design a system that … allows for independent communication across listeners and environments …

> [T]he goal of AAC intervention is to enhance communication between individuals and their outside world in the most efficient and effective means possible, creating as much independence as possible.[168]

Functional independence is as important a concept for individuals with CCN as it is for clients with mobility impairments. For example, funding sources will approve power wheelchairs and manual wheelchairs for young children, even those young enough to require close parental supervision. These children are not eligible only for dependent wheelchairs that require clients to be pushed. They will be approved for mobility aids that they can operate independently.

Clients Do Not Have Required Characteristics or Have Not Demonstrated Sufficient Ability to Use the Device: Prerequisites for Approval of Specific Speech-Generating Devices. Some health benefits sources demanded that clients have specific characteristics to be eligible for particular SGD models. For example, New York Medicaid once demanded that clients have "advanced language skills" to qualify for an SGD in the E2510 code. New York Medicaid also demanded that clients demonstrate they are "proficient," "competent," and "independent" in SGD use; that they "mastered" or are "very good at" SGD use—all *before any* SGD will be approved. Another example arises from a set of SGD coverage guidelines known as InterQual, which are used by several health benefits sources. The InterQual guidelines demand clients have a "large vocabulary" to be eligible for a synthesized speech output SGD.[169] When clients do not possess these characteristics or have not demonstrated these performance prerequisites, their SGD funding requests will be denied.

Demands such as these amount to prerequisites for SGD eligibility that are not consistent with speech-language pathology standards of practice and are not consistent with applicable laws and rules governing medical need. It is a longstanding professional practice principle that "there are no prerequisites for AAC intervention."[170] In addition, these prerequisites may be consistent with the client characteristics or performance skills stated in SGD coverage guidelines. As previously noted, those guidelines address different topics; for example, they ask whether clients have the cognitive, physical, and sensory ability or willingness to use the SGD and accessories effectively, whether they will benefit from use of the device, whether they have the ability to learn to use the device, whether they show potential abilities to use the device, and whether the SGD will allow the individual to improve their communication to a functional level not achievable without the ordered device.

The New York Medicaid example of "advanced language skills" to qualify for an E2510 SGD was challenged on several grounds. The phrase had no definition or generally accepted meaning. It did not originate in speech-language pathology practice, and it was not stated in the New York Medicaid SGD coverage criteria or other guidance. There was also no way to tell what language skills were "advanced" or how "advanced" would be measured. As a practical matter, whatever these skills may be, it is unknown how young children will have the opportunity to acquire or develop them. If young children cannot attain these skills, a demand for advanced language skills amounts to an age-based eligibility prerequisite (or an age-based exclusion) for this type of SGD. However, to date, no age-based access limits have been accepted as appropriate for AAC, for SGDs, or any particular type of SGDs.[171] Also, there is no accepted age threshold for access to eye gaze–controlled SGDs, which are available only on touchscreen SGDs in the E2510 code.

That clients may need SGDs controlled by eye gaze also justified rejection of the InterQual SGD criteria that limited E2510 SGDs to clients with large vocabularies. The determination that eye gaze is the most appropriate access method will be based on facts wholly unrelated to clients' language skills (whether advanced or not), their age, or their vocabulary size (whether large or small). These prerequisites are "wholly unrelated to the medical decision at hand."[172]

The performance prerequisites of "proficiency," "competence," "independence," "mastery," or being "very good at" are flawed because none is a reasonable criterion for SGD eligibility, that is, they must be achieved *before* an SGD will be approved. Common to all these abilities is that they may require years of training, support, practice, and most importantly, access to the device.[173] Moreover, for Medicaid recipients younger than age 21 years, these performance-based eligibility prerequisites are expressly forbidden.

> State Medicaid programs are permitted (but not required) to set parameters that apply to the determination of medical necessity in individual cases, but those parameters may not contradict or be more restrictive than the federal statutory requirements.[174]

The statute referenced here is the federal Medicaid Act.[175] It says that care will be medically necessary and must be provided to recipients younger than 21 years when it will ameliorate their conditions. To ameliorate means to improve or to lessen the adverse effects of a condition.[176] These performance prerequisites are far more restrictive than "improvement" or "lessening" adverse effects, and for that reason, they are prohibited.

Also, clients' communication skills can improve significantly, and they can derive great benefits from SGD use even if they never become "proficient," "competent," "independent," or "very good at" SGD use. The goal of treatment is to change clients' *status quo* levels of impairment and performance. That goal can be achieved even if the funding source's demands are not.

Health Benefits Source Special Rules Related to Speech-Generating Devices

The last of the four questions required to establish health benefits programs' duty to include SGDs as a benefit and to approve requests for them asks whether SGDs meet all applicable "special rules." As used here, special rules include limitations on SGD access, such as place of service limits and warranty and useful life requirements. They also include exclusions for SGDs that are a characteristic of a small number of insurance policies and health benefits plans. Clients may be able to meet or satisfy applicable special rules by conforming to them or by challenging them to render them void and without effect.

Place of Service Limitations

The "place of service" is the location where medical services, including DME items, are delivered to the client. The Medicare Act imposes place of service limitations on items of DME, including SGDs. The program limits DME coverage to recipients living in their own homes. Residents of group homes and independent or assisted-living facilities are considered as living in their own homes. Medicare will make payment for DME for people living in these residential settings.

However, the Medicare Act excludes hospitals and skilled nursing facilities as places of service eligible for Medicare DME funding.[177] In simpler terms, if clients are living in a skilled nursing facility or are in a hospital at the time Medicare DME is delivered to them, Medicare will not pay for the DME item. Also subject to this limitation are Medicare recipients who are in receipt of hospice services, whether at home or in a residential hospice care setting. Residents of intermediate care facilities for individuals with developmental or intellectual disabilities are also not covered for Medicare DME.[178]

Speech-Generating Device Access for Medicaid Nursing Facility Residents. Medicaid program obligations are different. Medical equipment is a component of the Medicaid home health care services benefit.[179] That benefit includes, as a requirement, that the services are provided to recipients at their place of residence. However, Medicaid rules define "place of residence" to *not* include "a hospital, nursing facility, or intermediate care facility [for individuals with developmental or intellectual disabilities]."[180] Notwithstanding this limiting definition, nursing facility residents and residents of intermediate care for individuals with developmental or intellectual disabilities can obtain access to devices and equipment, such as SGDs, that would be classified as medical equipment if the clients lived elsewhere. Medicaid imposes obligations directly on the facilities to ensure that clients' needs for SGDs and other equipment items are met. Substantively, this means Medicaid recipients are eligible for SGDs wherever they reside.

Discussion about SGD access for Medicaid nursing or other facility residents often is couched in the context of coverage barriers, but this is incorrect. Instead, SGD access barriers for these Medicaid recipients is based on *payment*. Nursing and other facilities are paid by Medicaid programs on a *per diem*, or daily rate, basis. In many states, Medicaid policy had once been to pay directly (apart from the daily rate) for a limited number of equipment items used by nursing facility residents. Some states named specific items to which this exception applied, often including SGDs. Others described the characteristics of items available for direct payment, such as devices that are rarely needed, are for use by a single resident, are not typically provided by nursing facilities, are not able to be shared, or are customized. When this Medicaid direct payment policy was in effect, nursing or other facilities had little financial interest in whether residents sought and received SGDs. Speech-language pathologists conducted evaluations and made recommendations; they were sent to Medicaid, and Medicaid approved and paid for the SGDs.

However, since 2000, Medicaid programs have been shifting these costs to the nursing or other facility daily rate, thereby forcing the facilities to pay for these items, including SGDs. This payment policy change has had significant adverse consequences for nursing and other facility residents. It gave nursing and other facilities very powerful financial *dis*incentives to "see" SGD needs. Unfortunately, although not surprisingly, where these cost-shifts have been implemented, the number of SGD recommendations decreased significantly.

To be clear, changing payment procedures does not change the entitlement of Medicaid nursing and other facility residents to acquire necessary SGDs. Their rights remain the same. What has changed is the level of difficulty they will face when they try to exercise those rights and gain access to SGDs.

There is no basis for Medicaid nursing or other facility residents to challenge these payment practices directly. Instead, they can insist on the provision of necessary care and can challenge its denial. First, they need a speech-language pathology evaluation that identifies SGD need and recommends an SGD as treatment. As a practical matter, the speech-language pathologist will likely have to be independent of the nursing facility. After that, an independent doctor (not associated with the nursing facility) will likely have to sign a prescription. These documents must then be presented to the facility. If the prescription is not acted on, clients have appeal rights to challenge the denial of necessary equipment.

Warranty and Useful Life Requirements

It is common for health benefits programs to have special rules stating warranty and useful life requirements that apply to DME items, such as SGDs. In general, these are not controversial topics. A 1 to 3–year warranty and a 3 to 5–year useful life are common requirements for SGDs.

Because funding approval is contingent on the existence of a warranty, all SGD manufacturers and suppliers wanting to sell their devices with funding assistance must deliver them with this promise. During the warranty period, the costs of necessary repair (or device replacement) will be borne by the device manufacturer or supplier. At the end of the warranty period, further repair costs will shift to the funding source if device repair is a covered benefit. Meeting post-warranty repair costs will be clients' obligation if there is no health benefits source eligibility or if device repair is not covered. All public health benefits programs include device repair as a covered benefit. It is also very likely to be covered by insurance and by health benefit plans. When devices malfunction, funding sources may authorize the repair or replacement of the device, whichever is more cost-effective to the funding source.

A proposal that, if adopted, would have made SGD repair controversial stated that any repair—no matter how insignificant—must increase the useful life of the device as a whole. This expectation was found in draft SGD coverage criteria written by two Medicaid programs. Comments provided to both programs stated this outcome is unattainable. Replacement of a battery is among the most common SGD repair needs. The battery powers the device, but it does not have any ability to correct or ameliorate the wear and tear issues that will affect future device performance. The comments also noted that an alternative would be to impose warranty requirements on each repaired or replaced part, but the proposed useful life extension for the device as a whole is inappropriate. Both programs deleted this proposal.

Another controversial repair-related issue is a funding source's refusal to offer repair to equipment that it did not pay for or for equipment that does not meet its coverage criteria. This is a matter of particular significance to clients asked to consider using a personal or family-owned computer as an SGD. Clients must consider their ability to pay for device repair (or possibly replacement) when the device malfunctions. Funding sources may also learn this limitation on repair has no cost savings effect. Rather than cost-shifting repair costs for these devices to clients, clients may submit funding requests for a new device, which may result in greater costs to the funding source than repair of the existing device.

Useful life requirements are intended to postpone costs, namely device replacement costs. They force SGD manufacturers or suppliers to support their devices (i.e., have the parts and capability to repair the SGD) for the length of the useful life period, which is typically 5 years after purchase. These requirements are often based on the assumption that in most circumstances it is less costly to repair devices than to replace them.

Useful life periods can become a potential barrier when a device is still needed but the client's condition has changed, when the device has experienced something that renders it nonrepairable, or when it is lost *before* the useful life period has expired.

In general, the change in a client's condition that causes an existing device to no longer be appropriate will be treated as an exception to a useful life requirement. In this circumstance, speech-language pathologists must report and explain: (a) the change in condition, (b) the existing SGD or access method was beneficial before the change but is no longer able to be used effectively, (c) there is a different device or access method that will enable the client to continue to communicate effectively (i.e., meet current medical need), (d) the replacement device or access aid will continue to be an effective tool for the client for the foreseeable future (i.e., assure there will not soon be another replacement request due to additional condition change), and (e) the replacement items are the least costly, equally effective alternative.[181]

Far more common are replacement requests arising from irreparable damage to or loss of the device during the useful life period. In this circumstance, among the most important questions is whether the useful life requirement can justify denial of a replacement request; in other words, whether a useful life requirement can override a source's general duty to provide covered care when medically necessary. There are no universal answers. One mitigating factor may be the cause of the damage or loss. For example, was the client responsible for the loss or damage? If yes, programs may argue that the client does not qualify for a replacement, the device is not appropriate, or the damage or loss event may repeat. Whatever the factual circumstances of the damage or loss, they are important and must be documented.

Useful life periods are conclusions based on expected normal use patterns and device wear and tear. However, if the damage or loss circumstances have no relation to those expectations, then the useful life limitation should not apply. For example, if the cause of damage or loss was beyond the client's control, such as resulting from a motor vehicle accident (e.g., the device was mounted to a wheelchair and the client was riding in a van that was struck by another vehicle), the device was stolen,[182] or the device was left behind and lost during an emergency evacuation forced by a natural disaster, such as a fire or flood, useful life expectations are all but a *nonsequitur*.

Yet another issue related to useful life requirements is whether their expiration should be interpreted as an entitlement to a device replacement. The answer is no. As long as SGDs continue to work reliably and to provide benefits to clients, there is no need for them to be replaced. The useful life requirement may have been exceeded, but the passage of time alone does not create a medical need for a new device.

A final issue regarding device replacement is technology change. Health benefits programs may consider replacement requests based on change of technology, but there is no clear standard for how to qualify for this opportunity. It is clear that the features and performance of new equipment must be *substantially* different—better—than the current equipment and that these differences must be of *significant* importance to the client. Great care must be taken to describe these differences and how they will directly impact clients' communication functioning.

Speech-Generating Device Exclusions

Exclusions are statements by insurers or health plan sponsors that imply "we do not want anything to do with this type of care or equipment."[183] SGD exclusions are a categorical rejection of SGDs, regardless of what else the policy or plan may offer as covered benefits. Exclusions also represent the complete disregard of speech-language pathologists' skill and the thoroughness of the assessment and recommendation and of clients' need for and ability to benefit from the SGD. Exclusions may be coverage-based or medical need-based. They may apply to all SGDs or only in specific circumstances. Common among them is that their effect is to deny clients SGD access.

It is reasonable to assume that all policies and health plans have limitations and exclusions. Insurers and health plan sponsors have discretion regarding what they will and will not cover and none covers everything. There are some limits to that discretion, such as the nondiscrimination in plan design provisions of the ACA[184] and state laws that mandate coverage of specific types of treatment, but neither prohibits all SGD exclusions nor mandates SGD coverage and access for all who need them.

However, it is important to note that SGD exclusions are as rare as their effect is severe. SGDs are accepted as benefits by health benefits sources far more often than not.[185] Nonetheless, SGD exclusions will sometimes be found in health insurance policies and health benefits plans.

Another important point is that from the perspective of a policy or plan reviewer, exclusions are "easy" to apply. The only skill reviewers must possess is the ability to read: After noting one or a few general characteristics about a funding request (e.g., clients' impairment, benefit sought) and reviewing a list of exclusions in the policy or plan, a decision can be issued. Reviewers need no special knowledge or experience and none of the "messy" facts about clients' condition or the justification for the requested care or device must be considered. These "efficiencies" create strong incentives for reviewers to claim exclusions are the basis for SGD denials far more frequently than is justified.

When exclusions are cited as the basis for denial of SGD purchase requests, the key questions will be whether they have been applied properly, and if so, whether it will be possible to escape their adverse effects. Several strategies that have been applied successfully to "get to yes" despite the existence of policy or plan exclusions are discussed here.

Is There a Speech-Generating Device Exclusion in a Policy or Health Plan? Clients and speech-language pathologists will typically learn that an exclusion exists in policies or health plans when an SGD purchase request is denied. The notice will state that an exclusion is the basis for the adverse decision. When this occurs, clients and speech-language pathologists should seek help from a legal advocate.[186] Working together, the policy or health plan documents, typically called a "certificate of coverage" or "certificate of insurance" for health insurance policies and a "summary plan description" for health benefits plans, must be reviewed. The purpose of the review is to find the text on which the denial is based.

The text stating the exclusion may be located in several places in these materials. Policy and plan documents commonly include a section titled "Exclusions and Limitations" or "Things We Do Not Cover." These sections may identify several dozen specific treatments and devices, as well as categories of care (e.g., treatment that is "experimental," "investigational," "unproven," "for comfort or convenience," "not medical in nature," "available without charge from another source") that are excluded. Exclusions may also be found in the description of the DME or prosthetic device benefit categories, in the description of medical need, or in the description of coverage of specific conditions (e.g., autism treatment).

The focus of the search must be to determine whether there is specific mention of SGDs where the limitations and exclusions are stated. Rephrased in the form of a question: Does the policy or plan state *SGD* exclusions, or just *general* exclusions? The distinction is important: Denials based on SGD exclusions will present limited opportunity for successful outcomes on appeal. By contrast, denials based on general exclusions are just expressions of the personal opinions of policy or health plan reviewers. SGD denials that interpret general exclusions are like all the other opinion-based denials discussed in this chapter (e.g., "not covered," "not medical in nature," "not medically necessary," "not least costly"). Opinion-based denials have been overturned throughout the history of SGD funding to enable SGD access.

To be considered an SGD exclusion, the policy or plan text must clearly identify SGDs as excluded.[187] This is because exclusions in insurance policies and health plans are generally disfavored, and they will be interpreted narrowly (strictly).[188] This means that the language claimed to be an SGD exclusion must be specific. The text must state plainly that SGDs are excluded, must use a synonymous phrase for SGDs (e.g., communication devices or AAC devices), or must describe device characteristics that make clear that SGDs are the intended item to be excluded.

An example of a device description recognized as an SGD exclusion states, "devices and computers to assist communication and speech."[189] By contrast, a device description found not to be an SGD exclusion stated, "computer story boards or light talkers for communication impaired individuals." This text was rejected as an SGD exclusion for three reasons: because "computer story boards" had no clear meaning and no recognizable link to any actual SGD, because "Light Talkers" were a specific model of SGD that had never been a synonym for all SGDs, and because by the time this text was reviewed in late 2002, Light Talkers were no longer being sold.[190]

Can Speech-Generating Device Exclusions Be Written in Medical Policy or Coverage Guidelines? The search of the policy or plan documents may not identify any text that establishes an SGD exclusion. Instead, an SGD exclusion may be found in medical coverage guidance for SGDs, DME, or specific conditions, such as autism. However, denials that rely on guidelines will be accepted as an SGD exclusion in a policy or health plan *only* if the policy or health plan documents clearly state that the guidelines must be followed as if their text was part of the policy or plan. But such "incorporations by reference" of coverage guidelines are very rare.

In the much more common circumstance, insurer or health plan denials based on SGD exclusions in coverage guidelines will not have the definitive door-closing effect of a true SGD exclusion. In these circumstances, reviewers' reliance on the guidelines as the basis for the decision was *a choice*. But that choice must be justified. Denials based on nonbinding guidelines will be subject significant scrutiny, based on the following legal principles:

- An insurer or health plan can rely on guidelines (they can be the basis for a decision) as an administrative convenience but only if they reasonably interpret the policy's or plan's provisions.[191]
- To be a reasonable interpretation, the guideline must meet two criteria. First, the definitions, standards, or tests applied by the guidelines must be the same as those stated in the policy or plan. Second, the guideline's conclusions must be credible: They must be based on a complete investigation of the facts and the analysis of those facts must be correct.[192]
- Finally, when a benefits denial is based on an exclusion, the insurer or health plan has the obligation ("burden of proof") to establish the exclusion is being applied properly.[193]

In practice, a guidelines-based denial, claimed to be an exclusion-based denial, typically will include the following: The policy or plan documents (certificate of coverage, summary plan description) will cover DME items, and define them such that SGDs "fit" within the definition of this benefit. The policy or plan will also include exclusions, but none mentions SGDs. One category of excluded care is "convenience items," which is not further defined. There is also an SGD, a DME, or other coverage guideline issued by the insurer or plan administrator that says SGDs are convenience items. The guideline may have no further explanation of the basis for this conclusion. When a client presents a purchase request to the policy or plan, it is denied. The denial basis is stated to be the policy or plan exclusion for convenience items.

In response to a denial based on an exclusion, the insurer or plan administrator must meet the criteria stated above: It must bear the burden of proof to establish the exclusion is properly applied to this request. To meet this burden, it cannot show the policy or plan and the guideline are applying the same definition of "convenience items," because neither defines the phrase. But if such a definition existed in the policy or plan, such commonality would be required. Also, the insurer or plan administrator must establish a complete factual investigation was completed about SGDs, focusing on their purpose and their effectiveness. It must establish:

- That there is a persuasive foundation of objective evidence to conclude that SGDs *are* convenience items
- That the insurer or plan administrator has reached the same conclusion, consistently, if it has been presented with other SGD purchase requests under this or any other policy or plan which they issued or administered, or can explain, on the basis of objective evidence, why different conclusions were justified in those other cases or why they were erroneous
- That professional literature supporting the medical need and effectiveness of SGD use is not credible or is not as persuasive as professional literature stating conclusions to the contrary

- That other funding sources that conclude SGDs are not convenience items are applying a different definition or standard or on the basis of objective evidence, have reached the wrong conclusion

These findings will support the conclusion in the guideline that links SGDs to convenience items. Absent this factual investigation, as well as the body of evidence to support the conclusion stated in the guidelines, there is no basis or justification for the insurer or plan administrator to *choose* to rely on this guideline or to claim that the policy or plan excludes SGDs as convenience items.

Although this is but one hypothetical example, as a general matter it may be exceedingly difficult, if not impossible, for insurers or health plans to meet their burden of proof to justify reliance on a guideline-based exclusion as opposed to a policy- or plan-based exclusion. Further discussion about the all-but-impossible burden required to show SGDs are convenience items is presented below.

Speech-Generating Devices Are NOT Convenience Items. The most frequently cited basis for excluding SGDs has been that they are "comfort or convenience" items. This is a common category of excluded medical care. It may be stated as part of the DME definition (e.g., DME items must be "used primarily and customarily for a medical purpose *and not primarily for the comfort or convenience of the client or caregiver*") or as part of the medical need definition (e.g., medically necessary care is "*not solely for the comfort or convenience of the patient, their family, or the provider of the service or supplies*").[194] Or, it may be listed as a category of excluded care in an Exclusions and Limitations section of the policy or health plan documents, or stated in a DME guideline.

If in the policy or health plan documents there is (a) no specific mention of SGDs as an example of "comfort or convenience" items, or (b)(1) if the only place a specific link is made is in a DME or other guideline and (b)(2) application of the guideline is not expressly required, a denial on this basis is opinion-based and subject to all of the same rules and the same scrutiny as was just discussed.

To justify an opinion-based claim that SGDs are a comfort or convenience item, the insurer or health plan will have the burden of proof to identify a persuasive rationale that establishes SGDs in general or a specific SGD warrants this label. To date, no funding source has ever done so. One reason for this may be that there is overwhelming evidence that supports the conclusion that no SGD-convenience item link exists. This evidence is reviewed here.

Discussion of this response begins with Medicare, the largest health benefits program in the country. For more than a decade, it had guidance that stated SGDs were convenience items. However, after review of relevant facts Medicare reversed that conclusion, acknowledged SGDs are not convenience items, and it became the single largest funding source of SGDs.

Medicare SGD coverage dates back at least to 1981.[195] However, from the mid-1980s to April 2000, Medicare had a national coverage decision (a type of Medicare guidance) that stated SGDs were convenience items. It stated:

| Augmentative Communication Devices | *see* Communicator |
| Communicator | Deny: convenience item, not primarily medical in nature [§ 1861(n) of the Act][196] |

Medicare defined "convenience items" as "[e]quipment which basically serves comfort or convenience functions or is primarily for the convenience of the person caring for the patient, such as elevators, stairway elevators, and posture chairs,"[197] but it never explained why it had concluded that SGDs fit that definition or on what it was based. When asked, Medicare reported it had no records to explain what had been reviewed, who had been consulted, who had reached this conclusion, or even when the guidance was first issued.[198]

The credibility of the convenience item conclusion was weakened further because this Medicare guidance was of a type that was not binding on all Medicare decision makers. Between 1993 and 2001, approximately two dozen appeals were pursued by Medicare recipients following denial of SGD payment claims. All were successful; no Medicare appeals decision concluded the "convenience item" guidance was credible and a basis to uphold an SGD denial.[199]

In June 1999, Medicare agreed to reconsider this guidance. Medicare staff was presented with the *Formal Request*, which included a detailed review of the professional literature that established SGDs as a safe and effective treatment for severe communication impairments, the speech-language pathology evaluation and decision-making process leading to SGD recommendations, the characteristics and features of then-current SGDs, and how other health benefits programs covered SGDs.[200] The information about SGDs as effective treatment was also supported by leading medical professional societies.[201]

In April 2000, Medicare completed its reconsideration and announced it was withdrawing the convenience item guidance, it was acknowledging that SGDs will be covered as Medicare DME, and SGDs will be approved when medically necessary.[202] A few months later, Medicare published its revised guidance for SGDs that went into effect on January 1, 2001.[203] Since 2001, Medicare has been the single largest funding source for SGDs.

The evolution of Medicare SGD policy and the evidence it reviewed supplies a strong foundation for a response to any other health benefits source that attempts to link SGDs and convenience items. This response contains four points: (1) SGDs are safe, effective, and medically necessary treatment for complex and severe communication impairments and are a form of speech-language pathology treatment; (2) SGDs are accepted as benefits by all types of health benefits sources, including sources that expressly prohibit coverage of and payment for care that serves convenience purposes; (3) when programs identify other supplies, equipment, and other similar incidental services as convenience items, SGDs are easily distinguished, as they share no characteristics with these items and services; and (4) SGDs are essential to the individuals with complex and severe communication impairments who need and use them. Each is discussed in the following.

> SGDs are safe, effective, and medically necessary treatment for complex and severe communication impairments and are a form of speech-language pathology treatment.

That SGDs are accepted as safe, effective, and medically necessary treatment for complex and severe communication impairments and are a form of speech-language pathology treatment has been discussed elsewhere in this chapter.[204]

> SGDs are accepted as benefits by all types of health benefits sources, including sources that expressly prohibit coverage of and payment for care that serves convenience purposes.

That SGDs are accepted as benefits by all types of health benefits programs has also been discussed elsewhere in this chapter.[205]

In addition, from a historic perspective, insurance and Medicaid programs were the first to accept SGDs as benefits.[206] It is noteworthy that almost all Medicaid programs accepted SGDs as program benefits *after* they were given express authority to exclude care that was not medically necessary,[207] such as care that served convenience purposes.[208] By 2000, every Medicaid program covered SGDs. None ever refused SGD coverage by claiming they were comfort or convenience items.

Before 2010, more than 1,000 insurers and health plans covered and provided SGDs.[209] The widespread coverage of SGDs by insurers and health plans also reflects the conclusion that SGDs are not comfort or convenience items. The following insurance appeal decision states the generally accepted view:

> The [SGD] should be considered [DME] in this particular case because it is a piece of equipment that can be used as part of a treatment plan for a child who clearly has a medical condition. This device is not just an 'invention to make life easier' that 'does not treat the underlying problem.'

> Augmentative communication devices are not convenience items; in most cases, they would fit under the category of [DME] ... [210]

Medicare's rejection of SGDs as convenience items has already been discussed. Its acceptance of SGDs as DME is also noteworthy because Congress expressly prohibits Medicare from providing reimbursement for items or services "which constitute personal comfort items."[211]

Tricare, which provides health benefits to dependents of active-duty military personnel and military retirees and their dependents, has also long accepted SGDs as benefits. It too is prohibited from covering and paying for convenience items.[212]

The U.S. Congress has also voiced its opinion that SGDs are not convenience items. On four occasions, Congress addressed SGDs in legislation. Each time, it expanded the scope of coverage for SGDs or SGD accessories. The first mention of SGDs was in a law related to the Tricare program. Prior to 2001, Tricare SGD coverage was limited to dependents of active-duty military personnel through its Program for People with Disabilities. In the FY 2002 National Defense Authorization Act, Congress expressly authorized Tricare to expand its SGD coverage to all beneficiaries.[213] This authorization led to Tricare's issuance of SGD coverage criteria applicable to all beneficiaries in early 2005.[214]

The second Congressional reference to SGDs affected veterans' benefits. In the FY 2009 Military Construction, Veterans Affairs and Related Agencies Appropriations Bill, the Senate Report stated:

> Additionally, the Committee encourages the Department to increase funding for the treatment of severe communication disabilities through the use of speech communication aids and the speech and language therapists who prescribe them.[215]

Congress next addressed coverage of SGDs in the Steve Gleason Act of 2015.[216] In that law, Congress prohibited Medicare from assigning SGDs to a DME payment category known as *capped rental*. Had the assignment of SGDs to capped rental been allowed, some recipients would have been unable to have continued access to SGDs. The law also amended the Medicare definition of its DME benefit to include "eye tracking and gaze interaction accessories for SGDs furnished to individuals with a demonstrated medical need for such accessories."[217] The provisions of the 2015 law were temporary. In early 2018, Congress addressed SGDs once again, making the Gleason Act changes permanent. Obviously, Congress does not recognize SGDs as convenience items.

> When programs identify other supplies, equipment, and other similar incidental services as convenience items, SGDs are easily distinguished, as they share no characteristics with these items and services.

Table 17-1

Examples of Comfort or Convenience Items in Health Benefits Plans

TYPICAL EMPLOYEE HEALTH BENEFITS PLAN EXAMPLES OF COMFORT AND CONVENIENCE ITEMS	MEDICARE COVERAGE STATUS OF SAME ITEMS
Air conditioners	Not covered: presumptively nonmedical item Air conditioners [environmental control equipment]; see also Medicare Carriers Manual, § 2100.1
Beauty/barber service	Not covered: not treatment of any illness or injury 42 USC § 1396y(a)(1)
Air purifiers and filters	Not covered: environmental control equipment Electric air cleaners
Dehumidifiers and humidifiers	Not covered: environmental control equipment Humidifiers, dehumidifiers, Medicare Coverage Issues Manual, § 60-9
Ergonomically correct chairs	Not covered: comfort or convenience item Posture chairs
Home remodeling to accommodate a health need (including but not limited to ramps, swimming pools, elevators, handrails, and stair glides)	Not covered: comfort or convenience item Elevators, stairway elevators
Nonhospital beds and comfort beds	Not covered See Medicare Coverage Issues Manual § 60-18 [describing scope of *hospital* bed coverage]
Television	Not covered: personal comfort services 42 CFR § 411.15(j)
Telephone	Not covered: personal comfort services 42 CFR § 411.15(j)

The next element of this response is directed to health benefits programs that identify SGDs, as well as other equipment items or services, as examples of convenience items. As noted above, Medicare's definition of "convenience items" refers to elevators, stairway elevators, and posture chairs.[218] Other examples in Medicare guidance include bathtub lifts, bathtub seats, lounge [type] beds, carafes, emesis basins, overbed tables, raised toilet seats, and standing tables.[219] Two other examples are identified in Medicare regulations: "use of a television set or telephone."[220]

Tricare's convenience item definition is similar: "[p]ersonal, comfort, or convenience items" include items "such as beauty and barber services, radio, television, and telephone."[221] Insurance policies and health benefits plans often identify the same items as Medicare and Tricare as examples of comfort or convenience items. References to these other items provide an opportunity to show that SGDs are different and that their characteristics are not comparable. For this reason, SGDs should not be considered a convenience item.

One way to distinguish SGDs from these other items is by reference to the coding (categorization) system for DME items (known by its acronym HCPCS) that is required to be used by health care programs. There are six HCPCS codes for SGDs and additional codes for SGD software, mounts, and accessories.[222] Each has an E prefix denoting that they are categorized as DME items. By comparison, it is likely that some of the items on a policy's or plan's convenience item list will not have an HCPCS code designation. If not, the conclusion to be drawn is that items without codes do not have the required characteristics of DME items, such as being primarily and customarily used to serve a medical purpose, and generally not useful to an individual in the absence of an illness or injury.[223] For this reason, items without DME codes are fundamentally different than SGDs.

A second basis for comparison is whether the items on an insurer's or plan's convenience item list are covered by Medicare or other benefits programs. Table 17-1 compares common items considered comfort or convenience items by employer-sponsored health benefits plans with the Medicare coverage status of the same items. As shown in this table, none of the items commonly listed by health benefits plans as convenience items is covered by Medicare. By contrast, as already discussed, Medicare covers and provides funding for SGDs and is the largest single funding source for SGDs. That Medicare covers SGDs but none of these items provides another basis to distinguish SGDs from these other items.

A third point of comparison is the benefits that SGDs and these other devices provide, that is, their importance to individuals who need them.[224] SGDs are different in kind from the things listed as convenience items. SGDs serve a medical purpose; comfort or convenience items do not. Also, in contrast to SGDs, none of the examples of convenience items cited by Medicare, Tricare, or by insurers is vitally important,[225] none is treatment for severe functional impairment, and the absence of any of these items will not create risk of death, serious injury, or physical neglect or abuse.

Simply stated, by comparing SGD coding, SGD coverage, and the benefits SGDs provide, SGDs can be established as having nothing in common with items typically cited as examples of comfort or convenience items. These differences provide a basis to conclude that SGDs are not comfort or convenience items.

These differences are important because it is generally accepted that the provisions of insurance policies and health benefits plans should be interpreted consistently, meaning that dissimilar items should not be grouped together (i.e., within the same benefits category for coverage purposes or the same exclusion category for noncoverage purposes).

When a contract groups clauses under a common heading, like the exclusions listed under "comfort or convenience," *interpretation of one provision is informed by the company it keeps.*[226]

> SGDs are essential to the individuals with complex and severe communication impairments who need and use them.

SGDs do not serve convenience purposes for their users or their caregivers. To the contrary, SGDs restore a vitally important basic human functional ability lost due to illness or disease—expressive communication through oral speech. The vital importance of the ability to speak has been recognized by the courts and other decision makers when SGD coverage was at issue. Others have noted that the ability to speak and to use language is a defining characteristic of the human species.[227] ASHA and USSAAC have both asserted, as a matter of organizational policy, that "communication is the essence of human life."[228]

Risks of Death, Severe Injury, Abuse, and Neglect. One measure of the vital importance of SGDs is the life-threatening circumstances and outrageous injuries experienced by people who lacked the ability to speak and the

perceptions by others that they are nonsentient or even non-human. For example, a physician became "locked in" following a stroke. Initially, he was only able to communicate by blinking his eyes. Shortly after his stroke, he was asked whether, due to his condition, he wanted medical treatment to continue. However, the question was asked incorrectly: one blink for "yes," two blinks for "no." An involuntary twitch causing a second blink almost cost this man his life. The questioner recognized his error and asked the question again, reversing the meaning of the responses. The physician, with an SGD, returned to the practice of medicine.[229]

Another example is the outrageous injury experienced by a young adult New York Medicaid recipient. A speech-language pathologist reported the preventable tragedy that he experienced:

> Andrew has a burn scar on his hand which occurred because he couldn't tell his attendants at school that they had pushed him up against a radiator and locked his wheels in a position where his hand was trapped to sear until the flesh melted off.[230]

These may be worst-case scenarios of the harm that can arise from the lack of an ability to communicate, but the adverse impacts of a severe communication disability go far beyond these examples. All too common have been reports of broken bones that were not discovered for days,[231] infections that were not identified and treated until they had become extremely severe,[232] and sources of pain that were not localized and timely addressed.[233] Indeed, for some individuals, the frustrations associated with the inability to communicate increased to the level of a mental health impairment that required treatment.[234]

Other descriptions of the harm caused by the inability to communicate effectively are found in published memoirs by individuals who use SGDs. One was written by a woman with cerebral palsy. She was institutionalized unnecessarily for years due to her inability to communicate. While in the institutional setting, she experienced ongoing abuse and neglect. As she later wrote:

> I tried to tell the doctors and nurses about it, but I couldn't communicate with them. Nobody told them about my facial signals. The nurses didn't know if I was deaf, dumb, or what. The nicer ones spoke to me slowly and loudly, as if this would make it easier for me to understand them. I wanted to tell them that English was my native language and I understood them well, but I couldn't get that message across. The nurses kept telling each other 'I guess that she doesn't understand us' while I was flashing my 'yes' expression so hard that my face hurt … Without a doubt, my inability to speak has been the single most devastating aspect of my handicap. If I were granted one wish and one wish only, I would not hesitate for an instant to request that I be able to talk, if only for 1 day, or even 1 hour.[235]

Another memoir became a best seller and was adapted into a motion picture. Jean Dominique-Bauby was the editor of the French fashion magazine Elle. He had a severe stroke that left him "locked in" and unable to communicate except by eye gaze. Using this method alone, he wrote *The Diving Bell and the Butterfly* (1999), which included the following:

'On June 8, it will be 6 months since my new life began' … Those were the first words of the first mailing of my monthly letter … [T]hat first bulletin caused a mild stir and repaired some damage caused by rumor … The gossipers [in Paris had] left no doubt that henceforth I belonged on a vegetable stall and not to the human race … [In response,] I would have to rely on myself if I wanted to prove that my IQ was still higher than a turnip's.[236]

Another type of harm from the inability to communicate effectively is opportunity lost. This impact is most easily illustrated by the example of Professor Stephen Hawking, the British astrophysicist who was also the world's best-known SGD user. He had used an SGD since the mid-1980's to overcome the loss of speech caused by ALS. In mid-1985, Dr. Hawking was a physicist well known only to a small community of scientists. After he lost the ability to speak, he was extraordinarily restricted in his ability to communicate. As he later explained it through the use of an SGD:

For a time, the only way I could communicate was to spell out words letter by letter, raising my eyebrows when someone pointed to the right letter on a spelling card. It is pretty difficult to carry on a conversation like that, let alone write a scientific paper.[237]

Biographers further describe the impact of the SGD:

Hawking's new computer-generated voice completely transformed his life. He could now communicate better than before the operation, and he no longer needed the help of an interpreter when lecturing or simply conversing with people.[238]

With this AAC device, Dr. Hawking was able to complete *A Brief History of Time* (1988), which catapulted him to international fame.

Finally, no one will claim that the ability to speak—to deter or explain a physical or sexual assault—is a matter of convenience. An SGD user described her experience in a poem:

She denied giving me a communication board
Because I could tell about the abuse
That would send her husband to a prison ward.
Eventually I was thrown out of her home
After my Social Worker discovered what they had done
Through my first clear voice.
One clear technology voice
That allows me to make many
Life choices.[239]

Misperceptions of Deficits. Additional support for the conclusion that the ability to communicate effectively is not a convenience is found in the statement of an adult with cerebral palsy who described the ability to communicate as essential to being recognized as a human being:

[When a person who is unable to communicate is among other people,] people [will be] talking behind, beside, around, over, under, through, and even for you. But never with you. You are ignored until you feel like a piece of furniture.[240]

Another individual who lost her speech following an accident expressed a similar thought with her SGD:

Speech is the most important thing we have. It makes us a person and not a thing. No one should ever have to be a 'thing.'[241]

Finally, consider the analogy drawn by one Ohio physician who could not effectively obtain information from his communication-impaired patient:

Current inability to communicate has greatly limited his access to medical care and indeed has reduced it to approximately veterinary proportions.[242]

Sadly, this comparison was repeated 2 decades later by a physician trying to treat an Iraq War veteran with a catastrophic injury:

He compared caring for someone as noncommunicative as Shurvon to a veterinarian's guesswork.[243]

The United Cerebral Palsy Association coined a metaphor to describe, in general, all the adverse impacts caused by being unable to communicate. It stated a "cloak of incompetence" lies over the lives of those with severe communication disabilities and describes this as the "heaviest burden Americans with significant speech disabilities have always faced."

Americans with significant speech disabilities routinely experience isolation, discrimination, illiteracy, institutionalization, unemployment, poverty, and despair. Due to the lack of understandable speech, these individuals are perceived to be unable to direct their own lives; a perception that often leads to an erosion or outright deprivation of their most basic civil rights and liberties.[244]

These and other memoirs and anecdotes describing the importance of the ability to communicate effectively are supported by professional literature and policy. The most respected treatise on AAC intervention acknowledges that, at first blush, people without disabilities may reach the wrong conclusion about the importance of the ability to communicate. "Clearly, someone who has not 'been there' cannot understand the experience of having a severe communication disorder."[245] An earlier article explained why this statement is true:

For the normal adult who has spoken without difficulty since early childhood, the prospect of being unable to communicate through natural speech is incomprehensible. Efficient communication with colleagues, family, and friends is taken for granted.[246]

Maintenance of Social and Familial Roles and Responsibilities. Efficient and effective communication is essential and is not a convenience for the speaker or the communication partner. Being able to communicate health needs to obtain appropriate and timely health care, and to be able to direct the provision of care is claimed—wrongly—to be the "medical need" for speech.[247] In addition, being able to communicate effectively to maintain social roles after onset of an impairment, such as ALS, is recognized as one of the most challenging of all aspects of acquired communication disorders.[248]

> When I first realized that I would be unable to speak someday, I viewed it as losing my life. Communication was my life. Now, I realize that was a little overly dramatic, but not much. *Speechlessness is not a loss of life, but a loss of access to life* …[249]

For this client, the access to life he lost was to his friends, both to their friendly conversations and intellectual debates. With an SGD, that access was restored.

For another client with ALS, the loss of access to life as her expressive communication abilities were eroding was the ability to interact with her husband of 55 years and with her siblings, children, and grandchildren, to take care of her personal needs and health care, to maintain her home, and maintain social contacts. The loss of speech was profoundly disruptive to her role and responsibilities in her family and profoundly isolating both to her and her husband. Her anarthria precluded the very speech—about home, family, health, and social matters—that researchers have established is typical of the conversations of older women.[250] With an SGD, some of these functional abilities were able to be restored.

Similarly, an adult who had a stroke described, with an SGD, the extent to which the device enabled him to regain "access to life." He reported that his SGD:

> … had opened up his life to express himself, and that he had regained up to 95% of his prestroke vocabulary … My [SGD] has opened up my life again by allowing me to express my thoughts coherently to myself and others … Although the typing process is slow and laborious for me, the joy of expression and communication is unsurpassed.[251]

This client was the first Medicare beneficiary known to have had a Medicare decision maker refuse to rely on the "convenience item" SGD guidance. In the decision approving the claim, the administrative law judge observed:

> His introduction to the [SGD] and subsequent learning of the device has resurrected to a great measure his ability to communicate and become much more functional to the extent that he can maintain greater independent living … There is no question, given the evidence, that the [SGD] has restored and improved his life … Without this device, as the evidence points out, the claimant's life would continue to be severely restricted and his ability to enjoy the fruits of life would not be available.[252]

Related Activities and Services. The importance of the ability to communicate can also be demonstrated by Congress' support for the expansion of Tricare and Veterans Affairs coverage of SGDs, already noted, and by its creation and support of the National Institute of Deafness and Other Communication Disorders within the National Institutes of Health (NIH). This institute conducts and facilitates research into treatment methods for individuals with severe communication impairments, including AAC interventions and SGDs.[253] The NIH is the nation's premier medical and allied health research institution; it does not direct its research activities to conveniences.

The leading edge of NIH- and the Department of Veterans' Affairs–sponsored research also makes clear that communication is not a matter of convenience. Among the research now being conducted are experiments with neurotrophic implants and other interface technologies that will enable individuals with severe ALS or other similar conditions to communicate by creating a direct link between the individual's brain and a computer-based SGD. One will be hard-pressed to describe research to enable direct brain control of a tool to control a person's environment—a communication aid, a mobility tool, a computer—as a matter of convenience.

Finally, that SGDs are not convenience items is also established by the fact that speech-language pathology services are not a convenience. All types of health benefits sources cover and provide speech-language pathology services. Impairments to speech clearly are recognized as health concerns sufficiently important to warrant covered treatment. By contrast, if the ability to speak was no more than a convenience, speech-language pathology services would not be covered. Moreover, once coverage exists to enable a speech-language pathologist to improve or restore speech or other natural communication methods, comparable services provided to enable an individual with a more severe or complex communication impairment to speak through use of an SGD cannot be a matter of convenience. Clients with progressive impairments who lose the ability to effectively communicate by natural communication methods do not simultaneously lose the need to communicate effectively. The need remains the same; indeed, as the person's condition deteriorates, the need to communicate effectively may be seen as heightened. All that changes is the means or method of communication—from speech or other natural communication methods to use of an SGD. Although, in general, it is not appropriate to link medical necessity to specific messages, a specific sentence is an appropriate tool to illustrate this point. If a client is unable to say "I need help" sufficiently intelligibly to get help (i.e., oral speech is not effective), then speech-language pathology services will be provided. On what basis is it possible to conclude that this same message, expressed through an SGD, is a matter of convenience?

Speech-Generating Devices Are NOT Experimental or Investigational Treatment. Premera BCBS is an insurer in the northwest United States. It wrote an SGD guideline that supported coverage generally but carved out an exception for SGD use by individuals with autism. That use was stated to be "experimental" or "investigational" because:

> the published literature regarding the use of [SGDs] in autism and other pervasive developmental disorders does not establish scientifically reliable evidence for their effectiveness for the following reasons: (1) there are no controlled studies; (2) almost all studies are either single-subject studies or consist of very small sample sizes, and are therefore anecdotal; and (3) almost all studies have been conducted only in school settings and therefore provide no data outcomes in home and community settings.[254]

Premera relied on this guidance to deny several SGD purchase requests for children with autism. But when appeals of these denials were pursued, it became clear this guideline could not be relied on. The clients' health plans did not require the guidelines to be applied: Doing so was a matter of choice. For this reason, Premera BCBS had the burden of proof to justify that choice (its reliance on an exclusion to deny the request), but it could not do so. This guideline had so many flaws that it could not be established as a reasonable interpretation of the clients' health plans.

One flaw was that the definitions, standards, or tests applied by the guideline were not the same as those stated in one client's health plan. The plan documents included a definition of "experimental/ investigational" care that did not require consideration of only published literature or of studies with particular research designs, sample sizes, or settings.[255] In other words, Premera BCBS denied the SGD purchase request because SGDs did not meet criteria A, B, or C, but SGD coverage under the plan was not dependent on A, B, or C. In this example, applying these guidelines would have resulted in a change to the terms of the plan by adding criteria and tests not otherwise required, which is not permitted.[256]

These appeals also brought to light the lack of credibility of the guideline's conclusion that SGDs for use by individuals with autism is experimental or investigational: It could not be established to be correct. Premera BCBS could not satisfy either the requirement that a complete factual investigation must be conducted for all policy or health plan benefits requests, regardless of whether an exclusion is involved[257] or the requirement that there be a correct interpretation of the facts. The "experimental" or "investigational" care conclusion focused on professional literature related to SGD use by individuals with autism, but there was no assertion a complete literature search had been conducted. Instead, the guideline had a bibliography that listed only six relevant references.[258] Rather than conduct a complete investigation of the literature as required, the Premera BCBS guideline appeared to reflect a strategy of "don't look, don't learn."

In addition, even on the basis of its very limited investigation of the professional literature, Premera BCBS could not support its conclusion that the professional literature "does not establish" SGD effectiveness. Clients pursued their own investigation of the literature cited in the guideline. That effort discovered other professional literature Premera BCBS had not reviewed. It also included contacting the lead authors of the six articles cited in the guideline's bibliography and asking if their research had been interpreted properly: if it supported the exclusion of SGDs for use by individuals with autism and if the authors' knowledge of the relevant literature as a whole supported the guideline's conclusion. All responded "no" to each question.[259] These responses were irrefutable. No insurer or health plan could bring forth a witness to credibly claim to know more about these references than did their authors. In response, Premera BCBS withdrew the guideline and removed the SGD exclusion for individuals with autism.[260]

Another SGD guideline, issued by Regence Blue Shield, also a health insurer in the northwest United States, also stated an "experimental" or "investigational" care exclusion applied to SGD use by individuals with autism. Its SGD guideline asserted "the long-term effects of same [SGD use] on health outcomes for [individuals with autism] is not established in the peer reviewed scientific literature."[261] These adverse decisions were also appealed. Once again, it was clear that although the conclusion was based on flaws in the professional literature, no complete literature review had been conducted.[262] And once again, the guideline's conclusion could not be established to be correct. In response, the same outcome was achieved: Regence Blue Shield withdrew this guideline and removed the exclusion.[263]

A third guideline, issued by CIGNA, stated an SGD exclusion for individuals with autism and asserted:

> The quality and quantity of data in current peer-reviewed scientific medical literature is inadequate to establish the clinical utility, safety, and efficacy of this device [as] treatment for [autism]. The requested service is therefore excluded under your medical benefit plan as experimental/ investigational/unproven.[264]

This guideline shared several characteristics with those of Premera BCBS and Regence Blue Shield. They all excluded SGD access by individuals with autism. They all stated they were linked to the professional literature. They all were challenged, and none was defended. Upon review, the relevant professional literature very clearly supports the conclusion that SGD use by individuals with autism *is* effective. In response to these challenges, all these guidelines were withdrawn and reissued without the experimental or investigational care conclusion.

The CIGNA guideline did present one distinct issue. The Premera BCBS and Regence Blue Shield guidelines reached definitive conclusions based on a specific list of articles: Each said they "did not establish" SGD effectiveness. For this reason, the substantive basis for this conclusion was challenged: All the relevant information had been considered—or not, and the literature supported the exclusions—or not. But the exclusion stated in the CIGNA guideline was based on a different finding. It claimed the professional literature was "inadequate" or "insufficient" to reach a conclusion about the effectiveness of SGD use by individuals with autism. However, the CIGNA guideline left unanswered *what is enough*: What amount or type of information will establish that SGDs are an effective tool to improve the communication functioning of individuals with autism?

In response to appeals from SGD denials based on this guidelines-based conclusion, CIGNA would have to answer the *what is enough* question and also establish both that the answer was reasonable and that the professional literature about SGD use by individuals with autism did not meet this threshold. Rather than wait for CIGNA to address these points, in 2011, clients proactively conducted a literature review of their own and submitted its findings as part of their appeals. Several dozen experimental research articles and research reviews (e.g., systematic reviews, meta-analyses) were identified. All supported the effectiveness of SGD use by individuals with autism.[265] The author of one of those research reviews summarized the consensus of professional opinion at that time:

> To me and other clinical and research professionals in autism and AAC, the question of the effectiveness of SGDs for use as a treatment technique for people with autism no longer is an open question for which additional research is necessary. To the community of autism and AAC professionals, SGDs are one part of the standard of care to improve the functional communication and other outcomes for people with autism. Thus, we are turning our research attention to other questions.[266]

Clients also searched for other health benefits funding sources that supported SGD access by individuals with autism and presented this information to CIGNA as well. For example, two SGD approvals by Humana for clients with autism noted:

> We approved your appeal because based on a review of the current peer-reviewed English language medical literature, this technology would be medically appropriate for the members' medical condition.[267]

ASHA also added its voice. It recognizes that SGDs are effective treatment tools for individuals with autism.[268] So too, does the American Academy of Pediatrics.[269]

As a practical matter, this literature search and analysis significantly increased the difficulty for CIGNA to meet its burden of proof. Its staff would have had to review every article the clients identified and to explain the flaws or inadequacies of each, and then also explain why all of them together were "inadequate" or "insufficient." CIGNA also would have had to distinguish the conclusions of the other funding sources—especially those based on those sources' review of the professional literature—that SGD coverage for individuals with autism was justified.

Faced with having to rebut all this information, CIGNA reviewers at first mulishly applied the guideline's conclusion, notwithstanding there was no plan requirement that CIGNA guidelines be applied. Relying on these guidelines

was a matter of reviewer choice; a choice CIGNA had the burden to explain. But no explanation was produced. The reviewers ignored the literature search and analysis and all the other information that had been submitted, also legally impermissible.[270] Instead, they offered as an excuse that assessing the credibility of guidelines was not their job: It was the responsibility of other staff that developed and periodically reviewed guidelines. In their view, if an administrative guideline is potentially applicable to a benefits request, it must be applied, and its conclusions are binding and not reviewable through the appeal process. This position, too, was legally indefensible.[271] CIGNA then withdrew the guideline and reissued it acknowledging SGD coverage for individuals with autism.[272]

Because of the value of this literature search and analysis, it has been updated several times.[273] It will be available for use by clients, speech-language pathologists, and advocates who face professional literature- or "experimental" or "investigational" care–based denials of SGD access by clients with autism.[274]

Securing Speech-Generating Device Access Notwithstanding Speech-Generating Device Exclusions. As noted above, some policies and health plans have SGD exclusions clearly stated in their text. To date, clients have been successful in a limited number of circumstances in evading the adverse effects of these exclusions. Some of these opportunities are discussed here.

Autism Treatment Mandate Laws. An opportunity for SGD access exists for some individuals with autism notwithstanding that they are subject to an SGD exclusion. The two prerequisites for their SGD access are (1) their health benefits source is an insurance policy, and (2) they live in a state with an autism treatment mandate law. For more than 10 years, Autism Speaks worked to persuade state legislatures to enact autism treatment mandate laws. These laws require insurance policies issued in these states to cover treatment for autism and often for related conditions as well. All or nearly all states have adopted these laws.

The scope of these mandates include treatment for autism's adverse communication effects. The Kentucky statute, for example, states:

> Treatment for autism spectrum disorders includes the following care:
> - Habilitative care, including therapy, and treatment programs that are necessary to develop and maintain, to the maximum extent practicable, the functioning of an individual; and
> - Therapeutic care services provided by licensed speech therapists.[275]

The text of these laws varies somewhat from state to state. Some specifically mention *communication devices* as covered,[276] some refer to *equipment* as covered,[277] and others do not mention communication devices or equipment at all. Regardless, the intent of these mandated benefit laws is to include SGDs in the scope of autism treatment. Autism Speaks reported:

Autism Speaks believes that SGD use is an effective intervention to improve the functional communication for individuals with autism … In sum, Autism Speaks supports the broadest possible access by individuals with autism to all treatment programs that will be effective in improving their functional communication abilities. SGDs are one way to accomplish that goal. Autism Speaks believes no benefits or funding program is justified in erecting access barriers to the speech-language pathology evaluation that will determine whether the individual with autism will be best served by a treatment program directed toward oral speech development or one that implements [AAC] strategies; or to speech-language pathology treatment programs that seek to improve functional communication including those that rely on speech-language pathology services and use of an SGD.[278]

In all states where these laws have been enacted,[279] SGD exclusions in insurance policies (or in autism treatment or SGD guidelines) are void, without effect, and are not enforceable. A generally applicable legal principle is that "statutory provisions applicable to contracts of insurance are deemed to form a part of such contract and must be construed in connection therewith; policy provisions in conflict with the statute are void."[280] For example, in 2012, the Louisiana statute mandating autism treatment caused Humana to reverse the SGD denial for a child with autism notwithstanding a diagnosis-based exclusion in her policy.[281]

However, it is important to remember that these statutes apply only to insurance policies, and they only apply to autism and sometimes to other related conditions. Clients who are covered by health plans and who have conditions other than those identified in the treatment mandates will not benefit from these laws.

Speech-Generating Device Exclusions With Limited Scope or With Exceptions. The plain text of some SGD exclusions state they are of limited scope. They may apply only to particular conditions or to particular devices. Alternately, an exclusion may be worded to suggest it has omnibus or across-the-board scope, but its text also includes exceptions for specific conditions or device types. Exceptions to exclusions are interpreted as statements of coverage. "Exceptions to exclusions are typically construed broadly, since they are provisions extending insurance coverage."[282] Thus, clients who do not have the excluded condition or do not seek the excluded equipment, or who qualify under an exception, will have their SGD access governed by the general rules of eligibility, coverage, and medical need.

Condition-Based Exceptions. An example of an SGD exclusion that applies only to some conditions states:

- Limitations and Exclusions
  - Unless specifically stated otherwise, no benefits will be provided for, or on account of, the following items:

◊ Expenses for services that are primarily and customarily used for environmental control or enhancement (whether or not prescribed by a health care practitioner) and certain medical devices, including:

– Communication devices, except after surgical removal of the larynx or a diagnosis of permanent lack of function of the larynx

This example can be described either as a condition-based SGD exclusion or as an across-the-board exclusion with a condition-based exception. It is common in Humana insurance policies. It does not exclude SGDs or any *types* of communication devices. Its focus is directed to clients' conditions. Thus, clients with a larynx-related impairment will be eligible for an SGD if identified as needed. For example, clients with head and neck cancer who at one point of the disease process require a laryngectomy will be eligible for any needed communication device, which may be an artificial larynx or an SGD. If the disease progresses to require a glossectomy as well, an artificial larynx will no longer be appropriate, and an SGD will likely be needed. The initial procedure satisfies the exception to Humana's condition-limited exclusion; either procedure may support clients' medical need for an SGD.

The effect of this condition-based exception is that individuals with other conditions, whose SGD need arises independent of larynx-impairment, are not eligible for an SGD. However, there is one more exception to this exclusion: Because it is stated in insurance policies and will cause the denial of SGD access to individuals with autism, it will be pre-empted and rendered void and unenforceable by state autism treatment mandate laws.[283]

To date, no explanation has ever been provided for the larynx impairment focus of this exclusion or of the claimed link between communication devices to "environmental control or enhancement."

Device-Based Exceptions. An example of an SGD exclusion that applies only to some types of devices—because of an exception—states:

devices and computers to assist communication and speech, except for speech aid devices (or speech aid prosthetics) …

This text is common in United Healthcare insurance policies and in health plans it designed. The first part of this text, "devices and computers to assist communication and speech," is recognized as describing SGDs.[284] If this was the entire content of the exclusion, it would be an omnibus coverage barrier to SGD access. If an appeal from such a denial, the insurer or plan will be able to meet its burden of proof to establish the SGD denial—based on the exclusion—was appropriate.

But that is not the end of the matter. The exclusion also has an exception for *speech aid devices.* As noted above, exceptions to exclusions restore coverage and they are interpreted broadly. But it must first be established that the exception is applicable here. That burden will be on clients, their speech-language pathologists, and advocates. "Generally speaking, the party seeking benefits bears the burden of proving his entitlement to benefits ... [Where there is an exclusion with an exception]—the insured ... has the burden of proving that an exception to the exclusion restores coverage."[285] Thus, clients will be required to present as much persuasive evidence as can be found that supports the conclusion that SGDs are *speech aid devices*.

As a starting point, consider the plain meaning of the phrase *speech aid devices*. It supports the conclusion that SGDs are both "speech aids" and "devices." SGDs are most assuredly *devices*. Equally clear is that they are *speech aids*. The word "aid" can be a noun or a verb. Its plain meaning as a noun is as help or assistance; as a verb it is an item that helps, assists, or supports a person or thing to achieve something; *an assisting device*.[286] SGDs are assisting devices that serve as a functional complement to or replacement for an individual's speaking ability that is impaired by condition, illness, or injury.

There also are numerous health benefits sources, including United Healthcare, that define SGDs as *speech aid devices*.

Examples among publicly funded programs include Medicare. It defines SGDs as *speech aids*:

> [SGDs] are defined as durable medical equipment that provides an individual who has a severe speech impairment with the ability to meet [their] functional, speaking needs. [SGDs] are speech aids consisting of devices or software that generate speech and are used solely by the individual who has a severe speech impairment.[287]

So too does Tricare,[288] the Veterans Administration,[289] Georgia Medicaid,[290] and New Hampshire Medicaid.[291]

Numerous insurers also define SGDs as *speech aids*.[292]

United Healthcare has defined SGDs as *speech aids*, too. Oxford Health Plans is a subsidiary of United Healthcare. It issued SGD guidelines applicable to "Oxford Commercial Plan membership" effective December 1, 2011, that defined SGDs as speech aids.[293] United Healthcare has also approved at least six SGD purchase requests for clients whose policy or plan text includes the "devices and computers to assist communication and speech" exclusion and the exception for speech aid devices.[294]

There is no clear threshold stating how many examples or from which sources will be enough to establish that SGDs fit the speech aid device exception. Clearly, a greater number will be more persuasive than fewer. Thus, a search for and review of insurer and plan SGD guidelines that is as extensive as possible will be necessary. Also, requests to the insurer or plan for additional decisions approving SGDs as speech aid devices should be submitted. Ultimately, the strategy will be to require the insurer or plan to rebut as many examples from as many sources as possible that support the conclusion SGDs are speech aid devices.[295]

Health Plan Exclusions. There are two primary types of privately funded sources of health benefits in the United States: insurance policies and employer-sponsored health benefits plans. Health plans are authorized by a federal law known as ERISA.[296] One characteristic of health plans is that they are not governed by state insurance laws. This freedom makes it possible for companies with employees in more than one state to offer all employees a uniform menu of benefits. That outcome might be difficult and expensive to achieve or might not otherwise be possible because state regulation of health insurance policies is not uniform. Other employers may just find it less costly to create a health plan than to purchase one of the available health insurance policies.

Another characteristic of health plans is that employers may have no expertise to design, to estimate the costs, or to administer one (including review of benefits requests and appeals). To accomplish these tasks, employers may hire a consultant, often a health insurer. Once the plan is established, the plan designer—insurer—also may be hired to administer the plan. One outcome of this relationship is that insurers with a history of including SGD exclusions into their insurance policies, such as United Healthcare, have inserted these exclusions into the plans they design. As a result, several plans have been identified with an exclusion for "comfort or convenience items," one example of which is stated to be "devices and computers to assist communication and speech." This exclusion has then been cited as the basis for denial of SGD purchase requests by plan beneficiaries—often the young children of company employees.

A strategy has been developed and applied successfully to get past plan SGD exclusions such as this one. Clients, through their advocates, ask the employer to remove the exclusion from the plan. A "just ask" strategy has as its basis the following core facts:

- There is no factual and no cost-basis to exclude SGDs, and that except for the exclusion, SGDs would "fit" within the plan's existing scope of covered benefits
- It is unlikely any employer ever insisted that SGDs be excluded
- It is unlikely any employer ever discussed a factual basis for the exclusion with the plan's designer
- It is unlikely any employer had ever been told the additional cost to the plan if SGDs were covered, or the cost-savings to the plan because the exclusion is present
- It is unlikely any employer could identify a specific benefit to the plan served by the exclusion or could assert the benefit was greater than the harm it caused to a member of the plan sponsor's corporate family by not being able to communicate effectively

From this foundation, a report was written to persuade employers to erase-delete-remove the SGD exclusion. It began by conceding this was only a request. There was no *"or else."* There was no legal duty on the part of the plan to remove the exclusion. Instead, the report stated its intent was *to persuade* the employer this was an exclusion it will want to delete because it saved no dollars and made no sense, and its only effect was to impose gratuitous harm on a member of its corporate family, as noted, often a child, which clearly is *not* a goal or purpose of any health benefits plan.

The report was divided into five sections that were proposed as review criteria for the plan sponsor to use. If any was not met, the request to remove the exclusion should be denied:

- SGDs fit within the plan's DME benefit, and except for the exclusion, they would be covered when medically necessary

- The exclusion has no factual support: SGDs have been recognized for several decades as treatment for severe communication impairments, for those identified as needing an SGD, they will supplement or substitute for other methods of expression that by themselves have not enabled the person to meet daily communication needs, and there is no factual basis to conclude that SGDs are "comfort or convenience" items

- The exclusion most likely was inserted in the plan by the plan designer, not at the request of the employer, and it is likely its factual basis, cost, or impact on the plan or plan beneficiaries were never discussed. In addition, the exclusion does not represent the opinion about SGDs held and applied by the plan designer (United Healthcare, for example, is one of if not the largest health insurance funding source for SGDs), by more than a thousand other insurers and health benefits plans, or by every system of health benefits in the United States, including Medicare, Medicaid programs in every state, Tricare, and the Veterans Administration.

- If covered, SGDs will have no actuarial impact on the plan

- SGDs are not a "Trojan horse" for any other item or service to demand coverage under the plan

Since 2007, this "just ask" strategy has led to the elimination of SGD exclusions by a dozen employer-sponsored plans. These employers range in size from approximately 2,000 employees to more than 330,000 employees. As a group, they employ almost a million workers, and they provide health benefits to more than 2.5 million. It is clear the size of the plan does not affect the employer's willingness to eliminate SGD exclusions shown to be both without factual or cost foundation and harmful.[297]

Summary

This chapter illuminated the "path to 'yes'" to SGD funding and access that has been created over the past 4 decades through the efforts of speech-language pathologists, clients, their families, SGD manufacturers and suppliers, and advocates. As time passes, this path continues to become easier to navigate.

It has been said that "you know you've won when things become routine." *Routine SGD acceptance and access* might be the label assigned to the third phase of AAC intervention following its pioneering phase and public policy phase.[298] By that measure, AAC and SGD interventions are still transitioning to this third phase. While routine acceptance of SGDs as health benefits largely has been achieved, the process to achieve routine SGD access and funding by health benefits sources is still a work in progress. Some barriers remain and the funding process takes too long. Nonetheless, it is fair to say there is a strong presumption that requests for SGD funding from health benefits sources will be approved and needed communication tools will be provided. As this process advances to a period of routine SGD access, all interested parties must prepare to meet the challenges achieving this goal will create. The world is going to get a lot noisier.

Study Questions

1. How does "funding" for SGDs from health benefits sources overlap with speech-language pathologists' professional roles and responsibilities?

2. Why are health benefits sources pursued as the primary funding source for SGDs?

3. Why is it necessary to establish SGDs are "covered" by health benefits sources, and on what basis are they covered?

4. Why is it necessary to establish SGDs are "medically necessary" as defined by health benefits sources, and on what basis are they medically necessary?

5. Once SGD need is established, why must speech-language pathologists identify the least costly, equally effective SGD, and how is this device identified?

6. Can third party payers use exclusions to deny coverage for SGDs? If so, what criteria must these exclusions follow in order to have legal standing?

7. In what way(s) is funding of SGDs different between children and adults? In what way(s) is funding similar between the two?

8. Describe thoroughly the speech-language pathologist's role in the SGD funding process.

ENDNOTES

Documents referenced in this chapter will be provided by the United States Society for Augmentative and Alternative Communication upon request.

1. This chapter will only use the phrase "speech-generating devices," or SGDs. At present, speech-generating device is the generally accepted phrase among the funding programs discussed. Although several other phrases have been used to describe these devices (e.g., augmentative and alternative communication devices, augmentative communication devices, augmentative communication systems, and voice output communication aids), they are not used here and should not be used by speech-language pathologists when seeking speech-generating device funding on a client's behalf. More contemporary phrases, such as "mobile technology," and more generic phrases, such as "low-tech," "mid-tech," and "high-tech" devices, are also not used here and should not be considered appropriate for use in speech-generating device funding requests or appeals.

2. *See* 20 United States Code (USC) §§ 1412(a)(12)(A)(i); (B) (the financial duty of other public agencies "shall precede the financial responsibility of the local education agency" for the cost of developing students with disabilities' Individualized Education Programs).

3. *See e.g., Fred C. v. Texas Health & Hum. Serv. Comm'n*, 988 F.Supp. 1032, 1035n.3 (W.D.Tex. 1997) *affirmed per curiam*, 167 F.3d 537 (5th Cir. 1998) (discussing four-part test in the context of Medicaid); 68 Fed. Reg. 55,634, 55,635, 2003 WL 22213011 (F.R.) (Sept. 26, 2003) (discussing same in the context of Medicare).

4. 42 USC § 1396d(a)(12); 42 Code of Federal Regulations (CFR) § 440.120.

5. 42 USC § 1396d(a)(10)(D); 42 USC § 1396d(a)(7); 42 CFR § 440.70(b)(3)(ii).

6. 42 USC § 1396d(a)(11); 42 CFR § 440.110.

7. 42 USC § 1396d(a)(13); 42 CFR § 440.130.

8. 42 USC § 1396d(a)(4)(A); 42 CFR § 440.140; 42 CFR Part 483.

9. 42 USC § 1396d(a)(15); 42 CFR § 440.150; 42 CFR Part 483.

10. 42 USC §§ 300gg-6(a); 18021(a)(1)B); 18022(b)(1)(G); 45 CFR Part 156.

11. Other programs' use of Medicare's benefits descriptions are voluntary. Medicare guidance is likely followed because Medicare is the nation's largest health benefits program.

12. 42 USC § 1395x(n). By using the word "includes," the items listed in this text are being presented as examples of covered durable medical equipment items rather than as an exclusive list of covered devices. Also, in legislation commonly known as the Steve Gleason Act, "eye tracking and gaze interaction accessories for SGDs furnished to individuals with a demonstrated medical need for such accessories" were added as examples of covered durable medical equipment items. The Steve Gleason Act was enacted in 2015 as a temporary measure, Pub.L.No. 114-40 (July 30, 3015). Its text was made permanent in February 2018, Pub.L.No. 115-123 (Feb. 9, 2018)).

13. 42 CFR § 414.202. This definition has been amended to add a fifth criterion applicable to equipment items classified by Medicare as durable medical equipment after January 1, 2012. These items must have an expected useful life of at least 3 years. This criterion does not apply to speech-generating devices, but if it did, they would satisfy it.

14. Medicare also states that an item is considered durable if it is "the type of item which could normally be rented." Soc. Sec. Admin. Program Operations Manual System (POMS) § HI 00610.200(A) This characteristic can be cited when applicable (*i.e.*, when the speech-language pathologist can establish the equipment item sought is able to be rented). The ability of a device to be rented can be determined by asking its manufacturer or supplier. It can also be established by review of the funding program's durable medical equipment fee schedule. If the relevant code for the device is present and there is a line for this code with the prefix "RR," then the equipment in that code can be rented.

15. 76 Fed. Reg.70228 (Nov. 10, 2011) (amending 42 CFR § 414.202) (making a 3-year minimum useful life a criterion for equipment items to be classified as durable medical equipment after January 1, 2012); *see also* 78 Fed. Reg. 40836, 40877 (July 8, 2013) ("The 3 years MLR is designed to represent a minimum threshold for a determination of durability for a piece of equipment. The 3 year MLR is not an indication of the typical or average lifespan of DME, which in many cases is far longer than 3 years …").

16. *In re: Martin B.*, slip op. at 3, Soc. Sec. Admin. Office of Hrgs & Appeals (Nov. 29, 2001).

17. Therapeutic, according to Stedman's Medical Dictionary, means "related to treatment of disease," which is also the definition of "therapy."

18. *Blue v. Bonta*, 99 Cal.App.4th 980, 989 121 Cal.Rptr.2d 483 (1st District 2002).

19. By contrast, no health benefits source limits treatment to interventions that will cure or correct a condition.

20. To ameliorate means "to make better or more tolerable." *Collins v. Hamilton*, 231 F.Supp.2d 840, 849 (S.D. In. 2002), *aff'd* 349 F.3d 371 (7th Cir. 2003); *accord Ekloff v. Rodgers*, 443 F.Supp.2d 1173, 1180 (D. Ariz. 2006), or to lessen the severity of its effects: to reduce the disability associated with a condition. *K.G. ex rel Garrido v. Dudek*, 839 F.Supp.2d 1254, 1277 (S.D. Fla. 2011); *Dudek*, 864 F.Supp.2d 1314 (S.D. Fla. 2013).

21. "Habilitative services, including devices, are provided for a person to attain, maintain, or prevent deterioration of a skill or function never learned or acquired due to a disabling condition." Examples include "therapy for a child who is not walking or talking at the expected age." 80 Fed. Reg. 10811; 10871 (Feb. 27, 2015); 45 C.F.R. § 156.115(a)(5). *See also Mosby's Medical Dictionary* (8th Ed.)(2009) (Habilitation: "the process of supplying a person with the means to develop maximum independence in activities of daily living through training or treatment.").

22. "Rehabilitative services, including devices, … are provided to help a person regain, maintain, or prevent deterioration of a skill or function that has been acquired but then lost or impaired due to illness, injury, or disabling condition." 80 Fed. Reg. 10811 (Feb. 27, 2015).

23. Beukelman, D., Yorkston, K., & Garrett, K., An Introduction to AAC Services for Adults with Chronic Medical Conditions: Who, What, When, Where and Why 4, in Beukelman, Garrett & Yorkston Eds., *Augmentative Communication Strategies* (2007). *See also* Medicare Local Coverage Determination for Speech Generating Devices, L33739, "Coverage Indications, Limitations and/or Medical Necessity," 1(b); *Myers v. State of Mississippi*, 3:94 CV 185LN Slip op at 2-3 (S.D.Miss. 1995) (Speech-generating devices "are recognized as a form of speech-language pathology treatment which is used when other forms of treatment are unsuccessful in allowing the patient to organically produce speech").

24. ASHA, "Position Statement on Non-Speech Communication," 23 *Asha* 577-581 (August 1981).

25. Am. Speech-Lang.-Hearing Assoc., Scope of Practice in Speech-Language Pathology, at p. 7 (2007); Am. Speech-Lang.-Hearing Assoc., Preferred Practice Patterns for the Profession of Speech-Language Pathology: § 26 Augmentative and Alternative Communication Assessment; § 27 Augmentative and Alternative Communication Intervention; § 28 Prosthetic/Adaptive Device Assessment; § 29 Prosthetic/Adaptive Device Intervention, at pp. 75-88 (2004); Am. Speech-Lang.-Hearing Assoc., Roles and Responsibilities of Speech-Language Pathologists with Respect to Augmentative and Alternative Communication: Technical Report (2004); Am. Speech-Lang.-Hearing Assoc., Augmentative and Alternative Communication: Knowledge and Skills for Service Delivery (2002); Am. Speech-Lang.-Hearing Assoc., Scope of Practice in Speech-Language Pathology, at pp. 1-28, 30 (2001); Am. Speech-Lang.-Hearing Assoc., Preferred Practice Patterns for the Profession of Speech-Language Pathology, at § 12.3 Augmentative and Alternative Communication Assessment, § 15.2 Augmentative and Alternative Communication System and/or Device Treatment/Orientation, at pp. 1-142; 165-166 (1997); Am. Speech-Lang.-Hearing Assoc., Preferred Practice Patterns for Speech-Language Pathology, § 30.3 Augmentative and Alternative Communication Assessment,; § 31.1 Augmentative and Alternative Communication System Fitting/Orientation," at pp. 61-62; 87- 88 (1992); Am. Speech-Lang.-Hearing Assoc., Augmentative and Alternative Communication: Position Statement, 33 Asha (Suppl. 5), 8 (1991); Am. Speech-Lang.-Hearing Assoc., Competencies for Speech-Language-Pathologists Providing Services in Augmentative Communication, 31 Asha 107-110 (1989).

26. Zangari, Lloyd & Vicker, "Augmentative and Alternative Communication: An Historic Perspective," 10 AAC 27-59 (1994); G. Vanderheiden & D. Yoder, "Overview," in S. Blackstone, Ph.D., Ed. Augmentative & Alternative Communication: An Introduction 10-13 (1986); see also Hourcade, Pilotte, West & Parette, "A History of Augmentative and Alternative Communication for Individuals with Severe and Profound Disabilities, Focus on Autism and Other Developmental Disabilities 19:235-244 (2004). A literature review, current through 1999, was prepared for Medicare staff that was re-examining its speech-generating device coverage policy. It reviewed the professional literature regarding the effectiveness of augmentative and alternative communication interventions, including speech-generating devices, as treatment for dysarthria, apraxia, and aphasia. L. Golinker (Ed.) Formal Request for National Coverage Decision for Augmentative and Alternative Communication Devices, Section 3 (Dec. 1999) [hereafter, "Formal Request"].

27. Letter dated March 22, 2000 to Hugh Hill, M.D., from Francis I. Kittredge, Jr., M.D., President, American Academy of Neurology.

28. Letter dated March 21, 2000 to Hugh Hill, M.D., from J. Ratcliffe Anderson, Jr., M.D., Executive Vice President, American Medical Association.

29. Letter dated March 23, 2000 to Hugh Hill, M.D., from Ronald Henrichs, Executive Director, American Academy of Physical Medicine and Rehabilitation.

30. L. Desch, D. Gaebler-Spira, & Council on Children with Disabilities, Special Report: Prescribing Assistive-Technology Systems: Focus on Children with Impaired Communication, Pediatrics, 121:1271-1280 (June 2008).

31. 48 Fed. Reg. 53049 (November 23, 1983), codifying 21 CFR § 890.3710 (emphasis added).

32. 42 USC § 1395y(a)(1)(A).

33. U.S. Centers for Medicare & Medicaid Services Medicare & You, 2022, at p. 123 (defining "medically necessary").

34. Detsel v. Sullivan, 895 F.2d 58, 64 (2nd Cir. 1990); Skubel v. Fuoroli, 113 F.3d 330 (2nd Cir. 1997).

35. Beukelman & Mirenda, Augmentative and Alternative Communication 104 (1992). See also Beukelman, Garrett, & Yorkston, Augmentative Communication Strategies for Adults with Acute or Chronic Medical Conditions 4 (2007) ("The general definition for AAC used in most legal, educational and funding activities is similar to the following: AAC is needed by individuals with such complex communication limitations that they are unable to meet their daily communication needs through natural speech [and/or language]."); Medicare RMRP (now LCD) for Speech Generating Devices (2001); Myers v. State of Mississippi, No. 3:94- CIV- 185 LN (S.D. Miss. June 23, 1995) (Speech-generating devices are "electronic and nonelectronic devices that allow individuals to overcome, to the maximum extent possible, communication limitations that interfere with their daily activities.").

36. National Joint Committee for the Communicative Needs of Persons with Severe Disabilities. (1992). "Guidelines for Meeting the Communication Needs of Persons with Severe Disabilities," 34 Asha (Supp. 7) at 2-3.

37. H. Shane, "Goals and Uses [of AAC Interventions] in S. Blackstone, Ed. Augmentative and Alternative Communication: An Introduction 29, 40 (1986).

38. See e.g., L. Ball, D. Beukelman & L. Bardach, Amyotrophic Lateral Sclerosis, in Beukelman, Garrett, & Yorkston, Eds., Augmentative Communication Strategies at 287-316 (2007); L. Ball, Adults with Acquired Physical Disabilities, in D. Beukelman & P. Mirenda, Augmentative and Alternative Communication 435-447 (3rd Ed.) (2005); Ball, Beukelman & Pattee, "Acceptance of Augmentative and Alternative Communication Technology by Persons with Amyotrophic Lateral Sclerosis," 20 AAC 113 (2004) (study showed people with amyotrophic lateral sclerosis who used speech-generating devices continued to use them through the end of life); P. Mathy, K. Yorkston, & M. Guttmann, AAC for Individuals with Amyotrophic Lateral Sclerosis, in D. Beukelman, K. Yorkston & J. Reichle, Augmentative and Alternative Communication for Adults with Acquired Neurologic Disorders 183-232 (2000).

39. P. Mathy, K. Yorkston, & M. Guttmann, AAC for Individuals with Amyotrophic Lateral Sclerosis, in D. Beukelman, K. Yorkston & J. Reichle, Augmentative and Alternative Communication for Adults with Acquired Neurologic Disorders 183 (2000).

40. R. Miller, M.D., Amyotrophic Lateral Sclerosis Standard of Care Consensus, in ALS Consensus Conf., at p. S 35 (1997); R. Sufit, M.D., Symptomatic Treatment of ALS, in id. at S.15. See also Letter dated March 21, 2000 to Hugh Hill, M.D., from E. Ratcliffe Anderson, Jr., M.D., Executive Vice President and CEO, American Medical Association.

41. D. Beukelman & P. Mirenda, Augmentative and Alternative Communication 73 (2nd Ed.) (1998) (comparing rate of speech production using natural speech and with speech-generating devices).

42. Roget's Thesaurus (3rd Ed. 1962); Webster's New Collegiate Dictionary (1975).

43. Environmental control: the ability to control electronic mechanisms that will turn lights on or off; open or close windows, shades, or blinds; change the temperature of a thermostat; control the features of a television; turn an air conditioner or fan on or off; or open, close, lock, or unlock doors were novelties for the general public when speech-generating devices were first introduced in the late 1970s—a convenience. All these tasks could be performed by members of the general public with their hands, at no charge. No one would be expected to purchase a speech-generating device for thousands of dollars to accomplish the same outcomes.

44. See Medicare National Coverage Determination for Speech Generating Devices # 50.1 (2015); Medicare Local Coverage Determination for Speech Generating Devices # L33739 (2015); Medicare Local Coverage Article for Speech Generating Devices # A52469 (2015).

45. See Formal Request at 57.

46. *Id.* (referencing Maine Medicaid SGD guideline); *see also id.*, at 57-58 (discussing New Hampshire, New York and Ohio Medicaid SGD guidelines).

47. *See* Medicare National Coverage Determination for Speech Generating Devices, # 50.1 (2001).

48. Letter to Lewis Golinker from Thomas Hoyer, Director, Chronic Care Policy Group, Center for Health Plans and Providers, Health Care Financing Administration (May 4, 2001). A more complete discussion of Medicare's acceptance of computer-based speech-generating devices is posted at http://aacfundinghelp.com/funding_programs (Medicare history). In 2015, Medicare again updated its National Coverage Determination for speech-generating devices to clarify and expand the scope of acceptable speech-generating device features. Medicare National Coverage Determination for Speech Generating Devices, # 50.1 (2015).

49. *See* Medicare National Coverage Determination for Speech Generating Devices # 50.1 (2015). Medicare also stated: "We also believe the 'dedication' requirement is overly restrictive." *Id.* However, that statement amounts to a distinction without a difference. The modifications that will make a speech-generating device limited to use by people with severe speech impairment, and to be used primarily for speech generation, are not meaningfully different than what was required to make speech-generating devices dedicated.

50. Medicare Local Coverage Article for Speech-Generating Devices # A52469 (2015).

51. Suggesting that off-the-shelf tablet computers represent a new "type" or class of speech-generating devices is more than just a historic inaccuracy. It also represents indifference to potential speech-generating device funding barriers. If these devices are a new speech-generating device type or class, they will have to go through all the steps outlined in this chapter to establish they qualify for funding: that they meet the requirements to be covered, are medically necessary, and not otherwise excluded. If defined as a new speech-generating device type or class, existing professional literature about speech-generating devices may be deemed inapplicable, possibly delaying acceptance for speech-generating device funding purposes for years. In short, discussion of these devices as a new speech-generating device type or class in professional literature or in funding requests has great potential to cause totally preventable self-inflicted injury to people with complex communication needs. Speech-generating devices based on off-the-shelf tablet computers should only be discussed as new models within the existing class of SGDs coded E2510.

52. Funding issues related to Tablet + App + Case speech-generating devices have often been misstated as "coverage" issues when the actual basis is that there is no participating supplier. Health benefits sources have rules related to suppliers of services and devices. However, several possible sources of these devices, such as online vendors and department stores, have not gone through this process. For this reason, despite coverage of these devices, health benefits source funding for them may not be available.

53. Practice Note: Because these devices may be sold in either their "dedicated" configuration or "open," allowing access to all their computer and speech-generating functions, it is essential that speech-language pathologists always recommend that the dedicated models of these devices be provided. If clients are interested in accessing additional device features, they can be "unlocked" (i.e., those features can be restored to operational status) after the device is delivered and the funding procedure is complete.

54. *See* Medicare Local Coverage Article: Speech-Generating Devices (SGD) - Policy Article # A52469 (2015).

55. Also note that the key phrase is "designed for," which is not affected by the fact that speech-generating devices are also used in in-patient settings, such as hospitals and nursing facilities.

56. See 42 USC § 1395x(n).

57. A durable medical equipment definition may refer to examples of the types of devices that are covered by stating: "items such as" or "items including."

58. *In re: Donald S.* slip op. at 3-4 (Soc. Sec. Admin. Office of Hrgs & App. 1999) ("[M]any commonly recognized items that Medicare approves as durable medical equipment do not cure an illness but rather treat the effects of an illness. A wheelchair is an obvious example. It is the means to treat the effects of an illness and provides a substitute for the body part that is not functioning.").

59. The Food and Drug Administration, for example, placed speech-generating devices in the same category of medical devices as power wheelchairs. 21 CFR Part 890.

60. The origin of the communication chain metaphor can be traced to F. deSaussure *Course in General Linguistics* (1916). It is also used in C. Shannon & W. Weaver, *The Mathematical Theory of Communication* (1949); P. Denes & E. Pinson, *The Speech Chain: the Physics and Biology of Spoken Language* (1963) and more recently D. Crystal & R. Varley, *Introduction to Language Pathology* (4th Ed.) (1999).

61. *See* Letter to Lewis Golinker from Peggy Locke, President, Communication Aid Manufacturers Association (CAMA) (Oct. 23, 1999).

62. *E.g., In re: Donald S.* slip op. at 3-4 (Soc. Sec. Admin. Office of Hrgs & App. 1999); *In re: Anonymous-II* (Minn. Dept. of Hum. Serv. 1984) (Minnesota Medicaid); *In re: John P.*, No. 7454-82 (N.J. Office of Admin. Law 1982) (New Jersey Medicaid); *In re: Kevin K.*, No. 2938-81 (N.J. Office of Admin. Law 1981) (same); *In re: Anthony M.*, No. 1360-79 (N.J. Office of Admin. Law 1979) (same).

63. 42 CFR § 440.110(c).

64. *Wilder v. VA. Hosp. Assoc.*, 496 U.S. 498, 502 (1990) ("Although participation in the program is voluntary, participating States must comply with certain requirements imposed by the Act and regulations promulgated by the Secretary of Health and Human Services.")

65. *Meyers v. Reagan*, 776 F.2d 241, 243 (8th Cir. 1985).

66. *Conley v. Dep't. of Health*, 287 P.3d 452 (Utah App. 2012).

67. *Rush v. Parham*, 625 F.2d 1150, 1157n.12 (5th Cir. 1980).

68. *Hope Med. Grp. v. Edwards*, 63 F.3d 418 (5th Cir. 1995) (coverage limitations not based on medical need factors are impermissible); *Bristol v. R.I. Dept. of Hum. Serv.*, 1997 WL 839884 (R.I. Super. Jan. 30, 1997) (coverage policy that does not and cannot respond to medical necessity is arbitrary and capricious).

69. 81 Fed. Reg. 5539 (col 1.) (Feb. 2, 2016).

70. 42 USC § 1396a(a)(17).

71. Letter to State Medicaid Directors from Sally K. Richardson, Director, Center for Medicaid and State Operations, Health Care Financing Administration (Sept. 4, 1998).

72. *Slekis v. Thomas*, 525 U.S. 1098 (1999) *vacating DeSario v. Thomas*, 139 F.3d 80 (2nd Cir. 1998).

73. *Detgen v. Janek*, 752 F.3d 627, 632 (5th Cir. 2014).

74. 80 Fed. Reg. 5539 (col. 1) (Feb. 2, 2016).

75. 42 CFR § 440.70(b)(3)(v).

76. "[B]ecause of the unique nature of medical supplies, equipment, and appliances, scope limitations within the applicable federal and state definitions are not consistent with sufficiency of the benefit." 81 Fed. Reg. 5539 (col 1.) (Feb. 2, 2016).

77. *Fred C. v. Texas Health & Hum. Serv. Comm'n*, 924 F.Supp. 788 (W.D.Tex. 1996), *vacated and remanded on other grounds per curiam*, 117 F.3d 1416 (5th Cir. 1997); *on remand*, 988 F.Supp. 1032, 1036 (W.D.Tex. 1997), *affirmed per curiam* 167 F.3d 537 (5th Cir. 1998).

78. *See Hunter v. Chiles*, 944 F.Supp. 914 (S.D.Fl. 1996); *Conley v. Dept. of Health*, 287 P.3d 452 (Utah App. 2012).

79. National Joint Committee for the Communication Needs of Persons with Severe Disabilities (2002) Access to communication services and supports: Concerns regarding the application of restrictive "eligibility" policies [Technical Report] at page 6.

80. 20 USC § 1400 et seq.; 34 CFR § 300.17.

81. 34 CFR § 300.34.

82. 34 CFR § 300.105(a)(2).

83. 42 USC § 1396b(c).

84. *Hunter v. Chiles*, 944 F.Supp. 914 (S.D.FL. 1996).

85. Letter to Mary Jo Butler from Madeline Will, Assistant Secretary, Office of Special Education Programs (OSEP) (March 25, 1988), Individuals with Disabilities Education Law Reporter § 213:118-121 ("[T]he statute and regulations reflect the recognition that required related services for a child with a [disability] could include services traditionally regarded as health-related services, in circumstances where the child needs those services to benefit from special education.").

86. FY 2002 National Defense Authorization Act, Pub.L. No. 107-107§ 702(2) (Dec. 28, 2001), *amending* 10 USC § 1077(a)(15) (authorizing expansion of Tricare SGD coverage as prosthetic devices); FY 2009 Military Construction, Veterans Affairs & Related Agencies Appropriation Bill, S.Rep.No. 110-428, 110th Cong. 2nd Sess. 2008 2008 WL 2814665 (Leg.Hist.) ("[T]he Committee encourages the Department [of Veterans Benefits] to increase funding for the treatment of severe communication disabilities through use of speech communication aids and the speech and language therapists who prescribe them.")

87. Some health benefits sources describe their prosthetic device coverage by a declarative statement limiting coverage to specific items. This is the most restrictive way to offer this benefit category. Most frequently, the only items listed as covered are artificial limbs. Speech-generating devices will be covered as prosthetic devices when coverage is described in this manner only if they are specifically identified as covered.

88. 42 CFR § 404.202.

89. Medicare Claims Processing Manual, Ch. 20, § 10.1.2.

90. Medicare National Coverage Determinations Manual, Ch. 1, Part 1, § 50.2.

91. Medicare National Coverage Determinations Manual, Ch. 1, Part 1, § 50.4.

92. *See McKenzie v. Carolina Care Plan*, 2005 WL 6111629, * 2, * 6 (D.S.C. July 25, 2005); *aff'd in part* 467 F.3d 383, 386, 388 (4th Cir. 2006).

93. *See* comments to draft revised Medicare NCD for SGDs (2015) ("speech-generating devices are speech aids.").

94. 68 Fed. Reg. 18577 (April 16, 2003) (adding definition of "speech-generating devices" to 32 CFR § 199.2 [definitions]).

95. Anthem Clinical UM Guideline: Augmentative and Alternative Communication (AAC) Devices / Speech Generating Devices (SGD), CG-DME-07 (Discussion/General Information) (Sept. 27, 2017).

96. This is the New York Medicaid definition of medical need. 18 NYCRR §§ 513.0; 513.1(c).

97. That speech-language pathologists have been delegated responsibility to identify medical need is all but unique. The determination of medical need is almost exclusively reserved for physicians. But for speech-generating devices, there is general acceptance among health benefits sources that the physician's role is secondary; they review the speech-language pathology recommendation report and write a prescription for the speech-generating device and, as needed, mount and access aids. (See Medicare SGD Coverage Guideline, item 6.)

98. Practice Note: Complementing speech-generating device guidelines are templates that speech-language pathologists can use as aids to report writing. They can be found at speech-generating device manufacturers' web pages, and there is an augmentative and alternative communication Report Coach, posted at www.aacfundinghelp.com. These templates generally follow the report outline stated in the Medicare speech-generating device guidelines.

99. Medicare Local Coverage Determination for SGDs # L33739 (2015).

100. *See* Raghavendra, P., Bornman, J., Granlund, M., & Bjorck-Akesson, E. (2007) "The World Health Organization's international classification of functioning, disability and health: implications for clinical and research practice in the field of augmentative and alternative communication," AAC, 23(4): 349-361.

101. *See Formal Request*, at 18-37 (1999).

102. Letter dated March 21, 2000 to Hugh Hill, M.D., from J. Ratcliffe Anderson, Jr., M.D., Executive Vice President, American Medical Association; Letter dated March 22, 2000 to Hugh Hill, M.D., from Francis I. Kittredge, Jr., M.D., President, American Academy of Neurology; Letter dated March 23, 2000 to Hugh Hill, M.D., from Ronald Henrichs, Executive Director, American Academy of Physical Medicine and Rehabilitation. *See also* Miller, Sufit, Mitsumoto, Gelinas & Brooks, (1997) "ALS standard of care consensus," in Miller, R., Ed., "Amyotrophic lateral sclerosis standard of care consensus conference," *Neurology* 48(Suppl. 4): S33, 35; R. Sufit, "Symptomatic treatment of ALS," in *id.* at S 15. The American Academy of Pediatrics' support is stated in L. Desch, D. Gaebler-Spira, & Council on Children with Disabilities (June 2008), "Special Report: Prescribing assistive-technology systems: focus on children with impaired communication," *Pediatrics* 121: 1271-1280 (June 2008).

103. H. Shane, "Goals and Uses," in S. Blackstone, Ed., *Augmentative Communication: An Introduction* 35-36 (Rockville, MD: ASHA 1986).

104. D. Beukelman & P. Mirenda, *Augmentative and Alternative Communication* 154, 158 (4th Ed.) (2013) ("It is important to realize that thousands of successful AAC interventions have been instituted without formal documentation of cognitive abilities.")

105. Factors, such as whether the exchange is face-to-face, by phone, across a counter, or other barrier, in a noisy or quiet environment, whether there are sensory or language issues for the partner. See http://www.augcominc.com/index.cfm/social_networks.htm.

106. D. Beukelman & P. Mirenda. *Augmentative and Alternative Communication* 104 (1st Ed.) (1992).

107. National Joint Commission for the Communicative Needs of Person with Severe Disabilities, "Guidelines for Meeting the Communication Needs of Persons with Severe Disabilities," 34 *Asha* (Supp. 7) at 2-3 (1992).

108. *See In re: A.H.*, FH # 7319049Z Slip Op. at 11 (N.Y. Dept. of Health Sept. 14, 2016) ("The Agency claims that the documentation provided did not establish that the Appellant has mastered his lower tech/no-tech communication systems … The Appellant's attorney responded that there is no requirement in the Medicaid guidelines regarding SGD coverage that an individual 'has mastered his lower tech/no-tech communication systems' as a prerequisite for any SGD approval.")

109. J. Tavalaro & R. Tayson, *Look Up for Yes* 13, 33, 121 (1997).

110. Light, J. (1989) Toward a Definition of Communicative Competence for Individuals Using Augmentative and Alternative Communication Systems, *AAC* 5(2): 137-145; D. Beukelman and P. Mirenda, *Augmentative and Alternative Communication* 280 (4th Ed.) (Baltimore: Brookes Publ. 2013).

111. Health benefits sources can be expected to not object to a speech-generating device being part of a broader range of strategies and tools that may include speech, gesture, facial expression or eye gaze, and non–voice output augmentative and alternative solutions, such as a communication board or book that will be used for specific communication situations. But among this array of tools, it is common that they will limit funding to one speech-generating device at a time.

112. J. Light, "Shattering the Silence," In J. Light, D. Beukelman & J. Reichle, *Communicative Competence for Individuals who use AAC* 3-38 (2003).

113. Light, J., (1997) "Communication is the Essence of Human Life:" Reflections on Communicative Competence, *AAC* 13, 61-70.

114. One funding source characterized the most appropriate equipment as "The SGD and related accessories [that] must allow members to improve their communication to a functional level not achievable without an SGD or less costly device." New York Department of Health, Durable Medical Equipment, Prosthetics, Orthotics, and Supplies Procedure Codes and Coverage Guidelines: Speech Generating Devices, Coverage Guidelines: Speech Generating Devices (SGDs) and Related Accessories, ¶ 1(i) at 113-121.

115. A similar system exists for medical services, known as CPT.

116. By definition, non–voice output tools, such as communication boards, books, or cards, are not speech-generating devices. These items are coded E1902: Communication board, nonelectronic augmentative or alternative communication device. In general, health benefits programs do not provide funding for their creation or purchase.

117. In *BZ v. Zucker*, 16-CV-5593 (MKB) Mem. And Order (E.D.N.Y. Nov. 8, 2017). New York Medicaid claimed a child should use eye-gaze boards. However, Medicaid refused to provide a paid communication assistant responsible for holding and changing the eye-gaze boards so the client could access her messages. Medicaid could also not identify anyone else responsible to perform these tasks. The result: Medicaid could not establish that this non–voice output solution was an equally effective alternative to the speech-language pathologist's recommendation of an eye gaze–controlled speech-generating device. A court ordered Medicaid to provide the speech-generating device.

118. Bondy, Andy. 2001 PECS: potential benefits and risks. *The Behavior Analyst Today*, 1: 127-132, at 131.

119. D. Beukelman & J. Light *Augmentative and Alternative Communication* (5th Ed.)(2020) at 247.

120. Speech-language pathologists must also consider clients' ability to perform this task repeatedly. As part of this task, speech-language pathologists should not assume the overlay pages will be laminated for durability. Speech-language pathologists must inquire whether clients will have access to the device required to laminate pages. If not, speech-language pathologists must consider that the client will be responsible to carefully (and repeatedly) store, transport, sort, and remove and insert ordinary paper pages. Can the pages be handled without bending, tearing, or otherwise becoming unusable? The answer to this question will impact the decision whether multilevel digitized speech output devices should be ruled out.

121. *In re: A.S.*, FH # 7319049Z, Slip Op. at 11-12 (N.Y. Dept of Health Sept. 14, 2016).

122. *BZ v. Zucker*, 16-CV-5593 (E.D.N.Y.) (Transcript of Hearing on Plaintiffs' Motion for Preliminary Injunction, at 222) (October 11, 2017).

123. By contrast, speech-generating devices in the E2510 code do not support switch access for direct selection.

124. It is inappropriate to describe these speech-generating devices as able to produce an "unlimited" number of messages. No client has unlimited vocabulary; dictionaries have a finite number of entries. How then can a need be justified for a device with this feature? That there is no limit to the number of possible messages (and therefore, clients will be able to produce all they wish to express) is a more accurate description of this speech-generating device capability.

125. Medicaid recipients in particular are unlikely to have the financial resources to pay for this assistance, making the need for these services a very strong basis to rule out speech-generating devices that do not come with a full menu of postdevice delivery support.

126. The actual availability of these services is very important. Without them, it is reasonably foreseeable that the device will not be used effectively or possibly, at all. Stated another way, yes, some speech-generating device models have a lower purchase price, but for clients who need these services and may not be able to get them, there will be a steep price to pay if one of these lower-cost speech-generating device models is recommended. If speech-language pathologists conclude clients and their families will need but are not likely to receive these services, this should be reported as yet another reason to rule out lower-cost speech-generating devices.

127. D. Beukelman & P. Mirenda, *Augmentative and Alternative Communication* 148 (4th Ed.) (2013).

128. See Medicare National Coverage Determination for Speech Generating Devices # 50.1 (2015).

129. See Medicare Local Coverage Article: Speech Generating Devices (SGD) - Policy Article # A52469 (2015).

130. American Speech-Language-Hearing Assoc., "Position Statement on Non-Speech Communication," *Asha* 577-581 (Aug. 1981).

131. Letter to Donna Frescatore, Medical Director, Office of Health Insurance Programs, NY State Dep't. of Health, from Elise Davis-McFarland, Ph.D., CCC-SLP, ASHA President (Sept. 14, 2018).

132. Letter to Lewis Golinker from Wendy Quach, Ph.D., CCC-SLP, President and Pat Ourand, M.S., CCC-SLP, Vice President for Professional Affairs, USSAAC (March 20, 2017); Letter to Lewis Golinker from Jeffrey Riley, M.Sc. RSLP, Former President, International Society for Augmentative and Alternative Communication (March 18, 2016).

133. Speech-generating devices are expected to be useful to clients whenever and wherever the desire or need to speak arises. To meet this expectation, clients must be able to transfer the skills required to operate the speech-generating device to all typical communication environments. To establish this fact, actual use in all environments during the trial is not required. Speech-language pathologists can report instead that operational skills, once learned, are not setting-specific, and as a result, clients will be able to use the device in all typical communication settings. *See e.g., In re: J.T.* FH # 7232234Q, Slip Op. at 12 (N.Y. Dept. of Health July 19, 2017) ("However, the Appellant's [speech-language pathologist] asserted that there was no reason to believe that Appellant would not be able to successfully use the SGD at his group home. She asserted the staff at the group home could be trained as to how to calibrate the device so that the Appellant could use it there."); *see also In re: Anon.* FH # 6275526L, Slip Op. at 8 (N.Y. Dept. of Health March 27, 2013); *In re: Anon.*, FH # 5976412J, Slip Op. at 12 (N.Y. Dept. of Health May 9, 2012); *In re: Anon.*, FH # 5495700Z, Slip Op. at 7 (N.Y. Dept. of Health Nov. 15, 2010); *In re: Anon.*, FH # 5546540R, Slip Op. at 7 (N.Y. Dept. of Health Nov. 4, 2010).

134. New York State Medicaid Program, DME, Orthotics, Prosthetics and Supplies Manual: Procedure Codes and Coverage Guidelines: Speech Generating Devices, pp 104-112 (V. 2019-1) (Eff. Date August 1, 2019).

135. *See* https://en.oxforddictionaries.com/definition/mastery.

136. American Heritage Dictionary of the English Language (5th Ed 2016).

137. 137. Random House Kernerman Webster's College Dictionary (2010).

138. *See In re: JT, FH* # 7232234Q Slip Op. at 11 (N.Y. Dept of Health July 19, 2017) New York Medicaid provided no evidence to support "mastery" as an appropriate standard of post–speech-generating device trial performance or as a lawful speech-generating device eligibility standard).

139. D. Beukelman & P. Mirenda, *Augmentative and Alternative Communication* 11 (4th Ed.)(2013).

140. Light, J., (1997) "Communication is the Essence of Human Life:" Reflections on Communicative Competence, *AAC* 13, 61-70; J. Light, "Shattering the Silence," In J. Light, D. Beukelman & J. Reichle, *Communicative Competence for Individuals Who use AAC* 3-38 (2003).

141. The ability of children to develop strong performance skills using eye-gaze accessories has been studied and reported to require longer than a year. *E.g.*, Borgestig, M., Sandqvist, J., Parsons, R., Falkmer, T., & Hemmingsson, H., (2016), "Eye Gaze Performance for Children with Severe Physical Impairments Using Gaze-Based Assistive Technology–A Longitudinal Study," *Assistive Technology*, 28(2):93-102; Donegan, M., (2012), "Participatory Design: The Story of Jayne and Other Complex Cases," In Majaranta, P., et al., *Gaze Interaction and Applications of Eye Tracking: Advances in Assistive Technologies* 55-61; Donegan, M., & Oosthuizen, L., (2006), "The 'KEE' Concept for Eye-Control and Complex Disabilities: Knowledge-Based, End User-Focused and Evolutionary," In Proceedings of COGAIN 2006 "*Gazing into the Future*," 83-87.

142. 42 USC § 1396a(a)(17).

143. *Detsel v. Sullivan*, 895 F.2d 58 (2nd Cir. 1990); *Skubel v. Fuoroli*, 113 F.3d 330 (2nd Cir. 1997).

144. *See* U.S. Centers for Medicare & Medicaid Services *Medicare and You* 123 (2022)("Medically necessary—Health care services or supplies needed to diagnose or treat an illness, injury, condition, disease, or its symptoms and that meet accepted standards of medicine.").

145. Taken from the New York Medicaid definition of medical necessity. 18 NYCRR § 513.1.

146. 42 USC § 1396d(r) (federal Medicaid medical necessity standard is care that will "correct or ameliorate" conditions); U.S. Centers for Medicare & Medicaid Services, *EPSDT – A Guide for States* 23 (June 2014) ("States are permitted (but not required) to set parameters that apply to the determination of medical necessity in individual cases, but those parameters may not contradict or be more restrictive than the federal statutory requirements.").

147. 42 USC §§ 1396a(a)(4); 1396d(r). Additional services can be provided through The Individuals with Disabilities Education Act, 20 USC § 1400 et seq.

148. *See* https://www.medicare.gov/coverage/.

149. *See* https://www.tricare.mil/CoveredServices/IsItCovered/Speech Therapy.

150. *See* https://www.patientcare.va.gov/Rehabilitation/Services.asp.

151. Common experience reinforces the inappropriateness of such performance requirements. For example, people may set weight loss goals (e.g., 10 pounds by year's end), but if they lose only 8 pounds by January 1 or do not reach the 10-pound goal until March 1, then the conclusion is not that the effort was a failure or that the person lacks the ability to lose weight and further efforts to lose weight should be abandoned.

152. D. Beukelman & J. Light, *Augmentative and Alternative Communication* (5th Ed. 2020) at 11.

153. 20 USC § 1412(a)(1)(A); § 1412(a)(1)(B)(ii).

154. *See* 18 NYCRR § 513.1.

155. D. Beukelman K. Garrett, & K. Yorkston, *Augmentative Communication Strategies* 4 (2007) *citing* D. Beukelman & P. Mirenda, *Augmentative and Alternative Communication* 4 (3rd Ed.) (2005); *see also* D. Beukelman & P. Mirenda, *Augmentative and Alternative Communication* 4 (4rd Ed.)(Baltimore: Brookes Publ. 2013).

156. NY Dep't. of Health, Durable Medical Equipment, Prosthetics, Orthotics, and Supplies Procedure Codes and Coverage Policies, Speech Generating Devices (Version 2021 (July 1, 2021).

157. *Collins v. Hamilton*, 231 F.Supp.2d 840, 849 (S.D. In. 2002), *aff 'd* 349 F.3d 371 (7th Cir. 2003); *accord Ekloff v. Rodgers*, 443 F.Supp.2d 1173, 1180 (D. Ariz. 2006), or to lessen the severity of its effects: to reduce the disability associated with a condition. *K.G. ex rel Garrido v. Dudek*, 839 F.Supp.2d 1254, 1277 (S.D. Fla. 2011); *Dudek*, 864 F.Supp.2d 1314 (S.D. Fla. 2013).

158. *Fred C. v. Texas Health & Hum. Serv. Comm'n*, 924 F.Supp. 788 (W.D.Tex. 1996), *vacated and remanded on other grounds per curiam*, 117 F.3d 1416 (5th Cir. 1997); *on remand*, 988 F.Supp. 1032, 1036 (W.D.Tex. 1997), *affirmed per curiam* 167 F.3d 537 (5th Cir. 1998).

159. *In re: D.S.*, Slip Op. at 3-4 (Soc. Sec. Admin. Office of Hrgs & App.)(Oct. 14, 1999).

160. *Myers v. State of Mississippi*, No 3:94CV185LN (Slip. Op.)(S.D.Miss June 23, 1995).

161. The reviewing court ultimately concluded this "med-speak" objection "was arbitrarily applied, contrary to the overwhelming weight of the evidence, and manifestly wrong." Id. Slip Op. at 13.

162. *In re: A.S.*, FH # 1115201R, Slip Op. at 5 (N.Y. Dept. of Health Mar. 17, 1988).

163. *In re: M.D.*, FH # 4281016K (N.Y. Dept. of Health Sept. 25, 2005).

164. *E.g.*, Iowa Dept. of Human Services (Feb. 2017) Augmentative Communication Guideline (referring to "basic needs through oral speech" but providing no further information as to what constitutes "basic needs").

165. Ohio Administrative Code, § 5160-1—24(a)(1)(2018) (Ohio Medicaid Speech Generating Device Coverage Guideline).

166. J. Light, (1997) "'Communication is the Essence of Human Life:' Reflections on Communicative Competence," *AAC* 13, 61-70.

167. M. Morris & L. Golinker, *Assistive Technology: A Funding Workbook* 14n.9 (Washington, D.C.: RESNA Press 1991).

168. Letter to Lewis Golinker, Esq. from I. Oliff, D. Paul, B. Ogletree & A. Goldman, (June 7, 2017).

169. *See e.g.*, InterQual 2014 Durable Medical Equipment Criteria: Synthesized Speech [Output] Speech Generating Devices. Question 2 of these criteria directs speech-language pathologists to choose whether clients require (A) "only limited specific vocabulary" or (B) "extensive core vocabulary." The criteria then say only if (B) is selected will the client qualify for a synthesized speech output speech-generating device. These criteria have been updated, but this inappropriate choice remains. Its use has been challenged, and in a settlement, has been rejected and will not be followed by Medical Mutual of Ohio. *BVA and USSAAC v. Medical Mutual of Ohio*, 1:16-cv: 03010-PAG (S.D. Ohio) (Stipulation of Settlement and Dismissal filed Sept. 6, 2017). The InterQual criteria are used by other health benefits programs. Speech-language pathologists should insist that none apply this vocabulary size prerequisite for speech-generating device access, which is clearly erroneous.

170. National Joint Committee for the Communication Needs of Persons with Severe Disabilities. (2003) Position statement on access to communication services and supports: Concerns regarding the application of restrictive "eligibility" policies, at 2.

171. *See* National Joint Committee for the Communication Needs of Persons With Severe Disabilities (NJC), Relation of Age to Service Eligibility; *see also Fred C. v. Texas Health & Hum. Serv. Comm'n*, 924 F.Supp. 788 (W.D.Tex. 1996), *vacated and remanded on other grounds, per curiam*, 117 F.3d 1416 (5th Cir. 1997); *on remand*, 988 F.Supp. 1032, 1036 (W.D.Tex. 1997), *affirmed per curiam* 167 F.3d 537 (5th Cir. 1998) (rejecting SGD coverage limits on the basis of client age.); *accord Hunter v. Chiles*, 944 F.Supp. 914 (S.D.Fl. 1996); *Conley v. Dept. of Health*, 287 P.3d 452 (Utah App. 2012).

172. *Fred C. v. Texas Health & Hum. Serv. Comm'n*, 924 F.Supp. 788 (W.D.Tex. 1996), *vacated and remanded on other grounds, per curiam*, 117 F.3d 1416 (5th Cir. 1997); *on remand*, 988 F.Supp. 1032, 1036 (W.D.Tex. 1997), *affirmed per curiam* 167 F.3d 537 (5th Cir. 1998).

173. J. Light, (1997) "Communication is the Essence of Human Life: Reflections on Communicative Competence," AAC 13, 61-70; J. Light, "Shattering the Silence, in J. Light, D. Beukelman & J. Reichle, *Communicative Competence for Individuals who use AAC* 3-38 (2003).

174. U.S. Centers for Medicare & Medicaid Services, *EPSDT–A Guide for States* 23 (June 2014).

175. 42 USC § 1396d(r)(5) (Medicaid EPSDT medical need standard).

176. *Collins v. Hamilton*, 231 F.Supp.2d 840, 849 (S.D. In. 2002), *aff'd* 349 F.3d 371 (7th Cir. 2003); *accord Ekloff v. Rodgers*, 443 F.Supp.2d 1173, 1180 (D. Ariz. 2006), or to lessen the severity of its effects: to reduce the disability associated with a condition. *K.G. ex rel Garrido v. Dudek*, 839 F.Supp.2d 1254, 1277 (S.D. Fla. 2011); *Dudek*, 864 F.Supp.2d 1314 (S.D. Fla. 2013).

177. 42 USC § 1395x(n).

178. The Steve Gleason Act, initially enacted in 2015, Pub.L. No. 114-40 (July 30, 2015) was re-enacted, and its provisions were made permanent in 2018. Pub.L.No. 115-123 (Feb. 9, 2018). It bars Medicare from assigning speech-generating devices to a Medicare payment category called "capped rental." Capped rental durable medical equipment must be rented for a period of 13 months and then it becomes the recipient's property. That is significant for speech-generating devices because as a capped rental item, Medicare will make a payment determination each month and recipients must satisfy the general durable medical equipment place of service limitation each month for more than a year. If they do not satisfy this rule, Medicare payment for that month will not be made. In practical terms, clients who enter nursing facilities or begin receipt of hospice care during the capped rental period were at risk of having any durable medical equipment items in this payment category recalled by their manufacturer or supplier based on nonpayment for ongoing rental. By prohibiting speech-generating device classification as capped rental durable medical equipment, the Steve Gleason Act will keep speech-generating devices in a payment category that provides device ownership to clients at initial delivery. Once the device becomes the client's property, it can come and go with the client to a nursing home or hospital or during hospice without consequence.

179. 42 USC § 1396d(a)(7); 42 CFR § 440.70.

180. 42 CFR § 440.70(a)(1); (c).

181. A less certain response can be offered regarding a replacement request that is based on a "mistake." The purpose of speech-language pathology evaluations is to identify the most appropriate speech-generating devices and access methods that meet clients' daily communication needs. However, sometimes mistakes are made. Devices or access methods are requested, approved, and delivered but cannot be used effectively or at all. In this circumstance, as in the change of condition example, requests to replace the device are not based on malfunction of the equipment; in this example, it is also not based on a change in the client's condition. Instead, the device should never have been recommended, ordered, or provided in the first place. This error will likely be discovered during the warranty period, but warranties do not address this circumstance, and thus, the speech-generating device manufacturers or suppliers will not accept that it is their duty to absorb the cost of a replacement. A program may approve a replacement in this circumstance. It is recommended that at least the following information is provided: (a) a new speech-language pathology evaluation is conducted that confirms speech-generating device need and explains the error in the prior speech-language pathology report, (b) the speech-language pathology report explains the significant differences between the equipment that was provided and what now is being sought, (c) a lengthy trial period has been conducted and reported in detail that shows the replacement device or access method is appropriate, and (d) the replacement equipment are the least costly, equally effective alternative.

182. If the damage or loss was related to any action that may be criminal, a police report should be filed and a copy of that report should be submitted with the replacement request.

183. Speech-generating device exclusions are found only in health insurance policies and health benefits plans: they are not found in publicly funded health benefits programs (e.g., Medicaid, Medicare, or the Veterans Administration). **Medicaid** regulations expressly prohibit categorical exclusion of any item, such as speech-generating devices, that can meet the definition of "medical equipment" as speech-generating devices can. 42 C.F.R. § 440.70(b)(3)(ii)(defines medical equipment); § 440.70(b)(3)(v)(prohibits "absolute exclusions" of any items that meet the medical equipment definition). The absolute exclusion prohibition applies to Medicaid recipients of all ages. In addition, for Medicaid recipients younger than age 21 years, 42 U.S.C. § 1396d(r)(5)(describing the EPSDT benefit) mandates coverage and provision of any form of treatment able to be reimbursed by Medicaid, including speech-generating devices, when necessary to correct or ameliorate a recipient's physical illness or condition. **Medicare** expressly covers speech-generating devices. Medicare National Coverage Determination for Speech Generating Devices, # 50.1 (2015), as does **Tricare**, 10 U.S.C. Section 1077(a)(15); Tricare SGD Coverage Policy, Tricare Policy Manual, Chapter 7, Section 23.1, and **the VA**, https:// www.rehab. va.gov/PROSTHETICS/SLP/index.asp (accessed July 27, 2022).

184. The Patient Protection and Affordable Care Act (ACA or Obamacare) prohibits discrimination on the basis of disability in both benefits design and the implementation of benefits design. 42 U.S.C. § 18022(b)(4)(B); 45 C.F.R. § 156.125; Notice of Template Comments for 2023 Notice of Benefit and Payment Parameters Rule from Chiquita Brooks-LaSure, Administrator, Centers for Medicare & Medicaid Services and Ellen Moritz, Deputy Administrator and Director, Center for Consumer Information and Insurance Oversight, at 8 (Jan. 2023)(Coverage exclusions are an example of health plan benefits design.).

185. Publicly funded health benefits programs (e.g., Medicare, Medicaid, Tricare, U.S. Department of Veterans Affairs) do not have speech-generating device exclusions. All include speech-generating devices as covered benefits, either as durable medical equipment or prosthetic devices, and all will approve and provide funding for them when medically necessary. Also, more than 1,000 different insurers and health benefits plans include speech-generating devices as benefits. See SGD Insurance Approval Database, posted at aacfundinghelp.com.

186. For assistance, contact the United States Society for Augmentative and Alternative Communication at ussaac.org.

187. *E.g. Russell v. Bush & Burchett, Inc.*, 559 S.E.2d 36, 42 (2001), *cert. denied* 537 U.S. 819 (2002)("An insurer … must make exclusionary clauses conspicuous, plain, and clear, ….").

188. *E.g. Tower Ins. Co. of New York v. Horn*, 472 S.W.3d 172, 173-74 (Ky. 2015) *citing Kentucky Farm Bur. Mut. Ins. Co. v. McKinney*, 831 S.W.2d164, 166 (Ky. 1992)("Policy exceptions and exclusions are strictly construed to make insurance effective.").

189. *Carolina Care Plan v. McKenzie*, 467 F.3d 383 (4th Cir. 2006), *affirming in part*, 2005 WL 6111629 (D.S.C. July 25, 2005)(interpreting this phrase to refer to SGDs).

190. Letter to Lewis Golinker from D.A. Root, United States Office of Personnel Management (Feb. 12, 2003).

191. *Egert v. Conn. Gen'l Life Ins. Co.*, 900 F.2d 1032, 1036 (7th Cir. 1990).

192. For example: "BCBS first stated that Durgin did not show that the standing component was 'medically necessary' because there were no 'peer-reviewed clinically controlled studies' showing 'improve[d] net health outcomes' … But the Plan does not contain any requirement that a service be supported by 'peer-reviewed clinically controlled studies' before BCBS will provide coverage, and such a requirement is impossible to square with the lower standard that the Plan establishes for 'Medical and Scientific Evidence.' BCBS's atextual requirement therefore 'impose[d] a standard not required by the plan's provisions,' *McCauley v. First Unum Life Ins. Co.*, 551 F.3d 126, 133 (2nd Cir. 2008), and accordingly was arbitrary and capricious. *Durgin v. BCBS of Vermont*, 353 F.App'x. 538, 539 (2nd Cir. 2009) …"

193. *E.g. M.H. Lipiner & Son, Inc. v. Hanover Ins. Co.*, 869 F.2d 685, 687 (2nd Cir.1989); *Mario v. P&C Food Markets*, 313 F.3d 758, 765 (2nd Cir. 2002)(It is the claimant's burden to establish medical necessity, but the insurer's burden to establish an exclusion applies); *Zaccone v. Standard Life Ins. Co.*, 36 F.Supp.3d 781, 783 (N.D.Ill. 2014)(in ERISA action, "an insurer has the burden of proving an exclusion applies"); *Retkowski v. Met.Life Ins. Co.*, 417 F.Supp.2d 1040, 1048 (W.D.Wis. 2006)(*citing Jenkins v. Montgomery Indus., Inc.*, 77 F.3d 740, 743 (4th Cir. 1996)(same, citing *McGee v. Equicor–Equitable HCA Corp.*, 953 F.2d 1192, 1205 (10th Cir.1992); *Travelers Property Cas. Co. of America v. B&W Res., Inc.* 2006 WL 3068810 at * 4 (E.D. Ky. Oct. 26, 2006)(Under rules of insurance contract interpretation, the insurer bears the "burden of establishing that an exclusion bars coverage."). Assigning the burden of proof to the insurer or health plan means that they must present evidence sufficient to establish speech-generating devices meet the characteristics of the exclusion. Clients do not have to prove they do not.

194. *E.g.* Wisconsin Medicaid definition of 'medically necessary' requires that care "is not solely for the convenience of the recipient, the recipient's family or a provider." Wisc. Admin. Code, HFS § 101.03(96m)(b))7).

195. *See* aacfundinghelp.com/funding_programs (Medicare history).

196. Medicare National Coverage Decision 60-9, reprinted in *CCH Medicare & Medicaid Guide*, 27, 221 at p. 29,803 (Oct. 1992) (DME Reference List).

197. 1 *CCH Medicare & Medicaid Guide*, § 3144.14, at p. 1128.

198. Letter to Elizabeth Carder, Esq., from Philip Brown, Director, HCFA Division of Freedom of Information and Policy (July 8, 1998); Letter to Lewis Golinker from Philip Brown, Director, HCFA Division of Freedom of Information and Policy (August 24, 1999).

199. These decisions are posted at aacfundinghelp.com/funding_programs (Medicare history).

200. See http://www.augcominc.com/index.cfm/funding.htm.

201. Medicare's acceptance of speech-generating devices was supported by the American Medical Association, the American Academy of Neurology, and the American Academy of Physical Medicine and Rehabilitation, and by ASHA and the Cerebral Palsy Research and Education Foundation. Letter dated March 21, 2000 to Hugh Hill, M.D., from J. Ratcliffe Anderson, Jr., M.D., Executive Vice President, American Medical Association; Letter dated March 22, 2000 to Hugh Hill, M.D., from Francis I. Kittredge, Jr., M.D., President, American Academy of Neurology; Letter dated March 23, 2000 to Hugh Hill, M.D., from Ronald Henrichs, Executive Director, American Academy of Physical Medicine and Rehabilitation; Letter dated March 20, 2000 to Hugh Hill, M.D., from Jeri A. Logeman, Ph.D., President, American Speech-Language-Hearing Association; Letter dated February 24, 2000 to Hugh Hill, M.D., from Murray Goldstein, D.O., M.P.H., Medical Director and Chief Operating Officer, United Cerebral Palsy Research & Education Foundation. A more complete discussion of the history of Medicare's development of speech-generating device coverage is reported at aacfundinghelp.com/funding_programs/ (Medicare history).

202. Medicare Decision Memorandum Re: Formal Request # CAG00055 Augmentative and Alternative Communication Devices (April 26, 2000).

203. *See generally* aacfundinghelp.com/funding_programs (Medicare history).

204. *See* **Establishing SGDs are 'Medically Necessary.'**

205. *See* **Devices and Equipment are Covered Benefits.**

206. *See* D. Beukelman, K. Yorkston, & K. Smith, "Third Party Payor Response to Requests for Purchase of Communication Augmentation Systems: A Study of Washington State," *AAC* 1, 5-10 (1985).

207. *Harris v. McRae*, 448 U.S. 297 (1980) (Medicaid programs are not required to pay for care that is not medically necessary).

208. For example, Ohio Medicaid regulations state that "comfort and convenience devices" are examples of excluded items. Ohio Admin. Code (OAC) § 5101:3-10-02(C)(1)(b). In the same section, SGDs are stated not to fit in this exclusion. Id., § (C)(1)(f).

209. The insurer SGD approval database is posted at www.aacfunding-help.com/funding_programs (insurance).

210. Letter to Ms. Lisa F. from Sharon Sheppard-Jefferson, Insurance Investigator, Maryland Insurance Administration (October 31, 2000).

211. 42 USC § 1395y(a)(6); 42 CFR § 411.15(j). Medicare describes "personal comfort items and services" as items that "do not meaningfully contribute to the treatment of a beneficiary's illness or injury or the functioning of a malformed body member ..." CMS, Medicare Learning Network: Items and Services Not Covered Under Medicare 7 (Jan. 2017).

212. 32 CFR § 199.4(g)(64).

213. Public L 107-107, § 702(2) (Dec. 28, 2001) *amending* 10 USC § 1077(a)(15).

214. Tricare Policy Manual, Chapter 7, § 23.1 (2005).

215. S. Rep. No. 110-428, 110th Cong., 2nd Sess. 2008, 2008 WL 2814665 (Leg.Hist.).

216. Pub. L. No. 114-40 (July 30, 2015); Pub.L.No. 115-123 (Feb. 9, 2018).

217. 42 USC § 1395x(n).

218. 1 *CCH Medicare & Medicaid Guide*, § 3144.14, at p. 1128.

219. Medicare National Coverage Determination for Durable Medical Equipment Reference List § 280.1. 220. 42 CFR § 411.15(j).

220. 32 CFR § 199.4(g)(64).

221. The six speech-generating device–related codes and their definitions are stated in Figure 17-2. The HCPCS code for speech-generating device software is E2511 (Speech-generating software program, for personal computer or personal digital assistant); for speech-generating device mounts is E2512 (Accessory for speech-generating device, mounting system); and for speech-generating device access aids is E2599 (Accessory for speech-generating device, not otherwise classified).

222. 42 CFR § 414.202.

223. *Carolina Care Plan Inc. v. McKenzie*, 467 F.3d 383, 388 (4th Cir. 2006) The court rejected the health benefits plan's decision that cochlear implants were convenience items because the benefits they provide are far more profound than those provided by the other items cited as examples. Because the court found cochlear implants were dissimilar to the other items listed, it overturned the denial.

224. *See Fred C. v. Texas Health & Hum. Serv. Comm'n*, 924 F.Supp. 788, 792 (W.D.Tex. 1996), *vacated and remanded on other grounds per curiam*, 117 F.3d 1416 (5th Cir. 1997); *on remand*, 988 F.Supp. 1032, 1036 (W.D.Tex. 1997) *affirmed per curiam*, 167 F.3d 537 (5th Cir. 1998); *Hunter v. Chiles*, 944 F.Supp. 914, 920 (S.D.Fl. 1996). A Medicare administrative law judge in *In re: Jeanine F.*, reached the same conclusion: "The ability to communicate is one of the most vital physical functional abilities for an individual." *In re: Jeanine F.*, Slip op. at 5 (Social Security Admin. Office of Hearings & Appeals Nov. 21, 2000).

225. *Carolina Care Plan Inc. v. McKenzie*, 467 F.3d 383, 388 (4th Cir. 2006).

226. *E.g.*, D. Bickerton, *Language and Human Behavior* (1995); S. Pinker, *The Language Instinct* (1994); M. Batshaw & Y. Perrett, *Children with Handicaps: A Medical Primer* (2d Ed. 1986); M. Fisher, Ed., *Illustrated Medical & Health Encyclopedia* (1956); J. Wilford, "Ancestral Humans Could Speak, Anthropologists' Finding Suggests," N.Y. Times, April 28, 1998, at A:1.

227. ASHA, "Report: Augmentative & Alternative Communication," 33 *Asha* 9 (Suppl. 5) (1991); USSAAC, By-laws, Article II, § 1; *see also* J. Light, "'Communication is the Essence of Human Life;' Reflections on Communicative Competence," 13 *AAC* 61-70 (1997).

228. D. Wedemeyer, "His Life Is His Mind," *N.Y. Times Magazine*, at 22-25 (Aug. 18, 1996).

229. Affidavit of Judith Frumkin, Feb. 11, 1995, 80, *submitted in Myers v. State of Mississippi*, No. 3:94 CV 185 LN (S.D. Miss. June 23, 1995).

230. *In re: Keith C.*, No. 105146 (Ohio Dept. of Human Services May 31, 1991).

231. *In re: Anonymous*, No. 851-0107314 (Ohio Dept. of Human Services, Dec. 7, 1988).

232. *In re: Shannon*, No. 8084 (Ohio Dept. of Human Services, Sept. 13, 1990).

233. J. Crawford, "Individual Psychotherapy with the Nonvocal Patient: A Unique Application of Communication Devices," *Rehabilitation Psychology* 32, 93-98 (1987).

234. R. Sienkiewicz-Mercer & S. Kaplan, *I Raise My Eyes to Say Yes* (1989). Ultimately, when provided a speech-generating device, Ms. Sienkiewicz-Mercer took a lead role in advocating for the closure of that institution.

235. J-D. Bauby, *The Diving Bell and the Butterfly* 81 (1997). *See also* J. Tavalaro & R. Tayson, *Look Up for Yes*, 13, 33, 121 (1997); D. Martin, "When Paralysis is no Match for P-O-E-T-R-Y," *N.Y. Times* March 16, 1991.

236. S. Hawking, (1995), reprinted at http://www.hawking.org.uk/.

237. M. White & S.Gribben, *Stephen Hawking: A Life in Science* 236 (1992).

238. Whitney Lyons, "My Voice, My Choice," *reprinted in* M. Williams & C. Krezman, Eds., *Beneath the Surface* 51 (2000). *See also Hanby v. Faunce*, No. 01-CV-1328 (JAP) Slip Op. (D.N.J. Aug. 20, 2002) (rejecting motion to set aside conviction for sexual abuse based on speech-generating device–aided testimony of victim).

239. C. Musselwhite & K St. Louis, *Communication Programming for Persons with Severe Handicaps* (2nd Ed.) (Boston: College Hill Press 1988).

240. D. Joseph, "The Morning," *Communication Outlook* 8(2), 2 (1986).

241. *In re: Anonymous*, No. 851-0107314 (Ohio Dept. of Human Services, Dec. 7, 1988).

242. D. Bergner, "The Sergeant Lost Within," *N.Y. Times Magazine*, 41, 43 (May 25, 2008).

243. UCPA Policy on Communication Access & Free Speech Rights of Americans with Disabilities (1992).

244. D. Beukelman & P. Mirenda, *Augmentative and Alternative Communication* 7 (2nd Ed.)(1998).

245. D. Beukelman & K. Garrett, "Augmentative and Alternative Communication for Adults with Acquired Severe Communication Disorders," *AAC* 4, 104-121 (1988).

246. *E.g., In re: M.D.*, FH # 4281016K (N.Y. Dept. of Health Sept. 25, 2005); *In re: A.S.* FH # 1115201R (N.Y. Dept. of Health March 11, 1988).

247. *See* L. Fox & McK. Sohlberg, "Meaningful Communication Roles," in D. Beukelman, K. Yorkston, & J. Reichle, Eds., *Augmentative and Alternative Communication for Adults with Acquired Neurologic Disorders* (2000).

248. D. Beukelman & K. Garrett, "Augmentative and Alternative Communication for Adults with Acquired Severe Communication Disorders," *AAC* 4, 104-121 (1988).

249. S. Stuart, D.Vanderhoof & D. Beukelman, (1993) "Topic and Vocabulary Use Patterns of Elderly Women," *AAC* 9, 95-110.

250. *In re: Emyln J.* (Soc. Sec. Admin. Office of Hrgs & App.) (Aug. 18, 1993).

251. *Id.*

252. *See e.g.,* D. Beukelman & B. Ansel, "Research Priorities in Augmentative and Alternative Communication," *AAC* 11, 131-134 (1995).

253. Premera Blue Cross Corporate Medical Policy, CP.MP.RP.1.01.402 at 3 (Nov. 11, 2005).

254. In contrast to the characteristics of evidence Premera Blue Cross cited, the plan required only that "reliable evidence demonstrates that the service is effective, in … treatment of the condition … Reliable evidence includes but is not limited to reports and articles published in authoritative peer-reviewed medical and scientific literature … " Definitions such as this may be found in a Glossary or Definitions section of policy or health plan documents.

255. The scope of benefits of policies and plans is stated in their contracts of insurance and plan documents. Item- or treatment-specific guidelines can be used to aid decision making regarding benefits requests to the extent they reasonably interpret the policy or plan. *Egert v. Conn. Gen.' Life Ins. Co.*, 900 F.2d 1032, 1036 (7th Cir. 1990) but coverage guidelines cannot change the terms of the policy or plan by adding tests of eligibility or exclusions not stated in or required by the policy or plan. *Durgin v. BCBS of Vermont*, 353 F.App'x 538, 539 (2nd Cir. 2009). If the policy or plan does not identify speech-generating devices as excluded, denials based on an exclusion stated in a speech-generating device guideline are just the reviewer's opinion.

256. A complete factual investigation is a key element of the fiduciary duty imposed by ERISA on those who review health benefits plans' benefits requests and appeals. 29 U.S.C. § 1104(a)(1)(A) & (B); *Howard v. Shay*, 100 F.3d 1484, 1488 (9th Cir. 1996), *cert. den.* 520 U.S. 237 (1997); *Katsaros v. Cody*, 744 F.2d 270 (2nd Cir.), *cert. den.* 469 U.S. 1084 (1984). Also, "[t]he duty of good faith and fair dealing implied in every insurance contract includes a duty on the part of the insurer to investigate claims submitted by its insured." *Safeco Ins. Co. of Amer. v. Parks*, 88 Cal.App.4th 992, 1003 (2009); "[A]n insurer cannot reasonably and in good faith deny payments to its insured without thoroughly investigating the foundation for its denial." *Id.* (*quoting Egan v. Mutual of Omaha Ins. Co.*, 620 P.2d 141 (Cal. 1979).

257. Durand, VM. Functional communication training using assistive devices: Recruiting natural communication training using assistive devices: Recruiting natural communities of reinforcement. *Journal of Applied Behavior Analysis*, 1999; 32:247-268; Hetzroni OE. AAC and Literacy. *Disabil Rehabil* 2004; 26(21-2)2:1305-12; Mirenda, P. Forward Functional Augmentative and Alternative Communication for Students with Autism. *Am J Speech Lang Pathol* July 2003; 34:203-216; Mirenda P, Wilk D, Carson P. A retrospective analysis of technology use patterns in students with autism over a five-year period. *Journal of Special Education Technology* 2000; 15:5-16; Schlosser R., Blischak D, Belfiore P, et al. The effectiveness of synthetic speech output and orthographic feedback in a student with autism: A preliminary study. *Journal of Autism and Developmental Disorders*, 1998; 28:309-319; Sevcik RA, Romski MA. Issues in augmentative and alternative communication in child psychiatry. *Child Adolesc Psychiatr Clin N Am*, January 1999; 8(1):77-87.

258. Letter to Lewis Golinker from Orit E. Hetzroni, Ph.D., University of Haifa (Nov. 15, 2006); Letter to Lewis Golinker from V. Mark Durand, Ph.D., University of South Florida (Sept. 6, 2006); Letter to Lewis Golinker from Ralf W. Schlosser, Ph.D., Northeastern University (July 21, 2006); Letter to Lewis Golinker from Rose A. Sevcik, Ph.D and MaryAnn Romski, Ph.D., Georgia State University (July 15, 2006); Letter To Whom It May Concern from Pat Mirenda, Ph.D., University of British Columbia (July 10, 2006).

259. In 2004, Premera Blue Cross adopted speech-generating device guidelines stating that speech-generating device use by individuals with autism is investigational. In December 2006, it revised the guidelines to remove that statement. In October 2007, Premera Blue Cross reinstated the autism exclusion, citing a single new article. Once again, the new article's lead author was contacted. She responded as had her peers: Premera Blue Cross had misinterpreted her research. Once again an employer that had hired Premera Blue Cross to review benefits requests and appeals for its health plan ignored the Premera Blue Cross decision and approved the speech-generating device. And once again, in March 2008, Premera Blue Cross removed the autism-investigational care conclusion.

260. Letter to Dynavox Systems from Laurel Frank, R.N., Regence Blue Shield, at 1 (Aug. 2, 2007). The Regence Blue Shield SGD guideline stated "augmentative communication devices and systems for the treatment of autism, autism spectrum disorders, or mental retardation are considered investigational." Regence Blue Shield, Medical Policy: Durable Medical Equipment Section – Augmentative Communication Devices and Systems at 4 (April 3, 2007).

261. Both the Premera Blue Cross and Regence Blue Shield guidelines stated they had conducted a follow-up search to update their guidelines. Each reported one database had been searched for more current literature. Premera Blue Cross reported it had searched only the PubMed database; Regence Blue Shield searched only Medline. Each reported nothing was found. However, neither considered whether follow up through only a single database or use of the specific database was appropriate for the task (i.e., whether other search efforts would have produced different results). These limited inquiries were not good practice. "AAC is a multidisciplinary field with a literature that is scattered across more than 50 professional journals ... [I]n order to retrieve complete evidence from this scattered literature, it is imperative to search multiple databases ..." Letter to Lewis Golinker from Ralf Schlosser, Ph.D., Professor, Dept. of Speech-Language Pathology and Audiology, Northeastern University (July 21, 2006).

262. The challenged Regence Blue Shield speech-generating device guideline had been issued in April 2007. After a plan sponsor rejected a Regence decision based on that guideline, it was revised. In September 2008, Regence Blue Shield issued a revised guideline: In it, the autism– speech-generating device–investigational care conclusion had been removed. Health Alliance is an insurer based in Illinois. It had relied on the Regence guideline. When told that Regence removed the autism–speech-generating device–investigational care conclusion, it agreed to do so as well. Letter to Lewis Golinker from Lori Cowdrey, Vice President, Corporate Affairs and General Counsel, Health Alliance (Oct. 22, 2008).

263. Letter to John C. from Charles Buttz, M.D., CIGNA Healthcare (April 19, 2011).

264. Letter to Lewis Golinker from Pamela Mathy, PhD, CCC-SLP, The Johns Hopkins Medical School (June 15, 2011); Letter to Lewis Golinker from Oliver Wendt, PhD, CCC-SLP, Assistant Professor, Dept. of Speech Language & Hearing Sciences and Dept. of Special Education, Purdue University (Sept. 20, 2011).

265. Letter to Lewis Golinker from Oliver Wendt, PhD, CCC-SLP, Assistant Professor, Dept. of Speech Language & Hearing Sciences and Dept. of Special Education, Purdue University (Sept. 20, 2011).

266. Letter to Lewis Golinker from Brook Pretot, Specialist, Humana Grievance and Appeal Dep't. (Jan. 6, 2016) and Letter to Lewis Golinker from Tiffany Bentley, Specialist, Humana Grievance and Appeal Dep't. (Jan. 12, 2016).

267. Letters to Lewis Golinker from Diane Paul, PhD, CCC-SLP (July 21, 2006) and from Laurie Alben Havens, MA, CCC-SLP (February 28, 2011).

268. Desch, L., et al, (2008) "Prescribing Assistive-Technology Systems: Focus on Children with Impaired Communication," *Pediatrics* 121:1271-1280.

269. A plan "may not arbitrarily refuse to credit a claimant's reliable evidence ..." *Black & Decker Disability Plan v. Nord*, 538 U.S. 822, 834 (2003). For policies: "In discharging this duty [to thoroughly investigate benefits requests and appeals] the insurer may not ignore evidence which supports coverage. If it does so, it acts unreasonably toward its insured and breaches the covenant of good faith and fair dealing." *Fresno Rock Taco LLC v. Nat'l Sur. Corp.*, 2012 WL 3260418 at * 13 (E.D. Cal. Aug. 8, 2012)(*quoting Jordan v. Allstate Ins. Co.*, 148 Cal.App.4th 1062, 1073 (2007).

270. *Egert v. Conn. Gen'l Life Ins. Co.*, 900 F2d 1032, 1036 (7th Cir. 1990).

271. CIGNA issued autism treatment guidelines that identified speech-generating devices as investigational care in 2008. In December 2011, revised guidelines were issued. The revised guidelines included autism-specific speech-generating device coverage criteria, replacing the investigational care label.

272. Letter to Lewis Golinker from Carrie Kerr, MS, CCC-SLP, Easter Seals of Central Illinois (Nov. 5, 2015); Professional literature review by Lindsey Huckle, BA and Jennifer Seale, PhD, CCC-SLP, University of Maine (Nov. 14, 2017); Professional literature review by Allie Sievers, University of South Dakota (Oct. 26, 2017); Letter to Lewis Golinker from Jennifer Seale, PhD, CCC-SLP, University of Maine and Kassidy Seeley (Oct. 15, 2019).

273. This literature search and analysis will also be valuable to refute denials based on claimed failure to establish medical necessity. Some policies and plans define "medical necessity" with reference to professional literature. For example, a Premera Blue Cross plan stated that the requested treatment must be "appropriate for the medical condition as specified in accordance with authoritative medical or scientific literature ..." Several Regence BlueShield policies and plans stated that medical necessity requires the requested treatment to "not be investigational." These definitions create risks to speech-generating device access because it is clients' burden to establish medical need, in contrast to the insurer's or plan's burden to justify reliance on an exclusion.

274. KY Rev. Stat. § 304.17A-142.

275. *E.g.* N.Y. Insurance Law § 3216(i)(25)(C)(ix)("treatment of autism spectrum disorder shall include ... 'assistive communication devices'...")

276. KY Rev. Stat. § 304.17A-142(8).

277. Letter to Lewis Golinker from Stuart Spielman, Senior Policy Advisor and Counsel, Autism Speaks (Aug. 29, 2011).

278. To identify states with autism treatment insurance mandates, see https://www.autismspeaks.org/state-initiatives.

279. *See e.g., Harris v. St. Paul Fire & Marine Ins. Co.*, 618 N.E.2d 330, 333 (Ill App. 1993) ("Statutory provisions applicable to contracts of insurance are deemed to form a part of such contract and must be construed in connection therewith; policy provisions in conflict with the statute are void."). *Hubner v. Grinnell Mut. Reinsur. Co.*, 4 F.Supp.2d 803, 807 (C.D.Ill. 1998); *accord In re Doctors Hosp. of Hyde Park Inc.*, 337 F.3d 951, 959 (7th Cir. 2003); *Hesbol v. Bd. Of Educ. Of Laraway Community Consol. Sch. Dist 70-C*, 14 F.Supp.3d 1101, 1107 (N.D. Ill. 2014); 2 *Couch on Insurance* § 21:20 (June 2017).

280. *See* Letter to Humana Health Benefit Plan of Louisiana, Inc. from Lewis Golinker (Jan. 31, 2012) (appeal letter); Letter to Lewis Golinker from Barbara Schober, Specialist, Humana Grievance and Appeal Department (Jan. 31, 2012) (approval letter).

281. *Hughes v. State Farm Fire & Cas. Co.*, 2007 WL 2874849, * 4 (W.D. PA. Sept. 27, 2007); *accord TRB Investments v. Fireman's Fund Ins. Co.*, 40 Cal.4th 19, 27; 50 Cal.Rptr. 597, 603 (CA 2006)("As a coverage provision, [an] exception [to an exclusion] will be construed broadly in favor of the insured."); *American Fam. Mut. Ins. Co. v. American Girl, Inc.*, 673 N.W.2d 65, 73 (WI 2004)("Exclusions sometimes have exceptions; if a particular exclusion applies, we then look to see whether any exception to that exclusion reinstates coverage.").

282. The example previously mentioned regarding the Louisiana autism treatment mandate statute nullified a Humana insurance policy with this exclusion text.

283. *Carolina Care Plan Inc. v. McKenzie*, 467 F.3d 383, 388 (4th Cir. 2006).

284. *E.g. Zaccone v. Standard Life Ins. Co.*, 36 F.Supp.3d 781 (N.D.Ill. 2014).

285. Merriam-Webster Online Dictionary: Aid, posted at https://www.merriam-webster.com/dictionary/aid.

286. Medicare National Coverage Determination §50.1: Speech Generating Devices (2015).

287. *See* 68 Fed. Reg. 18,575, 18,577 (April 16, 2003)(adding definition of *speech-generating device* to 32 C.F.R. § 199.2 (Definitions)).

288. VHA Prosthetic Clinical Management Program (PCMP): Clinical Practice Recommendations – Augmentative and Alternative Communication Devices (AAC Systems) (2004).

289. GA Dept of Community Health, Division of Medical Assistance Programs, Policies & Procedures for Durable Medical Equipment Services: Part II, Policy # 1101 at p. 53 (October 2021).

290. Northwood Medical Policy Speech Generating Devices (2020).

291. A search of *all* insurers' speech-generating device coverage and definition is not possible. The following are examples of insurers and health plans that define SGDs as *speech aids* in coverage guidelines. Allways Health Partners (2021); Amerihealth (2019); Anthem Blue Cross Blue Shield, operating in California, Indiana, Kentucky, Nevada, New York, Wisconsin and Virginia (2021); Capital BCBS (2013); Health Care Service Corp., consisting of BCBS of Illinois; Montana; New Mexico Oklahoma and Texas)(2017); Highmark BCBS (Pennsylvania) (2019) Independence BCBS (Pennsylvania) (2021); MedStar Health (2017); Meridian Health Plan (2015); BCBS of North Carolina (2019); BCBS of North Dakota (2021); Paramount (2021); Total Health (2008); Tufts Health Plan (2021); University of Utah Health Plans (2021).

292. Oxford Health Plans, Clinical Policy DME013.11 T3: Speech-Generating Devices at p. 2 (Dec. 1, 2011).

293. Letter to C.R. from United Healthcare Services (Aug. 11, 2021) (interpreting Caterpillar Corp. health plan); Letter to J.J. from United Healthcare Services (March 8, 2021)(interpreting Caterpillar Corp. health plan); Letter to J.J. from United Healthcare Services (March 8, 2021)(interpreting Caterpillar Corp. health plan); Letter to Trenton O. from Detricia T., United Healthcare Appeals Coordinator (Oct. 24, 2014)(interpreting Shelter Mutual Insurance Co. health plan); Letter to Mark B. from Melissa H., United Healthcare Appeals Coordinator (Aug. 7, 2014)(interpreting Target Corp. health plan); Letter to Terry B. from Vonetta L., United Healthcare Resolving Analyst (May 14, 2012)(interpreting Noah Webster Basic School health plan); Letter to Richard P from Michelle P., United Healthcare Appeals Coordinator (June 8, 2011) (interpreting Brown Brothers Harriman health plan).

294. The strength of the assertion that speech-generating devices are reasonably interpreted to be speech aid devices will increase in parallel to the number of other funding sources that interpret or define speech-generating devices as speech aids. In an individual case, an insurer may reject this interpretation, but there is a legal rule governing contract interpretations that will settle the matter. Policy terms or phrases (such as "speech aid devices") that are subject to more than one reasonable interpretation (such as by United Healthcare and other insurers, and by other funding sources, such as Medicare) are considered, as a matter of law, to be "ambiguous." Legal rules of insurance contract interpretation state that when an ambiguity exists in a policy and at least one of the reasonable interpretations supports coverage, that interpretation will control. This rule of interpretation is known by the Latin phrase "*contra proferentem*" which means "against the offerer." *E.g.* Cal.Civ.Code § 1654 (when an uncertainty exists in an insurance policy and cannot otherwise be resolved, "the language of a contract should be interpreted most strongly against the party who caused the uncertainty to exist."); *Westfield Ins. Co. v. Galatis*, 797 N.E.2d 1256, 1262 (OH. 2003). *Contra proferentem* is a rule generally applicable to insurance disputes.

295. 29 U.S.C. § 1001 *et seq.*

296. Further information about the "just ask" appeal strategy can be obtained from USSAAC.

297. Collins, G., "Katie Couric Moves On," *N.Y. Times* (May 21, 2011).

298. D. Beukelman (1990) "AAC in the 1990s: A clinical perspective." In Proceedings of the Visions Conference: Augmentative and Alternative Communication in the Next Decade (pp. 109-113). Wilmington, DE: Alfred I. DuPont Institute; D. Beukelman & P. Mirenda, *Augmentative and Alternative Communication* 88 (2nd Ed.) (1992).

18

Intervention for Persons With Developmental Disorders

Georgina Lynch, PhD
and Gail M. Van Tatenhove, PA, MS

MYTH

1. Language acquisition for an augmentative and alternative communication (AAC) user does not follow the path of typical language development.

2. Assessment of AAC for persons with developmental disabilities lacks a systematic framework and is best done in a naturalistic dynamic manner.

3. Once the person with a developmental disability has access to AAC, aversive behaviors will diminish and language will blossom.

REALITY

1. For some persons with developmental disorders, the clinician may introduce AAC taking a developmental approach, in which the use of symbols and grammatical structure may follow the early stages of typically developing oral language acquisition.

2. Although dynamic assessment for AAC is extremely valuable for determining needs in relation to context, there is also a predictable trajectory of development from non-linguistic to linguistic communication that can be assessed along a continuum of early communicative intent. This is done based on observation of unconventional and conventional communicative behaviors to guide development of AAC competency. Observation checklists for functional communication and language acquisition guide the assessment process.

3. This may be true for some but not all, as in the case of autism spectrum disorder (ASD), in which there may be a need to rely on explicit intervention strategies rooted in principles of applied behavior analysis, considered an evidence-based practice to support use of AAC.

INTRODUCTION

Individuals who use AAC require assistance in developing **functional communication** and expressive language resulting from impairments that occur prior to adulthood during the **developmental period** in which language acquisition rapidly develops and influences learning and cognitive

Fuller, D. R., & Lloyd, L. L. *Principles and Practices in Augmentative and Alternative Communication* (pp. 351-371).
© 2023 Taylor & Francis Group.

TABLE 18-1
Contributing Factors Associated With Developmental Disabilities

PRENATAL	PERINATAL	POSTNATAL	ENVIRONMENTAL
Genetic disorders	Birth trauma	Asphyxia	Educational level/ socioeconomic status of parent
Maternal drug use	Hypoxia/asphyxia	CVA (i.e., stroke)	Ingestion of toxins
Maternal infection	Low birth weight	Head/spinal cord trauma	Lead exposure
Maternal trauma	Prematurity	Infection (e.g., encephalitis)	Limited access to pediatric care
Metabolic disorders		Progressive disease	
Neural tube disorders			
Radiation exposure			

CVA = cerebrovascular accident.

development. AAC may be needed either temporarily as verbal speech and language is developed or throughout the lifespan. Developmental disabilities are a group of conditions due to an impairment in physical, learning, language, or behavior areas of development (National Center on Birth Defects and Developmental Disabilities, Centers for Disease Control and Prevention, 2015). These impairments may be present at birth (congenital) due to genetic conditions or complications during pregnancy or during delivery; although, many disabilities may not be definitively diagnosed until after infancy. Other impairments are incurred later during the developmental period resulting in a loss of skills and significant developmental delay. This chapter uses the term "developmental disabilities" to refer to conditions, such as cerebral palsy, ASD, cognitive impairment, severe speech and/ or language impairment (including **childhood apraxia of speech**), and other physical impairments that interfere with typical development during the developmental period and adolescence.

Developmental disabilities are associated with a group of relatively chronic conditions that are a result of neurologic deficits or injury. Neurologic injury in childhood may result from trauma, asphyxia, disease, or stroke, which may cause physical, cognitive, and/or speech-language impairments resulting in communication disorders. Differences in neurologic functioning is also characteristic of metabolic disorders, genetic abnormalities, or progressive diseases. See Table 18-1 for a list of contributing factors associated with developmental disabilities that may result in the need for AAC to support communication and language acquisition.

The AAC intervention methods discussed in this chapter emphasize the early developmental period in which ongoing assessment and treatment capitalizes on early intervention and the developing brain in response to techniques promoting principles of motor planning, language acquisition, and adaptability for AAC use with caregivers. However, similar considerations are needed for the adult with significant developmental disability and questions posed to use AAC in the most optimal manner are also similar in approach to

treatment goals. Development of communicative competence is emphasized as part of a comprehensive AAC intervention plan with an eye toward establishing a foundation upon which to build skills and expand AAC use in social, educational, and employment settings.

DEVELOPMENT OF COMMUNICATIVE COMPETENCE

It is generally well agreed upon that communicative competence in relation to AAC describes sufficient knowledge, judgment, and skill in four areas: (1) linguistic competence, (2) operational competence, (3) social competence, and (4) strategic competence (Light, 1989). **Communicative mastery** is distinguished from **communicative competence** in that few individuals ever achieve communicative mastery in their own native language, demonstrating adequate to exceptional communication skills in some settings but varied depending upon the context. However, most people achieve communicative competence, demonstrating adequacy of communication needed across social contexts, communication partners, and environments. AAC users may have compromised communication ability depending upon the context which may or may not be conducive to AAC use. Therefore, the primary goal in treatment is building communicative competence across the key areas defined by Light (1989) and creating an AAC system in anticipation of potential challenges in setting, operational use, and adaptability.

Development of communicative competence begins almost immediately from birth. Typically developing children effectively communicate wants and needs using communicative strategies that are appropriate for their age and developmental level, rendering them competent communicators. A key construct in establishing communicative competence depends upon a match in the developmental level of the individual to the communication strategies used. For example, AAC users may not use expressive language fully; however, they may still be considered competent if they use AAC to communicate functionally and adequately. Expectations for expansion of expressive language and existing communication skills are important, but this progression may be different for the AAC user in comparison to typical development. Many AAC users do not acquire communication and language through progressive mastery of phonology, lexicon, syntax, and discourse. For example, the development of a phonological system may be based more on the perception of others' speech and less on their own articulation given the constraints on the vocal abilities of AAC users. By nature of the AAC system and the effect of system use on social interaction, AAC users also differ in the ability to engage in discourse as equal and active members of a communicative dyad (Dunst & Lowe, 1986; Light et al., 1985; Light & McNaughton, 2014a). Therefore, when evaluating an AAC user for identifying treatment goals and determining an AAC user's performance in receptive and expressive language, the individual should not be deemed less competent in language or communication skill, rather the manifestation of the impact of AAC use should be considered in the context of the evaluation to determine competency and linguistic skill.

A predictable pattern of infant behavior in the context of caregiver/infant interactions has been presented by Dunst and Lowe (1986), in which the "readability" of infant behaviors influences the attainment of language acquisition. This developmental progression is based on the following six criteria to classify the development of communicative behaviors beginning in infancy:

1. The degree to which the infant is aware of environmental events

2. The infant's ability to attain a goal or goal state through sustained interactions with the environment

3. The degree to which the behavior is culturally defined, and thus, has social and conventional readability

4. The extent to which the child intentionally uses objects to operate on adult attention or to use adults to obtain desired objects

5. The extent to which the communicative behaviors are linguistic in nature

6. The extent to which communicative behaviors are used as signifiers for something signified in the absence of reference-giving cues

Stremel-Campbell and Rowland (1987) provide a useful framework from which to view the development of communicative competence from early infancy to the development of linguistic communication for assessing functional communication. This framework has been adapted to an observational assessment tool called the Communication Matrix, which assists the evaluator in defining stages of communicative competence from the perspective of "conventional" vs. "unconventional" use of language, depending upon developmental level and communicative behaviors (Rowland, 2011a). This assessment tool incorporates a social interactionist definition of communicative competence based on dyadic interactions according to Dunst and Lowe's (1986) construct of communicative competency and readability of communicative behaviors. This tool is particularly useful in characterizing communicative competence, as well as assisting in the development of specific treatment goals using AAC.

Table 18-2 provides a modification and extension of the developmental models of Stremel-Campbell and Rowland (1987), Dunst and Lowe (1986), and Light and McNaughton (2014a). AAC examples that parallel "natural" communication methods at each stage are included. The framework outlined demonstrates the simultaneous development of linguistic, operational, and social competence. For example, an infant's use of vocalization eventually may be shaped to phonology, but in this early stage of development, serves a linguistic function to communicate a need within a social interaction with a caregiver (social competence) using operational competence (use of the vocal tract for communication purposes). Strategic competence may develop later depending upon the child's need to avoid and repair communication breakdowns. However, this illustration is used to mark the developmental stages at which these areas are emphasized in AAC use.

NON-LINGUISTIC COMMUNICATION

A distinction is made between linguistic versus non-linguistic communication. **Linguistic communication** involves using symbols and word combination rules of a naturally developed language (e.g., manual signs, spoken words, traditional orthography). In the first year of life, communication is exclusively **non-linguistic**, in which communication lacks abstract symbol use but needs are met through other means, such as vocalization, crying, or body movement. However, this form of communication is shaping in its form, incorporating gesture use and the early stages of symbol use. Linguistic communication emerges in the second year of life in typically developing children, in which communication involves combining verbal words following a predictable pattern of morphological structure as the linguistic repertoire develops further. Competent communicators, including AAC users, will use a variety of linguistic and non-linguistic modes of communication. The stages of development described represent somewhat arbitrary divisions because there may be considerable overlap among them, as is the case of the 2-year-old child beginning to integrate communication modalities of gesture use and complex verbalizations. Although the transition between transparent symbol use to arbitrary symbol use may overlap in typically developing children, this may not occur naturally in children with developmental disabilities due to the abstract nature of the symbol use and the cognitive complexity associated with stimuli used to represent communicative intent.

TABLE 18-2
Developmental Levels of Non-Linguistic and Linguistic Communication

LEVEL*	SYMBOLS	BEHAVIOR	EXAMPLES (INCLUDING AAC)	COMPETENCE**
Non-Linguistic				
Preintentional reflexive	Vocalization	Reflexive behavior indicating physical state	Grimacing, crying to indicate hunger or pain	Social (emerging)
Preintentional anticipatory	Vocalization, gestures	Anticipatory behavior not intentionally communicative; caregiver infers intent	Eye gaze, whole body movement, and vocalizations directed to desired object	Social
Intentional	Vocalization, gestures, cause-and-effect movement	Nonconventional and conventional gestures paired with intent to change behavior of others	Pushing, tugging, extending arms up for "pick me up"; switch-activated button	Social strategic (emerging) Operational (emerging)
	Transparent symbols	Use of symbols that share one or more perceptual features of the referent	Gesture (patting floor for "sit") Manual sign (DRINK) Pictographs and photographs	Social strategic Operational
	Arbitrary symbols	Use of symbols whose relationship to the referent is arbitrary	Gestures with symbolic meaning (yes = nod; no = head shake) First spoken words Manual signs Textured symbols Three-dimensional arbitrary symbols Lexigrams Written sight words	Social Strategic Operational Linguistic (emerging)
Linguistic				
	Arbitrary symbols	Use of language, a rule-bound symbol system	Natural languages (spoken, sign)	Social Strategic Operational Linguistic
	Some transparent symbols		Language codes (orthography/written, manual signs, fingerspelling, symbolic) AAC use combining symbols by rule-based codes	

*Based on levels of communicative behaviors described by Rowland and Strembel-Campbell (1987).

**Based on levels of communication competence as described by Light (1989) and Light and McNaughton (2014a).

AAC = augmentative and alternative communication.

Despite the divergent path in which the early developmental AAC user acquires language in comparison to the natural sequence of language acquisition, it is important to note that intervention with the AAC user with a developmental disability may, in some cases, follow a typical path of language acquisition as a model for developing communicative competency, albeit with modifications. Such modifications include the selection of symbols, introduction of core vocabulary, and use of visual stimuli, which can influence the level of stimulus complexity when introducing AAC, a challenge in the case of supporting an individual with cognitive deficits. A discussion on the use of a **natural language acquisition** model is discussed in more detail later in the context of selecting initial treatment goals. Throughout this chapter, the importance of symbol acquisition and functional symbol use is emphasized. Although typically developing children often require little explicit intervention to learn functional linguistic and non-linguistic communication, children with developmental disabilities often require intense and systematic intervention. Teaching approaches incorporating behavioral principles should be used to address acquisition of the first functional symbols. Such principles in teaching this early stage of communicative competence to the developmentally delayed individual include intervention techniques, such as prompting, reinforcing, shaping, and fading. These techniques will be emphasized as examples provided throughout the chapter.

Humans produce non-linguistic communication behaviors alone or in conjunction with language. These behaviors generally consist of vocalizations and gestures. The term **vocalization** refers to the use of vocal patterns that may be **idiosyncratic** but recognizable in certain contexts. The term **gesture** broadly refers to unaided, non-linguistic communication, including generalized body movement; facial expression; hand, limb, or eye movement; and pantomime. Other forms of aided and unaided communication that may be employed non-linguistically by AAC users include micro-switch technology, eye-tracking technology, objects or three-dimensional symbols, graphic symbols, and manual signs.

Gestures and Vocalizations

Considerable overlap exists among the early gestural stages of non-linguistic communication. Thus, discussion of assessment and intervention in the first three levels (preintentional reflexive behavior, preintentional anticipatory behavior, and intentional behavior) will be combined. Assessment and intervention techniques emphasize engaging and sustaining interactions, focusing attention on objects, and promoting consistent, readable gesture and vocal communication.

Preintentional Reflexive Behavior

Infants naturally produce preintentional reflexive communicative behaviors beginning with the birth cry. Crying is the first preintentional reflexive behavior to which caregivers contingently respond. Preintentional behaviors are initially produced without intent and are reflexive reactions to biological states (e.g., fussing or crying to indicate hunger, discomfort, or pain). When caregivers respond by providing attention and engage the infant in interaction, an important bond lays the foundation for emerging communicative competence as social interactions occur over time.

Preintentional Anticipatory Behavior

Preintentional anticipatory communicative behaviors emerge as typically developing children begin to recognize, focus attention, and anticipate desired objects, people, or events. For example, an infant may produce arm motions, sucking movements of the mouth, and vocalizations in response to viewing a bottle. These behaviors are reflexive in response to stimuli reflecting anticipation of some action to occur. The consistent, contingent, predictable responses by the caregiver focus the infant's attention and reinforce the beginning stages of social interaction and intentional communication.

Research indicates that infants who produce non-linguistic behaviors that are more readable evolving into early gesture use are more likely to elicit responses from caregivers than infants who produce non-linguistic behaviors that are less readable (Dunst & Lowe, 1986; Vallotton, 2009). These more readable behaviors lead to more frequent and sustained caregiver interactions and further development of communicative competence. By 6 months of age, infants engage in a communicative "dialogue" timing their preintentional anticipatory behaviors in relation to caregiver response (Feldman, 2003; Jaffe et al., 2001). In children with severe developmental disabilities, these behaviors may be weak, infrequent, or absent and may not elicit contingent, consistent caregiver responses. This early critical link in the chain of events leading to communicative competence through social interaction is missing and leads to reduced caregiver attention and interactions. Treatment effects targeting increasing contingent social interactions through focused intervention with at-risk infants demonstrates the importance of this stage of development in building communicative competence (Resnick et al., 1988). Most recently, this link has been established as a contributing factor in the deviant pattern of language development found in children at risk for, and later diagnosed with, ASD, in which caregivers demonstrated decreased infant attentiveness, and infant positive affect during interactions were notably reduced (Wan et al., 2012).

Intentional Behavior

Intentional communicative behaviors develop parallel to physical development when the child acquires the ability to isolate limb movements and vocalizations from whole body movement. With the emergence of communicative intent, a child's early preintentional communication (e.g., cries, approximation of gestures, vocalizations) gradually becomes overlaid with more conventional behaviors. Identifiable, intentional gesture use becomes apparent in this stage. For example, a child may vocalize or whine and extend the arms up to indicate "pick me up," which will set off a chain of actions occurring on the part of the communicative partner. Subsequently, the child may produce a scream and point downward indicating a desire to be released. Emerging strategic competence is evident here as the child may repeat, modify, or increase the intensity of communicative behaviors to affect caregiver behavior.

ASSESSMENT

Before the clinician can begin to build upon non-linguistic communication attempts to shape intentional language use, it is imperative that careful observation is done by recording communication attempts and states of physical need in relation to the function of behaviors expressed. Capitalizing on the use of physical behaviors and approximation of gesture use may be particularly expedient and effective for many users of AAC. This observational process helps identify unaided non-linguistic forms of communication that fulfill a variety of communication functions, such as getting and maintaining attention, requesting, indicating physical state (e.g., pain, hunger), or rejecting/protesting. Thus, assessment of communication abilities should always involve careful observation and documentation of non-linguistic communicative behaviors. These non-linguistic forms of communication may build a foundation for eventual use of linguistic AAC and may be maintained if effective, then shaped into more conventional linguistic structure using symbols and aided AAC.

Gestures involve consistent, recognizable body movements, and as discussed previously, many children produce gestures that elicit contingent responses from caregivers. Children with cognitive, physical, and/or sensory impairments produce gestures that can go unrecognized and elicit no response. Gestures produced with interfering behaviors, such as extraneous or reflexive body movement, can be difficult to interpret. Poor motor coordination may make it difficult for children to produce movements consistently, as in the case of ataxia, ASD, cerebral palsy, and severe physical impairments due to congenital or acquired brain injury. Therefore, one of the first tasks of an AAC assessment team is to determine behaviors that are potentially communicative, which can be shaped into functionally communicative behaviors for the child. Communication partners will also need to be trained to recognize these behaviors to be consistent in their contingent responses and assist with gradual shaping toward more functional communicative behaviors.

Establishing a Baseline: Unconventional to Conventional Communicative Behaviors

A critical prerequisite assessment procedure for introducing AAC involves a two-step process of understanding the unconventional forms of communicative behaviors (e.g., vocalization, screaming, crying, kicking) and conventional forms (e.g., reaching, gesture use, pointing). It is important to identify the child's level of communicative competence in terms of stages of progression from unconventional to conventional communication along a continuum of observable behaviors. These behaviors reflect the progression from reflexive, physical behavior to abstract symbolic language use and support identifying a baseline upon which to build treatment goals toward AAC use and assist in replacing maladaptive behaviors with more functional forms of communication (see Chapter 20). This assessment can be done by incorporating observation of the child interacting in the natural environment with familiar caregivers and through parent interview. Naturalistic, dynamic assessment may also be used, in which the clinician elicits communicative attempts for desired objects, activities, and social interactions.

Assessment tools specifically designed to guide parents and clinicians along this continuum from preintentional communicative behaviors to intentional communication and abstract language use are designed to support observational assessment and guide development of treatment goals. The Communication Matrix (Rowland, 2013) supports this analysis by defining communicative behaviors along a developmental progression toward communicative competency, as previously discussed, and is based on empirical research in AAC and developmental stages of communicative competency (Rowland & Fried-Oken, 2010). The stages of communicative behaviors and examples of those behaviors assessed using the Communication Matrix are outlined below and guide observational assessment to characterize communication attempts and guide treatment toward functional AAC use. This tool is particularly well-developed to assess baseline observable behaviors for children at the earliest stage of communication and may be very well-suited to assess more challenging cases of AAC assessment. Such cases may include assessment of older children with significant cognitive and motoric impairment demonstrating interfering behaviors or maladaptive behaviors, such as in cases impacted by ASD. Seven levels of communication are assessed using the Communication Matrix, including:

1. Preintentional behavior
2. Intentional behavior
3. Unconventional communication (pre-symbolic)
4. Conventional communication (pre-symbolic)
5. Concrete symbols
6. Abstract symbols
7. Language

Levels of communication are assessed across four domains, including categories of Refuse, Obtain, Social, and Information, which address stages of early development of communicative competence (Schweigert & Rowland, 1992).

During the assessment process, evaluators should also assess the child's physical abilities and not just movements or actions that tend to occur consistently as part of daily routines, such as when eating, playing, or when engaging in other activities of daily living. This assessment process is best done in conjunction with a specialist in motor development, such as an occupational and/or physical therapist. Naturalistic, dynamic assessment guides this process as the clinician engages the child in an activity known to be pleasurable, according to the following general sequence:

- Before beginning the activity, pause to allow the child time to anticipate and produce a movement that may be interpreted as anticipatory.

- Begin the activity and pause periodically to observe any changes in muscle tone, movement, touch, vocalization, and/or eye contact that may be interpreted as indicating a desire to continue.

- Acknowledge the child's responses by providing spoken feedback and eye contact, along with the natural consequence inherent in the activity (e.g., gaining desired object or social interaction). The evaluator may also model or gently physically prompt a gesture if none is noted, but again, guard against attempting to replace a child's natural movements in the initial stages of assessment and intervention.

The activity should be continued for a given length of time with periodic pauses and responses to the child's gestures. Further assessment should be conducted across multiple sessions with a variety of communicative partners, such as caregivers, family, friends, teachers, and therapists. Evaluators should also note the child's desire to discontinue an activity. Children may indicate rejecting/protesting in a variety of ways, from increased vocalization, tension, and activity to sudden withdrawal or passivity. Any of these behaviors may be a "stop" signal to indicate a desire to discontinue.

Transition From Non-Linguistic to Linguistic Symbols

Transparent and arbitrary symbols may be used in both non-linguistic and linguistic communication to serve as a transition or bridging symbols. In typical development, linguistic communication appears after a child has used symbols in non-linguistic ways. For example, single spoken words and manual signs are part of a linguistic system or language. However, this does not mean they are perceived and processed in a linguistic way (i.e., being combined according to syntactic rules). In these early stages, the child may process these symbols in routine activities where one symbol refers to the next event. The transition from non-linguistic to linguistic communication is apparent when a child begins to combine symbols. It is this drive to put ideas together in symbolic form that launches linguistic processing. The use of single words and signs has the potential of reinforcing this transition. Children have been observed to use the combination of a gesture and a spoken word prior to producing two-word utterances (e.g., pointing to a cookie and saying "more"; Paul & Nordbury, 2013). This example can be interpreted as being an intermediate stage between non-linguistic and linguistic communication. Speaking a two-word utterance may still be too complex, so the child instead fills the empty slot of one of the words with a gesture. However, linguistic communication is not only a matter of using symbols that belong to linguistic systems (e.g., words in a spoken language or manual signs in a sign language). Linguistic communication involves perceiving and processing symbols as phonologic and syntactic combinations. However, symbols that do not originate from a linguistic system can be processed in a linguistic manner. Graphic symbols, such as Blissymbols and graphic symbols from the Makaton program, for example, may be used in a linguistic manner if the user processes these symbols as configurations of sublexical elements and as part of a syntactic system. It is important to keep in mind that individuals who have reached the linguistic level of communication continue to use symbols in a non-linguistic way. Linguistic communication does not replace non-linguistic communication; rather linguistic communication provides the communicator a powerful way to organize symbols that can also lead to emerging stages of literacy. Most individuals will use symbols both in a linguistic and a non-linguistic manner. A simplistic current example of this approach is the use of cellphone technology and emoji icons to emphasize points made in linguistic text, such as adding a happy or sad face at the end of a text message statement (the symbol is used in a non-linguistic manner here), or these graphic features may be used by some cellphone users in a linguistic manner, putting emoji symbols together using a language code or in a syntactic manner in which each emoji represents some element of linguistic structure. An example of this is the use of a person, car, food, clock, and unhappy face to indicate "I am driving my car. I will be late for lunch." In this instance, the user is putting together symbols to form thought, such as agent + object + action, representing generally syntactic form and linguistic use of symbols but lacking precision.

Transparent Symbols

The use of transparent symbols represents that stage at which AAC intervention first begins to depart, at least according to some features, from typical communication development. A variety of symbols bearing perceptual resemblance to their referents may be used to encourage, supplement, or replace the use of gestures and vocalizations. Unlike these natural communication modes, AAC modes, such as manual sign and object or pictographic communication displays, must be developed and introduced by the intervention team. Introducing these AAC modes brings on the challenge of further developing operational competence.

TABLE 18-3

Advantages and Disadvantages of Manual Sign Use

ADVANTAGES	DISADVANTAGES
Unaided	Communication partners must learn sign
Quick, portable, accessible, flexible	Requires fine and gross motor dexterity
May be multimodal—auditory and visual	May not be well suited for constructing multiword utterances
Transparency of many signs	
May be physically prompted	Signs and language code may be too abstract for persons with developmental disabilities
Encourages face-to-face contact	
May be shaped from natural gestures	Does not allow for delayed message reception
Allows for communication at a distance and in noise	Does not provide a permanent record

At this stage of intervention, it is necessary to focus on the sensory/perceptual and motor skills necessary to competently and efficiently form the manual sign or to indicate a selection on a communication display (Light, 1989).

A major leap in communicative power can be realized with the introduction of transparent symbols. Whereas gestural communication is relegated to the "here and now" with familiar communication partners, the use of transparent symbols, such as sign and/or object or pictographic communication displays, allows the AAC user to expand the number of communication partners, communicative contexts, and provide greater potential to initiate communication, expanding the content of the message beyond referents that are immediately present.

Another important feature of transparent symbols is their potential for transitioning an AAC user into linguistic communication. These symbols may assist the AAC user in developing multiword utterances, creating the foundation for developing language. Object and pictographic communication displays, much like written language, are arranged in a visual-spatial format, which shares principles of ordering information. Where symbols are sequentially combined, as in most forms of communication, the same basic structure is found with visually displayed symbols, such as agent + object or topic + comment. Moreover, the use of left-to-right orientation for combining symbols fosters a foundation for early stages of literacy development supporting the AAC user's potential for later reading ability and adapted texts.

MANUAL SIGNS

Most linguistic communication uses arbitrary symbols; however, arbitrary symbols can be used in both non-linguistic and linguistic communication as discussed above. Manual signs, an unaided form of AAC, are often used in the early stages of developing communicative competence to bridge linguistic communication and the use of graphic/pictorial communication displays. Many manual signs are transparent or highly translucent, but the majority are arbitrary. Arbitrary manual signs are used in non-linguistic communication in the same way as transparent manual signs—one symbol at a time. The term **manual sign** may be used to describe the use of natural sign language, such as American Sign Language by members of a Deaf community or the borrowing of these signs by AAC users for use as a code for spoken language. In the context of this chapter, discussion is primarily limited to use of manual signs as a mode of communication by individuals who are not deaf, although some may have impaired hearing.

AAC users most often use manual signs in conjunction with spoken language and/or graphic symbols. The use of multiple modes of communication in the early stage of introducing AAC, promoting positive outcomes and effective teaching of AAC use, and increasing vocabulary is established in the AAC literature (Hanson et al., 2013). Both input (communication directed to the AAC user) and output (communication produced by the AAC user) are described as multimodal. Manual signs are used for the same reasons as other modes of AAC: to develop an organized, consistent mode of communication and/or to facilitate, supplement, or replace natural speech. Advantages and disadvantages of using manual signs are described in Table 18-3.

Manual signs may fill a variety of communication purposes. Some AAC users use a small number of single signs in limited situations in a similar way as gestures. Due to perceptual/motor difficulties, manual signs are often interpreted as idiosyncratic gestures by unfamiliar communication partners. However, the manner in which signs and gestures are learned by the AAC user can be used to distinguish the two. Gestures generally develop naturally; manual signs are most often modeled or directly taught to provide a consistency across communication partners and environments. Motoric limitations often limit the effective use of manual signing by AAC users with developmental disabilities, thus aided AAC is introduced.

Because manual signs are conventionalized, they are recognized by individuals who know manual signs more readily than gestures. However, replacing natural gestures with manual signs is not always advisable if gestures are functional. This may be the case when an individual's capacity for lexical expansion is restricted. For instance, if an AAC user's total number of learnable manual signs is limited, then switching to a sign vocabulary may add little communicative power. A second factor to consider is the number of people with whom the AAC user interacts. If the number of communication partners is expected to remain limited, then little is to be gained by introducing manual signs unless most communication partners know sign language. In these instances, teaching functional signs for basic daily needs may be expedient in the process of transitioning from non-linguistic to linguistic communication and introduction of an AAC device, but this mode of communication would become part of a multimodal system of communication in that context.

Contrary to prior assumptions, use of manual signs has not been found to have a negative impact on the development of speech production. When physical and oral-motor mechanism skills are functional, speech has often been observed to develop after a period of manual signing (Garrett et al., 2013). The environment and the communication partners with whom manual signs are expected to be functional and the capacity of the environment to support sign acquisition and use should also be evaluated. Assessment should focus on the ability of the individual to produce signs bimodally and the ability to produce complex utterances. Most individuals with significant cognitive impairment produce primarily single sign utterances; however, some produce two or more sign utterances, and the clinician may capitalize on this basic linguistic structure and expand this to include AAC use in a more functional manner with a broader group of communication partners. When evaluating the use of sign and considering the addition of AAC as a long-term goal, the team must carefully select the referents/messages, the signs that will represent them, and the source from which signs will be selected (Fristoe & Lloyd, 1980). Teams should adopt a developmental approach regarding selection of the referents for which signs should be selected and consider how often the opportunities occur for use of those signs in the individual's natural environment (e.g., home, school), providing meaningful vocabulary that is functional for daily living (Beukelman et al., 1991; Kopchick & Lloyd, 1976).

The importance of sign selection from one system supports greater social function of communication itself. The more the lexicon is individualized, the less likely it will be understood by others. A program used to support sign selection addressing this issue has been developed by the originators of the Makaton approach to manual sign instruction, used predominantly in Great Britain (Grove & Walker, 1990). Manual signs used in the Makaton approach stem primarily from British Sign Language, and hence, have naturally acquired linguistic strength. Makaton vocabulary is a collection of approximately 350 signs that have been selected to correspond with core vocabulary that is used by young children to cover a wide range of meanings.

Following a developmental approach, Makaton vocabulary is classified into eight categories that are presented as stages of approximately 35 items each. These stages support sign acquisition and use to reflect consecutive levels of functioning in daily life. For example, the first stage consists mainly of concepts that refer to physical needs (e.g., food, toileting, help) and to the immediate environment of a young child. Later stages allow for individualized personal adjustment of this structure in which additional concepts are added according to individual needs (e.g., adaptive equipment needs, favorite activities/items). Developmental aspects should be one consideration in planning an initial sign lexicon. Other criteria to consider are iconicity and motor characteristics. Also important is the degree to which a motor approximation of a manual sign is still recognizable by others in the environment that affects attitudes toward communication with people who sign or use Makaton (Pennington et al., 1986; Sheehy & Duffy, 2009).

Although signs often need to be taught within systematic training sessions using reinforcement techniques (Duker & Remington, 1991; Tincani, 2004), signs should also be introduced and used in natural environments as much as possible to facilitate spontaneous discovery. Manual sign use should be oriented toward opening more modalities, including speech and graphic symbol communication. The bimodal use of speech and manual sign is meant to strengthen the link between internal sign and word representation. This bimodal presentation can be simultaneous communication. There is evidence that simultaneous communication is more effective for developing receptive and expressive language. However, the research is somewhat limited in generalization of these findings due to small sample sizes (Gevarter et al., 2013). There is limited evidence, for example, on the use of sign language with children with ASD for promoting development of either oral or sign communication (Schwartz & Nye, 2007). This issue is discussed in the context of special considerations for introducing AAC with the ASD population later in this chapter.

OBJECT COMMUNICATION DISPLAYS

Whereas the use of bridging manual sign and iconicity of those signs with graphic symbol use for AAC can be beneficial with many children, other factors may contribute to a lack of benefit from the use of sign to support the introduction of AAC. Such factors may include physical limitations related to the visual or motor system in which there is vision loss or cortical visual impairment that prevents visual discrimination of abstract sign use, or there is limited fine motor control to support the use of sign. In addition to these considerations, cognitive ability may also play a factor in a child's successful use of sign and extension to AAC use. For some individuals with developmental disabilities, there is a need for teaching strategies that incorporate the use of objects, supporting the learner who requires concrete vs. abstract exemplars to form the association between the communicative message and the item or need. Object communication displays contain three-dimensional tangible symbols that bear varying degrees of physical relationship

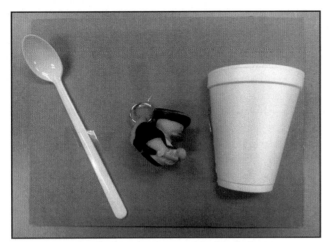

Figure 18-1. Example of an object communication display.

(i.e., iconicity) to the tactile or visual properties of a referent (Rowland & Schweigert, 2000a). At the transparent level are life-sized actual or artificial objects, such as a cracker, a cup, or a piece of plastic fruit. Miniature objects, such as a toy dish or spoon, are also considered to be transparent to some AAC users. Referents may be represented by attaching related objects to a communication display, such as a shoestring to represent "shoe" or a straw to represent "drink." These objects represent their referents by association.

Some objects may be represented by partial or miniature objects that share only one perceptual feature of the object. For example, a piece of basketball may represent the texture of the ball or a ping pong ball may represent its shape or simply be associated with the construct of "ball" based on the physical shape. Last, the relationship between a tangible symbol and object or event may be strictly arbitrary, as in three-dimensional abstract shapes or **textured symbols** (see subsequent section on arbitrary symbol communication displays).

Object displays are frequently used by individuals with visual impairment or sensory impairments but may also be used by individuals with severe cognitive impairments for whom two-dimensional symbols are not yet meaningful. Many individuals with significant cognitive impairment who communicate spontaneously through gestures are not able to shift this communicative act to communication using abstract symbols, such as spoken words or manual sign (McClean et al., 1999). The challenge lies in understanding the one-to-one correspondence between an arbitrary sound and or physical motion (i.e., manual sign) and its referent resulting from cognitive impairment involving memory and representational ability (Rowland & Schweigert, 2000a).

Object communication displays are effective for functional routines. For example, a communication partner may present a child with an object communication board containing a building block, a car, and a feather; each of these objects represent toys and play routines the child may engage with communicative partners through play and social interaction. This configuration allows the child to touch the object that matches the desired object/activity. Objects may also be attached on a board or wheelchair tray with Velcro, in which

the child removes the object and hands it to the communicative partner to initiate a request. This arrangement can be particularly beneficial as a transition communication display for individuals who have not engaged in the early communication behavior of requesting via extending an object. In the case where there are significant physical limitations, the introduction of eye-tracking technology, such as a Tobii Dynavox eye tracker (Tobii Dynavox, 2019) assists with selection of images and objects by matching and tracking pupillary activity and eye-gaze patterns of the individual to the object/symbol. When introducing object communication displays, as with other forms of AAC, it is important to consider the visual array that directly relates to the cognitive demand associated with its use. For example, it may be beneficial to begin with a visual array of only one or two objects to firmly associate the object with the intended item or activity, then gradually increase the array to a three- to four-object display (Figure 18-1). At this stage, tactile discrimination and associations with a variety of objects are needed to discern individual items from one another. This may prove challenging with individuals with more severe impairments and will likely require extensive, explicit practice and instruction to make functional use of this type of display. Table 18-4 outlines the steps and procedures for using an object communication display.

INTERVENTION AT EARLY STAGES OF COMMUNICATIVE COMPETENCE

As outlined within the steps for AAC evaluation, dynamic assessment is done in the context of a naturalistic interaction often with a familiar caregiver. Dynamic assessment is a way to assess baseline skills and to test the waters, so to speak, for potential targets of therapy. Using this approach, the clinician identifies ways to elicit and shape unconventional communicative acts into functional communication. Dynamic assessment takes a heterogenous range of approaches in which there is a blend of assessment and instruction within the evaluation process (Elliott, 2003). After establishing baseline communicative behaviors and determining the function of unconventional communicative behaviors, dynamic assessment should be used to bridge the evaluation with identifying treatment targets to support the introduction of AAC. Given the cognitive load associated with varied forms of visual stimuli used with AAC technology, it is prudent for the clinician to scale back the visual stimuli used to elicit responses and examine at what level the individual actively associates communicative intent with stimuli. A factor to consider in this approach is whether the stimuli should include—based on a hierarchy of difficulty—concrete objects, line drawings, photographs, or abstract symbols representing categorical constructs. In this process, the clinician considers the cognitive demand of the visual stimulus to help pair visual stimuli with an auditory cue or verbal message, so a strong learning association is made between objects, ideas, and symbols representing them.

TABLE 18-4

Case Example: Object Communication Display and Eye-Tracking Adaptation

Background: Bobby; age 6 years; limited verbal output, sensory impairment, developmental disability, limited gestural communication use secondary to physical limitations, difficulty communicating basic wants and needs, guides another's hand to request objects, extends object to request more.

PLAN	GOAL
1. Introduce symbols for items in classroom. 2. Analyze Bobby's preference for classroom activities/ toys/objects. 3. Design three-dimensional symbols that are tactually similar to three objects or pieces of equipment.	1. Bobby will touch an object or symbol to request or label desired objects. 2. Bobby will look to a symbol on his AAC device representing "stop" or "go" to maintain or terminate activities with a communication partner.

PROCEDURES	NOTE
1. Physically assist Bobby in tactually scanning each of three preferred objects (e.g., bubble wand, textured ball, paintbrush). 2. Following Bobby's rejection (pushing away) of nonpreferred object or selection (eye gaze toward object or touching object), present symbol WHAT? and speak WHAT while physically prompting Bobby to tactually scan symbol array. 3. Remove Bobby's hand from display and wait for him to select symbols by either touching or gazing at the symbol. 4. When the correct symbol has been selected, provide activity. 5. Intermittently stop the activity and wait for Bobby to physically indicate through touch, gesture, or eye gaze his desire to continue or stop the activity.	Initially only one meaningful symbol was presented along with a symbol for nothing (arbitrary shape); this provides information regarding discrimination, and if the child selected the arbitrary symbol, the activity did not occur, serving as a foil to assess whether the child associated the symbol with the activity correctly. As Bobby reached criterion, the symbol for nothing was replaced by the second, and eventually the third three-dimensional symbol.
	RESULTS
	Bobby achieved mastery (80% criterion) on 3 consecutive days for all three symbols. New staff and contexts were added to the instructional program. Bobby eventually used 20+ symbols across a period of 2 years. Eye tracking was incorporated on an SGD as associations were made between object and symbol, eventually allowing functional use of the device and ease of mobility by using eye gaze to select.

AAC = augmentative and alternative communication; SGD = speech-generating device.

Stimulus Complexity and Establishing Cause and Effect

Children with developmental disabilities require explicit teaching approaches that take into consideration the complexity of the stimuli using a hierarchy of communicative messages from concrete to abstract. If the visual stimuli are too complex, visual discrimination and associative learning may be jeopardized. A **"bottom-up" approach** requires the clinician to establish **visual attention** (a basic, bottom-up process involving perception of the desired object) and reinforces the child with verbal praise and attainment of the object when the child looks at or reaches for that object. The next stage of stimulus complexity in this approach involves **visual discrimination** between a preferred vs. nonpreferred object as a "foil" to ensure the child is attempting to request the desired object and that object is indeed what the child wants, not simply positioned in a manner that the child is orienting toward. This is done by changing the position of

objects in hands or by changing the position of a picture or symbolic representation of an object within an array of two objects, photographs, or symbols. Joint attention is necessary to establish this interaction and allows the clinician to begin to shape physical movement (e.g., eye gaze, reaching) into a conventional communicative act of requesting (e.g., pointing, touching a picture). If the clinician begins with stimuli that are too visually complex or too abstract for the individual, the connection between object and picture or symbolic representation may not be made. Once visual attention has been established and visual discrimination tested, pairing of the object to the photograph or symbol is done with reinforcement in the form of a **natural contingency**. In this context, the child obtains the desired item after reaching for the object, photograph, or icon. This may be paired with verbal reinforcement with strong intonation, such as, "You want the *bear* … here is the *bear*; nice asking for the *bear*!" The child hears the vocabulary term more than once, the word is emphasized, and the object is placed in the child's hands. Using this type of natural reinforcement strategy, the child's communicative act of reaching for the object may be shaped toward touching a picture, tapping an icon on a device, or touching an adaptive speech-generating switch that provides speech output. The natural contingency is gaining the desired object. This step is necessary to assist the child in establishing cause and effect, such that when the symbol, picture, or switch is touched, the child then receives the desired object. This association is strengthened each time this cycle of behavior and reinforcement occurs.

Schedules of Reinforcement to Support Learning

When cognitive challenges impact learning and language acquisition, a very structured teaching approach supports attainment of vocabulary based on repeated exposure with schedules of reinforcement rooted in principles of **applied behavior analysis**. Applied behavior analysis is the systematic study of behavior concerned with applying techniques based upon the principles of learning to change behavior of social significance (Baer et al., 1968). These principles are taken from a behaviorist theoretical perspective and support structured, explicit teaching of language. However, limitations in its use as the primary form of intervention for teaching language acquisition include challenges with generalization and difficulty helping the child develop abstract, novel language concepts. When these principles are applied within a naturalistic social interaction with reinforcement varied and eventually faded, spontaneous communication acts will occur. Moreover, when the clinician combines explicit, structured teaching with a developmental approach following the natural stages of language acquisition, language competency often emerges. The use of these principles relies on schedules of reinforcement that help firmly establish cause and effect and associative learning (Skinner, 1953).

Two main types of reinforcement schedules can be used to shape communicative attempts toward AAC use; one type is based on frequency of occurrence of the desired behavior in terms of a ratio and the other type is based on how much reinforcement is given over time. Examples of these types of reinforcement to use when introducing basic AAC include:

- Fixed ratio
- Intermittent or variable ratio
- Fixed interval
- Intermittent or variable interval

With a **fixed ratio reinforcement** system, the reinforcement is based on a predetermined number of responses. For example, the child may be reinforced verbally with "Nice job, here you go!" for every third attempt of touching the switch. This is a 3:1 fixed ratio reinforcement schedule. For every third attempt, there is one verbal reinforcement message given. When using an **intermittent/variable ratio reinforcement** schedule, the reinforcement is provided randomly, not based on a consistent number of attempts. During an interactive play session, the child may be rewarded verbally after the first attempt, fourth attempt, sixth attempt, seventh attempt,

etc. There is no preset number of attempts the child must make to be rewarded in a consistent manner. The choice to use intermittent reinforcement is often after a child has demonstrated some level of success with a particular skill, and the clinician is interested in maintaining that success in a more naturalistic context, so the reward is varied.

Whereas fixed and intermittent ratio schedules are based on the *number* of attempts at a skill, interval ratios are based on a *period of time* passing as those attempts are made. When using a **fixed interval reinforcement** schedule, the reinforcement is delivered after a set length of time and consistently provided for that set time period. For example, the clinician may verbally reward, "Nice asking with your device, Roberto" every 2 minutes, as the child is engaging in a task, play routine, or activity of daily living. Therefore, as the child is engaging with AAC use, the clinician is acknowledging positively the use of the device and the child begins to pair the context with positive reinforcement. This type of schedule is often chosen to help the child extend the duration with which they are engaged in active AAC use in a naturalistic context. When using an **intermittent/variable interval reinforcement** schedule, just as the name implies, the reinforcement is given intermittently or at varied times during engagement with the device. For example, verbal praise may be given at 2 minutes, then again at 5 minutes, then again at 7 minutes, then 3 minutes, then 12 minutes. This approach encourages extended engagement with a task and offers continued positive reinforcement after initial communicative competency is established.

When using structured, explicit teaching methods, as outlined earlier, it is important to consider how to encourage generalization or transference of the skill being practiced into more naturalistic environments and with multiple communicative partners. Often children with developmental disabilities may become prompt-dependent, in which they wait for the clinician to prompt before demonstrating a skill or using their AAC independently, so it is important to quickly fade verbal prompts and to extend AAC use to multiple settings and with multiple people.

NON-LINGUISTIC TO LINGUISTIC COMMUNICATION

The development of linguistic communication should be an important consideration in AAC intervention for individuals with developmental disabilities. Although an impairment may affect linguistic abilities, the development of linguistic skills should not be abandoned nor should it be assumed the individual does not have the capacity for acquiring a communication system based on structured language. Unfortunately, too often teaching functional communication takes the highest priority at the expense of establishing language structures within the AAC system, which will further expand communicative competence while concurrently developing language. Although behavioral intervention principles are often needed to introduce functional communication, as previously described, it is also important to consider a developmental model of language acquisition within that structured intervention approach as communication is established and the next steps toward language development are expanded upon using symbols introduced early in the assessment process.

An emphasis on developing language with the AAC user should always be considered for two reasons. The first reason relates to the unique characteristics of language that permit rapid processing of lexical items (e.g., words, symbols, signs) from a limited set of basic elements (e.g., sounds, icons, handshapes). This high degree of conventionalization makes language a superior means of expression, allowing for expression of novel ideas and infinite possibilities for combining thought and communicating this in a shared linguistic system with communicative partners. The second reason concerns the flexibility and apparent robustness of linguistic capacity even in individuals with limited access to language. Consideration must be given regarding the degree to which the AAC system provides the opportunity to enhance language development. This is typically done by creating an AAC interface that allows the user to first associate symbols with objects and ideas, then provide the ability for the user to combine two or more symbols together creating the basic linguistic structure needed to generate novel ideas. It is well documented that when given the structure and flexibility to generate novel ideas in this way, even individuals with complex communicative needs will demonstrate the natural human capacity to develop language (Light & Drager, 2007). Thus, the clinician does not focus solely on functional communication, particularly in the early stages of introducing AAC to children with developmental disabilities. The traditional approach to early language development assumes the child does indeed have the ability to explore language rules, that is, the ability to freely modify and combine linguistic symbols. However, demonstration of this knowledge of language by the AAC user may be extremely limited in the ability to use language naturally and productively. Nelson (1992) emphasizes the impact of environmental supports on fostering development of phonology, morphology, and syntax, which is not too different than its impact on typical language development such that the influence of communicative partners, communicative tasks, and intervention activities can help shape more complex language use expanded from functional communicative competence. Thus, the introduction of AAC should not be viewed as abandoning goals for developing speech and language but rather as bringing a new impetus for their development. The development of communicative competence (a primary goal of AAC use) serves to further expand linguistic competence in this model of context-driven knowledge and use of language.

Equally important in the consideration of environmental contextual supports on the development of language is the clinician's understanding that there exists a mismatch between the language input and the expected output involved in aided AAC use. In most cases of AAC intervention, the primary channel of language input to users of aided AAC is spoken language (Light, 1997b; O'Neill et al., 2017). However, given current technology used with aided AAC, speech-generating devices (SGDs) also uniquely affect the encoding of linguistic communication. There may be asymmetry between aided input and aided output not observed in typical language development. Factors related to human vocal components of language input vs. automated speech production components of language (i.e., SGDs) and their influence on the AAC user's linguistic communication create a novel intervention challenge. The term **aided AAC input** describes intervention in which the clinician or communicative partner points to or activates aided AAC symbols (on a communication board, SGD, or mobile technology application) while speaking with the AAC user. An analogous approach is the use of total communication in which manual sign, verbal speech, or aided forms of communication are provided simultaneously. Aided AAC input may be used to support language comprehension, as well as to model expressive language structure, in the context of everyday routines and activities. A recent meta-analysis examining the influence of aided AAC input on language outcome revealed a positive correlation between the use of aided AAC input on language comprehension and expressive language outcomes in children and adolescents (O'Neill et al., 2017), suggesting aided AAC input serves in a similar capacity as verbal modeling techniques used to promote development of oral language. Studies including the use of SGDs yielded slightly higher language outcomes in general, further supporting the use of aided AAC input to foster language development, given the paired auditory stimulus with visual stimulus (symbolic representation) and naturalistic contexts (O'Neill et al., 2017).

AAC service providers must understand typical language acquisition to evaluate an individual's linguistic competence. Although the developmental pattern of young AAC users may appear to be dramatically different from typically developing children, a developmental model of language acquisition can be useful in making decisions about the child's present linguistic competence and viable intervention strategies (Gerber & Kraat, 1992). This model is meant to be used as a guide to understand which language acquisition areas have been affected and to prioritize areas for intervention.

Challenges With Initiation of AAC and the Expansion of Language

Communication disabilities may disguise linguistic potential, as difficulty in speaking or reacting to spoken language may result in decreased quantity and quality of communication to which the child is exposed. This results in decreased exposure to vocabulary and often disproportionate exposure to directives from adults or their primary expressive language use consisting of requesting vs. generating novel statements, ideas, and comments. AAC intervention often seeks to restore interactions on par with the child's developmental level by providing symbols that are accessible according to the individual's sensory, motor, cognitive, and linguistic abilities and encouraging caregivers to communicate with AAC users in a more interactive way. Just as clinicians use recasting techniques to promote expansion of language in typically developing children or those with language impairment, the clinician can guide others to expand upon the AAC user's statements and questions and use open-ended questions to elicit more interactive exchanges. For example, the communication partner may ask, "Are you hungry?" and the AAC user may answer "Yes" and "What is for lunch?" thus requiring an expansion of language rather than simply answering questions.

Language Codes

Even if an individual has little or no access to primary linguistic expression, use of non-linguistic symbols (e.g., pictographs) can pave the way toward linguistic communication. Non-linguistic symbols can be used in ways similar to linguistic symbols. For example, pictographs or other graphic symbols can be used in the typical word order of spoken language. In this way, the symbols are used as language codes like the use of manual signs as a code for spoken language. Moreover, by using linguistic and non-linguistic symbols simultaneously, the more accessible non-linguistic symbols may serve as a bridge to language use. When speech and non-linguistic symbols are simultaneously presented to the user, all or part of the linguistic symbol will be processed by the receiver along with the non-linguistic symbol. Symbols that occur in earlier developmental stages (i.e., non-linguistic) function as a basis for higher-level symbols (i.e., linguistic). Many forms of direct communication tend to be multimodal where different types of symbols are incorporated. For example, people tend to enhance speech with gesture when communication breaks down or when a message needs to be emphasized (McNeill, 1985). AAC can be considered in the context of a multimodal system of communication. Attention should be given to (a) modes of communication relating to basic needs, symbols, or photographic representations to help the user connect ideas and access vocabulary for expression of novel ideas and (b) efficiency of access to these icons, words, and photographs/pictures, depending upon the need and goal related to language development.

Visual Scene Displays to Support Language Development

It is important to determine how best the individual with developmental disabilities processes visual, auditory, and tactile information and associates meaning in relation to building a language system. Often the language code relies heavily on visual orthographic representation or abstract symbolic representation to efficiently navigate the AAC system and organize vocabulary and messages. Although these modes of icon organization can assist many users of AAC in conveying thoughts more expediently, the individual with cognitive challenges and other visual/motor impairments may rely on other means for accessing the language code within a multimodal AAC system that is evolving as they are developing. In the early stages of building word knowledge and connecting ideas, the individual with a developmental disability may benefit from the use of a visual scene display (VSD). Emerging evidence for the benefits of the use of VSDs across developmental levels indicates positive outcomes for expanding language, improving comprehension, and building expressive vocabulary because of context-rich stimuli (Drager et al., 2017; Light & Drager, 2007; Wilkinson et al., 2012). A VSD is a picture, photograph, or virtual environment that depicts and represents a situation, place, or experience (Beukelman & Mirenda, 2005). There are many commercially available software applications for creating VSDs or using generic VSDs (see Figure 18-2 for an example of a VSD).

Because of its emphasis on context, a VSD is often a suitable choice for children with developmental disabilities because language can be developed using meaningful contexts that facilitate learning. In older individuals with developmental disabilities, a VSD serves as a concrete as opposed to abstract connection to the use of language and functional communication, such as a job site, a group home environment, and community services, such as transportation and restaurants.

A VSD embeds hotspots within a contextual scene. A hot spot is an object or person within the VSD photograph that can be activated to represent a target word. For example, a glass on the table in a kitchen scene may represent "drink" or "I am thirsty" when the person touches the glass on the display. VSDs are heavily contextual and can provide highly personable, individualized scenes using personally relevant vocabulary, or they can provide generic vocabulary to use across contexts once trained. Advantages of VSDs in comparison to grid displays for individuals with developmental disabilities is the lower cognitive demand associated with their use and their ability to engage the less motivated user to use AAC. Given the reliance of VSDs on photographs and embedded images, one disadvantage is they may not be very useful to persons with visual perceptual challenges. Focused visual attention and visual discrimination become prerequisites for their introduction just as they would with introducing grid displays. However, grid displays would hold more options for making icons salient and focusing attention by increasing size and decreasing cell numbers of the display to make the images visually salient. By design, VSDs are not meant to do that in the same way; although, scenes can be created to be more simplistic to facilitate their use. Therefore, the clinician should assess the user's basic perceptual skills and compare use of and competency with VSDs and grid displays, perhaps including a combination of the two for basic needs (e.g., VSDs) and to target early language structure (e.g., grid displays) simultaneously, depending upon the user's abilities.

FACILITATED COMMUNICATION: LACK OF SCIENTIFIC EVIDENCE FOR ITS USE

An approach that warrants cautious discussion in the context of AAC intervention with persons with developmental disabilities and significant cognitive impairments is what has come to be known as facilitated communication. Facilitated communication was developed in Australia in the 1970s by Rosemary Crossley for use by a child with cerebral palsy. It was later adopted in the 1990s by clinicians and educators in the United States for use with individuals with ASD and other communication disabilities. Facilitated communication involves the use of hand over hand physical support provided by an aide to facilitate a user of AAC in expressing ideas and thoughts, usually in the form of written communication via an alphabet board or SGD. As originally conceptualized, facilitated communication was intended to facilitate production of written language, and hence, communication by linguistically competent individuals. Early in its use, some believed the use of facilitated communication enabled individuals with severe disabilities to finally break through and express themselves. However, carefully controlled studies began to reveal the facilitator may have played a direct role in eliciting the messages conveyed (American Speech-Language-Hearing Association [ASHA], 2018b). Extremely discrepant outcomes between facilitators as "authors" of these messages, along with the entry of facilitated communication issues in social media and the courtroom, prompted professional organizations serving individuals with disabilities to provide position statements regarding limitations in treatment efficacy and lack of empirical evidence to support use of facilitated communication with individuals with severe disabilities. In a recent update to a 1995 position statement authored by ASHA (2018b), the organization takes a stronger stance and discourages the use of facilitated communication because of a lack of scientific validity and because facilitated communication does not foster independent communication. The most recent position statement provides the following board policy recommendations to practicing clinicians:

> Proponents of facilitated communication state that the technique reveals previously undetected literacy and communication skills in people with autism and other disabilities. However, these statements are made only on the basis of anecdotal reports, testimonials, and descriptive studies …

> The substantial and serious risks of facilitated communication outweigh any anecdotal reports of its benefit. The scientific evidence against facilitated

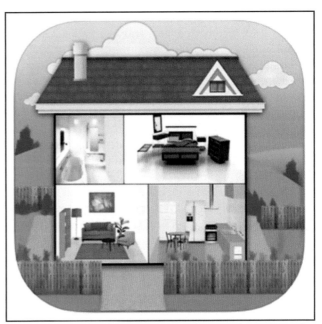

Figure 18-2. Example of a VSD. (Reproduced with permission from Tobii Dynavox, LLC © 2021 Tobii Dynavox. All rights reserved.)

communication, evidence of harms of facilitated communication, and potential for future harms to people who use facilitated communication and their families cannot be ignored in clinical decision making. Speech-language pathologists who use facilitated communication—despite being informed of and knowing these harms and risks—could face additional risks in terms of their own liability in the event of harms arising to people with disabilities or their families related to the use of facilitated communication.

Speech-language pathologists have a responsibility to inform and warn clients, family members, caregivers, teachers, administrators, and other professionals who are using or are considering using facilitated communication that:

a. Decades of scientific research on facilitated communication have established with confidence that facilitated communication is not a valid form of communication;

b. Messages produced using facilitated communication do not reflect the communication of the person with a disability;

c. Facilitated communication does not provide access to communication;

d. The use of facilitated communication is associated with several harms to individuals with disabilities, as well as their family members or teachers; and

e. ASHA's position on facilitated communication is that it should not be used. (ASHA, 2018, n.p.)

ASHA reports these recommendations are consistent with at least 19 other national and international advocacy organizations. To date, it is generally accepted that facilitated communication lacks validity and its use is considered unethical, posing potential harm. Although it is necessary to consider physical supports in the delivery of AAC intervention, the advancement of technology in recent years supporting the physical interface between SGDs and other forms of AAC allow an intervention team to identify modes of access that promote independence and do not rely on another person to engage with AAC. Thus, facilitated communication and its limitations and complications need not be considered, and moreover, as outlined very specifically above, should not be considered as part of an AAC treatment plan.

Special Considerations for Individuals With Autism Spectrum Disorder

As the prevalence of ASD has increased over the past decade—most recently cited as 1 in 69 in the United States (Christensen et al., 2018)—there is growing concern about the use of evidence-based practices to support early intervention, as well as identifying interventions shown to produce positive outcomes for individuals with ASD across the lifespan. Based on current prevalence data, it is estimated that approximately 55,000 individuals with ASD will enter the adult world annually over the next decade (Shattuck et al., 2012). Clinicians and educators are faced with the challenge of meeting unique needs of people with ASD at critical stages of development: from early acquisition of language and subsequently to the transition from adolescence to adulthood in which employment and quality of life are impacted significantly by intellectual disability and the need for an effective communication system to be independent after leaving the public education system. There is a need to draw upon the extensive body of research in this area that identifies evidence-based practice with respect to the use of visual supports and AAC with this population (Wong et al., 2015). There exist several intervention approaches designed to promote language development in persons with ASD, and parents frequently ask about AAC vs. sign language. Sign language is not considered an evidence-based practice for developing language in ASD due to a variety of reasons, such as lack of imitation, difficulty with fine motor control, lack of joint attention, and lack of initiating communicative attempts. Whereas other children with developmental disabilities have the desire to communicate and can benefit from both aided and unaided AAC, the child with ASD presents unique challenges with social communication that warrant a behavioral approach to teach fundamental skills needed to encourage social interaction using AAC. AAC is considered

evidence-based practice for treating ASD between ages 3 and 22 years based on meta-analyses of empirical studies examining treatment outcomes with AAC (National Autism Center, 2015; Wong et al., 2015). Clinicians must understand the path toward effective use of AAC with a person with ASD can be challenging and quite different from more conventional methods for introducing AAC. However, there is a predictable course of introducing AAC that has positive outcomes toward using AAC in a functional manner and mediation of maladaptive behaviors interfering with AAC use, often the most cited concern by clinicians. Often the question posed is, "How do I engage the child with ASD in using an AAC device for communication, not as a toy or reward?" Parents will also report that their child with ASD likes technology and the immediate visual feedback given but often uses a device as a self-stimulatory tool (i.e., repetitive behaviors associated with visual or sensory stimulation while interfacing with the device), not for effectively communicating wants and needs.

As previously mentioned in this chapter, often the clinician must make a distinction between use of behavioral principles to heavily reinforce appropriate interactions with AAC and encourage use of a device while concurrently making decisions about developing language drawing from a developmental framework. This is very true in the case of AAC intervention with people with ASD. Behavioral intervention including the use of **discrete trial training** and other forms of intervention relying on principles of applied behavioral analysis are also considered evidence-based practice (National Autism Center, 2015; Wong et al., 2015) and must be integrated with AAC intervention. Introduction of AAC often is done by a multidisciplinary team that includes a speech-language pathologist, a board-certified applied behavior analyst, an occupational therapist, the parent, and educators. Shared goals include developing joint attention, facilitating imitation, initiating requests, following daily routines, and building expressive vocabulary in naturalistic contexts of play and early intervention activities with other children and caregivers.

Establishing Basic Communicative Behaviors Using Non–Speech-Generating AAC First

Often the main issues contributing to a lack of AAC use by a child with ASD is the introduction of speech-generating AAC before establishing basic social interaction skills and use of conventional communicative behaviors. As discussed in relation to assessment, it is critical that the assessment identifies those preintentional communicative behaviors and treatment targets for replacing them with conventional communicative behaviors (e.g., grabbing a desired object vs. pointing to it). A comprehensive treatment plan would include a thorough assessment defining the levels of

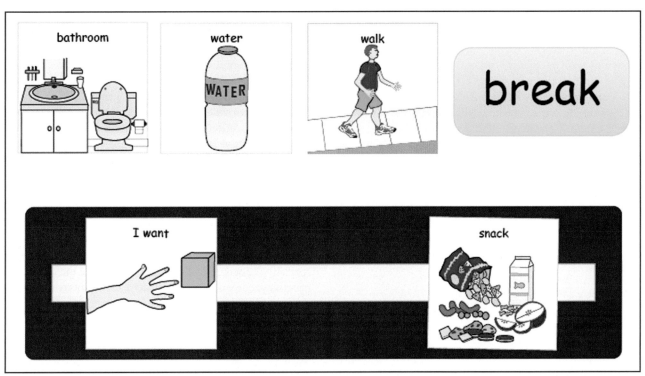

Figure 18-3. Example of a PECS communication strip. Vocabulary symbols can be combined on one tangible strip to give to the communication partner to express needs. (Images used with permission from Pyramid Educational Consultants [www.pecs.com]. All rights reserved.)

communicative behaviors and identifying communication goals to mediate any unconventional behaviors interfering with introduction of AAC. Often, assumptions will be made that AAC will resolve those issues because the child will now have a tool to communicate; however, one must remember that AAC is just that: a tool for communication. Without fundamental communicative behaviors in place, speech-generating AAC may not be helpful.

An evidence-based practice non–speech-generating option designed specifically to teach conventional communicative behaviors is the Picture Exchange Communication System (PECS; see Figure 18-3 for an example of a PECS communication strip). Originally designed to teach children with ASD and other developmental disabilities to express their needs and wants, over time it has been shown that a primary benefit of PECS is teaching the pre-linguistic behaviors needed for functional communication, which benefits not only the child who later develops verbal speech but also the child who may remain nonverbal but rely on AAC. Misperceptions about the PECS system continue to influence treatment with many clinicians applying its use either incorrectly or assuming the PECS system is the primary communication system to be used for a lengthy period of time, which results in a plateau in expressive language or functional communication.

The PECS system takes the child through six stages of functional communication, which builds from basic association of a symbol with an object and visual discrimination, to initiation of social interaction, to combining symbols to request and comment. The PECS program capitalizes on the child's need for tangible, concrete objects associated with a communicative exchange. As the child hands the PECS symbol card to another person, an exchange occurs, associating the visual cue with the object and the communicative act. Speech-generating AAC at this stage of teaching proves to be distractible to most children with ASD, and thus, this critical communicative behavior is lost in the teaching process. This very structured teaching program relies on reinforcement and gestural cues to gain and maintain the child's attention while also limiting language use to identifying the salient features of target words. The controversy surrounding its use when PECS was first developed was the heavy reliance on principles of applied behavior analysis and limited language stimulation. However, as our emerging understanding of the developing brain in ASD continues, the understanding there exists underconnectivity between regions of the brain supports the direct stimulation approach done with multiple trials based on principles of motor learning and language (Dawson et al., 2010). In addition, the body of intervention literature has grown, demonstrating practices considered evidence-based of which PECS is emerging (Wong et al., 2015). As a child attains consistency at Stage IV of PECS (i.e., combining symbols and initiating), this is often the stage at which the child either develops verbal speech (if physically capable) or early emerging language develops and successful transition from PECS to AAC occurs. AAC should be introduced at this stage once maladaptive behaviors have been mediated and conventional pre-linguistic behaviors have been established as occurs by Stage IV of PECS (Frost & Silverman-McGowan, 2014). When viewed as a stepping stone to AAC, the use of PECS can be a very efficient component of an AAC intervention plan for a child with ASD. It is imperative this step in the process is explained to parents, caregivers, educators, and team members working with the child daily. The use of PECS in this way should not take a lengthy period of time, and in fact, may facilitate AAC use within a few weeks of starting PECS if used with fidelity as outlined in the training guidelines. When done effectively and with appropriate schedules of reinforcement and shaping of behaviors, helping a child reach level IV in PECS can take as little as 8 to 10 sessions if done consistently and in the context of the natural environment in which the communicative interaction will occur. The transition from PECS to AAC becomes somewhat seamless as the child transitions from concrete exchanges of picture cards to the use of picture symbols on SGDs, in which language can then be further developed at a more advanced rate.

Increasing Motivation and Engagement: The Importance of Preference Assessments

Identifying objects and activities to promote engagement is noteworthy when discussing AAC use with persons with ASD and cannot be overstated. It is often difficult to establish if a child with ASD will engage with AAC functionally with others. Whereas it is intuitive to identify toys, games, and objects of interest to engage the child or rely on parent report to identify these things, often the choices are either ineffective or temporarily effective because the item has been used too much to attempt to mediate undesirable behaviors, thus the child has satiated on the reinforcing power of the object. A formal forced-choice preference assessment is recommended when considering the introduction of AAC with a child with ASD, as it will support the behavioral component of the intervention program and assist with maintaining engagement. When using a systematic preference assessment, often the clinician may be surprised by items that take priority of preference—this is done by placing 10 to 20 items in a box and randomly pairing the objects and identifying those most often chosen by the child. There are many forms of conducting this informal behavioral assessment and the reader is referred to Wright (2003) and Chazin and Ledford (2016) for protocols and demonstrations of the assessment. Appropriate selection of engaging items and activities provides the needed foundation for properly engaging in communicative exchanges that are meaningful to the child and productive within therapy sessions and generalizable outside the therapy room.

EDUCATIONAL ISSUES AND INCLUSION

Services within the public education system in the United States aim at providing a **"free, appropriate public education"** under the Individuals with Disabilities Education Act (2004). Free, appropriate public education describes the legal obligation of the public school system to aim toward providing the best options for challenges posed by use of AAC to access education. Special education law is intended to do just that: ensure a child's right to access general education. Special education is intended to provide specially designed instruction needed to benefit from general education, and the law also provides for reasonable accommodations to access one's education. A detailed analysis of the framework of special education law and education is beyond the scope of this chapter; however, fundamental to providing appropriate services for a student using AAC is an understanding of the AAC device as a *tool for access* as an accommodation, and the *specially designed instruction needed for learning how to use the device*, as well as the specially designed instruction needed for building language. The former concept is an access issue, the latter requires the skilled expertise required by specially trained educational staff to provide the instruction necessary to learn to use the system and adapt its use to general and special education.

Individualized Educational Program Development

Children with disabilities are best served when interventions are based on a collaborative team approach and systematic planning to increase functional skills while tapping into the developmental needs of the child. This approach is done through the **individualized education program** (IEP) team process required by law. In addition to identifying unique needs of the child, another high priority is attempting to include the child to the greatest extent possible in the **"least restrictive environment."** Inclusion (formerly, "mainstreaming") is a term used to describe a child's integration with typically developing peers within the general education classroom. Although a child may receive special education services, the IEP team must identify opportunities for inclusion so that the child is educated to the greatest extent possible with typically developing peers. This model is based on the idea that all students benefit from a heterogenous learning environment and that special education should be a service, not a place that isolates students from others or discriminates against them.

A guiding principle particularly useful when identifying educational goals and inclusion of the student using AAC is **"understanding by design"** (Wiggins & McTighe, 1998). Originally adapted from architecture and concepts related to access in physical environments, this framework is a "backward learning" design in which the end target is defined for all, and there may be different ways to achieve the goal, but in the end, all students have the same learning target. Just as a stairway helps a person get to the second floor, an elevator can accomplish the same thing for someone in a wheelchair, thus AAC can be used in innovative ways when the curriculum is modified with understanding by design in mind and AAC supports the child's participation.

The task of the IEP team is to develop objective, measurable goals that are reviewed at a minimum annually but may be modified at any time. Goals should focus on access to general education and inclusion and include academic, motor, and social goal areas incorporating AAC throughout. For inclusion to be successful for AAC users, IEP team members must be aware of the cognitive, linguistic, social, and emotional parameters of AAC use. As inclusion requires intense and frequent participation in all activities, AAC users must have sufficient knowledge, skills, and social sensitivity to actively take part in information sharing and social interaction. Given how familiar technology is in the classroom today in many modalities and among young children in day-to-day activities, the use of speech-generating technology is more generally accepted by school-age children today than the early days of AAC when the student with AAC was the only child using technology, setting them apart from their peers. Moreover, positive depictions of people with disabilities using AAC within the media have also contributed to its acceptance and the acceptance of differences in others, as well as to the understanding that AAC is used by many different people with varying strengths and limitations.

Although the child using AAC must learn to use the system effectively and efficiently, it is just as important that the classroom teacher also understands the system and its use. Others interacting regularly with the child, including their peers, must also understand how to communicate with the individual using AAC. These are starting points for the team to support in terms of training and education. Equally important is identifying opportunities throughout a child's school day that increase feasibility for the use of AAC with appropriate modifications of curricular goals and out-of-the-box thinking for creating social interaction opportunities. The tasks of inclusion, training, and teaching use of a device with adaptations for curriculum can be overwhelming to educators at first. A useful process to analyze needs and identify goals is for the IEP team to sketch out a child's daily schedule and identify the academic and social demands for each activity, persons with whom the child may interact as part of those demands, then develop specific measurable goals for using AAC in those contexts. This can be done concurrently with developing measurable IEP goals, documenting progress over time.

Attention should be given to actively involving peers to ensure frequent contact and interaction with the AAC user. Through games, activities, and structured routines (e.g., circle time, morning story reading groups, attendance taking, show and tell), a welcoming attitude toward the AAC user can be promoted. Empirical evidence supporting use of peer training programs as part of the AAC treatment plan have positive outcomes for increasing message use, initiations, and number of social interactions by the AAC user (Lilienfeld & Alant, 2005; Trottier et al., 2011). Under naturally occurring conditions, AAC use has been shown to decrease when there is not a peer-mediated or teacher training program in place to help others identify potential opportunities for communicating with the AAC user (Chung et al., 2012). Training programs help reduce over-dependency on familiar communication partners, promote increased independence, and decrease the amount of support needed from paraprofessionals as peer-mediated opportunities are identified.

VOCATIONAL ISSUES, TRANSITION, AND COMMUNITY-BASED INSTRUCTION

At all stages throughout the student's educational experience, transitions should be considered that will continue to support the user of AAC while also allowing steady progression to the next stage of academic experience without regression of skills related to AAC use. Proper training of staff should occur, which may change by educational level and by school as the child advances through grade levels. In addition, an essential element of a treatment program is assuring a plan is in place for unexpected transitions, such as loss of key personnel who know the AAC user very well. In these instances, the child may not yet have the self-determination to keep the daily program going independently and may therefore still rely on others for support.

The IEP plan is a written document outlining special education goals and accommodations. In addition to the written IEP plan should be an electronic or hard-copy reference folder outlining use of AAC and daily needs that also includes information, such as schedule, peer groups, teachers, modification of assignments, etc. This backup plan is very helpful to all who support and interact with the student who uses AAC. To support transitions, this compilation of information can be shared with the next team who will support the student as they move on to each stage of education.

Transitioning is a required component of the IEP, which should be addressed beginning at age 14 years. Long-term goals to support transition to the workplace become part of the IEP within a transition plan and prevocational activities are identified supporting these transition goals. For successful transition to prevocational experiences, an assessment is often needed in which the potential workplace setting is evaluated for daily needs, communicative opportunities, and key communication partners for the AAC user. This process is conducted by a team that may include an occupational therapist, physical therapist, and speech-language pathologist in conjunction with other key personnel, the student, and the parent(s). Once this part of the IEP process begins, goals on the IEP are addressed within the context of the prevocational environment, not the classroom or therapy room. Within this model of instruction, it is essential that IEP teams define success in a way that promotes independence, expands the number of communication partners the student interacts with using AAC, and allows the AAC user to demonstrate self-determination and self-advocacy. Ecological systems theory, developed by Urie Brofenbrenner in 1979, outlines a framework within which an individual may be influenced by factors in the community and identifies levels of community systems from the microsystem (i.e., the individual's immediate circle of community, such as the family unit) to the macrosystem (i.e., attitudes and ideology of the culture and systems affecting well-being of others), which affect an individual's ability to reach full potential developmentally. Through the transition process from late adolescence to early adulthood, this model helps teams identify levels of support in the community, the need for self-advocacy, and established policies affecting independent living and supported employment—all affecting outcomes for individuals with disabilities. An example of a macrosystem factor is the requirement that the device must be "educationally necessary" within the public education system but must be documented as "medically necessary" outside of that environment. These factors influence access to educational settings and workplace settings. The macrosystem of governmental support, insurance reimbursement, and educational needs converge in a way that may not be most optimal and could cause delay in the development and successful progression of the individual with AAC. Brofenbrenner's framework continues to be relevant today, and it is helpful for educators and clinicians to consider the needs of the AAC user in this context.

In line with ecological systems theory, the *Community Based Functional Skills Assessment for Transition Aged Youth with ASD*, developed by Autism Speaks (2014) is a tool intended to support young people transitioning into the "adult world" and categorizes eight skills according to the following:

1. Career path and employment
2. Self-determination/advocacy
3. Health and safety
4. Peer relationships, socialization, and social communication
5. Community participation and personal finance
6. Transportation
7. Leisure/recreation
8. Home living skills

The tool supports teams in identifying levels of independence in these categories, the AAC system needed, and physical supports and cueing needed. It also tracks the levels of prompting and support needed from a level requiring a good deal of support ("Life Aware") to a more independent level ("Life Explorer"), tracking the gradual release of support in a variety of community-based contexts. Although intended primarily for the ASD population, the *Community Based Functional Skills Assessment for Transition Aged Youth with ASD* is based on ecological systems theory and identifies systems of support, opportunities for teaching skills, and supportive employment needs that can be applied to any individual with a developmental disability. Success is defined by fading cues and levels of support, which help the individual achieve the highest level of independence.

Supported Employment

Meaningful employment is the goal of many AAC users just as it is for most able-bodied individuals, yet until recently, many individuals with disabilities faced extreme physical and attitudinal barriers in gaining employment outside of sheltered workshops. Barriers ranged from reduced expectations and inadequate preparation to difficulties accommodating the various communication, physical, and technological needs of individuals with disabilities. Although in recent years these barriers are receding, there is still a need to provide specially designed instruction and training to individuals with disabilities using AAC to support optimal conditions for access to supported or independent employment. Insights from AAC users help guide the development of appropriate long-term goal planning in relation to future employment. Individuals using AAC in supported employment contexts reported the main factors to success included access to appropriate prevocational experiences and positive supports, including community networks, government policies, supportive coworkers, and access to computer technology (McNaughton et al., 2002).

Summary

Future directions are positive for supporting individuals with developmental disabilities using AAC. When considerations are given to the broader contextual influences on development and education, a comprehensive treatment plan with flexibility and appropriate AAC technology helps establish a foundation for success. When training is provided to AAC users, as well as to their communication partners, persons with developmental disabilities develop the skills necessary to contribute in meaningful ways. Moreover, with the advent of technology permeating every aspect of daily life, AAC use and modifying traditional ways of doing things should no longer pose attitudinal barriers previously encountered when AAC technology was considered a unique or significantly different mode of communication. Technology is evolving at such a rapid pace that the evolution of AAC use to support persons with developmental disabilities may prove to help remove attitudinal barriers and promote the individual for strengths the person possesses but perhaps previously was unable to demonstrate. Thoughtful, purposeful training of professionals toward a team-based approach to treatment will serve to further change the landscape of service delivery in relation to AAC use with this population.

Although early AAC intervention for individuals with developmental disabilities is aimed at enhancing learning and developing opportunities, one of the most important issues to consider is improvement in quality of life and equipping individuals with skills that will enable, as much as possible, autonomy and self-fulfillment. Transition to adult life, vocational issues, and employment hold many challenges for AAC users but can be met appropriately if approached with long-term planning starting at an early age.

STUDY QUESTIONS

1. Describe five risk factors associated with developmental disorders.

2. Explain how communication mastery differs from communicative competence.

3. Contrast non-linguistic communication with linguistic communication, and describe how these stages of development occur in infancy and early childhood.

4. Describe the levels of communication that should be assessed when considering AAC, from unconventional to conventional forms of communication. What other physical considerations should be made as part of the assessment process?

5. Describe an object communication display and discuss for whom this type of AAC would be most beneficial.

6. Identify two types of reinforcement schedules that can be used to support intervention with AAC for individuals with cognitive challenges or challenging behavior.

7. Explain two factors contributing to ASHA's position statement associated with facilitated communication.

8. At what stage of PECS is it best to transition a child with ASD from PECS to an SGD?

19

Using AAC to Promote Literacy

Ruth Crutchfield, SLPD

MYTH

1. Augmentative and alternative communication (AAC) users do not learn to read because they cannot speak.

2. Age is a factor for acquiring literacy. AAC users can be too young or too old to acquire literacy.

3. AAC users do not need to learn to read and write because technology will do it for them.

4. Writing is particularly difficult for most AAC users and is best left until later.

5. There are some books and stories that may be too high level for AAC users to understand.

REALITY

1. Although AAC users are at increased risk for difficulty in developing reading and writing skills, mastery of spoken language is not necessary for literacy development. In fact, some individuals with no functional speech demonstrate competency in both reading and writing.

2. Early intervention is key for all individuals with communication disorders; therefore, initiating intervention as soon as possible regardless of age will impact the communication and literacy of AAC users.

3. AAC users absolutely need to learn to read and write, not just to participate more fully in daily life but to increase access to and use of AAC methods, including those that utilize technology.

4. Early experience in scribbling, coloring, and writing is important for AAC users as it is for any developing child.

5. It is crucial that the same opportunities for exposure to diverse books and stories be given to AAC users to provide them with the same language stimulation that is provided to typically developing children.

Fuller, D. R., & Lloyd, L. L. *Principles and Practices in Augmentative and Alternative Communication* (pp. 373-390).
© 2023 Taylor & Francis Group.

AAC and Literacy

Literacy is a skill acquired through a systematic learning process. Individuals learn to read from many avenues, including their teachers, parents, tutors, technology, and siblings. Once one has learned how to read, it is easy to forget those who struggle with learning how to read, and we forget how complex literacy skills really are. In April 2017, the U.S. Department of Education and the National Institute for Literacy completed a study where they found that 32 million adults in the United States cannot read. This is a total of 14% of the population. Additionally, their study reported 21% of American adults read below a fifth grade level along with the concerning find that 19% of high school graduates are unable to read as well. When comparing United States literacy rates to other developed countries, the United States ranked 12th according to the National Institute for Literacy. Additional statistics include 50% of adults cannot read a book written at an eighth grade level, 45 million Americans are functionally illiterate and read below a fifth grade level, 44% of Americans do not read at least one book per year, and 6 out of 10 homes do not purchase at least one book per year (Diemart, 2018). Understanding the need for increased literacy is a key factor when working with all populations. Literacy contributes to communication, maintenance of social interactions, assessment of different aspects of life, and simply entertainment. Having diminished or absent literacy impacts a person's life in many ways.

Considering how important literacy is and how it impacts life, it is imperative that individuals using AAC receive instruction in literacy and literacy concepts. Because of the complexity in etiologies of the population of AAC users, there are several major factors influencing the individual's life in the area of occupational choices. If severe physical impairments are present, possible vocational opportunities that rely more on literacy than on mobility are more viable options for AAC users. Individuals who use AAC will be able to participate, impact, and mold society with their literacy ability intact and feel connected to their community, as their reading and writing abilities are not hindered by their physical limitations.

Light and Kent-Walsh (2003) purport that literacy skills are important to users of AAC because they provide a channel for educational assessment and learning, enhance vocational opportunities, promote self-expression, and facilitate independent living. Despite this, most individuals who use AAC have difficulty with literacy development. Users of AAC have significantly less access to printed materials and seldom engage in early writing or drawing activities. Furthermore, despite the importance of emergent literacy skills, few early intervention plans emphasize them. Users of AAC do not have natural supports provided to them, and adults usually dominate their interactions with few opportunities for children to take communicative turns. Adults often focus too much on mechanical aspects of books and reading materials rather than their content, and access to AAC devices are not consistently provided to children. Intervention works best when adult partners modify their interaction patterns (Light & Kent-Walsh, 2003).

Mainstream Literacy Research

Historically, limited literacy and illiteracy continues to be a phenomenon that is consistent in Western society. For many, reading is a simple concept of decoding written material. Actually, it is a complex form of interpreting visual and auditory stimuli. When an individual has difficulty acquiring literacy, there are multiple factors contributing to their inability to learn a decoding skill. Visual acuity and visual perceptual problems could be a factor. However, it has become clearer that the language component is a larger contributing factor to impeding or hindering literacy growth. The processing of all components, such as semantics, syntax, metalinguistics, and phonology, all contribute to the presence or absence of reading difficulties. Phonemic and/or phonological awareness has been found to be a key factor for acquiring literacy; therefore, including phonemic awareness into AAC intervention is a must for every evidence-based practitioner. According to Wolf-Nelson (2010), phonemic awareness is the ability to recognize the sounds in spoken language and how the sounds can be segmented, blended, and manipulated. Wolf-Nelson (2010) identified phonemic awareness as a strong predictor of later reading success. More so, phonemic awareness is critical for those individuals identified as at risk for reading difficulties. What is important for those who work with individuals with complex communication needs (CCN) to know is that phonemic awareness can be taught, and when acquired, is related to significant gains in reading and spelling achievement (Wolf-Nelson, 2010).

What about the use of symbols? Light and Kent-Walsh (2003) stated that little is known about how AAC symbols may affect literacy development. Graphic symbols may facilitate the awareness that print carries meaning and can facilitate an understanding of directionality of print. Users of AAC can acquire reading skills despite impaired phonological awareness and limited speech production. While most phonological awareness intervention is not appropriate for users of AAC, the most successful interventions involve explicit, systematic, direct instruction (Light & Kent-Walsh, 2003).

Along with the visual demands of literacy, the rapidly developing world of technology presents itself. Technology has made AAC readily accessible in the form of apps. There are various AAC apps that are free to download, and therefore, easily accessible. Light and McNaughton (2012a) argued that technological advances in the avenue of apps have made AAC much more accessible, which makes the user feel they are moving forward with their communication. However, the accessibility of apps and/or technology does not necessarily signify an evidence-based system is being implemented. What impacts literacy most when working with individuals with CCN, according to Light and McNaughton (2012a), is a poor app design or poor technology design. While visual screen displays support early pragmatic and semantic development, they are not impacting more complex syntactic and morphological development. Literacy skills may be better taught to individuals with CCN around the ages of 4 to 5 years using grid display–based AAC devices instead of visual screen displays. Written language provides powerful visual support to show children the patterns of target syntactic/morphological structures (Light & McNaughton, 2012a).

Emergent literacy refers to the knowledge children have at an early age before beginning the process of learning how to read. It includes the skills, knowledge, and attitudes that are developmental precursors to traditional forms of reading (e.g., pictures) and writing (e.g., scribbling; Whitehurst & Lonigan, 1998). Galda and colleagues (1993) purported the following: literacy learning begins early in life, literacy develops concurrently with oral language, learning to read and write are both social and cognitive endeavors, literacy learning is a developmental process, and storybook reading, especially within the family, holds a unique role in young children's literacy development and literacy.

Research Note

Pufpaff (2008) investigated the development of emergent literacy skills of a child using AAC. She studied a 7-year-old student with AAC needs who qualified for special education services under the categories of communication disorder and intellectual disability and was integrated into a general education kindergarten classroom. This study was conducted within an interpretivist paradigm, using participant observation and unstructured and semistructured interviews. The participant was observed for 8 months in the kindergarten classroom and other educational settings. The participant experienced a kindergarten curriculum utilizing the Building Blocks reading program, which is a balanced approach to literacy instruction based on the Four-Blocks Literacy Model. The Four-Blocks Literacy Model includes self-selected reading, calendar, language board, and working with words. Results indicated that both access barriers (resulting from the participant's impairments) and opportunity barriers (i.e., practice, knowledge, and skill barriers imposed by others) limited the student's active participation in literacy instruction. Ultimately, findings revealed a lack of collaboration among key school personnel and appropriate supports and accommodations provided to the participant affected literacy outcomes.

Hetzroni (2004) completed a review of research regarding the use of AAC for promotion of literacy in children with special education needs across various populations relevant to emergent literacy and AAC. Results suggested AAC could provide strategies and structures to offset impairments and disabilities of individuals with CCN. Hetzroni's (2004) review indicated reduced access to literacy is caused by limited use of speech, lack of opportunities to interact in conversations, and limited access to print. Motor and sensory disabilities may cause access restrictions. Research suggests even without these skills or the ability to produce spoken words, children can develop reading skills. Using graphic symbols with AAC devices, using printed words, constructing sentences with symbols maintaining similar syntax to written text, and presenting written, text-based sentences with symbols promotes emergent literacy. When several symbols are added in conveying a complex message, individuals learn to maintain the message in a consistent manner presenting it in a consistent direction. Mastery of these practices is a predictor for emergent literacy. Rebus and Blissymbol systems combine and add elements into compounds. This combination initiates the idea that connecting symbols together can create new meaning. This can facilitate understanding that combining symbols can produce sentences (Hetzroni, 2004), which is an emergent literacy concept.

Models of Literacy Learning

There are three basic models of literacy learning that continue to be emphasized as the concept of teaching literacy progresses: top-down approaches, bottom-up approaches, and interactive approaches. Top-down approaches are also known as whole language approaches. A whole language approach emphasizes the meaning of messages holistically and relies on the reader's prior knowledge of the world to extract meaning from written text. What takes priority is the meaning of the text and not the written symbols. Concepts, such as phonics and phonological awareness, are part of the top-down process but not the focal point. A weakness of the top-down approach is when a topic is novel and the reader has no background to draw from. At this point, the reader is unable to extract meaning from a frame of reference because there is no frame of reference.

This leads us to a bottom-up approach, which focuses on the individual components of reading, such as phonics, letters, vowels, and syllables. These are viewed as the building blocks of reading. The learner scaffolds their learning by acquiring each individual component and then building their literacy from the bottom up. This can be called a linear model. A weakness of this model is it fails to give credit to the reader regarding their previous experiences or even their future expectations, which may assist them in moving along more quickly in the reading process (Ellis, 1993; Wolf-Nelson, 2010).

The interactive model combines both top-down and bottom-up approaches allowing the reader to extract from their world knowledge while building a sound foundation when learning the building blocks of literacy. There is an interaction that takes place from both the top-down and bottom-up theories that allows the learner to draw from both approaches and develop into a fluent reader. The interactive model provides for an emphasis on foundational concepts while still allowing for the implementation of background information (Reed, 2018; Wolf-Nelson, 2010).

Stages of Reading

There are several models for outlining the stages of reading. Chall's (1983) stages incorporate six levels:

0. Prereading
1. Initial reading
2. Confirmation and fluency
3. Reading for learning the new
4. Multiple viewpoints
5. Construction and reconstruction

Stage 0 (prereading) runs from preceding birth to age 6 years. In this stage, preliteracy or concepts of print are being learned. Stage 1 (initial reading) runs from ages 6 to 7 years (American grades 1 to 2) and is a decoding stage where the learner is acquiring graphophonemic relationships. Stage 2 (confirmation and fluency) runs from ages 7 to 8 years (American grades 2 to 3) where the learner is solidifying what has been learned in the previous two stages and is preparing to learn new skills. Stage 3 (reading for learning the new) runs from ages 9 to 13 years (American grades 4 to 8) and consists of learning new information from a specific point of view. Students are creating new semantic categories by adding to their vocabulary, learning where to find new information, and reading at the level of an adult reader. Stage 4 (multiple viewpoints) runs from ages 14 to 19 years (approximately American high school) and includes learning from different models and relying on prior knowledge to expand their comprehension to move toward analysis and critical thinking. Stage 5 (construction and reconstruction) runs from age 18 and up and is known as the worldview state where the reader is combining cohesively what is being read, joining prior knowledge and new knowledge fluidly, and entering the world of abstract thinking (Tompkins, 2010). According to Reade and Sayko (2017), these stages are the basis for the more current labeling of levels that are more commonly seen, which are exploratory reader, emergent reader, early reader, transitional reader, and finally, fluent reader (Chall, 1983; Dorn & Soffos, 2001; Fountas & Pinnell, 1996; Snow et al., 1998).

Stages of Writing

Writing or encoding skills follow a similar developmental sequence. Based on Gentry's (2007) conventions of writing development, the stages are as follows:

- Stage 1 is scribbling where the writings of the child on paper look random. At times, they are circular and large and can look like a drawing. This is an important stage because the child is using the scribblings to communicate their thoughts.

- Stage 2 is letter-like symbols where forms emerge but do not follow specific placement. Numbers may be included. The child will tell about what they are drawing.

- Stage 3 is strings of letters where the learner will write some letters that are legible, which communicate they are learning more about writing. Awareness of sound-to-symbol relationship is developing, but correct matching may not be occurring. Learners in this stage may write in all capital letters and will disregard spacing.

- Stage 4 is emergence of beginning sounds where the learner begins to differentiate between a letter and a word while not using consistent spacing. What they are writing typically correlates with the picture or topic they are discussing.

- Stage 5 is consonants represent words where the learner is now beginning to use spacing appropriately between words but will continue to mix capital and lowercase letters. Punctuation is beginning to emerge while their sentences typically communicate their ideas.

- Stage 6 is initial, middle, and final sounds where sight words are spelled correctly by the learners along with proper names of those in their immediate environment. Phonetic spelling is often exhibited, as the word is spelled in the way the child hears it.

- Stage 7 is transitional phases where learners are now approaching conventional spelling and their writing is legible. Standard letter patterns and forms are now seen in their writing.

- Stage 8 is standard spelling where the learner can now spell most words correctly and is beginning to develop comprehension of root words, contractions, and compound words.

These stages provide a foundation for understanding how the mind of a child works when acquiring new skills, such as reading and writing. They provide those who work with children a view of the stages as pivoting points for establishing intervention goals.

Literacy is a complex integration of both decoding and encoding skills. An understanding of how reading and writing develop is a key component for understanding where the breakdown is occurring when a child is not successful in acquiring either skill. There are many additional factors that come into play when viewing a child with CCN, such as culture, society, perception, linguistic background, and metalinguistic background. When engaging in an encoding task, the learner is selecting an idea they want to communicate to a specific audience. The learner will select their vocabulary and sentence format to reflect the intended audience. Linguistically, the learner is choosing words that communicate their thoughts, feelings, and ideas while building cohesive sentences and paragraphs. All this is occurring while the learner is engaging in motor planning to hold a writing utensil and complete writing tasks along with all the complexities they entail (Erickson & Clendon, 2009).

Research Note

There is a glimpse of the teacher's perspective when working with individuals with CCN based on research investigations. Ruppar and colleagues (2011) surveyed a sample of 69 special education teachers who were teaching students taking the Illinois Alternate Assessment. Findings revealed teachers prefer to provide life skills–linked literacy instruction in special education classrooms and consider student characteristics and features of the general education curriculum when making these decisions. The educational setting had a significant effect on teachers' rankings of preferred literacy skills to be taught. Ruppar and colleagues (2011) concluded that teachers may not understand how to adapt literacy content or how access to literacy instruction in a variety of contexts may benefit their students with severe disabilities. Sturm and colleagues (2006) surveyed 141 first and third grade teachers who ranged from 1 to 40 years in the field and came from seven school districts within six states. Teachers were asked to provide an overview of which activities they used for reading instruction, the focus of the reading activities, and adaptations made to the activities for individuals using AAC. The investigation had a 27% survey return rate. Findings indicated reading activities entailed automatic word recognition, decoding, text comprehension, and independent reading. Additionally, users of AAC typically required adaptation in shared reading, decoding, text comprehension, and independent practice activities. These researchers highlighted the importance of having the learner communicate by conversing and writing about what was read so they can fully participate in reading activities. Therefore, this should be a top consideration when helping AAC users learn to read.

What is the purpose of a literacy activity? Literacy activities are selecting to master a goal be it to establish a foundational concept of forming a simple sentence or to communicate a complex thought or idea. A goal-oriented literacy activity entails having the future of the learner in mind. In the general population, the goals of literacy include increasing communication to those in one's immediate environment while continuously broadening one's expanded network, widening world knowledge and world experiences, increasing exposure in educational experiences, providing vocational and recreational opportunities, and facilitating societal participation while promoting independence. Soto and colleagues (2009) purport the development of literacy for children who use AAC is crucial to the point that it may be the most important functional skill that can be taught to them. Literacy will provide users of ACC the means to direct their lives, establish and maintain relationships, and assist them in participating in everyday activities. Even with the wide range of communication that can be achieved by using symbols, the alphabet is the only true symbol system that allows users of AAC to communicate with precision across environments.

Literacy Development With AAC Users

Research with persons with CCN reveals that achieving functional literacy is a difficult task for most users of AAC. Van Balkom and Verhoeven (2010) highlighted the neurocognitive basis of literacy acquisition and provided new insights from neurolinguistics and neuroimaging studies on language and literacy and their relevance for verification and validation of assessment and intervention methods and techniques regarding literacy learning through AAC. They also provided additional information regarding the specific features of literacy in users of AAC. Comprehension of written material (whether presented orthographically, graphic-visually, or tactilely) involves bottom-up word recognition processes and top-down comprehension processes. No matter the form, the first steps in processing and gaining meaning from words/symbols/signs/tangible symbols are the same and interconnected. While it is assumed that the different coding systems for processing written text, pictures, or tactile information are all interconnected, it is unclear how the information from each gets integrated. Brain research results are providing information that may help improve literacy assessment with AAC users and validate early intervention programs that are currently in use with this population.

Research Note

Soto and colleagues (2007) completed a case study with an 8-year-old girl presenting with muscular atrophy. This participant used a speech-generating device (SGD) for communication. Specifically, these researchers were investigating the development of narrative skills. After a structured assessment, intervention proceeded with storybook reading and retelling, generation of personal stories, and fictional story generation. Intervention occurred each day for 20 to 40 minutes. The subject progressed from using single words at the beginning of the study to producing clauses and sentences for narrative purposes using her device. She also progressed from inconsistent use of story elements to increasingly consistent use of these elements. The authors were unable to infer causality between their intervention and the participant's progress due to a lack of experimental control; however, they indicated the intervention used may be helpful in encouraging narrative development in other users of AAC.

Intrinsic Factors

Intrinsic factors can be broadly separated into four general categories of impairment that impact literacy. The areas of impairment include: (1) physical, (2) sensory/perceptual, (3) language, and (4) cognitive. Individuals presenting with one, some, or all these impairments may present with decreased literacy development. Physical impairment is one of the initial areas seen as a larger hindrance, as it is foremost in the area of remediation when looking from the caregiver's perspective. A caregiver sees a physical/health problem and goes into problem-solving mode to assist their child in growth and development. Sensory/perceptual skills are affected in the presence of a visual impairment. Individuals with CCN may experience limited exposure to stimulation due to decreased vision or limited line of sight, which is directly connected to their physical impairment. Hearing loss may also be a factor that reduces stimulation in communication, much more so in basic language foundation impacting the type of learner the individual becomes. Top-down, bottom-up, or integrated, the individual with a hearing loss is developing in a different world than the hearing community. Language development may also be affected by the aforementioned areas of impairment. A language disorder and/or a language delay can impact literacy because the learner may be presenting with nontypically developing semantics, syntax, phonology, and metalinguistic skills in oral language. When a delay is present, literacy will be affected as well.

Cognitive impairments can be present in individuals with CCN as well and will hinder literacy, as the areas of memory and retention are critical when acquiring reading skills. Sturm and Clendon (2004) stated language is what connects all the modalities, such as reading, writing, listening, and speaking. Children who use AAC to participate in literacy learning in and out of the classroom need to have a solid foundation in language and a means of communicating. AAC users face difficulties in all domains of language (i.e., phonology, morphology, semantics, syntax, and pragmatics), any of which can have negative implications on the development of skills needed for reading and writing. Children who use AAC are also at a disadvantage when it comes to experience with language and literacy. They often have more restricted experiences and have not had rich opportunities to engage in these areas. It is important to find ways to maximize the access AAC users have to language and literacy experiences. Also, AAC users must be given access to contexts in which they will gain the language learning needed for literacy development (Sturm & Clendon, 2004). Ultimately, users of AAC may have reduced opportunities to practice and engage in literacy concepts because their physical, sensory, language, and cognitive needs take precedence for their quality of life.

Extrinsic Factors

Extrinsic factors include the home and school environments. In the home environment, the caregiver is pivotal in providing language stimulation by promoting active involvement in naturally occurring literacy activities, such as storytelling, book reading, and nursery rhymes. Trudeau and colleagues (2003) examined the impact of an interactive book reading program. Four mother-child dyads completed the study, two with typically developing children and two with children exhibiting impairment. Children participated in shared book reading activities at home with their mothers

and in a group setting. The mothers were not given any specific instructions. The groups met once a week for 6 weeks, for 60 to 90 minutes each session. Activities were conducted with a shared theme from the book being read. The children using AAC were given access to appropriate vocabulary from the books being used. The authors believed that more direct training with the mothers would have aided the generalization process, and that merely modeling is not enough for some adaptations. One mother expressed doubt about her child's intentionality with the device, which suggests a need to address parent beliefs about AAC (Trudeau et al., 2003). Exposing the child with CCN to reading concepts at an early age provides a stronger foundation for literacy, as is the case with typically developing children.

In the school environment, the educational team spearheads literacy stimulation for AAC users. Teachers, paraprofessionals, and itinerant staff provide the model and stimulation for literacy. Factors that may inhibit the educational team include lack of experience with AAC in general, lack of familiarity with the specific AAC device the child is using, and most importantly, a general lack of awareness of which strategies are most effective when working with users of AAC. Because the educational team uses explicit instruction for activities of daily living for a child with CCN, opportunities for practicing and teaching literacy concepts are reduced. The reduction of opportunities to practice impacts the child with CCN in that they are experiencing limited exposure to concepts of literacy foundationally.

Assessment

Assessment Principles

It is imperative that speech-language pathologists have pre-established principles to adhere to in order to obtain a balanced assessment in the area of literacy.

- Principle 1. Assessment must recognize that literacy involves an integration of many intrinsic and extrinsic factors. Literacy achievement reflects the complex interaction among the reader, the text, and the context. Above all, competence in literacy must not be viewed as static. Every reader adapts and accommodates to different situations and demands. Assessment must be conducted across a variety of situations and settings.

- Principle 2. Assessment must provide a guide to intervention rather than establish a list of deficits. Pumfrey and Reason (1991) referred to this as the symbiotic relationship between assessment and intervention. Within this framework, the strengths, abilities, and strategies being used by the individual are the focus of attention. This approach relies heavily on criterion- rather than norm-referenced assessment tools, and much of the information gathering is based on observation rather than direct formal evaluation.

- Principle 3. Assessment must be goal driven and reflect the varied functions of literacy in relation to current and future needs. On the one hand, AAC can be used to access literacy, such as using an SGD to allow a child to participate in group book reading. On the other hand, literacy skills may form the basis for use of an AAC method, such as **logical letter coding**, to produce spoken and written language. Thus, assessment must reflect current and future AAC and literacy functions.

- Principle 4. Assessment should, where appropriate, reflect the developmental nature of literacy attainment. Both the forms and functions of literacy change as individuals become more competent. Skills that are relevant at the emergent literacy stage, such as scribbling, turning pages, exploring pictures, and playing with sounds, have far less relevance at later stages. Assessing knowledge of grapheme-phoneme correspondence makes little sense when a child still does not understand that print, rather than pictures in a book, is the focus of attention. Task difficulty, whether in decoding or encoding, interacts in complex ways with the reader's/writer's abilities; thus, an individual may have certain skills but not be able to use them effectively in all contexts. Several developmental stages may be observed as text demands change. Therefore, a rigid application of developmental stages is often not the most appropriate framework for assessment or intervention.

- Principle 5. Assessment should consider the adaptations required by AAC users and the extent to which those adaptations may change task demands. Many tasks involved in reading assessment require a spoken response. Thus, for many AAC users obtaining a measure of letter or word identification is difficult. Although some AAC users may be able to produce a recognizable word approximation, others may not. Providing choices ultimately changes an identification task to a closed-set recognition task. The change in task demands plus the potential cognitive load imposed by use of AAC makes generalization by typically developing readers difficult. Assessment procedures that require the fewest adaptations are suggested (Blischak, 1994).

Balanced Assessment

Due to the variability of literacy assessment when working with individuals with CCN, it is imperative to consider the following components for a balanced assessment:

- Literacy is a small but important part of overall needs of the individual with disabilities. Literacy assessment may be accomplished by a multidisciplinary team and will always have at its focal point the needs of the person when establishing goals.

- Literacy assessment is ongoing as skills develop continuously throughout the individual's life. Literacy assessment may be affected by several factors, including state guidelines, educational curriculum requirements, common core, etc.

- Literacy assessment includes the consideration of other factors, such as physical impairments, vision concerns, and severe speech disabilities, such as apraxia. Assessment may need to be modified through material adaptation in order to accommodate individuals with CCN.

Components of a balanced literacy assessment provide essential information for forming an intervention. Each assessment needs to be tailored for the specific age group being assessed. General procedures include the use of norm-referenced assessments, criterion-referenced assessments, informal measures, questionnaires, interviews, and possibly, independently made inventories, to mention a few. According to Rush and Helling (2012), the goal for AAC assessment is to pinpoint where the person with CCN stands on the continuum from emergent to conventional literacy. Part of the AAC literacy assessment process is to be aware of modifications needed in existing assessment instruments along with speech-language pathologists accessing their expertise when interpreting results. Informal assessment is a consistent component when communication needs are complex in nature. A formal assessment may not be sensitive enough to determine the differences and variances in an AAC user's literacy levels.

The following are components of a comprehensive literacy assessment: reading inventory/word knowledge level, word identification, language comprehension, concept of print, comprehension/print processing, and the inclusion of differentiation of assessment according to age, such as young preschool, preschool–early elementary school, later elementary school, and adolescence-adulthood (Beukelman & Mirenda, 2005; Soto et al., 2009).

Reading Inventory/Word Level Knowledge

Completing a comprehensive reading inventory encompasses all areas that contribute to word identification. Components of word identification include alphabet knowledge, concept of word, phoneme awareness, and sight word recognition. Some inventories that are available include the *Basic Reading Inventory* by Johns (2005) and the *Qualitative Reading Inventory, Sixth Edition* by Leslie and Caldwell (2017). These two are informal reading inventories composed of word lists and various passages that scaffold in difficulty in order to assess the individual's level of performance. By identifying the level where the individual is performing, the evaluator can design an individualized intervention plan for increasing literacy skills.

Word Identification

This is also known as automatic word recognition or sight reading. There continues to be no consistently reliable source of assessment of this skill in individuals with CCN. This skill is assessed by accessing graded word lists and presenting them to the individual asking them to identify the words. Stimuli are presented with similar words holding minimal variances. The individual can respond in whichever manner they are able (e.g., eye gaze, pointing).

Language Comprehension

Formal assessment measures can be used to assess language comprehension, as is discussed in more detail in Chapter 11. These results are part of the literacy assessment process. Informally, a paragraph comprehension task requiring oral reading can be used to acquire additional differential data.

Concept of Print

When assessing concept of print, the evaluator is observing and documenting where the child with CCN stands in areas, such as book orientation (i.e., how to hold a book), where to begin reading a book, knowledge of the front and back of the book, where the story begins, where the story ends, left-to-right reading of the book, identification of a word in a book, identification of a sentence in a book, identification of punctuation on a page, and turning a page to continue story reading (Rush & Helling, 2012; Soto et al., 2009). Marvin and Ogden (2002) created a Home Literacy Inventory Form in the journal *Young Exceptional Children*, volume 5, issue 2, pages 2 through 10. This inventory works well for obtaining crucial information regarding all aspects of home literacy in the categories of nonprint and print knowledge.

Comprehension/Print Processing

Comprehension and print processing in literacy encompass identifying to what extent the individual is understanding what they are reading silently. An informal task to use when assessing this area is simply asking the child to read a grade-appropriate passage and asking them what they read to gauge paragraph comprehension. When working with a child with CCN, any mode of response is accepted, such as pointing to target responses from a field of choices.

Differentiation by Age

Assessment procedures are described according to general literacy requirements across age span for four groups: young preschool, preschool–early elementary school, later elementary school, and adolescence-adulthood. Suggestions for assessment include specific procedures and questions that relate to consideration of opportunities, needs, and barriers (both intrinsic and extrinsic), assessment of materials, consideration of present AAC use, and development of an individual performance profile. Clearly, this list provides only a starting point for developing a profile of abilities and potential intervention points for any one individual.

Young Preschool

Independent access to print materials is critical in developing an early enjoyment of literacy. Many literacy activities at this age revolve around storybooks, early drawing and scribbling, and independent handling of books and other print materials. Repetition of familiar stories is an important factor in determining the level of sophistication with which a young child engages in storybook activities, including the level of dialogue surrounding the activity (Clay, 1991). Table 19-1 provides a list of specific questions for use with young preschool children that may be answered via questionnaires, interviews, and observation of children across caregivers (e.g., parents, extended family, daycare providers, teachers) and environments.

Preschool–Early Elementary School

During this time, as some children are beginning to read, others are catching up on missed emergent literacy activities. As such, literacy experiences in formal preschool settings and early elementary school involve activities just described for young preschoolers, as well as explicit instruction in the specific skills involved in literacy. Needs become more evident as literacy is increasingly required for school and social participation. Assessment of skills, such as naming alphabet letters and knowing their associated sounds, often enters the assessment picture at this level of development. Table 19-2 provides questions for use with preschool–early elementary school children, bearing in mind that questions from Table 19-1 may apply as well.

Later Elementary School

It is during this period that students begin reading to learn. Those who are not fluent readers have a special need for concentrated, direct instruction and practice in reading and writing, although as emphasized throughout, instruction and practice are important at all stages of the journey toward literacy mastery. Assessment of this age group thus requires not only observation of opportunities to engage in literacy experiences but also documentation of both quantity and quality of literacy instructional time. Unfortunately, Koppenhaver and Yoder (1993) concluded that children of school age with severe disabilities tend to receive decreased instruction in literacy when compared to their peers without disabilities. They tend to be passive participants in instruction and rarely engage in interaction with peers during instruction. They are exposed to interruptions during their instruction even though it is being provided in small groups and individually. Given these findings, comparisons need to be made between scheduled literacy activities and actual time spent in literacy instruction. As part of the assessment process, teachers may themselves be encouraged to monitor the number of interruptions to their schedules, taking note of each interruption as it occurs during the school day. Alternately, Koppenhaver and Yoder (1993) suggested setting an alarm watch for regular intervals throughout the day. As the alarm goes off, the teacher notes exactly what is taking place in the class, paying particular attention to the AAC user. Over a set time, a profile of time organization should emerge. Allowing the teacher to

TABLE 19-1

Literacy Assessment of Young Preschool Children

OPPORTUNITIES	NEEDS	BARRIER REDUCTIONS
Are storybooks often read to the child at home? In other settings? By whom?	What are the literacy needs throughout the day?	Is literacy important in the home? Other environments?
Does the child have a favorite storybook? Do they reread stories?	How is the child encouraged during literacy activities?	Do caregivers believe the child can attain literacy?
Does the child participate in reading activities? Assist in turning pages? Ask questions?	Can the child differentiate between the front and back of books? Top from bottom? Turn pages?	Are there barriers for the child during reading and writing activities?
Does the child handle books or other printed materials?	Does the child differentiate between writing and drawing?	Is an assistive communicative device used? How do they typically communicate during literacy activities?
Does the child have various writing opportunities?	Does the child know that during reading, some elements are repeated?	Are tools, such as amplifications and magnifiers, available to the child?
Does the child have opportunities to observe adults engaged in literacy activities?	Does the child engage in finger plays, rhymes, and sound play?	Are activities interesting to the child? Relevant to their experiences? Are writing materials adapted?

monitor utilization of time is less intrusive than introducing an outsider or teaching assistant as the observer, and results of the observation may be more easily accepted. Questions for use with later elementary school children are provided in Table 19-3.

Adolescence-Adulthood

Typically, adolescents and young adults decide what independent literacy opportunities they wish to explore. At this major stage of personal development and conscious exploration of self-image, reading and writing may play an important role either through correspondence with peers or through journal writing and reading. Of crucial importance are opportunities for privacy in reading and writing. Therefore, although many of the opportunity questions raised in relation to younger age groups may be asked, AAC service providers must also explore the opportunities for and barriers to producing and reading private texts.

During adolescence and young adulthood, literacy for vocational and daily living needs becomes important, as well as for higher education where appropriate. Barriers that may arise at this time include an over-reliance on a developmental framework of literacy development with an insistence on orderly progression through each of the stages, ignoring the fact that typical development is characterized by overlapping abilities across stages. Persistence with such a rigid application of a developmental model may result in little functional gain for some students, leading to frustration and eventual rejection of all literacy-related activities. Furthermore, the student's self-perception as a potentially functional reader/writer may be seriously undermined. Here, again, individualized assessment is called for with careful evaluation of the student's current and future literacy needs and how they relate to total functioning in relevant situations and environments.

Individuals With Acquired Disabilities

Another group of potential adolescent or adult AAC users includes individuals with acquired disabilities occurring as a result of a cerebrovascular accident, traumatic brain injury, or neurological conditions, such as multiple sclerosis and Parkinson's disease. Much of the assessment information to be gathered will mirror that described previously, including consideration of opportunities, needs, and barriers to reading and writing. However, additional intrinsic factors must be considered; first and foremost, the individual's premorbid literacy skills should be considered. This information must be obtained to establish a point of reference from which to conduct the present assessment and determine appropriate AAC intervention. An individual for whom literacy was critical for employment and recreational participation presents quite a different challenge than an individual who experienced past difficulty in achieving even a basic level of literacy.

Some individuals with acquired disabilities, particularly those with stroke or traumatic brain injury, may have visual (Padula & Shapiro, 1993) or physical impairments such that application of technology is required for access to reading and writing. For further discussion of issues surrounding assessment of individuals with acquired disabilities, see Chapter 21.

TABLE 19-2

Literacy Assessment of Preschool–Early Elementary School Children

OPPORTUNITIES	NEEDS	BARRIER REDUCTIONS
Is the school environment print-rich?	Are reading activities language-themed, or do they occur independently of other school activities?	What is the general approach to literacy development in the school?
Does the school have a literacy center that provides reading and writing materials?	Does the child attend to print in the environment?	Are reading and writing materials accessible?
Is the child encouraged to watch educational television that includes exposure to literacy? By themselves or with an adult?	Does the child identify the alphabet, associate letters with sounds, identify sight words, or demonstrate beginning word-attack skills?	Is there access to technology in the school and/or the home?
Are children encouraged to engage in literacy activities in pairs, groups, or individually?	Does the child print letters, sounds, syllables, or words? Use invented spellings?	Can the child participate in literacy activities as well as their peers?
Are visits to the library part of the home or school curriculum? How often?	Can the child retell familiar stories? Remember or predict outcomes?	Are appropriate messages available via an AAC device? If not, how are changes managed?
Are books purchased or borrowed?		
Does the child have their own personal collection of books or a favorite?		
AAC = augmentative and alternative communication.		

In summary, of critical importance in literacy assessment is the recognition that the previously described general principles serve as a guide throughout the process. AAC service providers must recognize the complexity and nature of literacy development, the interaction between intrinsic and extrinsic factors that influence that development, the contributions of various types of AAC, and the reciprocal relationship between assessment and intervention.

Intervention

When working with users of AAC, the professional always seeks to implement evidence-based strategies. Why is this? If an approach or a method has been proven effective, then positive outcomes are likely to follow when the approach or method is implemented. As a professional working with individuals with CCN, there is a consistent desire to provide ethical and proven assessment and intervention. We are at a stage of developing a broad research base in AAC. Not all currently used methodologies have evidence as to their efficacy or effectiveness, so it is the responsibility of the professional to research and identify what approaches, methods, or techniques would be most effective to use with the individuals they are serving.

A balanced and comprehensive approach has proven to be successful in facilitating the development of literacy for the learner with CCN (Erickson & Koppenhaver, 2007). Educators are using skill-based and meaning-based literacy concepts to draw in the user of AAC (Orlando & Ruppar, 2016). When using a comprehensive approach, all aspects of literacy, such as listening, reading, writing, and speaking, are integrated into the child's educational domains. These authors stated that giving a general definition to literacy that includes communication invites all to participate in literacy, not just those individuals who show the prerequisite skill of speaking, which is what most people associate with learning to read (Downing, 2005).

Skill-Based Concepts

Skill-based and meaning-based concepts are delineated rather well in Erickson and Koppenhaver's (2007) Four-Blocks Literacy Model, which was formed with the purpose of working with individuals with cognitive impairments. The Four-Blocks Literacy Model is based on the premise that not all children learn the same way and educators need to be prepared to present their instruction in a variety of ways to meet the child's educational needs. The model includes guided reading, self-selected reading, writing, and working with words. Erickson and Koppenhaver (2007) defined the four blocks as:

TABLE 19-3

Literacy Assessment of Later Elementary School Children

OPPORTUNITIES	NEEDS	BARRIER REDUCTIONS
Does the child have opportunities to engage in various reading/writing activities?	What are the literacy needs of same-aged peers in relation to academics, social, and extracurricular participation?	Is AAC use linked to literacy activities in the classroom?
Does the child spend a majority of the time skill building at word or sentence level?	Does the child comprehend extended written text? Answer questions and discuss the reading?	Is technology integrated and expanded upon? Are backup devices provided?
How often does the child produce text longer than a paragraph?	Can the child compose coherent text with only a few spelling errors? Edit? Revise writing?	Are there appropriate adaptations for test taking, homework completion, independent study, and text production?
Does the child have opportunities to read text of their interest independently? Is adult guidance provided?	Can the child access dictionaries, encyclopedias or other reference materials?	
Does the child have opportunities for discussing literature and future reading?		

AAC = augmentative and alternative communication.

- Block 1—Guided reading: Helping students develop the skills to select reading materials they find interesting. Providing opportunities for students to share and respond to what they are reading.
- Block 2—Self-selected reading: Giving students experience with a wide variety of text types. Increasing student ability to self-select and apply purposes for comprehending.
- Block 3—Helping children learn high-frequency words needed for fluent, successful reading with comprehension. Teaching children the skills required to decode and spell words they will use for reading and writing.
- Block 4—Helping students develop the skills to independently write a variety of texts for real purposes on topics of interest. Providing opportunities for teachers to conference individually with children about the texts they are composing.

The beauty of Erickson and Koppenhaver's model is it provides examples for how to implement the Four-Blocks Literacy Model in a general classroom and in a self-contained classroom; therefore, educators are provided a clear view of what is expected of them. They also included in their model general education concepts that have evidence-based support, such as the Know, Want to Know, and Learned strategy. In the Know, Want to Know, and Learned strategy, students identify what they know before reading, what they want to know, and what they learned after reading (Cantrell et al., 2000; Mandewill, 1994).

Meaning-Based Concepts

Working under the umbrella of meaning-based concepts entails providing the learner with opportunities to engage in the stimulation of literacy as often as possible in naturally occurring settings that are implicitly meaningful. When literacy is targeted in a meaningful manner, the learner is provided with multiple opportunities to practice their literacy skills. Light and colleagues (2003) discussed the purpose literacy instruction has as the focal point in increasing students' motivation to learn reading and writing, increasing opportunities for carryover of skills learned, increasing the generalization of literacy skills to novel situations and settings, increasing fluency, and ultimately increasing the integration of reading and writing skills in their functional form.

Research Note

Machalicek and colleagues (2009) completed a systematic review of literacy intervention research related to users of AAC. They searched electronic databases and found 18 studies published between 1989 and 2009 that targeted literacy intervention. Systematic instruction that includes scaffolding, direct instruction, and least-to-most prompting with time delay appeared to be the most effective strategies for teaching literacy skills to users of AAC. Additionally, Sturm and Clendon (2004) highlighted the necessity to select vocabulary well, always thinking of the specific user and their needs when selecting an AAC system, not only keeping their wants and needs in mind when selecting vocabulary but also providing additional vocabulary that will give the user of AAC ample opportunities to communicate outside of the scope of basic wants and needs. Barker and colleagues (2012) completed a review of evidence-based literacy instruction of children with severe speech sound disorders who use AAC. They identified the following concepts as most used in controlled studies for teaching literacy to this type of user of AAC: sound matching, phoneme blending, letter-sound knowledge and word segmentation, spelling, and word identification. The teaching methods used in this single-subject multiple baseline design that were most effective included explicit and direct instruction in the areas of phonological awareness, reading and spelling, and a most-to-least prompt hierarchy.

What impacts most in the area of research is sample size and type of study. Recent studies continue to have smaller sample sizes and single-subject designs. In order to solidify and clarify which methods are most effective, longitudinal studies with larger sample sizes are necessary.

Language and Communication

Literacy skills draw heavily on the spoken language resources of the learner within the context of communication (Galda et al., 1993). Therefore, the related purposes of spoken and written language must be made explicit. AAC users may be advantaged in development of this concept, given their exposure to the use of graphic symbols for communication; however, caution is urged by Bishop and colleagues (1994) in accepting the blanket assertion that reading acquisition is facilitated by graphic symbols. The role of the graphic symbol system is discussed next in greater detail.

Use of Nonorthographic AAC

The transition to literacy from use of nonorthographic AAC must be given careful consideration, although research addressing this issue is only in its initial stages. Koehler and colleagues (1994) have suggested that the use of fingerspelling may be particularly beneficial in facilitating phonologic awareness, grapheme-phoneme correspondence, and spelling. Because assistive communication devices (both manual and electronic) often contain written words and the alphabet, their use requires careful advance planning to integrate communication and literacy intervention.

Language Structure

The term language structure is used here to refer to experience with and knowledge of the structural aspects of language—syntax, morphology, and phonology. For typically developing children, spoken language development provides a rich resource supporting top-down text processing. In later development, experience with written language has important benefits in increasing vocabulary (Nagy & Anderson, 1984) and encouraging complexity in sentence level language development (Gillam & Johnston, 1992).

Language Development

Although research into language development in AAC users is still in its infancy, certain trends have been suggested, including a tendency to rely on short utterances and restrictions in sentence structure with a predominance of simple syntactic structures (e.g., Kelford-Smith et al., 1989; Smith, 1994; Spiegel et al., 1993; Udwin & Yule, 1990). Distinguishing between such performance restrictions and potential underlying competence is extremely difficult. Use of reduced sentence length and simple structures may be a response to pragmatic constraints, reminiscent of pidgin language strategies (von Tetzchner, 1985). On the other hand, access to complete sentences through single keystrokes (e.g., via an SGD) may have implications for language development that have remained, as yet, relatively unexplored. Given the uncertainty surrounding these issues, expanding experience in communicative use with a range of syntactic structures and inflections may be an important focus in literacy intervention. Furthermore, the questions previously recommended in relation to intrinsic and extrinsic factors should help focus distinctions between underlying competence and performance limitations (see Intervention Principle 4).

Phonology

In relation to the role of phonology in literacy development, attention is given here only to the metalinguistic skill of phonologic awareness. For a review of the literature in this area with specific reference to AAC, see Blischak (1994) and Hjelmquist and colleagues (1994). Although a severe speech impairment does not necessarily inhibit the development of phonologic awareness, AAC users face greater challenges in developing this critical skill. For all beginning readers, Adams (1990) has concluded there is strong evidence-based support for implementing efficient and effective reading instruction, which results in the necessary skill of phonemic awareness. For young AAC users, instruction may focus on encouraging parents and caregivers to engage children in reading nursery rhymes, an activity that may be otherwise overlooked for children with severe speech impairments. For older learners, sound play activities specifically targeting manipulation of the phonologic structure of words should be an integral part of instruction. Such practice is more effective if the connection between phonologic segments and letters is made explicit (Blachman, 1991), and therefore, linking with print the final segment of Figure 19-1. Goswami (1994) stated for training programs to be successful, they must educate in phonology and orthography along with emphasizing the connection between rhyming and patterns in spelling for rimes. Specific suggestions for intervention at all levels of language are outlined in Table 19-4.

Print

However facilitative background information and spoken language proficiency may be, the reader is still faced with the task of decoding orthography and the writer with encoding messages into orthography. According to Stanovich (1986), beginning readers must have a pivotal discovery of the alphabetic principle, that is, units of print map onto units of sound. Thus, any effective instructional program must incorporate analytical elements that focus on the specific skills needed for both decoding and encoding. As mentioned above, explicit instruction in phonologic awareness is particularly relevant for AAC users who are typically restricted in their ability to engage in sound play in early development or in "sounding out" at a later stage (i.e., exploring the relationship between sounds, motor movements, and grapheme representations).

The value of writing is frequently overlooked, partly due to difficulties that may arise in providing access to independent writing. The reciprocal relationship between reading and writing is particularly critical in the early stages of development. Ellis (1991) suggested that knowledge gleaned from spelling contributes to reading in the early stages, but the reverse is not necessarily true. He attributes this to the fact that spelling acts as a mediator for the influence of explicit phonologic awareness on reading. Within this context, invented spelling plays a particularly important role. Therefore, access to written output must be provided as early as possible, whether this is achieved via an SGD, word processing, or non–speech-generating technological options, such as adapted writing materials. Few studies have been carried out on the differential effectiveness of instructional techniques and spelling for AAC users. McNaughton and Tawney (1993) compared a copy-write-compare method and a student-direct cueing method for two adult AAC users and found only minor differences in rates of acquisition, although a retention advantage for the student-direct cueing method was observed. This finding supports the position that effective instructional practice drawn from mainstream research is effective for AAC users; the primary challenge is to creatively provide practice for individual learners.

Concurrent with a focus on the analytical skills necessary for decoding and encoding orthography, AAC users must be encouraged to develop additional alternative strategies for word identification, such as a sight word vocabulary. Opportunities may be present in many school environments where names are placed on chairs and hooks for coats or labels are placed on play materials.

Just as no recipe consists of a single ingredient, no instructional approach is effective if it reduces the complexities of reading and writing to a specific set of skills. Of far greater importance is a focus on developing flexible strategies that accommodate both analytical and holistic components. Galda and colleagues (1993) suggested when children acquire certain strategies, skills automatically emerge as well. Unless such skills are specifically targeted, assuming certain skills have been developed by AAC users may be dangerous. Specific skill instruction, such as letter identification and sound-letter correspondence, is recommended in the context of meaningful literacy events. Frequently, criticisms of instructional approaches that incorporate analytical

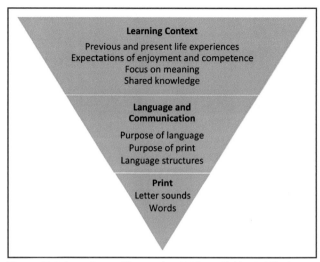

Figure 19-1. Ingredients of literacy. (© 1990 from *Children's difficulties in reading, spelling, and writing: Challenges and responses* by Peter D. Pumfrey & Colin D. Elliott. Reproduced by permission of Taylor and Francis Group, LLC, a division of Informa plc.)

components, such as explicit instruction in grapheme-phoneme correspondence, have arisen out of overzealous emphasis on the final segment in Figure 19-1, combined with inappropriate methods of instruction. However, as Blachman (1991) pointed out, in relation to phonologic awareness activities, no one has suggested that these activities provide a complete diet or encompass the child's entire day. Ideally, one would want phonologic awareness activities to be incorporated into a classroom where storybook reading was common-place, spoken language experiences were valued, basic concepts about print (e.g., how to hold a book) and the functions of reading and writing were developed, and children had opportunities both to talk and write about their experiences.

Balanced intervention requires consideration of all the components of Figure 19-1. For AAC users, certain aspects of intervention may be missing due to both intrinsic and extrinsic factors, and therefore, supplementary instruction must be provided, targeting particular risk areas, such as experience with print, expressive language development, and explicit instruction in phonologic awareness. Suggestions for intervention regarding print are described in Table 19-5.

Role of Technology

Technology can provide AAC users with opportunities for independent, active participation in all types of literacy experiences, overcoming many of the previously discussed barriers to literacy. Various types of technology to support literacy are readily available with new ones being developed almost daily. Indeed, keeping abreast of the latest developments in microcomputer hardware, software, and adaptations appropriate for AAC users can be difficult. Organizations, publications, educational software catalogs, and exhibits are available to assist members of the AAC team in product selection. As always, determining appropriate

TABLE 19-4

Language and Communication: Some Specific Suggestions for Intervention

PURPOSE OF LANGUAGE		
PRESCHOOL AGE/SCHOOL AGE/ADOLESCENT/ADULT		
Maximize opportunities to engage in communicative interaction with a range of partners, ensuring a range of communicative functions can be met.		

PURPOSE OF PRINT		
PRESCHOOL AGE	*SCHOOL AGE/ADOLESCENT/ADULT*	
Describe and demonstrate purpose; encourage caregivers' expression of reasons for reading.	Brainstorm, encourage students to list all the places where they see print in various environments, what that print means, reasons behind reading and writing, who they see reading and writing, when they themselves read and write.	
Recap the purpose following the task.	Provide the alphabet on communication displays, ensuring proper format of instruction is available.	
Label and indicate the printed message on an AAC display.	Highlight orthography on a communication display; use color emphasis to draw attention to the printed message.	
	Encourage use of orthographic strategies in communication to communicate messages otherwise unavailable through first letter cues.	

LANGUAGE STRUCTURES: SYNTAX-MORPHOLOGY		
PRESCHOOL/SCHOOL AGE/ADOLESCENT/ADULT		
Be aware of the expressive language level of the AAC user.		
Model a range of syntactic structures using the learner's own communication display; rephrase and expand on learner's own output to develop greater syntactic and morphologic complexity.		
Foster experience with a broad range of sentence types.		

LANGUAGE STRUCTURES: PHONOLOGY/PHONOLOGIC AWARENESS		
PRESCHOOL AGE	*SCHOOL AGE*	*ADOLESCENT/ADULT*
Encourage caregivers to engage in nursery rhyme activities as they would a typically speaking child, provide opportunities for the child to respond, and monitor responses.	Hide objects or pictures of rhyming objects around the room to foster rhyme recognition; present a target word and have the child eye gaze, point, or gesture to you the object or picture that rhymes.	Remember that building phonological awareness may not be an appropriate focus.
Segment words into onset and rime, prolonging initial phonemes starting with continuants.	Sort objects according to rhyme; have the student indicate by eye gaze or gesture where each object should go.	However, where indicated, similar activities to those suggested previously may be adapted to age-appropriate materials.
	Produce the target rhyme word and then list other words, have the child gesture when the adult provides a nonrhyming word.	
	Provide a spoken word and have the child indicate the rhyming word available on their AAC device.	
	Have the students sort objects in groups according to number of syllables, indicating by pointing or eye gaze to foster segmentation skills.	

(continued)

TABLE 19-4 (CONTINUED)
Language and Communication: Some Specific Suggestions for Intervention

PRESCHOOL AGE	SCHOOL AGE	ADOLESCENT/ADULT
	Have a bag for "sound of the day" to foster segmentation. Only words/objects that begin with the target sound will go in the bag. Student may indicate by yes/no response.	
	Choose one student's name, identify the initial phoneme, and have the children identify other objects in the room that share the initial phoneme. Use similar activities to practice segmentation-phoneme level, moving on to clusters, final, and medial phonemes; student's response may be adjusted through eye gaze, gestures, or yes/no responses.	

AAC = augmentative and alternative communication.

use of technology requires careful assessment of individual short-term and long-term needs, including opportunities afforded to typical peers and reduction of barriers experienced by AAC users.

Technology to support literacy—general computer hardware and software, as well as dedicated communication devices—can be divided into three broad categories with considerable overlap among them. These include technology that provides opportunities for: (1) early literacy experiences, (2) skill development, and (3) text composition, editing, and printing. Technology that consists of personal microcomputers and software for these purposes can be broadly referred to as computer-assisted instruction.

Technology for Young Children

The use of technology by young children should promote emerging literacy and provide reading and writing experiences through interactive learning with typical peers (Steelman et al., 1993). Preschool children who typically engage in emergent literacy experiences, such as independent book handling, rhyming and alliterative songs and poems, alphabet learning, and drawing/writing activities, may use both speech-generating and non–speech-generating technology, such as switches, tape loops, computers, synthetic speech output, enlarged keyboards, touch screens, and specialized software.

Experience With Books

Experience with books may be enhanced for young AAC users by various types of technology. A child must be provided a means to independently choose a desired book and the desired activity with the book via an appropriate AAC mode, such as a graphic symbol communication board or SGD. Preprogrammed messages, such as "Read to me," "I want to look at a book," and names of available books, should be readily accessible to the child. Some children with physical impairments may independently interact with books using modifications, such as page tabs, page separators, and/or thickened pages. Others with more severe physical disabilities may use switches to operate page turners, books on color slides (King-DeBaun, 1990) or videos, or computer software with graphics and synthetic speech output. Books on compact discs or other media commercially available for independent listening come with printed and illustrated text. For persons with visual and/or physical impairments, free books on audio are also available.

Active participation during storybook reading can be facilitated by use of an SGD or a computer with an adapted keyboard. An audio recording loop can be created to contain repeated or predictable text. SGDs with hybrid speech output are particularly useful in that they may be programmed quickly with any voice. Graphic symbols used to access voice output may be placed on pages of a book to assist the child in selecting appropriate utterances.

During storybook reading, typically developing children frequently comment and ask questions, later re-enacting the story alone or with another child. Unfortunately, these spontaneous uses of language are particularly difficult to provide for AAC users. Children who are afforded opportunities for extended interaction with typical peers are at a distinct advantage, as they can benefit from models of others' questions, comments, and protoreadings. Further, utterances produced by peers can be preprogrammed into SGDs for activation

TABLE 19-5

Print: Some Specific Suggestions for Intervention Using Letter Sounds

PRESCHOOL AGE	SCHOOL AGE
Name letters in the titles of their favorite books; attend to initial letter of their name and family members' names.	Incorporate letters onto communication displays; demonstrate access to letters in various devices; ensure appropriate formats.
Identify sections of communication displays for letters, adding letters as they are introduced in activities.	Encourage sound play by using SGDs; activate spell mode; encourage exploration of letter sounds, sequencing of letters, and activating the speaking function.
	Encourage invented spelling with voice output and explore spelling options.
	Provide word ending/rime; have students try different initial phonemes with an SGD and determine whether or not the output is a true word.
	Engage in "change a word" activity; providing a CVC word, then giving semantic clues to related words that require only one letter to change.

CVC = consonant-vowel-consonant; SGD = speech-generating device.

during both interactive and independent storybook reading. Preprogrammed SGD messages with accompanying graphic symbols should also be provided so that young AAC users can participate in a broad variety of imaginative play experiences that promote functional literacy, such as ordering food in a restaurant or writing tea party invitations (Koppenhaver, Coleman, et al., 1991; Pierce & McWilliam, 1993).

Technology may also be invaluable in providing opportunities for early drawing and writing experiences for AAC users—a challenging, yet critical aspect of literacy development. Non–speech-generating technology adaptations, such as splints that allow a child to hold a crayon or paintbrush independently, may be used, along with finger paints, rubber stamps, felt or magnetic boards, or unconventional drawing/writing materials (e.g., shaving cream). Children who have severe physical impairments may be limited to experiencing writing in a more indirect manner by using switch-activated or touchscreen software to draw, select graphic symbols (e.g., cartoon figures,

orthography), and compose lists of simple word/picture stories. Like early reading activities, drawing and writing activities may occur as part of an interactive group project (e.g., writing a language experience story after a cooking activity) or for independent exploration (King-DeBaun, 1990).

Skill Development

Classroom computers with appropriate software designed for vocabulary, word recognition, and spelling instruction, can be of benefit for many students in that they provide motivational opportunities for independent work with consistent, objective feedback (Beukelman & Mirenda, 1992). As previously emphasized, skill development should be used only in conjunction with interactive learning in meaningful contexts. Steelman and colleagues (1993) and Perez (2015) provide a list of desirable characteristics to guide software selection.

- Easy to use
  - Easy to install
  - Easy to update
  - Efficient
  - Able to quickly program
  - Aesthetically appealing
  - Easy to navigate
  - Easy to teach other service providers for carryover
- Differentiated software support
  - Online support (e.g., video tutorials, PDF files, remote login)
  - Technical support by phone
  - Personnel support (e.g., company representative availability for training)
- Flexible, allowing for individual modification
  - Allows for modification of the number of cells on the screen
  - Options for voices (gender-specific, options for accents depending on ethnicity)
  - Supports different languages for students who are English language learners
  - Allows for a variety of symbols (e.g., pictures, line drawings, photographs)
  - Allows for variations in the manner of physically selecting words/visuals for communication
    ◊ Direct selection (e.g., eye gaze)
    ◊ Scanning (e.g., joystick)
  - Allows for variations in positioning to meet physical needs
    ◊ Wheelchair
    ◊ Table
    ◊ Floor
    ◊ Different lap tray or display angles
  - Allows for adherence to color coding to reflect parts of speech (e.g., Fitzgerald keys)

- Supports classroom curriculum
    - Allows for the creation of page sets to support thematic-based literacy
    - Allows for commenting
- Language activity monitoring (e.g., maintaining a record of the words, phrases, and sentence structures used by the person with CCN can be useful to monitor outcomes, such as increases in utterance expansion and goal progress)
- Interesting to students (e.g., relevant to the age and background of the person with CCN)
- Appropriate for age and cognitive strengths (e.g., facilitating the ability to comment on age-appropriate topics)

Text Preparation

Beukelman and Mirenda's (1992) suggestions for text preparation for students with learning disabilities may certainly apply to many AAC users:

> Individuals whose progress with handwriting instruction has not matched their writing needs or who write very slowly may benefit tremendously from word processing programs operated through standard keyboards or alternative input devices. It simply does not make sense to deprive children or adults of the enjoyment of writing simply because of their poor handwriting. Unfortunately, however, many professionals are reluctant to allow access to a keyboard for young children in particular, possibly because they fear that the computer will become a permanent crutch and that handwriting will not develop as a result. As with all such decisions, this one need not be made on an either/or basis. (p. 240)

In the past, many literate AAC users with physical impairments tediously composed text letter-by-letter using one- or two-finger typing or a headstick. In this advanced age of technology, one can admire, if not marvel at, their perseverance in such a time-consuming and no doubt fatiguing and frustrating process. Communication acceleration techniques, such as semantic compaction (Baker, 1982) and word prediction (e.g., Newell et al., 1992), were designed to eliminate or save keystrokes in generating novel messages in conversation and text composition.

Semantic compaction is a specific semantic association approach. Chapter 9 discussed semantic association as a part of semantic and conceptual encoding in which individuals associate multiple meanings to graphic symbols (icons). These associations can result in keystroke savings.

Word Prediction

Word prediction, sometimes referred to as lexical prediction, is one of the most common methods for increasing speed of message preparation (see Chapter 9). Here, software in the assistive communication device is set up to provide the user with a group of likely choices after selecting (by using an input method, such as typing or scanning) the first letter(s) of the word. Some software programs also speak the predicted words via synthetic speech. The user then selects the whole word. For example, the user may select the letter D, whereby the words "Darlene," "David," "Dear," "Denny's," and "Denver" appear, usually in a window that is separate from the message. Most lexical prediction programs contain a stored dictionary of words, updated according to a specific user's most frequently used words. Entire messages, such as a name and address, may also be stored and accessed with a few keystrokes. However, keystroke savings is only one measure of efficiency of text generation. Extra time requirements (e.g., to scan a visual array, produce switch hits) and increased cognitive demands (e.g., memory) may work against acceleration for some individuals (e.g., Levine et al., 1986; Venkatagiri, 1993).

Most reported uses of communication acceleration techniques for text preparation have been by AAC users who had prior literacy abilities. As such, little is known about their effects on individuals who are developing literacy.

Role of Synthetic Speech

Although research continues to emerge regarding the benefits of synthetic speech in literacy development, opportunities to produce synthetic speech may foster the development of top-down and bottom-up reading processes and assist in text preparation. For example, Foley (1993) suggested that AAC users with poor decoding skills may make use of a talking word processing program to increase comprehension by independently listening to and reading previously entered text. Synthetic speech produced via an SGD or during computer-assisted instruction may also contribute to the development of word recognition (Romksi & Sevcik, 1993) and phonologic awareness skills (Barron et al., 1992; Foley, 1993), particularly when combined with print.

In producing text, synthetic speech feedback (with or without word prediction) may assist in selecting words for AAC users with poor reading and/or spelling skills. Teaching approaches to text preparation that emphasize process over product, often used with students with learning disabilities, make use of this technology so that the writer can devote greater cognitive energy to the actual process of composition. Here, software that allows pertinent vocabulary (e.g., science words) to be entered prior to student use may be employed (Beukelman & Mirenda, 1992; McGinnis & Beukelman, 1989). Synthetic speech feedback allows writers to hear their written work to assist in text editing.

Role of Graphic Symbols

One area specific to AAC that has just begun to be the focus of research and clinical interest is the role of graphic symbols employed by an AAC user (Bishop et al., 1994; McNaughton & Lindsay, 1995; McNaughton & Tawney, 1993; Rankin et al., 1994). Given the previous discussion on the importance of early language and communication experiences to literacy development, arguing against use of graphic symbols by prereading children to promote independent communication would be difficult. However, the specific processes involved when children produce language using nonorthographic means is currently unknown. McNaughton and Tawney (1993) described the holistic processing required when a young child is communicating with pictographic symbols and the visual analysis opportunities afforded by symbols containing sequenced components. They suggested that use of graphic symbols may differentially contribute to literacy development according to the type of symbol introduced at different developmental stages. McNaughton and Tawney (1993) regarded AAC users as having a vastly different development experience when compared to children without disabilities. However, the extent to which graphic symbol use may affect development of linguistic and metalinguistic underpinnings of literacy remains open to question. Bishop and colleagues (1994) speculated that the use of graphic symbols may support development of print awareness in young children, but that benefits may not extend to other processes involved in beginning reading.

Arguments against the contribution of graphic symbols to the development of print awareness, in particular for children with developmental disabilities, emerge from early work in reading instruction in which pairing pictures with written words actually impairs sight word acquisition (e.g., Blischak & McDaniel, 1995; Samuels, 1967; Saunders & Solman, 1984; Singh & Solman, 1990). In opposition to this, Romski and Sevcik (1993) reported results of a 2-year study involving graphic symbol and synthetic speech use by adolescents with severe developmental disabilities. In this study, without direct instruction in reading, participants recognized at least 60% of the words printed on their communication displays. Exposure to print in the context of meaningful communication interactions, along with the benefits of voice output, may have contributed to word recognition in contrast to previously cited studies in which sight words were taught in drill-type activities. However, until further research has been conducted, young AAC users should be provided with experiences that are known to promote the development of language and literacy.

SUMMARY

Throughout this chapter, the interrelationship between spoken and written language has been emphasized. For AAC users, this relationship is particularly critical because, to a great extent, aided AAC users are dependent on literacy for access to an open-ended communication system. Maintaining the delicate balance between a focus on encouraging communication and an emphasis on the development of literacy can be difficult. Using assistive communication devices to promote literacy development may lead to viewing the device as an academic rather than a communication tool. Thus, one aspect of communication may be overemphasized resulting in reduced opportunities to communicate across a broad range of settings and functions. Literacy development should not take precedence over more traditional communication intervention but rather the long-term impact of literacy on communicative competence should be recognized from the start. As with so many intervention issues with AAC users, a simple either/or position is ultimately disadvantageous to the AAC user. What is required is a holistic communication-centered perspective that recognizes the interdependence of communication and literacy without neglecting the unique demands specific to both. This requires consideration of the communication and learning environments of AAC users, as well as the resources they bring to the dual tasks of communication and literacy development.

STUDY QUESTIONS

1. What factors may impact the development of literacy in AAC users?

2. What is the complex integration of factors involved in learning to read and write?

3. What are the different stages of reading and writing that impact literacy and learning in AAC users?

4. Discuss the models of literacy and how knowledge of these models impact how intervention is planned.

5. What are the intrinsic and extrinsic factors that mold the communication and literacy needs of AAC users?

6. Name the variables that characterize effective literacy assessment.

7. Describe the differentiations that need to be made according to age when conducting assessment and intervention with AAC users (i.e., young preschool, preschool–early elementary, later elementary, and adolescence/adulthood).

8. Describe the differences between skill-based concepts and meaning-based concepts in literacy intervention for AAC users.

9. How can technology help in developing literacy skills in AAC users?

10. What are some desirable characteristics that can guide a clinician in software selection?

20

Communication–Based Approaches to Challenging Behavior

Lisa Beccera-Walker, MS

CHALLENGING BEHAVIOR

Challenging behaviors that are potentially affected by communication can take many forms. Emerson (2001) defined challenging behavior as "… culturally abnormal behavior(s) of such intensity, frequency, or duration that the

Fuller, D. R., & Lloyd, L. L. *Principles and Practices in Augmentative and Alternative Communication* (pp. 391-414).
© 2023 Taylor & Francis Group.

physical safety of the person or others is likely to be placed in serious jeopardy, or behavior which is likely to seriously limit use of, or result in the person being denied access to, ordinary community facilities" (p. 3). Challenging behavior can be categorized as destructive, disruptive, or distracting. Destructive challenging behaviors are harmful or threaten the safety of the individual or others, such as aggression directed toward themselves or other people (e.g., kicking, punching, scratching, biting, self-injurious behaviors [SIBs]) or things (e.g., property destruction). Disruptive behaviors do not immediately put the individual or others in danger but do interfere with activities of daily living. This can include disruptive verbal behaviors (e.g., tantrums with prolonged screaming and crying, loudly talking over others), verbal aggression, and disruptive physical behavior (e.g., flopping to the floor, running away from others). Distracting challenging behaviors deviate from typical age-appropriate behaviors and may include nonparticipation, ignoring teachers and peers, and stereotypical behavior. Examples of stereotypical or self-stimulatory behaviors include incessantly rocking back and forth, repetitiously moving fingers in front of the eyes, or flapping hands in the air. Challenging behavior varies in nature, frequency, and severity. Individuals with autism spectrum disorder (ASD) or intellectual disabilities may use challenging behavior as a form of expressive communication. Incorporating appropriate communication-based approaches promotes more adaptive behaviors and supports effective means to communicate wants, needs, and feelings.

THE COMMUNICATIVE NATURE OF CHALLENGING BEHAVIOR

The communicative nature of challenging behavior has a long-standing history. Typically developing children engage in challenging behavior for similar reasons as individuals with disabilities but gradually replace challenging behaviors as they acquire more acceptable and efficient forms of communication (e.g., speech). Individuals with intellectual disabilities and more severe communication issues seem to exhibit more challenging behaviors with increased severity than those with well-developed communication skills.

Because many individuals with little or no functional speech may never develop functional speech, AAC can play a role in replacing challenging behavior with functionally equivalent response alternatives, giving individuals an appropriate outlet to express their wants and needs.

Evidence From Typically Developing Children

Over time, typically developing children may learn that a behavior exhibited in the presence of a communication partner leads to a particular response by that partner. Eventually, the child will learn that behavior can be used to cause others to respond accordingly. For example, typically developing infants may cry to get their caregivers to fulfill their needs (Durand, 1990). However, there has long been discussion regarding the intentionality of such behavior. Evidence suggests that although challenging behavior may not be initially intentional, it may become intentional as a result of attributing meaning to these behaviors. For instance, a caregiver may interpret an infant's cry as hunger and respond by providing the infant a bottle. This pragmatic concept of perlocutionary behavior has been found useful in conceptualizing this stage toward intentionality. Challenging behaviors are "… perlocutionary in that their communicative value was more the result of the perceptions of the audience, than actual intent on behalf of the infant" (Day et al., 1986, p. 122). In reviewing the typical child development literature, the common conclusions are that challenging behaviors serve a purpose for the individual exhibiting them; moreover, as children acquire socially more appropriate ways to achieve their goals (e.g., speech), they tend to give up their old means (e.g., crying) of reaching those goals. It is also indicative of a behavioral instinct to increase use of spoken behavior (i.e., using words, phrases, sentences) with the simple **antecedent-behavior-consequence (ABC) model**. This model is a part of **functional behavioral assessment (FBA)** and serves in recognizing form and function of observable behaviors (see Figure 20-1 for an illustration).

Evidence From Individuals With Disabilities

Desrochers and Fallon (2014) state that an individual with a developmental disability shows functional limitations in "… three or more categories of: self-care, receptive and expressive language, academic learning, mobility, self-direction, independent living, and economic self-sufficiency" (p. 1). Among individuals with language disorders, developmental disabilities and psychiatric disorders, several findings suggest that the severity or frequency of challenging behavior is related to the severity of communication disability (Aram

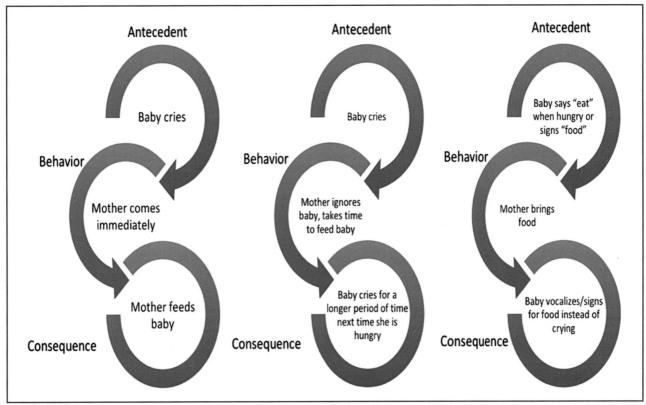

Figure 20-1. Sample of antecedent-behavior-consequence scenarios for infants.

et al., 1984; Baker & Cantwell, 1982; Cantwell et al., 1980; Caulfield et al., 1989; McClintock et al., 2003; Schlosser & Goetze, 1992; Shodell & Reiter, 1968; Stevenson & Richman, 1978; Talkington et al., 1971, Walker & Snell 2013). For example, Schlosser and Goetze (1992) found that 50% of the participants in intervention studies involving SIB had little or no functional speech, and 81% of the participants reportedly were not provided with AAC. In addition, McClintock and colleagues (2003) found individuals with deficits in receptive and expressive communication were more likely to exhibit aggression. Researchers conducted a meta-analysis of the risk markers for a variety of challenging behaviors. Self-injury was more common among individuals with a severe/profound degree of intellectual disability, a diagnosis of ASD, and deficits in receptive and/or expressive communication. Aggression was more common among males who had a diagnosis of ASD and individuals with deficits in expressive communication. Stereotypy appeared to be more common among individuals with a severe or profound degree of intellectual disability. Finally, destruction of property was more common among individuals with a diagnosis of ASD (McClintock et al., 2003). Trends suggest there is a possibility that severe intellectual disability, ASD, and poor communication ability could be interpreted as at-risk markers for challenging behavior but need further investigation.

A HOLISTIC VIEW OF INDIVIDUALS WITH DISABILITIES WHO EXHIBIT CHALLENGING BEHAVIORS

Before diving into a myriad of definitions and technical terms, it is important to state that as with any individual who is an early communicator (or early learner), it is paramount to ensure individuals who exhibit challenging behaviors are given a functional means to replace these behaviors with an effective means to communicate. While the following studies predominately involve education and organizational environments, it is essential to note that the same principles can be applied to this chapter. Psychologist Robert Rosenthal (2002) extrapolated the principles behind the Pygmalion effect (the idea that higher expectations lead to an increase in performance). While studies regarding the Pygmalion effect are difficult to conduct, results indicate there is a positive correlation between expectation and performance. Respectively, the Golem effect indicates when lower expectations are placed on individuals, lower performance follows. That being said, expectations (high or low) are critical when addressing challenging behavior and implementing communication-based approaches. Expectations are rooted in a fundamental understanding of the individual who exhibits challenging behaviors. While the term "expectation" is qualitative in nature, it serves as an underlying catalyst to ensure the presumed competence

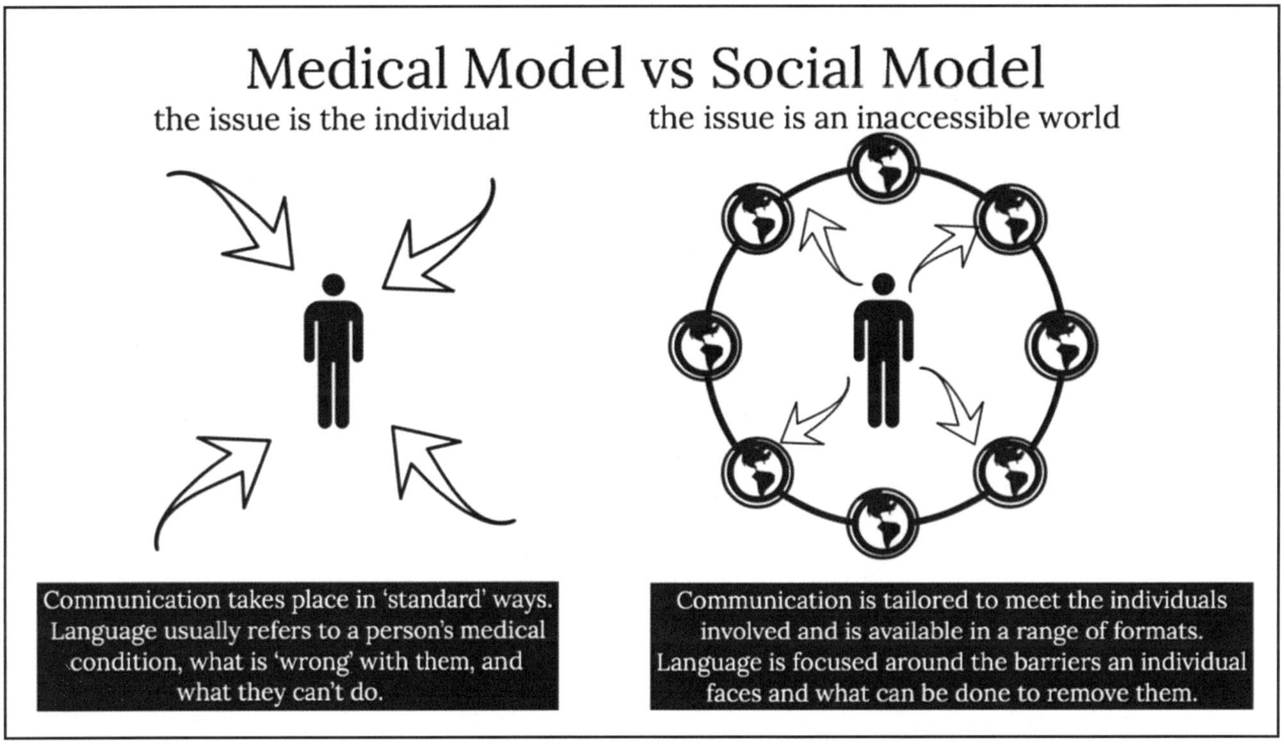

Medical Model vs Social Model
the issue is the individual   the issue is an inaccessible world

Communication takes place in 'standard' ways. Language usually refers to a person's medical condition, what is 'wrong' with them, and what they can't do.

Communication is tailored to meet the individuals involved and is available in a range of formats. Language is focused around the barriers an individual faces and what can be done to remove them.

Figure 20-2. A comparison of the medical vs. the social model of communication impairment. (Adapted from Parliamentary and Health Service Ombudsman. [n.d.]. *Introduction to the social and medical models of disability.* https://www.ombudsman.org.uk/sites/default/files/FDN-218144_Introduction_to_the_Social_and_Medical_Models_of_Disability.pdf)

is at the forefront of communication-based intervention. Often times, generalized statements regarding the individual's behavior, purpose, and even attitude are seen from a negative perspective. Reactive statements, such as "He's spoiled," "She doesn't understand," "He can't do anything," and "She attacked me," are biased in nature and often lead to low expectations and low outcomes. Proactive statements, such as "Let's try a different approach," "Let's see what I can do to help," and "How can I make this better?," are unbiased and lead to better expectations and outcomes. In order to set expectations high, one must see an individual who exhibits challenging behavior holistically. In doing so, we look beyond the challenging behavior to a child or adult with purpose, emotions, and the right to communicate. This type of social/neurodiversity model values the individual and differs from the disability model where the disability is typically seen as the problem (Figure 20-2). Individuals with disabilities "who embrace the social model view their disabilities as an additive identity, a positive trait which is an inextricable part of who they are. In this manner, the social model gives rise to the notion of disability pride and disability culture" (Disability Studies 101, n.d.). This shift in perspective will often result in a shift toward "presumed competence," a term used to describe an individual's level of competence to communicate effectively using communication-based strategies. Presumed competence indicates the belief that the individual exhibiting challenging behavior will develop the necessary skills required to access and use communication strategies to replace challenging behavior with an appropriate means to communicate. There is

a notion among practitioners that there are not any prerequisites for AAC. Individuals should have access to AAC systems or devices that promote effective communication (American Speech-Language-Hearing Association, 2018a).

COMMUNICATION-BASED APPROACHES TO CHALLENGING BEHAVIOR

There is a strong positive correlation between the severity of an individual's communication disorder and the frequency and intensity of challenging behavior exhibited. Prior to the widespread use of communication-based approaches, challenging behaviors were largely addressed through other interventions employed without consideration of the function of the behavior, including time out, medication, and restraint (Durand, 1990; Schlosser & Goetze, 1992). Matson and colleagues (2010) examined the relationship between communication skills, social skills, and challenging behaviors with children with ASD. These traditional approaches focused on reducing challenging behavior without considering what types of skills needed to be taught to bring about the permanent replacement of challenging behavior (Carr et al., 1994). Results from Walker and Snell's (2013) meta-analysis regarding the effects of AAC on challenging behavior indicated that if challenging behaviors of individuals with and without disabilities are left unresolved, these individuals will exhibit negative outcomes in the areas of educational achievement,

TABLE 20-1

Prevalence of Challenging Behavior in Persons With Certain Disabilities

POPULATION	PREVALENCE OF CHALLENGING BEHAVIOR	STUDY
Intellectual disabilities	Self-injurious behavior, 19.1% prevalence rate	Maclean & Dornbush, 2012
Autism spectrum disorder	Mild to severe aggression, 88% prevalence rate	Felce & Kerr, 2013
High-functioning children with autism spectrum disorder	Behavioral or emotional problems, 72% to 86% prevalence rate	Ooi et al., 2011

vocational success, and social relationships. Table 20-1 indicates prevalence rates regarding individuals with disabilities who exhibit challenging behaviors. The presence of communication deficiencies has often been linked to the presence of challenging behavior (Kevan, 2003; Matson et al., 2009). This chapter uses the term "communication-based approaches" rather than "communication approaches to challenging behavior." This distinction is made because communication-based approaches consider communication issues in the assessment and intervention processes but may also include other behavioral, or operant, strategies to address the challenging behavior (Carr et al., 1994). Communication-based approaches with an emphasis on behavioral intervention involve assessing the form, as well as functions, of the behaviors and subsequently replacing the challenging behavior by teaching an appropriate alternative behavior that serves the same communicative function, and in turn, affords the individual an opportunity to communicate appropriately.

Behavioral Contingencies That Affect Functional Communication

Behavioral contingencies state "if-then" conditions that prepare the stage for a *potential* occurrence of a particular behavior and its related consequences. Often times, challenging behavior can fall into "if-then" conditions. The contingency would then indicate the relationship between the child and the challenging behavior: If "A" (antecedent) occurs, then "B" (behavior) occurs, and if "B" occurs, then "C" (consequences) follow (see Figure 20-1). In an effort to change challenging behavior through the use of appropriate communication-based intervention, it is imperative to know the relationship between **reinforcement** and how it is contingent on the behavior. This relationship is illustrated in Figure 20-3. Desrochers and Fallon (2014) indicate that "[t]he main factors that contribute to the occurrence of challenging behavior include the immediate environmental consequences that follow that behavior and the cues or antecedents that signal those desired consequences" (pp. 6-7). Numerous studies demonstrate that **positive reinforcement**

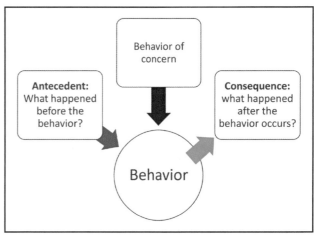

Figure 20-3. An overview of antecedent-behavior-consequence.

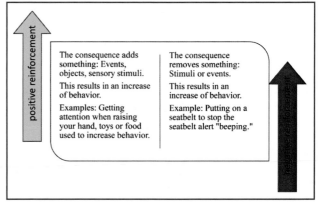

Figure 20-4. Positive reinforcement vs. negative reinforcement.

and **negative reinforcement** act as a precursor for an individual's challenging behavior (Beavers et al., 2013; Lancioni et al., 2012; Matson, 2009). A description of positive and negative reinforcement can be found in Figure 20-4.

The relationship of the contingency is directly related to the success of decreasing challenging behavior. It is the merging of communication-based approaches and establishing a behavioral contingency. Its success requires quick reinforcement, clear communication, and consistency. Students who do

TABLE 20-2

Topography of Behavior and Behavior Functions

FUNCTION	WHAT IS OCCURRING?	WHY IS IT OCCURRING?
Attention	Child pinches classmates during class without provocation. Teacher scolds child.	Child wants attention.
Tangibles or activities	Child screams when parents say "no" to buying a new toy at the store. Parents buy child the toy.	Child wants a toy (tangible).
Escape or avoidance	Child hits head against the desk when teacher tells them to finish their work.	Child does not want to complete work (escape).
Sensory stimulation	Child rocks back and forth throughout the day.	Child finds rocking enjoyable (internal sensation is pleasing).

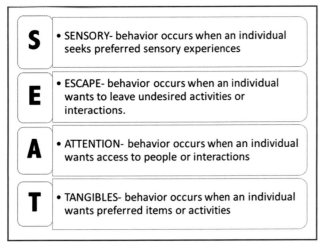

Figure 20-5. SEAT: An acronym for behavior functions. (Adapted from HonuIntervention. [2017]. Function-based intervention [PDF]. Retrieved from https://72aa752c-61fb-4cc4-a8c1-828003da22ee.filesusr.com/ugd/6ce87f_2fa2989c391e4b2a88977680ee7e9868.pdf)

not receive immediate reinforcement or are not clear about the relationship of contingency will not be as successful as those children who clearly understand the relationship or contingency (Webster, 2017). Understanding the consequences helps us to identify the function of the challenging behavior and how the behavior is being reinforced. When finding a communicative method to replace challenging behavior, practitioners need to understand the function of the original behavior.

Identifying Communicative Function of Challenging Behaviors

Four major areas of communicative function have been identified that can be addressed with communication-based approaches, including access to attention, access to tangibles, escape, and sensory stimulation (Durand, 1990). When challenging behavior is seen as a representation of an individual trying to transmit a message or a need instead of a response that needs to be reduced or extinguished, professionals are

able to identify the communicative function of the behavior, and in turn, offer an appropriate alternative that serves to increase communication skills and decrease challenging behavior (Bopp et al., 2004). Topography of behavior and behavior functions are noted in Table 20-2. An acronym for behavior functions can also be found in Figure 20-5.

Social Attention

Some challenging behavior may be positively reinforced by social attention, suggesting the behavior may be used to elicit or request attention (Carr & Durand, 1985a). For example, a student may engage in challenging behavior whenever the teacher directs attention away from the student to write on the blackboard or whenever the teacher divides attention between the student and a peer (Lalli & Goh, 1993). If the teacher redirects attention back to the student because of the behavior, the problem behavior is reinforced and likely to occur more frequently. If the student is taught to raise their hand to gain the teacher's attention, the challenging behavior might be decreased.

Access to Tangibles

Tangible consequences (e.g., food, toys, activities) may also serve as positive reinforcement for challenging behavior (e.g., Doss & Reichle, 1989). Individuals may engage in challenging behavior when they are denied access to a preferred item or activity, an item they had inappropriately manipulated or obtained is removed, or delays occur between a request and the actual presentation of a requested item (Lalli & Goh, 1993). For example, a resident in a group home liked to put on layers of clothing that belonged to other residents. When this was discovered by staff and he was asked to return the clothing items, he would engage in an episode of SIB. Frequently, staff did not follow through and the resident was allowed to keep the clothing. In another instance when a child wants a toy while shopping at a store, they may resort to flopping or screaming. If the parent complies and buys the toy, the behavior is reinforced.

Escape

Some challenging behavior may occur to escape demands and caregiver expectations for performance (Carr & Durand, 1985b; Mace & Roberts, 1993). This type of behavior serves as a request to terminate, postpone, or withdraw from ongoing activity or interaction. For example, a child may engage in aggressive behavior to terminate a personal care activity prematurely (Lalli & Goh, 1993). When the caregiver reduces expectations for the child to perform the personal care activity, the child may learn that by engaging in challenging behavior, the caregiver would stop making demands. In other words, the child's behavior was negatively reinforced for engaging in challenging behavior by the caregiver's withdrawal of aversive demands. Another example would be a child who is told to brush their teeth and then hits the caregiver in protest. The caregiver withdraws the demand and the child is not required to brush their teeth.

Sensory Consequences/ Automatic Reinforcement

In addition to these socially mediated functions, challenging behavior may be maintained by sensory consequences (e.g., auditory, visual, tactile) provided by engaging in the behavior (e.g., Rincover & Devany, 1982). For example, a student may obtain external stimulation as auditory feedback from banging objects against a hard surface or visual feedback from a spinning object (Rincover & Devany, 1982). A student engaging in stereotypic body rocking may be reinforced by such internal stimulation as kinesthetic feedback from the trunk and/or vestibular feedback from the inner ear (Lovaas et al., 1987). These scenarios are examples of automatic positively reinforced behavior because the student gets something without another person being involved (Cooper et al., 2007). Automatic negatively reinforced behavior can also occur in the event that an individual avoids something as a result of their own behavior (Miltenberger, 2008), such as an individual washes their hands because they wrote on them with a marker.

When Communicative Functions Cannot Be Honored

There will be situations when communicative functions can not be honored. For instance, caregivers may not always be able to provide attention or access to preferred objects every time the individual communicates appropriately. Staff in a group home cannot always provide a van ride whenever one of the residents requests one. Also, in community settings, it may be inappropriate for an individual to escape nonpreferred activities (e.g., brushing teeth, taking medicine) through communication because of missed learning opportunities (e.g., learning to brush teeth) or harmful consequences (e.g., seizures; Fisher et al., 1993).

In these situations, intervention strategies can be used in conjunction with teaching communicative alternatives. Teaching tolerance for delay is one such strategy that may be accomplished through demand fading and reinforcement fading (Bird et al., 1989; Fisher et al., 1993). In demand fading, the individual is required to complete one or a few task steps before communication will function to allow escape. For instance, an individual in a vocational program may be required to sort a predetermined number of items before signing FINISHED, which results in an escape from the task. The number of requested things to sort before escaping through signing FINISHED would then gradually increase. With reinforcement fading, the individual may be required to wait a few seconds after emitting the appropriate communicative response (e.g., signing FINISHED) associated with the positive reinforcer (e.g., escape). The length of delay would then gradually increase.

Functional Equivalence and Response Efficiency

When using communication-based approaches, appropriate communicative responses that serve the same function as challenging behavior are taught. For example, an individual may be taught to request objects by pointing rather than engaging in challenging behavior with the behavior of pointing being positively reinforced by obtaining the object more efficiently. An individual whose challenging behavior is motivated by escape may be taught to request a break or assistance by using manual signs (Fisher et al., 1993). The relationship between challenging behavior and desired replacement behavior is known as **functional equivalence** (Carr, 1988). The interventionist attempts to ensure that obtaining desirable consequences and reinforcers proves more successful through the use of appropriate communicative behaviors rather than the challenging behavior (Beukelman & Mirenda, 2012; Carr et al., 1994; Donnellan et al., 1984; Doss & Reichle, 1989; Durand, 1990; Durand & Berotti, 1991; Durand et al., 1993; Johnston & Reichle, 1993). Whether the replacement behavior can address the function of challenging behavior depends on its efficiency (Horner & Day, 1991).

Three variables affect **response efficiency**: (1) the physical effort required to perform the response (i.e., the energy that must be expended), (2) the schedule of reinforcement, and (3) the time delay between presentation of the discriminative stimulus for a target response and delivery of the reinforcer for that response (Beukelman & Miranda 2005; Horner & Day, 1991; Horner et al., 1990). Head hitting and signing may both serve as responses that result in the removal of a difficult task. Signing may be more efficient if it requires less effort than head hitting, is followed by a break each time the response is emitted, and the learner gets the break immediately after requesting. On the other hand, head hitting may be more efficient if signing must be done several times to get the teacher's attention and is followed by significant delays, whereas head hitting gets immediate results (Horner & Day, 1991). From the individual's perspective, the replacement behavior must be as good as or better than the challenging behavior at accomplishing the desired outcome. The challenging behavior will continue if the attempted replacement behavior is more difficult than the original behavior. This then renders the replacement behavior ineffective.

Functional Behavioral Assessment

To design and implement communication-based interventions, functional assessment techniques are required. These are the full range of strategies used to develop and test hypotheses regarding antecedents and consequences that control challenging behavior. FBA is an ongoing process for designing an initial intervention and continuously making adjustments based on changes in behavior during the implementation of intervention (Horner, 1994). Available techniques are reviewed only briefly here along with examples of their applications. The goal of an FBA is to determine the function of challenging behavior. For more comprehensive information, refer to *Instruction in Functional Assessment* (Desrochers & Fallon 2014).

Developing a Hypothesis About the Cause of Challenging Behaviors

Hypothesis development focuses on identifying the possible functional relationship between challenging behavior and naturally occurring environmental events. Hypotheses may be developed through indirect and direct methods. Indirect methods are typically completed by or with partners who are familiar with the individual rather than by the individual themselves. Indirect methods may include rating scales and interviews. Hypotheses developed from indirect methods may be further refined through direct methods. Direct methods involve gathering information by observing the individual who exhibits challenging behavior in a variety of environments. Some examples of commonly used methods for hypothesis development are outlined below. Ruling out medical reasons for challenging behavior should also be taken into consideration. Some examples of commonly used methods for hypothesis development are also outlined below.

Functional Analysis Screening Tool

The Functional Analysis Screening Tool (FAST) is a 16-item questionnaire that can be administered to individuals who know the person who exhibits challenging behavior. It serves to identify antecedents and consequences correlated with the behavior and organizes them into four functional categories based on contingencies that maintain problem behavior. Behavior is organized into the following functional categories: social (i.e., attention/preferred items), social (i.e., escape from tasks/activities), automatic (i.e., sensory stimulation), and automatic (i.e., pain attenuation; Iwata et al., 2013). FAST can be a quick means of obtaining preliminary

information about the nature of challenging behavior, but additional corroborating evidence about the function of the behavior is necessary (Desrochers & Fallon, 2014). A sample FAST form can be found in Figure 20-6.

Motivation Assessment Scale

The Motivation Assessment Scale (MAS) is a rating scale widely used to develop initial hypotheses regarding the functions of challenging behavior (Durand & Crimmins, 1992). The MAS is a 16-item survey with four questions within each of four groups of motivational factors (stimulus events): (1) sensory feedback, (2) escape, (3) social attention, and (4) tangibles. MAS is administered to many individuals who are familiar with the individual being assessed. Multiple assessments can be administered depending on the number of target behaviors and the number of different settings where the behavior occurs. Each question on MAS is scored on a scale from 0 (never) to 6 (always), and totals are derived for each of the four motivational factors. Higher scores for a particular factor establish the hypothesis that the challenging behavior may be maintained by this motivational factor. Overall, most researchers agree that MAS is useful in generating initial hypotheses, but it should only be used in conjunction with other assessment methods (Durand & Crimmins, 1992; Kearney, 1994).

Functional Assessment Interview

The Functional Assessment Interview is an example of a structured interview (O'Neill et al., 1990). The Functional Assessment Interview includes sections describing the challenging behavior, the events and situations that predict its occurrences, its possible functions, and a history of previous intervention attempts. Noteworthy from a communication perspective are the sections on the primary ways of communicating and the functional alternative behaviors known by the person. Included are questions regarding existing expressive communication strategies and their consistency, receptive communication (e.g., following verbal directions and gestural/signed instructions, making yes/no responses, and imitating models), and the behaviors used to express various communicative functions.

Antecedent-Behavior-Consequence Chart

The ABC chart is a tool used during direct observation of the individual to keep a continuous record of variables that affect challenging behavior (Alter et al., 2008). The goal of the observation is to witness the individual experiencing challenging behavior in natural settings where the events leading to and following the challenging behavior can be analyzed. The ABC chart is divided into three columns with each column used to collect information on antecedents leading to the behavior, the behavior itself, and consequences of the behavior, respectively. In order to get a clearer understanding of cause and effect, each behavior or stimulus is numbered

F A S T

Functional Analysis Screening Tool

Client:_____ Date:_____

Informant:_____ Interviewer:_____

To the Interviewer: The FAST identifies factors that may influence problem behaviors. Use it only for screening as part of a comprehensive functional analysis of the behavior. Administer the FAST to several individuals who interact with the client frequently. Then use the results to guide direct observation in several different situations to verify suspected behavioral functions and to identify other factors that may influence the problem behavior.

To the Informant: Complete the sections below. Then read each question carefully and answer it by circling "Yes" or "No." If you are uncertain about an answer, circle "N/A."

Informant-Client Relationship
1. Indicate your relationship to the person: ___Parent ___Instructor
___Therapist/Residential Staff _____(Other)
2. How long have you known the person? ____Years ____Months
3. Do you interact with the person daily? ____Yes ____No
4. In what situations do you usually interact with the person?
___ Meals ___ Academic training
___ Leisure ___ Work or vocational training
___ Self-care _____(Other)

Problem Behavior Information
1. Problem behavior (check and describe):
___ Aggression _____
___ Self-Injury _____
___ Stereotypy _____
___ Property destruction _____
___ Other _____
2. Frequency: __Hourly __Daily __Weekly __Less often
3. Severity: __Mild: Disruptive but little risk to property or health
__Moderate: Property damage or minor injury
__Severe: Significant threat to health or safety
4. Situations in which the problem behavior is <u>most</u> likely to occur:
Days/Times_____
Settings/Activities _____
Persons present _____
5. Situations in which the problem behavior is <u>least</u> likely to occur:
Days/Times_____
Settings/Activities _____
Persons present _____
6. What is usually happening to the person right <u>before</u> the problem behavior occurs?_____
_____
_____
7. What usually happens to the person right <u>after</u> the problem behavior occurs?_____
_____
_____
8. Current treatments_____
_____
_____
_____

1. Does the problem behavior occur when the person is not receiving attention or when caregivers are paying attention to someone else? — Yes No N/A

2. Does the problem behavior occur when the person's requests for preferred items or activities are denied or when these are taken away? — Yes No N/A

3. When the problem behavior occurs, do caregivers usually try to calm the person down or involve the person in preferred activities? — Yes No N/A

4. Is the person usually well behaved when (s)he is getting lots of attention or when preferred activities are freely available? — Yes No N/A

5. Does the person usually fuss or resist when (s)he is asked to perform a task or to participate in activities? — Yes No N/A

6. Does the problem behavior occur when the person is asked to perform a task or to participate in activities? — Yes No N/A

7. If the problem behavior occurs while tasks are being presented, is the person usually given a "break" from tasks? — Yes No N/A

8. Is the person usually well behaved when (s)he is not required to do anything? — Yes No N/A

9. Does the problem behavior occur even when no one is nearby or watching? — Yes No N/A

10. Does the person engage in the problem behavior even when leisure activities are available? — Yes No N/A

11. Does the problem behavior appear to be a form of "self-stimulation?" — Yes No N/A

12. Is the problem behavior <u>less</u> likely to occur when sensory stimulating activities are presented? — Yes No N/A

13. Is the problem behavior cyclical, occurring for several days and then stopping? — Yes No N/A

14. Does the person have recurring painful conditions such as ear infections or allergies? If so, list:_____ — Yes No N/A

15. Is the problem behavior <u>more</u> likely to occur when the person is ill? — Yes No N/A

16. If the person is experiencing physical problems, and these are treated, does the problem behavior usually go away? — Yes No N/A

Scoring Summary

Circle the number of each question that was answered "Yes" and enter the number of items that were circled in the "Total" column.

Items Circled "Yes"	Total	Potential Source of Reinforcement
1 2 3 4	____	Social (attention/preferred items)
5 6 7 8	____	Social (escape from tasks/activities)
9 10 11 12	____	Automatic (sensory stimulation)
13 14 15 16	____	Automatic (pain attenuation)

From Iwata, B. A., DeLeon, I. G., & Roscoe, E. M. (2013). Reliability and validity of the Functional Analysis Screening Tool. *Journal of Applied Behavior Analysis, 46*, 271-284.

Figure 20-6. FAST. (Reproduced with permission from Brian A. Iwata.)

in the order it occurs regardless of the column in which it is entered by the practitioner. The chart can then be used to identify patterns to develop a hypothesis about the function of the behavior (Bijou et al., 1968). The ABC principle is illustrated in Figure 20-3.

Testing and Confirming Hypotheses: Functional Analysis

The hypotheses developed from indirect and direct methods need to be tested through a functional analysis (Iwata et al., 1982). Functional analysis involves the experimental manipulation of environmental aspects that represent the hypothesized functions of challenging behavior. This model was developed by B. A. Iwata and identifies the function of the behavior with a success rate above 90% (Beavers et al., 2013). For example, if direct observation suggests that an individual engages in challenging behavior to escape difficult tasks, situations will be created that manipulate the difficulty of the tasks presented to the individual while assessing its effect on challenging behavior. Functional analysis can also be used to clarify the relationship between two differing events when indirect methods do not provide enough information. Because of ethical considerations, functional analysis should only be conducted with consent and by a trained, experienced professional. It is noted that prior to creating conditions for functional analysis, risk assessment should be determined by reviewing past or potential risks of the challenging behavior, obtaining informed consent, and including procedural safeguards if needed (Neidert et al., 2013). The safety of the client and professionals involved is always taken into consideration prior to testing hypotheses. Possible strategies for accomplishing this include consulting a board certified behavior analyst, using protective equipment, and determining a termination criterion ahead of time upon which the analysis would terminate for the safety of the participants.

Outlining Positive Behavior Supports

Once a hypothesis is confirmed, **positive behavior supports** (PBS) can be implemented to decrease challenging behavior. PBS focuses on "… the design of environments that promote desired behaviors and minimize the development and support of problem behaviors" (Dunlap et al., 2009, pp. 3-4). Problem behaviors are a major barrier to the social, vocational, and physical success of each individual. PBS emphasizes the "… (a) use of FBA to enhance the match between individual needs and specific supports; (b) prevention of problem behavior through environmental redesign; (c) active instruction of desired behaviors, especially desired behaviors that may serve the same behavioral function as problem behaviors; and (d) the organization of consequences that promote desired behavior, minimize rewards for problem

behavior, and if appropriate, provide consequences for challenging behavior" (Dunlap et al., 2009, p. 5). This section will outline PBS strategies that double as communication-based support for challenging behavior. PBS interventions related to communication rely on the simple notion that challenging behavior is a form of communication (Durand & Merges, 2001). Communication-based supports that are effective for the early communicator include visual schedules, contingency maps, and functional communication training (FCT).

Visual Activity Schedules

Visual activity schedules (VAS; e.g., activity schedules, calendar systems, event sequences) are used to sequence steps in a task and are useful for transitions between environments and activities (Bopp et al., 2004). VAS are part of a broader category known as visual supports (Mesibov et al., 2006). These types of supports include "… visually-enhanced physical environments, organization of materials (e.g., shoe box tasks), instructions (e.g., picture instructions, graphic organizers, structured worksheets) and instructional techniques (e.g., color highlighting, comic strip conversations; Gray 1994), as well as visual cues to support receptive and expressive communication (e.g., Treatment and Education of Autistic and Related Communication-Handicapped Children and Picture Exchange Communication System [PECS]; Kroupa 2013)" (Knight et al., 2015, p 158). Research has shown that visual supports can improve expressive and receptive communication skills for individuals with ASD and assist in decreasing challenging behavior. Visual schedules may utilize several different types of symbols, including photographs, videos, real objects, and line drawings. Studies indicate that positive outcomes were reported for 90% of participants with ASD in school settings and 100% of participants at home in which all participants were either "nonverbal" or had severe communication deficits (Lequia et al., 2012). Knight and colleagues (2015) evaluated VAS in a comprehensive review of the literature between 1993 and 2013 and found that "VAS can be used to increase, maintain, and generalize a range of skills of individuals from preschool through adulthood in a variety of settings (e.g., general education, community)" (p. 157). The purpose of a visual schedule is to introduce a sequence to prepare an individual for the next activity or next step of an activity. They are often used to decrease challenging behavior and improve transitions. Experts agree that part of the reason visual supports are successful for individuals with ASD is that they process visual information more efficiently than auditory information. Steps to creating a visual schedule should include the concept of symbolization, an overview of the sequence of activities across a day, and the necessary steps to complete a designated activity in a visual representation. Figure 20-7 illustrates a VAS morning routine. This type of visual schedule can have a variety of steps and be modified to include as many detailed events as needed for an individual's daily needs.

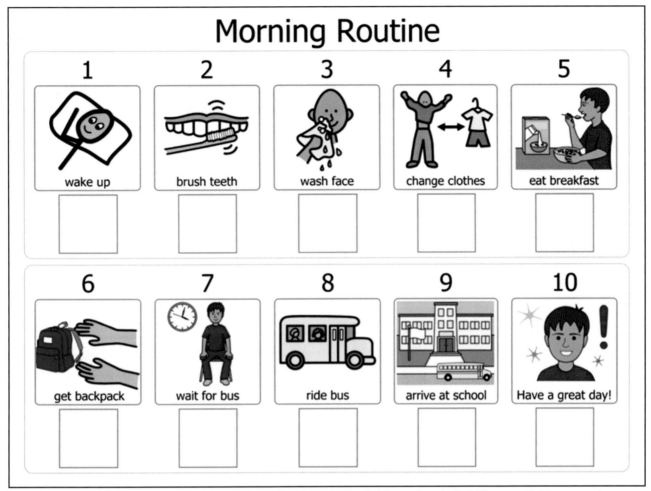

Figure 20-7. A visual schedule for a morning routine. (Picture Communication Symbols is a trademark of Tobii Dynavox. All rights reserved. Used with permission.)

Contingency Maps

Contingency mapping is a visual support strategy that uses graphic representations of the environment and behavior relationships. Contingency maps provide information regarding "current" (i.e., the challenging behavior) and "desired" behavioral pathways in an effort to help the individual understand what will occur if they engage in each pathway (see Figure 20-8 for a basic contingency map flowchart).

A contingency map provides a visual representation that lays out alternative ABC pathways related to the problem behavior. For instance, "[c]ontingency maps must represent all of—and the relationships between—the following components: (a) the common antecedent that precedes both the problem and the replacement behavior; (b) the topography of both the problem and alternative behavior; (c) the functional reinforcer that will be provided contingent on alternative behavior; and (d) the previously available functional reinforcer that will no longer be provided contingent on problem behavior" (Brown & Miranda, 2006, p. 156).

Figure 20-9 illustrates a sample behavior map used within a clinical setting for a 16-year-old girl with ASD who was exhibiting challenging behavior when asked to do her work.

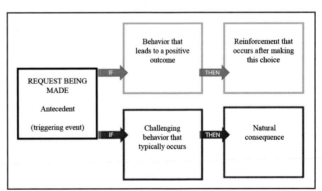

Figure 20-8. A basic behavior contingency flowchart. Green arrows indicate choices that will lead to a positive outcome, red arrows indicate a choice that leads to a natural consequence. (Reproduced with permission from Buie, A. [2013]. *Behavior mapping: A visual strategy for teaching appropriate behavior to individuals with autism spectrum and related disorders.* AAPC.)

The behavior map successfully redirected behavior after it was used in a variety of settings (e.g., school, home, private therapy). While there is still additional research needed to determine the effectiveness of contingency mapping, it fits within the framework of positive behavioral supports and provides an easy, convenient, and socially acceptable means

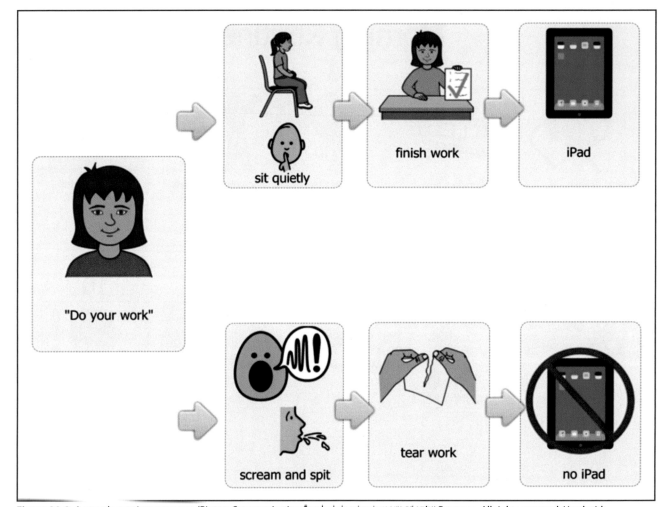

Figure 20-9. A sample contingency map. (Picture Communication Symbols is a trademark of Tobii Dynavox. All rights reserved. Used with permission.)

for promoting positive behavior change. Buie (2013) defines the term "behavior mapping" as a means to effectively reduce challenging behavior in children who have ASD and related disorders. An overview of evidenced-based practices correlated with behavior mapping is illustrated in Table 20-3 based on National Autism Center data.

Functional Communication Training

FCT was developed by Carr and Durand (1985b) as a proactive approach for reducing challenging behaviors in individuals with developmental disabilities (Miranda & Iacono, 2009). FCT reduces challenging behavior by teaching a more appropriate form of communication. Individuals are taught using communication-based interventions to replace challenging behavior with socially mediated consequences that serve the same function, such as seeking attention, gaining access to a desired object or action, avoiding or escaping an activity that seems aversive, or receiving **automatic reinforcement**. Hutchins and Prelock (2014) found evidence in nearly 200 studies to support positive outcomes for individuals with ASD or intellectual disability when FCT is used to address challenging behavior (e.g., Durand, 2012; Matson

et al., 2005; Mirenda, 1997; Petscher et al., 2009; Smith et al., 2007). FCT also meets the criteria for being considered a well-established treatment across a range of challenging behaviors. However, there are some potential unwanted effects when using FCT. Namely, overuse of the newly trained response or return of the unwanted behavior is possible if reinforcement is delayed or insufficient to meet the original communicative need (Hutchins & Prelock, 2014). Walker and Snell (2013) found that, in 54 studies involving 111 participants (ranging from less than 5 years to over 18 years of age), FCT was the most effective method of intervention to decrease challenging behavior. FCT interventions were most effective in younger participants.

FCT intervention must first identify the communicative function of challenging behavior through assessment (Mirenda, 1997). FBA is often conducted by an experienced individual in the area of applied behavior analysis. FBA determines the relationship between events (**antecedents**) in a person's environment that create the stage for the challenging behavior to occur and the **consequences** that reinforce or maintain said behavior (an ABC chart for data collection is presented in Figure 20-10). This behavior-analytic framework

TABLE 20-3

Evidence-Based Practices From the National Autism Center Correlated With Behavior Mapping:
A Visual Strategy for Teaching Appropriate Behavior to Individuals With Autism Spectrum Disorder and Related Disorders

STRATEGY	CORRESPONDING NATIONAL AUTISM CENTER EVIDENCE-BASED PRACTICE	BENEFITS SHOWN THROUGH RESEARCH
Choice making*	Antecedent package (changes in the environment before a problematic behavior occurs)	Communication skills; interpersonal (or social) skills; personal responsibility; play skills; self-regulation; and sensory and emotional regulation
Teaching alternative skills	Behavioral package (changes in the environment before and after a problematic behavior occurs)	Communication skills; interpersonal (or social) skills; personal responsibility; play skills; self-regulation; restricted, repetitive, nonfunctional patterns of behavior; sensory and emotional regulation; and reduction of problem behavior
Positive reinforcement	Behavioral package (changes in the environment before and after a problematic behavior occurs)	Communication skills; interpersonal (or social) skills; personal responsibility; play skills; self-regulation; restricted, repetitive, nonfunctional patterns of behavior; sensory and emotional regulation; and reduction of problem behaviors
Modeling	Modeling (adults or peers demonstrate a target behavior so it is imitated by the individual)	Communication skills; higher cognitive functions; interpersonal (or social) skills; play skills; and self-regulation
Differential reinforcement	Behavioral package (changes in the environment before and after a problematic behavior occurs)	Communication skills; interpersonal (or social) skills; personal responsibility; play skills; self-regulation; restricted, repetitive, nonfunctional patterns of behavior; sensory and emotional regulation; and reduction of problem behaviors
Social narratives	Story-based intervention package (written description of the situation under which specific behaviors are expected to occur)	Interpersonal (or social) skills and self-regulation
Self-monitoring	Self-management (teaching individuals to regulate their own behavior)	Interpersonal (or social) skills and self-regulation
Prompting*	Antecedent package (changes in the environment before a problematic behavior occurs)	Communication skills; interpersonal (or social) skills; personal responsibility; play skills; self-regulation; and sensory and emotional regulation
Social scripts	Story-based intervention package (written description of the situation under which specific behaviors are expected to occur)	Interpersonal (or social) skills and self-regulation
Special interests	Antecedent package (changes in the environment before a problematic behavior occurs)	Communication skills; interpersonal (or social) skills; personal responsibility; play skills; self-regulation; restricted, repetitive, nonfunctional patterns of behavior; sensory and emotional regulation; and reduction of problem behavior
Visual supports	Schedules (presentation of a task list that communicates a series of activities or steps)	Self-regulation

*Also behavioral package.

Reproduced with permission from Buie, A. (2013). *Behavior mapping: A visual strategy for teaching appropriate behavior to individuals with autism spectrum and related disorders*. AAPC.

Date:					Key: A-antecedent B-behavior C-consequence		
Client/Student:					Observer:		
Challenging Behavior(s):							
Location:							
Date	Time	A	B	C	Possible Function	Duration

Figure 20-10. ABC chart for data collection.

explains challenging behavior when its controlling variables have been outlined (Catania et al., 1988; Mirenda 2009). If the behavior can be explained, it can be interpreted as having a communicative function. FCT teaches new communication skills that replace challenging behavior. Clinicians select a communication-based intervention (e.g., PECS, manual signs, a speech-generating device [SGD]) that will function as a replacement for the challenging behavior under the same variables and in a more efficient way (Bopp et al., 2004; Carr & Durand 1985b; Horner & Day 1991). FCT requires systematic instructional production through the use of **differential reinforcement**, **errorless teaching**, and **prompting** (see Figure 20-11 for FCT steps from the National Professional Development Center on Autism Spectrum Disorders).

DEVELOPING INTERVENTIONS: REPRESENTING, SELECTING, AND TRANSMITTING FUNCTIONALLY EQUIVALENT RESPONSES

The development of AAC-based interventions involves several sets of considerations beginning with the outcomes of the FBA (e.g., Doss & Reichle, 1991; Durand, 1990; Mace & Roberts, 1993). The central consideration is selecting a response that is functionally equivalent and more efficient than the challenging behavior. For individuals with little or no functional speech, AAC is the key to functional equivalence and response efficiency. In selecting equivalent and efficient responses, interventionists must make important decisions regarding the means to represent, means to select, and means to transmit (Lloyd et al., 1990). Any response conveyed through AAC consists of these three components of the transmission process. The focus of this section is on selecting an appropriate mode of communication to replace challenging behavior. It is important to note that when dealing with challenging behavior, the speed and efficiency of the response tends to take precedence, especially when the behavior can result in the harm of the individual, peers, or caregivers. For this reason, it may be appropriate to consider an initial response that can be quickly and effectively implemented while also more patiently and deliberately developing a long-term strategy for a more robust communication system. An illustration of the AAC transmission process can be found in Figure 20-12.

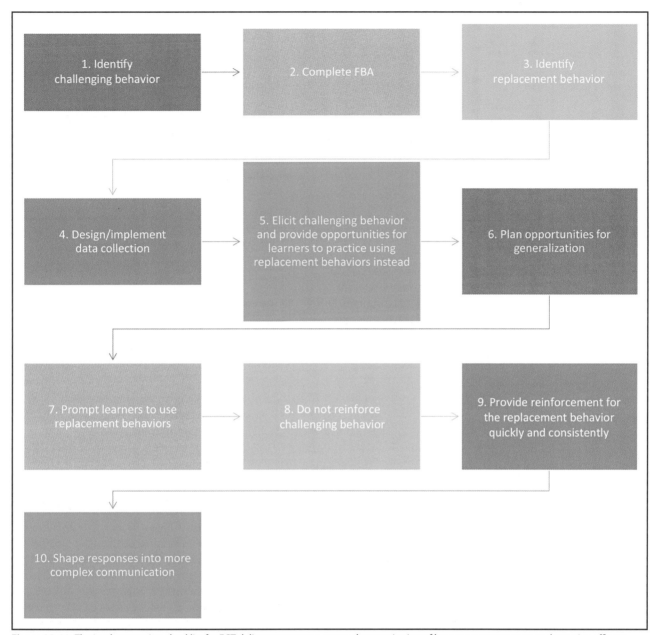

Figure 20-11. The implementation checklist for FCT delineates steps to ensure that monitoring of learner progress occurs to determine efficacy of a communication-based approach. (Adapted from Franzone, E. [2009]. *Implementation checklist for functional communication training [FCT].* The National Professional Development Center on Autism Spectrum Disorders, Waisman Center, University of Wisconsin.)

Considerations for the Use of Natural Speech

Natural speech is always the preferable and most acceptable means to represent ideas. However, poor intelligibility often does not permit reliance on residual speech in individuals with severe communication disabilities. Intelligibility refers to the comprehension of the communication signal, such as the natural speech or synthesized or digitized speech signal (Beukelman & Mirenda, 2012). The selection of an intelligible means to represent may be crucial if challenging behavior is to be replaced (Carr et al., 1994). With individuals

who have little or no functional speech, natural speech may not be a practical choice as the only means to represent because the lack of intelligibility may hinder partners from recognizing the response, and hence, hinder the success of the intervention. For instance, a child who hits themselves to get the attention of the teacher may be taught to request assistance through residual speech instead. However, if the teacher fails to respond to the child's requests for help because the teacher does not understand what the child is saying, then the SIB will likely continue (Durand & Carr, 1991). Although articulation training may lead to intelligible vocalizations and replacement of challenging behavior with some individuals (e.g., see Durand & Carr, 1991), frequently the

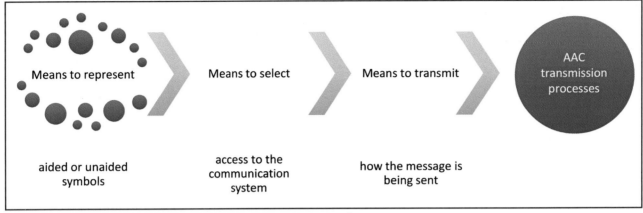

Figure 20-12. The AAC transmission processes: means to represent, means to select, means to transmit.

challenging behavior is dangerous and warrants faster solutions than extensive articulation training can provide. Thus, other means to represent, such as graphic symbols or manual signs, need to be given careful consideration as replacements for or supplements to the individual's residual natural speech.

One concern with using AAC is that it inhibits the production of natural speech. However, evidence suggests AAC does not inhibit natural speech, and in fact, may even facilitate it (Millar et al., 2006). AAC methods that involve speech production can actually serve as a consistent model for users leading to increased use of natural speech (Blischak, 2003). If AAC and natural speech are introduced and reinforced together, both will likely increase in frequency (Mirenda, 2003).

Unaided Versus Aided Symbols

Generally, the intervention team has the option of choosing between aided and unaided means to represent the message inherent in the functionally equivalent response. There are several important considerations that will be outlined in this section. It is possible to use a multimodal approach combining both aided and unaided means to represent. A wide range of AAC systems have been shown to reduce the rates of challenging behavior (Ringdahl et al., 2009; Winborn-Kemmerer et al., 2009; Winborn-Kemmerer et al., 2010). Typically, the more proficient a user is with a specific AAC system, the more likely the challenging behavior will be reduced (Ringdahl et al., 2009). From this perspective, there is evidence to suggest that practitioners may want to consider aided over unaided means because they result in quicker skill acquisition, are generally preferred by children, are more easily understood by communication partners, and are more appropriate for children with fine motor skill limitations (Gevarter et al., 2013; Nam & Hwang, 2016). However, especially when challenging behavior is involved, intervention teams should develop plans on a case-by-case basis that are tailored to the individual's abilities and context. A wide range of both aided and unaided AAC systems have been validated for their effectiveness with children with ASD and developmental disabilities (Ganz et al., 2012).

Intelligibility

As with natural speech, the **intelligibility** of symbols is important to the effectiveness of communication. Mirenda (2003) states that "[i]n order for communication to be truly functional, it must be understood by both familiar and unfamiliar communication partners" (p. 207). In some situations, unaided means, such as manual signs, may not be sufficiently intelligible to allow unfamiliar communication partners to understand and make appropriate responses (Durand et al., 1993). Communication partners, including parents and teachers, are often not proficient in the use of manual signs (Sundberg & Partington, 1998). For example, a child may learn a sign that is interpreted as MORE at home with their family, but it may be unrecognized by caregivers at school. The sign proves to be idiosyncratic because it is not recognized outside the context where it is effective. This example may result in a child exhibiting challenging behavior at school when teachers are unable to recognize the sign. If the trained means to represent is not easily recognizable by communication partners, then these partners will not respond, and challenging behavior will not be replaced (Durand et al., 1993). For the sign to reduce challenging behavior, it must be generalized to other environments (Mirenda, 2003). On the other hand, graphic symbols are consistent because they are selected rather than formed (Lloyd & Kangas, 1994). Rotholz and colleagues (1989) found that selecting graphic symbols transmitted via a communication book was more effective than manual signing in community settings that involve partners who are generally not trained in manual communication.

Learnability

Learnability refers to the ability of the individual to successfully learn how to use and implement a chosen method. Whether manual signs are easier to learn than graphic symbols depends on the background of the person exhibiting challenging behavior. With individuals who exhibit severe challenging behavior, intervention teams should spend as little time as possible teaching new communicative forms as replacements for the challenging behavior during the initial intervention. For example, for individuals whose challenging behavior is related to escape, introducing a means to represent escape may be difficult to learn, and therefore, may place an additional demand on the person, increasing the severity of the challenging behavior. Practitioners should consider selecting a means to represent that is easy to learn or already exists in the individual's communicative repertoire. Children with an intellectual disability can benefit from aided graphic symbols that function as prompts or reminders (Gervarter et al., 2013).

Existing Communicative Repertoire

The **existing communicative repertoire** involves those **receptive** (i.e., understanding of vocabulary and functions) and **expressive** (i.e., production of symbols and functions) skills that the individual has already learned. Because there is little conclusive evidence on the best AAC systems for addressing challenging behavior, the intervention team should consider building on the existing communicative repertoire of an individual when designing interventions, especially if those skills showed promise during the assessment and initial intervention (Sigafoos et al., 2007). In some situations, the team may decide that a different means to represent can provide a more efficient response for the student. However, the existing repertoire should still be included in the plan. For example, an intervention team might wish to build on an existing sign repertoire but also teach graphic symbols because of the shortcomings of using manual signs in an individual's particular environment. In such a situation, the intervention team might use the graphic representations of the manual signs, as found in the instructional book, *Signing Exact English* (Gustason, 1990). These representations permit an individual to build on an existing sign repertoire because the representations show both the movement and handshapes of the signs while providing a key to help caretakers understand messages.

Fine Motor Skills

Another consideration is that manual signs may require more physical effort than the pointing response often used with aided means (Mirenda & Erickson, 2000; Seal & Bonvillian, 1997). For children with fine motor limitations, manual signs may not be practical because each new sign requires a new motor response. By contrast, introducing new concepts through aided graphic symbols utilizes the same response form, such as pointing to a picture or pressing a button for each new concept introduced (Gevarter et al., 2013). If an individual struggles with poor motor imitation, the intervention team should consider using aided systems instead of unaided systems (Gregory et al., 2009; Tincani, 2004).

Portability

Portability is the ability of the user to bring the communicative means to different physical locations and contexts. Manual signs are more portable than graphic symbols (Mirenda, 2003). A child may be proficient with using an SGD to communicate, but the effectiveness of this communication technique is contingent on the availability, size, and weight of the device. If the SGD is lost or loses its charge regularly, it limits the ability of the individual to use it to communicate and for the intervention to provide a functionally equivalent response to challenging behavior. In addition, the type of device (i.e., a lightweight iPad [Apple] vs. a heavy SGD) can increase portability. Tablets are often chosen over SGDs because of their portability, but they are often less resilient. By contrast, manual signs are always available to an individual and do not require any specialized equipment beyond the parts of the human body.

Projectability

Projectability is the maximum distance at which one can immediately get the attention of their communication partner. Some techniques make it easier to communicate from a distance while others require the user to be in close proximity to the communication partner (Mirenda, 2003). Gestures and manual signs project better than graphic symbols if the latter are transmitted through a non–speech-generating communication board. For example, an individual can use manual signs to get the attention of a caregiver from across the room but would need to be positioned next to the caregiver to do the same with a book of graphic symbols (Doss & Reichle, 1991). However, if graphic symbols are converted to spoken words through SGDs, their projectability relative to manual signs is increased dependent upon the volume at which synthetic speech can be produced.

Required Specificity

A selection consideration that applies to both aided and unaided symbols is the required specificity of the means to represent (e.g., a symbol representing "pants" vs. one representing "jeans"). As a guiding principle, regardless of the means to represent, symbols should be sufficiently generic to allow the user to communicate in a large range of contexts while being sufficiently specific to minimize the communicative burden on the partner (O'Neill & Reichle, 1993). For example, a symbol for "coffee" may be sufficiently specific regardless of the context, but using the symbol SODA or POP (vs. PEPSI [PepsiCo]) in a fast food restaurant may not be sufficiently specific for the worker at the counter to provide the desired item. Different means to represent may have varied potentials to represent specificity. Unaided symbols may not be able to represent a particular type of pants because the subordinate sign does not exist. Such specificity may also be problematic with graphic symbol sets. For instance, most iconic symbol sets do not provide representations at the subordinate level of specificity, and if they are at all available, they are difficult to distinguish from the next higher level (Schlosser, 1993, 1997a,b). If specificity is required, product logos, such as Coca-Cola (The Coca-Cola Company), can be utilized (O'Neill & Reichle, 1993) or the symbols may be selected from a system that permits sufficient specificity (Schlosser, 1993, 1997a,b; Schlosser & Lloyd, 1997). Selecting the means to represent with the required degree of specificity may be guided by its implications for opportunities to teach an initial communicative repertoire to immediately reduce challenging behavior. General symbols, such as generic WANT or PLEASE, can be essential during initial intervention for many individuals. However, intervention teams should carefully consider the long-term implications of relying primarily on generic symbols for an overall communication program (Northup et al., 1991; Sigafoos et al., 1989).

Long-Term Expansion

More general responses may be appropriate during the initial intervention to reduce challenging behavior. However, intervention teams should consider future expansion capability of the selected means to communicate so that a long-term plan can be established to develop more robust communication for the individual. Graphic symbol systems, unlike symbol sets, have rules for expansion and allow the expression of virtually any thought. Manual signs also provide rules for expansion if they are taken from a system, such as American Sign Language (Fuller et al., 1994).

Unaided Means to Represent

Many studies concur that manual signs have a high rate of success as communication systems for individuals with ASD and other developmental disabilities (Gregory et al., 2009; Tincani, 2004). Manual signs are a potential option for individuals who have difficulty imitating sounds and words but can execute some fine motor movements (Sundberg & Partington, 1998). Several advantages exist, including that manual signs are always available to individuals, allow messages to be delivered quickly, and may serve as a prompt for natural speech vocalization (Mirenda, 2003; Sundberg & Partington, 1998). If the intervention team has opted for gestures or manual signs, a number of issues need to be considered in selecting the specific means to represent. A review indicates that although manual signs were selected in several studies, the specific type of manual signs selected were often not reported (Bird et al., 1989; Northup et al., 1991; Wacker et al., 1990). Specifically, the question arises: What sign or signs should be selected if several alternatives are available to represent the same referent, message, or function? This section considers this question from the standpoint of developing an initial intervention for challenging behavior rather than developing a complete communication plan, although this should be taken into consideration.

Learnability of Responses

The learnability of gestures or manual signs, especially within the context of developing a functionally equivalent response, seems to be a crucial consideration for selecting initial unaided symbols. In some situations, such as when challenging behavior has an escape function, the training of new gestures or manual signs may constitute a new demand further increasing the probability that the challenging behavior will occur (Fisher et al., 1993). Thus, for demand-escape situations, the intervention team should select manual signs that already exist in the person's repertoire, are approximations of actual signs, and are easy to produce. For instance, when selecting a sign approximation to represent requests for a desired item, a child might be introduced to the sign EAT to request food for an edible, positive reinforcer instead of CANDY if EAT is a sign already in his repertoire.

Physical Features

Physical features are discussed here as a consideration when choosing an initial sign vocabulary. Based on her review, Doherty (1985) recommended that **contact signs** be selected over **noncontact signs**. Bonvillian and Siedlecki (1996) suggest that signs acquired first by children of deaf parents are those that require contact between hands, are produced in a neutral space, and require single, simple handshapes, such as the open hand or A, B, or G handshapes. Karlan and Lloyd (1983) suggested that the number of opportunities to practice the chosen vocabulary may affect the success with which vocabulary is acquired. That is, the more opportunities the learner has to use vocabulary, the quicker the learner might acquire it and the greater the likelihood it will be maintained. Keogh and Reichle (1985) suggested that vocabulary representing items and events of great interest to the learner represent highly desirable initial intervention targets.

Further, symmetric manual signs should be selected over asymmetric signs. In addition, Doherty (1985) suggested translucent manual signs be selected over opaque signs for those produced with one hand. Finally, she suggested that one-handed signs be selected over two-handed signs because they are easier to produce. With respect to the handshapes that are used to produce manual signs, Doherty (1985) made a number of recommendations. First, she suggested selecting signs with handshape features that are less difficult to produce. Signs at Boyes-Braem's (1973) stages I (i.e., A, S, L, baby 0 [zero], 5, C, G) and II (i.e., B, F, 0 [zero]) of handshape difficulty are believed to be acquired more readily than those at stages III (i.e., I, D, Y, P, 3, V, H, W) and IV (i.e., 8, 7, X, R, T, M, N, E). Second, Doherty recommended that motoric capabilities to form handshapes and conduct movements be tested to determine which signs should be avoided initially and which signs would be acceptable to approximate.

Iconicity

The iconicity of individual manual signs as perceived by partners may be crucial if the functionally equivalent communicative behavior is to be recognized by partners. The literature (see Doherty, 1985; Chapters 8 and 13) overwhelmingly supports the facilitative effect of iconicity on sign comprehension by individuals with cognitive impairments (e.g., potential peers) and individuals without disabilities (e.g., potential caregivers). In addition, because they are usually not accompanied by the referent, manual signs must remain highly guessable.

The degree to which a response is recognized has been purported as a precondition to response success, which refers to whether partners respond to the trained communicative responses (Durand et al., 1993). Thus, the selection of highly guessable signs as the means to represent is suggested to increase the probability that partners will recognize and respond to communicative attempts. Other researchers have examined whether children more readily learn arbitrary gestures or iconic ones (e.g., a thumb peeking out of one fist to represent a turtle). Brown (1977) found that 4-year-old children learned iconic gestures more easily than arbitrary gestures. Namy and colleagues (2004) found that 18-month-old and 4-year-old children were equally successful at both.

Physical and Mental Effort

Manual signs needed to produce a message involve no external aids but rather recall memory. On the other hand, with graphic symbols, recognition memory may be sufficient. For aided symbols, selection is facilitated by the display of symbols on an aid or device that requires only recognition, not recall. Because individuals must rely primarily on more difficult recall memory in using signs expressively, an important consideration is whether to use manual signs for an entire English sentence (sentence signing) or only one or a few representative manual signs via key word signing (BREAK standing for "I want to go, please") or generalized requests (e.g., MORE PLEASE).

Horner and Day (1991) examined the effects of sentence signing (I WANT TO GO, PLEASE) vs. key word signing (BREAK) on challenging behavior, on attempts to complete tasks, and on requesting with one of their participants. Results indicated that key word signing, in contrast to sentence signing, resulted in increased requesting, increased attempts to complete tasks, and decreased aggression. In addition, during the key word signing, the individual never resorted to sentence signing. Horner and Day (1991) concluded that only key word signing could compete with aggressive behavior in terms of the physical effort required to perform the response. Although this conclusion is accurate from the perspective of applied behavior analysis, a cognitive perspective may add to the understanding of this phenomenon. From such a perspective, sentence signing may also have placed a greater mental effort on the individual because they needed to select several signs in correct order from memory.

However, in key word signing, they have to select only one sign (BREAK). Aggressive behavior, in this case, was already established as an effective means of escaping, thus it already had response efficiency. Therefore, the mental effort required of key word signing, as a new response, could compete with the response efficiency of the aggressive behavior.

Although generalized requests have been shown to be effective when establishing functionally equivalent responses, consideration should be given to what happens if the desired object or consequence of the generalized request is unclear to the communication partner. What, for example, would happen in community environments when more than one object is present and the partner is unaware of the individual's known preferences? Also, what would happen if an unfamiliar partner were to respond to the use of PLEASE as though it were a request for an object and not a request for a break? In these instances, the individual might revert to the challenging behavior, largely as a result of the lesser specificity of the generalized request. Thus, clinicians need to scrutinize empirically the relative physical and mental effort associated with using briefer, more generalized means of selecting (e.g., key signs or generalized requests) vs. lengthier, more specific responses (e.g., sentence signing or combining a generalized want and the sign for the object) relative to the challenging behavior.

Aided Means to Represent

In recent years, aided systems have become more popular, as evidenced by the increase in attention in academic research (Lancioni et al., 2007). In some situations, aided systems of communication are more readily learnable because the often-utilized graphic symbols can serve as a reminder to users (Gevarter et al., 2013). If the intervention team has decided to employ aided means, a number of issues need to be considered in choosing the specific means to be used. As with unaided means, decisions must be made by the intervention team concerning which aided symbols (i.e., sets vs. systems) to choose and which particular symbols within the chosen aided sets and/or systems to select to represent the various referents, messages, or functions to be used by an individual who exhibits challenging behavior.

Existing Communicative Repertoire

Some individuals with challenging behavior may have an existing communicative repertoire that goes unacknowledged by caretakers or clinicians. Individuals may manipulate objects in the environment as attempts to communicate. The challenging behavior may occur if the attempts to communicate go unrecognized or unacknowledged. For example, if a student grabs a magazine to indicate a desire to escape from a demand and flips through the magazine during the time spent away from a demand task, the partner may not recognize this as a request to escape and takes the magazine away, resulting in aggressive behavior (which, in turn, temporarily ends the demand task). This repertoire must be taken into consideration and has the capacity to provide a platform for building up core vocabulary or fringe vocabulary to communicate appropriately. The aforementioned student is likely to learn "go" (core vocabulary) or "magazine" (fringe vocabulary) more quickly if it is paired with their existing communicative repertoire (via a variety of modalities, such as manual signs, pictures, and an SGD), and in turn, decrease the likelihood of challenging behavior occurring.

Iconicity

The intervention team may choose a specific aided means to represent from an array that varies in the degree of iconicity present to promote both the degree of recognition and learnability. Iconicity is a powerful variable in graphic symbol learning in that more iconic symbols (across and within symbol sets and systems) are more readily learned than opaque symbols. Therefore, as a general guiding principle, intervention teams should select iconic symbols over opaque symbols for the initial repertoire of communicative alternatives to challenging behavior.

There are some situations when iconicity may be superseded by other considerations regarding the learnability of symbols and degree to which they are recognized. The reinforcing value (motivation) of the referent might have a greater effect on the rate at which a symbol is acquired than its iconicity (Reichle, 1991). For example, a child who has a desired toy may more readily learn the symbol representing the toy—even if it is opaque—than a highly iconic symbol for a newspaper, which has little meaning to the child. Individuals lacking receptive knowledge of the referent may not benefit from iconicity in associating a symbol with its referent (Sevcik et al., 1991).

Selection Techniques

The major techniques involved in selecting aided symbols are direct selection and scanning (Reichle, 1991). To compete with challenging behavior, the symbols representing the desired consequences must be selected as quickly as possible with minimum physical and mental effort, yielding a functionally equivalent and more efficient response. The means to select should also place as little burden on the communication partner as possible. Direct selection involves directly pointing to a sentence or picture with a body part (e.g., a finger) or tool, such as a computer mouse. Direct selection for a non–speech-generating communication board requires adequate visual acuity and the physical capability required to point to symbols (Reichle, 1991). Direct selection via an SGD requires the physical abilities to perform a key-activation response. Direct selection tends to be more efficient than scanning because it is cognitively less difficult (Mizuko et al., 1994; Ratcliff, 1987) and quicker than scanning (Reichle, 1991). Various techniques can be used to select. For example, a child who can point can use their hands to select, but a child who has difficulty using their hands could use a

head pointer (Durand, 1993). Visual scanning is the use of a visual display that can highlight each option on a screen and the individual selects via a switch or eye-gaze technology. Auditory scanning involves a communication partner presenting choices using natural speech or a device where a synthetic voice announces vocabulary choices. Items are communicated one at a time until the individual hears their preferred vocabulary item and makes their selection using a switch. Partner-assisted scanning is the use of a partner or aide who accesses symbols on a communication device that includes either auditory scanning, visual scanning, or both. The partner or aide points to, shows, or speaks the names of items in a sequential order for the individual who engages in challenging behavior (Burkhart & Porter, 2006).

Encoding

Encoding allows an individual using AAC to produce an entire word, sentence, or phrase using only one or two activations of their communication system. Encoding techniques may provide a viable option to further increase the efficiency of direct selection. Horner and colleagues (1990) compared the effects of a no-encoding condition with a color-encoding condition on escape-motivated challenging behavior exhibited by one individual with moderate cognitive impairment. Using an SGD, the first condition involved spelling out the complete message by pressing one key for each letter ("H-e-l-p-p-l-e-a-s-e"), whereas the second condition involved activating a single colored key representing the pre-stored message ("Help, please"). An underlying assumption was that spelling the message was less efficient than the challenging behavior, and that challenging behavior was less efficient than pressing one key that resulted in assistance. Results demonstrated that the low-efficiency response (spelling a message) did not replace aggression in the long term, whereas the high-efficiency response (activating one key) seemed to decrease aggression and increase use of appropriate communication. As mentioned earlier for manual sign selection, the differences may also be due to the varying levels of mental effort required, as the no-encoding condition required greater recall memory (recall of the phrase and recall of how to spell the words in the phrase) than did the color encoding (recall of the phrase and recognition of one color associated with the phrase). It is noted that while encoding provides an opportunity to produce sentences or phrases with the push of a button, providing AAC users with a robust communication system is paramount to ensuring that communication needs of all types are met. Zangari (2021) outlines what comprises a robust communication system into seven areas:

1. Multiple components (different elements that work together to offer a variety of options for expression)
2. Multimodal ("all forms of communication are valid and should be acknowledged and treated respectfully")
3. Alphabet access
4. Vocabulary access (core vocabulary, fringe vocabulary, prestored messages)

5. Flexibility in word forms (the ability for AAC users to change word forms, such as plurals or verb tenses)

6. Organization (language tools [communication books, SGDs, apps, etc.] are organized to support linguistic expression)

7. Evolution (in a robust system, "communicative growth is expected and planned for" and "the architecture of the communication system easily accommodates new words, phrases, and longer messages")

Speech-Generating Devices

One consideration when selecting aided systems is whether to use non–speech-generating or speech-generating means. Typically, most students in research studies are successful with either type of aided system (Lancioni et al., 2007). However, speech-generating aided communication systems offer some unique advantages worth noting. First, the output for an SGD is spoken messages produced through electronic speech generation, which allows individuals to easily gain the attention of their communication partners (Lorah et al., 2013). In addition, when graphic symbols (e.g., lexigrams) received augmented input and feedback through speech output from an SGD, they were learned more efficiently by two of three individuals with severe to profound cognitive impairments than when the SGD was turned off (Schlosser et al., 1995). The efficacy of the SGD transmission was attributed to the provision of auditory stimuli in the form of augmented input and feedback during training. Thus, one might expect that individuals who exhibit challenging behavior and whose characteristics are similar to those of the participants in this study may learn the means to represent more readily with an SGD. A second consideration is that technological advances in SGDs have made them more socially acceptable, less stigmatizing, and more readily available (Lorah et al., 2015).

Picture Exchange Systems

Picture exchange (PE) systems use pictures to communicate. A basic PE system involves the exchanging of an individual picture of an object for the actual object or an action associated with the object. For instance, if the child wants a ball, they would get a picture of a ball and give it to their communication partner in exchange for a ball. PE systems require the same topography for each word, which facilitates instruction. The individual using the PE system points to the specified pictures in the same way and complex motor movement is unwarranted. PECS is a PE system that begins with requesting preferred items via pointing. PE systems are seen as beneficial to individuals with ASD, given that they might prefer visual stimuli over auditory stimuli (Boesch et al., 2013). Mirenda (2003) states that the most significant disadvantage of PE systems is that successful communication is dependent upon supplementary equipment, such as a communication book or board, which may be difficult to carry at all times. If the board is not available, the response

cannot occur. Sundberg and Partington (1998) also note that PE systems require a large amount of response time for the student and can be limited when it comes to representing words or phrases increasing in complexity.

Perhaps the main advantage of PE systems is that the communication partner does not need any special training to understand what the child is saying. Also, PE systems are easier for the instructor because the response topography (i.e., motor movement) is the same for each word. The child always points to (i.e., touches, exchanges) specified pictures, so complex motor movement and training differential responses is not necessary. It is also noted that PECS starts with the teaching of requesting for preferred items by pointing to pictures. As previously mentioned, many individuals with ASD prefer visual stimuli over auditory stimuli, thus PE systems may be advantageous for use with these children (Boesch et al., 2013).

Assertiveness

The selected means to transmit may also alter the projectability of the means to represent (i.e., symbols), and therefore, alter the user's potential assertiveness. Assertiveness is defined as the degree to which the means of communication allows the user to influence communicative interactions, such as getting someone's attention, interrupting, or protesting. Doss and Reichle (1991) suggested that graphic symbols require that the partner be fairly close to the user to be understood, and therefore, this mode of communication may be less suitable for individuals whose challenging behavior has an escape function and who might be aggressive toward others. Under such circumstances, they recommend using a system with greater projectability, such as gestures (e.g., STOP), that can be discerned from a distance. To increase projectability when graphic symbols are transmitted via non–speech-generating systems, O'Neill and Reichle (1993) recommended using a separate response to obtain the partner's attention (e.g., activating a buzzer) before emitting a more complete response. Another option may be to transmit the selected message via an SGD. With individuals who are taught appropriate means to request attention, acoustic symbols transmitted through an SGD may project better than either non–speech-generating communication devices or manual signs because the communication partner does not need to face the individual to receive and respond to the request. This may be crucial in classroom situations where teachers cannot face a particular student all the time because their attention needs to be distributed among many students.

Assertiveness can also be affected by time delay and schedule of reinforcement. In one study, Horner and Day (1991) instructed a partner to systematically vary the delay (1 second or 20 seconds) between the participant handing over a card (with the word "break") or engaging in aggression and the delivery of the break. The 20-second delay condition may be viewed as a simulation of low assertiveness, that is, the communicative behavior is not assertive enough to yield a more immediate response from the partner. Results indicated that the 20-second delay not only increased aggression but also resulted in decreased use of the card. On the other hand, the 1-second delay resulted in increased use of the card and a marked decrease in aggression. Horner and Day (1991) concluded that the longer delay could not compete with the challenging behavior; the challenging behavior resulted in quicker receipt of the break than the use of the card. In other words, the learner did not perceive it as a good deal to have to wait 20 seconds for the break after communicating appropriately. Horner and Day (1991) demonstrated what might happen relative to signing, task completion, and challenging behavior if an individual is required to sign several times to receive teacher assistance. They provided teacher assistance on a picture-matching task any time the participant engaged in SIB or if they signed HELP either once or three times. This scenario considered the schedule of reinforcement, which refers to the number of appropriate communicative responses required to obtain the requested consequence. Repeating the same sign simulates a situation in which the partner responds to a request only after an appropriate communicative behavior is repeated. When the individual only had to sign once to get assistance, they signed for help on nearly every trial, attempted the tasks in every trial, and engaged in no SIB. When the individual had to sign three times to get assistance, there was a decrease in attempts to complete the task, a substantial increase in challenging behavior, and a dramatic reduction in the use of the manual sign. Horner and Day (1991) concluded that signing three times was less efficient than challenging behavior in that the participant needed to sign several times to obtain teacher attention whereas SIB resulted in immediate attention. This study demonstrates that the intervention team needs to select a means to transmit that permits partners to respond quickly and frequently to the appropriate communicative behavior for appropriate communication to compete with challenging behavior.

User Preference

User preference for a certain means to transmit is a selection consideration frequently ignored. However, communication effectiveness research indicates that preference may be an important consideration, especially when there are no effectiveness advantages for possible means to transmit. Research suggests that personal preference and other characteristics (e.g., visual acuity, motor abilities) are seen as more influential than a system's effectiveness (Nam et al., 2018). Van der Meer and colleagues (2012) suggest that learning and maintenance are better with a person's preferred communication method. More importantly, when systems are deemed equally effective, incorporating preference choices may allow individuals to use self-determination and exert more control over their environment. Overall, user preference plays a significant role in communication effectiveness and should be considered when establishing long-term

communication-based interventions. In addition, consulting with experienced AAC users also provides a unique perspective for user preference, families, and professionals. When possible, AAC facilitators should consult with AAC users or have an AAC mentor to gain understanding, knowledge, and first-hand experience. Blackstone and colleagues state that "AAC should enable people to communicate what, how, and with whom they wish all day, every day, as they fulfill their desired societal roles. If the work of researchers and practitioners is successful, then AAC stakeholders will value it, adopt it, use it, and thus, demonstrate its social validity. In addressing outcomes, the viewpoints of multiple stakeholder groups, who have different perspectives and needs, are considered" (p. 200).

Durability and Ability to Replace

Durability and the ability to replace are another set of variables to consider when selecting devices for communication-based intervention for challenging behavior. Durability refers to the ability of a device to withstand damage and wear while ability to replace refers to the ease with which a device can be replaced if it is lost or broken. It may be difficult to justify purchasing an expensive device if the challenging behavior is likely to result in damage to it. However, this has become less of an issue in recent years with the availability of more durable devices, devices with warranties, and protective cases. When utilizing electronic devices, it is good practice to have a non–speech-generating communication board available in case the electronic device is not available for any reason. This can help prevent regression of the challenging behavior during the period of time the electronic device is unavailable.

Physical Effort

When using SGDs for communication, physical effort may be another important consideration when selecting these systems. Especially for young children, the weight of an SGD and the physical skill needed to pick it up and use it may be prohibitive (Beck et al., 2008). SGDs require individuals to activate a key or icon, which can cause frustration if the individual struggles to apply the required amount of pressure to register the response (Cannella-Malone et al., 2009). In contrast, non–speech-generating communication boards and books only require pointing to the appropriate cell containing the desired graphic symbol. An individual should be comfortable carrying the device with them for long periods of time or it will be likely that the AAC system will be abandoned.

Multimodal Means to Represent

In some situations, utilizing a combination of AAC systems may result in favorable outcomes for individuals (Sundberg & Partington, 1998). Most people utilize a variety of communication techniques based on context and many of these techniques could be considered aided or unaided (Mirenda, 2003). Multimodal means to represent may incorporate any combination of aided means (e.g., graphic symbols and objects), unaided means (e.g., pointing, reaching, leading, gestures, manual signs), or aided and unaided means to represent (e.g., a combination of graphic symbols and manual signs). Multimodal approaches provide the team with ways of combining several of the considerations discussed above within the same intervention. For example, an individual could be taught to use a handclap to get the attention of the communication partner (unaided), and then use a PE system to relay a more specific message (aided). This approach is noteworthy because it successfully addresses the low projectability of using a book of graphic symbols to communicate. A multimodal approach is based on the notion that individuals who are using AAC can more efficiently communicate with different communication partners in a variety of environments using a combination of modes. Differential means to represent may be required when partners or settings change from familiar to unfamiliar ones. For instance, familiar partners may understand a user's idiosyncratic manual signs whereas unfamiliar partners may not. Differential means to represent may also be necessitated by the changing availability of an aided system, such as an SGD. Horner and colleagues (1990) provided initial data of such multimodal use (i.e., SGDs, gestures, manual signs) within the realm of communication-based approaches to challenging behavior. They reported a collateral increase in an untrained means to represent (i.e., gesturing and signing) in situations when the trained means to represent could not be used because the SGD was unavailable. Thus, the selection of multiple means to represent and training their differential use are important considerations if communication-based approaches to challenging behavior are to be generalized to community settings with unfamiliar partners.

SUMMARY

A communication-based approach to addressing challenging behavior considers that an individual may be participating in challenging behavior because they do not possess more functional means to communicate their needs. The intervention team should consider identifying the function of the challenging behavior and developing a plan to replace it with a more efficient, functionally equivalent behavior that is socially appropriate. An overview of approaches to challenging behavior is seen in Figure 20-13. This can be done by completing a functional behavioral assessment and then developing an intervention plan that utilizes practical approaches for replacing the challenging behavior. There are many AAC systems that have proven to be successful with individuals with developmental disabilities. The intervention team must weigh their strengths and weaknesses when

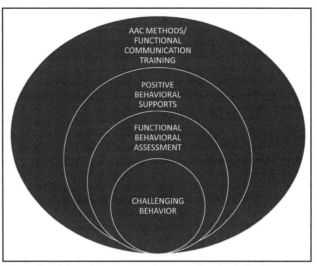

Figure 20-13. Overview of approaches to challenging behavior.

selecting between aided and unaided systems. The team should utilize an AAC system that compliments the prior abilities of the individual and best fits the context. Figure 20-14 illustrates important considerations for addressing challenging behavior. In order to be effective, the replacement communicative system should provide the same function as the challenging behavior in a more efficient manner.

STUDY QUESTIONS

1. How is behavior communication?
2. Define challenging behavior.
3. Explain the ABC chart.
4. Name the four most common behavior functions.
5. What is the best way to determine the function of a behavior?
6. What are the three components of the AAC transmission process?
7. Consider the following scenario. AB is a 7-year-old diagnosed with ASD who enjoys listening to children's music and being pushed on a swing round and round. He often erupts into laughter when he listens to his favorite songs. AB is an early learner and does not have a functional means to communicate. He does not have any spoken words in his repertoire at this time. When an unfamiliar sound or a nonpreferred song is played, he becomes aggressive toward himself and others around him. He scratches clinicians and himself, cries, bites himself, and hits his head until the unwanted song stops. When the challenging behavior occurs, the clinician stops the song and the challenging behavior stops. Challenging behavior also occurs when his favorite song stops playing. He begins to hit himself after his favorite song stops; the clinician plays his preferred song again, and AB then stops hitting his head. Indicate how you would determine the functions of behavior and develop appropriate positive behavior supports that provide opportunities to enhance core vocabulary and communication skills in this scenario.

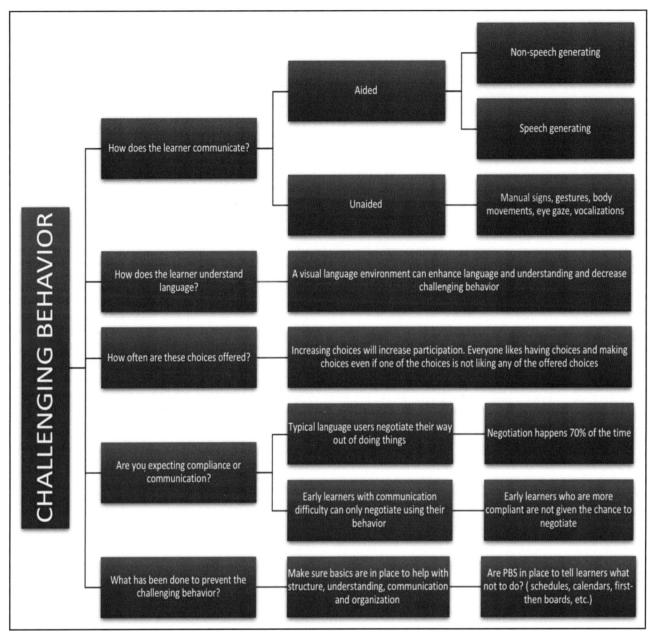

Figure 20-14. Considerations for addressing challenging behavior. (Adapted from Parker, R. [2013]. PrAACtical thoughts on challenging behavior: Things to think about. Retrieved from https://praacticalaac.org/praactical/praactical-thoughts-on-challenging-behavior-things-to-think-about/)

AAC Intervention for Persons With Acquired Disorders

Michelle L. Gutmann, PhD and Rajinder Koul, PhD

MYTH

1. Since each person's aphasia is different, general principles of augmentative and alternative communication (AAC) intervention do not apply.

2. If cognitive decline is part of a neurodegenerative disease, it precludes AAC intervention. Most people become nonverbal and do not interact that much with those around them as the disease progresses.

3. If a person did not embrace technology before having a stroke or being diagnosed with a neurodegenerative disease, they will certainly not do so for the sake of AAC intervention.

4. A person with Alzheimer's disease cannot use AAC options in a meaningful way.

REALITY

1. Although language profiles and levels of impairment differ across various types of aphasia, general principles of AAC intervention can and should be applied to persons with aphasia.

2. It is ideal to intervene before there is a precipitous decline in cognition so that people can rely on procedural memory and therapeutic supports to facilitate learning and mastery of AAC. However, if that does not happen, it is still possible to introduce AAC supports to facilitate maintenance of existing communication skills.

3. Demonstration and evaluation of AAC options, and all communication supports, may sway a potential user's opinion. Adoption of AAC is a multifactorial decision.

4. Research indicates that people with Alzheimer's disease can use AAC strategies and supports to participate in both communication and decision-making situations.

Fuller, D. R., & Lloyd, L. L. *Principles and Practices in Augmentative and Alternative Communication* (pp. 415-437).
© 2023 Taylor & Francis Group.

INTRODUCTION

For adults who lose the ability to speak either temporarily or permanently, the instinctual drive is to regain natural speech, the default system for communication (Fried-Oken, 2001). This drive pervades much of the rehabilitative effort that targets restoration. If, despite consistent effort, restoration of speech does not work, some people reluctantly change course from restoration to compensation (Frankoff & Hatfield, 2011; Lasker & Bedrosian, 2001). The field of AAC is composed of and dedicated to the development and implementation of compensatory strategies and techniques for both written and spoken communication. Yet it sometimes has been considered a method of last resort by clinicians, users, and other stakeholders with respect to both pediatric (e.g., Cress & Marvin, 2003; Romski & Sevcik, 2005) and adult (e.g., Beukelman & Ball, 2002; Frankoff & Hatfield, 2011; Koul, 2011; Lasker & Beukelman, 1999) populations. With adults, this meant that use of AAC was only broached as an option when therapy had failed to meet the elusive goal of restoration of speech and language skills back to premorbid levels. Recent research indicates that with a focus on communication, rehabilitative efforts can encompass both restorative and compensatory elements, and compensation may be viewed as an integral part of therapy from the outset (Baxter et al., 2012; Frankoff & Hatfield, 2011; Russo et al., 2017; Taylor et al., 2019). Indeed, the scope of use of AAC in the rehabilitative endeavor has expanded and been refined with the evolution of technology, policy, and research (Baxter et al., 2012; Beukelman & Ball, 2002; Taylor et al., 2019). The fuller integration of technology into the everyday lives of ordinary people provides promise for people affected by neurologic or neurodegenerative diseases and makes the topic of this chapter relevant for clinicians.

AAC FOR PERSONS WITH ACQUIRED NEUROGENIC COMMUNICATION DISORDERS

Aphasia

Research indicates approximately 40% to 60% of people with aphasia do not recover sufficient speech and language skill to be independent communicators (Laska et al., 2001). Rather, they will have a chronic aphasia and be more limited in terms of their communicative interactions (Holland & Beeson, 1993; Van de Sandt-Koenderman, 2004).

The history of the use of AAC options with people with aphasia suggests that this has been an active area of endeavor. Early efforts included the use of non–speech-generating technology options, such as communication displays and books (e.g., Garrett et al., 1989; Ho et al., 2005), drawing protocols (Lyon, 1995; Lyon & Helm-Estabrooks, 1987), and early speech-generating devices (SGDs) and software (e.g.,

Aftomonos et al., 1997; Katz & Wertz, 1997, Koul & Harding, 1998). Although much of this early work relied on single case studies or studies with very small sample sizes, it provided an important foundation for later advancement.

Kraat (1990) summarized the application of various modes of AAC with people with severe aphasia from the 1960s through the 1980s. Overall, Kraat (1990) reported mixed results; despite success by people with aphasia in learning both technical and nontechnical alternative modes of communication, functional use of these alternative modes did not generalize to use outside the clinic environment. Kraat (1990) further highlighted some of the problems in the application of AAC techniques and early AAC devices, including the very heterogeneous population of people with aphasia and not enough attention to the various linguistic and cognitive variables that commonly manifest in aphasia.

Fox and Fried-Oken (1996) extended Kraat's work by outlining an agenda for how AAC and aphasiology could work together to advance the state of intervention and research about the use of AAC for people with aphasia. Critically, Fox and Fried-Oken (1996) made the case for comprehensive AAC assessment in addition to standard aphasia assessment and for careful reporting of outcomes of intervention. The heterogeneous nature of the population of people with aphasia precluded large-scale group studies at the time. Rather, the authors stressed the need to investigate treatment effectiveness and efficiency, as well as generalization from the clinic to the community.

A variety of AAC needs assessments were developed, many of which are still in use today (e.g., Beukelman et al., 1985; Lasker et al., 2007a). Additional tools for AAC assessment include *Social Networks* (Blackstone & Hunt-Berg, 2003) and the development of the *Multimodal Communication Screening Tool for Persons with Aphasia* (Garrett & Lasker, 2005; Lasker & Garrett, 2006). The *Multimodal Communication Screening Tool for Persons with Aphasia* is designed to help clinicians differentiate between individuals who may be able to learn to use AAC options to communicate independently and those who are more partner-dependent, and therefore, more reliant on partner-assisted communication strategies.

Lasker and colleagues (2007b) provide comprehensive coverage of AAC supports for people with severe aphasia. In their work, they outline a categorization system for people with aphasia who use AAC. This categorization rubric includes three levels of partner-dependent communicators and three levels of independent communicators. Partner-dependent communicators are those who rely on their communication partners to continuously structure and scaffold communication exchanges aside from very general communicative efforts (e.g., to acknowledge a greeting, answering simple yes/no questions with an appropriate head nod/shake, or pointing to a referent). Partner-dependent communicators are more likely to use non–speech-generating communication technology strategies and supports. In contrast, independent communicators do not rely on their communication partners to structure and scaffold their communicative interactions. Those at the highest of the three levels of independent communicator can retrieve and encode messages on their own. Both types of communicators may use various forms of AAC, with independent communicators being able to use speech-generating technology options, such as an SGD with stored messages and/or multilevel SGDs requiring navigation to access messages. This categorization scheme for people with aphasia provides a backdrop for outlining some of the communication supports described in their work and that of others.

Non–Speech-Generating Technology Options for Use by People With Aphasia

Non–speech-generating technology AAC supports for people with aphasia cover a range of options from graphic and/or symbol-based communication displays or books (Bellaire et al., 1991; Garrett et al., 1989; Ho et al., 2005, Shakila et al., 2019), signs and/or gestures (Conlon & McNeil, 1991; Daumuller et al., 2010), drawing (Lyon, 1995; Lyon & Helm-Estabrooks, 1987), or a combination of drawing and gesture (Rao, 1995). Additional non–speech-generating communication technology supports include the use of rating scales and partner-assisted communication strategies, such as written choice communication. Shakila and colleagues (2019) observed that supporting narrative auditory comprehension tasks with high-context images and no-context Picture Communication Symbols images may facilitate auditory comprehension of narratives for persons with chronic aphasia. They suggest clinicians evaluate the potential benefits of augmented input and partner involvement in enhancing comprehension of people with aphasia.

Written Choice Conversation

Written choice communication (Garrett & Huth, 2002; Garrett & Lasker, 2007) is a technique that involves providing the person with aphasia with a spoken (and possibly written) question and written options for answers, much like a multiple-choice question. The conversation partner is responsible for identifying the key words and printing the question (if needed) and potential answers for the person with aphasia. The person with aphasia then responds by pointing to, underlining, or circling the desired written text. Variations on the written choice technique exist (Lasker et al., 1997) in that clinicians may vary whether they provide both verbal and graphic input with respect to the answers provided (e.g., reading the written choices aloud) or they may provide just the written cues. Lasker and colleagues (1997) comment that success with variation of the written choice technique varies with the linguistic impairment profile of each person with aphasia. Graphic supports to supplement written text may include rating scales with text and/or numeric anchors, maps, travel brochures, and timelines. Examples of rating scales are in Figure 21-1.

Importantly, use of written choice conversation can be a primary means of communication for someone with severe aphasia and relatively intact reading ability or as an adjunct to other non–speech-generating technology options. See Figure 21-2 for an example of written word choice communication.

Identification and Communication Cards

A basic but important non–speech-generating technology option to communication supports of any person with aphasia is a card outlining their name, the nature of communication impairment, and strategies that are helpful for communication. These "aphasia identification cards" are widely available online. Some national organizations (e.g., the National Aphasia Association, http://www.aphasia.org; the Aphasia Center, http://theaphasiacenter.com/pocket-card) have free downloadable and customizable options. The "how to" or "what helps me" section of this type of card is critical and should be customized as part of intervention. If communication strategies change, another card can be created readily. These cards may be laminated so the edges do not fray. See Figure 21-3 for an example of an aphasia identification and communication card.

Speech-Generating Technology Options for Use by People With Aphasia

Due to rapid advances in computer technology, AAC aids, such as SGDs and software programs (i.e., apps) for handheld multipurpose electronic devices (e.g., iPod or iPad [Apple]), have become increasingly available to people with aphasia (Koul et al., 2010). The AAC literature indicates that significant effort has been expended designing speech-generating options specifically for people with aphasia. An early example was computerized visual communication, which had icons representing parts of speech (e.g., nouns, verbs, prepositions) for sentence formulation. Studies indicated moderate success with computerized visual communication (Steele et al., 1989; Weinrich, 1991), which was commercialized by Lingraphica and reported to be successful (Aftomonos et al., 1997). Results of this initial work were extended with a larger cohort of people with chronic aphasia, most of whom demonstrated improvements in both language and communicative function (Aftonomos et al., 1999). The TalksBac (Waller et al., 1998) was another option. It ran on a Macintosh Powerbook [Apple] with a built-in speech synthesizer. When trialed with four people with Broca's aphasia, researchers noted communicative gains in terms of topic initiations and fewer communicative breakdowns. Finally, an international team of software specialists, aphasiologists, and AAC specialists designed the Portable Communication Assistant for Dysphasic People (van de Sandt-Koenderman et al., 2005), a forerunner to the current TouchSpeak app (van de Sandt-Koenderman et al., 2007). Results of implementation with a cohort of 22 people were

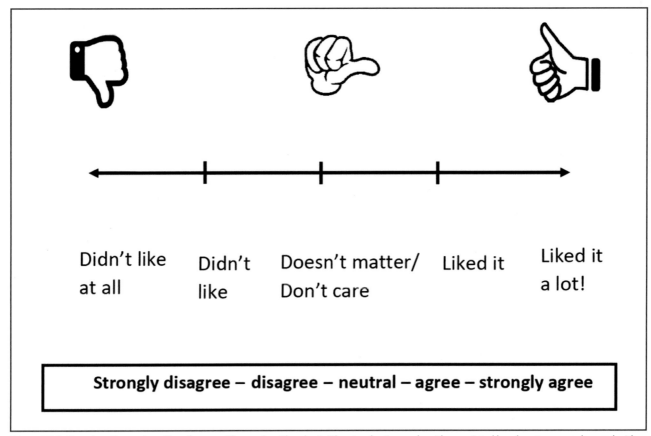

Figure 21-1. Sample rating scale options for use with people with aphasia. The visual rating scale with associated hand gestures may be used with or without the associated text. Some people may prefer to have the scale labeled with numbers instead of words. Another option is to use a written rating scale from "strongly disagree" to "strongly agree." These could all be adapted for conversation.

largely positive; most research participants used the device for a variety of communicative functions, and some continued to use the system after the research was completed (van de Sandt-Koenderman et al., 2005).

Most commercially available SGDs provide options that allow the AAC user to access messages from grid displays. There are three types of grid displays: taxonomic, semantic-syntactic, and visual-scene (Beukelman & Mirenda, 2013). Results from studies that have used a taxonomic grid display indicate that persons with severe chronic aphasia are able to access, manipulate, and combine symbols across several screens to produce simple sentences and phrases (Koul et al., 2005; Koul et al., 2008; Koul & Harding, 1998).

The landscape of speech-generating options for people with aphasia changed dramatically with the introduction of visual scene displays (VSDs; Dietz et al., 2006; McKelvey et al., 2007). VSDs leverage the retained ability of people with aphasia to relate to highly contextualized and personally meaningful pictures paired with the technology of SGDs to create an interface that supports communication. Research indicates that the combination of contextualization and personal meaningfulness of photos is important to the facilitation of communication for people with aphasia (Beukelman et al., 2015; McKelvey et al., 2010). For instance, a picture of a sunset does not provide a lot of personal information; it is largely decontextualized. In contrast, a picture of the sun

setting behind a cabin in the mountains with family members of a person with aphasia making s'mores over a small campfire provides both contextual information and personal relevance. The relation of the person with aphasia to the context and the people, places, or objects in a photo provide the foundation for communication. The written text that accompanies photos should support a variety of relevant linguistic functions (e.g., labels, short sentences, questions, comments) to engage a conversation partner. When selected, each message is spoken by the SGD.

To provide people with aphasia a compilation of visual scenes that comprise more of a system than a single VSD, researchers needed a way for people with aphasia to access multiple visual scenes on a single device. Although traditional navigation tools, such as buttons labeled "Back" or "Home Page," worked for people with aphasia under study conditions, researchers found that a **navigation ring** was more transparent and better facilitated navigation for people with aphasia. A navigation ring is a D-shaped layout where thumbnails of the other available visual scenes surround the currently active VSD. The person with aphasia selects from among the thumbnails to navigate between pages on the device rather than having to sort through words and/or icons, as is the case on some devices with dynamic displays (Beukelman et al., 2015; Wallace & Hux, 2014).

Conversation between grandparents about grandchild attending an out-of-state college because he won a scholarship.

"What do you think about Tim attending college out-of-state instead of the local state college?"

- Good for him
- Stay in state
- He must go
- Up to him

> PWA indicates their response by selecting from among the written choices presented.

Follow-up question, "So you think it's good for him to go, yes or no?"

PWA answers with head nod for 'yes'.

> PWA answers verbal question. Then written choice communication continues.

Follow up comment: "He'll be far from home."

- Show map of U.S. with an 'X' on Tim's hometown and a circle around location of out-of-state college. Maybe draw a line connecting the two marks.

> Supplement written word choice with other graphics (e.g., map of the United States).

Additional comment: "Even though he'll be far away, you still think he should go?"

- He's a good student
- Won a scholarship
- I'll miss him
- Regret staying here

> PWA indicates their response by selecting from among the written choices presented.

Comment: "Yes, I agree. He might regret staying here. He won that scholarship and should go. I'll miss him, too."

Figure 21-2. Example of a written word choice conversation for a person with aphasia (PWA).

The paradigmatic shift wrought by the introduction of VSDs has dominated the speech-generating intervention landscape for people with aphasia and has been the focus of much current research. The advent of smartphones with better cameras, the ever-increasing facility of transfer of photos between devices, refinements in space-saving technologies to support libraries of photos on a single device, and the technical ability to add text and speech output capacity to selected photos has changed the scope and horizon for the implementation of VSDs. The proliferation of mobile tablets and apps to support communication extends now to encompass apps that support VSDs (Caron et al., 2016; McNaughton & Light, 2013).

Initial research comparing VSDs to traditional grid-based SGD layouts indicates a clear advantage for VSD-type layouts with respect to efficient and accurate navigation (Wallace & Hux, 2014) and ease of use and greater number of communicative turns taken (Beukelman et al., 2015; Brock et al., 2017; Koul, 2011). Importantly, as is true for all AAC options, VSDs require training in their use. People with aphasia and other stakeholder input is necessary in their development and customization. Communication partner training is key to successful implementation since the goal of any communication intervention is to facilitate communicative interaction between the user and their conversation partners.

Since mobile tablets support VSDs, as well as apps for therapy, communication, and possibly for entertainment, clinicians must consider models for app selection (e.g., Holland et al., 2012; McCall, 2012; Munoz et al., 2013). For people with aphasia, prior to app selection, there needs to be consensus about use of a mobile tablet for agreed-upon purposes (e.g., to use with apps to support therapy, apps to support

My name is _____. I had a stroke. I have APHASIA which means I have trouble communicating.

To help me please:
1) **Speak clearly and simply.**

2) **<u>Don't</u> talk louder** – I can hear you.

3) Give me **time to respond.**

4) **Ask me a question I can answer with 'yes' or 'no'** if I'm having trouble finding the right word.

5) **Ask me before you repeat** what you said.

Figure 21-3. An identification and communication card for a person with aphasia.

communication, apps for other purposes). To establish buy-in, the person with aphasia and significant other(s) have to agree to learn how to use the system (i.e., the tablet and one or more apps). Buy-in to the use of AAC is a critical issue (Holland et al., 2012; Hustad et al., 2002) and is not always an easy sell. One approach is to target a communicative function valued by the person with aphasia and to introduce an app that supports that function. For instance, video chatting with children or grandchildren may be identified as an important goal. Introducing an app that will support that function may provide the impetus for the person with aphasia to learn how to operate the device and app. To scaffold video chatting with children or grandchildren, therapeutic goals to address impairment-level issues can be embedded within therapy with a view to facilitating communication. Using apps to support therapeutic goals may be enough for some people with aphasia; however, they may not wish to use an app or apps for all communicative functions.

Holland and colleagues (2012) note that in addition to portability, cosmesis, commercial availability, and durability of a mobile tablet, additional factors influence adoption of a tablet by a person with aphasia. These factors include the ease of finding, selecting, and purchasing apps, the purpose(s) the person with aphasia has identified for using a device, and the acceptance and support available to the user by family and friends. Although their study was not conducted with a mobile tablet and a communication app, Lasker and Beukelman (1999) reported that families of people with aphasia preferred natural speech vs. a digitized voice on an AAC device for storytelling. In contrast, less familiar conversation partners preferred AAC strategies for storytelling. Buy-in to the use of AAC can be tenuous (Lasker & Bedrosian, 2001; Lasker & Beukelman, 1999); clinicians can encourage use of AAC by supporting people with aphasia to engage successfully in their valued and self-identified communicative functions.

Although apps are ubiquitous in the personal lives of many clinicians, it is important to remember that introduction of each app is akin to introduction of an entirely new device (Zimmerman & Vanderheiden, 2008), especially for people with aphasia who are not familiar with mobile technology. Many rubrics are available to assist with app selection (e.g., Fonner & Marfilius, 2011; Gosnell et al., 2011; Lee & Cherner, 2015) and should be consulted as aids to the clinician.

Cognition as it Relates to AAC for People With Aphasia

Implementation of AAC for people with aphasia requires careful consideration of the many speech, language, and cognitive issues that often accompany aphasia. The cognitive sequelae of aphasia include deficits in **nonverbal cognition**—areas of cognitive functioning that are not language-based, such as attention (Murray, 2012), cognitive flexibility (Chiou & Kennedy, 2009; Vallila-Rohter & Kiran, 2015), executive function (Frankel et al., 2007; Mayer et al., 2017; Murray, 2012; Nicholas & Connor, 2017; Purdy, 2002), and memory and visuospatial functioning. These nonverbal cognitive functions influence the type of AAC with which a person with aphasia may be successful. Based on two models of executive function that use slightly different terminologies, Nicholas and Connor (2017) suggest that executive attention, which includes working memory, as well as the ability to simultaneously update memory, shift attentional set, and inhibit competing thoughts or responses, are all important cognitive components related to the successful use of AAC by people with aphasia (Brock et al., 2017; Nicholas et al., 2011).

Petroi and colleagues (2014) investigated the ability of people with aphasia to identify single symbols and simple subject-verb-object sentences presented using an SGD in the presence or absence of competing stimuli. Results indicated that the number of symbols on the screen and complexity of navigation had a significant effect on accuracy and latency of correct responses. For the single-symbol identification task, about 14% of the variance in results was accounted for by navigational complexity and 9% by the number of symbols presented on screen. This indicates that navigation puts greater load on cognitive processing, and thus, navigational demands should be reduced. Additionally, people with aphasia perceived tasks to be more difficult than persons in the control group.

In an interesting study, Koul and colleagues (2005) investigated the ability of nine individuals with severe Broca's aphasia or global aphasia to produce sentences of varying syntactical complexity using graphic symbols organized across multiple screens using a taxonomic interface display. The sentences ranged in complexity from simple two-word phrases to those with morphological inflections, transformations, and relative clauses. Although individuals with aphasia were able to access, identify, and combine graphic symbols to produce phrases and sentences of varying degrees of syntactical complexity, the underlying linguistic impairment observed in individuals with aphasia also affected their ability to produce grammatically complex sentences using graphic symbols.

In summary, the use of AAC for people with aphasia has a history that is replete with efforts by researchers and clinicians to provide both speech-generating and non–speech-generating technology options. The introduction of VSDs for use by people with aphasia represents a paradigmatic shift in speech-generating AAC options available for people with chronic and severe aphasia. Research indicates that people with aphasia prefer VSDs to traditional grid layouts and that VSDs lend themselves to communication that is more efficient. Additional research indicates that nonverbal cognition issues may interact both positively and negatively with the ability of people with aphasia to use AAC. Clinical decision making regarding AAC options for someone with aphasia must include consideration of nonverbal cognition issues.

AAC FOR PERSONS WITH NEURODEGENERATIVE CONDITIONS

Neurodegeneration is the progressive loss of structure or function of neurons, including death of neurons. Many neurodegenerative diseases, such as Alzheimer's disease (AD), amyotrophic lateral sclerosis (ALS), Huntington's disease (HD), multiple sclerosis (MS), and Parkinson's disease (PD), occur because of neurodegenerative processes in the brain and spinal cord. The clinical features of this diverse group of neurological disorders differ depending on the regions of the central and/or peripheral nervous system involved and the mechanism(s) of degeneration. Neurodegenerative diseases are progressive and terminal. Most cause systemic motor problems, many of which affect the speech mechanism, resulting in a variety of motor speech-based symptoms that together yield a disorder-specific profile. Either a single or mixed type dysarthria is typically associated with each disease, the severity of which ranges from mild to severe. In some diseases, the dysarthria may become so severe that the person becomes anarthric. In other situations, the dysarthria may be less severe yet still significantly compromise communication. See Table 21-1 for a summary of the dysarthrias and associated diseases.

Aside from bulbar onset ALS in which the disease manifests itself with speech and swallowing symptoms (Duffy, 2013), most neurodegenerative diseases do not present themselves with motor speech symptoms. Rather, effects on speech are part of the disease's progression, not its presentation.

To address the speech, language, and communication compromises that accompany neurodegenerative disease, it is incumbent on the speech-language pathologist to be knowledgeable about a broad range of AAC options so they can intervene in a timely and appropriate manner. It is further helpful to adopt a **systems approach** to the assessment and implementation of AAC for people with neurodegenerative disease. A systems approach is a concept often used in business management and engineering, which considers the multidimensional and interrelated nature of all factors and aspects of an entity and how these factors interact with the environment in pursuit of a designated goal (Churchman & Churchman, 1968; Frederiksen & Collins, 1989; Kerzner, 2017). Systems both influence and are influenced by external environments. Within a systems approach, goals are defined as "the result or achievement toward which effort is directed" (*Merriam-Webster's Collegiate Dictionary*, 1999, p. 499) and are often associated with necessary preconditions that must be satisfied along the way. In this line of thinking, goal attainment is a process in and of itself.

With respect to neurodegenerative disease, a systems approach provides a way to consider the unique profile of each disease alongside the commonalities among the diseases. Pairing this thinking with the need to provide communication supports across the continuum of a disease allows the clinician to consider the known trajectory of each disease, its speech, language, and cognitive sequelae, and current best practices for staging AAC intervention (Fried-Oken et al., 2015). A systems approach leverages the known progressive nature of neurodegenerative diseases to the clinician's advantage. Thus, although each disease is unique, fundamental similarities exist such that speech, language, and often cognitive skills decline across the duration of each disease, although not always in tandem or in a linear manner. Likewise, most neurodegenerative diseases can be divided into three stages: an early, middle, and late stage. As part of the systems approach to neurodegenerative disease, it is important to

TABLE 21-1

Summary of Speech, Language, Cognitive, and Behavioral Characteristics Associated With Amyotrophic Lateral Sclerosis, Huntington's Disease, Multiple Sclerosis, and Parkinson's Disease in Early, Mid, and Late Stages of Each Disease

	ALS	HD	MS	PD
Commonly Associated Motor Speech Impairment (dysarthria type)	Mixed spastic-flaccid	Hyperkinetic	Mixed spastic-ataxic	Hypokinetic

Language Deficits
• Word retrieval
• Latency of response
• Difficulty with
  ◦ Topic maintenance
  ◦ Discourse comprehension
• Preservation
• Decreasing
  ◦ Length of utterance
  ◦ Syntactic complexity
	Early	Early ✓	Early	Early

	Mid ✓*	Mid ✓	Mid ✓*	Mid ✓
	Late ✓*	Late ✓	Late ✓	Late ✓

Cognitive Impairments
• Executive dysfunction
• Difficulty with
  ◦ New learning
  ◦ Delayed recall
  ◦ Abstraction
  ◦ Concentration
  ◦ Sustained attention
  ◦ Decision making
• Social cognition deficit
  ◦ Recognition of emotion
  ◦ Theory of mind
	Early ✓*
	With ALSci
		Early ✓	Early	Early ✓

	Mid ✓* With ALSci	Mid ✓	Mid ✓	Mid ✓
	Late ✓* With ALSci	Late ✓	Late ✓	Late ✓
Behavioral Changes • Apathy • Irritability • Depression • Delusions • Psychosis • Disinhibited behavior	Early ✓* With ALSbv	Early ✓	Early	Early ✓
	Mid ✓ With ALSbv	Mid ✓	Mid ✓* Typically do not demonstrate delusions, psychosis, or disinhibited behavior	Mid ✓
	Late ✓ With ALSbv	Late ✓	Late ✓*	Late ✓

(continued)

TABLE 21-1 (CONTINUED)

Summary of Speech, Language, Cognitive, and Behavioral Characteristics Associated With Amyotrophic Lateral Sclerosis, Huntington's Disease, Multiple Sclerosis, and Parkinson's Disease in Early, Mid, and Late Stages of Each Disease

	ALS	HD	MS	PD
Presence of Emotional Lability	Early	Early	Early	Early
	Mid ✓	Mid	Mid ✓	Mid
	Late ✓	Late	Late ✓	Late
Maintenance of Literacy Skills (ability to read)	Early ✓	Early ✓	Early ✓	Early ✓
	Mid ✓	Mid ✓ (visual disturbances may disrupt)	Mid ✓ (visual disturbances may disrupt)	Mid ✓
	Late ✓	Late (✓) (visual disturbances may disrupt)	Late ✓ (visual disturbances may disrupt)	Late ✓

✓ = presence of disorder/impairment; ✓* = may be present and would appear during the stage of disease noted if present; ALSci = ALS with cognitive impairment; ALSbv = ALS behavioral variant; ALS = amyotrophic lateral sclerosis; HD = Huntington's disease; MS = multiple sclerosis; PD = Parkinson's disease.

Color Coding: blue = early stages; yellow = mid stages; green = late stages. Exceptions noted.

note that although use of AAC strategies and options may begin as supplementary to natural speech, they may assume an increasingly central role with progression of the disease.

Themes central to a systems approach to AAC intervention in neurodegenerative disease are energy conservation and access to a variety of communication options at each step along the disease continuum to best meet the individual's needs. Basic principles of intervention in the systems approach include the need to intervene early and often (Gutmann & Gryfe, 1996; Brownlee & Bruening, 2012; Fried-Oken et al., 2015), the iterative nature of the AAC assessment and intervention process, the need to educate all stakeholders about AAC in general and the specific AAC options being implemented at each point, and the importance of planning ahead for anticipated needs based on the disease trajectory.

Customization of the systems approach for each disease and for each patient is necessary, although the overarching principles and themes remain constant. An example of customization might be the timing of the introduction of end-of-life vocabulary to a given individual. People with neurodegenerative diseases often need and want to discuss end-of-life issues with family members, friends, lawyers, accountants, and others. If the person is using non–speech-generating AAC technology options and does not spell, the clinician may need to broach the topic and provide the necessary symbols, pictures, or full words and phrases to support conversation on this important topic. Figure 21-4 illustrates a systems approach to AAC for ALS.

The utility of a systems approach is that the goal—providing communication supports, such as AAC strategies, devices, and techniques, to the person and their identified significant others across the course of a degenerative disease—inherently acknowledges the multidimensional nature of this process and that it is not a one-and-done type of endeavor. Rather, this process subsumes all the necessary "moving parts" that must work in tandem to realize this goal. The exigency of time impinges on the intervention schedule in neurodegenerative diseases. Time is a crucial variable in both the type and scope of AAC intervention across these disorders.

The Five Cs

As part of a systems approach to conceptualization of AAC assessment and intervention in neurodegenerative disease, clinicians will want to consider the five Cs: caregiver burden, cognitive decline, conservation of communicative competence, counseling, and cultural considerations. The five Cs, as depicted in Figure 21-5, represent a cycle of clinical considerations for each aspect of assessment and intervention. Importantly, there is an evidence base for each C with respect to its applicability to each disease or disorder. The five Cs are outlined next in alphabetic order.

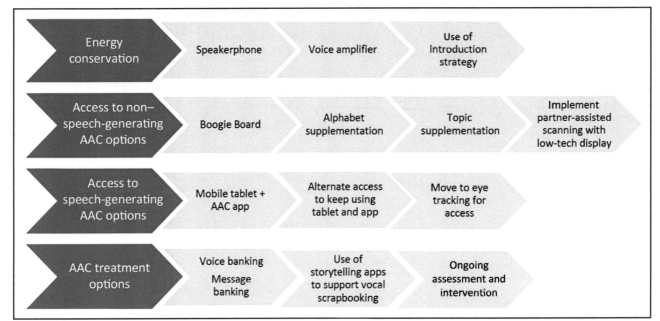

Figure 21-4. Central themes in a systems approach to AAC for patients with ALS. Energy conservation undergirds all AAC intervention in ALS. The steps may be interchanged in terms of their order of implementation. For instance, a person with spinal onset ALS may find it fatiguing to hold a phone while they talk. To attenuate that fatigue, use of a speakerphone obviates the need to hold the phone. Similarly, if vocal fatigue and/or hypophonia are issues, use of a voice amplifier lessens the need to project one's voice. Use of an introduction strategy (e.g., using a business card or a brief prerecorded message on a cellphone) urging communication partners not to hang up and that the person has some trouble with their speech but understands everything saves the effort of repeating this introduction with each communication partner and/or for each phone conversation. For non–speech-generating technology options, if the person has use of their hand to write, they may find use of a Boogie Board, an electronic magic slate, handy and easy to use. Alphabet and/or topic supplementation can be implemented as compensatory strategies for dysarthria on a non–speech-generating display and/or via an app that supports them.

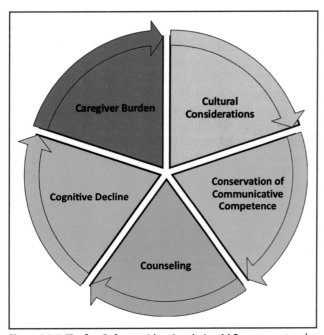

Figure 21-5. The five Cs for consideration during AAC assessment and intervention. The cycle is iterative and there is no fixed entry or exit point. The ultimate goal of providing AAC supports is to conserve communicative competence. The other Cs are factors that influence how and to what extent AAC supports may be implemented.

Caregiver Burden

Across diseases, caregiver burden and its expression are important considerations for the speech-language pathologist. Although the concept of caregiver burden itself is complex with a lack of agreement surrounding the exact meaning of the terminology, it is intimately related to cultural considerations, such as veneration of elders, care for the sick, view of disability, and filial responsibility (Bastawrous, 2013). Despite the lack of clarity around the concept itself, researchers typically operationalize the term "caregiver burden" with respect to a particular scale or metric. Research indicates that cognitive decline typically exacerbates caregiver burden (e.g., Chiò et al., 2010; Lillo, Mioshi, et al., 2012), sometimes even more so than physical disability. Increasing caregiver burden can lead to caregiver burnout, a serious problem in the landscape of caregiving (e.g., Adelman et al., 2014). Adding one more thing to a caregiver's seemingly already overwhelming load may be perceived as a gross imposition. For this reason, if/when AAC is needed, caregiver(s) may be unable and/or reluctant to support its implementation; this may be expressed as a fear of learning new technology, especially some of the speech-generating options. Since successful implementation of AAC relies on caregiver support and buy-in, lack of it presents a serious obstacle (Gona et al., 2014; DeCarlo et al., 2019). Potential workarounds are to identify another family member or friend who is willing to take responsibility for learning, set-up, and maintenance of a client's AAC supports. It is not a perfect solution since if the designated person is sick, away, or decides they can no longer undertake the responsibility, the AAC user may be unable to use their system. Another option is to promote use of AAC as a way for the user to exert some communicative independence, especially in light of the patient's growing dependence on others for an increasing number of tasks. For people who use AAC to be able to express themselves is of utmost importance and may relieve some small portion the work associated with communication if it has become problematic, and this may lessen perceived caregiver burden. Clinicians may also suggest external sources to mitigate caregiver burden; these might include but are not limited to attendance in support groups, the need to arrange respite care, the importance of regularly scheduled social activities away from the person with the disease, and the overall importance of self care.

Cognitive Decline

As noted above, cognitive decline can exacerbate caregiver burden. It can also obstruct implementation of AAC since cognitive skills are required to learn how to use an AAC strategy or device (e.g., Purdy & Dietz, 2010). The presence of cognitive impairment, as well as the very real potential of further cognitive decline with progression of the disease, are touchstone points to be acknowledged and addressed with empathy. Further, the interface of cognition and AAC cannot be underestimated (Nicholas & Connor, 2017; Purdy & Dietz, 2010). Although procedural memory may be relatively well-preserved for some of a disease's trajectory, sometimes AAC is not needed until later in the disease process when new learning is difficult. This presents a conundrum for the clinician since some viable options may need to be tabled in favor of simpler options. However, the best AAC option is the one that is used regularly, even if it is not the most sophisticated option. That said, every speech-generating option requires a non–speech-generating technology back up for use when speech-generating technology cannot be used, such as in the bath/shower, the event of a power outage that outlasts a system's power reserve, or if the system is not working for whatever reason.

Conservation of Communicative Competence

Supporting patients' communicative competence is at the core of all clinician efforts to provide AAC options (Light & McNaughton, 2014a). This overarching theme subsumes all aspects of clinical function with respect to AAC: assessment, planning intervention, implementation of AAC supports, caregiver and/or facilitator training, system(s) customization, and ongoing revision. Given the nature of each communication disorder and the trajectory of each disease discussed in this chapter, it is necessary to consider the interaction of the five Cs. Treating dysarthria associated with a neurodegenerative disease or stroke-induced aphasia may also involve addressing concomitant cognitive deficits. As

a field, speech-language pathology has a growing literature about the use of AAC supports for people with cognitive-communication disorders and a growing literature related to outcomes associated with the use of AAC supports for people with cognitive decline (e.g., Purdy & Wallace, 2016; Wallace & Diehl, 2017). The presence of a cognitive component to an existing disorder complicates both assessment and intervention and obligates the clinician to anticipate additional cognitive challenges to planned interventions. As research indicates, communication disorders can lead to social withdrawal and social isolation (Dietz et al., 2013; Holland & Beeson, 1993; Shadden, 2005). As such, preservation of communicative competence, arguably the most central of the five Cs to speech-language pathologists, is of primary importance. The overlap of preserving communicative competence with the other identified Cs supports this flexibility in service provision. Using evidence-based practices, speech-language pathologists can provide communication supports that help patients maintain social engagement in spite of constrained or waning cognitive and communicative abilities.

Counseling

Across neurodegenerative diseases, counseling plays a pivotal role in assessment and intervention. A major theme with respect to the diagnosis of a neurodegenerative disease is **violation of expectation** (Luterman, 2008). Violation of expectation is the feeling that results from violation of the implicit or explicit expectations in a given situation. In the realm of neurodegenerative diseases, the diagnosis itself is a violation of expectation; it is something nobody planned for and is unwelcome, even if it is a relief to have a name and a validation of the constellation of symptoms that have been occurring over time. Even in the case of inherited disorders, there is always the hope that the disease may not express itself. People often rail against the unfairness of the diagnosis, which may strike them in the prime of their lives during peak earning years, when beginning a family or when relishing the freedom of retirement. The main sentiment is, "It wasn't supposed to be like this." The person with the disease, as well as family members, friends, and caregivers, may express this sentiment in a myriad of ways. For clinicians, this is a very important consideration on the time horizon of intervention. Each loss or decrement in ability, cognitive and/or physical, reinforces the feeling of violation of expectation. A particularly potent example of this relates to the need for AAC. The loss of natural speech, or the loss of the viability of natural speech as one's primary mode of communication, is a particularly emotional touchstone in any disease process. The primordial importance of voice to personal identity underscores the enormity of this loss and may explain, in part, why some people are reluctant to adopt AAC options.

Another important concept in counseling as it relates to progressive diseases is that of **ambiguous loss** (Boss, 1999; 2010; Boss & Couden, 2002). Boss defines ambiguous loss as loss that is unclear, indeterminate, and unresolved for some period of time (1999). Boss identifies two types of ambiguous loss, one of which is particularly relevant to neurodegenerative disorders. This type of ambiguous loss is labeled as "goodbye without leaving," that is, the person is still physically present but increasingly psychologically absent. With respect to neurodegenerative disorders, people are alive but no longer function as they once did due to physical, cognitive, psychological, and communicative changes (Blieszner et al., 2007; Boss, 1999). This type of loss is particularly poignant. Clinicians need to be aware of the stress involved in ambiguity for all involved—the patient, family members, and caregivers. The other type of loss is "leaving without goodbye," which captures what happens after a sudden catastrophic event (e.g., motor vehicle accident) whereby the person dies without opportunity to say goodbye. With respect to goodbye without leaving, patients may experience significant ambiguity around loss of self (Holland & Beeson, 1993; Shadden, 2005) and some confusion around new roles and changes in the family and the living environment. Similarly, family members experience significant ambiguity with each loss because each loss underscores the progression of decline. Part of our work as clinicians is to continue to support communication in whatever form—be it speech and/or AAC—as best we can, to support people to continue to engage communicatively.

Cultural Considerations

Addressing any of the already identified Cs must be suffused with cultural considerations in the broadest sense of the term. Consideration of culture mandates that clinicians learn about a patient's culture on a deeper level—more than a passing familiarity with the holidays, rituals, and religion of a given patient. It requires a willingness to learn and to expose one's vulnerability. It means being open to taking another's perspective and arriving at an understanding of their worldview. Soto (2018) broadens the concept of culture to include development of a deep understanding and appreciation of the multiple factors that create and perpetuate the marginalization of people with complex communication needs. This is a critical in-service provision for people with acquired neurologic and/or neurodegenerative disorders. The proliferation of mobile tablets in the mainstream makes use of this commercially available technology less stigmatizing than use of SGDs of previous generations. However, it does not change the fact that someone with severe communication impairment, even one who uses mainstream technology, may still be considered different from their peers and family members. Use of AAC is not yet mainstream. To that end, AAC service providers need to continue to advocate for acceptance of AAC and to educate all involved stakeholders on the value and validity of all forms of communication, particularly as it relates to acquired communication disorders for adults who are likely to have used natural speech prior to the onset or progression of the disorder.

This framework lends itself well to clinical function since it is iterative; at each point in the process, these considerations should be revisited and reimagined. There is no designated entry or exit point; rather, clinicians should use it

to ensure that they are addressing all necessary aspects when interacting with clients and their caregivers. All five Cs are integrally related. One C may predominate as a concern at one appointment whereas another C may be a prevailing concern at the next. The framework is flexible and yields to the clinician's needs.

AAC Assessment

With both a systems approach and the five Cs in mind, the following section provides a brief overview of general AAC considerations for clinicians treating individuals with neurodegenerative conditions.

The starting point for AAC is a comprehensive assessment of the person's speech, language, and cognitive status to serve as baseline. For any of the neurodegenerative disorders, the following is an example of what a comprehensive speech, language, and cognitive evaluation should include:

- Oral mechanism examination
- Assessment of speech and speaking
   ○ Measure of intelligibility (e.g., *Sentence Intelligibility Test*, as indicated; Yorkston et al., 2007)
- Language assessment (e.g., *Boston Naming Test*; Kaplan et al., 2001; reading a standardized passage; comprehension measure)
- Hearing screening
- Cognitive screening (e.g., *Montreal Cognitive Assessment*; Nasreddine et al., 2005; *ALS Cognitive Behavioral Screen*; Woolley et al., 2010; a short form *Montreal Cognitive Assessment*; Roalf et al., 2016)
- Cognitive testing (e.g., *Repeatable Battery for the Assessment of Neuropsychological Status*; Randolph et al., 1998)
- Information about the patient's literacy level
- Information about the patient's and others' familiarity with technology

Results of this assessment provide baseline measures for ongoing comparison. At this assessment, the speech-language pathologist will begin to establish rapport with the patient and family. This is a critical step in the process since the speech-language pathologist is likely to have ongoing involvement in the patient's care. This is also a good opportunity to share information regarding the speech-language pathologist's role in intervention. The speech-language pathologist must gauge the patient's readiness to hear information about how the disease may affect communication. Some patients ask questions based on information gleaned from the internet and/or other sources whereas others may not know what the future portends with respect to communication.

Once baseline speech, language, and cognitive information is collected, it is appropriate to collect basic AAC-relevant information. This might include options, such as *Social Networks Inventory* (Blackstone & Hunt-Berg, 2003) and other communication inventories, such as the

Communicative Participation Item Bank (Baylor et al., 2013), the *Communicative Effectiveness Index—Modified* (Ball et al., 2004b), and the *Levels of Speech Usage* categorical rating scale (Yorkston et al., 2013). These tools provide ways to capture critical information about current and potential communication partners, communication environments, and communication challenges.

Alternate Access

A critical aspect of any AAC assessment is determination of access method. In neurodegenerative disease, assessment of access takes on even greater importance since it is likely to change with physical and/or cognitive decline. To this end, it is important to verify the patient's current method of access and consider AAC options that support the patient's current method of access. All else being equal, if a patient is a direct selector, then they will have the greatest number of AAC options available to them—both non–speech-generating and speech-generating technology. The need for alternate access constrains the number of options available, as not all speech-generating technology options support all modes of alternate access. Many options for alternate access are currently available. Research and development of new and more refined access options continues such that previously unfathomable access solutions have become reality. Eye tracking is now widely available as an access option. New switches that leverage materials science, such as the NeuroNode (Control Bionics), or those that provide one portal that supports multiple options for access, such as the Noddle (Voxello), are now available. An active area of research in terms of alternate access for AAC is in brain-computer interfaces (BCIs). Although a thorough discussion of BCIs is beyond the scope of this chapter, it is important to mention them in the context of alternate access since this is an active area of research. BCIs "… are assistive technology interfaces that directly interpret brain activity to enable a person to control (another) technology. In AAC applications, a BCI can be conceptualized as a system of four basic components: sensors to record brain activity, signal analysis methods to extract desired control signals from the brain activity, communication rate enhancement techniques to improve the efficiency of each selection, and the output that results from the process, often on a display" (Huggins & Kovacs, 2018, p. 13). At present, use of BCIs as modes of access for people with neurodegenerative diseases is extremely limited and still largely confined to use in research settings or protocols (e.g., RSVP Keyboard BCI; Fried-Oken et al., 2015). Neurodegenerative conditions themselves may present challenges for the use of BCIs since both physical and cognitive status may change with disease progression and may influence one's ability to use a BCI. More research is required to determine what type(s) of BCIs will support continued access to AAC systems in the face of cognitive and/or physical deterioration, and how to provide the user with the most robust communication options.

Consideration of AAC Options

Using information from speech, language, cognitive, and access assessments, coupled with information from other inventories, it is appropriate to consider the range of available AAC options. Assessment techniques, such as feature matching (Shane & Costello, 1994) and matching person to technology (Scherer & Craddock, 2002), figure prominently in any AAC assessment. The ultimate goal of feature matching is to match the client's current AAC needs with system(s) that support the necessary features. Trial of each system is necessary as is evaluation of which system(s) best meet the client's needs. With respect to SGDs or mobile tablets with AAC apps, navigation skills need to be assessed and consideration given to various layouts and types of system organization.

AAC IN SPECIFIC NEURODEGENERATIVE CONDITIONS

Amyotrophic Lateral Sclerosis

ALS is a progressive neurodegenerative disease that affects motor neurons in the brain and spinal cord, and by extension, muscles throughout the body. Progressive degeneration of the motor neurons in ALS results in death. Once the motor neurons die, the brain loses its ability to direct voluntary muscle movement and muscle control.

Two major types of ALS are sporadic and familial or genetic. According to the Amyotrophic Lateral Sclerosis Association website (http://www.alsa.org), sporadic ALS is the most common form of the disease in the United States, accounting for approximately 90% to 95% of all cases. Familial ALS accounts for approximately 5% to 10% of all cases in the United States and is often determined by patient ancestry. Since 1993, there has been an explosion of information about the genetic mutations associated with ALS. For this reason, familial ALS is sometimes replaced by the term "genetic," which better captures what is known about genetic aspects of ALS; specifically, mutations in 37 genes that predispose someone to ALS have been reported (e.g., see Forsberg et al., 2019). In Caucasian individuals, the most commonly reported mutation is in C9orf72, found in 8% to 10% of patients with ALS. Mutations of various types in the genes encoding superoxide dismutase-1, TAR-DNA-binding protein 43, and other mutations are found in 2% to 6% of European patients (Forsberg et al., 2019). Mutations may be causally associated with ALS (Andersen & Al-Chalabi, 2011; Rosen et al., 1993) or may be disease modifiers (e.g., Andersen et al., 1997).

Patterns of upper and lower motor neuron involvement result in phenotypic classifications of ALS. The two most common phenotypic presentations of ALS are (1) spinal onset, in which limbs and extremities are affected first, and (2) bulbar onset, in which the speech and swallowing mechanism is affected first. Other presentations exist, as does a mixed presentation where there are elements of both spinal and bulbar onset.

ALS typically strikes between the ages of 40 and 70 years with an estimated 16,000 to 18,000 Americans having the disease at any given time (http://www.alsa.org). Military veterans, particularly those who participated in the first Gulf War in 1991, tend to be diagnosed with ALS twice as often as members of the general public. This has increased the number of younger people diagnosed with the disease. In general, ALS is 20% more common in men than in women, although this trend equals out with increasing age (Manjaly et al., 2010). Life expectancy with ALS is variable; 2 to 5 years after diagnosis is average, although some people live 5 and even 10 years beyond diagnosis (http://www.alsa.org).

Although there is no known cure for ALS, four U.S. Food and Drug Administration–approved drugs are used in its treatment—Rilutek, Nuedexta, Radicava, and Tiglutik (http://www.alsa.org/als-care/fda-approved-drugs.html). These drugs may alleviate symptoms and mitigate disease progression in the short term; none of these drugs is curative.

Cognitive Impairment Associated With Amyotrophic Lateral Sclerosis

In addition to motor symptomatology, cognitive impairment in ALS has been recognized and well-characterized (e.g., Lomen-Hoerth et al., 2002; Murphy et al., 2016; Ringholz et al., 2005; Woolley et al., 2010). Approximately 40% to 60% of patients with ALS exhibit mild to moderate cognitive impairment (e.g., Lillo, Savage, et al., 2012; Woolley et al., 2010). In a systematic review and meta-analysis, Beeldman and colleagues (2016) reported that the cognitive profile of ALS consists of deficits in executive functions, fluency, language, social cognition, and verbal memory. The behavioral issues often associated with ALS include apathy, inflexibility, increased irritability, poor frustration tolerance, and a tendency to be more withdrawn. Both cognitive and behavioral components of ALS contribute to increased burden of disease for patients and affect their caregivers as well (Murphy et al., 2016; Woolley et al., 2010).

Strong and colleagues (2017) corroborated these findings and revised the criteria for the diagnosis of frontotemporal dysfunction in ALS. Strong and colleagues (2017) reported that the neuropsychological deficits in ALS are very heterogeneous, affecting more than 50% of people with ALS. These deficits significantly and adversely affect survival. Recognition of the clinical heterogeneity of the neuropsychological deficits in ALS and the data supporting this claim led to the reconceptualization of neuropsychological deficits along a spectrum named the frontotemporal spectrum disorder of ALS. This finding has implications for AAC intervention at every stage of the disease, especially since it is related to shorter life span.

Therapeutic interventions are the mainstay of symptomatic treatment in ALS. Multidisciplinary clinics where providers are seen in a centralized location are associated with greater patient satisfaction (e.g., Van den Berg et al., 2005). An apt quote from Steve Gleason about ALS, "Until there is a cure, technology is the cure" (https://teamgleason.org/technology-equipment) is a clarion call to clinicians providing AAC, and all types of assistive technology, to people with ALS.

AAC in Amyotrophic Lateral Sclerosis

One of the most pernicious aspects of ALS is the loss or anticipated loss of speech (Hecht et al., 2002; Körner et al., 2013). Research indicates approximately 95% of people with ALS will have speech disturbances at some point during their disease, and many will lose their speech entirely (Ball et al., 2004a; Beukelman, Fager, et al., 2007; Beukelman et al., 2011). Timing of intervention is critical given the speech deterioration in ALS (Makkonen et al., 2018; Yorkston et al., 1993).

One way to begin to address this aspect of ALS is the introduction of **voice banking** and **message banking**. Voice banking is the process whereby large inventories of a person's speech sounds are electronically recorded and stored to be used in the creation of a synthetic voice for later use (Creer et al., 2013; Yamagishi et al., 2012). Although voice banking may be a time-intensive endeavor, it is an important aspect of intervention since a synthetic voice can be created from banked speech samples for use in an AAC device (Mills et al., 2014). In contrast, message banking is a process whereby the person with ALS records whole phrases and/or messages that are stored electronically. This type of banking can be emotionally intensive since often people will create a vocal legacy for family members while doing this. Message banking also supports the creation of a corpus of messages for later use in an AAC device.

Timing of the introduction of this aspect of intervention is crucial. Introduced too early in the disease when the diagnosis is fresh and raw, some people may find the idea offensive. If not introduced until the patient is severely dysarthric, it will be too late to engage meaningfully in this process. Some patients may read about this via online sources and bring it to the speech-language pathologist's attention whereas others may not know about it. Regardless, speech-language pathologists who work with this population should be knowledgeable about the differences between voice and message banking, the procedural how-to for each type of banking, the equipment needed, and the relevant research (Costello, 2014; Creer et al., 2013; Oosthuizen et al., 2018; Yamagishi et al., 2012). AAC has gained significant traction in the ALS population (Ball et al., 2004b; Richter et al., 2003). This may be attributable to the fact that for a long time, ALS was considered primarily a motor disorder that affected people in middle to older age, long after they had acquired literacy skills that are preserved throughout the disease. Preservation of literacy skills against a backdrop of motor speech disorder rendered AAC intervention relatively straightforward from a language perspective. Options that supported text-to-speech and rate enhancement features, such as abbreviation expansion, were the mainstay of AAC intervention for persons with ALS for many years. These included dedicated devices, such as the Lightwriter and scanning Lightwriter, as well as the Epson Alternative Communication System, that supported a variety of access options. These options worked well until the person's access needs surpassed the access options available.

Non–Speech-Generating Technology Communication Supports

For some people with ALS, an early problem is difficulty projecting one's voice due to low voice volume (i.e., hypophonia) exacerbated by stress, fatigue, or exertion. To address this, one option to consider is a voice amplifier. Even for someone with a mild dysarthria, voice amplification can be helpful as a tool for energy conservation. The amplification scaffolds the user to concentrate on communication rather than to expend additional effort on projecting their voice. However, as dysarthria becomes more severe, voice amplification is less helpful since it amplifies the dysarthric speech signal without disambiguation.

Subsequent to voice amplification, additional AAC options are likely to be needed. Further assessment is required to determine the most appropriate options. Both non–speech-generating and speech-generating technology options should be addressed and trialed during an assessment. It is also important to conduct an evaluation of access to determine whether alternate access is necessary. For any system chosen, **adaptability** is a must-have feature, that is, the system should support a range of access options (e.g., direct selection, eye gaze, scanning) so it remains useful even if access modes change. Adaptability is especially important for people with progressive diseases since being able to use the same system, only via a different means of access, can facilitate continuity of use and decrease the need for new learning.

The range of communication options should continue to include both non–speech-generating and speech-generating technology options. Among non–speech-generating options are items, such as alphabet displays, topic displays, and communication displays (some options may be prefabricated and commercially available). An alphabet display may be helpful as an aid for **speech supplementation**. Research indicates that speech supplementation is an effective technique to enhance intelligibility for dysarthric speakers (Hanson et al., 2013; Hanson et al., 2011; Hustad, 2001, 2005). By having the speaker point to the first letter of each word prior to saying it, the speaker's rate is effectively slowed, and the linguistic constraints introduced by a word's first letter narrow the range of potential lexical items from which the communication partner must choose when they hear what the speaker is saying. For instance, if the speaker wants to say, "It's pouring rain today," they would point first to the letter I, then say "it's," followed by

pointing to the letter P, then saying "pouring," then pointing to the letter R and saying "rain," and end by pointing to the letter T and saying "today." This method of speech supplementation supports the speaker's use of novel utterances while providing the communication partner an alphabetic avenue for clarification. If the speaker has difficulty pointing, an alphabet board may be accessed via partner-assisted scanning, a technique that must be taught to communication partners.

In conjunction with speech supplementation or separately, a topic board may be used for **topic supplementation**. Much like the principle of alphabet supplementation outlined earlier, a topic board consists of a list or lists of topics to which a speaker frequently refers (e.g., family, health, baseball, banking, friends, doctor's appointments, politics) and is used for the speaker to indicate the topic of conversation. In this way, a speaker can efficiently indicate a change of topic without having to use alphabet supplementation to spell out this shift in conversation. For instance, the speaker may be talking about baseball and then point to "banking" when wanting to shift topics and discuss finances. Within a given topic, alphabet supplementation may be useful to ask questions, specify comments, etc. When used together, alphabet and topic supplementation provide a powerful way to supplement natural speech in the face of intelligibility challenges.

Speech-Generating Technology Communication Supports

In terms of speech-generating AAC options, many people with ALS will look toward SGDs. When eye-tracking technology became available on communication devices, it provided a much-needed addition to the access options available to people with ALS (Ball et al., 2010; Beukelman et al., 2011). Since ocular muscle movements are typically preserved even in late-stage ALS, eye-tracking access supports use of AAC beyond the boundaries imposed by other access options. Currently, both dedicated SGDs and tablet-based options support eye-tracking access. People with ALS continue to leverage their literacy skills with AAC systems to engage in both spoken and written communication. In an increasingly information-based society, people need continued access to the internet and various modes of communication (e.g., email, text messaging, video chats) to establish and maintain social closeness and gainful employment.

Mobile tablets with AAC apps provide another speech-generating option. This type of system may be particularly useful to individuals with ALS who are still ambulatory and have use of their upper extremities. Thus, people with bulbar onset ALS may begin by using a tablet and an AAC app for communication because of its portability and commercial availability. Although physical access and mobility concerns may preclude continued use of a portable system, mobile tablets and AAC apps figure prominently in AAC intervention in ALS.

Important Technology Considerations in Amyotrophic Lateral Sclerosis

The Gleason Act

Steve Gleason, a former football player for the New Orleans Saints, was diagnosed with ALS in 2011. He soon recognized that access to AAC was critical for continued connection to the world and communication with friends, family, and medical personnel. The Gleason Act, enacted in 2015, applied only to Medicare-funded SGDs. Prior to this act, Medicare had implemented a **capped rental** system for SGDs. This capped rental system required that the beneficiary pay a rental fee for an SGD up to the point where full Medicare payment for the device occurred. At that point, the device would become the client's device to own. The Gleason Act changed the situation entirely; it eradicated the capped rental of Medicare-funded SGDs so they became the client's property upon delivery. This brought Medicare-funded SGDs in line with other durable medical equipment (DME).

Importantly, the Gleason Act allowed individuals with ALS to receive and *keep* a Medicare-funded SGD even if they moved to a nursing facility, entered hospice care, or began a long-term hospital stay within a year of acquiring the SGD. Under the previous capped rental system, the client was required to return the SGD even if their need for it had stayed the same or increased. Medicare would not continue to subsidize ongoing rental of any DME in the various care settings previously mentioned. This change supported continued access to SGDs across the settings in which a person with ALS might live.

The Steve Gleason Enduring Voice Act, enacted in 2018, replaced the Gleason Act that had been in place from 2015 and was set to expire in 2018. The Steve Gleason Enduring Voice Act permanently enshrines changes to Medicare funding of SGDs for people with neurodegenerative diseases. This provision means that Medicare will continue to fund SGDs for people with ALS (and other diseases) regardless of the care setting, even if the person has had the SGD for less than a year. Further, this act provides coverage for any accessories needed to allow SGDs to work most efficiently and to meet the user's needs.

Technology Recycling Programs/Loan Closets

A disease, such as ALS, in which needs change and a range of technological options is required across its duration, lends itself well to the concept of recycling. People with ALS can return to a predetermined person and place a prescribed piece of technology when it is no longer useful to them. They may then access other technology to meet their changing needs. To support such an endeavor, many local and regional ALS programs support a loan closet for DME, such as wheelchairs, automated recliners, Hoyer lifts, and shower chairs. AAC systems are often included in loan closets. In this way, some AAC technology can be recycled for use by people who

need it. As with all technology, it must be well-maintained, inventoried, and stored appropriately. Organizations, such as the Amyotrophic Lateral Sclerosis Association and Muscular Dystrophy Association, may maintain loan closets. To access an organization's loan closet, a person typically must register with that association. Loan programs may differ by city, state, and region. However, the principle of recycling usable assistive technology by way of a loan closet supports one sustainable way of meeting peoples' needs and is appropriate across neurodegenerative disorders. This principle also supports a counseling need, so that after a person with ALS dies, the family has a clear path for disposal of the assistive technology. Family members often welcome having a plan for equipment they no longer need and may not want in the home. Further, donating previously used equipment to a loan closet provides a way to "pay it forward" and help others with ALS.

Parkinson's Disease

PD is a chronic progressive movement disorder that is most closely associated with basal ganglia dysfunction. Approximately 1 million Americans live with PD and more than 10 million people live with the disease worldwide (American Parkinson Disease Association; https://www. apdaparkinson.org/). PD is characterized by resting tremor, rigidity of the muscles, bradykinesia, and postural instability, the latter having been added to the classic triad of symptoms in the early 2000s (Chaudhuri et al., 2006; Williams-Gray et al., 2007). A well-documented cognitive disorder often accompanies or may predate the diagnosis of PD (Dubois & Pillon, 1997; Owen, 2004; Zgaljardic et al., 2004). The cognitive disorder associated with PD is a **dysexecutive syndrome** affecting predominantly frontal lobe, executive-type cognitive skills, such as planning, initiation, set shifting, decision making, disinhibition, organization, and monitoring of goal-directed behavior, while memory remains intact (Zgaljardic et al., 2006). Later in the disease, this may develop into a full-blown dementia known as Parkinson's disease dementia. Parkinson's disease dementia subsumes the dysexecutive syndrome and includes problems with memory and depression.

Research indicates people with PD also have difficulty with processing of prosody (Dara et al., 2008; Pell et al., 2006; Stirnimann et al., 2018), comprehension of facial expression (Gray & Tickle-Degnen, 2010; Pell & Leonard, 2005), and high-level language functions. These high-level language functions include discourse comprehension, processing of syntactically complex sentences (Altmann & Troche, 2011; Murray, 2000; Pell & Monetta, 2008), and pragmatic language deficits that include processing of metaphors (Monetta & Pell, 2007) and drawing inferences (Murray & Stout, 1999).

Although hypokinetic dysarthria is the most closely associated motor speech problem in PD, it is not the only communication problem associated with the disease. Early in the disease, hypophonia may be a problem, as well as **masked facies** that often accompany PD.

An evidence-based speech therapy program, such as Lee Silverman Voice Therapy (LSVT LOUD; Fox et al., 2006) can address this issue using principles of motor learning and neuroplasticity. To derive benefit from this program, patients must be invested in the process. LSVT LOUD is a time-intensive therapy regimen that requires commitments for attendance and practice for the duration of the program, followed by continued practice once therapy is completed. LSVT LOUD can be administered in the clinic or via telepractice (Constantinescu et al., 2010; Theodoros et al., 2016; Theodoros & Ramig, 2011). Gains made can be maintained with continued practice; however, research indicates that many people are unable to sustain the gains made in therapy in the long run (Edwards et al., 2018).

Non–Speech-Generating Communication Supports in Parkinson's Disease

Once dysarthria worsens, AAC supports may be necessary to scaffold communication. Relatively new on the horizon is the **SpeechVive**, which looks somewhat like a hearing aid and presents white noise in the form of multitalker babble to the user's ear when it senses speech-related jaw movements. The SpeechVive exploits the **Lombard effect**, which is the natural propensity of speakers to increase vocal volume when speaking in a noisy environment. Development of the SpeechVive for use by people with PD included careful attention to the motor and cognitive impairments associated with the disease. As such, the SpeechVive is designed to be easy to wear and use. Since the device is based on the Lombard effect (a reflexive action), there is no cognitive load associated with its use. This is critically important since cognitive impairment in PD typically worsens over the course of the disease. Research indicates most speakers with PD experience significant gains in vocal volume, more natural-sounding speech patterns, increased utterance length, and better intonation contrasts when using the SpeechVive (Richardson et al., 2014). The device is U.S. Food and Drug Administration–registered (SpeechVive website: http://www.speechvive.com/) and is currently undergoing further testing with a view to seeking insurance coverage in the future.

The progressive nature of the movement disorder, coupled with PD-associated cognitive and language impairments, presents a challenge for AAC intervention. As with MS and HD, intervention is staged with respect to the early, middle, and late stages of the disease.

People with PD may also need assistance with computer access early on to support written communication. This can take the form of various keyguards or activation of the accessibility features available on personal computers or mobile tablets to alter input rates and/or sensitivity of key selection. These assistive technology supports are widely available, and a knowledgeable clinician should be able to implement them easily. An occupational therapist should be consulted with respect to trials and acquisition of a keyguard.

AAC needs may increase as dysarthria and communication issues worsen. Methods, such as speech supplementation and topic supplementation, may be implemented to bolster intelligibility. Adjustments to the organization and layout of these traditionally non–speech-generating technology communication aids can mitigate issues related to tremor and physical access. AlphaTopics-AAC (https://tactustherapy.com/app/alphatopics-aac/), a customizable app, exists that supports both speech and topic supplementation. This technology also supports speech output, which provides additional communicative support to both the user and their conversation partner(s). Since both gait and balance are affected in PD, the issue of portability of any AAC options is a serious consideration. The SpeechVive is lightweight and worn on the ear, similarly to a hearing aid.

Paper versions of speech and/or topic supplementation displays are lightweight and may be carried in a pouch or pocket or attached to the person's clothing with a retractable badge holder. If the person with PD uses a walker, paper versions could be attached to the walker using basic non–speech-generating technology methods. If the person uses a mobile tablet or smartphone, they may be able to carry the phone in a pocket or a pouch hung on the walker or wheelchair. A mobile tablet may need to be mounted to a walker or wheelchair using a mount that pivots and can release the device, if desired. These issues would all be addressed during assessment and intervention.

Along with any AAC options supported by a mobile tablet or an SGD (see next section), communication partners should be trained in the use of partner-assisted scanning with non–speech-generating communication technology displays. The importance of having a well-learned non–speech-generating technology option, especially later in the course of the disease, cannot be overstated. Since there are few reports of AAC implementation for people with PD, Figure 21-6 provides an outline of steps to maximize communication in PD.

Speech-Generating AAC in Parkinson's Disease

Given the ongoing motor and cognitive decline in PD, assessment and prescription of speech-generating communication aids has not been that common. The proliferation of mobile tablets and the apps that run on them may open up new avenues for scaffolding both cognitive and communication problems for people with PD. For instance, an app that supports topic and speech supplementation and provides speech output may help if tremor can be addressed via accessibility settings. Similarly, robust speech-generating AAC apps may be applicable for people with PD if they support tremor mitigation via accessibility settings and if they include features, such as adjustable layouts, easy navigation, and operational aspects, that can be learned with relative ease. Although no published reports in the literature were found, use of VSDs may be a viable communication option for people with PD and awaits further research.

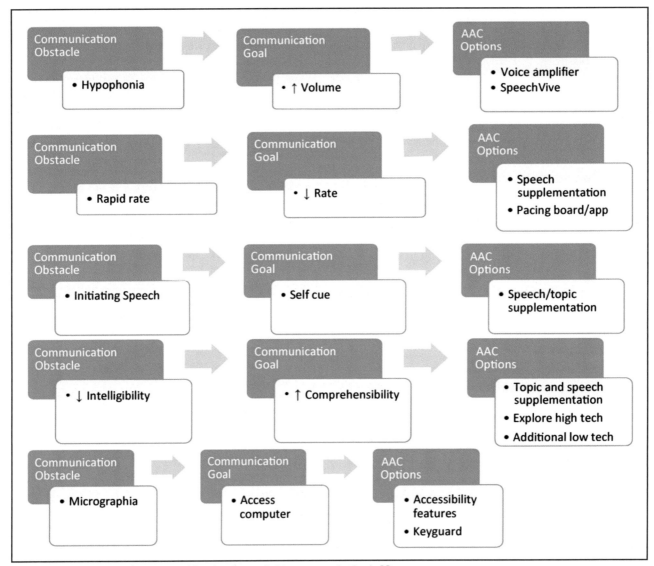

Figure 21-6. An overview of various considerations for maximizing communication in PD.

Huntington's Disease

HD is an inherited autosomal-dominant neurodegenerative disease. Originally referred to as **Huntington's chorea**, HD results from a cytosine-adenine-guanine triplet repeat expansion in the Huntington gene (Chao et al., 2017; Pringsheim et al., 2012). HD is characterized by chorea, cognitive decline, and behavioral changes that may vary in presentation depending on age of onset (Kirkwood et al., 2001). Average symptom onset occurs around 35 to 40 years of age with an average life expectancy of 10 to 20 years post-diagnosis (Klasner & Yorkston, 2000; Pringsheim et al., 2012). Juvenile onset (i.e., prior to age 20) of the disease may occur, as does late onset (after 50 years of age; Pringsheim et al., 2012). Since HD is inherited, each child of an affected parent has a 50% chance of inheriting the disease. In some cases, people may already have had children by the time they receive a diagnosis, setting the stage for potential continuation of the disease in the new generation. A parent may be symptomatic and experiencing the disease concurrently with a young adult offspring who begins to experience symptoms.

The speech, language, cognitive, and communication issues associated with HD have been delineated by many authors (e.g., Hartelius et al., 2003; Hartelius et al., 2010; Murray, 2000). Speech impairment is characterized most typically by hyperkinetic dysarthria and reflects the degeneration of the basal ganglia and its attendant circuitry. Language impairments in HD include word retrieval issues, long latency of response, difficulty with topic maintenance, perseveration, decreasing length of utterances and use of syntactic complexity, and difficulty with discourse comprehension and drawing inferences (Hamilton et al., 2012; Klasner & Yorkston, 2000). Cognitive impairments include executive dysfunction, impulsivity, difficulty with new learning, perceptual problems, apathy (Zakzanis, 1998), and difficulty with social cognition, such as emotion recognition deficits, particularly for negative emotions (Bora et al., 2016).

Addressing the communication needs of the person with HD requires that the speech-language pathologist be aware of the breadth and depth of the person's motor, cognitive, language, and behavioral symptoms, as well as communication needs across home, residential, work (if appropriate), and community settings.

Non–Speech-Generating Technology Options in Huntington's Disease

Limited literature about AAC intervention in HD indicates that the arc of the disease complicates it. Klasner and Yorkston (2000) outlined the staging of speech, language, and AAC intervention in their chapter, emphasizing increasing reliance on **external memory aids** (e.g., calendars, memory binders, or personal digital assistants) or small, portable writing aids (e.g., notebooks, magic slates) in the early stages, along with the need to acknowledge triggers for communication breakdowns (e.g., stress and exertion). As the disease progresses, natural speech continues to decline and becomes increasingly less reliable as a primary means of communication, necessitating the introduction of additional AAC strategies and techniques, such as speech and/or topic supplementation (Klasner & Yorkston, 2001), designating a specific time and place for a given conversation and reducing ambient noise. When speech is no longer viable, AAC strategies and techniques begin to take center stage. Non–speech-generating technology options continue to play a central role in intervention. Partner-assisted scanning may become necessary as involuntary movements may preclude direct selection for non–speech-generating technology boards or displays. Speech-generating options may be appropriate, but it is inappropriate to wait until late in the disease to assess for and prescribe these options, as the cognitive, behavioral, and motor aspects of the disease eclipse any residual ability to learn to use a speech-generating technology system.

Klasner and Yorkston (2001) outlined the use of linguistic and **cognitive supplementation strategies** in a case report about a person with HD. Linguistic strategies involved use of non–speech-generating technology aids, such as index cards and a binder, as well as scripts for common interactions and key words to trigger use of a specific script. Cognitive strategies included compensation for executive function and memory deficits using non–speech-generating technology aids. Strategies included itemizing each step within a given task, posting a list of to-be-completed tasks in a central location, and deciding on a method for indicating task completion.

Additional evidence for the use of non–speech-generating technology options for people with HD can be found in the work of Hamilton and colleagues (2012) who reported that AAC can compensate for some of the communication problems associated with HD and may increase the individual's ability to participate in daily life. These authors caution that strategies need to be implemented while motivation and learning capacity are still present and that communication partners must be invested and involved in the process. Use of **Talking Mats** to support the communication of people with HD (Ferm et al., 2010) and in group discussions for people with HD (Hallberg et al., 2013) showed that individuals with HD were more successful communicating using the Talking Mats framework than when communication was unaided. Extension of this work showed that people with HD and their care providers used a Talking Mats framework with moderate success during an interaction with a dental hygienist (Ferm et al., 2012).

Speech-Generating Technology Options in Huntington's Disease

The implementation of speech-generating AAC options with people with HD has met with limited success, as reported by Diehl and de Riesthal (2019). Factors beyond the clinician's control, such as variable levels of caregiver and family support and a paucity of funding for AAC devices in long-term care facilities where individuals with HD may reside, constrained the success of planned interventions. Likewise, the variability in age-related symptom presentation of people with HD and the often-limited access to high-quality AAC services in their local communities presented challenges to the full implementation and integration of speech-generating AAC devices into their communication repertoires.

Late in the disease, individuals with HD often become mostly nonvocal. They still need access to communication strategies to indicate "yes," "no," and "maybe" and may depend on non–speech-generating technology options, such as a two-step switch device or a communication display with bold, large font for text and different colored backgrounds for each word to make them more readily distinguishable. Some people may retain the ability to spell and/or use pre-spelled words and phrases, so these should continue to be available to the person with HD. Care provider training is crucial at all stages of intervention but particularly for this late phase of the disease since the care provider may be the one who has to initiate communication and support all communicative attempts.

Multiple Sclerosis

MS is a chronic progressive inflammatory disease of the central nervous system (CNS) that typically presents in young and middle-aged adults (i.e., ages 20 to 50 years). MS is universally more prevalent in women than in men (Harbo et al., 2013), in a ratio of approximately three-to-four to one (National Multiple Sclerosis Society, http://www.nationalmssociety.org). MS is globally the most prevalent chronic autoimmune inflammatory disease of the CNS (Kawachi, 2019). Historically, there was limited consensus regarding geographic latitudinal variation in MS frequency, such that higher latitudes were correlated with increased prevalence, incidence, and mortality (Simpson et al., 2011). However, exceptions to this geographic gradient exist (e.g., in Italy and northern Scandinavia) rendering the debate unresolved.

In terms of presentation, MS may present as a **clinically isolated syndrome** (CIS) which is a first episode of neurologic symptoms caused by inflammation and **demyelination** in the CNS. A person who presents with CIS whose magnetic resonance imaging shows lesions similar to those seen in MS is likely to experience a second episode of neurologic symptoms and may then be diagnosed with relapsing-remitting MS. If MS-like lesions do not accompany CIS on magnetic resonance imaging, the person is less likely to develop MS (National Multiple Sclerosis Society, http://www.nationalmssociety.org).

Most often, MS causes relapsing-remitting attacks of inflammation, demyelination, and axonal damage resulting in various neurological symptoms and levels of disability. The relapsing-remitting variant of the disease is the most frequently observed at onset and is the most common course of the disease. This form of the disease may remain dominant for the initial decades and then the disease course may change to secondary progressive MS. In secondary progressive MS, there is progressive worsening of neurologic function and level of disability. For some people, MS may not present as relapsing-remitting; rather, it presents in the primary progressive format in which both neurologic function and level of disability worsen from the onset.

Symptoms of MS vary depending on the locations of lesions and amount of demyelination. Common symptoms include gait difficulties; optic disturbances; bowel and bladder problems; numbness or tingling in the face, body, or extremities; spasticity; fatigue; cognitive changes; depression; sexual dysfunction; and emotional lability. Less common symptoms, according to the National Multiple Sclerosis Society, include speech and swallowing issues, seizures, hearing loss, and respiratory compromise. Given the pervasiveness of symptoms of MS across motor and cognitive domains, it is easy to appreciate how MS can interfere with many activities of daily living and compromise quality of life.

Since not all people with MS experience dysarthria severe enough to totally disrupt communication, the role of AAC in MS is more variable than it is in other neurodegenerative diseases. The mixed spastic-ataxic dysarthria associated with MS may or may not be a significant symptom of the disease. However, research indicates that fatigue is one of the primary symptoms of the disease (Yorkston et al., 2001) that exerts significant impact on a patient's quality of life (e.g., Garg et al., 2016; Manjaly et al., 2019; Moghaddam Tabrizi & Radfar, 2015). The concept of fatigue as it relates to MS is heterogeneous and its definition remains elusive. Induruwa and colleagues (2012) describe fatigue as "… a subjective feeling of tiredness that is disproportionate to the performed activity" (p. 9). Others describe MS-related fatigue as "… difficulty with initiation and sustaining voluntary effort" (Chaudhuri & Behan, 2004, p. 978).

Kluger and colleagues (2013) outline two dimensions of fatigue: the perception of fatigue, which is subjective and difficult to quantify, and performance fatigue, which is objective and can be measured by a decrement in performance during a cognitive or motor task. Other researchers continue to investigate the pathophysiological and cognitive underpinnings of fatigue in MS (e.g., Manjaly et al., 2019). These dimensions of fatigue are important considerations with respect to AAC intervention since they may govern or influence to some degree a patient's willingness and ability to engage in learning and using AAC options.

As with ALS, adults with MS who are literate when diagnosed with the disease tend to maintain their literacy skills throughout the course of the disease. Vision problems may compromise reading ability, but reading skill is typically maintained throughout the course of the disease. However, language skills are more variable in MS. A systematic review of language disorders in MS (Renaud et al., 2016) indicated that the language impairment profiles associated with MS are highly variable and may involve anomia, difficulty with higher level language tasks, such as discourse cohesion and comprehension, and pragmatic functions. Anomia is composed of both word retrieval deficits and overall slowed cognitive processing (Svindt et al., 2019).

Although debate about the nature and extent of language impairment in MS continues, there is consensus about cognitive impairment associated with MS. Cognitive impairments are detected in 40% to 70% of persons with MS (Chiaravalloti & DeLuca, 2008; Di Filippo et al., 2018; Kawachi, 2019; Rocca et al., 2015; Saji et al., 2013). Cognitive dysfunction has been reported at all stages and in all presentations of the disease (Langdon, 2011; Prakash et al., 2008; Ruet et al., 2013). Identified cognitive impairments include decrements in sustained attention, information processing speed, episodic memory, visuospatial learning, executive function, verbal learning, and verbal fluency (e.g., Chiaravalloti & DeLuca, 2008; Feinstein et al., 2015). Recently, deficits in **social cognition**, or the cognitive operations and underpinnings of social interactions, have been identified in people with MS (Cotter et al., 2016; Pottgen et al., 2013). Thus, cognitive impairment in MS is far-reaching and has implications for AAC intervention. Specifically, diminished capacity in both visuospatial learning and executive function could negatively affect learning to navigate an AAC system. Similarly, diminished information processing speed and sustained attention could affect participation in AAC assessment and intervention, the type of intervention prescribed, and the schedule for implementation.

Although cognitive impairment in MS is pervasive, research indicates that **cognitive reserve** may mitigate some of the effects of cognitive impairment. Cognitive reserve refers to the active compensation mechanisms by which brain damage may be offset across individuals. Proxies, such as educational level, occupational attainment, leisure activities, and vocabulary knowledge (Stern, 2012), index cognitive reserve. Data about the mitigation of cognitive impairment by cognitive reserve in MS is variable. A recent meta-analysis indicated that cognitive reserve was protective against decline in cognitive flexibility, but this limited protective effect is subject to decay with disease progression (Santangelo et al., 2019).

The motor and nonmotor symptoms (e.g., ataxia, cognition, depression, emotional lability, fatigue, spasticity) that characterize MS contribute to an overall decrement in quality of life (Lobentanz et al., 2004; Mitchell et al., 2005) and influence both the amount and type of AAC intervention patients with MS may accept.

As with other neurodegenerative diseases, energy conservation is important. Fatigue is a hallmark of MS and dictates each patient's daily schedule. Thus fatigue, cognitive impairment, motor concerns, and language issues must be considered when designing intervention for the patient with MS. To optimize any AAC intervention, it has to work within the constraints imposed by these concomitant impairments (Yorkston et al., 2005; Yorkston et al., 2001).

Ideally, baseline levels of speech, language, and cognitive function will be obtained via formal and informal assessment, as outlined earlier in this chapter. In MS, a careful AAC needs assessment should be completed to facilitate identification of communication needs across relevant work, home, and community settings, as warranted.

The AAC literature does not contain many reports of intervention for people with MS. The few existing reports indicate the need for comprehensive evaluation and coordination with other disciplines (e.g., occupational therapy, physical therapy) and other medical specialties, such as neuro-ophthalmology. AAC intervention in MS typically follows three identified phases reflecting the early, middle, and late stages of the disease (Beukelman et al., 2007; Blake & Bodine, 2002; Honsinger, 1989; Porter, 1989). Intervention in the early stage may consist of AAC to support written communication (e.g., keyboard and software adaptations, armrests to counteract fatigue while using a computer, accommodations for visual disturbances). Both a speech-language pathologist and occupational therapist knowledgeable about assistive technology may address these needs. In terms of face-to-face communication, a mixed ataxic-spastic dysarthria typical of MS may present with symptoms, such as slowed rate of speech, slurred speech, **scanning speech**, hypernasality, and decreased vocal volume. To address decreased vocal volume, a voice amplifier may be helpful. Other compensatory strategies to address dysarthria include topic and alphabet supplementation.

Cognitive issues may be present even in the early stages of the disease and may be addressed with software adjustments to smartphone calendars, use of technology to interface with a smartphone or mobile tablet, and introduction of audible books or magazines to accommodate both fatigue and visual disturbances that may interfere with reading.

In the middle stage of the disease, options that are more sophisticated may be needed. In addition to the AAC options outlined previously, people with mid-stage MS find that their

dysarthria has compromised speech such that it interferes with face-to-face communication, especially in adverse listening situations (e.g., ambient noise, conversation partners with hearing impairment) and when compounded by fatigue. To offset some of this difficulty, use of a voice amplifier may not be enough, and use of speech and topic supplementation may support participation in communication contexts. Visual constraints and cognitive impairment may interfere with implementation of speech and topic supplementation requiring adjustments, such as optimizing the size and layout of alphabet and topic displays, modifying font size and background colors, and using a technique, such as errorless learning, to facilitate correct acquisition of necessary skills.

In late-stage MS, the severity of the dysarthria may render natural speech ineffective for almost all communication purposes. At this point, non–speech-generating and possibly speech-generating AAC options may be necessary. Careful assessment is critical, as motor, visual, fatigue, and cognitive issues will all influence the person's ability to use AAC options. Physical access and cognitive burden will be central in decision making regarding which communication supports to use. Using what worked during mid-stage intervention, with appropriate modifications, may decrease the need for new learning. As suggested for use with people with aphasia, a multimodal communication program for adults (e.g., first attempt, use speech; second attempt, use gesture; next attempt, use an SGD; Wallace & Diehl, 2017) may be helpful in this regard. A multimodal approach would require instruction and practice, and written materials would need to be designed with visual accommodations to meet the user's needs.

Partner-assisted auditory scanning may be used with both non–speech-generating and speech-generating options. All communication partners must be trained in any system(s) implemented along with ways to troubleshoot when problems inevitably arise. Whereas eye-tracking systems predominate in AAC intervention in ALS, the visual disturbances common in MS may preclude their use with this population.

Alzheimer's Disease

AD is a degenerative brain disease characterized by a progressive decline across domains of cognitive function, including memory, attention, language, and problem solving that have a profound effect on the ability to carry out activities of daily living (Alzheimer's Association, https://www.alz.org). AD is the most common form of dementia.

Worldwide, approximately 50 million people are living with AD and other dementias (Alzheimer's Association, https://www.alz.org). According to estimates, approximately 6 million Americans are living with AD, and by 2050, 14 million Americans over the age of 65 will have AD (Alzheimer's Association, 2018). This increase in numbers foreshadows a clear threat to public health and untold costs in terms of the need for paid and unpaid caregivers.

Memory impairment in AD underlies some of the difficulties with language and communication. Difficulty with word-retrieval, sentence formulation, and language comprehension are pervasive and progressive in AD (e.g., Bayles et al., 2000; Bourgeois, 2014; Wilson et al., 2012). Toward the end stage of AD, many people are nonverbal and may not communicate at all. Reading skills remain intact until relatively late in the disease, although reading comprehension is affected by the deterioration of language skills. Writing ability may be preserved with respect to drafting one's signature, but writing of longer messages or as a mode of communication is not well-preserved later in the disease. Visuospatial skills also tend to be affected in people with AD. In sum, both written and face-to-face communication are negatively affected by AD.

As language and cognitive skills begin to disintegrate, people with AD need increasing levels of support to engage in communicative interactions. Different types of communication supports have been found to be helpful for people with AD, all of which are some form of AAC.

AAC Supports in Alzheimer's Disease

Bourgeois conducted seminal research and identified the utility of external memory aids for people with AD (1992, 1993, 1994; Bourgeois et al., 2001). An external memory aid can be anything from a calendar, an erasable white board, a **remnant book**, a small memory wallet, and an itemized shopping list with steps for meal preparation to a memory binder or life history book (Bourgeois, 1992, 1993; Ho et al., 2005; Hopper et al., 2015; Koul & Corwin, 2003). All these are easily customizable non–speech-generating communication supports. Use of a white board to list an upcoming appointment or visit by a friend can serve as a reminder that the person can read when shown to them, and then as a reminder and focus for conversation after the event.

A **remnant page**, often in a plastic page protector or in a binder, is a sheet of card stock or paper composed of remnants of events, places, or occasions. The purpose of a remnant is to evoke a memory and to serve as a focus for conversation. For instance, a ticket stub from a Broadway play, a cocktail napkin from a favorite restaurant, or the program from a relative's graduation ceremony could all serve as remnants. The communication partner can elicit conversation by helping the person with AD label the item(s) and scaffold reminiscence about the event.

An extension of remnant books is a non–speech-generating external memory aid called a **memory binder** or **life history book**. As the name suggests, a life history book is a collection of pages, each of which contains a picture (or pictures) and syntactically simple text that relates the picture to the person with AD. For instance, a page may be dedicated to the person's family and siblings. Additional pages may depict graduation from high school, military service, weddings, having children, family trips, family lore, favorite prayers, or anything of importance to the person with AD. Often created on card stock for endurance, each page is encased in a page protector and all pages are housed in a binder that may be tabbed into sections or labeled per the individual's preference. The purpose of a life history book is to provide a visual and textual compilation of a person's life events. The combination of text and graphics serves to scaffold reminiscence and conversation. Importantly, the aim of using a life history book or memory binder as a communication support is for it to serve as a bridge to communicating about a given event or person depicted in a picture and text. Its purpose is not to be as a quiz asking the person with AD to identify each picture from memory (Bourgeois, 2014).

To help people with AD communicate, researchers have implemented a Talking Mats framework. These are essentially non–speech-generating fabric-based mats with carefully selected commercially available communication symbols (e.g., Picture Communication Symbols) arranged purposefully to facilitate communication and attached with Velcro. Murphy and colleagues (2007) reported greater success on a communication task (e.g., "Tell me what you did today.") using Talking Mats than in two other conditions—unstructured and structured interviews. An extension of this research revealed that use of the Talking Mats framework was effective in helping people with dementia express their views on wellbeing (Murphy et al., 2010), and in a subsequent study, to participate in decision making about life and care transitions (Murphy & Oliver, 2013). This growing body of work indicates that use of non–speech-generating communication aids can facilitate communication and participation in the decision-making process by people with dementia.

Additional research supports the use of non–speech-generating AAC to support conversation in persons with moderate AD. Fried-Oken, Rowland, and colleagues (2012) reported that use of an AAC option that supported voice output did not facilitate conversations between the researchers and participants. However, when voice output was removed from the protocol and learning strategies included the use of both spaced-retrieval training in how to use the AAC aid and standardized prompts during conversations between the researcher and the person with AD, results indicated greater use of target words.

With the proliferation of mobile tablets, it is possible that additional avenues for use of AAC supports will emerge. For instance, use of apps that support storytelling with pictures from the person's life and digitized recordings of them telling the story by reading the text accompanying each picture may provide a way to use technology to facilitate conversation about a familiar story or event from the person's life. Other options include the adaptation of visual schedules for use with a mobile tablet depending on the user's visuospatial perception.

It is important to note that most of the research conducted to date has been with older adults (i.e., 65 years of age and older, with an average participant age in many studies of 75 years) who have AD. Going forward, people diagnosed with early-onset AD who are typically in the 40- to 60-year age range may more readily embrace the use of assistive technology as part of intervention given they are likely to have been technology users for a majority of their lives, if not digital natives outright. Further, people who may be part of the predicted increase in cases of AD by 2050 may be more familiar with technology, such as smartphones and tablets, and more willing to accept assistive technology interventions than many older adults today.

To address the anticipated AAC needs of people with AD, we will need to implement AAC for people with dementia in person-centered ways (Lanzi et al., 2017) that capitalize to the extent possible on preserved procedural memory and optimize training strategies for caregivers and facilitators (Hopper, 2001; Thiessen & Beukelman, 2019). Clinicians and individuals with mild dementia may also play a role in informing the evolution of technology with a view to simplification of both interfaces and navigational schema that could facilitate use of assistive technology by people with more advanced AD.

SUMMARY

Neurologic and neurodegenerative diseases in adults often adversely affect communication to the extent that AAC may become a primary mode of communication for them. To ensure patients receive AAC services to meet their communication needs, it is helpful for speech-language pathologists to consider a systems approach. This approach incorporates the known trajectory of disease progression, the variable rate of decline across domains of function, acknowledgement that all individuals will need access to vocabulary and scaffolding for end-of-life conversations, and the recognition that cognitive deficits and decline may accompany all diseases. Themes that apply across neurodegenerative disorders are to intervene early and often, to be familiar with the iterative nature of the AAC assessment and intervention processes, to recognize the need to educate all stakeholders about AAC and the specific options being implemented at each point, and to plan ahead for anticipated needs based on disease trajectory.

The five Cs—caregiver burden, cognitive decline, conservation of communicative competence, counseling, cultural considerations—are broadly applicable as a framework for both assessment and intervention across disorders. This framework is helpful in situating the individual and their changing needs, as well as those of their care providers, in the larger context of the World Health Organization model as it relates to activity and participation.

Advancements in the use of AAC and the role of assistive technology in the management of communication impairments are encouraging. For example, message banking, which is most frequently associated with ALS, can be applied more widely with patients with other neurodegenerative diseases, particularly with a view to creating a vocal legacy for family and friends. VSDs, researched most widely in the aphasia population, may prove to be useful as a communication strategy for people with neurodegenerative diseases. Perhaps a non–speech-generating technology adaptation of VSDs for use by people with dementia could be an adjunct to a life history book to facilitate communication and scaffold reminiscence. Use of VSDs instead of grid-based communication layouts could also serve as a rate enhancement strategy for people who use scanning as their mode of access regardless of disease. Simplification of navigational schemes and organizational layouts may increase the applicability of AAC options to people who need communication supports but whose cognitive deterioration has precluded their use until now. Establishment and maintenance of loan closets for AAC equipment and communication supports for a broad range of communication impairments would be helpful across neurodegenerative diseases.

Speech-language pathologists who can provide AAC options and communication supports for patients with neurologic or neurodegenerative diseases have the potential to contribute to the preservation of communicative function for these individuals.

STUDY QUESTIONS

1. Describe a communication system that may be appropriate for an individual with severe aphasia.

2. Discuss how a systems approach is helpful when considering AAC for people with progressive neurodegenerative disorders.

3. Discuss communication supports that can be used to facilitate communication in individuals with AD.

4. Discuss the differences in AAC strategies for individuals with dementia and individuals with acquired physical disabilities.

5. Describe the five Cs and how the framework could be applied to intervention with a person with ALS.

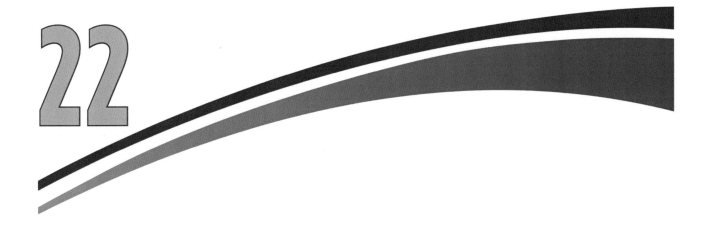

AAC in Acute Care Settings

Richard Hurtig, PhD
and Debora Downey, PhD

MYTH

1. Augmentative and alternative communication (AAC) is only for individuals with developmental or acquired communication disorders.

2. Hospitalized patients will overcome communication barriers and/or will likely be discharged before they can learn to use AAC strategies.

3. Intensive care patients are too sick to be able to learn and use AAC strategies.

4. Best practice dictates that AAC strategies are to be used only with communication-vulnerable patients who cannot speak.

REALITY

1. Many hospitalized patients face communication barriers that can be addressed by implementing AAC strategies.

2. AAC strategies can be quickly implemented and effectively used in intensive care settings.

3. Patients who are intubated and physically unable to move can use AAC strategies to effectively communicate with caregivers and participate in medical decision making.

4. AAC strategies can increase patient-provider communication for patients with limited English proficiency.

COMMUNICATION NEEDS OF HOSPITALIZED PATIENTS

Effective **patient-provider communication** is critical to the well-being of patients regardless of their medical condition and age. For patients to be able to fully participate in

their care, they must be able to summon help and effectively communicate about symptoms and treatment preferences. Likewise, it is critical that patients be able to understand what they are being told about their condition and the treatment plan. It has been estimated that 16 million Medicare beneficiaries report some level of communication disability (Hoffman et al., 2005). While there are no estimates of

Fuller, D. R., & Lloyd, L. L. *Principles and Practices in*
Augmentative and Alternative Communication (pp. 439-452).
© 2023 Taylor & Francis Group.

the number of persons with a disability who face barriers to communication, persons with a disability are over six times more likely to face barriers to effective patient-provider communication (Bauer et al., 2016). There are also 25 million people in the United States who face communication challenges due to their limited fluency in English (Betancourt et al., 2012). Meeting the needs of all these individuals presents a significant challenge to the United States health care system, its patients, and its providers.

Every year over 35 million individuals are hospitalized in the United States (American Hospital Association [AHA], 2017). Some of these individuals are admitted with pre-existing complex communication needs (CCN) that will impact their ability to communicate with their physicians, nurses, and other health care providers. Likewise, a large proportion of emergently hospitalized patients find themselves unable to communicate effectively because their admitting diagnosis or its treatment make their use of speech and writing a challenge (Zubow & Hurtig, 2013). Finally, approximately 8.6% of the U.S. population is at risk for experiencing an **adverse medical event** due to their limited English proficiency (Betancourt et al., 2012).

REGULATORY REQUIREMENTS AND ETHICAL CONSIDERATIONS

Patient's Bill of Rights

AHA developed a Patient's Bill of Rights that has since been replaced by a common language brochure (http://www.aha.org/advocacy-issues/communicatingpts/pt-care-partnership.shtml) that informs patients of their rights and responsibilities. The document lays out what patients can expect during their hospitalization and what their rights are with regard to their care and **medical decision making** and end-of-life decisions. While the document is available in several languages, it makes no specific reference to meeting the needs of patients with CCN or patients who have limited English proficiency.

Communication Bill of Rights

The National Joint Committee for the Communication Needs of People with Severe Disabilities (NJC) has developed a Communication Bill of Rights that specifically addresses the communication rights of individuals with disabilities but is equally applicable to all patients (Brady et al., 2016). The NJC has identified the fundamental rights necessary for communication across all environments and the "right to have access to functioning AAC and other assistive technology services and devices at all times" (Brady et al., 2016, item 11).

Americans with Disabilities Act

The **Americans with Disabilities Act, Title III** specifies that hospitals, along with other places of public accommodation, address the communication needs of individuals with disabilities. The Department of Justice Civil Rights Division's highlights for Title III emphasize the importance of addressing the needs of individuals with communication impairments (Table 22-1).

Joint Commission Hospital Accreditation Standards

In 2010, **The Joint Commission** (JC) recognized the criticality of effective patient-provider communication and the increased number of potentially communication-vulnerable patients and stipulated that health care organizations make effective communication a priority during all points of care (The JC, 2010). The JC accreditation standards require hospitals to assess the communication needs of every patient upon admission. The JC also require hospitals to address their patients' communication needs and monitor those needs throughout the patients' hospitalizations to ensure patients can effectively communicate with caregivers regardless of their medical status. The JC explicitly requires hospitals to address barriers due to medical conditions, as well as those due to linguistic and cultural barriers.

To a large extent, The JC's communication standards, as well as their other patient safety standards, reflect a recognition that to improve medical outcomes it is essential that hospitals establish a culture of communication that will endeavor to meet the communication needs of all their patients.

TYPES OF COMMUNICATION BARRIERS

The JC's standards have caused health care facilities to identify barriers that may adversely impact patient-provider communication. Communication barriers can result from:

- An inaccessible nurse call
- A permanent or temporary lack or limitation of oral speech production
- An inability to write
- Cognitive-linguistic issues relating to comprehension and expression
- Cultural-linguistic differences
- Literacy barriers due to poor proficiency in reading, vision impairment, or being a non-native speaker

TABLE 22-1
Highlights of the Americans with Disabilities Act, Title III

"The purpose of the effective communication rules is to ensure that the person with a vision, hearing, or speech disability can communicate with, receive information from, and convey information to, the covered entity." (p. 1)

"Covered entities must provide aids and services when needed to communicate effectively with people who have communication disabilities." (p. 4)

"The ADA uses the term 'auxiliary aids and services' ('aids and services') to refer to the ways to communicate with people who have communication disabilities." (p. 2)

(This includes such services or devices as qualified interpreters, assistive listening headsets, television captioning and decoders, telecommunications devices for deaf persons, videotext displays, readers, taped texts, brailled materials, large print materials, paper and pencil, and communication boards.)

"Entities are **encouraged** to consult with the person with a disability to discuss what aid or service is appropriate. The goal is to provide an aid or service that will be effective, given the nature of what is being communicated and the person's method of communicating." (p. 6)

"Covered entities should teach staff about the ADA's requirements for communicating effectively with people who have communication disabilities." (p. 7)

"Covered entities are required to provide aids and services unless doing so would result in an 'undue burden,' which is defined as significant difficulty or expense. If a particular aid or service would result in an undue burden, the entity must provide another effective aid or service, if possible, that would not result in an undue burden." (p. 6)

ADA = Americans with Disabilities Act.

Data Source: https://www.ada.gov/effective-comm.htm

Access—Being Able to Summon Help

Effective patient-provider communication cannot be accomplished if a patient is unable to summon help. To that end, every hospital bed must have a working call pendant. Similarly, patient bathrooms and examining rooms must also be outfitted with a switch or pull cord to enable patients to summon help. A key component of a hospital's patient safety protocol involves ensuring that each patient has access to the nurse call system. The traditional call pendants and pull cords require that the patient have the strength and dexterity necessary to use them. Most facilities will have a selection of alternative call switches that can be used by patients who cannot use the standard call pendant due to physical limitations.

Access—Being Able to Communicate Using Speech or Writing

Once a caregiver is at the bedside, it is equally important that patients are able to communicate with their caregivers and family members about how they feel and what they need. Being unable to speak or write severely limits the patients' ability to participate in their care. This barrier is encountered when the patient's attempts to speak or write result in incomprehensible spoken or written messages. The experience of an inability to communicate can cause great anxiety for the patient that may last well beyond the hospitalization.

Cognitive Linguistic Barrier

When a pre-existing condition or the admitting condition impacts the neural substrate of language, patients may be unable to comprehend what their caregivers are telling them, and they may likewise be unable to formulate utterances to communicate effectively.

Linguistic/Cultural Barrier

For a growing number of individuals admitted to U.S. hospitals and nursing homes, the inability to speak and understand their caregivers poses a significant barrier to effective care. While The JC's 2010 communication standards mandate hospitals address these barriers by making interpreters available, it remains a challenge to ensure that non–English-speaking patients can actively engage their caregivers at the bedside throughout their hospitalization. Even when linguistic barriers are addressed, cultural differences can also contribute to barriers to effective patient-provider communication. This latter barrier can lead to disastrous consequences (Fadiman, 1997).

Literacy Barrier

Much of the information provided to patients about their care is presented in written form. This includes consent documents, documentation of advanced directives, and discharge instructions. For some individuals, chronic or temporary sensory deficits make reading a challenge, while for others, premorbid illiteracy poses a significant challenge in dealing with medical and legal terminology. Finally, patients who have sustained damage to the neural circuits involved in being able to read also face a literacy barrier.

TYPES OF OPPORTUNITY BARRIERS

Opportunity barriers are more likely to be more pervasive in health care settings. Opportunity barriers reflect more top-down attitudes within the facility. They include:

- A lack of existing protocols for the identification and treatment of patients with impaired communication across the patient's care continuum
- The attitude and practice of perpetuating the existence of untrained medical professionals in the area of patient-provider communication and the deployment of the AAC strategies and solutions
- The failure to provide the patient with the necessary equipment or tools to improve communication (i.e., the full range of communication aids)

Facility Policy and Attitude Barriers

Often, opportunity barriers, such as staff training, are not appreciated by health care administrators, as they inaccurately believe such training, if necessary, would have occurred within the medical professional's pre-service training program. Unfortunately, this belief perpetuates this opportunity barrier.

Practice/Training Barriers

Nurses are the frontline staff who communicate vital information to their patients multiple times per day, yet they often find themselves unable to communicate effectively with their patients. However, a review of the literature suggests critical care nurses reported acquiring communication strategies with nonspeaking intensive care unit (ICU) patients by trial and error and reported being frustrated due to lack of their preparedness (Bergbom-Engberg & Haljamae, 1993; Leathart, 1994; Magnus & Turkington, 2006). These feelings of unpreparedness elicited avoidance behavior by nurses toward nonspeaking patients whose nonvocal messages were difficult to understand (Bergbom-Engberg & Haljamae, 1993; Hemsley et al., 2001; Leathart, 1994; Magnus & Turkington, 2006; Radtke et al., 2012). Nurses identified a lack of appropriate training, availability of communication materials, and access to communication experts (e.g., speech-language pathologists) as barriers to meeting patients' communication needs in the ICU (Leathart 1994; Hemsley et al., 2001). A 2017 survey of University of Iowa Hospitals and Clinics ICU nurses revealed that nurses identified more training on how to communicate with patients demonstrating communication vulnerability as one of their top three training needs. These findings are likely commonplace for other health care providers, too.

Equipment Barriers

The absence of a wide range of communication tools, proper mounting equipment, and staff training create an equipment barrier to effective patient-provider communication. While providing a nurse call pendant is considered a necessary standard of care, Zubow and Hurtig (2013) reported that many hospitalized patients are physically unable to use the nurse call pendant to summon help. Although alternative call switches are available, many nurses are unaware of their availability and may not have been sufficiently trained to use them. For patients with sensory deficits that require them to use glasses or hearing aids, having access to their aids is often a challenge. These sensory aids may have been put away for safe keeping and not all of the patient's caregivers may be aware of the sensory deficits or that the patient uses sensory aids. For patients who cannot speak, providing them with the means to express themselves using written communication is often considered. While providing paper and pens/markers or writing tablets can work well for literate patients with sufficient manual dexterity and the ability to sit up, it is a real challenge for patients who must remain supine or who may be restrained to prevent treatment interference (i.e., self-extubation or pulling out of intravenous [IV] lines). The use of communication boards with nonspeaking patients has also been implemented with moderate success. They work reasonably well for patients who can sit up, point, and directly select intended messages on the board. Again, for supine patients and patients who cannot point, accessing the boards can be a challenge. While speech-generating AAC solutions have been implemented at some facilities (Costello et al., 2015; Hurtig et al., 2015), most facilities have not yet implemented them with patients with communication vulnerability.

Populations Who Face Barriers and Are Candidates for AAC

The JC defines communication-vulnerable patients as presenting with:

- Poor vision, resulting in an inability to read hospital consent forms or patient-education materials despite the use of corrective lenses
- Poor hearing, resulting in an inability to understand loud speech despite the use of hearing aids
- Poor speech intelligibility, resulting in inability to be understood by the health care team
- Poor or altered mental status
- Poor literacy skills, resulting in an inability to comprehend patient instructions and consent forms
- Poor motor control due to disease that limits oral speech abilities
- Limited English proficiency and different cultural expectations about medical care

It is clear that The JC's definition of communication-vulnerable patients extends beyond individuals with chronic communication disorders secondary to neurological or linguistic compromise, which traditionally are thought of as individuals presenting with CCN and/or patients with linguistic compromise. The JC's definition is more expansive and encompasses patients with sequelae from newly acquired traumatic injuries that lead to a chronic inability to use normal modes of communication. Finally, it extends to individuals with sensory deficits, individuals for whom English may be a second language, and those with cultural beliefs that are less commonplace in Western medicine. Deaf individuals whose primary mode of communication involves the use of American Sign Language (ASL) or other sign systems clearly can experience communication barriers similar to those of non–English-speaking patients. The inclusion of such patients significantly increases the number of patients who may exhibit communication vulnerability during a hospital encounter. Arguably, this is not a population most health care professionals and agencies are equipped to support. What The JC wants hospitals to do is ensure that optimal patient-provider communication occurs across all points of the care continuum. Table 22-2 provides an overview of the medical conditions that can render patients communication-vulnerable.

Patients Who Suffered a Trauma Causing Communication Vulnerability

A range of traumatic injuries can impact an individual's ability to form utterances and express those utterances orally or in written form. Injuries to cortical structures involved in speech and language will severely restrict a patient's ability to

TABLE 22-2
Medical Conditions Associated With Communication Vulnerability

MEDICAL CONDITION AND/OR ETIOLOGY	TYPE OF COMMUNICATION COMPROMISE
ALS Cerebral palsy CVAs (chronic) Muscular dystrophy	Chronic neurogenic speech/language compromise
ASD CVAs (acute) Intellectual disabilities Other developmental disabilities TBI	Cognitive/language compromise
Sequela that lead to intubation • Brain injury • Guillain-Barré syndrome • Spinal cord injuries	Acute speech/language compromise

ALS = amyotrophic lateral sclerosis; ASD = autism spectrum disorder; CVA = cerebral vascular accident; TBI = traumatic brain injury.

describe their symptoms and to express their wishes. Injuries that impact the motor control circuits necessary for phonation and articulation will also limit the patient's ability to effectively communicate with caregivers. Patients who have experienced spinal cord trauma may also lose control of their upper limbs, rendering them unable to use written modes of communication.

Patients With Chronic Communication Issues Who Used AAC to Communicate Prior to Admission to Hospital

AAC strategies are often developed for individuals with developmental disorders or with acquired conditions that preclude normal use of speech and writing. Typically, the programming of content for their communication boards or speech-generating devices (SGDs) does not include the vocabulary the AAC user may need during an acute care stay. At best, content may have been programmed to support communication in outpatient medical contexts. For individuals to fully participate in their medical care and to exercise autonomy in medical decision making, they need to be able to characterize symptoms, ask questions about their condition and treatment, and express their wishes regarding their care. Another significant challenge AAC users face when they are hospitalized is that either their AAC system is not brought to the hospital or that it cannot be easily positioned so they can have access to the system when they are in a hospital bed. The range of medical conditions that lead to their hospitalization may also preclude their use of the system's access strategies they had been using prior to being hospitalized. Additionally, the health care team's lack of familiarity with patients' communication aids and/or the operational deployment of the AAC system/solution may impact the user's communication effectiveness negatively.

Patients Who Cannot Communicate Using Speech/Writing Because of a Temporary Medical Intervention

Critically ill patients may be intubated or trached and mechanically ventilated. The placement of the endotracheal tube or tracheostomy will render them unable to produce speech. The endotracheal tube and tracheostomy pass through the vocal folds and preclude phonation, and the former will make it physically impossible to move the oral structures appropriately for speech production purposes. Thus, for patients with an endotracheal tube, even mouthing words is a challenge. Producing intelligible speech is also a challenge for patients who are receiving ventilatory support with an oral or facial mask.

For head and neck cancer patients, the surgical procedures they have undergone may significantly impact both phonation and articulation. While laryngectomy patients may eventually be able to use voice prostheses, they will not be able to take advantage of them in their immediate post-surgical hospitalization. Speech articulation is impossible for patients who have glossectomies, radical excision of the mandible, or other oral-pharyngeal structures.

In addition to limitations on producing oral speech, many patients in acute care may have limited use of their hands, and as such, are unable to communicate with their caregivers using written modes of communication. Patients may be unable to write because they are unable to raise their arms and use a pen or pencil. This can be a consequence of:

- Their arms or hands are in a cast
- Their arms or hands are in traction
- Their arms or hands are in physical restraints to prevent treatment interference (i.e., self-extubating or pulling out IV lines or catheters)
- Placement of IV lines limits movement of arms and hands
- General weakness or paralysis

Patients Who Do Not Speak the Language of the Caregivers

Twenty percent of people living in the United States speak a language other than English in the home. Among these, it has been estimated that 25 million individuals or 8.6% of the U.S. population have **limited English proficiency** (LEP) and are, as a consequence, at risk of experiencing adverse medical outcomes (Betancourt et al., 2012; Ryan, 2013). While over 50% of the population who has LEP are speakers of Spanish, the remainder are speakers of over 40 different languages (Ryan, 2013). The JC has recognized the risk that non–English-speaking patients face and has included accommodating the patients' preferred languages in the patient-centered communication standards (The JC, 2010).

Deaf and Hard-of-Hearing Patients

Approximately 3.3% of the U.S. population is deaf or has significant problems hearing (Schoenborn & Heyman, 2008). For these individuals, communication with caregivers may be limited and may also put them at risk for experiencing adverse effects. For individuals who are deaf and whose primary mode of communication is ASL, communicating with medical care providers would require an interpreter. Since the use of ASL or other sign language is not recorded in census data, it is difficult to estimate the number of individuals in the United States for whom ASL is the primary language. However, an examination of the use of interpreters in hospital settings suggests there is a substantial number of requests for sign interpreters (Hurtig et al., 2015).

PROVIDING UNIVERSAL ACCESS TO THE NURSE CALL SYSTEM

Patients being able to summon their nurses is critical to patient safety and effective medical care. Each hospital in-patient room, patient bathroom, and outpatient treatment room is required to have a nurse call system in place. These include call pendants at each bed and call buttons or pull chains in the bathrooms and clinic rooms. Hospital patient safety protocols require that every patient have a working nurse call, that nurses make sure their patients can use them, and that they are appropriately positioned where patients can reach them. Unfortunately, many conscious patients cannot use the nurse call system as a function of either weakness, paralysis, or because they are in traction or on a restraint protocol (Zubow & Hurtig 2013).

Assistive Technology Options to Overcome Barriers

Most hospitals have an auxiliary jack on the headwall behind each bed. This allows patients who cannot use the standard call pendant to use alternatives, like the Curbell soft touch, pressure bulb, or breath call (Table 22-3). These alternatives can work for patients who have some use of their hands and are not intubated. At some institutions, specialized assistive technology switches (see Table 22-3 for links to sources) have also been deployed successfully to address the needs of patients for whom the Curbell alternatives will not work.

SIMPLE SOLUTIONS TO ENHANCE PATIENT-PROVIDER COMMUNICATION

Yes/No

At the very least, patients need to be able to indicate whether they understand what they are being told and to indicate their preferences when given choices. This typically may involve posing yes/no questions that the patient can respond to by producing a recognizable intentional gesture. To that end, it is essential that the clinician identify some intentional gesture that the patient may be able to produce on command. This could be a gaze shift, a wink, a tongue click, a thumbs up, a foot tap, or a hand squeeze. For example, one might instruct a patient to look up for "yes" and down for "no," or blink once for "yes" and twice for "no," or squeeze the caregivers hand once for "yes" and twice for "no." It is essential that in addition to the patient being able to produce the gestures reliably, all individuals working with the patient understand how to communicate with the patient and be able to recognize the gesture's meaning. Using yes/no questions works well in situations in which the patient is given a binary choice of confirming or rejecting, as when asking, "Are you in pain?" However, the situation is more complicated when the caregiver is trying to obtain more information as in, "Where is your pain?" To get an answer to that question, the caregiver must ask a series of yes/no questions, such as, "Is your pain in your head?" or "Is your pain in your leg?" Trying to determine what a patient wants to communicate by going through a "20 questions" routine can be stressful for both the patient and caregivers (Hurtig et al., 2015).

Yes/No Is Not Enough

Consider the situation of a patient who is receiving medications for pain and anxiety. One consequence of getting the medication may be that the patient would be sedated and unable to interact with family and visitors. So, if the

TABLE 22-3

Alternative Nurse Call and Assistive Technology Switch Sources

AbleNet Inc	https://www.ablenetinc.com/
Curbell Medical	http://www.curbellmedical.com/products/nurse-call
Voxello	www.voxello.com

nurse comes in and asks the patient if they want to get the medication and the patient only has the option of indicating yes or no, the patient may be placed in a bind. If the patient responds with a "no" gesture because they want to continue interacting with guests, they may worry that they will not be able to get a dose after the guests have left. Likewise, if the patient is tired and is asked, "Do you want us to get your family from the waiting room?," they may worry that if they respond "no," that might be interpreted as indicating they do not want to see their family. The better alternative is for the nurse to give the patient the added option(s) to indicate "maybe" and "later" in response to yes/no questions. The challenge is how to provide those options. If each response option has to be tied to a unique gesture, then the patient must be able to produce multiple gestures that communication partners can recognize. For example, a patient might use looking up for "yes," down for "no," and blink for "maybe". Alternatively, if a patient may only be able to produce a single gesture, one might pair a yes/no question with the set of response options deploying the technique of partner-assisted scanning (see Communication Boards section). Thus, the patient would gesture when the communication partner provides the option. For example, "Would you like something to drink, yes—no—maybe—later?"

Regardless of what options a patient is given for responding to questions from nurses and other health care providers, it is essential that health care providers make every effort to ensure patients understand what they are being asked and that the response is correctly understood. To that end, it is essential that everyone use the same response strategy with a patient.

Communication Boards

It is possible to address some of the communication needs of patients by implementing low-cost, non–speech-generating technology solutions. Relying on written communication strategies can work well for patients on ventilator support who are intact cognitively, linguistically, and have the motoric skills to use them. In place of paper and pencil, an inexpensive digital notepad (e.g., Boogie Board) can be used, which can eliminate the need for a supply of paper (Table 22-4).

TABLE 22-4
Free and Inexpensive Low-End Technology Communication Solutions for Acute Care Use

SOURCE	WEB LINK	COST (AS OF 2022)
Bedside communication board from Widgit, UK (28 languages)	http://widgit-health.com/downloads/bedside-messages.htm	Free
PatientProviderCommunication.org	http://www.patientprovidercommunication.org/	Free
SpeakBook	https://vimeo.com/25812980	Free
AliMed, Critical Communicator Board in 21 languages	http://www.alimed.com/the-critical-communicator.html	$41.50
Boogie Board	https://myboogieboard.com/	$20 to $45
Green House Publications: Pack of 50 health care communication boards	http://www.greenhousepub.com/hecacobo.html	$20

Preprinted communication boards can be used by patients to address their needs in a variety of medical settings. Such non–speech-generating technology solutions are readily available and are either free or available at minimal cost. Typically, such boards are two-sided. Commonly used statements and questions are on one side of the board while the other side of the board may contain letters of the alphabet to allow the patient to spell out novel words or sentences. These communication boards can be printed and stored in large quantities so they are on hand and can be deployed quickly to patients with communication needs. Customized communication boards can be created easily using software tools, such as BoardMaker or LessonPix, and then printed out and laminated for patient use. While generic boards may address basic common patient communication needs, tailored communication boards can be produced to address the communication needs of patients in a particular medical unit or to address patient-specific communication needs. It is recommended that all boards provide patients with the means to respond to questions and that the boards provide yes/no/maybe/later options.

The use of communication boards requires that patients have functional vision and sufficient motor skills to point to items on the board. For patients who cannot use their hands but have sufficient control of head movements, using a head-pointer or a light-pointer can enable them to use a communication board effectively with limited assistance. It is crucial caregivers be aware that the patient is using the boards to communicate, the boards are accessible, and the boards be placed so the patient can effectively make selections.

For patients who have limited motoric abilities, non–speech-generating communication boards can be implemented using a technique called partner-assisted scanning (PAS). To use the PAS technique, patients must be able to produce a recognizable gesture indicating they have made a choice. The communication partner directs the process by pointing to or verbalizing the items on the communication board. The patient uses the voluntary gesture to indicate that the communication partner has identified the intended target. The partner may present the options by pointing or by speaking. The message options can be presented either in a serial or row-column scanning sequence. The latter scan pattern can be used to move quickly to identify the intended message (Beukelman, Garrett, et al., 2007). Because messages can be presented either visually, by pointing, or by speaking, PAS is a technique appropriate for use with patients who have motoric problems, as well as with patients who are visually impaired. PAS requires that the patient have intact cognitive, linguistic, and attention skills, that communication partners are trained to use PAS, and that they can recognize the patient's selection gesture.

Another non–speech-generating solution for patients who have limited motoric abilities involves the use of an eye transfer (E-TRAN) or eye-gaze board. E-TRANs are typically constructed with a central opening with communication options displayed around that opening (Figure 22-1). Patients indicate their desired message by directing their gaze to the desired message. This technique also requires a trained communication partner who can track the patient's gaze shifts and provide verbal feedback. Communication options may include either words or whole phrases. There are a variety of E-TRAN boards that can be deployed with patients; some simple E-TRANs may have a single message at each location while more complex systems can be created to give the patient a greater number of options. With such boards, patients use encoding to indicate what they want to say. The first gaze identifies the set in which the intended word or message resides and the patient's gaze then shifts to identify which specific letter, word, or message of that set is the desired choice. An example of such an eye-gaze system is the Speakbook developed by Patrick Joyce (see Table 22-4). Essentially, it is a non–speech-generating eye gaze system that is available online as a free download.

The University of Iowa's Assistive Devices Laboratory, using feedback from hundreds of patients, their nurses, and family members, has created a set of communication boards for use with adults and children in acute care settings. They have also developed bilingual boards that can be used with LEP patients. Other communication boards, such as those from Widgit Health, are available in 28 languages and can also be downloaded for free. Most of these boards pair text with icons to address both linguistic/cultural differences and to make them useful with preliterate children and adults who may have difficulty reading. Table 22-4 provides names and links from which communication boards may be downloaded.

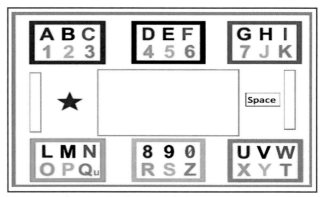

Figure 22-1. An example of a color-coded E-TRAN.

EXPRESSIVE AIDED SPEECH-GENERATING TECHNOLOGY SOLUTIONS

Some hospitals have implemented use of expressive aided speech-generating technology AAC systems with patients in acute care who are unable to speak or write (e.g., Boston Children's Hospital, Costello et al., 2015; University of Iowa Hospitals & Clinics, Hurtig & Downey 2009; Hurtig et al., 2015). These implementations have utilized a wide array of AAC systems ranging from proprietary SGDs to tablet-based AAC apps. The key to the successful use of AAC in the acute care setting is that whatever technology is used must be easy for the patient and caregivers to learn quickly. Unlike the use of AAC in the traditional outpatient setting, the evaluation of the patient's communication needs, the selection of the appropriate device, and the programming of the device must be accomplished very quickly. It is not as easy to conduct the individualized feature matching and device selection that is used in outpatient clinical settings for individuals with long-term AAC needs. The AAC devices belong to the hospital, and as such, will be less individualized systems and will need to be as *plug-and-play* as possible. In this setting, AAC systems are used to allow individuals who, in all likelihood, had fully functioning language prior to their hospitalization. Thus, the main challenge for the patient is learning how to use the AAC device to communicate rather than having to learn language. The challenge for nurses, physicians, and other health care professionals will be learning to deploy the AAC devices and support the patient's use of them.

Digitized Versus Synthesized Speech

Devices and apps currently on the market allow for the use of both digitized and synthesized speech. Devices that utilize digitized speech allow a patient's own voice to be used. This option should be considered when the patient can be seen prior to being hospitalized or being placed on mechanical ventilation. A key to this approach is being able to guide the patient in deciding what messages they may want to be able to produce once they are in the unit and unable to speak.

This approach has been very successfully implemented by John Costello's team at Boston Children's Hospital (Costello, 2000). A challenge of this approach is how to address the patient's need to communicate novel messages.

Devices that utilize a text-to-speech engine to produce synthesized speech allow patients to utilize a wide array of communication templates and provide the patient with an on-screen keyboard option(s) to be able to produce novel utterances as the need arises. The quality of the synthesized voices currently available has made for greater acceptability of the synthesized speech option. The key for patients is that their communication partners understand that it is the patient that is communicating. Thus, while a close match of the synthesized voice to the patient's voice is important, conveying the patient's personality is also a function of how the utterances are constructed. While in the past, one had to choose between devices that produced digitized and synthesized speech, there are many devices that allow the use of both.

Dedicated Speech-Generating Devices Versus iPad and Android Apps

The decision to select a dedicated device over an app that can run on an iPad (Apple) or Android (Google) tablet in the outpatient setting is in part constrained by the source of funding of the AAC system. Thus, to obtain Medicare/Medicaid funding for an AAC device, clinicians have to generate detailed evaluations that identify the most clinically appropriate SGD systems that are locked so they can only run the AAC application. In the hospital setting, the devices are purchased by the hospital as capital expense items, much like IV pumps, ventilators, and other medical equipment. Thus, a hospital's decision to purchase a particular type of device will more likely be influenced by a determination that the device can be used to meet the needs of a wide range of patients who will face communication barriers. Thus, ease of installation, necessary staff training, and compatibility with other technologies also play a significant role in purchasing decisions.

Eye-Gaze Systems

For patients who are *locked in*, eye gaze may be the only way they can respond to their caregivers. In addition to the non–speech-generating gaze options previously described, the MegaBee (http://www.megabee.net/) is an electronic version of an E-TRAN. It permits the patient to either select among phrases or construct a novel phrase. However, it still requires the communication partner to determine the patient's selections. The device's ability to visually display feedback and track the patient's choices reduces the memory burden on both the patient and communication partner. Given the need for all communication partners to be trained on how to use the MegaBee and the challenge of positioning it for some bedridden patients, it may not serve as a universal solution.

Early attempts to utilize SGDs with built-in eye trackers at the University of Iowa Hospitals and Clinics also presented challenges. First of all, positioning a fairly large device at bedside in the ICU was a challenge, particularly for patients who could not sit up. Secondly, because of changes in room lighting, as well as positioning issues, it was sometimes difficult to calibrate eye-tracking SGDs. With recent advances in eye-tracking technology, including a significant reduction in the size of the devices, some of the earlier challenges of positioning and calibration may be overcome. To date, there have been only a limited number of reports on the use of eye-gaze SGDs in acute care settings (Hurtig & Downey, 2009; Hurtig et al., 2015) and none using the latest eye-gaze systems.

Mounting and Access Issues

Regardless of how well any particular SGD can satisfy the communication needs of patients in acute care, access to the device will determine how successfully it can meet the patient's needs. Just as with the nurse call pendant, the SGD is useless if the patient cannot see or access it. To that end, it is essential that device mounting equipment that can work at the bedside be in place. It is likely that the selection of mounting equipment will in large part be a function of institutional preference. At the University of Iowa Hospitals and Clinics, devices have been mounted primarily on flexible arms attached to IV poles. By contrast, at Boston Children's Hospital, devices have been typically placed on bed trays that can be positioned over the bed.

For patients who have the ability to either point with their hands or with a head stick or use a mouse or trackball, direct selection access allows for the most rapid selection of communication messages and use of the on-screen keyboard. This will require that the devices accept either touchscreen input or a USB pointing device. For patients who have more limited motor skills, it will be necessary to select the specific switches that will allow them to utilize scanning selection modes on the devices. Some patients may be able to use two-switch scanning to take advantage of the faster row-column scanning method. Regardless of how many switches the patient uses, it will be essential to ensure that the switches be mounted so that patients will always have access to them.

Recently, Voxello, with support from the National Institute of Nursing Research of the National Institutes of Health, has developed an integrated system that provides hospitals with a tablet-based SGD that can be mounted to either an IV pole or bed tray and can be controlled by the noddle switch, which allows patients who can only produce a single gesture to nevertheless take advantage of row-column scanning (www.voxello.com[1]).

THE IMPACT OF COMMUNICATION BARRIERS IN HOSPITAL SETTINGS

Adverse Medical Outcomes

The publication of the Institute of Medicine's report (*To Err Is Human: Building a Safer Health System*; Kohn et al., 2000) directed our attention to the pervasive problem of adverse medical events in our health care system. Even with the heightened awareness concerning patient safety, a decade later 18% of admitted patients were harmed by a medical intervention (Landrigan et al., 2010) with 63% of those being judged to be preventable errors. A report from the Health and Human Services inspector general indicated that 13.5% of Medicare patients experienced an adverse medical event and 1.5% of those resulted in death (Levinson, 2010). Additional studies suggest that the rate of adverse medical events may have been underestimated by a factor of 10 (Classen et al., 2011). Preventable adverse medical events may contribute to over 100,000 deaths a year (James, 2013). The prevalence of preventable adverse medical events is unfortunately seen in other countries as well (Davis et al., 2002; de Vries et al., 2008; Neale et al., 2001; Wu et al., 2013). The additional costs associated with treating patients who have experienced an adverse medical event has been estimated to run into billions of dollars (Hurtig et al., 2018; Hurtig et al., 2020).

Patients who experience barriers to communication that impact their ability to communicate with health care providers are three times more likely to experience an adverse medical event (Bartlett et al., 2008). Communication barriers also impact health outcomes in the pediatric population (Cohen et al., 2005). Poor patient-provider communication has also been found to increase patient and provider stress and lead to poorer patient satisfaction with care (Balandin et al., 2007; Hemsley et al., 2007; Helmsley et al., 2011; Hoffman et al., 2005; Rodriquez et al., 2016).

---

[1] Full disclosure: The senior author of this chapter developed this system.

Meeting the Needs of Non–English–Speaking Patients

Given the changes in the demographics of the U.S. population, many hospitalized patients experience a communication barrier due to their limited proficiency in English. Hospitals are required to address the needs of LEP patients and provide interpreters and written materials in the patient's primary language. While that is fairly straightforward for the most commonly spoken languages, there are many languages for which an individual hospital may not have a certified medical interpreter. Currently, hospitals can access interpreter services remotely via phone or internet. While interpreter services for inpatients are used for admissions processing, consent processes, and discharge planning, it is a challenge even with the availability of online interpreting to provide interpreters for routine bedside care interactions.

Bilingual AAC Solutions

As mentioned previously in the section on non–speech-generating technology solutions, communication boards that address the needs of hospitalized patients are available for a whole host of languages (see Table 22-4). Hurtig and colleagues (2013) have developed bilingual communication templates and apps to support bedside communication between LEP patients and their nurses. These prototype apps provide a patient the ability to select items labeled in the patient's language that produce speech output in English and provide the nurse the ability to select items labeled in English that produce speech output in the patient's language. They also developed a prototype for use by deaf patients who use ASL to communicate that provide video clips of the signed messages. A commercial version was developed by Voxello with support from the National Institutes of Health.[2]

AAC Service Delivery Models for Acute Care Settings

Assistive Technology Team/ Interprofessional Practice Issues

Care of hospitalized patients has traditionally called for health care professionals to collaborate. Today, that collaboration is expanding to all points of care and structured to increase the involvement of patients in their care. The increased emphasis on health care outcomes has also prompted a paradigm shift from "sick care" to "health care promotion" (Pickering & Embry, 2013). With the growing realization of the connection between patient-provider communication and medical outcomes and patient satisfaction, everyone on a patient's health care team has a vested interest in helping patients overcome barriers to communication. Everyone must work to ensure patients can summon help and they can effectively communicate with care providers. Therefore, a patient's needs must be assessed dynamically, and the patient's medical record should reflect not only the patient's needs but also the accommodations made to overcome a specific barrier. This process begins with the patient's nurse but will require the involvement of the speech-language pathologist, occupational therapist, and other care providers as needed.

Nurse Call Decision Tree

Hurtig and colleagues (2015) identified a process for ensuring that patients be able to summon help. Figure 22-2 illustrates how the dynamic assessment of access to the nurse call would work.

While the responsibility for this lies with the patient's nurses, speech-language pathology and occupational therapy services may work collaboratively to design or adapt a nurse call system to ensure the patient can elicit help. The speech-language pathologist working alone may not have the necessary skill set to solve this access problem. Similarly, the occupational therapist working in isolation may not consider the patient's need to communicate with their nurses.

Communication Decision Tree

Hurtig and colleagues (2015) also identified a process for ensuring that patients be able to communicate with their caregivers. Figure 22-3 illustrates the dynamic assessment of the patient's ability to communicate. While the initial responsibility for this lies with the patient's nurses, it is essential that speech-language pathology services provide adequate training to ensure that the nursing staff understands the nature of the communication barrier and what tools are available to address the patient's needs. As with provision of AAC solutions in the schools and outpatient settings, an active collaboration of speech-language pathologists, occupational therapists, and assistive technology professionals will be necessary to implement a system that meets the patient's communication needs and addresses the key issues of overcoming physical barriers that may limit access.

Supporting Medical Decision Making and End-of-Life Conversations

While patients must be able to communicate they are in pain and experiencing other symptoms, they also have a right to be more actively engaged in their care. To that end, they must be provided with the means to participate actively

[2] Research was supported by the National Institute of Nursing Research of the National Institutes of Health under Award Numbers R43NR016406 & 2R44 NR016406 - 02. The content is solely the responsibility of the authors and does not necessarily represent the official views of the National Institutes of Health.

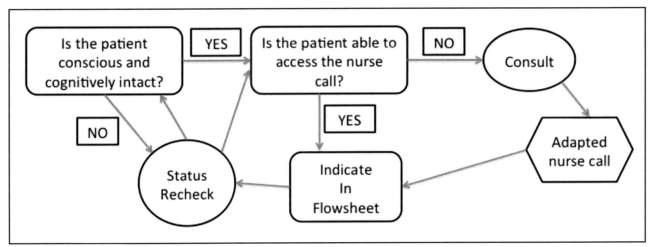

Figure 22-2. A nurse call decision tree.

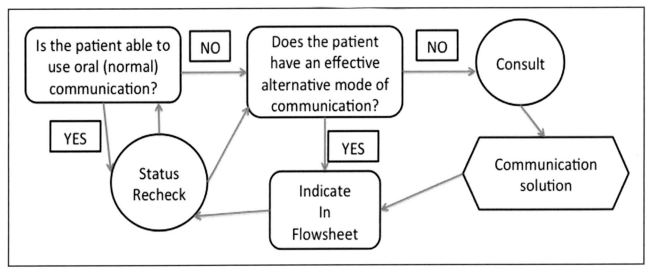

Figure 22-3. A communication decision tree.

in their care. This means that they must be able to ask questions about their condition and treatment options, as well as express their preferences. Without this ability, it is not clear what it would mean for a patient to give informed consent for a particular medical procedure. This is all the more crucial when decisions have to be made about maintaining or withdrawing life support. End-of-life conversations are difficult for everyone but even more of a challenge for the patient and family members facing communication barriers. Standard non–speech-generating communication boards and default user templates on speech-generating technology devices do not provide patients with the necessary content to engage in medical decision making and end-of-life communication. The University of Iowa's Assistive Devices Laboratory and Voxello (Hurtig & Slayman, 2016) have developed template page sets to provide patients with the means to be able to demonstrate they are competent and can have a degree of autonomy in the critical decisions about their care. There is no reason that patients who are cognitively intact but effectively locked-in should be left out of medical decision making (see

Dominique Bauby, *The Diving Bell and the Butterfly*, 1997). AAC tools and solutions enable patients autonomy in medical decision making, including the ability to more fully engage with family and friends at the end of life.

Staff Training

For institutions to meet The JC standards, they must develop interprofessional training materials so all members of the health care team participate in removing the barriers to effective patient-provider communication. Given the size of staff at most hospitals, the development and implementation of staff training can appear overwhelming. To achieve real change, an organization must pair staff training with continual modeling, testing, and reinforcement of the desired practice change. The NJC has also identified the need for interprofessional education and practice as essential to meeting the communication needs of individuals with disabilities (Brady et al., 2016). Health care staff must be trained and tested on new skill sets and be provided with the necessary tools to prepare for the implementation of AAC solutions across patients' hospital stays and to address the needs of patients who exhibit communication vulnerability. To that end, hospitals have to determine the balance between live training and e-learning. The benefit of online training is its enhanced economic and flexible features allowing managers the means to deal with time constraints for their employees. However, caution must be taken to allow for adequate time to engage in e-learning and to preclude the problems of online training fatigue. It is unreasonable to expect that e-learning will be effective if staff attempt to do it at the same time as caring for their patients. Regardless of the medium for training, the training should include elements of the following (Downey & Happ, 2013):

- Easy access (if online instruction is used, slide sets should be no more than 5 to 10 in length with a maximum time of 5 minutes to avoid online training fatigue; full training may be accomplished using several short module sets)

- Skill modeling for the development of a yes/no/maybe response

- Skill modeling for the use of the full continuum of AAC technology and strategies

- Introduction to available AAC tools or equipment to be used in the unit for use with patients with CCN

- Understanding that health care team members are always in a state of monitoring as an individual patient's needs vary as treatment protocols unfold and change to ensure that medical needs are met

- A unit champion to serve as the go-to person for assistance when the speech-language pathologist is not available to answer questions

- Standardized training appropriate for all health care providers

- Testing to measure established learning

It is essential training be incorporated into the hospital's ongoing training regime and nurse educators and unit champions be key players along with the content experts from speech-language pathology and occupational therapy. The end goal must be to empower patients to remain able to communicate with all their health care providers as they navigate medical encounters that may include a high amount of anxiety, near-death experiences, unexplained setbacks, and even end-of-life care. Enhanced patient-provider communication can be a reality if health care facilities and administrators embrace interprofessional care standards and ensure that all health care staff develop the knowledge and skills to implement the range of AAC solutions for patients who exhibit communication vulnerability.

How AAC Services for Inpatients Are Reimbursed

Speech-language pathologists are providing AAC services to inpatients in some hospitals and have been using the Current Procedural Terminology codes for AAC evaluations and therapeutic services (92607 and 92609). The reimbursement hospitals receive is based on the patient's diagnosis (diagnosis-related group), so it remains unclear how professional services provided by speech-language pathologists get factored into the per diem charge established by the Centers for Medicare and Medicaid Services prospective payment system. For patients who have exhausted their Medicare inpatient benefit, hospitals may be able to bill for professional speech-language pathology services (personal communication, Neela Swanson, Director, Health Care Coding Policy, American Speech-Language-Hearing Association).

The new **International Classification of Diseases, Tenth Revision Procedure Coding System** codes for inpatient billing also include "billable codes" for inpatient AAC services, but an informal survey of hospital speech-language pathologists who provide AAC services indicated they have not yet been used to code professional services provided to inpatients. The lack of consistency of how inpatient AAC services are documented and billed has contributed to an administrative barrier limiting speech-language pathologists' ability to address the communication barriers faced by hospitalized patients.

SUMMARY

A substantial percentage of the roughly 35 million patients who are hospitalized in the United States annually (AHA, 2017) face barriers that limit their ability to summon help and effectively communicate with their caregivers (Hurtig et al., 2018). These barriers expose these patients to an increased risk of experiencing a preventable adverse medical event (Bartlett et al., 2008) and increases health care costs by approximately $29 billion annually (Hurtig et al., 2018). The inability to communicate also increases patient and caregiver stress that contribute to both poorer outcomes and staff burnout. The speech-language pathologist has a crucial role to play in building a culture of communication that helps mitigate the adverse effects of communication barriers.

All patients should be able to express their needs and feelings, actively participate in their care, and if they are competent, to participate in medical decision making. The costs associated with meeting the assistive technology and AAC needs of patients are minimal by comparison to the costs associated with having to treat patients who experience adverse medical events (Hurtig et al., 2018).

It is the ethical responsibility of the speech-language pathologist to address the communication barriers faced by patients regardless of the cause of those barriers or whether the patient has a short- or long-term need. The needs of hospitalized patients must be addressed quickly. The speech-language pathologist must be able to rapidly assess the patient's needs and abilities to implement AAC strategies that both the patient and the health care team can effectively use. To ensure that good patient-provider communication can be achieved, the speech-language pathologist must engage the entire health care team and provide the necessary support and training for AAC strategies being implemented.

STUDY QUESTIONS

1. Characterize the barriers to communication encountered by hospitalized patients.

2. Identify the types of patients who face barriers to communication.

3. Describe non–speech-generating solutions that can be used at the bedside.

4. Describe speech-generating solutions that can be used at the bedside and how one would address mounting and access issues.

5. What is the relationship between communication barriers and adverse medical outcomes?

6. How can AAC tools be used to address the needs of non–English-speaking patients?

7. Provide a description of an AAC service delivery model for acute care settings.

23

AAC for Persons With Sensory Impairments

Vineetha S. Philip, PhD; Susan M. Bashinski, EdD;
Samuel N. Mathew, PhD; Donald R. Fuller, PhD; and Lyle L. Lloyd, PhD

MYTH

1. Individuals with little or no functional speech have hearing and visual impairments in about the same proportion as the general population.

2. Most individuals with multiple impairments will not benefit from amplification or corrective lenses.

3. When an individual is described as having dual sensory impairment (DSI), it typically conjures up the impression that the individual sees or hears absolutely nothing.

4. A lay person's initial response to hearing about dual sensory loss is to believe that individuals with this condition must also experience an intellectual disability.

5. An individual experiencing dual sensory loss is unable to speak or communicate effectively.

6. Many people automatically assume an individual who experiences dual sensory loss cannot live independently as an adult.

REALITY

1. Individuals with impairments, including those that contribute to severe speech impairment, are at increased risk for hearing and visual impairments.

2. All individuals with sensory impairments, including those individuals with multiple impairments, should have an opportunity to try hearing and vision assistive technologies. Many individuals with multiple impairments will experience considerable success in the use of sensory technology.

3. It is estimated that only approximately 5% of the population with DSI do, in fact, experience total vision and hearing loss. The vast majority of individuals who experience dual sensory loss do retain at least some degree of functional (i.e., residual) vision and hearing abilities. DSI simply means that an individual experiences both a vision and a hearing impairment of some type, to some degree.

(continued)

Fuller, D. R., & Lloyd, L. L. *Principles and Practices in Augmentative and Alternative Communication* (pp. 453-498).
© 2023 Taylor & Francis Group.

REALITY (CONTINUED)

4. Nothing could be further from the truth. Approximately 87% of children and youth identified as having DSI (birth to 21 years) do experience at least one other disability (National Center on Deaf-Blindness, 2020). In a 2012 investigation, Dammeyer found that language delay and/or intellectual disability occurred in 82% of children with CHARGE syndrome (*N* = 17) and among 42% of children with Usher syndrome (*N* = 26). Despite these statistics, a majority of individuals with this condition *across the lifespan* demonstrate average or above-average intelligence. Approximately 50% of individuals in the United States who experience DSI have Usher syndrome (American Association of the Deaf-Blind, 2009). The range of intellectual ability in individuals with Usher across the lifespan mirrors the distribution of intelligence of the entire U.S. population. Even in the case of individuals who experience most of the conditions commonly associated with DSI discussed later in this chapter, a percentage (albeit sometimes small) demonstrates average or above-average intelligence as well. The condition of DSI itself has no direct association with intellectual ability. More important to the determination of intellectual ability is the etiology or syndrome that resulted in the individual's impaired visual and auditory sensory systems.

5. Dual sensory loss unquestionably presents barriers to the accessibility of data from the external world because it affects two of the individual's three information-gathering senses (i.e., visual and auditory). Therefore, acquisition of communication and language skills is more challenging for such individuals and is typically delayed. However, through effective augmentative and alternative communication (AAC) programming implemented by interprofessional teams, individuals who experience sensory loss learn how to effectively utilize their residual vision and/or hearing skills in functional ways. Additionally, a majority of individuals learn to use various forms of AAC, which include tactile and technology-aided components, to attain fluent levels of various forms of both receptive and expressive communication, including speech.

6. As described immediately above, DSI unquestionably presents unique challenges for learning to work competitively and live independently. However, these challenges can be overcome with specialized training in orientation and mobility and application of 21st century technologies and hands-on learning. They can often travel independently and/or with support service providers. Many individuals use public transportation—buses or subways—if they live in an area where public transportation is available. Persons with DSI may receive specialized training at local and state rehabilitation agencies or through the Helen Keller National Center for Deaf-Blind Youths and Adults located in Sands Point, New York. This center provides rehabilitation services for youth and adults who experience DSI. For several examples of youth and adults who have successfully completed training at Helen Keller National Center for Deaf-Blind Youths and Adults and are using their skills to live/work independently, the reader is referred to https://www.helenkeller.org/hknc.

THE SENSE OF HEARING

Sound is a pressure wave characterized by frequency, amplitude, and phase parameters that, upon interaction with the human auditory system, results in its perception. This ability to perceive sound is known as "hearing." The sound is measured in terms of frequency in Hertz (Hz) and amplitude/intensity in **decibels** (dB). A typical human ear can perceive sounds in the frequency range of 20 to 20,000 Hz and within the intensity range of 0 to 120 dB.

Anatomy of the Ear

The human ear is divided structurally into three fundamental parts: outer ear, middle ear, and inner ear (Figure 23-1). The outer ear consists of the pinna (i.e., auricle) and the external auditory canal. The middle ear houses the tympanic membrane (i.e., eardrum) and an air-filled middle ear cavity that includes the ear ossicles and the eustachian tube. The ear ossicles are three tiny bones that bridge the outer and inner ear. The first bone, the malleus (i.e., the hammer), is attached to the tympanic membrane; the second bone, the incus (i.e., the anvil), is attached to the malleus on one end and to the third bone, the stapes (i.e., the stirrup), on the other end. The stapes at its distal end makes an attachment to the inner ear through a structure known as the oval window. The inner ear houses the **cochlea** (i.e., the organ of hearing) and the vestibular system (i.e., organ of balance). The cochlea consists of membranous ducts that have sensory hair cells immersed in a surrounding fluid medium. The base of the sensory hair cells is in contact with the terminal fibers of the cochlear nerve (cranial nerve VIII), which conveys auditory sensory information from the peripheral hearing organs to the central auditory pathway located from the level of the brainstem up to the auditory cortex in the brain.

The Hearing Mechanism

For a better understanding of the physiology of human hearing, the ear can be functionally divided into two parts: a part that conducts sound and a part that perceives sound. The pinna, the external auditory canal, and the middle ear structures serve to function as the conducting apparatus for sound. Specifically, the pinna collects sound waves that get delivered to the tympanic membrane through the external auditory canal. As these waves strike the tympanic membrane, it vibrates, which in turn causes the ear ossicles to vibrate as well. The movement of the stapes causes the oval window of the inner ear to move like a piston, which sets the fluid inside the cochlea into motion. This fluid motion causes energy from the sound waves to get transferred from the oval window to the sensory hair cells within the cochlea (a process known as transmission). The sensory hair cells then convert this hydraulic energy into chemoelectrical impulses (a process known as transduction), which gets conducted to higher auditory structures via the auditory nerve. The sound is then perceived and interpreted at different levels along the **central auditory nervous system**, which extends from the medulla to the auditory cortex situated in the temporal lobe of the brain.

HEARING IMPAIRMENT

Definition and Overview

Hearing is a primary involuntary sensory function that allows us to monitor our environment, provide a social connection, and facilitate the process of communication (Peterson & Bell, 2008). The primary function of communication gets significantly affected when hearing loss occurs. The most commonly used terms to describe hearing loss are "hearing impairment," "hard of hearing," and "**deafness**" (Cole & Flexer, 2016). According to the Individuals with Disabilities Education Act (2004), "[h]earing impairment means an impairment in hearing, whether permanent or fluctuating, that adversely affects a child's educational performance, but that is not included in the definition of deafness" (Section 300. 8[c][5]). Hearing impairment is also viewed as a generic term, and it implies that hearing is not within the normal range and involves a number of types and degree of hearing loss. The terms "deaf" and "hard of hearing" describe subcategories within the context of hearing impairment based on the use of residual hearing and the ability to hear and develop speech.

"Deafness means a hearing impairment which is so severe that the child is impaired in processing linguistic information through hearing, with or without amplification, which adversely affects educational performance" (Individuals with Disabilities Education Act, 2004, Section 300, 8[c][3]). Individuals with deafness have an extensive amount of hearing loss, and hence, tend to use the visual mode as their primary modality for language learning and receiving environmental information. The visual inputs used by them include speech reading, cued speech, manual communication, or sign language (Flexer, 1999). There is a difference in the usage of the word "deaf" in the latter part of the 20th century and in the first quarter of the 21st century, which is primarily due to the difference in the context of occurrence (Cole & Flexer, 2016). This is because a child who is deaf but who is given appropriate early intervention using hearing devices or implants today will be able to hear enough to perceive and understand spoken language and function using their oral language skills in mainstream society. This means that such a child does not function like a deaf child who did not have access to such technology and interventions in the 1970s.

At this point, it is essential to clarify the difference between the terms "deaf" and "Deaf." According to Tye-Murray (2015), "[p]eople who are born deaf or who grew up with

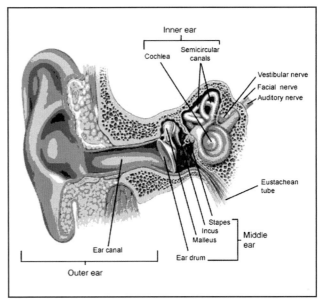

Figure 23-1. Parts of the auditory system. (Artwork by R. V. Shiju & P. S. Rakesh, National Institute of Speech and Hearing, India.)

deaf family members may refer to themselves as Deaf" (p. 14) and such individuals tend to belong to the Deaf community and identify themselves as part of a Deaf culture, which is denoted as "Deaf" with a capital D. On the other hand, the term "deaf" simply denotes the fact that the individual has a profound hearing loss.

Hard of hearing means an individual has a hearing impairment but even then has access to loud conversational speech without the use of amplification. Such individuals can use the auditory mode as their primary modality of language learning irrespective of the degree of hearing loss or its time of onset (Flexer, 1999). Each of these usages mentioned above has different physiological, psychological, and cultural implications. The meaning of these usages will be relevant in considering AAC strategies for the user.

CLASSIFICATIONS OF HEARING IMPAIRMENT

Hearing impairment can be classified in terms of degree of hearing loss, type of hearing loss, time of onset of hearing loss, whether one or both ears is affected, and with respect to the nature of its progression. Each of these are described below:

- Degree of hearing loss: Hearing impairment can be of a mild, moderate, moderately severe, severe, or profound degree depending on the amount of hearing loss as measured in dB (Table 23-1).
- Type of hearing loss: Depending on the location and structure(s) within the hearing mechanism affected, hearing impairment may be of conductive, sensorineural, or mixed type.

TABLE 23-1

Communication Difficulty and Handicapping Effects of Different Degrees of Hearing Loss as Measured in Decibels

HEARING AS MEASURED IN DB HL	DEGREE OF HEARING LOSS	ABILITY TO HEAR AND UNDERSTAND SPEECH WITHOUT AMPLIFICATION	HANDICAPPING EFFECTS (IF NOT TREATED EARLY)
0 to 25	Within normal limits	Able to hear even soft sounds	No handicapping effects for hearing range from 0 to 15 dB HL
25 to 40	Mild	Demonstrates difficulty in understanding soft-spoken speech	Auditory learning dysfunction, mild language delay, mild speech problems, inattention
41 to 55	Moderate	Demonstrates an understanding of speech at 3 to 5 feet	Speech problems, language delay, learning dysfunction, inattention
56 to 70	Moderately severe	Speech must be loud for auditory reception; difficulty in group settings	
71 to 90	Severe	Loud speech may not be understood at 1 foot from the ear; may distinguish vowels but not consonants	Severe speech problems, language delay, learning dysfunction, inattention
91 and above	Profound	Does not rely on audition as primary modality for communication; cannot hear any speech sounds	

db HL = decibels hearing level.

Adapted from Northern, J. L., & Downs, M. P. (2014). *Hearing in children* (6th ed.). Plural Publishing and Roeser, R. J., Valente, M., & Hosford-Dunn, H. (2007). *Audiology diagnosis* (2nd ed.). Thieme Medical Publishers Inc.

○ **Conductive hearing impairment** occurs when the outer and/or middle ear is affected, which results in reduced conduction of sound. The major causes of conductive hearing loss include accumulation of foreign bodies or wax in the outer ear, congenital deformities of the pinna and external auditory canal, collapsed ear canal, middle ear fluid (i.e., **otitis media**), or various ossicular disorders. Conductive hearing loss is reversible by addressing the underlying problem through medical management.

○ **Sensorineural hearing impairment** is caused by irreversible damage to the inner ear (cochlea and/or auditory nerve). Bacterial and viral infections, noise exposure, ototoxic medications, age-related changes (i.e., presbycusis), or a tumor of the auditory nerve or cerebellopontine angle can cause sensorineural hearing impairment. Abnormal functioning of inner hair cells of the cochlea and/or auditory nerve fibers can lead to the faulty conversion of acoustic impulses into neural discharges. This abnormal functioning is often termed as auditory neuropathy spectrum disorder, which can also show sensorineural impairment of any degree.

○ In some individuals, various factors may combine to produce both conductive and sensorineural components leading to a **mixed hearing impairment**. For example, the presence of noise-induced hearing loss and otitis media in the same ear can lead to mixed hearing impairment. If the underlying issue of the conductive component can be corrected, the conductive loss will be abated but the sensorineural loss will remain permanent and irreversible.

○ Apart from these three common types of hearing loss is another type known as central hearing loss. The most common causes of central hearing loss include infarction, hemorrhage, tumor, and infections affecting the auditory pathway and the auditory centers (Zahnert, 2011). "Central hearing loss" was more of a term used in the past to describe a condition now known as **central auditory processing disorder** (CAPD). In CAPD, **central auditory processing**, especially at the level of the brainstem or the brain, may be affected, which results in symptoms, such as difficulty in speech perception, localizing a sound source, poor understanding of language, and difficulty in perceiving speech in noise. Thus, CAPD makes interpreting or understanding of speech and language through the auditory modality virtually impossible despite individuals with CAPD having an otherwise normal peripheral hearing mechanism (Keith, 1999).

• Configuration of hearing loss: The amount of loss varies across the frequency range leading to different configurations or shapes of the frequency spectrum revealing the configuration of hearing impairment. Three common configurations are flat, sloping, and rising. A flat configuration is one in which **hearing thresholds** are at the same level for most test frequencies (250 Hz to 8,000 Hz). In a sloping configuration, hearing thresholds may be better at lower frequencies than higher, but the opposite condition may occur where the slope is reversed with a rising configuration that features poorer thresholds at lower frequencies than higher (Hall, 2014).

- Time of onset of hearing loss: Hearing impairment can be classified as pre-lingual or post-lingual and congenital or acquired based on the time of onset of hearing loss. Pre-lingual vs. post-lingual categorization is based on the onset of hearing impairment with respect to language acquisition in early childhood. Pre-lingual denotes a hearing impairment that occurred before the acquisition of language, and post-lingual implies an onset of hearing loss after the development of spoken language. The congenital vs. acquired categorization usually refers to hearing impairment that occurs at the time of birth in contrast to that which is acquired later in life. Congenital hearing impairment typically occurs before, at, or shortly after birth but before learning of speech and language, usually around 3 years of age (Northern & Downs, 2014). It is often due to hereditary/genetic factors, abnormality in the development of anatomic structures of the outer, middle, and/or inner ear, or due to maternal infections, such as **TORCH** (toxoplasmosis, other infections, rubella, cytomegalovirus [CMV], and herpes). TORCH complex is known to cause both hearing and vision impairments, as well as brain damage (Holvoet & Helmstetter, 1989). Some other risk factors for hearing impairment are listed in Table 23-2. Acquired hearing impairment usually occurs after speech and language development and may occur in isolation as a result of noise or drug exposure, accidents, diseases of the ear, or aging.

- Classification based on the ear(s) affected: Unilateral and bilateral hearing impairment are terms used to indicate if the hearing is impaired in one or both ears. Cole and Flexer (2016) state that "[a] person with normal hearing in one ear and at least a mild permanent hearing loss in the other has a unilateral hearing loss" (p. 43). Unilateral hearing impairment is mostly caused due to viral infections, trauma, or even as a result of surgery to remove tumors.

- Classification based on the progression of hearing loss: Progressive hearing impairment occurs when an individual's hearing ability worsens over time. On the contrary, nonprogressive losses do not progress over time (i.e., the loss plateaus and progresses no further). Vestibular aqueduct, perilymphatic fistula, CMV, meningitis, congenital syphilis, ototoxicity, endolymphatic hydrops, autoimmune disorders, and delayed hereditary hearing loss are some of the known causes for progressive hearing impairment (Cole & Flexer, 2016).

IMPACT OF HEARING IMPAIRMENT ON COMMUNICATION

The global prevalence of hearing impairment appears to be gradually increasing with an estimate of 0.9% (42 million) of the world's population in 1985, to 2.1% (120 million) in 1995 to 5.3% (360 million) in 2011. Of the 360 million people thought to have disabling hearing impairment in 2011, approximately 32 million (9%) were children younger than 15 years of age (7.5 million of these were younger than 5 years) and 328 million (91%) were adults. Improved technology for identification and diagnosis of hearing loss, widespread use of ototoxic medications, and common lack of regulations on environmental and occupational noise are some of the reasons for this upward trend in the estimates of hearing impairment (Olusanya et al., 2014). With an ascending pattern of hearing impairment prevalence, a much larger segment of the population will suffer its far-reaching negative consequences on opportunities for linguistic, social, educational, and vocational independence. However, the primary and most devastating effect of hearing loss is its impact on verbal (oral) communication (see Table 23-1). Moreover, the impact will vary considerably depending on some personal and environmental factors and also due to the presence of other serious disabilities, such as visual impairment, physical limitations, or intellectual disability (Schow & Nerbonne, 2013). The International Classification of Functioning, Disability and Health developed by the World Health Organization (2001) identifies communication difficulty as the primary consequence of hearing loss (i.e., activity limitation) along with social and vocational problems as secondary consequences (i.e., participation restriction).

Approximately 50% of persons in their seventh decade and 80% of those in their 8th decade of life are estimated to have hearing loss that is severe enough to affect daily communication (Cunningham & Tucci, 2017). The consequence of hearing loss in adults includes difficulty in interpreting speech, reduced ability to communicate, decreased participation in social activities leading to social isolation and stigmatization, and stress on intimate relationships (Kochkin & Rogin, 2002). This may be worsened by age-related changes in cognition and decline of other sensory systems (Thorslund, 2015).

The effect of hearing loss on children is quite different from that of adults due to its direct impact on speech and language development and, in turn, on their communicative competence. In a typically developing child with normal hearing, spoken language is learned rather effortlessly due to the presence of a language-rich environment along with an intact hearing mechanism. However, in the case of a child with hearing loss, accessing and utilizing this language-rich environment becomes a hurdle in the absence of an adequately functioning hearing system. The adverse effects of bilateral hearing impairment of different degrees on oral language development and overall communication are well documented (Arlinger, 2003; Tharpe, 2008).

TABLE 23-2
Risk Factors for Hearing Impairment

HIGH-RISK FACTORS (HIGH-RISK REGISTER) FOR NEONATES

- Birth weight less than 1,500 grams
- Craniofacial anomalies (including cleft palate)
- Family history of permanent childhood hearing loss
- *In utero* infection (e.g., CMV, herpes, toxoplasmosis, rubella, syphilis)
- Low **APGAR scores**
- Neonatal intensive care stay of more than 5 days or any of the following irrespective of the length of stay—hyperbilirubinemia (increased bilirubin concentration in blood; greater than 20 mg/100 mL serum) that requires a blood transfusion, exposure to ototoxic medications, assisted ventilation
- Prematurity

OTHER RISK FACTORS

- Caregiver concern regarding hearing, speech, and language or developmental delay
- Chemotherapy
- Head trauma
- Neurodegenerative conditions (e.g., Hunter syndrome, Friedreich ataxia, Charcot-Marie-Tooth syndrome)
- Physical findings associated with syndromes known to have hearing loss
- Postnatal infections associated with hearing loss (e.g., bacterial and viral meningitis, HIV)
- Recurrent and persistent **otitis media with effusion** for at least 3 months
- Syndromes involving chromosomal abnormalities (e.g., Down, Hurler, Treacher-Collins, Turner, Waardenburg, Usher, neurofibromatosis)

INDIVIDUALS WITH OTHER DISABILITIES WHO ARE AT RISK FOR HEARING IMPAIRMENT

- Attention deficit disorder/attention deficit hyperactivity disorder
- Autism
- Cerebral palsy
- Developmental delay
- Emotional disturbance
- Intellectual disability
- Learning disability/specific learning disability
- Visual impairment

APGAR = Appearance, Pulse, Grimace, Activity, Respiration; CMV = cytomegalovirus.

Adapted from Bess, F. H., & Humes, L. E. (2008). *Audiology: The fundamentals* (4th ed). Wolters Kluwer; Joint Committee on Infant Hearing. (2007). *Year 2007 position statement: Principles and guidelines for early hearing detection and intervention programs. American Academy of Pediatrics, 120*(4), 898-921; Katz, J. (2015). *Handbook of clinical audiology* (7th ed.). Wolters Kluwer; Northern, J. L., & Downs, M. P. (2014). *Hearing in children* (6th ed.). Plural Publishing; and Roush, J., & Wilson, K. (2013). Interdisciplinary assessment of children with hearing loss and multiple disabilities. *Perspectives on Hearing and Hearing Disorders in Childhood, 23*(1), 13.

Although hearing loss does not preclude speech, language, and communication development in children, it can seriously impact their overall language competence (Blaiser & Culbertson, 2013). All aspects of language development including phonology, morphology, semantics, syntax, and pragmatics seem to be significantly affected as a result of bilateral hearing loss, especially those of moderate, severe, and profound degrees (Stredler-Brown, 2014). These children tend to exhibit a delay in language acquisition and vocabulary development, limited receptive and expressive repertoire, use of simple sentences with shorter mean length of utterances, restricted use of communicative intents, limited knowledge, and use of conversational conventions and communication repair strategies and speech deficits in terms of suprasegmental and articulatory precision (Blaiser & Culbertson, 2013; Culbertson, 2007). Contradictory to the earlier belief that minimal and mild degrees of hearing loss, unilateral hearing loss, or single-sided deafness has little or no impact on speech, language, and communication aspects, evidence is mounting that states otherwise (Cho Lieu, 2004; Holstrum et al., & Ross, 2009; Kiese-Himmel, 2002; Kiese-Himmel & Ohlwein, 2003). The biggest issues posed by unilateral hearing loss are difficulty in localizing sound, poor understanding of speech in noise, and reduced ability to listen from a distance, which interferes with incidental learning and acquisition of information. Their impact on the academic, social, and behavioral domains are also documented (Alpiner & McCarthy, 2000; Traxler, 2000). Further, the earlier the onset of hearing impairment, the more it interferes with language, learning, and development of auditory brain function, unless the child receives effective auditory/linguistic intervention (Cole & Flexer, 2016).

Detection and Assessment of Hearing Impairment

The impact of hearing impairment may be devastating, and if left unidentified, magnifies the effect. Hence, detection of hearing impairment, even if the level of loss is only mild and/or unilateral, is required as early as possible to reduce its consequences on the individual's speech, language, cognitive, and social skills (Oyiborhoro, 2005). A hearing screening program can reveal the presence of hearing loss and is often a short process that distinguishes a person who requires further evaluation from those who do not. On the other hand, "[a] diagnostic evaluation involves a 'gold standard' test to confirm the nature, type, and degree of hearing loss" (Johnson, 2012, p. 9). As with any assessment, the initial step is gathering a case history, including personal and family history, and when appropriate, a description of the onset and symptoms surrounding the hearing loss. A comprehensive auditory assessment involves administering a series of tests in a sound-treated room to reduce the interference of any noise on the individual's ability to detect sounds.

Detection of Hearing Impairment

The gold standard test for evaluating an individual's hearing is pure tone audiometry. Pure tone testing includes **air conduction testing** and **bone conduction testing** to determine the hearing threshold across a range of test frequencies (typically 250 Hz to 8,000 Hz). The results of the testing are displayed in a graphic form known as an **audiogram** (Figure 23-2), which gives an estimate of the type and degree of hearing impairment. Hearing thresholds below 25 dB are considered **within normal limits** and any value above 25 dB is classified into various levels of severity of hearing impairment ranging from mild to profound (see Table 23-1). In the case of children, reliable test results using pure tone audiometry may not always be possible, and hence, test procedures may need to be modified to enable easy administration. Such tests are known as behavioral audiometric tests and include **behavioral observation audiometry**, **visual reinforcement audiometry**, **tangible reinforcement operant conditioning audiometry**, and conditioned **play audiometry**.

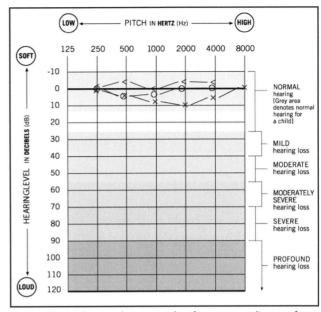

Figure 23-2. Audiogram showing results of pure tone audiometry from 250 Hz to 8,000 Hz.

Assessment of the impact of hearing loss on detection and understanding of speech in an individual is critical because the ability to perceive and interpret speech is essential to establish everyday communication. Test procedures that utilize speech as test stimuli to assess auditory abilities are known as speech audiometry and are often used in conjunction with other diagnostic tests. It has also found usefulness in the evaluation of difficult-to-test populations, such as children with multiple disabilities. This is because such individuals may not respond consistently to pure tones but may respond to speech as it is more meaningful. Speech audiometry testing usually involves obtaining three measures:

1. Speech awareness threshold: the minimum level at which an individual can detect speech stimuli as measured in dB. It is also known as **speech reception threshold** or speech detection threshold.

2. Speech recognition threshold: the minimum level at which an individual can recognize speech as measured in dB.

3. Word recognition score: an estimate of the number of correctly identified monosyllabic words, recorded as a percentage. It is also known as a speech discrimination score or speech identification score.

Other diagnostic tests can be used when an individual is unable to respond consistently to behavioral measures of hearing sensitivity and include impedance or immittance audiometry, **otoacoustic emissions** (OAE) testing, and **auditory brainstem response audiometry** (ABR). These tests provide information about physiological function and are not a direct test of hearing sensitivity. They are often administered along with behavioral tests to bring objectivity to the results. Impedance audiometry includes common procedures, such as tympanometry and **acoustic reflex testing**.

Tympanometry involves introducing air into the ear canal via an inserted probe to provide an indirect measure of the mobility of the eardrum and ossicles. Acoustic reflex testing measures the movement of the stapedius muscle, which contracts in response to loud sound. **Acoustic reflexes** should occur when tones are presented between 65 and 90 dB in individuals with normal hearing (Bess & Humes, 2008). Impedance audiometry thus provides information on the function of the middle ear and often helps in identifying various pathologies, such as otitis media, eustachian tube dysfunction, or ossicular chain discontinuity. OAE testing evaluates the integrity of sensory hair cells (i.e., **outer hair cells**) located in the cochlea and test results assist in differentiating sensory and neural components of a sensorineural hearing loss. ABR measures the electrical activity of the auditory nerve in response to sound stimuli. Auditory sensitivity of each ear can be inferred from the ABR tracing. For further reading on diagnostic audiological tests, the reader is referred to Bess and Humes (2008), Katz (2015) and Roesera and colleagues (2007).

Audiologic Assessment for AAC Users

The auditory status of all AAC users should be periodically monitored throughout their lifespans, even if a prior hearing loss has not been documented. However, identification of hearing loss in individuals with little or no functional speech may be difficult. Although pinpointing exact hearing abilities may not always be possible in some individuals, AAC teams should try to "… rule out moderate-profound, bilateral hearing impairments involving the speech frequencies (500 to 2,000 Hz inclusive)" (Gans & Gans, 1993, p. 128). Presence of additional disabilities might make audiological testing quite difficult. However, a test battery approach will help in establishing the individual's hearing thresholds. In situations where behavioral audiological test procedures cannot be used, physiological measures can be relied upon to give an estimate of hearing.

Specific Adaptations in Audiological Assessment

To complete a reliable audiological assessment, special adaptations to accommodate the communication, cognitive, physical, and behavioral needs of AAC users should be made by the AAC team. No person is too young or too impaired for such an assessment (Lloyd & Cox, 1972; Young, 1986). AAC users should prepare for and participate in the assessment process to the fullest extent possible. Preparation may involve creating and rehearsing vocabulary items for asking and answering questions, describing a problem, or responding to auditory stimuli. Contact should be made with the audiologist before the initial examination to prioritize tests among a battery of tests and to determine what will be required of the AAC user for the selected test procedures. This initial contact informs the audiologist of the unique communication needs and behaviors of the individual who will be assessed. It also allows the audiologist to collaborate with the AAC user, caregivers, and AAC service provider to determine the preferred response mode and select and prepare stimuli before the audiological assessment. Additional considerations are provided in Table 23-3.

Not all audiological test procedures require adaptations. Those tests, which are mostly objective and do not require an active subject response, such as OAE, ABR, and impedance audiometry, are examples of them. Adaptations are more often sought for tests where the individual is required to produce a behavioral response or those tests that use complex stimuli. Adaptations of a few test procedures are discussed briefly in sections below.

Pure Tone Audiometry

Pure tone audiometry involves measurement of hearing thresholds by presenting pure tone stimuli either through standard headphones (a procedure known as close field testing) or through standard loudspeakers (a procedure known as free field or sound field testing) in a sound-proof booth. In many cases, children are reluctant to wear headphones during the procedure or sometimes it is not possible to wear them due to reduced head circumference. In such cases, free field testing is a more appropriate solution. Once the mode of presentation of stimuli is decided, the response modality of the individual being tested should be determined. Production of a voluntary motor response (e.g., a hand raise) is the most common type of response to sound stimuli in pure tone testing. For AAC users with physical impairments, any consistent voluntary motor response that is observable, repeatable, and resistant to fatigue while not promoting abnormal posture or movements, may be used. Use of adapted switches that activate a light or buzzer may also be appropriate. The audiologist needs to determine an appropriate motor response and prepare adaptations (e.g., switches) as needed themselves or with the help of a physiotherapist or occupational therapist (depending on the availability of such service providers). The AAC user must be given adequate practice to produce the desired motor response before testing. For children with cerebral palsy, appropriate seating to maintain correct and comfortable posture is necessary to endure the slightly lengthy testing procedure. Even with comfortable seating arrangement and provision of adaptations to yield a motor response, if the individual's response to pure tone stimuli appears unreliable, the sound stimuli may be changed to pulsed tones, warbled tones, noise, or speech. This is done to determine if a change in stimulus might improve the consistency of responses. For young children who are unable to perform pure tone testing even with adaptations, behavioral testing mentioned earlier may be used to estimate hearing sensitivity.

TABLE 23-3
Adaptations for Audiologic Assessment

GENERAL CONSIDERATIONS

- Be aware of attention span and physical stamina. Frequent breaks may be necessary or the assessment may need to be conducted over several sessions.
- Remember to establish eye contact, use gestures, simplify speech, repeat, and rephrase as necessary. Allow adequate pause time for all responses.
- Communicate with the AAC user and not with an accompanying caregiver exclusively. Actively involve the AAC user in the evaluation and counseling process by explaining procedures.

PLAN AHEAD

- Prepare the AAC user and accompanying caregiver by explaining, demonstrating, and roleplaying what will happen during the audiologic assessment.
- Work with the AAC user and desensitize as needed to improve tolerance for otoscopic examination, insertion of probe tips, and headphone placement.
- Determine the AAC user's preferred mode of communicating for this situation. Preprogram and/or practice message items before the assessment session.
- Determine and practice an appropriate motor response and prepare adaptations (e.g., switches) as needed.
- Prepare materials, such as objects, pictures, or written words, for **speech reception** testing and speech identification testing. Practice the indicating response (e.g., eye gaze, pointing, switch).
- Ensure all assessment locations are physically accessible and safe.
- Ensure the AAC user can be positioned appropriately to maximize concentration and comfort and inhibit reflexive movement.
- Be aware that pure tones or sudden flashes of light may trigger seizures in some individuals. Find out whether an AAC user is at risk, what precautions to take, and how to manage a seizure.

AAC = augmentative and alternative communication.

Adapted from Bennet, T. L. (1992). *The neuropsychology of epilepsy.* Plenum Press; Byers, V. W., & Bristow, D. C. (1990). Audiologic evaluation of nonspeaking, physically challenged populations. *Ear and Hearing, 11,* 382-386; McEwen, I. R., & Lloyd, L. L. (1990). Positioning students with cerebral palsy to use augmentative and alternative communication. *Language, Speech, and Hearing Services in Schools, 21,* 15-21; and Young, C. V. (1986). Developmental disabilities. In J. Katz (Ed.), *Handbook of clinical audiology* (3rd ed., pp. 689-706). Williams & Wilkins.

Speech Audiometry

In speech audiometry testing for an AAC user, both the test stimuli and the response-eliciting methods may require adaptations. For speech awareness threshold testing, adaptations of test material are generally not necessary, as the individual does not need to interpret the spoken word but is only required to detect the presence of speech stimuli. However, the responses of the individual may need to be adapted due to motor or sensory issues similar to that discussed in the Pure Tone Audiometry section. Behavioral techniques, such as visual reinforcement audiometry or play audiometry, may be used for obtaining a response to speech detection testing.

For speech recognition testing and word discrimination testing, the individual's receptive and expressive language skills need to be considered along with their motor capacity (Katz, 2015), as it plays a vital role in the selection of test stimuli. **Spondee** words (e.g., cupcake, ice cream, toothbrush) are the standard test stimuli for speech recognition threshold and can be used with the AAC user if those words are within the receptive repertoire of the individual. In response to the stimuli presented, the individual under testing is expected to repeat back the spondee words. For some AAC users, production of such natural speech responses may be appropriate given the high predictability of the word list used. Another option is to use familiar words that the AAC user can indicate via an established communication mode (e.g., manual signs). Similarly, an AAC user may also indicate responses using common objects, line drawings, or written words via eye gaze, pointing, or adapted switches.

Speech identification (i.e., word discrimination) testing requires repeating **phonetically balanced** words (e.g., rat) and is often problematic for many AAC users even with interpreting by a familiar partner. Although most speech identification tasks use open-set material, two closed-set adaptations—the *Word Intelligibility by Picture Identification* (Ross & Lerman, 1970) and the *Northwestern University-Children's Perception of Speech* (Elliot & Katz, 1980)—may be appropriate (Katz, 2015). Closed set material provides the individual with a limited set of response choices, and hence, is easier than open set stimuli (Tye-Murray, 2015). Here, the individual may point or use eye gaze to make a selection from a set of pictures, objects, or written text. For more detailed information regarding test adaptations for AAC users see Byers and Bristow (1990), Katz (2015), Penrod (1985), and Wasson and colleagues (1981).

MANAGEMENT OF COMMUNICATION IMPAIRMENTS IN HEARING IMPAIRMENT

Communication impairment in children with congenital hearing impairment is mostly a result of poor development of speech, language, and literacy skills; in the case of individuals with an acquired loss, it may be due to poor understanding of speech. For both children and adults with hearing impairment, management of communication impairment is necessary to establish their connection to the world around them—family, friends, community, and the wider world.

For children diagnosed with pre-lingual bilateral profound hearing impairment, three general modes of communication that may be used during management are: (a) oral methods—use of devices that enhance and assist listening along with auditory training in order to utilize residual hearing to develop speech and language skills; (b) manual methods—use of manual signs (e.g., American Sign Language [ASL]), which is an alternate language in itself; and (c) simultaneous communication (i.e., total communication) methods—a combination of oral and manual methods. Luckner and colleagues (2016) are of the opinion that no mode has been demonstrated to be superior to the others. Even then, the oral method of communication tends to be the chosen first option of parents as a majority of them wish to integrate their children into the hearing world. This method focuses on developing sufficient auditory and verbal skills in order to function in mainstream society. This will require hearing and assistive listening devices to be prescribed early in life in order for the AAC user to be taught to receive information through the auditory mode and improve their receptive and expressive verbal language skills. Hence, the following discussion begins with the importance of early intervention and the use of amplification devices and **assistive listening devices** for individuals with hearing impairment. Subsequently, the relevance of AAC in the management of communication impairment in individuals with hearing impairment will be discussed.

Early Intervention to Develop Communication Skills in Hearing Impairment

The importance of early identification and intervention for children with hearing loss becomes clear as we understand the consequences of hearing loss in children and later into their adolescence and adulthood. The consequence of hearing impairment is significantly more detrimental when it occurs early in life. The first 3 years of a child's life are the critical period for developing the cognitive and linguistic foundation from which all further development unfolds, and also the time for learning to communicate with family and acquire new information (Nicholas & Geers, 2006). Thus, early intervention when applied during this critical period of development can prevent delays in language, speech, communication and literacy in children with hearing loss of any degree (Moeller, 2000). The goal of early intervention is to prevent or at least minimize the effects of hearing loss on auditory development and subsequent language learning (Harrison, 2017). A positive outcome of early intervention on language development is well documented over the years, especially among those for whom intervention was provided before 6 months of age (Moeller, 2000; Nicholas & Geers, 2006; Shojaei et al., 2016; Yoshinaga-Itano, 2003).

Advocates of early intervention emphasize the optimal use of this critical period of development in children with hearing impairment which is made possible by today's technological advancements, as well as evidence-based early intervention strategies. Technological developments have played a significant role in early intervention in terms of early fitting of amplification and assistive listening devices. This early enhancement of hearing abilities has immense potential to mitigate the effects of hearing loss on speech and language development. Hence, this becomes the first and foremost step toward management of hearing loss as it enhances communication competence.

Using Technology for Improving Communication

Recall that the classification system for technology proposed by Fuller, Pampoulou, and Lloyd in Chapter 3 includes a superordinate classification of expressive vs. receptive. For the first time, it is suggested that classification of technology include *receptive* aids and devices. Under the broad category of receptive technology is the subordinate level of aided vs. unaided. As there presently are not any fully developed receptive unaided aids or devices on the market, the focus here will be on receptive aided technology.

Hearing Devices

To reduce the effect of hearing impairment on speech, language, and communication, it is essential to enhance effectively the residual hearing abilities of the affected individual. Thus, fitting an individual with an appropriate amplification device—the primary step in aural rehabilitation—is a major leap to minimizing the communication deficits caused by hearing impairment. Hearing aids and implantable hearing devices are the two commonly available options to improve hearing abilities.

Electronic amplifier hearing aids were first introduced in the 1950s; technology has advanced significantly since the introduction of digitally programmable hearing aids in the 1990s. Implantable hearing devices were invented in the 1970s and have advanced considerably with a better understanding of the audiological system and also the development of miniaturized speech processors with advanced programmable features. Both of these technological options are advancing at a very rapid rate and are expected to bring revolutionary progress for use in mitigating communication impairments.

Conventional hearing aids acoustically stimulate ears with amplified sounds that are transmitted via air conduction. Today's conventional hearing aids use digital technology to enhance audibility, improve the signal-to-noise ratio, and reduce steady background noise with the help of sophisticated directional microphones and efficient digital signal processing algorithms. The most advanced aids utilize artificial intelligence to automatically adjust the aids to the wearer's environment (e.g., a movie theatre vs. a lecture room). This enables improved communication performance in different listening situations and environments. Rather than just merely amplifying the sound signal, modern-era hearing aids also allow direct connectivity via Bluetooth wireless technology to a variety of devices, such as telephones, televisions, and personal music players for enhanced listening. Wireless technology allows communication between the two hearing aids for persons with bilateral hearing loss, provides a higher quality sound that improves speech understanding, reduces technical difficulties when using telephones and televisions, allows increased mobility while using a telephone, and is of greater convenience while watching television with others (Hall, 2014).

The most common types of conventional hearing aids include (a) Receiver-in-the-Ear, (b) In-the-Canal, (c) In-the-Ear, (d) Behind-the-Ear, (e) Completely-in-the-Canal, and (f) open fit mini Behind-the-Ear (see Figure 23-3 for examples of these aids). Other styles of hearing aids include contralateral routing of signals hearing aids and bone conduction hearing aids. Contralateral routing of signals technology allows individuals with single-sided deafness to regain access to sounds in the impaired ear by transferring it to the better hearing ear, thereby reducing the impact of the acoustic head shadow (Snap, 2019). Bone conduction hearing aids based on the principle that skull vibrations can transmit sound are used for individuals with conductive or mixed hearing loss who are unable to use conventional hearing aids. Conventional bone conduction devices or bone conduction hearing devices have an actuator that vibrates the skull attached to the individual using a headband, a softband, adhesive, or eyeglasses (Maier et al., 2022). Examples of conventional bone conduction devices include ADHEAR (MED-EL, Austria), which uses an adhesive to couple the device to the skull, and Baha (Cochlear), which uses a softband for coupling the device.

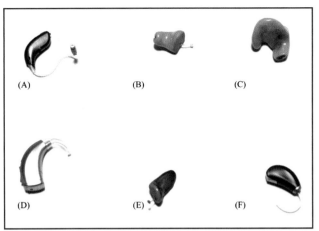

Figure 23-3. Common types of hearing aids: (a) Receiver-in-the-Ear, (b) In-the-Canal, (c) In-the-Ear, (d) Behind-the-Ear, (e) Completely-in-the-Canal, and (f) open fit mini Behind-the-Ear.

Implantable hearing devices include bone conduction implantable devices (BCID), implantable middle ear devices, **cochlear implants**, and auditory brainstem implants. BCIDs or surgically implanted bone conduction devices are used for individuals with outer ear malformations, chronic middle ear disease, and/or unilateral hearing loss/single-sided deafness. BCIDs can be of percutaneous and transcutaneous types. Percutaneous BCIDs use a skin penetrating abutment to couple the device to the skull. Baha and Ponto (Oticon Medical) are examples of percutaneous BCIDs. Transcutaneous BCIDs use magnetic coupling to keep the device in place with the help of an implanted subcutaneous magnet. Baha Attract (Cochlear) is an example of the same. For further information on BCIDs, refer to Ellsperman and colleagues (2021) and Maier and colleagues (2022).

A noninvasive prosthetic bone conduction device for persons with conductive hearing loss and unilateral hearing loss, known as the Sound-Bite Hearing System by Sonitus Medical, is an advancement in the management of hearing loss. It consists of a behind-the-ear component with a microphone deeply located in the ear canal along with a removable in-the-mouth device that is custom fitted to the patient's teeth. The external behind-the-ear component captures sound, which is transmitted wirelessly to the oral device, and the vibrations are transmitted transcranially from the teeth to the cochlea. This hearing prosthesis is shown to enhance the ability to localize sound (Murray et al., 2011), improve ease of communication, and enhance hearing in background noise (Gurgel & Shelton, 2013).

Middle ear implants, which were approved by the U.S. Food and Drug Administration in 2002, are options for individuals with hearing impairment who cannot benefit from conventional hearing aids. The Soundbridge (Vibrant) and the Esteem (Envoy Medical) hearing implant systems are examples of such an implantable middle ear device. The Soundbridge is a semi-implantable active middle ear device (Liu et al., 2018) that can be used with adults having

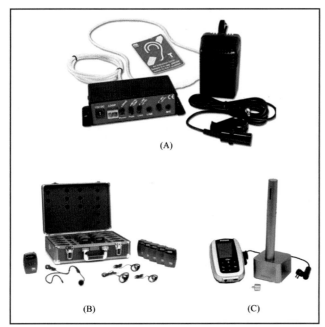

(A)

(B)   (C)

Figure 23-4. Assistive listening devices. (A) CL1/US fixed counter induction loop system (Reproduced with permission from SigNET, United Kingdom), (B) LS-07-072, 15-person portable radio frequency system (72 MHz; Reproduced with permission from Listen Technologies Corporation, Bluffdale, Utah), and (C) Phonak Roger Inspiro transmitter and pen (Reproduced with permission from Phonak, Warrenville, Illinois.)

moderate to severe conductive, sensorineural, and mixed hearing loss (Katz, 2015). The device consists of an external processor that is fixed to the skin on the patient's head using a magnet (Mondelli et al., 2016) and an internal component that is mounted on one of the ossicles in the middle ear. The external processor has a microphone that picks up the sound and transmits to the internal processor thus working similarly to a hearing aid. The internal processor is generally attached to the stapes and converts vibrations from the tympanic membrane and middle ear ossicles into electrical signals. These are then sent to the sound processor, which amplifies and filters the sound based on the patient's hearing.

The Esteem is a totally implantable hearing system that is indicated for use in individuals with moderate to severe stable sensorineural hearing losses who are 18 years or older with a minimum discrimination score of 60% and a middle ear which is anatomically and functionally intact (Gerard et al., 2012). This system consists of two components, a sensor, which picks up natural vibrations from the body of the incus bone, and a driver, which transfers the signal processed by the receiver to the head of the stapes bone.

Cochlear implants are one type of implantable hearing device that has gained popularity due to its immense ability to improve the hearing and communication abilities of individuals with profound bilateral hearing impairment, especially for those who receive early intervention. It consists of an external sound processor like other implantable devices along with a receiving coil/internal processor and an electrode array that is implanted. The microphone sends sounds

to the speech processor which converts the sound into digital form to be transmitted into the internal device. The integrated circuit within the internal processor converts the digital input to electrical impulses which are delivered to the inner ear through the array of electrodes.

A development in cochlear implants are hybrid cochlear implant devices (Woodson et al., 2010). They provide high-frequency information in an electrical form and low-frequency information in an acoustic form to the same ear to preserve and enhance residual hearing that might otherwise be lost following insertion of the electrode array into the cochlea. When surgical placement of electrode arrays into the cochlea is not possible due to cochlear malformations or ossifications or due to bilateral lesions of the auditory nerve, the option of brainstem implants has been approved since 2000 by the U.S. Food and Drug Administration for individuals more than 12 years of age (Monsanto et al., 2014). For additional information on implantable hearing devices, see Katz (2015) and Valente and colleagues (2008).

Assistive Listening Devices

Even with the use of a hearing aid, an individual with a hearing impairment might encounter difficulty while communicating in certain public areas, such as auditoriums, meeting halls, cafeterias, and classrooms or while using the telephone, watching TV, or riding in a car. In such cases, assistive listening devices/hearing assistance technology can be used in conjunction with hearing devices to restore effective communication. These devices include a microphone that is positioned close to the targeted sound source (e.g., another person's voice, a telephone receiver, or TV speaker) to capture sound and then transmits it wirelessly over frequency modulation, infrared induction loop transmission, and/or other transmission techniques (Kim & Kim, 2014; Figure 23-4). Development of wireless technologies, such as Bluetooth and radio frequency transmissions, have a significant impact on focused listening by providing an improved signal-to-noise ratio in a crowded environment. This streaming technology allows direct communication of assistive listening devices to hearing aids, resulting in improved listening due to little or no amplification of extraneous sounds (Katz, 2015; Kim & Kim, 2014).

Apart from technologies that enhance hearing in adverse listening situations, various telecommunication and related technologies have been evolving over the years to assist individuals with hearing impairment. A brief overview is provided below:

- Telephone amplifiers, accessories, and telecommunication devices: These technologies support effective understanding of spoken messages from partners who are only remotely available by making information from a telephone readily available to the person with hearing impairment. Telecommunication devices for the Deaf or teletypewriters are text-based telephones that have been in use by the Deaf since the 1980s. Teletypewriters are most useful when individuals with hearing impairment or deafness are unable to use a conventional telephone due to extremely poor speech perception. Teletypewriter systems modified to communicate with a computer are also now available (Katz, 2015). A voice-carryover phone is a hybrid of a teletypewriter and a regular phone, wherein a relay operator types everything that the hearing individual says. However, these devices might phase out rapidly with the introduction, prevalence, and increased availability of high-speed internet. For those communicating using sign language, video-based internet and mobile phone communication tools are the current trend. Video relay service features in some smartphone applications make mobile phones more accessible to Deaf sign language users allowing them to communicate with voice telephone users. This is made possible through a video relay service operator with whom the deaf person connects using internet-based video conferencing. The operator then places a voice telephone call to the other party and translates the conversation from sign language to speech and vice-versa (Alnfiai & Sampali, 2017).

- Text-based access technology: Captioning technology allows individuals with hearing impairment to better access information imparted through television by providing subtitles called captions. Closed captioning is mandated on all TV broadcasting in the United States and is enforced with Federal Communications Commission regulations. Captioning is made available for different types of media, such as prerecorded programs that use an offline captioning option and live programs that use real-time captioning. Captions are also available for programs on the web and even in public cinemas. Text-to-text communication in the form of cellular-based text messages and web-based instant messaging have become immensely popular to enable easy communication.

- Alerting devices: These technologies are designed to alert individuals with hearing impairment to situations that require them to respond to environmental sounds (e.g., when a doorbell or telephone rings or when a warning alarm goes off) but are unable to do so due to their inability to hear them. The alert systems for individuals with hearing impairment promote independence and improve their quality of life. These devices tend to use signals in one or more forms of sound, light, and vibration. A few examples include special alarm clocks, emergency alert signalers, sound monitors, and motion detectors. With advances in technology, there is a shift from such devices to software/mobile applications that serve the same purpose as that of the alerting devices but are more easily accessible.

AAC in Communication Management for Hearing Impairment

Early identification and intervention are being successfully implemented around the world to prevent the incapacitating consequences of hearing loss and improve overall language and communication competence in individuals with hearing impairment. Even then, many factors adversely affect the extent to which individuals with hearing impairment achieve this goal. Overcoming some factors related to hearing loss, such as the level of involvement of family in intervention and the presence of coexisting anatomical, sensory, medical, or developmental conditions that pose as barriers to listening and speech development, can be very challenging (Harrison, 2017; Moeller, 2000). Significant language gaps and communication deficits are being reported in a considerable number for children with hearing impairment even after receiving early intervention, probably due to the presence of such factors. Moreover, children with hearing loss tend to experience reduced communicative interactions if adaptations, such as modifying the environment, using hearing enhancement technology, and selecting appropriate communication modes are not made (Luckner et al., 2016). Thus, the need for augmentation of speech becomes all the more critical for individuals with hearing impairment in order to reduce language gaps and overcome communication barriers and reduce communication breakdowns (Davis et al., 2010; Meinzen-Derr, 2018). Further, improving communication access for the Deaf also has the potential to improve their educational level and work performance while generally increasing independence and improving self-confidence in performing daily life tasks (Alnfiai & Sampali, 2017).

When spoken language cannot be relied upon solely to fulfill various communicative functions, individuals with hearing impairment and their communicative partners tend to rely additionally on other well-established unaided communication options, such as manual-visual systems (e.g., sign languages, like ASL, British Sign Language, Indian Sign Language, International Sign Language, and other gestural systems). Sign language is considered the most popular mode of communication for individuals who are deaf (Koenigsfeld et al., 1993). While sign language is an unaided form of AAC, when used by the Deaf as a primary mode of communication, it is not viewed as AAC (Pennington et al., 2007). To elaborate, Loncke (2014) stated that,

Although 'AAC' is usually not the term used for the most obvious and well-known solutions for individuals with severe hearing impairment, the use of manual signing (sign language, such as [ASL]) in educational programs for deaf individuals is nevertheless based on the same principle of AAC: Identify and use the most accessible modality (visual-gestural) to enable cognitive-linguistic and academic development. (p. 2)

Why AAC Beyond Sign Language?

Individuals with hearing impairment often use sign language to communicate with their peers effectively, but they also tend to rely on writing, speaking, gestures, pointing, and mouthing of words to communicate with hearing individuals who do not understand or use sign language (Cohen et al., 2001). These strategies are considered unaided AAC and have been in use for the rehabilitation of individuals with hearing impairment for several decades.

Communication breakdowns are common when a deaf individual interacts with those not familiar with sign language. The breakdown at the receiver's end could be due to difficulty in understanding signs by an unfamiliar communication partner (Mirenda, 2003), lack of functional use and generalization abilities of signs (Lee et al., 2013), or lack of ability to understand mouthing of words or lack of literacy. Communication breakdowns on the sender's end could be due to an inability to speech read efficiently, to the lack of literary skills to use writing to communicate, or to the presence of any coexisting disability that hampers the use of signs and gestures. Data from the Gallaudet University Research Institute in 2011 indicated that 40% of individuals with hearing loss have an additional disability (Roush & Wilson, 2013). These additional disabilities have the potential to further burden the communication abilities of the individual with hearing impairment. For example, an additional disability, such as physical impairment, can limit the motor abilities needed by a person to use sign language, and an additional intellectual disability may limit the individual's capacity to learn communication in any mode—verbal, sign language, or written. Moreover, at times the comorbid condition itself can have communication impairment as a characteristic symptom, such as in autism spectrum disorder. Hence, in order to overcome these communication barriers, individuals with hearing impairment need to be taught to switch to other augmentative or alternative forms of communication and to use them accurately.

In today's world, AAC solutions have come way beyond the use of manual signs, gestures, and writing. Gestures and signs that were developed originally for use with individuals with hearing impairment have recently found their application into various other developmental and acquired disorders. Similarly, several aided AAC approaches used successfully with persons exhibiting other communication disorders is now providing assistance to individuals with hearing impairment. They include non–speech-generating technology (e.g., communication boards, picture books, simple battery-operated communication devices), or speech-generating technology (e.g., dedicated speech-generating devices [SGDs], smartphones and tablets, mobile applications, or AAC software). These aided forms of AAC are becoming more popular and show promise in use with individuals having hearing impairment due to their inherent capacity to transmit messages, which are often easily perceived by communication partners and by their ability to quickly accommodate receptive vocabularies (Lee et al., 2013).

APPLICATION OF TECHNOLOGY IN AAC FOR HEARING IMPAIRMENT

Koenigsfeld and colleagues (1993) report that in the past, most individuals who were deaf or hard of hearing had minimal experience using technology-based AAC devices other than those used for assistive listening, such as telecommunication devices for the Deaf or teletypewriters, portable typewriters and computers, closed captioning, or paper and pencil. The interest in owning a portable AAC device to communicate with nonsigning hearing people was rare and AAC devices were viewed to be more useful in work settings than other settings, such as home or shopping. The limited use of AAC technology in the past for individuals with hearing impairment was found to be due to a lack of knowledge about available technology, attitudinal barriers, and/or the cost of the device (Koenigsfeld et al., 1993). However, this has changed considerably in the new millennium because of the explosive growth of technology, its availability, and its user-friendliness. Artificial intelligence and machine learning allow the devices to be self-configuring and adaptable based on user needs and limitations. The decreasing cost of technology has reduced the high cost associated with proprietary technology for AAC devices.

Non–Speech-Generating Technology

In situations where individuals with hearing impairment who use sign language as their primary mode of communication are not able to communicate solely using manual signs due to limitations imposed by the communication partner, an aided AAC approach, such as non–speech-generating technology, can supplement communication. Non–speech-generating technology might also be used to supplement functional speech abilities in individuals with hearing impairment to a lesser degree. Such aids might range from pen and paper to simple battery-operated devices.

Photographs, line drawings, printed words, pictures, or symbols displayed on communication boards, books, and picture dictionaries are examples of some of the non–speech-generating options that can be used for individuals with hearing impairment. Writing down messages is practiced commonly by individuals with hearing impairment when others do not understand sign language. Writing may be on paper, a computer, a tablet, or a smartphone (Power et al., 2006). Telecommunication devices mentioned earlier in this chapter are also considered non–speech-generating communication devices.

Speech-Generating Technology

The development of various communication applications on iPads (Apple), Android (Google) tablets, and smartphones after 2010 had a different impact on the use of aided

AAC systems across the range of individuals with different disabilities. These new devices are loaded with applications for video conferencing and texting, which allows communication to be much easier and faster for individuals with hearing impairment.

Speech-to-text applications, which use automatic speech recognition (ASR) technology, and text-to-speech applications are gaining popularity among individuals with hearing impairment who have necessary literary skills. Major players in the technology field, such as Google, Microsoft, and Apple, have speech-to-text and text-to-speech engines built into their operating systems for multiple languages and regional accents. These are under continuous development and a lot of open-source resources are available on the internet. Numerous apps are available in Apple's popular App Store and Android's Play Store. A search with keywords, such as "AAC apps for the Deaf" or "communication apps for Deaf" will bring up applications that are both free of cost or purchasable. It is safer to download apps from authorized and reliable resources to avoid dangers associated with virus and other malware issues. The number of downloads and the overall rating of the app could be indicators of the usefulness of the app itself.

Dialogue on reliability and security issues of apps is beyond the scope of this chapter. An example of a speech-to-text mobile app that has gained recent popularity is Ava by Transcence, Inc. Ava, an iOS-based app, allows a deaf individual to participate in and understand a conversation involving hearing individuals in a group situation. It uses real-time captioning based on artificial intelligence to transcribe live speech to make it readily available to the Deaf. There are smartwatches that display emails with their original formatting and utilize speech-to-text to transcribe messages. The Apple Watch Series 6 is an example of such a smartwatch. These technologies are constantly in a state of evolution and current developments are made available to the general public on an ongoing basis.

For a deaf individual who uses an unaided form of AAC (such as sign language), successful use of aided AAC (such as any of the devices mentioned) or communication apps will depend on whether they will effectively supplement communication in real life. Consider a situation when a deaf person who uses sign language meets a communication partner who does not understand sign language at all. Aided AAC device technology can bridge this gap and enable communication. One concern would be the speed of interaction being as close as possible to natural communication while using such a device. At least a partial solution comes in the form of word prediction software and sign language-to-text conversion technologies.

Word prediction software assists in completing words or phrases contextually by predicting the word as initial letters are keyed in. This feature can be a valuable tool for individuals with hearing impairment who have difficulty with spelling, vocabulary, and grammar. Predictions can be based on spelling, syntax, and recent use. When used with speech-generating software, it serves as a speech-generating communication device for the individual who is nonspeaking. Windows 10 has a built-in on-screen keyboard emulator that uses word prediction, which is available free of cost.

Technologies that allow automatic translation of sign language to text or spoken language has been continuously developing since the last 2 decades. Research on the conversion of different sign languages using machine translation around the world is being documented (Kouremenos et al., 2018; Luqman & Mahmoud, 2018; Verma & Srivastava, 2018). Sign language translation requires recognition of sign language, which is mostly enabled through a gesture recognition system. "Gesture and sign language recognition includes the whole process of tracking and identifying the signs performed and converting them into semantically meaningful words and expressions" (Cheok et al., 2017, p. 131). Hand gestures are recognized either using a vision-based or a sensor-based approach or using a hybrid approach (Ahmed et al., 2018). Vision-based approaches acquire images or videos of hand gestures using a video camera, whereas sensor-based approaches require the use of sensors to capture the motion, velocity, and position of the hands. Within these vision- and sensor-based approaches, some of the technologies that readily capture gesture information include electromyography, Leap Motion controller, and Kinect (Microsoft). Electromyography measures electrical pulses from human muscles and utilizes this bio-signal to detect fingers movements. On the other hand, Leap Motion controller uses two monochromatic cameras and three infrared light-emitting diodes to collect information regarding the fingertips, center of the palm, and hand orientation to aid recognition of sign language (Cheok et al., 2017). The Kinect device (released in 2010) also uses a depth camera along with a color sensor and an infrared emitter to collect color and depth information to create a three-dimensional motion trajectory database (Amatya et al., 2018; Mustafa & Dimopoulos, 2014; Suvagiya et al., 2016).

Sign languages are analyzed for translation in ways similar to that of spoken languages, wherein the software uses knowledge of components of signs just as it uses knowledge of grammar and other linguistic variables to understand a spoken sentence. The features of sign language, such as hand configuration, hand orientation, the relation between hands, and the direction of hand movements can be coded using a notation system. An example of a notation system is the Hamburg Notation System developed in the 1980s. It is an alphabetic system describing signs at the phonetic level (Hanke, 2004). "The transcriptions using this system are precise but long and cumbersome to decipher" (Parton, 2006, p. 97). Moreover, sign recognition systems that make use of this notation system are only a few in number (Hanke, 2004).

Advances in sign language translation technologies are also making real-time conversion of sign-to-text possible. KinTrans, Inc is a U.S.-based machine learning software company that is building a suite of human movement and gesture recognition application program interfaces and three-dimensional datasets that are now licensed annually under special projects to corporate partners and governments. They were expected to be made available to the global developer community through a subscriber-based platform in 2019. KinTrans Hands Can Talk is one of their applications that translates sign language to voice and text in real time, with embedded third-party speech-to-text software in the corresponding language. They have also developed a KinTrans multilingual signing avatar for use in the translator application itself to translate speech or text data into sign language (C. Bentley, personal communication, January 24, 2018).

In children with hearing impairment who have not acquired spoken or sign language, technology can be useful to teach sign language–based communication. On the foundation built by sign language, spoken and written languages can be further taught (Yorganci et al., n.d.). Video-based representations of sign languages are used by teachers to teach signs in context and allow for replaying of signs whenever required. Virtual Conversation Agent (Avatar) is a technology application developed for signed conversation that uses three-dimensional animated models. These signing avatars can also be used by children with hearing impairment to receive early exposure to language for better communication. Mobile applications that allow easy learning of sign languages for individuals with hearing impairment (from young children to adults) or their communication partners (e.g., parents, teachers) are also available now. Other applications that allow systematic learning of grammar and facilitate a visual way of learning syntax and language are available in English. Such apps can be explored for use in individuals with hearing impairment after its efficacy has been researched.

Technological evolution has also made it possible to enable the successful participation of individuals with hearing impairment in the classroom environment. Apps that provide remote computer access and screen mirroring for all students' devices is also now available. This enables the teacher to replicate content from a whiteboard to an individual student's device. Speech-to-text technologies can be used in classrooms for a better understanding of lectures delivered. Atcherson and colleagues (2015) discussed a number of speech-to-text technologies that may be used for educational and other purposes. They include communication access real-time translation, text-interpreting (e.g., C-Print or Typewell), and ASR. Communication access real-time translation is generally used for captioning during live events and uses a verbatim approach that captures and types every spoken word regardless of relevance to the lecture. Text interpreting uses a meaning-to-meaning approach rather than verbatim interpretation and is similar to receptive key word signing. C-Print and TypeWell can be projected on a laptop so students have the option of editing lecture notes, and transcriptions can be received on mobile devices, such as an iPhone (Apple), iPad, and Android-based devices, using an internet connection. ASR involves automatic transcription using computer software.

Even though smartphone apps that facilitate various types of communication are abundant in the marketplace, communication apps with features necessary to accommodate the needs of individuals with hearing impairment are limited. Apps, such as Skype, FaceTime and WhatsApp, in smartphones have established their niche as the most popular video and text chat programs and are immensely popular among the Deaf population. Certain core features that make communication apps accessible to the Deaf include:

(1) Comprehension (text, sound, and video streaming); (2) speech-to-text; (3) text-to-speech (4) joining social network application; (5) notification; (6) support several languages; (7) real-time communication; (8) internet connection (offline); (9) sign language (speech reading, hand movement, and facial expression); (10) size readability (large font size); (11) size of buttons; (12) provide a card or image library; and (13) enabling privacy. (Alnfiai & Sampali, 2017, p. 123)

AAC Use by Persons With Hearing Impairment

In AAC intervention, implementation of AAC is often a step that follows after the selection of an appropriate AAC system and vocabulary. Effective AAC implementation is often based on intervention goals, the individual's age, and the type of AAC system selected, and it often involves AAC user, as well as communication partner, training.

Context of AAC Use in Early Childhood

For children using aided AAC as an alternative form of communication, intervention will likely focus on facilitation of acquisition and use of language and development of literacy. On the other hand, for children and adults who are using it to augment their speech, the implementation of AAC will be to facilitate communication. Aided AAC, such as SGDs, can be used for children with hearing impairment who have undergone cochlear implantation but show insufficient oral communication skills. The use of an SGD tends to improve their speech perception, production, receptive vocabulary, and communicative skills. AAC intervention using an SGD will involve training to operate the device and instruction for learning symbols (beginning with requesting for a preferred object). Modeling, imitation (with physical guidance, if required), questions or mands, and elicitation of symbols can be used hierarchically through parental prompting to teach communicative skills during the intervention (Lee et al., 2013). Although SGDs may be useful for individuals with hearing impairment, if the user exhibits an inability to hear auditory output, a barrier toward independent usage of the SGD will likely result, and it will negatively influence the individual's ability to provide conversational repairs (Davis et al., 2010).

The possibility of using AAC technology on an iPad to enhance language development in individuals who are Deaf and hard of hearing is under research. Meinzen-Derr and colleagues (2017) used an iPad application known as TouchChat HD-AAC With Wordpower having both synthesized and digitized speech options for intervention with individuals with hearing impairment and found a significant increase in the mean length of utterance and different words spoken irrespective of the cognitive abilities of the participants. They concluded that the use of AAC technology on iPads shows promise in supporting rapid language growth among elementary school–age children who are deaf or hard of hearing. Subsequent studies, including a single-case experimental design (Meinzen-Derr et al., 2019) and a randomized controlled trial (Meinzen-Derr et al., 2021), also showed positive impact of AAC intervention on language outcomes in children with bilateral hearing loss.

In the case of individuals with hearing impairment and coexisting intellectual disability, use of picture dictionaries tends to promote expressive communication and spelling of words (Allgood et al., 2009; Cohen et al., 2001). Training using picture dictionaries initially can involve discussing the intent of the picture dictionaries and teaching symbol meanings. Strategies, such as modeling, guided practice, and independent practice, can be used to teach communicative skills.

The structured training protocol used in the Picture Exchange Communication System has also found its application for individuals with autism and hearing impairment (Malandraki & Okalidou, 2007) to improve spontaneous communication skills. Until recently, AAC intervention for individuals with hearing impairment has been focused more on such individuals having an additional disability. However, in order to understand which AAC strategy should be implemented for individuals with hearing impairment with no other concomitant disability, more focused research on aided AAC implementation in deaf and hard-of-hearing individuals is required (Meinzen-Derr, 2018; Meinzen-Derr et al., 2018, Meinzen-Derr et al., 2017). This calls for systematic incorporation of AAC strategies into traditional aural rehabilitation programs for individuals with hearing impairment to build on evidence of the use of AAC, such as those available for other individuals with complex communication needs. It is worth noting here that each AAC user presents a unique combination of sensory, motor, cognitive, social, and communication abilities; hence, the effective implementation of AAC requires a thorough prior assessment and documentation of user abilities and appropriate selection of the AAC system. General intervention suggestions are provided in Table 23-4.

Importance of Communication Partner Training in AAC

Since communication is a two-way process where message transmitters and receivers are involved, the AAC user needs to have communication partners who understand the alternative or augmentative methods employed. For some individuals, AAC uses mainly strategies, techniques, and devices that are not used by the typical person who uses communication methods, such as speech or written communication. Hence, training the communication partner (especially those who regularly communicate with the AAC user) will be beneficial for effective communication and continued use of AAC. This stands true in the case of individuals with hearing impairment as much as for any other disability.

The communication partner is labeled "good" if they are motivated, interested, and comfortable with all methods of communication. However, becoming a good communication partner requires skills and strategies that may require training and practice. Partners often include those who use speech as a primary mode of communication, and hence, they unknowingly tend to take the majority of conversational turns, provide fewer opportunities for the AAC user to respond, or focus more on the technology used than the message being communicated or the individual with the communication impairment (Blackstone, 1999). Even though communication partner training is a less focused area in AAC intervention, it appears to be the most cost-effective part of intervention (Kent-Walsh & McNaughton, 2005). The communication partner takes the role of a facilitator for communication and maximizes use of the alternative or augmentative system by the AAC user. As a facilitator, communication partners are expected to use certain strategies, such as structuring the environment to support communication, providing varied and meaningful opportunities for communication, prompting only when required, and modeling appropriate use of AAC techniques and strategies (Blackstone, 1999).

In general, communication partners of individuals with hearing impairment may be informally or formally trained to use compensatory measures to enhance communication and avoid communication breakdowns. Some compensatory strategies that can be adapted by communication partners while communicating with an individual with hearing impairment include: (a) getting the attention of the person with hearing loss, (b) facing the individual with hearing loss while speaking, (c) providing a topic, (d) rephrasing, (e) using keywords, (f) asking for confirmation of information, (g) speaking slowly and clearly, (h) eliminating noise and reducing distractions, (i) improving lighting, and (j) using assistive technology to enhance real-time conversations (Alnfiai & Sampali, 2017; Atcherson et al., 2015). Communication partners of young children with hearing impairment may

---

TABLE 23-4

Intervention Suggestions for Working With AAC Users With Hearing Impairment

- Use appropriate assistive technology and monitor equipment functioning daily.
- Reduce background noise as much as possible in the home and classroom.
- Realize that hearing may not be optimal in noisy cafeterias, gymnasiums, or crowded public areas.
- Seat the child as close as possible to the speaker (e.g., teacher), away from distractions.
- Gain the child's attention before giving instructions or engaging in conversation.
- Encourage the child to respond to the sound of the child's name.
- Look at the child when communicating and maintain eye contact as much as possible. Position the child at eye level or move/bend to maintain eye contact. This is particularly important for children whose position is frequently varied from wheelchair to adapted stander to sidelyer.
- Speak in single words, phrases, and short sentences using natural pitch, rhythm, and intonation. Vary intonation naturally for conversation, reading aloud, and expressing emotions. Use natural facial expressions and body movements to supplement speech. Keep hands and papers away from the face when speaking.
- Help the child notice environmental sounds (e.g., telephone, dog barking) by calling attention to them. Point out the direction from which the sound came to encourage localization skills. Provide toys, activities, and experiences that make noise and encourage auditory attention to them. Match the referent to a representation on the child's AAC device.
- Provide a variety of sensory experiences involving touch, taste, smell, sound, and other meaningful experiences within which language and communication can develop. Describe these using short meaningful sentences and model them with the child's own AAC device. Respond to what interests the child and provide appropriate spoken and AAC models.
- Associate a spoken word or phrase with the child's AAC representation and the actual referent. Use the word/phrase many times in varying contexts. Alternately speak then indicate the referent to allow the child to shift visual attention between the two.
- Read aloud facing the child, giving the child the opportunity to alternately look at the pictures and the reader's face. As books become familiar, occasionally read from behind the child and follow the print with an index finger.
- Give the child a chance to listen and then respond to encourage turn-taking communication. Allow sufficient time for the child to process and respond.

AAC = augmentative and alternative communication.

Adapted from Bigge, J. L. (1982). *Teaching individuals with multiple disabilities* (2nd ed.). Charles E. Merrill and Gdowski, B. S., Sanger, D. D., & Decker, T. N. (1986). Otitis media effect on a child's learning. *Academic Therapy, 21,* 283-289.

---

be required to model manual signs or gestures along with speech during natural routines (Moeller et al., 1987). Use of aided methods employing graphic symbols, by nature of their static presentation, can enhance comprehension as well.

It may be appropriate to provide structured training at the time of initiation of AAC use by the user followed by necessary documentation for training. This documentation can serve as training guidance for future communication partners when the AAC user shifts to newer environments and when professional help is unavailable.

CHALLENGES/BARRIERS IN IMPLEMENTATION OF AAC

AAC ranging from simple manual signs to complex SGDs is used across a variety of communication disorders of different etiologies. However, clarity on the type of AAC system or intervention method that is more successful for a

person is a question that must be determined individually (Pennington et al., 2007). AAC devices are a subset of assistive technology, but AAC devices are different in several ways from other straightforward assistive technology, such as wheelchairs or hearing aids. Communication by a person is a much more complicated process that requires a different set of skills for its effective use, and hence, the barriers associated with AAC use are also unique. Communication requires thoughts to be converted into words and sentences and brought out in a such way that it will be easily received and understood by the communication partner.

While the AAC user's environment may impose opportunity barriers, access barriers are imposed by the individual's abilities (i.e., cognitive abilities, perceptual abilities, physical abilities) and needs. Opportunity barriers can be explained in terms of policy, practice, attitude, knowledge, and communicative barriers (Beukelman & Mirenda, 1992; Glennen & DeCoste, 1997). In the United States, federal laws, such as the Communication Bill of Rights (National Joint Committee for the Communication Needs of Persons With Severe

Disabilities, 1992), revised Communication Bill of Rights of 2016 (Brady et al., 2016), Individuals with Disabilities Education Improvement Act (2004), and Americans with Disabilities Amendment Act of 2008, advocate for the use of assistive technology and AAC in particular. These laws assist individuals with disabilities—especially those with hearing impairments—to receive necessary services and support for effective use of AAC devices. However, other countries around the world may not have equally strong advocacy for individuals with a disability, creating policy barriers in using AAC.

An attitudinal barrier is often found to have a severe impact on the selection and use of AAC. Special educators and speech-language pathologists who might be loyal toward introducing sign language as a mode of communication for individuals with hearing impairment might not be comfortable in introducing picture-/symbol-based communication strategies to accommodate the child's needs. Also, when professionals and caregivers are not "tech-savvy," they may create a knowledge barrier for implementing AAC. One responsibility of the communication partners of individuals with hearing impairment is to create a conducive and barrier-free environment to communicate. However, this ideal situation may not be a possibility, especially in a public place. A hypothetical example would be a deaf person using an SGD to communicate in a noisy environment, wherein the noise prevents the synthesized speech from being heard by the AAC user, thus causing a communication barrier.

It becomes a necessity to identify environmental barriers right at the beginning of the selection of an AAC system for the individual with hearing impairment. An International Classification of Functioning, Disability and Health–based tool called *Communication Supports Inventory-Children and Youth* (Rowland et al., 2016) is a viable option for identifying barriers specific to a particular individual with hearing impairment who is using AAC. Minimizing barriers forms a major step in the successful implementation of AAC in any population with a disability, including the Deaf and hard of hearing.

Considerations for Success of AAC Use in Hearing Impairment

Defining success of AAC use is dependent on the goals set for a particular AAC user. As discussed in earlier chapters, successfully feature matching the AAC system to the abilities and needs of the user is as critical as identifying the facilitators and barriers that positively or negatively affect its implementation or use. Some of these factors that determine the success of AAC use in individuals with hearing impairment are discussed in the following:

- Selection of appropriate AAC system: Appropriate selection of AAC should always be made after an objective and thorough assessment. Even when sign language is chosen and implemented as the primary mode of communication for an individual with hearing impairment, the individual's communicative competence should be monitored and other necessary AAC options should be provided, if required. For individuals with a lesser degree of hearing impairment and having functional speech and language skills, AAC may be used to augment their speech in conversation or in an environment demanding interaction. For such individuals, speech alone may suffice in familiar environments. An individual may be provided and trained for different forms of aided and unaided AAC as per their communication needs to meet ultimate success in communication. While selecting an appropriate system, factors, such as availability, affordability, sturdiness, and upgrading of the AAC system, should be considered. Acceptance of the AAC system by the user is needed for successful use along with ease of use. This is especially true of persons with hearing impairment with additional disabilities. Selection of appropriate vocabulary is also an equally important step in the selection of an AAC system. This should consider inputs from various communication partners of the individual with a hearing impairment and consider the individual's age, culture, educational background, and communication environments. In a world where technology is changing at an explosive pace, selection of an appropriate AAC system also means updated technology. Since artificial intelligence and machine learning are embedded in most devices available today, suitably updated technology will be a main factor for the appropriateness of the AAC system.

- Acceptance of the selected AAC system: Selection of the appropriate AAC system must be based on user needs and abilities. Despite the successful use of symbol-based AAC systems in general, individuals with deafness do not prefer it, as they are not typical forms of communication for individuals who are deaf, and they fear others may perceive those who use these systems as having an intellectual disability (Allgood et al., 2009; King, 1999; Koenigsfeld et al., 1993). However, individuals with hearing impairment now have many choices with the introduction of more non–speech-generating and speech-generating AAC devices and software. Even then, a careful selection of AAC from an array of options is essential for acceptance by the AAC user. Also, acceptance of significant others (e.g., family and peers) of the chosen AAC system is equally important as acceptance by the AAC user.

- Setting of appropriate goals for intervention: The selection of appropriate goals for using the identified communication mode (AAC) is also essential. A few suggested principles to guide a holistic approach to AAC intervention includes: (a) building the individual's strengths and focusing on integration of skills to maximize communication; (b) focusing on the individual's participation in real-world contexts; (c) addressing psychosocial

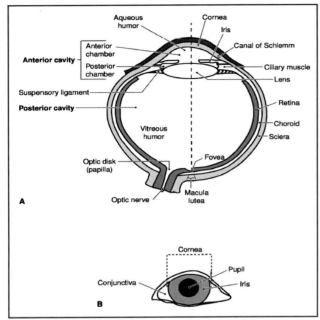

Figure 23-5. Anatomical structures of the eye: (A) the eyeball, (B) the outer, visible surface of the eye. (Reproduced with permission from Bhatnagar, S. C. [2017]. *Neuroscience for the study of communicative disorders* [5th ed.]. Wolters Kluwer Lippincott Williams and Wilkins.)

factors and skills; and (d) attending to extrinsic factors related to the individual who requires AAC (Light & McNaughton, 2015). The overall goal of AAC intervention has been to enhance quality of life and participation in everyday life and to augment spoken language with additional means of communication (Granlund et al., 2008). Hence, goals for AAC intervention for each individual need to be tailor made while keeping in mind the previously mentioned concrete aims of AAC intervention to ensure success.

- AAC user and communication partner training: Owing to the vast differences in the levels of communication barriers among individuals with hearing impairment due to the severity of the impairment, it is essential to classify these individuals based on their communicative skills before initiating AAC intervention. This includes both individuals with hearing impairment with functional hearing and speech for primary communication but require AAC to supplement communication in particular situations, and individuals with hearing impairment with limited functional hearing and speech who require AAC as an alternate mode of communication in almost all situations.

Approximately 95% of children who are deaf or hard of hearing in the United States are born to hearing parents who have little to no prior knowledge or experience of how to communicate effectively with a child having a hearing impairment (Mitchell & Karchmer, 2004). Hence, for communication partners (e.g., parents, siblings, and peers), training in AAC becomes crucial, as they are the most important interaction partners for the individual who uses AAC and also the primary interventionists after the speech-language pathologist.

THE SENSE OF VISION

Definition and Prevalence

Vision is the ability to see with clarity over a wide visual field. As such, proper vision requires both acuity (the ability to see the detail, contours, and borders of an image) and visual field (the spatial range of vision typically expressed in degrees). In terms of visual acuity, the standard for "normal" vision is 20/20, which means a person can see at 20 feet what should be seen at 20 feet (Cline et al., 1997). The normal or typical monocular visual field consists of a central visual field, which includes the inner 30 degrees of vision and central fixation, and the peripheral visual field, which extends 100 degrees laterally, 60 degrees medially, 60 degrees upward, and 75 degrees downward (Walker et al., 1990). Any impairment of visual acuity or field that deviates from these norms results in low vision or visual impairment (up to and including total blindness).

According to 2016 data (Erickson et al., 2017), approximately 7.66 million noninstitutionalized people in the United States (2.4% of 320 million Americans) have a visual disability. If this figure is indicative of visual disabilities worldwide, the total number of humans with visual disability exceeds 175 million. Prevalence of visual disability is slightly higher for females, persons over 65 years of age, and American Indians/Alaska natives. The number of noninstitutionalized persons aged 21 to 64 years with a visual disability in the United States who were employed full-time for the full year in 2016 was 1.12 million, or 29.5%. Indeed, 1.05 million (27.7%) of Americans between 21 and 64 years of age with a visual disability live below the national poverty line.

The visual system is obviously important to language function in regard to reading comprehension and oral reading, as well as perceiving and interpreting the nonverbal visual signals relied upon to supplement a communicator's message. Vision begins peripherally with light acting as the stimulus entering the eye and ends centrally with the processing of visual information in the single-modality association cortex and even beyond to multimodal association areas of the brain.

Anatomy of Vision

A brief review of the structure of the eyeball will serve to assist in understanding the input from the visual fields to our retinas. The different parts of the eyeball are labeled in Figure 23-5. The cornea is the transparent covering of the eye that bends and focuses the incoming light rays. The sclera is the lateral continuation of the cornea and is often referred to as "the white of our eye." The lens of the eye inverts the visual image projection onto the retina. The iris is the colored ring that surrounds and controls the size of the pupil, the opening through which light enters. The choroid layer is deep to the sclera and provides vascularization to the eye. The innermost layer of the eye is the retina, which we will return to shortly.

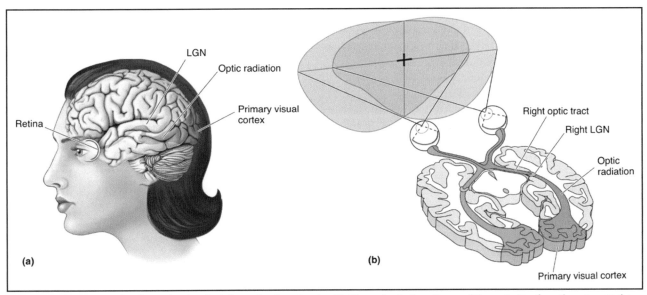

Figure 23-6. Primary visual pathway showing the information from the visual fields coming to the retinas and the projection from the retinas to the primary visual cortex in the occipital lobes: (A) the visual pathway within the brain, (B) the visual pathway in greater detail. (Reproduced with permission from Bear, M. F., Connors, B. W., & Paradiso, M. A. [2015]. *Neuroscience: Exploring the brain* [4th ed.]. Wolters Kluwer Lippincott Williams and Wilkins.)

The eye maintains its spherical shape via a liquid filling; the anterior cavity of the eye is filled with aqueous humor (a watery substance) and the posterior cavity is filled with vitreous humor (a jelly-like substance). Furthermore, the anterior cavity has two chambers: an anterior chamber between the cornea and iris and the posterior chamber between the iris and the lens. The canal of Schlemm connects these two chambers for regular drainage of aqueous humor into the venous system; this is a critical system that regulates intraocular pressure. Glaucoma is a condition of increased intraocular pressure that results from problems with either overproduction of aqueous humor or dysfunction of this canal.

Returning to the retina, it is here that the nervous system's involvement in vision begins. The retina develops from diencephalic tissue; therefore, it acts, in a way, like a "mini brain." The retina is multilayered with three nuclear layers and two synaptic layers. The focus here is on the outer nuclear layer of the retina that houses the sensory receptors for vision—the rods and cones. Returning to Figure 23-5, it can be seen that the retina is interrupted by the optic disc—a "hole" in the back of our eye. The optic disc is the exit point for the axons making up cranial nerve II (the optic nerve), as well as the entry point for blood vessels supplying the eye. Due to the lack of sensory receptors at the disc, any image falling there will not be perceived, and hence, we have a blind spot. Interestingly, this blind spot goes unnoticed as our brain makes up for the missing information through perceptual processes in the visual cortex at the occipital lobe. Another key feature of the retina is the fovea. At the fovea, intervening neural layers are shifted to the side so that light focuses directly on the sensory receptors there for increased resolution.

The rods and cones are referred to as **photoreceptors**. Rods are sensitive to light and are found in most abundance lateral to the fovea. There are around 100 million rods in each retina. Rods assist us greatly in "night vision," helping us to see shades of gray and perceive movement and shapes. The retina also contains cones, found in greatest abundance at the fovea; nonetheless, cones are much less in number as compared with rods. There are around 6 million cones, the photoreceptors responsible for perceiving form and color. Thus, cones are responsible for visual acuity. Light is transferred to neural information by the photoreceptors and passed on to axons making up the optic nerve via the nuclear and synaptic layers of the retina. The optic nerve transmits this neural information toward the central nervous system.

Physiology of Vision

The Primary Visual Pathway

The primary visual pathway is our system for sight and begins with the optic nerve, as illustrated in Figure 23-6. The optic nerve from each eye transmits visual information from left and right visual fields (what you see with your eyes straight forward) toward the optic chiasm. At the chiasm, the outer fibers of the optic nerves stay ipsilateral while the inner fibers cross, or decussate, to the contralateral hemisphere. It is at the optic chiasm that fibers get "sorted out" so that the fibers carrying information from the right visual field are destined for the left hemisphere, and the fibers carrying information from the left visual field are destined for the right hemisphere. From the chiasm, the fibers continue back as the optic tract to synapse at the lateral geniculate nuclei of the thalamus. Fibers fan out from the thalamus as they project back toward the occipital lobe as the optic radiations. Finally, synapses occur at the primary visual cortex, Brodmann area 17, at the occipital cortex surrounding the calcarine fissure. The surrounding single-function association areas, 18 and 19, further process visual information.

Small secondary visual pathways exist that send axons to the hypothalamus and midbrain. Those going to the hypothalamus play a role in the sleep-wake cycle by relaying information regarding the amount of light in our environment. Other axons diverge from the optic tract to synapse with the nuclei of the superior colliculi found in the midbrain. Visual reflexes important to maintain the position of our eyes and control the fixation of the eyes to keep objects focused on the fovea for the best resolution are part of this system.

Oculomotor Control

Our eyes move in synergy to draw attention to visual fields and focus light on our fovea. The cranial nerves responsible for these eye movements are the oculomotor, trochlear, and abducens. Each of these cranial nerves innervates muscles associated with a particular eyeball movement. The oculomotor is responsible for moving our eyes upward, downward, and medially. Importantly, oculomotor also innervates the muscle responsible for elevating the eyelid (i.e., levator palpebrae superioris). Damage to this cranial nerve then results in a droopy eyelid called **ptosis**. The oculomotor nucleus for oculomotor is located centrally in the midbrain and its nerve fibers exit from the ventral surface of the brainstem. The trochlear cranial nerve enables our eyes to move downward and outward. The trochlear nerve is engaged when we walk downstairs. The motor nucleus for the trochlear is found just caudal to the oculomotor nucleus at the junction of the midbrain and pons. The abducens' fibers emerge from the dorsal surface of the brainstem where they immediately decussate to curve around the brainstem and join the other cranial nerves on the ventral side. The abducens cranial nerve innervates muscles associated with moving the eye laterally (i.e., abduction—away from midline). This is tested easily by visually tracking an object from one side of the visual field to the other. The abducens motor nucleus is found in the caudal pons with its fibers emerging from the ventral surface of the brainstem.

Cranial nerve III, the oculomotor, also has an autonomic nervous system component. It is part of the parasympathetic system innervating smooth muscle to adjust the lens of the eye for accommodation to focus and adjust for moving targets and distances. It is also involved in pupil constriction; this is tested by the pupillary light reflex. Any autonomic nervous system component of a cranial nerve has its own nuclei in the brainstem, and oculomotor is no exception. The Edinger-Westphal nucleus found next to the motor nucleus of oculomotor gives rise to parasympathetic fibers that exit as part of the oculomotor nerve. These cranial nerves are also related to the vestibular system associated with balance and equilibrium.

Visual Impairment

"Blind" is a term used frequently to denote an individual who has no visual perceptual ability at all. However, this is not completely true. Visual impairment—a term that is perhaps more accurate—is a highly variable disorder that ranges from low vision to complete loss of ability to see light. The visual impairment can be either unilateral or bilateral and can be congenital or acquired. Visual impairment can be used to describe impairments in visual acuity or visual field, and these will be addressed separately in sections that follow. Poor oculomotor or other cranial nerve control can also result in visual impairment, usually **diplopia**.

Impairment of Visual Acuity

Visual acuity is the sharpness or clarity of vision. The standard for normal or typical vision is 20/20. By comparison, a person who has 20/300 vision must be within 20 feet of an image a person with typical vision can see clearly at 300 feet.

Impairments of visual acuity are determined by the corrected acuity of the better eye. Let's return to the individual who has 20/300 vision in their better eye after correction with eyeglasses. To put this in perspective in terms of impairment of visual acuity, values in the range of 20/70 to 20/200 are characterized as "partially sighted." A visual acuity impairment that extends beyond 20/200 is considered legal blindness in the United States. For our example of 20/300 then, this individual would be considered legally blind. To be legally blind, a person does not have to have complete loss of vision.

Impairment of Visual Field

The normal or typical visual field includes the central visual field (i.e., the inner 30 degrees of vision and central fixation) and the peripheral visual field (i.e., 100 degrees laterally, 60 degrees medially, 60 degrees upward, and 75 degrees downward [Walker et al., 1990]). Any restriction of this field, whether central, peripheral, or both, will result in a visual field impairment. As was discussed under the physiology of the visual system, visual field perception is quite complex. There could be a host of visual field deficits depending specifically on where along the visual pathway a lesion or other damage occurs. The two visual field impairments most readily understood are tunnel vision and peripheral vision. With tunnel vision, the entire peripheral visual field is impaired so the individual can see only those things directly in front of them. With peripheral vision impaired, the individual's vision would be analogous to looking through a tunnel. Opposite this would be peripheral vision, where central vision is impaired and the individual can only see objects, people, and images to the sides, above, and below. In the United States, the legal definition of visual field blindness is a visual field restricted to 20 degrees or less.

Cortical Visual Impairment and Blindness

In a relatively small number of cases of visual impairment, the individual's visual system appears to be normal in terms of anatomy and physiology, and yet, the individual reports an inability to perceive by sense of sight. For such individuals, the most likely cause is cortical blindness. A lesion will likely be found along the visual pathway and most likely within the visual cortex in the occipital lobe of the brain. The most common etiology of cortical blindness is loss of oxygen to this region of the brain either due to loss of blood flow (especially via the posterior cerebral artery) or as a result of cardiac surgery. Cortical visual impairment or blindness is highly variable from person to person who exhibits the disorder. In some individuals, cortical blindness is not permanent, and the patient may regain some of their vision at some point. Regardless of the etiology or course of this disorder, visual cortical impairment or blindness can adversely affect the AAC system one employs with an individual who exhibits this impairment.

TYPES OF VISUAL IMPAIRMENTS

Similar to hearing impairment, many different types and degrees of visual impairment exist. Loss of visual acuity may range from slight to profound. Visual field loss may also range from slight to profound and may be predominantly peripheral, central, or both (Jan & Groenveld, 1993; Morse, 1990). A number of specific impairments of the peripheral and central visual system are associated with specific visual structures (Table 23-5).

Eye Muscle Disorders

Strabismus, a general term referring to abnormal ocular alignment due to disorders of any of six extraocular muscles, interferes with the eye's ability to fixate (Trief & Morse, 1988). Although not uncommon in children within the general population (3% to 4%), it occurs more frequently in preterm infants (15%; Nelson et al., 1987) and in persons with cerebral palsy (40%; Batshaw & Perret, 1992). Several conditions related to strabismus exist. Esotropia describes the turning inward of one or both eyes (a person who has bilateral esotropia would be "cross-eyed," to use common vernacular), whereas exotropia refers to the turning outward of one or both eyes. Treatment may involve eye patching, wearing of prescriptive lenses, surgical correction, and/or visual exercises. Amblyopia, characterized by a reduction in vision despite optimal visual management, is closely associated with and directly caused by strabismus (Trief & Morse, 1988). Early management of strabismus is important in preventing the development of amblyopia.

Corneal Disorders

Corneal disorders result in blurred or reduced visual acuity. Causes include herpes simplex, swelling of the cornea, inherited and degenerative disease, and toxic drug/chemical exposure (Batshaw & Perret, 1992; Erhardt, 1990; Hayes, 1985). The most common corneal disorder, refractive errors, affects more than 100 million Americans and is caused by misshaped corneas (Smith, 1982). Refractive errors range from mild to profound and include myopia (nearsightedness), hyperopia (farsightedness), and blurred vision due to astigmatism. Refractive errors are commonly corrected by prescriptive eyeglasses or contact lenses.

Corneal clouding may occur as a consequence of glaucoma, metabolic disorders, trauma, or riboflavin deficiency (Batshaw & Perret, 1992; Hayes, 1985). In severe cases, corneal transplantation is performed to yield rapid correction (Hayes, 1985).

Glaucoma

Glaucoma, a collection of diseases resulting in increased pressure in the anterior chamber of the eye, can lead to optic nerve damage, vision loss, and blindness. Although vision loss is usually peripheral, glaucoma can also affect central vision. It is predominantly age-related, yet it may occur at any time. Glaucoma is commonly associated with diabetes mellitus and with syndromes that include anatomic underdevelopment (Rosenthal, 1993). It may also develop as a consequence of cataracts, congenital infections, retinopathy of prematurity (ROP), trauma, or chronic inflammation. Both drug and surgical management of glaucoma may be appropriate. Although no specific cause or cure is currently known, early detection and management can preserve remaining vision for many individuals (Batshaw & Perret, 1992; Rosenthal, 1993).

Impairments of the Lens

Two common disorders, presbyopia and cataracts, relate to a loss of lens clarity and flexibility. Presbyopia, which occurs in many persons as a part of the aging process, involves reduced flexibility and accommodation of the lens resulting in blurred near vision. Prescriptive eyewear is often recommended.

A cataract is any opacity or clouding of the lens. Although small, stable cataracts may not impede light transmission, dense ones severely impair vision. Cataracts can develop at any time (even prenatally) as an isolated disorder or as part of a larger syndrome (e.g., Down syndrome, diabetes mellitus; Batshaw & Perret, 1992; Ponchillia, 1993; Rosenthal, 1993). Successful surgical removal is often completed on an outpatient basis.

TABLE 23-5

Visual Abnormalities Associated With Select Conditions and Syndromes

CONDITIONS/SYNDROMES	VISUAL ABNORMALITIES
Aging	Cataracts, macular degeneration
Brain damage	Amblyopia, cortical visual impairment, strabismus
Cerebral hypoxia	Cortical visual impairment
Cerebral palsy	Amblyopia, ocular motor dysfunction, optic nerve atrophy, refractive errors, retinal abnormalities, strabismus
CHARGE	Coloboma, iris choroid, optic nerve atrophy
Diabetes mellitus	Cataracts, glaucoma, optic neuropathy, retinopathy
Fetal alcohol syndrome	Optic nerve hypoplasia, retinopathy, strabismus
HIV	Retinopathy
Hurler syndrome	Clouded cornea
Lowe syndrome	Cataracts, glaucoma
Marfan syndrome	Dislocated lens
Maternal rubella	Amblyopia, cataracts, nystagmus, pigmentary retinopathy, strabismus
Prematurity	Retinopathy
Pre- or postnatal drug exposure	Strabismus
Tay-Sachs disease	Cherry red spot on macula, optic nerve atrophy
Trisomy 13, 18	Astigmatism, cataracts, coloboma, corneal opacities, hyperopia, microphthalmos, myopia, nystagmus, strabismus
Trisomy 21 (Down syndrome)	Astigmatism, cataracts, hypermetropia, myopia, nystagmus, strabismus
Turner syndrome	Cataracts, ptosis, strabismus
Zellweger syndrome	Cataracts, retinitis pigmentosa

Adapted from Alexander, P. K. (1990). The effects of brain damage on visual functioning in children. *Journal of Visual Impairment and Blindness, 84,* 372-376; Batshaw, M. L., & Perret, Y. M. (1992). *Children with handicaps: A medical primer* (3rd ed.). Paul H. Brookes Publishing Co; Chalifoux, L. M. (1991). Macular degeneration: An overview. *Journal of Visual Impairment and Blindness, 85,* 249-252; Morse, M. T. (1990). Cortical visual impairment in young children with multiple disabilities. *Journal of Visual Impairment and Blindness, 84,* 200-203; Nelson, L. B., Ehrlick, S., Calhoun, J. H., Matteucci, T., & Finnegan, L. P. (1987). Occurrence of strabismus in infants born to drug-dependent women. *American Journal of Diseases of Childhood, 141,* 175-178; Ponchillia, S. V. (1993). Complications of diabetes and their implication for service providers. *Journal of Visual Impairment and Blindness, 87,* 354-358; Regenbogen, L. S., & Coscas, G. C. (1985). *Oculo-auditory syndromes.* Masson Publishing; Trief, E., Duckman, R., Morse, A. R., & Silberman, R. K. (1989). Retinopathy of prematurity. *Journal of Visual Impairment and Blindness, 83,* 500-504; and Trief, E., & Morse, A. R. (1988). Strabismus and amblyopia. *Journal of Visual Impairment and Blindness, 82,* 327-330.

Retinopathy

Most cases of visual impairment in the United States can be attributed to disorders of the retina and choroid, the underlying tissue layer containing blood vessels (Trief et al., 1989). One type of retinopathy, retinitis pigmentosa, is a progressive disease that may initially cause night blindness eventually leading to severe vision loss.

Another type of retinopathy, retinoblastoma (retinal tumor), is usually diagnosed early in life. Often the affected eye is removed; however, a continued risk does exist for development of additional tumors in other areas of the body (Batshaw & Perret, 1992).

ROP was once thought to be directly attributed to high levels of oxygen administered to preterm infants shortly after birth. However, recent research indicates that birth weight and gestational age also factor into the occurrence and severity of ROP (Batshaw & Perret, 1992; Dekker & Koole, 1992; Trief et al., 1989, Wang et al., 2014). Given preterm infants are at risk for multiple impairments and ROP is incurable, early detection and management of visual impairments in preterm infants are critical.

Diabetic retinopathy is a retinal disorder closely related in occurrence and severity to the duration of diabetes. Medical management includes drug therapy, laser procedures, and surgery. As with ROP, diabetic retinopathy is incurable, and some individuals are nonresponsive to medical intervention (Rosenthal, 1993).

TABLE 23-6

Characteristic Differences Between Ocular and Cortical Visual Disorders

CHARACTERISTIC	OCULAR DISORDER	CORTICAL DISORDER
Appearance	Appears visually impaired	Usually appears normal
Close viewing	Common, used as means of magnification	Common, used as a means of magnification, to reduce crowding, or both
Color perception	Dependent on particular eye disorder	Preserved
Compulsive light gazing	Rarely	Common
Eye examination	Usually abnormal	Normal
Eye pressing	Especially noted in congenital retinal disorders	Never
Light sensitivity	Dependent on particular eye disorder	In one-third of cases
Peripheral field loss	Occasionally	Nearly always
Poorly coordinated eye movements	Present when congenital and early onset	Usually normal
Presence of additional neurological impairments	Fairly common	Nearly always
Rapid horizontal head shaking	Occasionally	Never
Sensory nystagmus	Present when congenital and early onset	Not present
Visual attention span	Usually normal	Markedly short
Visual function	Consistent	Highly variable

Adapted from Batstone, S., & Harris, G. (1990). *Questions regarding the functional vision of people with multiple disabilities with reference to communication needs*. Arbitrus Society for Children; Erhardt, R. P. (1990). *Developmental visual dysfunction*. Therapy Skill Builders; and Jan, J. E., & Groenveld, M. (1993). Visual behaviors and adaptations associated with cortical and ocular impairments in children. *Journal of Visual Impairment and Blindness, 87,* 101-105.

Other types of retinal disorders are associated with the macula. Because it is situated in the center of the retina, the macula provides the most acute vision and is particularly susceptible to damage. Macular damage will likely result in an individual having an impaired ability to perform visual tasks requiring close work (Chalifoux, 1991). Early warning signs include mild blurring in one eye; later, a central vision field blind spot may develop. Rapidly progressing wet macular degeneration occurs when blood vessels beneath the macula hemorrhage. This condition is treated with laser therapy. Dry macular degeneration (i.e., without hemorrhage) progresses at a slower rate and may stabilize at a level that allows the retention of some functional vision. However, it is generally unresponsive to treatment.

Visual Pathway Disorders

When the visual neural pathway, as opposed to the eye itself, is damaged anywhere from the lateral geniculate body up to and including the visual cortex (i.e., a central neurological disorder), cortical visual impairment will likely occur (Alexander, 1990; Jan & Groenveld, 1993). The damage may be localized within the brain's visual landmarks or generalized to various other cerebral areas (Morse, 1990). Individuals with cortical visual impairment often present unique visual, as well as general, behavioral characteristics. To assist AAC team members in differential diagnosis, Table 23-6 compares these characteristics with those that may typically be displayed by individuals with ocular (i.e., peripheral) visual disorders.

VISUAL ASSESSMENT

Visual assessment should be completed any time an AAC user is suspect for visual impairment even when testing cannot be conducted through usual methods (Hall et al., 1991). Although the primary criteria for determining visual impairment are visual acuity scores, additional standards are necessary because visual impairment is considerably more complex than what acuity scores or categories of scores might indicate (Sobsey & Wolf-Schein, 1996). Further, "[t]he use of vision is not an isolated phenomenon. It is one behavior within a large constellation of behaviors, all of which are influenced by interactions with the environment" (Morse, 1992, p. 77). Thus, no single test or approach is sufficient for examining the functional capacity of the visual system (Alexander, 1990; Bishop, 1988). Areas of both physiological functioning and functional visual use must be considered (Batstone & Harris, 1990; Erhardt, 1987; Sobsey & Wolf-Schein, 1996), and as is true in all areas of AAC service delivery, the efforts of many team members must be pooled to ensure appropriate identification and management. Just as the audiologist becomes a key member of the team serving the needs of AAC users with known or suspected hearing impairments, the vision specialist (e.g., optometrist and/or ophthalmologist) becomes a key member of teams working with AAC users with known or suspected visual impairments. Effective service delivery requires this collaborative effort because individuals who know the AAC user well may be unskilled in visual assessment whereas vision specialists may not know the unique needs and behaviors of the AAC user.

Areas of Assessment

Several sources provide detailed discussions of the essential components of visual assessment for individuals with multiple impairments (e.g., Atkinson, 1989; Bane & Birch, 1992; Bishop, 1988; Hall et al., 1991; Macht, 1971; Morse, 1992; O'Dell et al., 1993; Sacks et al., 1991, Sobsey & Wolf-Schein, 1996). Most of these procedures are specifically applicable to evaluating AAC users or can be effectively adapted.

Screening

A small number of formal and informal procedures are available to screen AAC users who are suspect for visual impairment (for example, see Atkinson, 1989). The first step in any of these screening procedures involves visual inspection of the eye and its typical behaviors to detect obvious cosmetic and/or motor manifestations of visual impairment (e.g., esotropia, exotropia, or nystagmus). Trief and Morse (1988) recommend systematic repetition of this visual inspection because many disorders of ocular alignment may change over time.

Although "[s]ubjective acuity tests are the single most effective tools available to screeners to determine the need for professional vision care" for individuals with multiple impairments (Cress et al., 1981, p. 43), several commercially available acuity tests recently have been criticized as being time-consuming, unreliable, and difficult to administer (O'Dell et al., 1993). However, screening procedures can and should be adapted to fit particular individual abilities, as demonstrated by Sacks and colleagues (1991) in their screening of adults with moderate to profound cognitive impairments. Subjects were able to perform subjective acuity tasks using the conventional Snellen chart, "E" chart, Allen picture chart, finger counting, and/or perception of a handlight.

When traditional methods of assessing visual acuity are not effective, one may use forced-choice preferential looking (FPL) procedures (Orel-Bixler, 1999). O'Dell and colleagues (1993) successfully screened individuals with severe to profound cognitive impairments using visual acuity cards in an FPL task. Further, Geruschat (1992) reported successful use of the Acuity Card Procedure in screening children with multiple impairments. Finally, Sobsey and Wolf-Schein (1996) developed a more recent FPL procedure using a microcomputer split screen that displays various images or patterns. The test taker's fixation on particular images or patterns provides an estimate of their visual acuity. Such FPL tasks can be used for visual screening with many AAC users because FPL places few communication demands on the individual (Bane & Birch, 1992; Birch & Bane, 1991).

Assessment

When an individual manifests behaviors during screening procedures or when general behavioral observations indicate that further diagnostic procedures are needed, more extensive evaluation should be carried out by the assessment team using both objective and subjective assessment tools (Bishop, 1988; Hall et al., 1991). Potential assessment tools (e.g., electrophysiological testing and more extensive FPL tasks) can be adapted by vision specialists or others under their guidance for use with AAC users. As part of the assessment, emphasis should be given to information gained from case histories, functional checklists, and behavioral observations (Atkinson, 1989; Hall et al., 1991; Jan & Groenveld, 1993; Sobsey & Wolf-Schein, 1996). Table 23-7 provides a summary of a visual assessment protocol that includes both formal and informal assessments.

A vision specialist who works collaboratively with other primary and secondary team members will likely be the primary member on the AAC assessment team for an individual with visual impairment. The speech-language pathologist may provide information regarding the visual demands of current and projected aided AAC methods, including information regarding the importance of illumination, size, space, contrast, color, and placement of graphic symbols. Team members may assist in preparing AAC users for assessment sessions by readying materials, adapting current AAC methods to facilitate responses or roleplaying the assessment scenario. Educational and/or vocational specialists can assess current skills and needs in educational and/or work environments and assist others in determining how unique visual and communication characteristics affect participation in functional activities (Dekker & Koole, 1992).

The orientation and mobility specialist is often an underused member of assessment teams (Bailey & Head, 1993), including those serving AAC users with visual impairment. The orientation and mobility specialist gathers data regarding the individual's current ambulatory and travel skills in the context of demands of the environment and then assists in developing and monitoring orientation and mobility recommendations (Joffee & Rikhye, 1991; Kelley et al., 1993). In reality, orientation and mobility services for AAC users may be difficult to obtain. As noted by Chen and Smith (1992), "[t]ypically, a more capable student will receive orientation and mobility instruction more frequently than the child who is multihandicapped. The assumption is that the more capable student will attain the skills and will become an independent traveller" (p. 134).

The ophthalmologist may conduct specialized assessment procedures to gather information about specific types of visual impairments, their potential etiology, and projected course. These procedures may include assessment of visual acuity, awareness, orientation and location, attention, fixation, and pursuit. Here, several forms of electrodiagnostic testing can augment subjective assessments (e.g., FLP tasks). These include electro-oculograms, electroencephalograms, visual evoked responses, visual evoked potential mappings, electroretinograms, and computed tomography scans (Alexander, 1990; Bane & Birch, 1992; Hall et al., 1991; Sacks et al., 1991).

Visual assessment may occur over an extended period and should be repeated as necessary throughout an AAC user's life span. Prior exchange of information between core AAC service providers and vision specialists who will be involved only on an intermittent basis will ensure optimal assessment. Various team members may assist with assessment adaptations, such as client and materials preparation, adapting seating/positioning, and acquiring and administering specialized tests similar to those described for AAC users with hearing impairments. Some of the adaptations AAC team members and vision specialists may consider in preparing for and conducting a functional visual assessment are listed in Table 23-8.

The necessity of ongoing visual assessment cannot be overemphasized. Too often, once a team has determined that no follow-up is possible or necessary, or that implemented management procedures (e.g., acquisition of prescriptive lenses) are adequate, an "abandoning attitude" develops (Hofstetter, 1991). Team members must observe an individual's functioning after management procedures are implemented or modified (Kelley et al., 1993). When no management has been initiated and there is still concern regarding visual functioning, the team should remain intact and continue to investigate other management strategies, as outlined in the next section.

FUNCTIONAL MANAGEMENT OF VISUAL IMPAIRMENT

AAC users with visual impairments require special considerations to facilitate maximal development of functional communication. The service delivery team must bear in mind AAC users' unique sensory, motor, concept development, social-emotional, academic, orientation and mobility,

TABLE 23-7
Summary of Vision Assessment Protocol

PROCEDURES/ PROCESSES	TYPE OF INFORMATION PROVIDED
Caregiver interview	Preferred items or activities; current and preferred visual patterns; current travel and mobility skills; muscle balance; motivation for intake of visual information; current visual needs
Case history	Family history; possible etiology; current estimates regarding auditory, cognitive, motor, tactile, and visual abilities; current AAC system use
Elicited observation	Discrepancies in current and potential skills in cognitive, motor, and visual abilities
Environmental assessment	Sensory demands of materials and routines
Natural observation	Preferred items or activities; current and preferred visual patterns; current travel and mobility skills; muscle balance; motivation for intake of visual information
Seating and positioning	Relationship between motor functioning and visual functioning
Visual ability testing	Presence or absence of refractive errors; near and far acuity; central and peripheral visual field; visual localization, fixation, and tracking

AAC = augmentative and alternative communication.

Adapted from Alexander, P. K. (1990). The effects of brain damage on visual functioning in children. *Journal of Visual Impairment and Blindness, 84,* 372-376; Bishop, V. (1988). Making choices in functional vision evaluation: "Hoodles, needles, and haystacks." *Journal of Visual Impairment and Blindness, 82,* 94-99; and Hall, A., Orel-Bixler, D., & Haegerstrom-Portnoy, G. (1991). Special visual assessment techniques for multiple handicapped persons. *Journal of Visual Impairment and Blindness, 85,* 23-29.

and vocational needs (Hazenkamp & Huebner, 1989). These needs, as related to receptive and expressive communication in general and to AAC use in particular, will require careful and ongoing attention. Because most aided and unaided AAC modes have a heavy visual component, issues related to illumination, size, space, color, contrast, and placement must be addressed. The AAC user's physical positioning, position in relation to an AAC device or display, visual demands entailed in using graphic symbols, and potential adaptation of both non–speech-generating and speech-generating devices all become important issues in AAC intervention when vision loss is suspected or confirmed.

TABLE 23-8
Adaptations for Visual Screening and Assessment

GENERAL CONSIDERATIONS

- Be aware of attention span and physical stamina. Frequent breaks may be necessary.
- Simplify procedures and materials to accommodate for the individual's level of functioning.
- Talk to and involve the person who uses AAC directly.
- Talk to and involve the accompanying caregiver directly.

PLAN AHEAD

- Inquire as to what specific information is desired from the assessment.
- Schedule ample time to complete the assessment and be prepared to break up the assessment over several appointments.
- Determine all assessment sites to be accessible and safe.
- Prepare or adapt materials to fit the functional needs of the person who uses AAC.
- Involve caregivers in training necessary examination behaviors, such as sitting in particular positions (if possible), tolerating the shining of light into the eyes, and fixating on a distant target.
- Determine the AAC user's preferred mode of communication and be prepared to allow responses in that mode.

AAC = augmentative and alternative communication.

Adapted from Atkinson, J. (1989). New test of vision screening and assessment in infants and young children. In J. H. French, S. Harel, & P. Casaer (Eds.), Child neurology and developmental disabilities. *Review, 25,* 57-66; Bane, M. C, & Birch, E. E. (1992). Forced-choice preferential looking and visual evoked potential acuities of visually impaired children. *Journal of Visual Impairment and Blindness, 86,* 21-24; Batshaw, M. L., & Perret, Y. M. (1992). *Children with handicaps: A medical primer* (3rd ed.). Paul H. Brookes Publishing Co; and Cress, P. J., Spellman, C. R., DeBriere, T. J., Sizemore, A. C., Northam, J. K., & Johnson, J. L. (1981). Vision screening for persons with severe handicaps. *Journal of the Association for the Severely Handicapped, 6,* 41-50.

A Framework for Intervention

AAC users with visual impairment are not a homogeneous group. Each individual represents a unique blend of strengths and needs, successes and failures, and cultural-ethnic backgrounds. Although AAC intervention must be individualized, three guiding principles that frequently shape service delivery for individuals with visual impairments can be applied to AAC users as well. They include: (1) optimizing residual visual abilities, (2) optimizing visual characteristics of stimuli (e.g., the AAC system), and (3) stimulating and/or training residual vision to maximal functional levels (Beevers & Hallinan, 1990; Boyd et al., 1990; Erhardt, 1987; Mann et al., 1993; Sobsey & Wolf-Schein, 1996; Sonksen et al., 1991; Tavernier, 1993; Uslan, 1992).

Optimizing Visual Abilities

An individual may receive less than the maximal possible visual signal due to undercorrection. Although approximately three-fourths of the general population makes use of some sort of corrective eyewear (The Vision Council, 2015), a much smaller proportion of individuals with multiple impairments seems to be fitted with corrective eyewear (O'Dell et al., 1993; Sacks et al., 1991). One possible reason for this may relate to the speculated inability of such individuals to independently manage their eyewear. Newer corrective lenses and procedures, such as extended-wear contact lenses and radial keratonomy, may hold merit for the management of certain visual impairments in AAC users because they require one-time or infrequent care and maintenance. Members of the AAC team must be persistent advocates for the prescription of appropriate visual correction devices. Team members must also ensure the ongoing monitoring of existing eyewear and advocate that a proper replacement schedule be followed (Tavernier, 1993; Trief & Morse, 1988).

Optimizing Visual Characteristics of Stimuli

AAC service providers hold a key role in optimizing the visual characteristics of stimuli relevant to an AAC user. For AAC users who rely on unaided forms of communication, the obvious factor to consider is proximity to partners in environments relatively free of visual and auditory noise. For AAC users who rely on aided methods, a whole host of issues becomes relevant. Enormous amounts of cognitive and motor energy may be expended when materials are not optimally designed and placed in a supportive visual environment (Erhardt, 1987, 1990; Tavernier, 1993). Maximizing the salient features of graphic symbols may facilitate more efficient processing of visual input, allowing voluntary attention to be directed elsewhere (Erhardt, 1987). Design, size, spacing, color, and illumination of graphic symbols must be considered for each AAC user and must be addressed concurrently with issues of motor functioning, cognition, audition, and tactile skills.

TABLE 23-9

Intervention Suggestions for Working With AAC Users With Visual Impairments

VISUAL
• Ensure maximal visual correction.
• Train localization to symbol display.
• Maximize ability to shift gaze from display to partner.
• Adjust display as needed for most comfortable viewing distance.

DISPLAY
• Use appropriate size, design, spacing, arrangement, color, contrast, and distance between symbols.
• Minimize visual noise and glare.

MOTOR
• Adjust trunk and head position to facilitate maximal intake of visual information.
• Allow for frequent positional changes to accommodate for motor fatigue.
• Ensure optimal distance between AAC user and display.

ENVIRONMENT
• Ensure appropriate seating and positioning for trunk support and head control.
• Provide sufficient illumination, without glare.
• Present stimuli within the AAC user's field of vision, at an appropriate angle and distance.
• Provide tactile and/or auditory supports.

AAC = augmentative and alternative communication.

Adapted from Batstone, S., & Harris, G. (1990). *Questions regarding the functional vision of people with multiple disabilities with reference to communication needs.* Arbitrus Society for Children; Downing, J. E., & Eichinger, J. (1990). Instructional strategies for learners with dual sensory impairments in integrated settings. *Journal of the Association for Persons with Severe Handicaps, 15,* 98-105; and Van Hedel-Van Grinsven, R. (1989). Communication and language development in a child with severe visual and auditory impairments: A case study and discussion of multiple modalities. *Review, 26,* 153-162.

Assessment of trunk and neck position, head control, and range of motion should be conducted to determine symbol position(s) to optimize motor movements (see Batstone & Harris, 1990, as well as Chapter 16). Because many AAC users demonstrate motor fatigue over time, the assistive communication device itself, as well as the size and structure of its symbols, may need adjustment to accommodate coordination between motor and visual movements and most comfortable viewing distance. Although many service providers attend to issues of comfortable loudness level in regard to auditory stimuli, far too few are aware of the need to adjust for a similar component in the visual system (consider, for example, the natural adjustments individuals without disabilities make during reading or TV viewing). Thus, an important part of AAC service delivery for individuals with visual impairments is to offer multiple symbol arrangements, distances, and positions.

An additional issue regarding position is worth noting. To achieve a steady visual gaze, some individuals (e.g., those with nystagmus or central vision deficits) may actually shift the head away from the viewed object. This is usually a functional, self-taught compensatory behavior and should not be discouraged (Batstone & Harris, 1990; Blischak, 1995).

AAC service providers working with individuals with documented or suspected visual impairments may learn critical skills from the efforts of individuals who work with the general population of individuals with low vision. For example, early Braille instruction can be optimized when the size and vertical and horizontal spacing of Braille symbols has been customized (Pester et al., 1994). Customizing the size, spacing, contrast, color, and illumination of graphic symbols may similarly facilitate optimal use of residual vision in AAC users. Table 23-9 details several intervention suggestions.

Simple tactile enhancements, such as texture, may be provided to add a third dimension to graphic symbols. More sophisticated tactile enhancements, such as the inclusion of Braille features as part of an overall symbol set/system or the use of Braille as the sole symbol system, may also be considered. Other sources of technology or technology features (e.g., the auditory scanning feature of several SGDs) that may benefit AAC users with visual impairments are well reviewed (e.g., Blischak, 1995; Boyd et al., 1990; Coleman & Meyers, 1991; Locke & Mirenda, 1988; Noyes & Frankish, 1992; Rowland, 1990). Although "[a]ssistive technology is recognized as key to independence for individuals with disabilities because it provides a means of access to the mainstream society" (Uslan, 1992, p. 402), acquiring such technology is a challenge for members of AAC teams working with AAC users with visual impairments. One example of AAC and other assistive technology used by a child with physical and visual impairments was described in a case study of Thomas by Blischak (1995). Thomas successfully used a switch-activated SGD with auditory scanning, corrective lenses, and magnification in his elementary school classroom.

Stimulating and/or Training Residual Vision

Research has documented that typically developing children up to age 10 years have the capacity to strengthen the neurological processes responsible for vision (Gellhaus & Olson, 1993). Because 90% of the population with visual impairments retains some degree of usable vision, the logic behind early and aggressive visual stimulation and training is obvious (Morse, 1990; Tavernier, 1993). A rich environment that includes varying sensory stimuli and experiences is crucial if individuals with visual impairments are to reach maximal skill levels. Without visual stimulation, irreversible underdevelopment of the visual system may occur (Potenski, 1993; Sonksen et al., 1991).

Visual stimulation denotes presentation of visual stimuli to individuals who have little or no reaction to objects in the visual environment, whereas vision training refers to attempts to enhance the skills of individuals who demonstrate some involvement with objects (Tavernier, 1993). Typically, stimulation is implemented using operant conditioning strategies or by the presentation of highly contrasting visual stimuli (e.g., under black light conditions; Sonksen et al., 1991). A gradated program involving scanning, recognition, and perception has been beneficial in vision training. Both procedures may hold merit for individual AAC users to stimulate interest in visual information, particularly when functional consequences are tied to the procedures (Batstone & Harris, 1990).

INTRODUCTION TO DUAL SENSORY IMPAIRMENT AS A DISABILITY

The heterogeneous nature of the population of individuals who experience DSIs cannot be overstated. Dual sensory loss is a disability that is exponentially more than a hearing loss plus a vision loss; it is a unique disability (Bashinski, 2011b). DSIs may be due to **congenital**, developmental, and acquired (i.e., **adventitious**) factors. Historically, individuals who experience dual sensory loss have constituted one of the lowest incidence categories of disability; this trend continues to the present day.

Four Primary Categories of Dual Sensory Impairment

For purposes of instructional intervention, including the determination of needs for communication augmentation, four functional categories of DSI are crucial for consideration. The primary determinant that differentiates these four categories is the time in the individual's life when the loss occurred. Congenital hearing and/or vision loss is generally defined as occurring prior to the age of *approximately* 2 years (Munroe, 2001). First, some children may experience both vision and hearing losses congenitally (e.g., complications of prematurity, CHARGE, trisomy 13). Second, other individuals might acquire both a vision and a hearing loss later in life (e.g., Usher syndrome type III, traumatic brain injury, or an individual who acquires both glaucoma and a hearing impairment as part of the aging process). Third, some children experience congenital vision loss, but develop a hearing loss later in life (e.g., meningitis, Meniere's disease). Fourth is a child born with hearing loss who acquires a vision loss later in life—even at differing rates (e.g., Usher syndrome types I and II).

In regard to hearing impairment, the most critical question to be answered is whether or not the child had developed language prior to their loss of hearing ability. In regard to vision loss, the key is whether or not the child had developed visual memory prior to their loss of vision.

COMMON ETIOLOGIES OF DUAL SENSORY IMPAIRMENT

More than 70 specific etiologies are listed as identified causes of DSI in the National Center on Deaf-Blindness' 2019 census report, which includes individuals from birth to 21 years of age (National Center on Deaf-Blindness, 2020). At least 13 unique etiologies are cited as the cause of at least 100 cases of dual sensory loss, across all four primary etiologic categories that have been identified (i.e., hereditary syndromes, prenatal/congenital complications, postnatal complications, and complications of prematurity) in the population of children and youth 21 years of age and younger. Other identified etiologies are extremely rare with fewer than five cases (e.g., Alport syndrome, Marfan syndrome, Hunter syndrome) reported nationally across the United States. It is estimated that 17.22% of individuals with identified dual sensory loss, birth through 21 years, have no determined etiology for their DSI (i.e., 1,830 of 10,627 nationally; National Center on Deaf-Blindness, 2020).

Specific etiologies of DSI present unique challenges and characteristics for interprofessional teams planning AAC programs for individuals who demonstrate each diagnostic category of dual sensory loss. A few of the most common etiologies are discussed in the following.

Complications of Prematurity

Premature birth is associated with a wide variety of both short-term and long-term problems for the baby. Not all babies born prematurely experience complications, but generally speaking, the earlier a baby is born the greater the risk of difficulties. Not only does timing of a premature infant's birth affect their potential for developing sensory problems, birth weight plays an important role as well. Particularly at risk for dual sensory loss are infants born "very prematurely" (i.e., at less than 32 of the typical 40 weeks of pregnancy) and those described as "extremely preterm" who are born at or before the 25th week of pregnancy (Mayo Clinic, 2017b).

ROP, formerly called retrolental fibroplasia, is a condition that develops when blood vessels in the back of the eye show excessive growth and swelling in the retina. The result of this overgrowth might be retinal scarring or detachment; if untreated or not treated sufficiently promptly, these conditions can result in vision impairment. Premature babies are also at increased risk of hearing loss to some degree (Mayo Clinic, 2017b). ROP occurs primarily in babies born between 23 and 28 weeks gestation or who weigh less than approximately 2 pounds, 3 ounces—though ROP is not limited to infants in these categories. In as many as 90% of babies who evidence ROP, the disorder resolves itself with no treatment (Texas School for the Blind and Visually Impaired, n.d.).

For the past several years, the single most commonly identified cause of DSI of children and youth on the national child count maintained by the National Center on Deaf-Blindness has been and continues to be complications of prematurity (i.e., 1,050 children and youth, 9.88% of total; National Center on Deaf-Blindness, 2020).

Generally speaking, individuals whose DSI is attributable to complications of prematurity demonstrate greater degrees of loss in vision than in auditory skills; most retain at least some functional hearing ability. Augmentative communication intervention for individuals with this etiology is influenced significantly by the presence or absence of additional disabilities—many of which are also correlated with premature birth (e.g., cerebral palsy, intellectual disability, attention-deficit/hyperactivity disorder). AAC programming teams for an individual with dual sensory loss due to prematurity must consider their motor abilities (particularly of the upper extremities) and intellectual skills in order to design an appropriate intervention plan. Individuals with this diagnosis should have ongoing, regularly scheduled vision checks.

CHARGE

CHARGE is an exceptionally complex, highly variable genetic condition that presents uniquely in the individuals it affects—across multiple ethnicities and approximately equally in males and females. Though individuals with CHARGE do share similar characteristics and areas of need, there is no such "typical" individual with this condition.

The incidence of CHARGE is estimated to be one in every 8,000 to 10,000 births (CHARGE Syndrome Foundation, 2022). CHARGE is the principle hereditary/syndromic cause of congenital dual sensory loss in the United States. On the national child count maintained by the National Center on Deaf-Blindness, the prevalence of CHARGE has shown a consistent upward trend in recent years. The most recent deaf-blind census reported 1,033 individuals with CHARGE syndrome—9.72% of the total population identified, birth through 21 years of age (National Center on Deaf-Blindness, 2020).

In the majority of cases, CHARGE results from mutation in at least one gene, *CHD7*, which impacts development of the neural crest very early in embryonic development. Many of the 12 cranial nerves that innervate the head and neck (thereby controlling the auditory, visual, and olfactory sensory systems, as well as muscle functioning in the face, mouth, throat, and neck) are affected by the *CHD7* mutation. As a result, "[m]ore than 90% of individuals with CHARGE have both vision loss and hearing loss (classified as deafblindness)" (Hartshorne et al., 2011a, p. xii). In 2017, Bashinski and colleagues found that 92.59% of their study participants with CHARGE (25 of 27 children and youth ages 3 to 29 years) experienced DSI. The majority of participants retained some functional vision though hearing losses occurred in the severe to profound range.

Though the communication profiles of individuals with CHARGE vary tremendously, it is generally accepted that both receptive and expressive communication abilities are delayed (Bashinski, 2011a). "The biggest barrier to ultimate success for individuals with CHARGE is communication. Those children who are able to establish abstract communication in childhood ultimately do far better than those who do not. The barriers to communication are legion" (Hartshorne et al., 2011a, p. xi).

AAC intervention is particularly challenging with individuals who exhibit CHARGE not only because of their dual sensory losses but also due to their lack of facial muscle control and general motor weakness. However, it is projected that approximately 60% of these individuals do eventually develop symbolic language skills (Miller et al., 2011; Swanson, 2011). It is not unusual for individuals who experience CHARGE to require lengthier periods of time to process language (Bruce et al., 2018).

Usher Syndrome

Usher syndrome, a rare inherited condition, is the most common genetic cause of dual sensory loss across the lifespan in the United States. Evans (2017) estimates that approximately 3% to 6% of individuals in the United Kingdom who are born deaf will develop Usher syndrome in their lifetimes. The Usher Syndrome Coalition (2019) estimates that more than 400,000 people worldwide experience one type of Usher syndrome. It is approximated that Usher syndrome accounts for almost one-half of all people who experience acquired

DSI (Moller, 2003). The condition involves hearing loss or deafness and the progressive loss of vision due to **retinitis pigmentosa**. Three discrete types of Usher syndrome have been identified; each is characterized by a unique profile of hearing, vision, and balance characteristics.

An individual who has Usher syndrome type I typically is born with a bilateral, severe to profound, sensorineural hearing loss. During the early elementary school years, a visual field loss is usually identified (i.e., retinitis pigmentosa results initially in night blindness, followed by a narrowing of the visual field—tunnel vision); the vision impairment typically progresses to total blindness in adulthood. In almost all cases, the individual's sense of balance is affected because of dysfunction of the **vestibular** system.

A person with Usher syndrome type II experiences a bilateral, moderate to profound sensorineural hearing loss at birth. The progressive loss of vision is typically noted during the middle to late teenage years but might not appear until adulthood. Generally, this loss does not result in total blindness even in adulthood. The majority of individuals with Usher syndrome type II do not experience significant balance problems.

Individuals who experience Usher syndrome type III are usually born with normal hearing or only a mild, bilateral hearing loss. Sensorineural hearing loss begins in the majority of cases during late childhood or the adolescent years; the impairment becomes progressively more severe, generally to a profound level. These individuals' vision loss usually develops in late childhood or during the teen years (similar to Usher syndrome type II). A portion of individuals with Usher syndrome type III develops vestibular and balance problems (Genetics Home Reference, 2017; Minnesota DeafBlind Project, n.d.; Usher Syndrome Coalition, 2019). Usher syndrome type III is the rarest, accounting for approximately 2% of all Usher cases (Genetics Home Reference, 2017).

Infants and toddlers with Usher syndrome type I consistently demonstrate language delay due to their significant hearing loss. Recent studies estimate that 8% to 10% or more of children who are congenitally deaf or hard of hearing exhibit Usher syndrome (Usher Syndrome Coalition, 2019), but because these children are the first in their families to be diagnosed with a hearing loss, their diagnoses of deafness and Usher syndrome are often delayed. Due to their impairments in the vestibular system, these children also demonstrate delayed motor skills (e.g., crawling, walking). For these reasons, these children are frequently labelled as having developmental delay or intellectual impairment (Minnesota DeafBlind Project, n.d.).

Implications of Usher syndrome for AAC intervention vary dramatically by type. With children with Usher syndrome types I and II, one foundational concern is the reliability of intelligence testing; these children's intellectual ability is often underestimated. The potential impact on expectations for both communication achievement and education in general can be significant. Because individuals with type I experience deafness at birth, the most appropriate communication augmentation for them is going to be similar to those AAC interventions discussed previously in this chapter under Hearing Impairment. By stark contrast, individuals who experience Usher syndrome type III do not generally experience sensory loss until after the development of speech, so they will likely not require AAC intervention during their school years and will continue to utilize verbal expressive communication.

Other Syndromic Conditions

A recent deaf-blind census by the National Center on Deaf-Blindness (2020) reports etiologic data regarding a wide variety of hereditary syndromes and disorders. In addition to those syndromes discussed in detail here (i.e., CHARGE and Usher syndromes), the following four represent the next most frequently identified genetic syndromes among the 10,627 individuals with DSI included in that census. Along with the frequencies with which each was reported, the syndromes included: (1) Down syndrome (3.29%), (2) Stickler syndrome (1.29%), (3) Dandy Walker syndrome (1.14%), and (4) Goldenhar syndrome (1.02%). In total, approximately 47.45% of the children and youth represented in this most recent census experience DSI due to some identified hereditary syndrome.

Cytomegalovirus

Babies who are infected with CMV before birth are at higher risk for manifesting a variety of long-term developmental disabilities. However, it is important to note that not all infants born with CMV demonstrate signs at birth, and approximately only one in five babies with congenital CMV infection will manifest long-term health problems (Centers for Disease Control and Prevention, 2018). However, for this small group of infants, long-term health consequences may be significant.

Babies who are sick at birth because of CMV tend to show significant symptoms. Not only are hearing and vision impairments commonly associated with congenital CMV, so too are premature birth, low birth weight, microcephaly, and seizure disorders (Mayo Clinic, 2017a). General developmental delays across all skill domains often characterize individuals with a diagnosis of dual sensory loss associated with CMV. A few babies with congenital CMV appear typically healthy at birth; however, they can develop symptoms over time, sometimes not for months or years after birth (Mayo Clinic, 2017a). Hearing loss in the moderate to severe/profound ranges is one of the most common of the late-occurring signs of congenital CMV—even for infants who pass a newborn hearing screening exam. Some babies also experience late onset vision loss due to retinitis.

The most recent deaf-blind census reported CMV as the second most frequently occurring prenatal/congenital complication that resulted in DSI in the population birth through 21 years of age (National Center on Deaf-Blindness, 2020).

This report cited 307 children and youth (2.89% of total) who experienced dual sensory loss due to CMV. The total percentage of individuals included in this census, whose DSI is attributed to prenatal/congenital complications, was reported as approximately 13.79%.

Generally speaking, individuals whose DSI is attributable to congenital CMV infection demonstrate greater degrees of loss in hearing than in visual skills; most retain at least some functional visual ability. AAC intervention for individuals with this etiology is influenced significantly by the presence or absence of additional disabilities, many of which are also correlated with premature birth (e.g., microcephaly, seizure disorder, muscular discoordination, and/or intellectual disability; Mayo Clinic, 2017a). AAC programming for an individual with dual sensory loss due to CMV must consider the presence or absence of additional disabilities in order to design intervention appropriately. Individuals with a diagnosis of congenital CMV, whether or not they showed characteristics at birth, should have ongoing, regularly scheduled hearing checks.

Cephalic Disorders

Hydrocephalus is the excessive accumulation of cerebrospinal fluid within the skull. The most common causes of hydrocephalus in infants and young children include complications of prematurity, including brain hemorrhage. Though most cases of hydrocephalus are diagnosed in children 2 years of age and younger, in older children and adults, traumatic head injury, meningitis, and tumors can result in this condition (National Institute of Neurological Disorders and Stroke, 2019).

As a result of the accumulation of excessive cerebrospinal fluid in hydrocephalus, pressure on the brain continually increases unless the condition is treated (most commonly by the surgical insertion of a shunt that drains the fluid to another part of the individual's body to be absorbed through the typical circulatory process). Left untreated, the increased intracranial pressure can result in blindness and a continuing loss of intellectual function (National Organization for Rare Disorders, 2007). In some cases, hearing loss may also result.

Microcephalus is a condition in which the circumference of the head is smaller than is typically expected because the brain prematurely stopped growing or did not develop properly. Microcephaly is often present at birth, but the condition may develop during the first few years of life (MedicineNet, n.d.). The most common causes of microcephalus include a variety of genetic syndromes, some viruses (including CMV and rubella), and environmental toxins or drugs to which a fetus may be exposed during pregnancy. Often, atypical brain development leads to the smaller head size. As a result of abnormal brain growth and development, losses in vision and/or hearing may result, as well as impairment of intellectual function and motor development. The extent and degree of impaired function are associated with the location(s) of the underdeveloped/abnormally developed brain tissue.

The National Center on Deaf-Blindness (2020) census reported cephalic disorders (i.e., hydrocephaly and microcephaly combined) as the most frequently occurring prenatal/congenital complications, which resulted in DSI in the population birth through 21 years of age. This report cited 475 children and youth (4.47% of total) who experienced dual sensory loss due to hydrocephaly ($n = 243$, or 2.29%) or microcephaly ($n = 232$, or 2.18%). Though approximately one to two children in 1,000 live births are diagnosed with hydrocephalus, the vast majority benefit from medical treatment and/or rehabilitation therapies and show no signs of sensory impairment. The majority of children diagnosed with microcephalus will demonstrate some sort of developmental disability primarily associated with the syndromic cause of the condition. A portion of this population will experience DSI.

Generally speaking, individuals whose DSI is attributable to hydrocephalus demonstrate greater degrees of loss of vision than auditory skills. AAC intervention for individuals with this condition is influenced significantly by the presence or absence of additional disabilities, particularly seizure disorder, a lack of muscular coordination, and/or intellectual disability (National Organization for Rare Disorders, 2007). AAC programming for an individual with dual sensory loss due to hydrocephalus must consider the presence or absence of additional disabilities in order to design intervention appropriately.

AAC programming for an individual who experiences DSI due to microcephaly will need to take into account the presence or absence of comorbid disabilities. Most common among these are generally delayed motor function (including speech), facial distortion, motor coordination problems, seizure disorder, and/or intellectual disability. A small percentage of children diagnosed with microcephaly will demonstrate intellectual skills within the expected developmental range (MedicineNet, n.d.).

Trisomy 13 and 18

Trisomy 13 and trisomy 18 are separate genetic conditions, both of which result in a significant communication disability associated with impairments of the eyes and ears. Trisomy 13, also known as **Patau syndrome**, occurs with an incidence of approximately 1 per 5,000 births (Petry et al., 2013). It is estimated that less than 20% of infants born with trisomy 13 survive beyond the first month of life (National Institutes of Health—Genetic and Rare Diseases Information Center, 2015). Vision and hearing impairments are typically moderate to severe. The majority of children who do live beyond 1 month of age (a few reports exist of children with trisomy 13 surviving into adolescence) generally communicate at a pre-linguistic level—most have no expressive speech but do utilize expressive gestures. Their auditory comprehension typically exceeds these individuals' expressive abilities (Braddock et al., 2012; Bruce et al., 2015).

Trisomy 18, also known as **Edwards syndrome**, also occurs at a rate of approximately one per 6,000 to 8,000 live births. It is estimated that only 5% to 10% of infants born with trisomy 18 survive beyond 12 months of age (Cereda & Carey, 2012; Simpson, 2013). Hearing impairment is typically moderate to severe; vision impairment is more variable. Children with trisomy 18 usually retain some functional vision though they do experience both anatomic and physiologic differences in their vision system. Cortical vision impairment is not unusual in this population. The majority of children who do live beyond 1 year generally communicate in ways previously described regarding trisomy 13 (Braddock et al., 2012; Bruce et al., 2015).

Characteristics of Individuals Who Experience Dual Sensory Impairments

Two key questions to ask when assessing whether or not a learner experiences dual sensory loss are: (1) Does the individual have sufficient vision to allow them to fully function as an individual who experiences only a hearing impairment? and (2) Does the individual have sufficient hearing to allow them to fully function as an individual who experiences only a vision impairment? If the answer is not "yes" to "... both these questions without reservation, the individual should be considered Deafblind" (McInnes, 1993, p. 223).

DSI is a disability associated with information gathering. Access to information about the external world is limited for an individual diagnosed with this condition. Because dual sensory loss affects two of an individual's three distance senses (i.e., vision, hearing, smell), it necessitates that the individual uses their impact senses (i.e., taste, touch, kinesthesis) to gather information about the world external to their body.

General Characteristics

Depending on the degree and type of a particular individual's vision and hearing losses, most individuals with this condition require direct teaching as opposed to secondary or incidental learning to benefit from instruction (Bashinski, 2011b; Brown et al., 2020). Partnering with a learner with DSI involves building connections with them and inviting the individual out of their body to join the external world. Individuals with DSI need to have the opportunity to learn and interact in an enhanced context in order to know what is happening around them. The individual's interaction partners need to consider the immediate physical, visual, and auditory environmental contexts of every activity in which they will engage. Due to the extra energy required to process sight and sound stimuli, many individuals with DSI fatigue more rapidly than their peers.

Individuals with dual sensory loss often demonstrate inconsistent responses to sounds and/or visual images. They may demonstrate difficulty interacting with things in the environment in a meaningful way and/or a distorted perception of the world due to lack of nondistorted information from the distance senses. Many individuals in this population perceive time very differently. A percentage of individuals who experience DSI demonstrate heightened tactile sensitivity or tactile defensiveness (Chen & Downing, 2006) particularly around the face; several display an overactive startle response. Many individuals with DSI exhibit various stereotypies to minor or major degrees out of fear, confusion, and/or sensory deprivation. They may experience challenges counteracting boredom (Bashinski, 2011b).

Specific Characteristics Regarding Communication Development

As noted previously, individuals who experience DSIs are incredibly heterogeneous. This condition is exponentially more than a hearing loss plus a vision loss; it is a unique disability. The communication development and programming needs of any given individual are going to vary according to three critical variables: (1) the time of onset of the individual's vision and hearing losses, (2) the type(s) of vision and hearing impairment, and (3) the degrees of vision and hearing loss. That said, some characteristics are shared across a majority of the population of individuals who exhibit DSI.

An individual with DSI needs to be alerted to the availability of a partner to begin a communicative interaction, as well as the identity of the person. Conversely, when the partner leaves the immediate area of the individual who exhibits DSI (i.e., becoming unavailable for further interaction), the individual with DSI needs to be told the interaction is about to end.

An individual who has DSI needs to understand concepts through more than one sensory/communicative mode; that is, they need communication partners to use multimodal communication. Most individuals with DSI require extended time to respond during a communicative interaction.

Many individuals, particularly those with early onset DSI, experience difficulty communicating with others in a meaningful way. They require support to learn to establish and maintain interpersonal relationships. These individuals also often experience difficulty with generalization and so must be taught to utilize their language and communication skills across partners and communicative environments. Deliberate instruction on how to make choices is an important communicative skill many individuals with dual sensory loss require (Bashinski, 2011b).

AAC NEEDS OF INDIVIDUALS WHO EXPERIENCE DUAL SENSORY IMPAIRMENTS

The first, most essential characteristic of an AAC program for a person who exhibits DSI is that it be individualized. Due to the extreme range of visual skills (e.g., acuity, field, onset of impairment), hearing abilities (e.g., degree of loss, dB range of loss, conductive vs. sensorineural loss, onset of impairment), and motor skills (e.g., hand dexterity, facial expression, ambulation) that characterize persons with this diagnosis, the AAC program must be customized for each individual.

Second, it is crucial that the AAC program be designed to enable the individual who exhibits DSI to clearly communicate in functional ways across a variety of authentic, natural environments.

Third, the AAC system designed for the individual with dual sensory loss should facilitate concise, efficient communication exchanges without bombarding the person with extraneous, nonessential information. However, this caveat should not be interpreted to mean that all small talk should be avoided! AAC programming should equip the individual who has DSI to engage in meaningful conversations that address the full range of communicative functions.

Finally, the team responsible for designing an AAC program for an individual with DSI should take into account whether or not they have, or could benefit from, the support of an **intervener**. An intervener, typically a paraeducator, provides consistent one-on-one support to a learner with DSI (3 to 21 years of age) through their instructional day. Certification standards for interveners have been adopted (Council for Exceptional Children, 2015) to guide interveners' specialized training in DSI. The purpose of an intervener is to provide access to environmental information gained by learners who are typically developing through vision and hearing, but which might be unavailable or incomplete for an individual who has impaired vision and hearing. Additionally, an intervener provides support to help the learner with DSI to form reciprocal relationships with others, increase the learner's social and emotional well-being and communication skills, and facilitate the learner's participation in a variety of activities (Beukelman & Mirenda, 2013; National Consortium on Deaf-Blindness, 2013).

Contrast of Total Communication and Multimodal Communication

Total communication was proposed in the late 1960s to make spoken language structures more visually transparent, and hence, easier for deaf children to understand and acquire. Total communication involves the simultaneous presentation of manual signs and speech throughout a complete communication exchange. This approach (also referred to as simultaneous communication) allows parallel production and processing of manual signs and speech.

Multimodal communication, on the other hand, refers to the selective use of various modes of communication, including verbal/vocal, aided, and unaided forms. Particular forms are chosen for a specific expression, dependent on environmental context, content, and availability, in an effort to ensure maximally successful information exchange. Multimodal communication is more the rule than the exception in typical everyday communication exchanges. Especially when a given situation makes both visual and auditory reception possible, as in most face-to-face interactions, communication partners typically tend to combine speech, gestures, pointing, and handling of objects. Multimodal functioning is highly natural (Beukelman & Mirenda, 2013).

Mode Selection for Receptive and Expressive Communication

For many individuals who experience DSI, modes for both receiving and expressing information may be the same. For example, an individual with Usher syndrome type II (i.e., congenital, bilateral, moderate-profound sensorineural hearing loss and late onset of progressive vision loss typically not resulting in total blindness) might use manual signs for both receptive and expressive purposes. However, for many individuals who experience DSI, the way in which the individual receives information might necessarily be different from the way in which that individual expresses information.

Determinations of optimal modes for each communication channel should depend on both the type of vision and hearing losses an individual experiences and the relative strengths of their visual, auditory, and motoric skills. For example, an individual with congenital, bilateral, sensorineural hearing loss but with moderate visual acuity might first be considered a candidate for an AAC system focused on manual signs. However, when the interprofessional team planning for this individual considers the fact that they have extreme muscle weakness and limited fine motor control (due to CHARGE), the recommendations of the team should change. In this instance, a key word signing approach would be very appropriately adopted for this young person's receptive mode of communication, but an appropriate expressive communication system for them may consist of a variety of aided forms (e.g., objects, pictures, speech-generating technology). For an individual who has only light vision (due to complications of prematurity) but who experiences only mild-moderate hearing loss, the most appropriate recommendations of the team might include tactile sign for receptive communication but verbal speech for expressive communication needs.

Major Categories of AAC With Individuals Who Experience Dual Sensory Impairments

Manual Signs

A comprehensive discussion of the use of manual sign as an unaided AAC system was provided in Chapter 8 of this textbook. In this section, only those aspects unique to manual sign use in communication programming for individuals who experience DSIs as an AAC intervention will be discussed. In particular, five variables will be addressed:

1. Distance of the communication partner from the individual with dual sensory loss
2. The size of the physical space in which manual signs are produced
3. The location of the space in which signs are made
4. Distance of sign production from the face of the individual with DSI
5. The role visual feedback plays in the production of manual sign

Due to tunnel vision as a result of retinitis pigmentosa (which is associated with all three types of Usher syndrome), the individual's visual field narrows as their vision loss progresses (Genetics Home Reference, 2017; Usher Syndrome Coalition, 2019). As this occurs, it is very common for the individual's communication partners to need to *increase* their distance from the individual with DSI in order for them to be able to visually perceive all manual signs. Concomitantly, the sizing of the partner's signs might also need to be reduced to enable the individual with significant tunnel vision to see them all. In the cases of individuals with dual sensory loss who do not experience a visual field loss but whose visual acuity is diminishing, the communication partner might need to *decrease* the distance between the two of them in order for the manual signs to be seen clearly.

Generally speaking, the size of the manual signing space used by individuals who experience dual sensory loss is more restricted than the signing space utilized by individuals who are deaf (Emmorey et al., 2009). Evans (2017) describes this use of smaller space in British Sign Language as "visual frame signing." She goes on to explain that the restricted sign space keeps the individual's manual signs within their own visual field "… to enable utilization (sic) of residual vision" (p. 2330). Individuals with DSI due to Usher syndrome and those who experience functional blindness due to other etiologies both

> … produced signs within a smaller signing space … but we hypothesize that they did so for different reasons. Signers with tunnel vision may align their signing space with that of their interlocutor. In contrast, blind signers may enhance proprioceptive

feedback by producing signs within an enlarged signing space for monologues, which do not require switching between tactile and visual signing. (Emmorey et al., 2009, p. 99)

Further, Emmorey and colleagues (2009) found that the signing space of the individual with DSI increased when the person became totally blind, possibly because at that point the individual was released from the need to visually monitor their own sign productions.

Depending on the nature of the vision loss of the individual who experiences DSI, the signing position of the communication partner might need to be changed from the standard, which is directly in front of the person. If the individual's central visual field is lost and only peripheral vision remains, the partner will need to stand to the side of the individual with DSI. Consequently, the communication partner's use of space will necessarily be altered as well. Emmorey and colleagues (2009) observed that a significant number of individuals with Usher syndrome produced manual signs at a raised level from the standard positions for many signs (e.g., the sign for "introduce," typically made near the waist, was shifted to shoulder level).

Emmorey and colleagues (2009) also observed differences in the distance of the production of manual signs from the faces of individuals with DSI. Signers with tunnel vision (e.g., those individuals who experience Usher syndrome) produced a greater proportion of their manual signs near their faces than did manual sign users who were normally sighted or blind and did not differ from one another. It is hypothesized that perhaps this practice was developed to keep an individual's own manual sign production from disappearing and then reappearing within their own visual field.

Finally, Emmorey and colleagues (2009) investigated the role of visual feedback during ASL conversations. They concluded that visual feedback does play some role during the production of manual signs. These researchers hypothesized that manual signers utilized "… visual feedback to phonetically calibrate the dimensions of signing space, rather than to monitor (their) language output" (p. 99).

Gestures

"Communication occurs long before language is developed with prelingual communication often expressed through body movements, vocalizations … and gestures" (Bruce et al., 2016, p. 74). During the earliest stage of nonsymbolic communication development, children use unconventional/idiosyncratic gestures, including body posturing, to express their needs. Gestures constitute a natural target for instruction since they are readily understood by numerous partners, no equipment is needed to utilize them, and gestures can be used across many different contexts. It is important to remember that appropriate gestural use is very heavily influenced by the individual's culture, age, environmental context(s), and their motor skills (Bashinski, 2012). Chapter 8 goes into this topic in greater detail.

In a hallmark advancement regarding the development of communicative gestures, Wetherby (2014) demonstrated in a number of studies that typically developing children should use at least 16 gestures by 16 months of age (16by16). She and her colleagues have demonstrated that the development of gestures between 9 and 16 months of age predicts language level 2 years later (Caselli et al., 2012; Watt et al., 2006; Wetherby, 2014). During this critical period for gesture development, children's expressive gestures shift from idiosyncratic to conventional forms.

A pilot study by Brady and Bashinski (2009) attempted to develop an efficacious adaptation of pre-linguistic milieu teaching (PMT) for use with children who experience dual sensory loss. PMT is a well-established intervention approach for a variety of learners with developmental disabilities or language delay (Fey et al., 2006; Warren et al., 2006; Warren & Yoder, 1998), though participants in none of these cited studies experienced sensory loss. Brady and Bashinski's adaptation (2009), referred to as A-PMT, targeted the instruction of natural gestures (with or without accompanying vocalizations) in child-focused, one-on-one activities with children with DSI. Gestures targeted for instruction were, for the most part, drawn from Wetherby's 16by16 (2014) with the adaptation of some to "eye gestures" for those learners who experienced concurrent severe motor disability (e.g., purposefully closing eyes, turning head away, visually fixating on an object). Overall adaptations included using more physical prompts than in other forms of PMT and using means other than directed eye gaze to determine directionality of gestures. All nine participants increased their rates of self-initiated, intentional communication during the course of intervention. The children who experienced significant motor disability in addition to DSI made less substantial gains as a group. All nine participants acquired both new forms of gestural communication ($x = 6$; e.g., gives to partner, reaches, extends open hand, points) and the functions for which both previously used and new forms served ($x = 7$), though a majority of functions involved protesting or requesting of some sort (e.g., object, action, attention, assistance, continuation). Most importantly, the self-initiated communication rate of the participants who did not also experience significant upper extremity motor disability averaged an increase of 59 communication acts in a 45-minute period. Brady and Bashinski (2009) demonstrated that gestures both provide effective augmented comprehension support and constitute a viable mode of communication expression for individuals who experience dual sensory loss. The participants' gestural gains also contributed to facilitating the progress of individuals who experience dual sensory loss from preintentional to intentional communication (another cited benefit of Warren and Yoder's initial work regarding PMT [1998]). The reader is referred to Chapter 8 for additional information.

Tactile Communication Approaches

For individuals who experience DSI, tactile communication approaches are sometimes the forms of choice for augmenting receptive and/or expressive communication. A carefully selected tactile mode can serve as an alternative communication channel to compensate for information typically received and expressed through auditory and visual means. Many communication approaches used with individuals who exhibit DSI (e.g., object cues, tangible symbols, touch cues) are broadly applicable for persons with severe developmental disabilities. No singular sequence for introducing various types of tactile communication approaches has been identified. Each individual has unique strengths and needs. Each situation is different.

Object Communication

Concept development associated with objects occurs naturally with infants who are typically developing because of the constant flow of information they experience. However, for the vast majority of children who experience congenital dual sensory loss, object concepts must be directly taught. The degree to which object concepts must be learned is tempered by the degrees of each child's sensory losses, but particularly vision. Basic object concepts many children learn include the facts that objects exist in the world (i.e., are external to their own bodies), have permanence, are different from one another, have names and a variety of characteristics, and serve a function or use. In addition to learning these basic object concepts, many children with DSI will need to learn and rely on objects as formal cues to the people, places, things, and activities that occur in their various environments (Bashinski, 2013a).

An object cue is defined as "… an object or part of object used to refer to a person, place, object, or activity … to provide a concrete means of supporting conversational interactions and language development" (Chen et al., 2005a, p. 1). Object cues may consist of whole objects or parts of objects (e.g., whole object—cup to mean "time for lunch"; partial object—section of backpack strap to mean "time to go home"). Object cues have obvious relationships to their referents and are therefore generally easily understood. Care needs to be taken to differentiate an object cue from the actual object to which it refers by mounting the cue on some sort of firm background (Bruce et al., 2011; Rowland & Schweigert, 2000a). Object cues as components of an individual's communication system should have an obvious tactile relationship with their referents (whenever possible) and be small in size to enhance portability (Bashinski, 2013a; Chen et al., 2005a).

When an interprofessional team is considering the use of objects to enhance an individual's comprehension of communication, several questions need to be asked. Does the individual have sufficient motor ability to actively explore and interact with the object in a meaningful way? Do they have sufficient sensory ability to process the object's features? Additionally, the team should consider the individual's preferences when selecting object cues. Miniatures should always be avoided because they are visually based referents (Chen et al., 2005a; Miles & Riggio, 1999). When using object communication, partners should share the object cue with the learner, that is, touch and handle the cue with the learner and engage in interaction about the object cue's referent (Bashinski, 2013a).

Textures

A majority of individuals who experience DSI respond positively to enhanced textures; the sense of touch is generally an important avenue for gathering information. Although textured symbols are less complex than other AAC symbols based on tactile information (e.g., braille, tactile sign), they are definitely more abstract than object cues and tangible symbols (Murray-Branch & Bailey, 1998). Textured symbols are artificial; they are generally not visually associated with their referents in any way (Beukelman & Mirenda, 2013). Typically, textured symbols are created from pieces of bubble wrap, various grades of sandpaper, plastic netting, pipe cleaners, felt dots, corrugated cardboard, various types of fabric, or glue dots arranged in various patterns on small cards.

"A textured symbol is permanent, tactually unique, and instantly recognized when in contact with the skin surface or when touched" (Murray-Branch & Bailey, 1998, p. 5). Each texture should be distinctive so it can be associated with a unique object, person, place, or activity. The textured symbols should each have a uniform surface and be recognizable from any orientation (Chen et al., 2005c; Murray-Branch & Bailey, 1998). They may be utilized for both receptive and expressive communication.

When an interprofessional team is considering the use of textures/textured symbols to enhance an individual's communication development, it is critical to select textures that are tactilely salient and developed with a particular individual's tactile preferences in mind; they are unique to each individual. It is essential that the individual be able to tactilely discriminate textured symbols. When introducing these to the individual who experiences DSI, it is important that team members use tactile modeling and "… create conversations through mutual tactile attention" (Chen & Downing, 2006, p. 117).

Tangible/Tactile Symbols

Rowland and Schweigert (1989, 2000a) first used the term "tangible symbol" to refer to symbols that are permanent, highly iconic, two- or three-dimensional, easily manipulated through simple motor movements, and tactilely discriminable. They are used to represent people, places, objects, activities, and concepts; tangible symbols are obviously related to the properties of their referents. For referents that do not automatically lend themselves to a visual or textural representation (e.g., concepts, locations, some activities), the individual's team must artificially create a symbol.

Highly similar to object cues, the purpose of tangible symbols is to provide concrete support for an individual's language development and social interactions. Like object cues and textured symbols, they are discriminated by touch—shape, consistency, and texture. Unlike object cues and textures or textured symbols, tangible symbols may be two-dimensional (Flener & Nygard, 2015; Rowland & Schweigert, 2000b).

Tangible symbols have become widely accepted as a communicative intervention for individuals who have DSI, particularly those with complex and multiple disabilities (Trief et al., 2010). Rowland and Schweigert (1989a) first demonstrated that tangible symbols positively impact the communication development of learners with DSI, even bridging a few of their participants' communication from nonsymbolic to symbolic.

Over the last 30 years, some residential schools for the blind in the United States have developed their own standardized sets of tangible symbols. The most well-known of these is the directory of symbols created at the Texas School for the Blind and Visually Impaired, which includes more than 300 symbols (Hagood, 1992). The efforts of the state schools for the blind network "… led to the development of more commercial (tangible) symbol programs. In recent years the American Printing House for the Blind developed the Tactile Connections Kit and Guidebook" (Flener & Nygard, 2015, p. 18). In 2009, Trief and colleagues developed a standardized set of 55 tangible symbols and topics at the request of educators and related services professionals for use in public schools. These symbols were shown to be efficacious in a follow-up field study (Trief et al., 2013) conducted with 43 learners with DSI who attended four different schools and received services in 21 classrooms.

To this day, various researchers continue to argue the relative benefits of an individualized tangible symbol system (Chen et al., 2005b) and a standardized system (Trief, 2013). Advantages and disadvantages of each system design can be identified. Therefore, when considering tangible symbols for incorporation in the communication program for an individual with DSI, the team should consider not only the type and degree of the individual's sensory losses but also the individual's age and the number of major environmental and residential settings the individual is likely to experience in the future. Use of a standardized system is likely to transfer to new communication contexts more smoothly.

Touch Cues

Scientists recognize that human beings require touch from others. Touch has been shown to yield benefits for both physical and mental health (Cohut, 2018; Keltner, 2010). The saying, "To touch can be to give life" has long been attributed to Michelangelo.

During his work in The Netherlands in the 1960s, Jan van Dijk developed a movement-based approach with children who experience DSI. He concluded (1966) that touch and movement assist learners with dual sensory loss to come out into the world and engage with others. Three of the primary themes of van Dijk's work were to view a child holistically, reverse a child's inwardly directed behavior, and develop reciprocal turn-taking skills. Through clearly articulated stages, van Dijk suggested strategies that systematically integrated touch in his interactions with these children. He encouraged touching/feeling early on, as well as close proximity to the learner (to enable the determination of muscle tone) and maintenance of high levels of physical contact. Van Dijk suggested teachers use hand-under-hand strategies for exploration. This work forms the foundation for the systematic use of touch cues today. In addition to learning basic tactile skills, many learners with DSI need to learn to use touch as a formal cue for understanding the people and events in their various environments (Bashinski, 2013b).

A touch cue is defined as "… a physical prompt made in a consistent manner directly on the body to communicate with a child" (Chen & Downing, 2006, p. 33). Touch cues are used to communicate a variety of purposes (e.g., greeting, requesting, seeking information). "Touch cues may reduce startle or inappropriate behaviors by helping the child anticipate what is about to happen. Touch cues signal the communication (partner's) intent" (Chen et al., 2005d, p. 1) to the individual with dual sensory loss. Examples include gently pulling on the individual's upper arms (i.e., "Get ready to stand"), touching the adolescent's left elbow (i.e., "This is the way I say 'Hi,'" so the learner knows the partner's identity) or rubbing the middle of a child's back (i.e., "I like that!").

When an interprofessional team is considering the use of touch cues to enhance an individual's comprehension of communication, several important variables must be considered. Identify any severe neurological disability that might affect the individual's ability to perceive a touch cue. Carefully select the type and placement for a touch cue (i.e., generally speaking, a firm touch cue is preferred by more individuals than a light stroke). Choose touch cues that should be easy for the individual to differentiate from routine physical contact. Consider the individual's preferences when selecting both the type of, and placement for, a touch cue. Most importantly, never force an individual to accept a touch cue or engage in mutual "touch conversations" (Bashinski, 2013b; Chen & Downing, 2006).

Specific assessment of the ways in which an individual with DSI uses touch must be completed (e.g., how they use hands and for what purpose, what forms of touch they use, how the individual uses muscle tone and gross body movements). Assessment should also be conducted regarding ways in which the learner responds to touch, whether with signs of awareness, reflexive behavior, attention, alerting, recognition, discrimination, and/or comprehension of the touch or tactile stimulus. The individual's responses to both the provision of mutual tactile attention and tactile modeling by a communication partner are both important as

well (Chen & Downing, 2006). Finally, the interprofessional team considering the use of touch cues with an individual who experiences dual sensory loss should assess their tactile environments:

- How and when does the child have physical contact with others (e.g., at recess, playing with peers)? How does the child respond to these physical interactions?
- How and when does the child have opportunities to explore, handle, and use materials (e.g., during a lesson on the ocean, were shells examined)?
- How is the environment organized to encourage movement and tactile exploration (e.g., does the room have specific activity areas; is the floor uncluttered; are materials available or accessible to the child)?
- What supports and adaptations are needed to facilitate the child's exploration and manipulation of objects (e.g., how does the assistant or peer introduce materials to the child's hand)? (Chen & Downing, 2006, pp. 55-57)

Tactile Sign Language

One of the most basic forms involving a tactile sign approach to communication is "signs on body." "*Signs on body* [italics provided] are different from *touch cues* [italics provided] because they are standard manual signs that are produced on the child's body" (Chen & Downing, 2006, p. 125). As previously explained, touch cues consist of very individualized prompts made on the body of an individual who experiences dual sensory loss to enhance the individual's comprehension. Signs on body are abstract symbols used to represent objects, activities, persons, places, etc., and involve one distinct touch or movement; signs on body are utilized for communicative expression. Using signs on a child's body as an introductory stage for tactile communication is an excellent starting point for a child who is being considered a candidate for tactile communication because this approach "… helps the child obtain tactile information about the hand shape and other characteristics of the sign by allowing time for the child to explore the hand shape" (Chen & Downing, 2006, p. 126).

A second tactile sign language approach is co-active signing. This approach consists of "… physical guidance of a child's hand or hands to facilitate production of a standard manual sign for expressive communication" (Chen & Downing, 2006, p. 33). The use of co-active signing may be interspersed throughout an interaction with an individual who exhibits DSI and used in conjunction with touch, object, and movement cues, as well as speech. The primary purpose of co-active signing is instructional, to help an individual learn how to produce a new manual sign. Co-active signs (as well as tactile signs) are much more complicated than signs on body for the individual with dual sensory loss to decipher since they involve multiple, complex movements and touches.

"The term *co-active signing* [italics provided] is derived from van Dijk's terminology 'coactive movement' or moving together" (Chen & Downing, 2006, p. 126). It is critical when implementing co-active signing with an individual that all manual signs be produced from the perspective of the individual with dual sensory loss and not inadvertently reversed (i.e., produced from the partner's perspective). A co-active signing approach might not be effective with individuals who demonstrate tactile defensiveness, who simply do not like their hands to be manipulated, or who have limited upper extremity movement (MacFarland, 1995). If this approach is adopted, communication partners need to take care to decrease the amount of physical guidance as soon as possible to reduce the likelihood of the individual becoming dependent on physical assistance in order to produce manual signs (Chen & Downing, 2006).

After an individual with dual sensory loss has been introduced to co-active signing, the natural progression for instruction would be to begin to expose the individual to formal tactile sign language. An individual with DSI who opens their hands, makes minimal hand movements, accepts tactile input, and is able to maintain physical contact with another person's hands or object for at least a few seconds should be considered a candidate for tactile sign language instruction.

In this method, the individual who experiences DSI places either one or both hands on the communication partner's dominant signing hand and traces the signing motion to tactually receive information. An individual with dual sensory loss may learn to use tactile sign language for both receptive and expressive communication or produce sign language visually for expression but receive communicative information via tactile sign language.

Tactile sign language is "… commonly used by individuals with DSI who acquire their knowledge of sign language before becoming blind" (Beukelman & Mirenda, 2013, p. 50). This statement was affirmed in a recent investigation by Checchetto and colleagues (2018). These researchers studied Italian Sign Language and found that facile users of tactile Italian Sign Language most often competently utilized a visual sign system first before transferring to a tactile system because of an acquired vision loss.

Research suggests that tactile sign language users do have the potential to become conversationally competent, especially in cases of individuals who build tactile sign skills on a previously existing knowledge base of visual sign (Checchetto et al., 2018). Tactile sign language users demonstrate only slightly slower rates of receptive communication. Beukelman and Mirenda (2013) found that tactile sign reception approximated 1.5 signs per second, a favorable comparison with the 2.5 sign-per-second rate of sighted signers' reception of manual signs. Finally, tactile fingerspelling should be mentioned here, although this technique is explained later under "Other Tactile Methods."

Print-on-Palm

The print-on-palm method involves tracing numbers or letters of the alphabet, one at a time, on the palm of one hand of the individual who experiences DSI. It is this method of message transmission that resulted in the method's name. In some cases, the individual with DSI prefers the tracing be conducted in the center of their back. Functionally, this alternative serves the same purpose.

Regardless of the method of delivery (i.e., to a palm or the center of an individual's back), the communication partner of the individual with DSI must be aware of and take into consideration the cultural traditions of the individual with DSI. Cultures around the world embrace different social customs, particularly regarding ways in which touch is viewed and especially between individuals of different genders and age groups.

Tadoma Method

Tadoma is an approach to communication that is unique to individuals who experience DSI. In this method, the individual who exhibits DSI places their thumb on a speaker's lips and their fingers along the speaker's jaw. The middle three fingers of the person with DSI rest along the speaker's cheek and their little finger is in contact with the speaker's throat to pick up vibrations of the speaker's vocal cords. Through these vibrations, physical contact, movements of the speaker's jaw, and facial expression, the individual with DSI is able to decipher the speaker's spoken words. Though learning to communicate through the Tadoma method is difficult and very time-consuming, fluent Tadoma users have demonstrated the ability to comprehend up to 40 words per minute (Tabak, 2006).

Other Tactile Methods

Generally speaking, these additional tactile methods for communication require that both the individual with dual sensory loss and their partners have good literacy skills. In addition to the specific tactile communication approaches discussed here, AAC programming for individuals who experience dual sensory loss might include gestural Morse code (i.e., tapping out the dits and dahs that make up the alphabetic letters or other characters on any part of the person's body) or **Braille hand speech** (i.e., positioning the fingers to represent the configurations of the braille alphabet then touching the arm or hand of the individual with DSI with these finger configurations).

Use of an **alphabet glove** requires the individual who has DSI to wear a thin glove that has numbers and letters of the alphabet printed across the individual fingers. The communication partner then touches the appropriate areas of the fingers to spell out words to comprise a message. Once the individual with DSI and their communication partners memorize the positions of the composition elements, this method can be utilized without the glove.

Cards embossed with braille or raised alphabet letters may be utilized by persons who exhibit DSI. The communication partner places the finger of the individual with DSI on each raised symbol to spell a message for them to receive. Conversely, the individual with DSI touches the raised braille or printed letters for the communication partner to read.

Social haptic (Sense, 2019) consists of the presentation of tactile signs commonly made on the back of an individual with DSI (though they may be made anywhere on the individual's body) to supplement information they receive through other modes of communication. The signs utilized in haptic communication are used to enhance descriptions of the physical environment, people and their emotional responses, and other information typically provided through vision.

The **Lorma alphabet** is the alphabet used by persons with DSI in Poland. It was developed by Heinrich Landesmann under the pseudonym Hieronymus Lorm in the 19th century. Use of this alphabet involves drawing lines or points on the hands of communication partners, one to the other. A few examples of this alphabet include the vowels (i.e., A, E, I, O, U) corresponding to the tips of the four fingers and thumb, in order. The letter Y is a horizontal line that crosses the fingers; the letter S involves drawing a circle in the palm of the hand (M. Książek, personal communication, September 8, 2017). Using this system, the individual with DSI may be either the sender or receiver of information.

Tactile fingerspelling may also be utilized to communicate with individuals who exhibit dual sensory loss. In this approach, the hand of the person with DSI is placed over the hand of the partner who is formulating a message using the alphabetic letters of a manual alphabet (Beukelman & Mirenda, 2013). An individual who experiences DSI may function as both the receiver and the sender of information using the tactile fingerspelling method (Evans, 2017).

IMPLEMENTATION OF AAC PROGRAMMING WITH INDIVIDUALS WHO EXPERIENCE DUAL SENSORY IMPAIRMENTS

Most vital to AAC intervention is the tenet that all AAC programming with individuals who exhibit DSI occurs within authentic, natural contexts. AAC intervention activities should be embedded within meaningful, functional routines in the person's home, school/work environment, and community (Bruce & Bashinski, 2017; Downing et al., 2015; Luckner et al., 2016; Rødbroe & Janssen, 2006; Trief et al., 2013).

Challenges

The challenges that confront the families and educational teams of individuals with DSI vary quite significantly based on the severity and time of onset of an individual's vision and hearing losses. Several characteristics a majority of children and young adults with congenital DSI demonstrate may also be representative of adults who experience intellectual and other disabilities in addition to their sensory losses. Many of these characteristics present challenges for families of these individuals and for educational teams trying to develop effective AAC programs for them. Individuals with congenital DSI are likely to be deprived of many of the most basic intrinsic motivations (i.e., curiosity), which lead to exploration within their environments. Auditory and visual stimuli are distorted to the point they are ineffective sources of motivation. Typically, these children and young adults are not likely to benefit from being left alone for long periods of time even with so-called motivating toys and materials. They generally do not independently learn from their mistakes due to an inability to understand the results or impact of their actions on others. Most individuals who experience congenital sensory losses and/or DSI in combination with other disabilities cannot benefit from incidental learning. Their families and interprofessional teams must directly teach AAC skills through consistent, systematic instruction. Similarly, group instruction likely will not be beneficial because these individuals typically cannot learn from watching and listening to others. Many individuals with DSI lack the ability to anticipate events (Bashinski, 2011b).

In general, the challenges associated with developing and implementing AAC programs for individuals who exhibit adventitious DSI and Usher syndrome (particularly types I and II) are very different in nature. Challenges facing families and teams of children with Usher syndrome types I and II are associated with teaching communication and language skills to a child who experiences severe/profound bilateral hearing loss. Additionally, these families, teams, and children themselves face practical and emotional challenges associated with the inevitable progressive loss of vision in the future. Proactive AAC decision making involves knowing when to begin to implement strategies and materials to teach the child to compensate for the increasingly limited visual function they will experience. Not only is timing an issue here. Families and children with Usher types I and II must deal with the emotional upheaval that is very frequently associated with this condition.

Even individuals with Usher syndrome who experience postlingual DSI report challenging situations associated with work, recreation, and routine daily activities. The majority of participants in an investigation by de Andrade Figueiredo and colleagues (2013) responded that their DSI interfered with interpersonal relationships, even relationships with family members and their circle of friends. The most frequently mentioned challenges experienced by study participants were dealing with feelings of isolation, the impossibility of continuing employment, and experiencing mobility problems in and outside their homes. The emotional challenges (including fear, anxiety, and depression) faced by these individuals, their families, and their educational/rehabilitation teams should not be underestimated (Genetics Home Reference, 2017; Usher Syndrome Coalition, 2019).

Finally, one of the most pragmatic challenges facing interprofessional teams responsible for designing and implementing AAC programming with individuals with DSI is simply the very wide range of AAC options that must be considered. Several of these options are unique to the population of individuals with DSI (e.g., tactile approaches), but teams should not limit their consideration to only these possibilities. Team members are challenged by time and the need to keep their personal knowledge current in regard to available AAC technologies.

Individual Presentation of Vision and Hearing Losses

The DSI section of this chapter began with the assertion that the heterogeneous nature of the population of individuals who experience this condition cannot be overstated. As the chapter begins to draw to a close, it is important the reader be reminded of this certainty. As families and educational teams meet to plan the most effective AAC systems possible for individuals who have DSI, they are requested to take into account all the information presented in the two major previous sections of this chapter—"The Sense of Hearing" and "The Sense of Vision." Deaf-blindness is unquestionably much more than a hearing impairment plus a vision impairment. Nonetheless, information regarding the types (e.g., conductive, sensorineural; unilateral, bilateral; CAPD) and degrees (e.g., mild to profound, frequencies within the speech range) of hearing loss and the types (e.g., acuity, field, cortical visual impairment) and degrees (e.g., fluctuating, night blindness) of vision loss presented in those two sections is critically important. Families and teams of individuals who exhibit DSI are well advised to consider all such information when planning for implementation of AAC programming with individuals who experience DSI.

A number of specific etiologies associated with the condition of DSI are discussed in this chapter. It is important for an interprofessional team to be aware of the etiology of an individual's DSI since many syndromic and pre-/perinatal conditions do share common characteristics. However, the team should simultaneously bear in mind the variability of individuals who share the same diagnosis.

For example, awareness that a child has a diagnosis of Usher syndrome type I affords the family and team the opportunity to prepare for what is likely to be a fairly rapid onset of progressive vision loss (a common characteristic of this syndrome). No one can predict, though, how a particular child will respond emotionally to their changing vision,

how receptive they and the family will be to the introduction of tactile supports for language and learning, or the rate and pattern with which the vision loss will present itself and proceed. An infant born with CHARGE is likely to spend 3 to 6 months in a hospital by the time they are 2 years of age. Approximately 50% of these infants will eventually catch up with developmental milestones (M. Hefner, personal communication, July 28, 2017). A percentage of these individuals with CHARGE demonstrate above-average intelligence, will graduate from college, hold professional jobs, and self-manage the complex medical and psychological issues associated with this condition. AAC intervention for these individuals needs to focus only on strategies for supplementing their residual auditory and visual skills to enhance their communication effectiveness and satisfaction. However, the developmental rates and patterns of the remaining 50% of infants and young children who experience CHARGE are very likely to be extremely variable. A portion of these individuals is likely to never successfully bridge to symbolic communication. AAC intervention for these children will hardly resemble AAC intervention for the group of individuals with CHARGE first described here.

A discussion of the individual presentation of vision and hearing losses in individuals with DSI would be incomplete if it did not highlight the percentage of etiologies of DSI that are associated with progressive sensory loss(es). Usher syndrome comes to mind as the primary example of this phenomenon. Usher is associated with both progressive vision and hearing loss. CMV (discussed in this chapter) is often associated with progressive hearing loss, as are Mondini syndrome and age-related effects of persons who already experience a vision loss of some sort. In addition to Usher syndrome, glaucoma and macular degeneration are age-related conditions that can result in a later-in-life diagnosis of DSI.

One final point regarding consideration of the individual presentation of hearing and vision losses of individuals with DSI deserves mention. Professionals with wide-ranging areas of expertise must be involved in assessment and program planning for AAC with individuals who experience DSI. Professionals with particular expertise in sensory (e.g., teacher of students with visual impairment, deaf/hard-of-hearing educator) or motor development (e.g., physical therapist, occupational therapist) must lead modification of environments to ensure the individual's needs are considered and their ability to use residual sensory and motor skills is maximized. A teacher of students with visual impairment, speech-language pathologist, and classroom teacher may contribute ideas about iconic, concrete, or abstract representational options, size of options, and arrangement of the array for a learner's choice-making activities. An audiologist or teacher of the Deaf may contribute information regarding appropriate amplification, enhancement of auditory stimuli, and preferred positioning for an interpreter or intervener. Physical therapists and occupational therapists may contribute ideas about proper body positioning and how to best present options in choice-making routines in the most physically accessible manner, as well as appropriate positioning of all AAC displays, switches, representations, and SGDs. DSI is a very complex disability; appropriate AAC intervention requires the participation of multiple family members and professionals working together as a collaborative team (Bruce & Bashinski, 2017).

Preparation of Communication Partners for Interaction

Generally speaking, typically developed motor, language, and literacy skills are required of individuals who will serve as effective communication partners for persons who exhibit DSI. Most importantly, all persons who are communication partners for an individual with DSI need to expect them to be able to communicate! Potential communication partners for the individual need to maintain a positive attitude and attune themselves to even subtle cues from the individual with DSI. Attunement can be described as the process of the communicative partner "… drawing forth and enhancing the (individual's) attention and involvement, pacing and modifying her acts in coordination with signs from the (individual)" (Janssen & Rødbroe, 2007, p. 14). The importance of partners' responsiveness cannot be overrated. However, partners do need to remember that it will take some time for the individual with DSI to establish a sufficiently trusting relationship with them before communication initiation is likely to occur.

Individuals who have DSI demonstrate different levels and types of communication skills with familiar and unfamiliar partners. Typically, these individuals will demonstrate more frequent and more effective communication with familiar communication partners in familiar environments because they are likely to feel less anxious, less stress, and more comfortable to ask for assistance or a break (Bashinski, 2018).

When partnering with an individual with DSI who communicates primarily at a nonsymbolic level (see Chapter 8 for details), the responsibility for a successful communicative interaction rests with the partner. The partner must interpret the idiosyncratic forms expressed by an individual who is performing at this level, treating these as if they were intentional by drawing from the communicative context and their knowledge of the individual. Partners' acknowledgement of even potentially communicative signals shows respect for the dignity of the person who has DSI. It is equally important that the partner, and all other potential partners for the individual, respond as consistently as possible over time. Partners' repeated interpretations of an individual's unconventional communicative signals over time will shape both intentionality and conventionality. As the individual with DSI begins to communicate using more conventional expressive signals, the magnitude of the partner's role diminishes, though some interpretation will likely still be required (Bashinski, 2018; Bashinski & Bruce, 2018).

When the individual who experiences DSI understands and expressively uses conventional expressions consistent with their culture and primary language, they have achieved a symbolic level of communication. At this stage, equal communication partnership in which both partners share responsibility for successful interaction can be achieved.

Communication partners should address the individual with DSI directly, not through an interpreter, intervener, or anyone else. Partners need to be in close, yet respectful, proximity to the individual who experiences DSI. They might enhance the individual's receptive communication development by describing things that are happening or are about to happen (individuals who experience more severe sensory losses often experience difficulty anticipating events). The nature of DSI requires an individual's partner to deliberately plan how the individual with DSI will receive information in every activity and what that individual will do in every activity in order to express themselves (Bashinski, 2011b).

Criticality of Interprofessional Collaboration

"Effective IPCP [interprofessional collaborative practice] in communication intervention considers the learner's characteristics, the knowledge and skills required of communication partners, and effective environmental arrangements to support communication" (Bruce & Bashinski, 2017, p. 162). Family members and service providers who participate on an interprofessional team tasked with designing an effective AAC system for an individual with DSI have very different interpersonal experiences with the individual, as well as different areas of expertise. Exemplary interprofessional collaborative practice involves team members, including both hearing and vision specialists, building a more extensive base of collective knowledge by sharing their diverse perspectives and engaging in collaborative problem solving. These practices, directed toward the goal of optimizing the individual's participation, constitute the basic tenets of interprofessional collaborative practice (Bruce & Bashinski, 2017). For these reasons, it is essential team members engage in ongoing interprofessional collaboration in regard to planning and implementation of an AAC program, particularly early intervention teams and teams of individuals who experience multiple, complex disabilities—including DSI (Braddock, 2015; Ogletree, 2017).

Benefits

Without support of their families and an invested interprofessional team, individuals who experience DSI are likely to experience feelings of anxiety and isolation. Even when provided with ongoing support, many communicatively competent persons with Usher syndrome report such feelings along with challenges in establishing and maintaining interpersonal relationships, finding and holding a job, and even performing the routine activities associated with daily living (de Andrade Figueiredo et al., 2013).

The vast majority of individuals who experience DSI would not reach their maximum communicative potential without appropriate AAC intervention and programming. The earlier the onset and the greater the severity of an individual's sensory disabilities, this likelihood only increases. Particularly in the case of children who experience congenital DSI, the need for AAC intervention is intensified. Without intervention—even minimally appropriate communication augmentation—this group of children is likely to struggle to interact meaningfully with the external world (of which they are likely to be generally unaware).

At the very least, educational and rehabilitation teams for individuals who experience DSI should strive to implement AAC programming that targets the development of functional communication skills. The American Speech-Language-Hearing Association defines this basic level of communicative achievement as "… forms of behavior that express needs, wants, feelings, and preferences that others can understand" (n.d.d, https://www.asha.org/NJC/Definition-of-Communication-and-Appropriate-Targets/). One very noteworthy benefit of AAC teams striving to establish at least functional communication skills with individuals who exhibit DSI is that this achievement frequently results in the individual being able to express themselves without having to resort to challenging behaviors.

Stated simply, the benefit of AAC intervention is central to quality of life, as well as meaningful participation in activities of everyday living, for an individual with DSI and their family. Other than the treatment of any potentially life-threatening health conditions, communication is consistently identified as the top-ranking priority for persons who experience DSI. Individuals with DSI "who are able to establish abstract communication in childhood ultimately do far better than those who do not" (Hartshorne et al., 2011b, p. xi). It is the responsibility of AAC interprofessional teams to exert their best efforts to help individuals achieve this success.

CONSIDERATIONS FOR SUCCESS IN THE IMPLEMENTATION OF UNAIDED COMMUNICATION COMPONENTS

The achievement of successful unaided AAC implementation with an individual who has DSI must begin with consideration of the types and degrees of their vision and hearing losses but also take into account the individual's motor abilities and intellectual skills.

Unaided AAC predominates neither receptive nor expressive communication intervention with the population of individuals with DSI as an entire group. Some individuals will use unaided forms to receive information from communication partners (e.g., touch cues, signs on body, manual sign, the Tadoma method, tactile sign language); others will utilize gestural forms and/or manual signs to express information. Some individuals who experience DSI will rely on unaided communication modes for both their receptive and expressive needs; others will require or prefer aided forms of AAC (see next section).

When considering unaided AAC elements as components of an individual's receptive communication repertoire, one of the first assessments to be completed is of the individual's level of symbolization (i.e., does the individual demonstrate understanding that one thing can stand for another?). If the answer to this question is "no," as is often the case with children and youth who exhibit DSI, unaided AAC elements designed to build the individual's comprehension of communication will need to be concrete and place low demand on the individual (e.g., touch cues, signs on body). If communication partners are to employ such AAC strategies, it is crucial the interprofessional team evaluate the individual's tactile sensitivities and skills (e.g., how does the individual respond to being touched; do they demonstrate tactile defensiveness?). In addition, any time interpersonal touch is going to be involved in an individual's communication system, it is crucial that person's cultural mores be taken into account by the team designing the AAC system.

If the individual with DSI does understand abstract symbols, then receiving information from communication partners via manual sign, the Tadoma method, or tactile sign language are reasonable AAC considerations for the team and family. In this instance, assessment will address the ways in which the individual with DSI uses touch and the levels of their tactile recognition and discrimination skills (e.g., for Tadoma and tactile sign language). If manual signing is to be considered as the primary vehicle for the individual's receptive communication, it is crucial the AAC team evaluate their visual skills, in terms of both acuity and visual field. The team should prioritize the individual's use of their residual vision skills and include long-range plans for transitioning the individual's mode of receptive communication from visual to tactile manual sign in the case the individual's DSI entails a progressive vision loss.

For consideration of unaided AAC elements as components of an individual's expressive communication repertoire, the first assessment of their level of symbolization is important as well. If the individual with DSI does not demonstrate clear understanding that one thing can stand for another, unaided AAC elements designed for communication expression should be more iconic and less abstract. Mastery of conventional gestures could be reasonable goals for such individuals.

For persons who do understand abstract symbols, then expressing information to communication partners via manual sign could be a reasonable unaided AAC goal. However, in this instance, a thorough assessment of the individual's motor abilities is necessary, including bilateral fine motor skills, dexterity, facial expressions, and general body movement and motor control.

Considerations for Success in the Implementation of Aided Communication Components

As is the case in regard to the adoption of unaided AAC communication elements, the achievement of successful aided AAC implementation with an individual who exhibits DSI must also begin with consideration of the types and degrees of their vision and hearing losses. Assessment must also take into account the individual's motor abilities and intellectual skills.

Considering the population of individuals with DSI as an entire group, aided AAC predominates neither receptive nor expressive communication intervention. Some individuals will use aided forms to receive information from communication partners and the environment (e.g., objects, textures, tactile symbols, vibrotactile aids). Some individuals will utilize aided components for the purposes of communicative expression: object systems (e.g., calendar systems), non–speech-generating AAC technology (e.g., communication book/board), and speech-generating technology (e.g., SGDs, apps, and ever-changing technologies, such as the Screen Braille Communicator). Some individuals who experience DSI will rely solely on aided communication modes to meet both their receptive and expressive needs; others will require or prefer unaided forms of AAC.

Similarly to assessment for unaided AAC communication system design, one of the first assessments to be completed to determine aided elements of the individual's receptive system is their level of symbolization. With many individuals who experience DSI, regardless of their age, it might well be that the individual does not understand that one thing can stand for another. In this case, aided AAC elements designed to build the individual's comprehension of communication will need to be concrete and place low demand on the individual's memory and cognitive skills (e.g., object cues, iconic textures). It is important that object cues be accessible to all communication partners and that these be used consistently.

If the individual with DSI demonstrates understanding of abstract symbols, then using textured symbols or tactile symbols to receive information from communication partners are reasonable AAC considerations for the team and family. In this case, assessment will necessarily address the individual's levels of tactile recognition and discrimination skills. Textured and tactile symbols created for use should be durable, in order that they will endure over time.

For consideration of aided AAC elements as components of an individual's expressive communication repertoire, the first assessment of their level of symbolization is important as well. If the individual with DSI does not demonstrate clear understanding that one thing can stand for another, aided AAC elements designed for communication expression should be more iconic and less abstract. Utilization

of a calendar system could be a reasonable goal for such individuals. A calendar system is a communication strategy that incorporates the linear arrangement of objects or tangible symbols to let the learner know what to anticipate next (Blaha, 2001; Rowland & Schweigert, 2000a). This approach has been identified by alternative names, including anticipation shelf, concrete calendar, and calendar box (Bashinski, 2014a).

A calendar system is developed from a sequence of objects chosen to correspond with the individual's level of symbolization development, arranged in the order of their daily routine. One object or tangible symbol is associated with each activity and is separated from the others by dividers. A communication partner assists the individual with DSI to physically move to the calendar's location, check it, pick up the object or tangible symbol for the next activity, then move to that activity's physical location. At the activity's conclusion, the object or tangible symbol is deposited in some sort of "finished" container. This routine is repeated throughout the sequence of the activities planned for the individual with DSI (Bashinski, 2014a; Bruce & Bashinski, 2017). Over time, it is hoped that the partner's physical assistance can be faded as the individual develops some understanding of symbolic representation.

For persons who do understand abstract symbols, expressing information to communication partners using sophisticated software/apps or an SGD could be reasonable aided AAC goals. In this instance, an assessment of the individual's motor abilities should be completed, particularly if the individual with DSI also experiences significant motor impairment (i.e., assessments for positioning of the AAC display and placement for any necessary switches would be crucial). Assessment of the individual's visual abilities would be essential for the appropriate design and layout of the aided AAC display so that image size, proximity, color, and contrasts will be well-matched to the individual's skills and needs. The team should prioritize the individual's use of their residual sensory skills, both visual and auditory, and include long-range plans for transitioning the individual's mode of receptive communication if progression of their vision and/or hearing loss might impact use of expressive AAC system components.

Considerations for Success in the Implementation of Multimodal AAC Systems With Individuals Who Experience Dual Sensory Impairment

A majority of individuals with DSI will likely benefit more significantly from a multimodal AAC system, which includes both aided and unaided elements. Regardless of the receptive and expressive modes an AAC team, the individual with DSI, and their family are exploring, several considerations are important.

First and foremost, the elements of the AAC system being considered for adoption must be acceptable to the potential user. If the individual with DSI does not welcome and embrace both receptive and expressive modes, achievement of communicative competence is not likely, even if the system is exceptionally well-designed to match the user's needs and abilities.

Second, it is very important that significant individuals in the potential AAC user's life find the proposed multimodal system acceptable as well. Parents, children, other family members, peers, and friends will need to embrace the proposed AAC system if they are expected to function as communication partners with the individual who experiences DSI. Related to this point is the reality that individuals who will serve as the AAC user's partners must have deep knowledge of elements of the AAC system and how these work together to function as an effective vehicle for their communication. A plan must be in place to provide the individual's communicative partners with training regarding how to implement all components of the system reliably (e.g., where to place signs on body, how to position hands for tactile signing, how to utilize components of a calendar system, ways to navigate a multilevel SGD). Detailed plans for teaching the individual who exhibits DSI and their most likely communication partners are crucial to the successful implementation of an AAC system.

Beyond these two important considerations, another point crucial to successful implementation of an AAC system with an individual who has DSI is the appropriateness of *all* system components to the individual's age and the environments in which they will most frequently need to communicate. A portion of the individual's AAC lexicon, particularly emergency vocabulary and words that represent the individual's strongest preferences and personal interests, should be available to them in both aided and unaided modes.

SUMMARY

This chapter explored and explained the relevance of AAC for persons with sensory impairments, primarily visual and hearing deficiencies and DSI. Because hearing has a significant impact on a person's communication ability, early use of AAC is important.

The challenges are doubled when a person with DSI uses AAC. Though exceptions exist to every generalization, the majority of individuals who experience DSI require intensive, ongoing assessment and intervention efforts if they are to become successful augmented communicators. As noted in previous sections of this chapter dedicated to individuals who experience either vision loss or hearing impairment, team members are advised to vigilantly assess the sensory status of the person with DSI. Educational programming for children and youth, as well as intervention for adults beyond school age, should be designed to preserve the individual's current vision and hearing abilities and make use of the individual's residual vision and/or hearing skills, taking particular advantage of the stronger sensory channel.

Much more information regarding augmenting communication for individuals who experience DSI can be accessed through texts devoted specifically to the education of children and youth with DSI (e.g., Chen & Downing, 2006; Downing et al., 2015; Hartshorne et al., 2011a; Janssen & Rødbroe, 2007; Miles & Riggio,, 1999; Riggio & McLetchie, 2008; Rødbroe & Janssen, 2006; Souriau et al., 2008; Souriau et al., 2009).

Technology is beginning to play a significant role in AAC because of the lowering cost of devices, quick availability of new technology on the market, and explosive innovations in devices that have artificial intelligence built into them. Overall, the future looks very bright for augmentative and alternative methods of communication by persons with sensory impairments.

STUDY QUESTIONS

1. Why are adaptations required for AAC users to undergo audiological evaluation? Describe some adaptations that may be made for AAC users in responding to pure tone audiometry or speech audiometry.

2. What groups of individuals with multiple disabilities are at risk for hearing impairment?

3. What are the recent technological advancements to improve communication in individuals with hearing impairment?

4. What factors may account for the high correlation between visual impairment and other disabilities?

5. What three approaches are appropriate in the management of visual impairment?

6. What types of AAC systems are available for persons with DSIs?

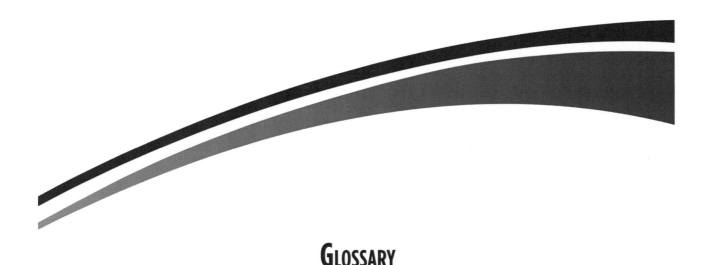

GLOSSARY

AAC: See *augmentative and alternative communication.*

AAC-based approaches to problem behavior: Communication based approaches that use AAC as alternative behaviors to less desirable behaviors, such as hitting, screaming, and self-injurious behavior.

AAC facilitation: An activity designed to assist an AAC user in developing and maintaining communicative competence in a variety of communication contexts.

AAC facilitator: Any person who aids, assists, or in some way, frees individuals from their severe communicative difficulties related to physical, linguistic, and/or cognitive impairments.

AAC interface: A component of the AAC transmission process of the AAC model proposed by Lloyd and colleagues (1990). The interface refers to the aid or device (e.g., communication board, speech-generating device, pen) that is used to transmit a message.

AAC processes and interface: A component of the Lloyd and colleagues (1990) AAC model that describes the unique way persons who require or rely upon AAC communicate with others; it consists of the means to represent (i.e., symbols), the means to select symbols, and the means to transmit a message (i.e., non–speech-generating or speech-generating technology).

AAC service delivery: The provision of direct or consultative assessment and intervention services to individuals with little or no functional speech.

AAC strategy: A learned or self-realized method of employing AAC aids, symbols, and/or techniques to facilitate communication or communication potential.

AAC system: The totality of aided and unaided means to represent (symbols), means to select, and means to transmit, and the strategies, techniques, skills, and devices that an individual uses to communicate. A system involves the integrated use of many components for communication; a.k.a., *communication system.*

AAC transmission processes: A component of the AAC model proposed by Lloyd and colleagues (1990) referring to the means to represent, means to select, and means to transmit a message. The means to represent (i.e., symbols), the means to select (e.g., direct selection, eye blink codes, scanning), and the means to transmit (i.e., the aid, device, or parts of the body) can be aided or unaided.

AAC user: An individual with little or no functional speech who is currently using or is a candidate for an AAC system.

AAIDD: See *American Association on Intellectual and Developmental Disabilities.*

AAROM: Common medical abbreviation for active assisted range of motion.

ABA: See *applied behavioral analysis.*

abbreviation expansion: The process by which an individual uses typical or idiosyncratic abbreviations (e.g., contractions, truncations) to represent words, phrases, or sentences. The net effect of the process is the transmission of complete messages with a reduced number of keystrokes.

ABC: See *activity-based curriculum* and *antecedent-behavior-consequence.*

ABCD: See *Arizona Battery for Communication Disorders of Dementia.*

abd: A common medical abbreviation for abduction.

Fuller, D. R., & Lloyd, L. L. *Principles and Practices in Augmentative and Alternative Communication* (pp. 499-578).
© 2023 Taylor & Francis Group.

abduction: Lateral movement of the limbs or fingers away from the midline of the body, or side bending of the head and trunk.

abex: See *abbreviation expansion*.

ABI: See *activity-based instruction*.

abnormal muscle tone: Refers to an increase (hypertonia) or decrease (hypotonia) in tension within a muscle to resistance depending on the type, location, and severity of neuromotor damage.

ABR: See *auditory brainstem response audiometry*.

abstract: A term used to describe intangible referents, such as beliefs, concepts, emotions, and ideas. For graphic symbols, abstract referents are difficult to depict by pictographs and are more typically depicted by ideographs or arbitrary symbols (e.g., traditional orthography).

abstract concept: An idea or image that can be selected from any of the specific attributes of a situation, symbol, or object (e.g., shape [squareness] is an abstraction [abstract concept] from a physical object); may also refer to complex ideas that are generally symbolic.

academic expectations: (1) Competitive: academic requirements are similar to those of regular education students. The amount of work may be reduced, but students are expected to learn concepts comparable to peers. No adjustment in evaluation expectations is required. (2) Active: reduced academic expectation. The workload is adjusted, and students are evaluated based upon their capabilities. Modifications to the grading system are made. (3) Involved: minimum requirements for meeting academic standards. Students may attend classes for subjects they are interested in but are not evaluated with the same criteria as their regular education peers and are graded on participation and involvement.

acalculia: Difficulty using mathematical symbols, often following brain injury, where mathematical skills existed prior to injury. Less severe forms may be referred to as dyscalculia.

acceleration: Increasing rate or speed, as in message transmission.

accentuation: Modification of alphabet letters or other graphic symbols to make words or symbols more closely resemble their referents; a.k.a., *elaboration, embellishment*.

acceptability: A selection consideration pertaining to how acceptable symbols or communication devices are to an AAC user, family members, caregivers, peers, and the general community.

ACCESS: See *adapted communication concepts for the education of severely impaired students*.

access software: Software that accepts input to the computer by devices other than the standard keyboard or supports output from the computer in formats other than those normally provided by the standard monitor.

access strand: Refers to the individual's ability to compensate for physical or communication barriers in order to participate more fully in meaningful life activities.

accessibility: (1) The ability to approach, enter, or communicate. Accessibility allows an individual with a disability to enter a building, participate with others in an activity, gain an education, and/or communicate with others. (2) Ability to select or activate components of an AAC system (e.g., retrieve vocabulary from a communication device). The term accessible is often used to describe components that a person can physically manipulate, such as a computer keyboard or a switch activated scanning system.

accommodation: (1) In Piagetian theory, one of the processes of adaptation in which the individual has to revise their internalized view of the world due to the evidence that is presented. (2) In special education, any adaptation or modification of the curriculum or environment that will allow an individual with a disability to effectively participate.

acculturation: (1) The process of modifying one's original identity and belief system to become more like those of another culture. (2) The process that results in population-level changes due to contact with other cultures.

accuracy: Having sampling statistics without bias within sampling studies (contrasted with *precision*).

accurate system: A system that allows the AAC user to produce intended messages with a minimum number of communication breakdowns or errors.

achondroplasia: A genetic condition characterized by short limbs, bowed legs, shortened stature, and a large head. The condition is typically not accompanied by hydrocephalus (excess fluid in the brain) or developmental disorders.

acoustic reflex: The protective reflex that occurs at the level of the cochlear nucleus when a high intensity sound that exceeds threshold (i.e., stimulus) is presented to either ear. The stimulus triggers the stapedius muscle within the middle ear to contract in both ears, which then causes the ossicular chain (i.e., malleus, incus, and stapes) to stiffen. This stiffening of the ossicular chain produces a change in acoustic immittance (i.e., decreased mobility of the tympanic membrane due to increased stiffness) that results in reduced transmission of sound through the middle ear.

acoustic reflex testing: An audiometric testing procedure in which a loud tone or noise that exceeds threshold is presented in the test ear in an attempt to activate an acoustic reflex; any change in immittance is then measured.

acoustic reflex threshold: An audiometric test performed to determine the lowest stimulus level that results in a reflex response and, consequently, a change in acoustic immittance.

acquired disability: A disability not present at birth that usually occurs as a result of disease or injury.

acquired immune deficiency syndrome (AIDS): A chronic, fatally progressive disease caused by infection from a retrovirus (HIV-1). The most acute symptom of this disease is a suppression or deficiency of the immune system, which in turn increases the likelihood of the individual developing infections and malignancies.

acrocephaly: A malformation of the skull caused by premature fusion of the skull sutures (craniosynostosis) that results in an elongated skull.

ACT: See *adapted cueing technique*.

action research: A form of applied scientific investigation or experimentation on educational curricula and processes. The main objective of action research is to utilize research methods to change or improve educational practice in an educational setting.

activation force: The minimal and maximal amount of force that an individual can exert using a given anatomic site.

activation sites: The areas on a device that control its operation when pressed, touched, or otherwise accessed.

active assisted range of motion: The range of movement of a joint that an individual can perform with assistance.

active matrix screen: Laptop computer monitor technology in which each pixel element has its own transistor. This technology provides a larger number of colors, better color depth, and quick screen refreshing. Screen graphics are also sharp without ghost images.

active range of motion: The range of movement of a joint that an individual can perform without assistance.

activities of daily living: The basic skills that are required for independence in everyday living (e.g., personal care, mobility, food preparation, homemaking, telephone use).

activity-based curriculum: An educational or academic curriculum that is based on or revolves around activities of daily living.

activity-based instruction: An instructional method based on teaching the fundamentals or daily life skills in the educational and academic setting.

activity-based overlay: An overlay designed with vocabulary that allows the user to participate in a specific activity.

activity participation inventory: An inventory that measures the level of participation for each skill or task necessary to complete an activity within an environment by comparing a target student to a peer and determining discrepancies that may exist between them. Barriers due to lack of opportunity or inability to access are identified. The activity participation inventory was developed and modified by Zangari and members of the Purdue AAC Group based, in part, on the Beukelman and Mirenda participation model and activity/standards inventory.

activity/standards inventory: An inventory developed by Beukelman and Mirenda that measures an AAC user's level of participation and identifies possible barriers to participation across a wide variety of activities.

acute flaccid myelitis: A rare, polio-type illness that affects the motor neurons in the gray matter of the spinal cord, resulting in sudden weakness in the arms or legs, loss of muscle tone, and loss of reflexes. It is seen most often in young children.

AD: See *Alzheimer's disease*.

ADA: See *Americans with Disabilities Act of 1990 (PL 101-336)*.

ADA Accessibility Guidelines: Guidelines drawn from standards of the United Federal Accessibility Standards and American National Standards Institute that include guidelines for restaurants and businesses not specified in the American National Standards Institute standards and are focused on individuals who have hearing, speech, or vision impairments.

ADA and ABA Accessibility Guidelines for Buildings and Facilities: A set of federal guidelines for addressing accessibility to federal buildings implemented in 2006 by the General Services Administration, to replace the *Uniform Federal Accessibility Standards*. The new guidelines are an attempt to better meet the mandates of the Americans with Disabilities Act of 1990 and the Architectural Barriers Act of 1969.

ADAAG: See *ADA Accessibility Guidelines*.

adaptability: The ability of an AAC system to support a range of access options or other functions so that the system remains useful when changes occur within the system or AAC user.

adaptation: (1) In Piagetian theory: the manner in which an individual's awareness of the outside world is internalized, consisting of two processes: *accommodation and assimilation*. (2) In special education: a documented process that allows a student with special educational needs to participate in the prescribed curriculum with changes in format, instructional strategies, or assessment procedures that retain the learning outcomes of the curriculum.

adapted communication concepts for the education of severely impaired students: A pictographic set of aided symbols composed primarily of simple line drawings with words printed below them (from the United States).

adapted cueing technique: Manual cues that are transmitted along with speech sounds in conversation. Each cue reflects the shape of the oral cavity, the articulatory placement and movement pattern, and the manner in which a sound is produced.

adapted play and recreation: The use of technology to assist individuals with disabilities in participating in fun, non-vocationally related activities for the purpose of leisure and learning.

adapted technology: A modification that is made to a device or a service that allows it to be usable or accessible for a person with a disability.

adaptive behavior: The process of modifying a less desirable behavior to promote a target behavior.

adaptive computer access: Computer hardware or software that is created or modified to allow individuals to use a computer with or without its standard input or output devices.

adaptive firmware card: A keyboard emulation device manufactured by Adaptive Peripherals, Inc that allowed Apple IIe or IIGS software to be operated with a variety of input methods (e.g., expanded keyboards, scanning, switches).

adaptive positioning: The use of specialized supports and adaptive equipment (e.g., for seating) to optimize the functional abilities of persons with physical impairments.

adaptive site: A website that customizes personalized pages for the user based upon an analysis of that individual's habits.

ADB: See *Apple desktop bus port.*

ADD: See *attention deficit disorder.*

add: A common medical abbreviation for adduction.

adduction: Movement of an extremity toward the midline of the body.

adenoid facies: A clinical condition having symptoms that include hanging the mouth open, breathing through the mouth, and generally exhibiting a dull and listless expression; snoring typically accompanies this condition.

ADHD: See *attention-deficit/hyperactivity disorder.*

ADLs: See *activities of daily living.*

adolescent: Typically refers to individuals in the 12- to 17-year-old age range.

adoption: The incorporation of changes into educational practices (including instatement, trial, and institutionalization) as part of the knowledge implementation and use processes.

adult: (1) Typically refers to individuals who are 18 years of age or older. (2) A skill level based on an individual's ability to successfully apply skills associated with the 18-or-older age group.

adventitious: Occurring or acquired at birth.

adverse medical event: An unanticipated medical outcome that negatively impacts the patient's health.

AE: See *age equivalent scores.*

AEPs: See *auditory evoked potentials.*

AFC: See *adaptive firmware card.*

age equivalent scores: Scores that are determined by the averages obtained on a test by children of different ages. Age equivalent scores allow the assessor to determine how much the individual's performance varies from their chronological age by comparison to other individuals of the same chronological age.

agglutination: The process of forming new concepts by combining symbols in sequence (e.g., in Amer-Ind, the gestures "taste" and "reject" are produced sequentially to represent the concept "bitter"). Basically, the new concept is the sum of its parts (i.e., the symbols).

aggression: Negative behavior that is directed toward other persons (e.g., biting, kicking, punching, scratching) or things (i.e., property destruction).

agnosia: A loss of the ability to recognize sensory input, usually due to brain injury. Agnosia is typically specific to a modality (e.g., auditory, tactile, visual).

agraphia: A difficulty in writing as a result of central nervous system damage. In a less severe form, agraphia may be referred to as dysgraphia.

AI: See *artificial intelligence.*

Aicardi syndrome: A syndrome characterized by a combination of generalized seizures, vertebral defects, retinal defects, growth failure of the corpus callosum, and severe intellectual impairment.

aid: An assistive device or interface (e.g., communication board, speech-generating device) that augments or serves as an alternative to natural speech and/or writing.

aided: A term used to refer to communication symbols, strategies, or techniques that require something external to the body to represent, select, or transmit messages.

aided AAC input: Describes interventions in which partners point to (or activate) aided AAC symbols while speaking with an individual who uses AAC; this form of language input models the use of AAC as the speaking communicative partner is interacting with the AAC user; aided AAC input balances language input/output for the AAC user.

aided approach: The use of aided symbols and techniques to accomplish effective communication.

aided communication: Communication in which aided symbols and some type of external aid or assistive device are used.

aided communication technique: A communication technique that uses some type of external aid or assistive device.

aided language stimulation: A technique in which the AAC user's partner combines the use of AAC with natural speech during communication. This technique has the dual purpose of augmenting spoken input to enhance an AAC user's comprehension and providing a model of effective AAC use; a.k.a., *augmented input* or *augmented communicative input.*

aided symbol: A symbol that requires an external aid or assistive device for display and transmission (e.g., Blissymbols, pictures, Sigsymbols, synthetic speech, letters of the alphabet).

AIDS: See *acquired immune deficiency syndrome* and *Assessment of Intelligibility of Dysarthric Speech.*

air conduction testing: A general term applied to audiological testing in which sound is presented to the listener via earphones or a sound field.

AKA: See *Alphabet de Kinèmes Assistés.*

ALD: See *assistive listening device.*

alexia: A difficulty in reading, especially as a result of neurological impairment. In a less severe form, alexia may be referred to as dyslexia.

allomorph: Any of the variant forms of a morpheme (e.g., the plural "-s" can be pronounced as /s/ as in cats, /z/ as in dogs, or /ɪz/ as in bushes).

AllTalk: An archaic, portable, dedicated speech-generating device that featured natural speech output recalled by direct selection of up to 128 one-inch cells. Standard memory for an AllTalk device was 600 words with memory expansion available for up to 1,200 words. An unlimited number of programs could be stored using a standard cassette player.

alphabet board: A non–speech-generating communication aid or device that displays the letters of the alphabet. An AAC user points to the letters to spell words in order to communicate a message.

alphabet board supplementation: A procedure in which a speaker with reduced intelligibility points to the first letter of each word as it is spoken. This method of augmentation enhances communication by forcing the speaker to slow their speaking rate while providing the communication partner with extra information in the form of the first letters of words spoken.

Alphabet de Kinèmes Assistés: A hand cued system designed by Wouts (1987) and used in Belgium.

alphabet encoding: A process of language formulation that uses letters and numbers or symbols that represent letters and numbers (e.g., Braille, fingerspelling, Morse code, traditional orthography); a.k.a., *letter encoding.*

alphabet glove: Also known as the "Braille glove." The glove may be utilized in a non–speech-generating format, in which a thin glove with numerals and letters of the alphabet printed across the individual fingers is worn by a person with dual sensory impairment and are touched by a communication partner to comprise a message, or a more sophisticated version (known as the "Lorm glove"), which allows real-time translation between texting and Braille.

alphanumeric encoding: A process of language formulation based on the systematic organization of information/messages for storage and retrieval using letter and number codes (e.g., G 3 can be used to represent "Good morning," the third message in the greeting category).

Alport syndrome: A genetic syndrome characterized by progressive chronic kidney disease (starting by about age 6 years) and progressive hearing loss (starting at about age 10 years).

ALS: See *aided language stimulation* and *amyotrophic lateral sclerosis.*

alternative access: Refers to how an AAC user interacts with their AAC system as related to the individual's motor skills and message composition ability.

alternative communication: A communication approach that is a substitute for (or alternative to) natural speech and/or writing.

alternative input device: A device that enables access to technology through means other than direct selection (e.g., single or multiple switches, expanded keyboards).

alternative keyboard: A computer hardware device that replaces the standard keyboard and can be reconfigured to meet the needs of the user (e.g., IntelliKeys, Unicorn Keyboard).

Alzheimer's disease: The most common cause of primary, degenerative dementia. Stage I is characterized by deterioration of recent memory, disorientation, mood disturbances, and difficulty in dealing with day to day tasks. Stage II involves rapid intellectual deterioration and symptoms resembling aphasia, apraxia, and agnosia. Stage III is when a person is highly demented and bed bound.

amb: Common medical abbreviation for *ambulation* or *ambulatory.*

ambiguous loss: A loss that is unclear, indeterminate, and unresolved for an extended period of time. This is seen often in persons with progressive neurological disorders where the patient is physically present but cognitively or emotionally distant.

amblyopia: Visual impairment in the absence of apparent disease.

ambulation: The process of walking.

ambulatory: Having the ability to walk.

American Association on Intellectual and Development Disabilities: An interdisciplinary association of administrators, educators, occupational therapists, physical therapists, psychologists, speech-language pathologists, social workers, and others concerned with intellectual (i.e., cognitive) impairment and developmental disabilities. The association has several professional divisions; of particular importance to AAC is the Communication Disorders Division. Formerly known as the American Association on Mental Retardation.

American Manual Alphabet: Representation of the 26 letters of the English alphabet in American Sign Language. Varying hand shapes and finger positions are used for the purpose of spelling words not represented by manual signs.

American National Standards Institute: A private organization established in 1959 that issues standards for construction guidelines in the private sector. In 1961, the American National Standards Institute published standards for physical accessibility to buildings and facilities. The American National Standards Institute has also established standards for the calibration of certain electronic equipment, such as audiometers.

American Sign Language: The natural sign language used by the Deaf community in the United States and certain regions of Canada.

American Speech-Language-Hearing Association: The primary professional organization for audiologists, speech language pathologists, speech and hearing scientists, and others interested in human communication and human communication disorders. The American Speech-Language-Hearing Association has several special interest groups; of particular relevance to AAC is Special Interest Group 12: AAC.

American Standard Code for Information Interchange: An eight-bit standard code that lets characters (e.g., letters, numbers, punctuation, and other symbols) be represented by the same eight bits on many different kinds of computers. Prior to the American Standard Code for Information Interchange, the various computer manufacturers tended to use their own code. This prevented computers from different manufacturers to communicate with each other. The American Standard Code for Information Interchange is the code used on the internet. In the 1990s, a 16-bit code (called Unicode) was developed that would handle alphabets of many nations. It contains the American Standard Code for Information Interchange sequence.

Americans with Disabilities Act of 1990 (PL 101-336): Federal legislation that prohibits discrimination in the hiring of individuals with disabilities and mandates modification of the work environment to accommodate individuals with disabilities.

Amer-Ind: An unaided set of gestures created by Madge Skelly, based somewhat on the gestures that Native American tribes used for intertribal communication.

Ameslan: A term used for *American Sign Language.*

amniocentesis: A medical procedure in which amniotic fluid from a pregnant woman's uterus is extracted and used to diagnose possible chromosomal disorders in the fetus.

amputee: An individual who has had a limb surgically removed or who had a limb absent at birth (congenital amputee).

amusia: A difficulty in producing or comprehending music, often as a result of brain injury.

amyotrophic lateral sclerosis: A progressive, degenerative neurological disease of unknown etiology that affects motor neurons of the brain and spinal cord, eventually resulting in total loss of muscle function and death; often referred to as *Lou Gehrig's disease,* named after a professional baseball player in the early 1900s who had the disease.

analog: A continuous representation, in real time, of light or sound waves.

analysis of variance: A statistical analysis procedure used for determining possible differences for a dependent variable that has two or more levels, and therefore, two or more means (averages).

anarthria: The inability to articulate (i.e., speak) because of neuromuscular involvement.

anencephaly: A defect in neural tube closure that takes place during the first 28 days of embryonic development. This leads to failed development of the forebrain, incomplete development of the skull, and a variety of facial abnormalities. Babies with anencephaly do not survive.

Angelman syndrome: A syndrome characterized by severe intellectual impairment, an ataxic, "puppet-like" gait, convulsive laughter, and characteristic facial features (e.g., large mouth, protruding jaw); often referred to as "happy puppet" syndrome.

anomaly: Any deviation from the normal or expected structure, form, or function in an individual.

anomia: A difficulty in recalling and recognizing the names of persons, places, or things, usually due to brain injury. In a less severe form, anomia may be referred to as dysnomia.

anomic aphasia: A type of aphasia where the individual has difficulty remembering or recognizing names which they should know well. The individual speaks fluently and grammatically and has normal comprehension; the only deficit is trouble finding appropriate words. The individual may often use circumlocutions in order to express a certain word they cannot find the name for. Sometimes the individual can recall the name when given clues.

ANOVA: See *analysis of variance.*

anoxia: An inadequate supply of oxygen in the body that may result in brain injury with concomitant impairments (e.g., intellectual impairment, physical impairment).

ANSI: See *American National Standards Institute.*

antecedent-behavior-consequence: A principle of behavioral theory that can be applied to behavior assessment and intervention. When using this approach, one would observe and manipulate what happens prior to a behavior (antecedent), observe the behavior itself (behavior), and observe and manipulate what happens after the behavior occurs (consequence).

antecedents: Actions or events that lead to a behavior (i.e., what happens before the behavior occurs, often described within the ABC chart as what triggers challenging behavior).

anterior: In or toward the front.

anterior superior iliac spines: Front (anterior), upper (superior) protrusions (spines) of the ilium (upper part of the bony pelvis above the hip joint); commonly called the "hip bones."

anthropological research: The study of social and cultural patterns within education relative to educational operations (including classrooms, school systems, teachers, etc.), revolving around values, attitudes, behaviors, role expectations, and modes of personal relationships.

anticipation shelf: An AAC strategy whereby objects or pictures are used to inform a learner of upcoming activities and as a context and method for conveying information.

Apert syndrome: A genetic syndrome characterized by a premature fusion of skull sutures, an odd-shaped skull, and webbed fingers or toes.

aphasia: Impairment in the comprehension and/or formulation of language symbols resulting from damage to certain areas of the brain. Aphasia is frequently caused by focal brain lesions in the cortical and subcortical areas of the left hemisphere as a result of hemorrhage or thromboembolic clots. Modalities of communication other than speaking may also be deficient (e.g., gesturing, reading, writing) either singly or in combination.

aphonia: A complete loss of voice-production ability.

aphonic: Exhibiting a lack of voice or phonation.

API: See *activity participation inventory.*

APIB: See *Assessment of Preterm Infant Behavior.*

Apple desktop bus port: A low-speed computer input port that allowed a person to daisy chain (string together) up to 16 peripheral devices.

application software: Computer programs that are designed for a particular purpose, such as education, gaming, word processing, database management, finances, drawing, graphics, etc. Referred to as "apps."

applied behavioral analysis: A program involving application of behavioral principles that may be used to treat children with autism spectrum disorder or related disorders; often referred to as *Lovaas Therapy* in reference to the work of Dr. Ole Ivar Løvaas. See also *discrete trial therapy.*

apraxia: A disorder of motor planning caused by damage to the motor control areas of the brain; inability to execute volitional movements. Limb apraxia and apraxia of speech are characterized by difficulty sequencing and coordinating movements in the absence of paralysis or weakness of muscles, usually resulting in highly inconsistent performance.

AR: See *acoustic reflex.*

arachnodactyly: A condition where an individual's fingers and toes are long and thin; commonly called "spider fingers."

arbitrary: A term used to describe symbols that bear little or no discernible relationship to their referents, and therefore, tend to be more opaque in terms of iconicity.

Arc: See *Arc of the United States, The.*

Arc of the United States, The: A parent organization that plays a role in identifying children with intellectual impairments considered to be good candidates for AAC. This organization was instrumental in securing educational opportunities for children with intellectual impairments and paving the way for the provision of special services in the public schools. Originally founded as the National Association for Retarded Children in 1953, the organization has had a few name changes: National Association for Retarded Citizens in 1973, Association for Retarded Citizens of the United States in 1981, and finally, its current name in 1992. Also referred to as The Arc.

arena assessment: An assessment in which all team members (e.g., occupational therapist, physical therapist, rehabilitation engineer, speech-language pathologist) are present throughout the entire evaluation.

Arizona Battery for Communication Disorders of Dementia: An assessment instrument used to measure the effects and severity of Alzheimer's disease.

Arnold-Chiari malformation: A brain malformation in which structures of the brainstem are extended and project into the part of the skull where the spinal cord resides.

AROM: Common medical abbreviation for *active range of motion.*

arousal: Alertness, which is necessary to interact with the environment. The reticular formation in the brainstem functions in maintaining normal wakefulness.

array: A selection of pictures, letters, numbers, punctuation marks, or computer commands commonly used with scanning input.

ART: See *acoustic reflex threshold.*

arthrogryposis multiplex: An apparently hereditary disorder (chronic but nonprogressive in nature) characterized by an absence of fetal movement. This rare congenital disorder is manifested by joint immobility, weak or absent limb muscles, and spinal curvature. Functional use of the upper extremities is minimal, even with medical intervention. Individuals with this disorder usually develop normal language skills but require alternative supports for reading, writing, and computer operation.

articulation: (1) The production of speech sounds through movement of the structures of the speech production mechanism (e.g., tongue, teeth, lips, soft palate). (2) The production of manual signs (with the parameters of location, movement, handshape, and orientation).

artificial intelligence: (1) The ability of a computer or other machine to perform activities that are normally thought to require human intelligence. (2) The branch of computer science that is concerned with the development of machines that can perform activities thought to require human intelligence.

artificial larynx: Any device that uses either pulmonary airflow directed through a vibrating reed or an electronic vibrating source to produce speech; used by an individual who has had their larynx surgically removed (i.e., laryngectomee). See also *electrolarynx.*

artificial sign system: A pedagogical tool created for the purpose of signed communication within the Deaf community (e.g., manually coded sign).

ASCII: See *American Standard Code for Information Interchange.*

ASHA: See *American Speech-Language-Hearing Association.*

ASIS: See *anterior superior iliac spines.*

ASL: See *American Sign Language.*

Asperger's syndrome: A pervasive developmental disorder classified as an autism spectrum disorder, seen most often during the early school years, characterized by impairments in social interactions and repetitive behavior patterns.

asphyxia: An interruption of oxygen to the blood that leads to loss of consciousness and possible brain damage.

aspiration: (1) A desire to excel beyond one's current level of functioning. The "level of aspiration" is the maximum goal that an individual or a group wishes to reach at any given moment during a specific activity. (2) A release of breath during the production of some speech sounds. (3) The taking in of foreign matter, such as food or liquid, into the respiratory system, typically causing gagging or coughing.

assertiveness: An attribute of the means to transmit that allows the AAC user to influence interactions by initiating a request or interrupting a partner, warding off interruptions from others or protesting something.

assessment: A process whereby data are collected and information is gathered to make intervention or management decisions.

assessment—cognitive: Instruments and processes, whether standardized or informal, that evaluate behaviors within the cognitive domain (e.g., conception, imagination, intelligence, judgment, memory, perception, and reasoning) for the purpose of making intervention or management decisions.

assessment—interaction: Instruments and processes, whether standardized or informal, that evaluate an individual's ability to interact effectively during the process of communication in a variety of contexts and with a variety of communication partners. Data are collected for the purpose of making intervention or management decisions.

assessment—language: Instruments and processes, whether standardized or informal, that evaluate behaviors within the linguistic domain (e.g., articulation and phonology, expressive language, receptive language) for the purpose of making intervention or management decisions.

assessment—physical ability: Instruments and processes, whether standardized or informal, that evaluate behaviors within the physical domain (e.g., ambulatory ability, fine motor skills, gross motor skills) for the purpose of making intervention or management decisions.

Assessment of Intelligibility of Dysarthric Speech: A standardized test that assesses single-word and sentence intelligibility and speaking rates of individuals with dysarthria.

Assessment of Preterm Infant Behavior: An adapted version of the Brazelton Neonatal Behavioral Assessment Scale. It is used with preterm infants (i.e., under 37 weeks gestational age) and examines behaviors in several developmental domains.

assigned variable: See *attribute variable.*

assimilation: (1) In Piagetian theory, one of the processes of adaptation in which the individual accepts what they perceive from the external world without changing their internalized view (in some cases, this could lead to pigeon-holing or stereotyping). (2) The process where minority groups or persons with disabilities are absorbed into a generally larger community. In the strictest sense of the word, this presumes a loss of all characteristics that make the newcomers different.

assistive communication device: Any electronic or non-electronic device that assists an individual in communication.

assistive device—high-tech: Any type of communication, environmental, or other assistive device or equipment that is electronic and uses a computer chip or integrated circuit.

assistive device—light-tech: Any type of communication, environmental, or other assistive device or equipment that is nonelectronic, or if electronic, does not use a computer chip or integrated circuit.

assistive device—speech output: Any communication or other assistive device or equipment that has speech output. See *speech-generating device.*

assistive device—text composition: Any type of communication or other assistive device or equipment that allows an individual to compose, edit, and send written messages.

assistive listening device: An amplification device that improves the signal-to-noise ratio so the important sound source is delivered to the ear at an advantage over background noise.

assistive technology: (1) Any technology that is used to enable an individual with a disability to perform tasks that are otherwise difficult or impossible to do. (2) The field or discipline that pertains to the development and provision of assistive technology.

assistive technology device: Any device or system that is used to increase, maintain, or improve the functional capabilities of individuals with disabilities. The device or system can be acquired commercially off the shelf, modified, or customized. This term comes from the Tech Act (PL 100-407, 1988) and Individuals with Disabilities Education Act (PL 101-476, 1990).

assistive technology service: Any service that directly assists an individual with a disability in selecting, acquiring, or using an assistive technology device. This term comes from the Tech Act (PL 100-407, 1988) and Individuals with Disabilities Education Act (PL 101-476, 1990).

associative play: The fourth stage of play development in which children make brief contact with one another while playing.

astigmatism: An irregular curvature of the cornea of the eye, resulting in an aspherical surface and blurred vision.

asymmetrical: A characteristic of manual signs and gestures in which the hands take different motor pathways on or in relation to the body of the signer. Asymmetrical signs and gestures generally pose a higher degree of difficulty than symmetrical signs and gestures.

asymmetrical tonic neck reflex: A postural reflex often seen in children with cerebral palsy. When the head is rotated, the asymmetrical tonic neck reflex causes an extension in the arm and leg on the side to which the face is turned, while the opposite site increases in flexion. The asymmetrical tonic neck reflex is considered normal for typically developing young infants and usually disappears during the first 6 months of an infant's life.

asynchronous: Therapeutic services and/or learning contexts in which information, images, video, or data are saved and transmitted for viewing or interpretation at a later time. Examples include transmission of voice clips, audiologic testing results, patient education materials, or outcomes of independent client practice. Store-and-forward or chat-based interactions are examples of asynchronous services.

AT: See *assistive technology.*

ataxia: A total or partial inability to coordinate volitional muscular movements, typically due to cerebellar pathology. Gait and ambulation may be uncoordinated, with the individual frequently falling or walking into obstacles, such as furniture.

athetosis: A type of cerebral palsy characterized by repetitive, involuntary movements. A more severe form of this is called choreoathetosis.

atresia of the choanae (also, choanal atresia): A blockage or narrowing of the nasal passageways by bone or tissue that results in breathing difficulty.

At-Risk Institute: See *National Institute on the Education of At-Risk Students (At-Risk Institute).*

A-Tronix Morse code translator: A device used to translate Morse code into English traditional orthography.

atrophy: A decrease in size or wasting away of body tissues or organs (e.g., muscles) often as a result of flaccid paralysis.

attention: Concentration or direction of the mind to objects or people in the environment.

attention deficit disorder: A syndrome, usually seen in childhood, that is characterized by a persistent pattern of impulsivity, short attention span, and, in some cases, hyperactivity. Persons with attention deficit disorder typically have difficulty with academic, occupational, and social skills.

attention-deficit/hyperactivity disorder: A disorder that is characterized by a short attention span, high susceptibility to distraction and impulsivity, and accompanied by hyperactivity. Attention-deficit/hyperactivity disorder may also be accompanied by various learning disabilities.

attitude barriers: Opinions and beliefs people have that adversely affect an AAC user's full participation in society.

attribute variable: In research, an independent variable that cannot be changed, influenced, or otherwise manipulated. Gender, age, and disability are examples of attribute variables.

auding: See *aural reading.*

audiogram: The graph onto which the results of an audiometric evaluation are charted to indicate an individual's ability to hear pure tones at each of the test frequencies. Red circles are used to indicate hearing sensitivity for the test frequencies for the right ear, while blue Xs are used to indicate hearing sensitivity for the test frequencies for the left ear.

auditory brainstem response audiometry: A noninvasive audiometric procedure that measures electrical responses along the auditory pathway at the level of the brainstem. An auditory brainstem response reflects neural activity of cranial nerve VIII; the response is triggered within 10 msec of the introduction of a stimulus presentation; a.k.a., *auditory evoked response, brainstem response,* and *brainstem auditory evoked response.*

auditory evoked potentials: Electrical potentials (i.e., sound energy conducted and transmitted by the inner ear to the brain) recorded over a broad period of time following the presentation of a stimulus tone during an auditory brainstem response procedure. Auditory evoked potentials are used by audiologists to determine the functioning of specific areas along the auditory pathway.

auditory scanning: A selection technique in which the potential message choices are sequentially presented to the AAC user through earphones or in a free field. When the wanted message is presented, the AAC user interrupts the scan (usually with a switch) to make the selection.

aug com: A shortened term for augmentative and alternative communication that is not widely used. See *augmentative and alternative communication.*

Augmentative and Alternative Communication: The professional journal published by the International Society for Augmentative and Alternative Communication that contains peer-reviewed clinical, educational, and research papers.

augmentative and alternative communication: (1) The supplementation or replacement of natural speech and/or writing using aided and/or unaided symbols. Blissymbols, pictographs, Sigsymbols, tangible symbols, and electronically produced speech are examples of aided symbols. Manual signs, gestures, and fingerspelling are examples of unaided symbols. The use of aided symbols requires a transmission device, whereas the use of unaided symbols requires only the user's body. (2) The interdisciplinary field or area of clinical/educational practice that seeks to improve the communication skills of individuals with little or no functional speech.

augmentative communication: A communication approach that augments or serves as an addition to natural speech and/or writing. The term is used correctly when some natural speech and/or writing ability in the individual is present.

augmentative communication device: A term that is too often used to describe an AAC user's system. It is a poor term to use because the system that many AAC users rely upon for communication includes not only a non–speech-generating and/or speech-generating device but gestures and, in some cases, vocal activity. Similarly, many AAC users have functionally little to no speech and/or writing ability, and therefore, their system is an alternative to these modes of communication as opposed to an augmentation. A better term to use is AAC system.

augmentative communication system: The total communication system of an individual who uses AAC as an augmentation to speaking and/or writing. The system includes methods for message transmission, representational means (e.g., symbol system or set), and techniques for the social interchange necessary to transmit and receive messages. Most AAC users use more than one method and means of communicating. It is important not to use this term in describing the system of an individual who must rely on AAC as an alternative to speech and/or writing.

augmentative components (of a communication system): The components of communication that enhance communication effectiveness. Standard augmentative components (such as ordinary gestures, facial expression, writing) are used by most individuals to supplement speech and enhance communication effectiveness. Special augmentative components are those that have been developed for individuals with severe communication impairments to enhance functional communication and include special gestures, symbols, and electronic devices, as well as special communication techniques (e.g., scanning).

augmented input: See *aided language stimulation*.

augmented input communicator: In AAC intervention, one of the five categories of persons with aphasia described by Garrett and Beukelman (1992); an individual who requires their communication partner to use graphic symbols and/or gestures in addition to natural speech during conversation. The individual with aphasia typically exhibits a significant impairment in auditory comprehension, necessitating the use of other modes of communication by their communication partner.

aural reading: For persons who cannot efficiently read printed text, a supplement that involves the process of hearing, listening, recognizing, and interpreting previously recorded language. It relies on the individual's ability to process auditory and linguistic information efficiently and accurately; a.k.a., *auding*.

authoring program: Computer software that enables individuals to construct programs for specific uses (e.g., interactive lessons, multimedia presentations).

autism: See *autism spectrum disorder*.

autism spectrum disorder: A developmental disorder that may be characterized by problems in social interaction and communication, restricted or repetitive behaviors or interests, attention deficits, and differences in learning by comparison to peers without autism spectrum disorder.

autistic leading: A non-linguistic form of requesting in which an individual with autism takes a communication partner by the wrist, leads the partner to a desired object, and then places the partner's hands on the object. Autistic leading is sometimes perceived as socially unacceptable behavior.

Auto-Com: An archaic AAC device that was developed at the Trace Research and Development Center. As words were inputted to the Auto-Com from the keyboard, they were displayed on an LED display and printed onto a strip of paper. The user was able to use the Auto-Com in various environments and could program and correct messages.

automated data logging: The automatic recording of data that can be analyzed to produce a time-stamped transcript of what has been generated on a speech-generating device.

Automatic, Appropriate: Minimal Assistance for Daily Living Skills: Level VII of the *Rancho Los Amigos Levels of Cognitive Functioning Scale-Revised*, characterized in part by consistent orientation to person and place, minimal supervision for new learning, superficial awareness of their condition, minimal supervision for safety in routine home and community activities, moderate assistance for orientation to time, and unrealistic planning for the future.

automatic linear scanning: A message selection technique in which the movement of the cursor is automatic and continuous according to a preset pattern. The user activates a switch to stop the cursor and make a selection; a.k.a., *automatic scanning*.

automatic reinforcement: Sensory consequences (e.g., auditory, visual, tactile) that increases a behavior by engaging in the behavior.

automatic-reinforcement-motivated problem behavior: Problem behavior that may be maintained by sensory consequences (e.g., auditory, tactile, visual) and are provided automatically by engaging in the behavior; a.k.a., *sensory-consequences-motivated problem behavior*.

automatic scanning: See *automatic linear scanning*.

autosomal dominant: The non–sex-related chromosomal inheritance pattern for a genetic trait that is passed from generation to the next by a person with the affected chromosome. The trait can never be transmitted from an unaffected person.

autosomal recessive: The chromosomal inheritance pattern for a genetic trait that is passed from one generation to the next when a child receives one gene for the trait from each parent. Both parents must carry the gene for that trait, although they may not necessarily be affected by it.

averaged activation: Switch activation that requires a preset specified duration or pressure in order to operate. This is done to reduce false hits; a.k.a., *filtered activation*.

awareness of contingencies: The knowledge that certain actions and behaviors can directly lead to specific outcomes, including social outcomes. The understanding of this cause-and-effect relationship often leads to intentional communication.

Babbelplaatjes: Developed in Belgium, a pictographic set of aided symbols composed primarily of simple line drawings with words printed above them.

Baker's basic ergonomic equation: A formula that demonstrates how success or failure with assistive technology may be related to time constraints, as well as the user's motivation and physical, linguistic, and cognitive effort.

balance: The normal state of action and reaction between two or more organs or body parts.

bandwidth: The amount of data that can be passed along a communications channel in a given period of time.

barrier: (1) Any characteristic of the workplace that functions to inhibit or prevent a worker from performing job duties in an efficient and orderly manner. (2) Any characteristic of people (e.g., attitudinal barrier) or the environment (e.g., physical barrier) that functions to inhibit or prevent a person with a disability from fully participating in society.

barrier game: A communication game in which a speaker knows something that is not known by the listener. The speaker has to successfully communicate a message to the listener related to that something in order to accomplish a specific task.

baseline: The natural level of occurrence of a behavior before intervention. The results of an intervention or program are judged in reference to the baseline.

BASIC: See *Beginner's All-Purpose Symbolic Instruction Code.*

basic choice communicator: In AAC intervention, one of the five categories of persons with aphasia described by Garrett and Beukelman (1992); an individual who requires maximal assistance (e.g., cues, prompts) from communication partners to make basic choices (usually related to activities of daily living) often as a result of persisting global aphasia and severe neurological impairment.

basic rebus: Originally a component of the *Peabody Rebus Reading Program*, an aided set of graphic symbols composed primarily of pictographs and some ideographs and relational symbols; a.k.a., *simple rebus.*

battered child syndrome: A specific pattern of injuries evident on the bones of a child who has been severely beaten. Also called *Caffey syndrome* or *Caffey-Kempe syndrome.*

baud: In telecommunications and electronics, it is the measure of the signaling rate, or the number of changes to the transmission media per second in a modulated signal (e.g., 200 baud means that 200 signals are transmitted per second; if each signal carries four bits of information, then in each second, 800 bits are transmitted [800 bps]).

BCI: See *brain-computer interfaces.*

B-DAC: See *Brady-Dobson Alternative Communication.*

beam/light sensor: A method of direct selection that uses a light beam and light sensor for environmental control and for making selections on communication displays. For example, a device that creates a light beam is attached to a cap that the AAC user wears; the AAC user guides the beam by movements of the head to symbols on a communication board, thereby illuminating them to indicate their symbol choices.

Beeldlezen/de Dikke van Roepaan: Developed in The Netherlands, a pictographic set of aided symbols composed primarily of simple line drawings with words printed below them.

Beeldspraak: Developed in The Netherlands, a photographic symbol set with words printed below the photos.

Beginner's All-Purpose Symbolic Instruction Code: A simple computer programming language for beginners that resembles broken English. One of the first programming languages created so that the novice computer user could create their own simple programs.

behavior chain interruption technique: A technique that uses a predictable routine to increase early developing intentional communication. An established sequence is interrupted, and the learner is expected to indicate that the sequence should be continued.

behavioral contingencies: State "if-then" conditions for the potential occurrence of a specific behavior and its related consequences (i.e., *if* a student raises their hand in class, *then* the teacher calls on them).

behavioral genetics: A field of study that examines how genes affect the expression of behavior.

behavioral intervention plan: A part of the individualized education program that outlines the steps that will be taken to alter a student's specific behavioral patterns. The plan should include a description of what skills will be taught, identification of positive behavioral intervention strategies that will be used, and a description of any educational environment alterations that will be needed. Development of the plan is based on information gathered during a functional behavior assessment.

behavioral observation audiometry: A type of audiological test performed on children that requires subjective observation of a child's unconditioned response to sound stimuli to measure their hearing threshold.

benign in MS: A form of multiple sclerosis wherein the affected individual demonstrates little or no progression of disease and appears to have a normal lifespan.

Betaprentenboek/Beeldtaal: Developed in Belgium, a pictographic set of aided symbols composed primarily of simple line drawings with words printed above them.

bicultural: Simultaneously belonging to two cultural groups.

BID: Common medical abbreviation for *bis in die* (twice daily).

bilat: Common medical abbreviation for *bilateral*.

bilateral: Referring to both sides of the body, as in bilateral hearing impairment.

Bild-grundwortschatz fur sprach-undsprechbehinderte: Developed in Germany, a pictographic set of aided symbols composed primarily of simple line drawings with words printed below them.

bilingual: (1) Being fluent in two languages. Bilingualism is balanced when an individual has equal competence in both languages. If the bilingualism is not balanced, the language in which the individual is more competent is referred to as the dominant language. (2) In education, the term describes the process in which two languages are used to foster general development and language acquisition. For example, bilingualism is often used in the education of immigrant children whose home language is different from the dominant community language.

bimanual: (1) A skill or activity requiring the use of both hands. (2) The ability to use both hands with essentially equal dexterity.

binary code: Any system that is based on the representation of things through various combinations of two symbols, such as one and zero, true and false, and the presence and absence of voltage; a.k.a., *binary logic*.

binary logic: See *binary code*.

birth defect: An impairment or disorder that is present at birth.

biserial correlation: See *correlation*.

bit: A binary digit; a single digit (0 or 1) that represents the basic unit of information used by computers.

Blissymbolics/Blissymbols: Originally designed as a graphic means of international communication, Blissymbolics is an aided symbol system composed of a finite set of meaning-based elements (semantic elements), some iconic and some opaque, which are combined according to generative rules and logic to create a virtually unlimited vocabulary.

block grants: Monies provided to the states by the federal government that have no mandates or restrictions as to how they must be spent.

block/group scanning: A message selection technique in which a relatively large block or group of items is initially selected (e.g., one-half, one-fourth, or one-eighth of the entire display), and then progressively smaller blocks or groups are selected within the larger ones until the target item is selected; a.k.a., *group item scanning, multidimensional scanning*.

blood pressure: The pressure that is exerted on the walls of the blood vessels as blood travels through the body. Expressed as two values, one value over the other: systolic, the upper value, represents blood pressure as the heart beats; diastolic, the lower value, represents blood pressure when the heart is between beats. Normal blood pressure is a systolic value of 120 or less and a diastolic value of 80 or less (i.e., 120/80 or less). Values above 120/80 are indicative of hypertension (high blood pressure).

Bluetooth technology: Wireless technology in the IEEE 802.15.1 protocol. Bluetooth technology has slightly slower data transfer speeds than WiFi but requires less power, making it ideal for small appliances, such as cellular telephones and personal digital assistants.

bone conduction testing: A general term applied to audiological testing in which stimuli (pure tones) are presented to the listener via a vibrator that is placed on the mastoid process of the skull, thereby bypassing the air conduction channel.

Borel Maisonny: Developed in France, a hand coded alphabet system used to provide psychomotor support for children with learning disabilities who are learning to read.

bottom-up strategy: A cognitive style of information processing (linguistic or non-linguistic) in which an individual identifies simple, basic elements and proceeds to identify and comprehend more complex and meaningful wholes. Low level elements (e.g., sounds, printed letters, strokes in a picture) are typically identified first, with the individual then discovering how these lower-level elements relate to each other in terms of order, spatial, and temporal configuration in higher-level structures (e.g., words, pictures) and, eventually, in still higher structures (e.g., sentences, discourse).

bound morpheme: In morphology, a unit of language that cannot stand alone as a word, but instead is attached to an unbound (free) morpheme to change its meaning. Affixes are examples of bound morphemes (e.g., *un-, -ly, -ing*).

box-and-whisker plot: A graphic representation of the variability that exists in a set of scores.

BP: Common medical abbreviation for *blood pressure*.

Brady-Dobson Alternative Communication: A symbol set of pictographic black-and-white line drawings numbering approximately 1,250 symbols arranged in 10 categories. Brady-Dobson Alternative Communication symbols have reportedly been used successfully with individuals with aphasia, cerebral palsy, cognitive impairments, and other developmental disabilities.

Braille: A system of reading and writing for individuals with visual impairments that uses letters, numbers, and punctuation marks made up of raised dot patterns. Braille software can translate English words into Braille, Braille into English, or can function as a Braille training program.

Braille hand speech: A tactile communication mode utilized by persons who experience dual sensory impairment; this method involves positioning the index, middle, and ring fingers of both hands to represent the configurations of the Braille alphabet, then touching the arm or hand of the individual with dual sensory impairment with these finger configurations.

Braille input: A computer hardware device that allows input to the computer via a Braille-style keyboard or specific keys on a standard keyboard that function in Braille patterns.

Braille output: A computer hardware device used to produce a hard copy of Braille or refreshable Braille output.

brain-computer interfaces (BCIs): Refer to a growing group of technologies that capture brain signals via either direct (i.e., invasive) or indirect (i.e., noninvasive) ways, analyze the signals, and translate the signals into commands to run devices such as a wheelchair or a keyboard. With respect to AAC, a brain-computer interface would allow a user to select directly from a visual or auditory array presented to them without need of additional switches or other means of access.

brain injury: Damage to brain tissue resulting in impairment of central nervous system functioning with concomitant impairments in cognitive, physical, or other functioning.

brain stem: The lower part of the brain located between the cerebrum and the spinal cord that controls basic life functions.

brain stem lesions: Tissue damage or loss of function in the brain stem.

British Sign Language: The natural sign language used by the Deaf community in Great Britain.

brittle bone disease: See *osteogenesis imperfecta*.

Broca's aphasia: A type of aphasia characterized by nonfluent speech, few words, short sentences, and many pauses. The words that the patient can produce come with great effort and often sound distorted. Intonation tends to be flat and monopitched. Speech has the general appearance of being telegraphic in nature because of the deletion of function words and disturbances in word order. On the other hand, comprehension for conversational speech is relatively intact.

BSE: Common medical abbreviation for *bedside swallowing evaluation*.

BSL: See *British Sign Language*.

bubble jet printer: A nonimpact computer printer that produces characters on paper by bubbles of ink that burst when they are heated.

BUILLDer: See *Therapy Material BUILLD*.

bulbar amyotrophic lateral sclerosis: A form of ALS where dysarthria is a symptom early in the disease process; deterioration of speech and swallowing functions may occur rapidly. Motor impairments of the extremities are usually less extensive until much later in the disease process; thus, the individual is usually able to use direct selection AAC techniques by using their hands or fingers.

buses: Electrical circuits that allow transmission of data from one part of a computer to another or from the computer to its peripherals.

byte: Equal to eight bits; in order to be stored in a computer, a single alphanumeric character requires a byte of information.

CA: See *chronological age*.

Caffey syndrome: See *battered child syndrome*.

Caffey-Kempe syndrome: See *battered child syndrome*.

CAI: See *computer-assisted instruction*.

calendar box: A box or other container used for the purpose of cueing an individual to their daily or weekly routine. Objects that present activities are placed in the cells of the box in a particular sequence to indicate the temporal order of the activities.

CAMA: See *Communication Aid Manufacturers Association*.

Canon Communicator: A portable, dedicated communication aid featuring a small alphabetically arranged keyboard with a paper strip printout. It can store messages up to 95 characters long.

CANS: See *central auditory nervous system*.

canthus: The corner where the upper and lower eyelids meet (the "eye slit").

CAP: See *central auditory processing*.

capability assessment: The portion of an AAC evaluation in which motor control, language, cognitive, visual, and hearing capabilities of the individual are assessed.

capability profile: A profile obtained during a thorough assessment that accurately details a person's level of functioning across various areas of interest.

capability profiling: A comprehensive approach to assessment that involves identifying an individual's maximum level of performance across critical areas of interest.

CAPD: See *central auditory processing disorder*.

capped rental: Typically used when a new speech-generating device is prescribed, the receiver of the device pays a rental fee up to what it would cost to purchase the device, at which time the device becomes the property of the receiver.

captive portal: A default webpage typically used for WiFi hotspots that is downloaded to everyone who logs onto the internet.

cardiac functional evaluation: An evaluation of cardiovascular response done during functional activities and therapeutic exercises, performed by a qualified physical or occupational therapist with a doctor's order.

case conference committee: A committee whose purpose is to identify the abilities and needs of an AAC user. The committee is typically composed of family members or caregivers, general education teachers, special education teachers, speech-language pathologists, school psychometrists, and occupational and physical therapists.

case management: A system for managing activities for individuals who need many types of services and/or long-term services; a case manager is usually appointed to coordinate the services for an individual. Case management can either be done on an individual agency basis or community level.

case study: A research approach that describes a single individual for the purposes of generating hypotheses for research and sharing information/experiences with others. Although data may be presented, case studies generally lack the experimental control required of single-subject design research.

case study design: The one observable fact selected by the experimenter to study in depth, regardless of the number of settings, social scenes, or participants involved in the study.

cataract: An eye abnormality that is characterized by opacity of the lens.

categorical variable: In research, a variable that is used to separate subjects, objects, etc. into multiple mutually exclusive groups.

categories test: A subtest of the Halstead-Reitan Neuropsychological Test Battery that measures abstracting ability, where figures of varying size, shape, number, intensity, color, and location are grouped by abstract principles. Subjects identify the principle by responding on a simple keyboard.

category: The organization of human experience into general concepts with associated linguistic labels.

cathode ray tube: A display device (e.g., computer monitor) in which streams of electrons are projected onto light sensitive material to create a visible image.

causality: A sensorimotor scheme in which an individual demonstrates the ability to search for a source behind a problem.

cause and effect: A relationship between two events in which one is the cause of the other (e.g., turning the key in the ignition causes the car engine to start).

CBI: See *community-based instruction* and *computer-based instruction*.

CD: See *compact disk*.

CD ROM: See *compact disk read only memory*.

CE: See *continuing education*.

CEC: See *Council for Exceptional Children*.

center-based program: A program where the AAC user travels to agency settings where assessment and/or intervention services are provided.

centering: A feature option for scanning that automatically returns the scanning indicator to the center of the scanner display after each selection.

central auditory nervous system: Specific neural pathways and nuclei (bundles of cell bodies at which nerve fibers synapse) within the central nervous system that relay auditory information from the cochlea and cranial nerve VIII to other nuclei within the auditory, sensory, and motor neural pathways. Specific nuclei within the central auditory nervous system include the cochlear nucleus, superior olivary complex, lateral leminiscus, inferior colliculus, and medial geniculate body.

central auditory processing: The level of efficiency with which the auditory system processes incoming auditory input and stored auditory information simultaneously.

central auditory processing disorder: A disorder of the central auditory processing system that may be manifested by difficulty with understanding speech in noisy environments.

central field loss: A type of visual impairment in which an affected individual experiences difficulty in seeing a vertical target presented at the midline of the body.

central nervous system: The part of the nervous system, comprised of the brain and spinal cord, involved in voluntary movements and thought processes.

central processing unit: The "brain" of the computer that processes information, executes software commands, and coordinates input and output functions.

cerebral palsy: A central nervous system disorder that occurs at or about the time of birth, prior to the achievement of muscular coordination. Primarily characterized by impaired motor control, cerebral palsy may also include concomitant intellectual impairment, seizures, and visual and auditory impairments.

cerebrospinal fluid: Fluid that surrounds the brain and spinal cord. It is often extracted from the body in order to do diagnostic testing for central nervous system diseases.

cerebrovascular accident: An interruption of blood supply to brain tissue due to ruptured blood vessels or clots; a.k.a., *stroke*.

certification: A process by which individuals are recognized for meeting certain minimum standards held by an agency or organization (e.g., state department of education, Council for Clinical Certification of American Speech-Language-Hearing Association). Certification is often used by agencies to determine eligibility for employment or reimbursement.

cerumen: A wax-like substance found in the external ear canal.

cervical spinal cord injury: Injury occurring at the cervical (neck) level of the spinal cord frequently resulting in paresis or paralysis of the upper limbs with possible involvement of the lower limbs.

CGA: See *color graphics adapter*.

challenging behavior: A term coined in the 1980s as a euphemism for problem behavior, disruptive behavior, and/or aberrant behavior. See *problem behavior*.

CHARGE association: See *CHARGE syndrome*.

CHARGE syndrome: A congenital syndrome that includes coloboma (incomplete fusion of the retina or iris), heart disease, atresia of the nasal passage, hearing loss, developmental/growth delay, genital and/or urinary abnormalities, and sometimes cleft of the lip and/or palate; a.k.a., *CHARGE association*.

chart-based encoding: An encoding technique in which the AAC user refers to a chart while sending messages. The chart can be used by the communication partner to decode messages, eliminating the need to memorize codes.

Chatterbox: A portable speech-generating device featuring a QWERTY keyboard, a 12-character display screen, and memory for 74 phrases and sentences.

cheremes: Minimal morphological units that signify differences in meaning between specific manual signs (e.g., hand shape, location, and movement).

CHF: Common medical abbreviation for *congestive heart failure*.

CHI: See *closed head injury*.

childhood apraxia of speech: A speech sound disorder present from birth in which motor planning affects the sequencing and coordination of speech sounds, impacting intelligibility; childhood apraxia of speech is distinct from delayed speech in that it does not follow a developmental progression and is characterized by sound distortions, omissions, and inconsistent speech sound substitutions.

children: Typically refers to individuals under 12 years of age.

chin stick: A device worn on the head with a pointer that extends at the level of the chin, which allows the individual to use head movement to independently point toward a symbol or object.

chi-square: A statistical analysis procedure that uses nominal data to demonstrate relationships between two variables.

chorea disorder: A disorder characterized by irregular, spasmodic, involuntary movements of the limbs and/or facial muscles.

chronemics: The study of the temporal aspects of communication (e.g., the rate of communication exchanges, timing between responses, and/or the amount of time it takes to express ideas).

chronic progressive: A common aspect of multiple sclerosis among older affected adults where motor and neurological signs and symptoms gradually worsen.

chronological age: The natural age of an individual. It is frequently compared to an age-equivalent score during the assessment process.

circle of friends: A strategy used to facilitate inclusion of school-aged individuals with severe disabilities into regular classroom settings. This dynamic process of including persons with severe disabilities in activities involves family members, principals, teachers, and most importantly, classroom peers.

circular scanning: A message selection technique in which a pointer (e.g., clock hand) moves sequentially in a clockwise or counterclockwise direction to select items or messages displayed in a circular format.

circumlocution: A roundabout expression or use of indirect language, typically seen in persons with anomic aphasia or other expressive language disorders.

civil case: A lawsuit initiated by one party against another to seek compensation for a legal injury for which there are civil remedies.

classification: The arrangement of people or objects into groups or categories according to specific criteria.

classification systems: Means of categorizing or organizing phenomena into meaningful groups or divisions. Taxonomy is an example of a classification system, but there are more classification systems than taxonomies.

cleft palate: A partial or complete fissure in the hard and/or soft palate(s) caused by failure of the palatal elements to fuse during embryonic development.

clinically isolated syndrome: Seen in multiple sclerosis, the first episode of neurological symptoms that lasts at least 24 hours, caused by inflammation or loss of the myelin sheath that covers the axons of nerve cells.

clock communicator: A switch-activated communication aid featuring adjustable-speed scanning with a clock-like dial. Words, pictures, or symbols may be attached to the panel; these items are selected via circular scanning.

clonus: Rapid involuntary alternations of muscle contraction and relaxation, which causes repetitive flexion and extension.

closed head injury: A type of head injury resulting from blunt trauma to the skull, not including injury secondary to penetrating head wounds, strokes, or tumors. A closed-head injury generally results in diffuse rather than focal brain injury.

Cloverleaf skull syndrome: A syndrome characterized by premature closure of the cranial sutures which causes upward and lateral growth of the skull into a three-leaf clover shape. Also known as *Kleebattshadel syndrome*.

cluster sampling: In research, the selection of, and focus on, a representative portion (or cluster) of a group that is being studied.

CMV: See *cytomegalovirus*.

co-active movement: One of the components of Van Dijk's (1966) Movement Based Approach. The learner and caregiver engage in activities to promote anticipatory behavior within predictable steps increasing in physical distance. Gestures and tactile cues may be used, but support should be faded as progress toward the goal (independence) is made.

co-active signing: A tactile communication approach in which the communication partner physically manipulates the hand(s)/arm(s) of the individual who experiences deaf-blindness to form standard manual signs or fingerspelling for expressive communication.

COBOL: See *Common Business-Oriented Language.*

cochlea: The snail-shaped structure in the inner ear containing the end organ of hearing (organ of Corti).

cochlear implant: An electronic device with electrodes that are surgically implanted into the cochlea to improve hearing for individuals with profound sensorineural hearing loss.

cockayne syndrome: A chronic genetic syndrome, degenerative in nature, characterized by cachectic (starvation) dwarfism, intellectual impairment, premature senility, retinal degeneration, sensorineural hearing loss, and skin photosensitivity.

coding: (1) The systematic organization of information or messages for storage and retrieval. (2) A code or system of signals (e.g., eye blink codes) used for the purpose of communication.

coding system: The process or system of assigning codes, abbreviations, or labels to represent letters, items, or messages.

Coffin-Lowry syndrome: A genetic syndrome characterized by severe intellectual impairment, abnormal facial features (e.g., bulbous nose, antimongoloid slant, pouting lower lip), tapering fingers, and short stature.

Coffin-Siris syndrome: A syndrome characterized by intrauterine and postnatal growth deficiency, intellectual impairment, abnormally small head size, course facies but very full lips, underdeveloped fifth-digit nails, and excessive hair growth (hirsutism) combined with sparse scalp hair growth; a.k.a., *fifth-digit syndrome.*

cognition: (1) The general concept embracing all the various models of knowing, including perceiving, remembering, imagining, conceiving, judging, and reasoning. (2) Awareness and ability to understand and process information.

cognitive ability: The ability of a person to learn and retain information.

cognitive development: Progressive and continuous growth of intelligence, perception, memory, imagination, conception, judgment, and reasoning.

cognitive effort: The level of complexity and intensity of cognitive processes that are required to complete a task.

cognitive impairment: An impairment of any number of the cognitive processes, including but not limited to intelligence, perception, memory, imagination, conception, judgment, and reasoning. This term is sometimes used interchangeably with intellectual impairment, but they are technically not the same. Intellectual impairment is only a type of cognitive impairment, as are aphasia and dementia, for example.

cognitive load: The amount of cognitive processing that is necessitated by a task, activity, or event.

cognitive processes: The components of cognition (e.g., intelligence, perception, memory, imagination, conception, judgment, and reasoning) that assist an individual in understanding their environment and to interact effectively within it.

cognitive reserve: Cognitive proxies, such as educational level, occupation, leisure activities, and vocabulary knowledge, that tend to compensate for cognitive loss caused by brain damage (e.g., in multiple sclerosis).

cognitive supplementation strategies: Aids and strategies used to assist an individual with cognitive decline to orient to and complete tasks (e.g., using a non–speech-generating device as a means to show a chronological sequence of events in which the patient is to engage).

Cohen syndrome: A genetic syndrome characterized by a peculiar facies, prominent incisors, long slender fingers and toes, decreased muscle tone, short stature, and onset of obesity during mid-childhood.

collaboration: The sharing of information and expertise for the purpose of generating plans, programs, and solutions to problems.

collaborative consultation: The close interaction among team members with diverse backgrounds and expertise to generate solutions to problems; most commonly associated with transdisciplinary service delivery.

collaborative learning: Learning that takes place through participation in small diverse groups. Students exchange information and use the contributions of individual group members to complete a learning task; a.k.a., *cooperative learning.*

collaborative teamwork model: A model of transdisciplinary service delivery characterized by collaboration among team members.

College of Speech Therapists: The professional body that organizes speech therapy services in the United Kingdom.

colloquial: Pertaining to familiar and informal conversation.

coloboma: An incomplete closure in one or more structures of the eye (e.g., lens, iris, retina), which appears as a cleft, gap, or keyhole; coloboma may or may not cause visual deficits.

color coding: The use of color as a basis for the systematic organization of information or messages for storage and retrieval; used in color encoding.

color graphics adapter: A monitor (e.g., computer screen) that allows a 320 x 200 dots per inch display in four colors.

Com Board: A communication aid with an adjustable-speed clock dial face that uses switch-activated scanning, with single or dual-switch input (for both clockwise and counterclockwise movement). Pictures, words, letters, or symbols may be attached to the panel.

coma: A state of unconsciousness in which there is little or no sign of mental or physical response to external stimulation; level of response is typically rated on normed objective scales.

Common Business-Oriented Language: An early computer programming language developed for use in business.

common gestures: Gestures that are used and readily recognized by members of the same culture. Examples in the American culture include thumb up meaning "perfect" or "good job"; head shake meaning "no"; and head nod meaning "yes."

communication: The linguistic or non-linguistic transmission or exchange of thoughts and information from one individual to another, regardless of the means (e.g., speech, manual sign, gestures, letters of the alphabet, or other graphic symbols).

communication act: The act of communicating, including such functions as requesting, answering, making statements, or providing descriptions.

communication aid: A physical object or device that assists an individual in communicating (e.g., partaking in conversation, writing, expressing basic needs). Communication aids are commercially available (e.g., mechanical or electronic devices) or can be individually constructed (e.g., boards, charts).

Communication Aid Manufacturers Association: An organization of manufacturers of assistive communication devices, specialized AAC materials, and software. The chair of the organization is not elected but rotates from one manufacturer to another.

communication based approaches to problem behavior: Any approach that assesses the communicative functions of problem behavior and then teaches alternative behaviors that serve the same communicative function as the replaced problem behavior.

Communication Bill of Rights: A set of guidelines developed by the National Joint Committee for the Communication Needs of Persons With Severe Disabilities that states individuals' basic rights to communication.

Communication Bill of Rights (2016): A set of guidelines that outline 15 rights designed to facilitate the AAC user's impact on the environment. These rights reflected a social mandate to improve communication and increase participation in social, educational, and vocational settings.

communication board: A non–speech-generating device used for the purpose of displaying aided symbols for communication (e.g., Picture Communication Symbols, photographs, line drawings).

communication breakdown: A communication failure between partners during a communicative interaction.

communication competence: See *communicative competence.*

communication context: See *communication environment.*

communication device: A mechanical or electronic communication aid, with or without speech output. See also *dedicated communicator* and *assistive devices—speech output.*

communication display: A general term that refers to sets of organized graphic communication symbols, including printed words. Communication displays appear in non–speech-generating and speech-generating devices.

communication efficacy: The effectiveness of communication (i.e., the ability of the individual to successfully get an intended message across to a communication partner).

communication environment: The physical and social environment of the message sender and receiver during communication. The communication environment is affected by such variables as distance between communication partners, noise level, and variations in lighting; a.k.a., *communication context.*

communication mode: The modality in which communication occurs. Gestures, facial expressions, vocalizations, reading and writing, and speech are examples of communication modes.

communication participation model: A model that provides a systematic process for conducting AAC assessments by examining the participation requirements of peers without disabilities of the same chronological age, and then using this information to design the assessment and/or intervention for a person with a disability. The four areas examined include: identification of participation patterns and communication needs, assessment of barriers, plan and implementation for interventions, and evaluation of intervention effectiveness.

communication partners: The actual and potential persons who engage in communication exchanges with an individual.

communication repair: The ability to restore and/or compensate for a conversation once a breakdown has occurred.

communication system: See *AAC system.*

communication system (multicomponent): A collection of speech, symbols, strategies, and skills that are integrated and used by an individual to communicate.

communication wall chart: A wall-mounted aid that allows several children in a classroom to make use of the same display (but in a larger format) as is available on their communication devices to communicate with their peers in the classroom.

communication wallet: A wallet-sized booklet in which an individual's communication symbols are housed.

communicative competence: The ability to communicate functionally and effectively in most or all situations. In AAC, communicative competence includes linguistic, operational, social, and strategic competence.

communicative mastery: An ability to communicate effectively at the highest level of skill in most or all situations; seldom achieved even by native speakers of a language.

Communiclock: A switch-activated communication aid featuring scanning with a clock-like dial. Words, pictures, or symbols may be attached to the panel.

community-based employment: Training programs that typically provide individuals with basic skills training, workplace-readiness, career counseling, and job search and placement services.

community-based instruction: A special education and rehabilitation approach in which functional, daily living goals are met in the actual context in which skills are required (e.g., learning to count and handle money in a department or grocery store setting); a.k.a., *community-referenced instruction.*

community language: The vernacular language that is used by the majority group in a community. Mastery of and access to the community language is a critical factor for full participation in the economic and cultural life of a community.

community-referenced instruction: See *community-based instruction.*

compact disk: A media disk in which audio and/or video information is digitally recorded and stored then played back via optic technology.

compact disk read-only memory: A media disk with storage of up to 800 MB of data. The data stored on a compact disk read only memory can be read and copied but not modified or deleted.

compatibility: (1) The ability of hardware and software devices to work together. (2) The ability of an AAC system or communication aid to meet an AAC user's abilities and needs.

competence: The quality or state of being functionally adequate or having sufficient knowledge, judgment, or skill.

complex communication needs: The needs of individuals who face barriers to effective communication. This term is often used to describe persons who rely on or use AAC.

complex rebus: See *expanded rebus.*

complexity: The physical complexity of a graphic symbol or manual sign. For graphic symbols, complexity may be related to the number of strokes or semantic elements that are required to create a symbol. The degree to which the figure of a graphic symbol may be discriminated from its background may also be an indicator of complexity. Complexity of manual signs is related to handshape difficulty, number of different movements, and type of movements.

component: An element or part of a whole. For example, the means to represent, means to select, and means to transmit a message are major components of the AAC model proposed by Lloyd and colleagues (1990).

compound symbol: In Blissymbolics, a symbol that is created from two or more semantic elements that are either sequenced or superimposed. The meaning of the compound symbol is based on the meanings of its semantic elements.

comprehension: The process whereby speech and language are understood.

comprehensive capability profiling: The gathering of maximal information about an individual in various areas for the purpose of developing a comprehensive profile of abilities and disabilities.

comprehensive communicator: In AAC intervention, one of the five categories of persons with aphasia described by Garrett and Beukelman (1992); the individual with aphasia enjoys an independent lifestyle and is typically able to augment limited spoken language with graphic and manual symbols to communicate in a variety of communication contexts.

comprehensive language assessment: An evaluation in which comprehension, expression, and communication skills are assessed. Within these three areas, single words, morphological units, syntactic structures, and connected language are assessed.

computed tomography: An imaging technique that uses X-rays to create a computerized representation of a structure (typically the brain). Computed tomography images are not as clear as magnetic resonance imaging scans but are better at pinpointing some tumors and calcified areas.

computer: An electronic device that can store, retrieve, and process data and then send the data out in a specified manner.

computer-assisted instruction: A method of instruction in which tasks or lessons are presented through the use of a computer.

computer-based communication augmentation system: A computer-hosted approach or device that can be used to augment or substitute for human speech.

computer-based communication system: A computer system that uses special software and input modes for the purpose of communication.

computer-based instruction: A method of instruction where computers are used to teach students via word processing, database, or graphic design programs.

computer system: The computer and all peripherals (e.g., monitor, printer, scanner, external drives) connected to it.

computerized visual input communication system: A computer system that contains a lexicon of linearly sequenced iconographic symbols the user accesses via a mouse. Researchers can determine whether individuals with severe aphasia can access, manipulate, and combine the visual icons according to the grammatical structures of the system.

concept: (1) An idea or meaning usually represented by a word, graphic symbol, gesture, or manual sign. (2) An idea that joins several elements from multiple sources into a single general thought.

conceptual encoding: A process of language formulation in which an individual's own association of meanings with symbols is used as the basis for the systematic organization of information or messages for storage and retrieval.

concordancer: A software tool that searches large collections of texts and creates an alphabetical list of every individual word in that collection, along with examples of how each word is used in context.

concrete: A term that describes tangible referents, such as people, places, and objects. For graphic symbols, pictographs are used to represent concrete referents; ideographs are used to represent less concrete (i.e., abstract) referents.

concrete concept: An idea or notion of a situation, symbol, or object that is characterized by actual tangible experiences, whether physical, sensational, or emotional.

concreteness: (1) A term tied to Paivio's Dual Coding Model and used in the psychology literature, defined as the ability of a word to form a mental image. A word with high concreteness is easy to visualize while a word with low concreteness (an abstract word) is difficult to visualize. (2) In AAC, concreteness is used as a descriptor for referents. Concrete referents are relatively easy to depict graphically, usually as pictographs. Less concrete referents require depiction through ideographic or arbitrary symbols.

concurrent validity: The relationship between a valid measurement that already exists and a measurement that is under development. In developing formal assessment tools, measures obtained from the assessment tool under development are compared to measures from an established assessment tool that presumably assesses the same phenomena. A high positive correlation between the two assessment tools serves as an indicator of concurrent validity for the assessment tool under development.

conduction aphasia: A relatively rare type of aphasia caused by damage to the nerve fibers in the arcuate fasciculus that connects Wernicke's and Broca's areas. The disorder is characterized by generally fluent speech and good language comprehension, but poor oral reading and verbal repetition, and metathesis of sounds within words (e.g., "ephelant" for "elephant").

conductive hearing impairment: A reversible hearing loss caused by impairment or loss of function in the outer and/or middle ear structures. Once proper function returns to these structures (e.g., due to medical intervention), prepathological hearing acuity returns.

confidence interval: A statistical term most often used in sampling studies; the distance determined by confidence limits wherein a population value is most likely to be found.

confidence limits: The range wherein a population value is most likely to be found, set off by confidence intervals.

configure: The changing of hardware and software settings to optimize usage.

Confused/Agitated: Maximal Assistance: Level IV of the *Rancho Los Amigos Levels of Cognitive Functioning Scale-Revised*, characterized in part by very brief and usually nonpurposeful moments of sustained alternatives and divided attention, poor short-term memory, possible aggressive or flight behavior, inability to cooperate with treatment efforts, and verbalizations that are frequently incoherent and/or inappropriate to the activity or environment.

Confused, Appropriate: Moderate Assistance: Level VI of the *Rancho Los Amigos Levels of Cognitive Functioning Scale-Revised*, characterized in part by inconsistent orientation to person, time, and place, ability to attend to highly familiar tasks in a nondistracting environment, vague recognition of staff members, moderate assistance for problem-solving obstacles to task completion ability to consistently follow simple directions, and verbal expressions that are appropriate in highly familiar and structured situations.

Confused, Inappropriate Non-Agitated: Maximal Assistance: Level V of the *Rancho Los Amigos Levels of Cognitive Functioning Scale-Revised*, characterized in part by possible agitation in response to external stimuli, lack of orientation to person, place, or time, severely impaired recent memory with confusion of past and present, inappropriate use of objects without supervision, inability to learn new information, and verbalizations about present events that become inappropriate and confabulatory when external structure and cues are not provided.

congenital disability: A disability that is present at birth and usually the result of disease or injury.

congenital disorder: A disorder that is present at birth and possibly caused by hereditary or other problems occurring before or during the birth process.

congestive heart failure: A potentially fatal condition resulting from venous stasis and reduced outflow of blood from the heart, characterized by weakness, breathlessness, abdominal discomfort, and edema in the lower body.

consensus building: A service delivery process whereby information is shared and processed by members within a transdisciplinary team. Decisions are made by agreement of team members.

consequences: Actions or events that occur after a behavior occurs, often described within ABC charts to determine the function of the behavior.

constant light cue: A cue consisting of a flashing light for 5-second intervals or a continuously shining light on the target symbol(s); used when the augmented speaker fails to respond to a momentary light cue.

construct validity: In research, the concern that a test or instrument is measuring the theoretical variables it claims to be measuring.

consultant: An individual (usually a professional) who provides "expert" information to another individual (e.g., another professional or a lay person).

consultee: An individual who receives "expert" information from a consultant and often implements programs based on this information.

consumer: See *AAC user*. A family member of an AAC user may also be referred to as a consumer.

contact gesture: A category of gesture in which some part of the individual's body (e.g., finger, thumb, hand) is touching a real object/person that is within reach to establish shared attention.

contact guard: The placing of hands on a patient to assist with thorough and safe completion of a task.

contact signs: Manual signs in which the hands make contact with each other or one or both hands make contact with another body part during production.

content validity: In research, indicates the representativeness of a variable being measured.

context: The social, linguistic, and/or physical circumstances in which spoken or written communication occurs that generally aids comprehension of meaning.

contingency mapping: A visual representation of two choices to a situation, representing the consequence for each choice.

continuing education: In-service education (e.g., conferences, seminars, workshops) that provides practicing professionals opportunities to acquire updated information on relevant topics, develop new skills, and meet ongoing continuing education requirements for certification or licensure. Continuing education activities serve to maintain and upgrade the skills of professionals who have AAC training and develop new skills in professionals who do not.

continuum of developmental disabilities: A categorical method of examining developmental disabilities by emphasizing how they are similar. Oftentimes children with one disorder exhibit characteristics of one or more other disorders.

continuum of services: The entire range of services and programs that are available to individuals with AAC needs.

contoured seats: Chairs and other seats that have curved surfaces to approximate the shape of the body.

contraction: The shortening of a muscle, thereby creating tension. Without this tension, one would not be able to maintain and control upright posture and resist the force of gravity.

contracture: Tightening of soft tissues around a joint resulting from restricted joint movement.

control display: A communication system display that enables the user to observe message choices and monitor message preparation.

control groups (or subjects, or participants): The group(s) or individual(s) in an experimental study who do not receive the experimental treatment or condition. Control groups serve as a means of comparison for the various experimental groups on which a study is focused.

control series: An experimental design wherein the research groups are not the same, so comparisons among the groups are made based on differences that are greater or lesser than the original differences.

control site: An individual's point of contact with a device, used to activate its switches or controls. Control sites can include body surfaces or the end of a pointer (e.g., a head pointer).

controlled situation communicator: In AAC intervention, one of the five categories of persons with aphasia described by Garrett and Beukelman (1992); the individual typically exhibits severe chronic Broca's aphasia and does not typically initiate communication but rather needs a great degree of assistance to engage in routine conversational exchanges. The individual can usually indicate their needs by spontaneously pointing to items and objects.

Convaid: An archaic, portable speech-generating device that features a 64-square keyboard and a choice of male, female, or child voice.

conventionality: In AAC, the acceptance and adoption of a symbol as a representation of a specific referent or group of referents. Conventionality occurs through widespread use of symbols.

conversational competence: The knowledge and skills that are needed to transmit and receive information and messages sufficiently for conversation.

conversational control: The method by which an individual manages communication interaction. It involves a number of behaviors that occur during interaction, such as turn taking, topic initiating, interrupting, and role changing (between the initiator and responder).

conversational controllers: Words and phrases that facilitate an individual's ability to maintain conversational control, including turn taking, topic initiating, interrupting, and role changing (between the initiator and responder).

Converse with Claudius: "Calling Line Announcement Using Digitally Integrated Voice Synthesis" (named for the Roman Emperor who suffered from a speech defect); a device that can be attached to a telephone, consisting of a 16-button keypad that can produce 64 synthesized speech messages, including emergency (911) messages; it can also be used during face-to-face interactions. Claudius was developed by British Telecom and is manufactured by A. P. Besson.

cooperative learning: See *collaborative learning*.

cooperative play: The fifth stage of play development in which children begin to take turns and play together cooperatively.

core vocabulary: Words or messages with universal utility across individuals; includes commonly used structure words.

Cornelia de Lange syndrome: A severe intellectual impairment accompanied by abnormally small head growth (microcephaly), short stature, small arms and legs, excessive hair growth, and facial abnormalities.

correlation: A statistical measurement of the relationship between or among two or more variables; a correlation coefficient shows the strength and direction (positive or negative) of the relationship.

cortical visual impairment: A loss of sight, yet with preserved pupillary reflexes, caused by bilateral lesions in the visual sensory cortex.

cosmesis: The aesthetic quality (as defined by the user and others) of symbols and communication devices.

COTA: Common medical abbreviation for *certified occupational therapy assistant.*

cotreatment: Service delivery model in which professionals from more than one discipline provide treatment at the same time (e.g., an occupational therapist works alongside a speech-language pathologist to facilitate communication for an AAC user during lunch).

Council for Exceptional Children: A national association having a focus on improving services for exceptional individuals (e.g., gifted individuals and individuals with intellectual impairments, emotional disturbances, learning disabilities, and physical impairments). Professionals in special education and related fields, parents, and individuals with disabilities make up the larger proportion of its membership. Several Council for Exceptional Children divisions are of particular relevance to AAC: Division for Children's Communication Development, Division for Culturally and Linguistically Diverse Exceptional Learners, Division for Physical and Health Disabilities, Division on Mental Retardation and Developmental Disabilities, and Technology and Media Division.

course facies: A term synonymous with masked facies, a blank facial expression due to neurological involvement of the facial muscles.

covariance: A process of statistical analysis where a criterion variable is mathematically changed to compensate for the preliminary difference(s) in the groups being compared.

coverage vocabulary: The limited number of words or messages that enable an individual to communicate on a wide range of topics.

CP: See *cerebral palsy.*

CPT: See *current procedural terminology.*

CPU: See *central processing unit.*

cranial nerves: Twelve pairs of nerves originating from the brainstem that provide sensory and motor innervation primarily to the facial, head, and neck regions; visceral organs are also provided with innervation from the autonomic nervous system.

craniofacial: Referring to the bones of the skull, including the cranial (i.e., "brain case") and facial bones.

craniostosis: See *craniosynostosis.*

craniosynostosis: A premature closing of the skull sutures that prevents brain growth and usually leads to developmental disabilities; a.k.a., *craniostosis.*

credentialing: Professional recognition accomplished through certification by professional organizations and licensing by state agencies. It assures the public that professionals have met certain minimum standards (academic coursework and clinical experiences) needed to deliver appropriate services.

credibility: In evaluation studies, the belief in the competence and integrity of those administering the evaluation.

cri-du-chat syndrome: A genetic syndrome characterized by lack of growth and a mewing, cat-like cry in infancy; also results in abnormally small head growth (microcephaly) and a rounded, moon-shaped face with widely spaced eyes, elongated upper eyelid folds (i.e., epicanthic folds), and downward slanting eye slits.

criteria-based assessment: Assessment that is designed to determine whether skills are sufficient to support particular AAC strategies and techniques based on predetermined criteria.

criteria-based profiling: The judging of an individual's abilities against a set of criteria considered essential to that particular area of investigation.

criterion (criteria): A pre-established reference that serves as a point of comparison or as a means for inclusion or exclusion during assessment or research activity.

cross modal: Simultaneous use of more than one mode of communication (e.g., the concurrent use of speech and manual signs as occurs in manually coded English).

Crouzon syndrome: A genetic syndrome characterized by premature fusion of skull sutures that leads to an irregular, flat head shape (brachycephaly), atypical facial tissue development (hypoplasia), shallow eye orbits (resulting in a pop-eyed look), a parrot beaked nose, and a relatively prominent jaw (prognathism).

CRT: See *cathode ray tube.*

CSF: See *cerebrospinal fluid.*

CT: See *computed tomography.*

CTG: Common medical abbreviation for *contact guard.*

cued speech: An unaided symbol system developed in the 1960s by Orin Cornett that utilizes hand cues produced simultaneously with speech to assist a person with profound hearing impairment in speechreading (lipreading).

cued systems: Communication systems in which partial phonemic or phonologic information is represented by symbols, usually hand cues (i.e., various handshapes and placement locations). The symbols are presented simultaneously with speech to provide visual cues for the person with a profound hearing impairment as they attempt to "read" the speaker's lips.

cues: (1) Naturally occurring stimuli in the environment that may prompt a response (e.g., the sight and/or smell of a cookie may cause an individual to ask for it). (2) Artificially created stimuli that are used in the educational setting as a part of certain teaching strategies (e.g., embellishment, prompting and fading, expectant time delay).

cultural background: The totality of an individual's beliefs, values, traditions, behaviors, language institutions, technologies, and survival systems, formed by the individual's identity and life experiences.

cultural competence: A set of congruent behaviors, attitudes, and policies that come together in a system, agency, or among professionals that enable that system, agency, or profession to work effectively in situations that cross cultural boundaries.

culture: The beliefs, values, traditions, behaviors, and communication patterns members of a community share as a function of social membership.

current procedural terminology: Code used in audiology for audiograms and hearing aid examinations and selections.

curriculum research: Experimental methods used to evaluate courses and methods of instruction. It involves making statements of theory, conditions, and hypotheses and identifying necessary data to be collected to test the hypotheses.

cursor: A special dynamic screen character that marks the location of the mouse or where the next keyboard character will appear. Cursors may be arrows, blinking bars, underlined letters, or any other type of special character.

cursor keys: Specified keys on a keyboard (usually arrow keys) that can be used to move a cursor up, down, left, or right on the computer screen.

custom contoured seats: Customized chairs and other seats with surfaces shaped to conform to the individual's body.

custom-encoded speech: See *linear predictive coding*.

CVA: See *cerebrovascular accident*.

C-VIC: See *computerized visual input communication system*.

cytomegalovirus: A herpes-type virus that may be transmitted to the fetus in utero, during delivery, or from breast milk. In-utero transmission results in the most severe congenital defects. Cytomegalovirus may result in symptoms resembling mononucleosis or may result in no symptoms at all (i.e., asymptomatic). Cytomegalovirus is the most common viral etiology of congenital hearing loss, resulting in various types of sensorineural hearing losses (e.g., bilateral or unilateral, progressive or stable).

dactylology: Hand and finger movements as a means of communication (e.g., fingerspelling).

daily routine diary: A tool for identifying the vocabulary needed for communication and participation in daily routines. Words, phrases, and sentences that an AAC user may need to engage in various activities are recorded.

daisy wheel printer: An impact printer in which letters and other characters are on individual spokes on a daisy wheel and are pressed through an inked ribbon. The characters are of higher quality that those in dot matrix printers.

Dandy-Walker syndrome: A syndrome resulting from a malformation of the brain where the fourth ventricle enlarges so much that it pushes into the cerebellum, prohibiting normal formation of the cerebellum's central portion. It is often associated with hydrocephalus, as well as other brain and body malformations.

Danish Mouth-Hand System: A Danish cued-speech system that disambiguates the movement patterns of the mouth, lips, cheeks, and face during speech to assist a person with a profound hearing impairment to speech-read.

database: A collection of data or information that is arranged for ease and speed of search and retrieval.

database program: A computer program (software) that enables the user to organize, store, and retrieve data according to specified fields or categories (e.g., alphabetical, numerical, topical).

day clock: A device that resembles a clock, used to display information about an AAC user's daily routine or schedule.

dB: See *decibel*.

deaf (deafness): A condition in which the auditory system is not used as the primary sensory means for learning speech and language and the sense of hearing is so lacking or drastically reduced that it prohibits normal functioning as a hearing person.

Deaf-blind: A term used to describe an individual whose vision and hearing are so impaired that they require specialized methods of communication different from those used by the Deaf or the blind. Instead, residual vision and hearing are used in conjunction with the sense of touch. Such individuals may not be equally handicapped in each modality, and in fact, might not meet the legal definition of either deafness or blindness. The term *dual sensory impairment* is used more commonly today.

decibel: The unit of measure for sound intensity. The range of human audibility is measured on a Bel scale (named in honor of Alexander Graham Bell) that represents the difference in pressure from a sound that is just barely audible to a sound that reaches the threshold of pain (this magnitude is approximately 10^{14}); each unit of the Bel scale is an exponent of 10, so that range of human audibility is expressed on a scale from 1 to 14 units. Since this scale is too narrow, the decibel is used instead of the Bel. "Deci-" means one-tenth, so that each Bel is equal to 10 decibels, making the range of human audibility 0 to 140 dB (0 dB represents a sound that is just barely audible; 140 dB represents the threshold of pain).

decoding: The cognitive process of interpreting a sender's message (i.e., converting the sender's symbols into the message).

DECtalk: Digital Equipment Corporation's synthetic speech that is a combination of text-to-speech synthesis and digitization. It includes nine factory-made voices (e.g., Beautiful Betty, Kit the Kid, Perfect Paul) and one user-definable voice.

dedicated augmentative and alternative communication system: An AAC device or piece of equipment that is designed specifically to operate as a communication aid.

dedicated augmentative communication device: A device that is specifically designed to be used for communication but may also be interfaced to a computer, printer, or environmental control unit.

dedicated communication aid: A communication device designed specifically to operate as a communication aid.

default: The standard factory settings for hardware or software that remain in effect until specifically changed by the user. Defaults are preset to those choices most commonly chosen or that require the minimal time for setup or operation.

deferred imitation: One of the components of Van Dijk's (1966) Movement Based Approach. Initially, the caregiver physically prompts the learner to produce a target movement, then the prompts are gradually faded so the learner begins to imitate the movement in response to a model separated by space and time (e.g., rolling a ball back to the caregiver after the caregiver has rolled the ball to the learner).

degenerative: A term that is used to describe conditions or diseases that progressively worsen over time (e.g., amyotrophic lateral sclerosis).

degree of ambiguity: The number of concepts one can encode for a single symbol. As the number of different meanings for a symbol increases, ambiguity becomes greater as well.

degrees of freedom: A statistical phrase implying the lack of restraints on a set of scores. Degrees of freedom are closely associated with the number of observations in a set of data (e.g., n-1).

deictic: A type of natural gesture, generally pointing with the index finger extended (although other body parts can be used), to call attention to a specific referent and single it out from other possible ones; deictic gestures vary across cultures.

dementia: An acquired progressive deterioration of cognitive function.

demographics: The characteristics of human populations and population segments, including such variables as age, disability, education, family life cycle, family size, gender, home ownership, income, nationality, occupation, religion, sexual orientation, and socioeconomic status.

demyelination: A breakdown or loss of myelin, the protein and lipid-rich matter that surrounds, protects, isolates, and insulates the axons of nerve cells in the brain and spinal cord, seen in degenerative neurological disorders such as multiple sclerosis.

Department of Health and Human Services: An agency of the federal government that is concerned with the health and welfare issues of U.S. citizens. The Department of Health and Human Services oversees the Social Security Administration, Office of Human Development, Health Care Financing Administration, Family Services Administration, Developmental Disabilities Administration, and Public Health Service.

deposition: A written or videotaped statement taken under oath used as testimony in a due process hearing or a court of law.

dermatome: A localized area of skin that has its sensation via a single nerve from a single nerve root in the spinal cord.

design attributes: A component of aided and unaided AAC symbols and refers to how the symbols are presented or transmitted. There are six design attributes for aided symbols (object, pictorial, line drawing, phonemic- or phonetic-based, alphabet-based, electronically generated) and seven design attributes for unaided symbols (gestures, sign languages, pedagogical sign systems, tactile or vibrotactile, phonemic- or phonetic-based, alphabet-based, vocal).

design characteristics: See *design attributes*.

designation: One of the basic parameters of manual sign, along with handshape, location, and movement.

desktop: The area on a computer monitor screen where icons for application software (computer programs), files, and trash usually appear.

developmental aphasia: A childhood language disorder characterized by complete or partial impairment of language comprehension, formulation, and use, excluding disorders associated with primary sensory deficits, general mental deterioration, or psychiatric disorders. See also *specific language impairment*.

developmental apraxia: A term used to describe apraxia during childhood, characterized by unintelligible speech in the absence of any known neuromuscular pathology (e.g., dysarthria) or other obvious organic impairment.

developmental delay: A persistent delay in the process of development occurring in one or several areas (e.g., cognitive, language, motor, or social skills).

Developmental Disabilities Assistance and Bill of Rights Act Amendments of 1975 (PL 94-103): Federal legislation that further expanded the definition of developmental disabilities to include persons with autism spectrum disorder and select types of dyslexia. This law also mandated that states and territories design a system of protection and advocacy for persons with developmental disabilities as a condition of receiving federal funding.

Developmental Disabilities Assistance and Bill of Rights Act Amendments of 1987 (PL 100-146): Federal legislation that was an amendment to the Community Mental Health Act of 1963 (PL 88-164). This law included persons with intellectual impairments, autism spectrum disorder, cerebral palsy, and seizure disorders under the definition of developmental disabilities and included a Bill of Rights for people with developmental disabilities. Funding was also authorized for a wide variety of programs and services affecting these individuals.

Developmental Disabilities Assistance and Bill of Rights Act Amendments of 1990 (PL 101-496): Federal legislation that amended PL 88-164 and PL 100-146 by adding goals of interdependence, community acceptance, and inclusion for all people with developmental disabilities. Grants were also authorized to support planning, coordination, and delivery of specialized services to people with developmental disabilities.

Developmental Disabilities Services and Facilities Construction Amendments of 1970 (PL 91-517): Federal legislation that expanded the Community Mental Health Act of 1963 (PL 88-164) by including services for people with cerebral palsy and seizure disorders. The concept of developmental disability was introduced in this law.

developmental disability: A disability affecting the development of cognitive, communication, motor, or social-emotional skills that is present prior to adulthood. See *acquired disability.*

developmental disorder: Any disorder that occurs after birth, during childhood (as opposed to a congenital disorder).

developmental dysphasia: A less severe form of developmental aphasia. See also *specific language impairment.*

developmental language disorder: See *specific language impairment.*

developmental period: The period from birth to approximately 18 years of age when cognitive, communication, motor, and social-emotional skills are developing.

developmental vocabulary: Vocabulary that an individual is acquiring but may not be able to read.

df: See *degrees of freedom.*

DHHS: See *Department of Health and Human Services.*

Dial Scan: A dedicated communication aid that uses rotary scanning and has a clear face that allows for interactive communication. The user uses an adjustable-speed switch to stop a clock-like dial on the appropriate item on the overlay.

dialogue method: A vocabulary selection method that considers several factors, including age and cognitive appropriateness, colloquialism, vocabulary richness, reusability, and intelligibility of synthesized speech.

differential reinforcement: The idea that appropriate behaviors (e.g., not displaying challenging behavior, using an effective and socially acceptable communication strategy, choosing a positive responsive) will be reinforced while reinforcement will be withheld for inappropriate behaviors.

digital: The storage and retrieval of data in binary code.

digitized speech: Natural speech that is electronically recorded and digitized (i.e., converted into a binary code).

diplegia: Paralysis of corresponding parts on both sides of the body, more often referring to the lower extremities.

diplopia: Double vision.

direct method: Any method (e.g., antecedent-behavior-consequence charts, scatterplot analyses, direct observations) that identifies the natural covariation between problem behavior and environmental events occurring prior and subsequent to the problem behavior.

direct selection: A message selection technique in which the AAC user indicates choices on a display using a body part or prosthetic device interfaced with a body part (e.g., touching with a finger, gazing with the eyes, touching with a headstick).

directed scanning: A message selection technique in which the movement of a cursor is directed by a multidirectional switch (e.g., joystick) that allows movement in four or more directions.

disability: A limitation, due to an impairment, to engage in activities or perform skills that the typical person can do (e.g., a motor impairment might result in a walking disability).

discourse: The continuous exchange of ideas or information during communication; the pattern of conversation.

discourse analysis: The analysis of conversational patterns.

discrete trial therapy: A component of applied behavioral analysis in which skills are broken down into discrete elements and then taught in a series of steps using behavioral principles.

disjuncture: Transition that occurs during conversation.

disk drive: A computer hardware device that can store information. The disk drive can use removable media or may be hard disk storage.

disk operating system: Software that exercises direct control and management of computer hardware and basic system operations. Additionally, it provides a foundation upon which to run application software, such as word processing programs, web browsers, and others. See also *MS-DOS.*

display: The housing of aided AAC symbols (e.g., communication book, board, wallet, computer overlay).

display-based encoding: Encoding that involves the use of a display with a control device that allows the AAC user to send a message without the need to memorize a code or refer to a chart.

display permanence: A symbol selection consideration that refers to aided symbols that can be mounted on a communication device external to the body.

disruptive behavior: Behavior that disrupts instruction (e.g., throwing oneself on the floor, manipulating lights in the classroom).

distal: Removed in location to the point of origin or attachment. Opposite of *proximal*.

distal gesture: A category of gesture in which the individual uses some part of their body to call attention to a referent that is distant and out of reach, often with the index finger extended (e.g., pointing).

DME: See *durable medical equipment*.

DOE: Common medical abbreviation for *dyspnea on exertion*.

dopamine: A neurotransmitter released by neurons in the basal ganglia of the brain; a deficiency of its production has been linked to Parkinson's disease.

dorsal: Posterior or pertaining to the back or backside.

dorsiflexion: Flexing the foot upward, toward the knee.

DOS: See *disk operating system*.

dot matrix printer: An impact printer that forms patterns of tiny dots to create characters on a page when pressed through an inked ribbon.

dots per inch: Used to describe the resolution of computer monitors (the greater the dots per inch, the better the resolution of the screen).

Down syndrome: A congenital condition (trisomy 21) typically resulting in cognitive impairment and also characterized by any number of the following: hypotonia, short stature, speckling of the iris, short fingers, flat facial profile, epicanthal folds, upslanting eye slits, small ears, cardiac and thyroid disorders, duodenal atresia, atlantoaxial instability, and hearing loss.

dpi: See *dots per inch*.

DS: See *Down syndrome*.

DSI: See *dual sensory impairment*.

DTT: See *discrete trial therapy*.

dual classification: A term used to describe symbols that may be viewed as either pictographs or ideographs in Blissymbolics.

dual rocker lever: A general purpose dual switch in which a lever rocks back and forth on a fulcrum.

dual sensory impairment: Simultaneous impairment of both hearing and vision. One impairment may come on before the other or they both may come on at the same time.

durability: The ability of symbols and communication devices to withstand the rigors of daily use.

durable medical equipment: Equipment that is primarily and customarily used to serve a medical or therapeutic purpose, is built for repeated use, generally does not benefit a person in the absence of illness or injury, and is appropriate for use within the home.

Dvorak keyboard: A variation of the standard typewriter keyboard, where the most frequently occurring letters are arranged in the "home" or middle row where they tend to be most accessible.

dx: Common medical abbreviation for *diagnosis*.

dyad: The relationship between two persons who are engaged in a communicative exchange.

dynamic: (1) A symbol in which movement or change is necessary to understand its meaning (e.g., most manual signs). (2) Symbols that are animated on the display of a device (e.g., DynaSyms).

dynamic displays: (1) A method of vocabulary selection where activation of a spot on a touch-sensitive screen will cause related vocabulary items to appear; the images or symbols on the screen continuously change with subsequent activations. (2) Screens on speech-generative devices that display animated symbols or images.

dynamic symbols: Symbols whose meanings are conveyed by change, transition, or movement, and because of this, cannot be considered permanent and enduring. Examples are speech (both natural and synthetic) and most gestures and manual signs.

DynaSyms: Graphic symbols used on DynaVox devices, created by Faith Carlson.

dysarthria: A general term used to denote a motor impairment in the production of speech due to damage to the central or peripheral nervous system, resulting in paralysis, weakness, and lack of coordination of the muscles involved in speech. Any number of the processes of speech (i.e., articulation, phonation, prosody, resonance, respiration) can be adversely affected.

dysexecutive syndrome: A dysregulation of executive functions (e.g., defining and achieving goals, flexibility, emotion control, organization, planning and prioritization, time management, self-restraint) associated with damage to the frontal lobe of the brain.

dyscalculia: Typically associated with a pattern of learning disabilities, it is an impairment of the ability to calculate or manipulate number symbols.

dysphagia: A disorder of any step in the process of swallowing, including bolus preparation, bolus movement, and the mechanics of the swallow.

dysphasia: See *aphasia*.

dysphonia: A voice disorder characterized by faulty phonation or resonation and pitch deviations, usually a result of vocal hyperfunction (abusive vocal behaviors) but may also have an organic etiology.

dyspnea on exertion: Abnormal shortness of breath during physical activity, usually a sign of cardiac pathology.

early communication process: Consists of four levels of communication: gaining attention, making requests or expressing interests, making choices or expressing preferences, and using symbols to make choices or express preferences.

early intervention: Educational and other services provided to children of school age or younger who are discovered to have or be at risk of developing a handicapping condition or other special need that may affect their development. Early intervention can be remedial or preventive in nature.

early intervention service coordinator: The individual who is responsible for coordinating the various services that are provided to a child who is engaged in early intervention.

EBP: See *evidence-based practice.*

echolalia: Speech that is characterized by a parrot-like echoing of words spoken by others. See also *unconventional verbal behavior.*

ecological inventory: A tool for gathering information for identifying vocabulary needs through systematic task analyses of routines and activities; similar to an environmental inventory.

ECU: See *environmental control unit.*

Education Amendments of 1974 (PL 93-380): Federal legislation that amended the Elementary and Secondary Education Act of 1965 (PL 89-10). One of the amendments renamed Title VI of the Elementary and Secondary Education Act to the Education of the Handicapped Act Amendments of 1974. This law required states to establish a timeline for implementing complete educational opportunities for all children with disabilities. The second major amendment, the Family Education Rights and Privacy Act, gave parents and students the right to examine their child's school records.

Education for All Handicapped Children Act of 1975 (PL 94-142): Landmark federal legislation that mandated free and appropriate public education for all children with disabilities. Its primary provisions included a process for evaluating children to determine their disabilities, developing individualized education programs, and requiring that students be placed in the least restrictive environment.

Education for All Handicapped Children Act Amendments of 1983 (PL 98-199): Federal legislation that expanded programs for individuals with disabilities to include transition services, parent training, and financial incentives for research into preschool education and early intervention programs.

Education for All Handicapped Children Act Amendments of 1986 (PL 99-457): Federal legislation that mandated services for children with disabilities from 3 years of age and also provided incentives for states to provide early intervention services for children (birth to 3 years).

Education for All Handicapped Children Act Amendments of 1990 (PL 101-476): See *Individuals with Disabilities Education Act of 1990.*

educational/regional center: A center created primarily to train personnel, assess equipment, and provide assistance with intervention and follow-up. Regional centers establish an "umbrella" agency that ensures AAC services are provided to individuals and staff members.

Edwards syndrome: Also known as Trisomy 18; Edwards syndrome is a serious genetic disorder associated with a third copy of a portion or the entirety of chromosome 18. Individuals born with this condition are very likely to experience severe multiple disabilities; only a very small minority survive to reach 1 year of age.

efficacy: A term meaning effectiveness and used to describe approaches, services, systems, methods, and techniques in general and communication specifically.

efficiency: A term meaning productivity and used to describe AAC symbols or systems.

efficient system: An AAC system that enables the user to produce messages in an acceptable amount of time without the need for extensive training or practice.

EGA: See *enhanced graphics adapter.*

EHA: See *Education for All Handicapped Children Act of 1975 (PL 94-142).*

e-helper: An aide who assists a person who uses AAC to help them access tele-practice services. This electronic helper (e-helper for short) may assist with some or all the following tasks or issues: technical setup of cameras, web connectivity/ensuring access to the internet is available, positioning the person who uses AAC so they can readily see the screen and be picked up by a camera, and attend to all manner of technical issues before, during, and after a session. This person may also have a role in training support personnel and extenders (e.g., rehabilitation technicians, family members, community workers, speech-language pathology assistants and audiology assistants) appropriately when delivering services.

EHF: See *extremely high frequency.*

EI: See *early intervention.*

elective mutism: An emotional disorder characterized by an unwillingness to speak, usually in certain situations or environments (e.g., speaking to an authority figure, speaking in front of class at school).

electrolarynx: A type of battery operated artificial larynx that generates a buzzing sound by means of a vibrating head. When the device is placed against the neck or in the mouth, sound is transmitted to the oral-pharyngeal cavity, which can be modified into phonemes for speech by movement of the articulators.

electronic book: A computer input system that allows alternate access to a BBC microcomputer, consisting of an A4 ring binder that is connected to the computer with 12 touch-sensitive cells at the back. An overlay is placed on top and when the operator touches the required picture, the computer responds accordingly.

electronic scanning: A message selection technique in which an electronic device is used to select items from a display.

electronics: The science or use of electron-flow devices that have no moving parts, such as vacuum tubes and transistors.

elementary: The level of skill associated with the 5- to 13-year-old age group.

Elementary and Secondary Education Act Amendments of 1969 (PL 91-230): Federal legislation that consolidated a number of federal grant programs for the education of children with disabilities.

elfin facies: An elf-like facial appearance often observed in a number of syndromes, such as leprechaunism and Williams syndrome.

elicitation techniques: Any intervention technique used in an attempt to increase the likelihood that certain behaviors will occur (e.g., modeling, expansion, prompting, and questioning).

embedded skill: A specific behavior or ability that occurs within the context of a larger, more encompassing activity.

emblem: Gestural behavior that can be translated or defined by a few words or a phrase without using speech to convey the message.

emergent literacy: A theory developed from research in child development, psychology, education, linguistics, anthropology, and sociology that is gradually replacing the notion of reading readiness. Emergent literacy suggests that the development of literacy (i.e., speaking, listening, reading, writing) is a gradual process that takes place over time within the child, based upon the child's own natural learning ability and upon the right conditions being in place. Emergent literacy theory requires a shift away from the traditional approaches that have been used to teach literacy in early childhood programs.

emojis: Various icons, images, or symbols typically used in electronic communication (e.g., text messages, emails) usually confined to emotions but can also represent other concepts graphically instead of by using words.

emulator: A device that simulates the action of another device, thereby providing an alternate to the device being emulated (e.g., a mouse simulates the function of a keyboard when it is used to select letters from a screen).

encephalitis: An inflammation or infection of the brain, having either a bacterial or viral etiology.

encoding: The formulation of language. In AAC, encoding refers to the systematic organization of information or messages for storage and retrieval and the process by which signals or symbols are used to express messages.

encoding system: Any system in which an object, sound, vocalization, or other cue is used as a form of code to produce communication (e.g., dits and dahs are used to represent the letters of the alphabet in Morse code).

endogenous feedback: Feedback that originates from within the organism. Proprioceptive feedback is a form of endogenous feedback for humans.

endurance: The ability to sustain an activity for a certain amount of time (e.g., sustain muscle forces necessary to direct select).

enhanced graphics adapter: A high-quality color computer monitor that allows a 640 x 360 dots per inch display in 16 colors.

enhanced natural gestures: Intentional behaviors present in an individual's gesture/motor repertoire or that can be easily taught on the basis of extant motor skills; selected for ease of interpretation by others.

enhancement: The addition of visual cues to clarify the meaning of graphic symbols. Enhancements are usually faded so that the individual learns the meanings of the original (nonenhanced) symbols.

environmental control unit: An electronic device that allows the user to exercise control over objects in the environment (e.g., fan, lights, television).

environmental inventory: A tool for gathering information for identifying vocabulary needs related to the interests and activities of individuals; similar to an ecological inventory.

EOB: See *explanation of benefits.*

epicanthus/epicanthal fold: A semilunar (crescent-shaped) fold of skin that extends downward from the side of the nose to the lower eyelid and partially covers the inner canthus of the eye. It is associated with Down syndrome and other genetic syndromes.

epidemiology: The study of diseases and their distribution, determinants, and deterrents.

epilepsy: See *seizure.*

Epson HX-20 computer: An archaic, portable, battery-powered microcomputer that had a built-in mini-printer, screen, and microcassette drive to allow uploading and downloading of vocabulary.

ergonomics: A term used more often in Europe, it is the study and practice of the interaction and interrelatedness of humans with technology. The term *human factors* tends to be used more in North America.

error analysis: The process of examining an individual's incorrect responses to gain insight into their use of ineffective strategies or productions.

errorless learning: Learning in which few or no errors are made. The clinician or educator uses procedures, such as stimulus shaping, fading, and most to least prompting, so that the learner has minimal opportunity for errors. For example, if the learner begins to reach toward an incorrect symbol, the clinician or educator may provide a physical prompt directing the learner to the correct symbol.

escape motivated problem behavior: Problem behavior in which the purpose is to terminate, postpone, or escape demands.

esophageal atresia: A congenital condition in which the esophagus terminates in a blind pouch and is not continuous with the stomach.

esophageal speech: Speech that is produced by vibration of the upper portion of the esophagus, rather than the vocal folds, usually by a person who has undergone laryngectomy.

esotropia: The movement of turning inward (e.g., an eyeball turning towards the nose).

ethics: Principles that are related to acceptable behavior, based upon precepts of morality.

E-TRAN: Eye transfer; a transparent communication board (usually constructed of plexiglass) with the center cut out that enables an AAC user to sit opposite a communication partner and send a message by gazing at symbols on the board. The communication partner follows the user's eye gaze to the selected symbols.

EvalPAC/Epson: An archaic, portable, dedicated speech-generating device that featured a variety of input modes for evaluation purposes. It included the SpeechPAC, a connection panel activated by a light pointer, gross motor scanning, a joystick, and Morse code. It could also function as a keyboard with the Apple IIe emulator or with the Unicorn Keyboard. It used both alphabet and picture overlays, and programs could be stored on a microcassette.

EvalPAC with RealVoice: An archaic communication device that was similar to the EvalPAC/Epson (Adaptive Communication Systems Technology, Inc.) but featured the RealVoice speech synthesizer that was available in both male and female voices.

evaluation: The process of assessing an individual's abilities through the use of formal and informal procedures to determine the nature, extent, and impact of a problem.

evidence-based practice: The establishment of best practice in a discipline that occurs when clinicians work in partnership with their clients and use research evidence along with clinical knowledge and reasoning to implement interventions that are most effective in terms of their costs and outcomes for the client.

ex parte communication: Undisclosed communication between a judge or impartial hearing officer and one of the two parties involved in a legal action. This type of communication is considered illegal and applies to hearings, as well as civil and criminal cases.

Exacttalk: A synthetic speech code that allowed for novel and spontaneous messages.

existing communicative repertoire: Receptive and expressive communication skills that an individual has already learned.

exogenous feedback: Feedback originating from outside the organism. For example, in the process of communication, a listener may use a head nod or other signal to indicate to the speaker that they understand the speaker's message.

exotropia: The movement of turning outward (e.g., an eyeball turning away from the nose).

expanded abbreviation: See *abbreviation expansion.*

expanded keyboard: A keyboard with touch sensitive membrane cells that can be adjusted to different sizes to meet the needs of individuals with severe motor impairments (e.g., Unicorn Keyboard).

expanded rebus: An aided graphic symbol system that includes pictographs and ideographs combined with the letters of the alphabet to represent referents. It also includes symbols with names that rhyme with referents or sound the same as intended words (e.g., a symbol depicting logs [wood] is used to represent the word "would"); a.k.a., *complex rebus.*

expansion capability: The capability of a set of symbols to be expanded beyond its initial lexicon through the use of well defined rules and logic for expansion, thereby converting the symbol set into a symbol system.

experiential background: The collective knowledge an individual possesses from all previous experiences throughout their life.

expert consultation: Consultation services of fixed duration in which a professional (i.e., expert) provides assessment and intervention information but does not implement programs. Instead, program recommendations are implemented by the consultee, and no set procedures exist for follow up.

explanation of benefits: A form that details an insurance company's response to a funding request.

exploratory play: The first stage of play development that consists of sensory and causative exploration with toys.

express communication system(s): A family of communication systems that features speech and printed output and multiple interface options, such as direct selection and scanning. Messages can be selected through letter-by-letter spelling or message retrieval strategies.

expressive communication: The symbolic or nonsymbolic conveying, sending, or transmitting of a message.

expressive language: An individual's ability to use language to transmit or send messages to others.

expressive vocabulary: In AAC, words and messages that are available to an AAC user for the purpose of expressing ideas, information, wants, or needs to a communication partner.

extended keyboard: A keyboard that has function keys in addition to the keys of a standard keyboard (e.g., a computer keyboard).

extension: The straightening of a joint, thereby increasing the joint angle.

extensor thrust/hyperextension: Seen in individuals who have neuromuscular impairments, a forceful, involuntary extension of the lower extremities that may result in the individual sliding out of their seat.

external memory aids: Speech-generating and non–speech-generating displays used to assist an individual with impaired memory to engage in activities of daily living or to remember past events (e.g., calendars, daily planners, photographs, remnants).

external rotation: Movement that occurs when the anterior surface turns outward (e.g., when an arm or leg turns outward).

external scaffolding: Information representation and activity structure that is external to the individual (e.g., using sticky notes as reminders of upcoming activities).

extraneous movement: Any irrelevant or inappropriate movement, typically seen in individuals with neuromuscular disorders.

extrapyramidal: A term that refers to the descending motor nerve tracts that do not cross over at the pyramids of the medulla; these tracts serve to coordinate and refine motor activity.

extremely high frequency: Radio waves with frequencies above 30 GHz.

extrinsic message: Involving the use of devices that results in a message that is different than the mode that was used to send it (e.g., a written-word message [visual modality] sent by use of a pencil [manual modality]).

eye blink codes: Any code in which agreed upon sequences of eye blinks are used to send messages. Each set of eye blinks has a specific meaning.

eye contact: The natural, although not constant, interaction of a speaker's eyes with those of the listener during conversation.

eye gaze: A method of direct selection in which an individual looks toward a specific location, symbol, or thing for the purpose of communication; a.k.a., as *eye pointing* (a misnomer because of the inability of eyes to point).

eye pointing: A technically incorrect term. See *eye gaze*.

EyeLink: Communication that takes place by using eye-to-eye contact through a see-through alphabet board.

Eyetyper model 200: An archaic, portable speech-generating device that was operated by direct eye gaze to a control panel. A variety of eye-gaze sensors and overlay combinations could be used. The device could be interfaced to a computer, modem, printer, or used for environmental control.

Eyetyper model 300: An archaic, portable speech-generating device that featured an eye gaze–controlled keyboard to type messages for synthetic speech output. The device also functioned as an alternate keyboard for the Apple II, IIe, and IBM PC computers.

facies: Facial expressions that are associated with a variety of disabilities and syndromes.

facilitated communication: An intervention technique that provides physical and emotional support to individuals with severe communication disabilities to facilitate expressive communication via an alphabet board or keyboard. The efficacy of facilitated communication as a legitimate technique has not received widespread support in the field of AAC. Several professional organizations (e.g., American Association on Intellectual and Developmental Disabilities, American Psychological Association, American Speech-Language-Hearing Association) have passed resolutions questioning the validity of this technique.

facilitation: The use of a technique, method, or strategy to enable an individual to learn or perform a particular skill more easily or with less effort.

facilitator: (1) An individual (e.g., a communication partner) who assists the AAC user in effectively and successfully using their AAC system to communicate. (2) An individual who assists an AAC user or their family in obtaining services or making adjustments.

fading: The gradual reduction in the strength, frequency, or duration of a prompt that assists an individual to produce a response. When fading is accomplished, an individual produces a response without prompts.

FAE: See *fetal alcohol effect*.

FAPE: See *free, appropriate public education*.

FAS: See *fetal alcohol syndrome*.

Fast ForWord program: An intensive CD-ROM and internet-based adaptive training program that targets language comprehension and phonological awareness skills. Exercises include acoustically modified sounds to simultaneously cross train many phonological skills. Areas in which gains have been seen include phonological awareness, working memory, syntax, grammar, oral language comprehension, and listening comprehension.

FC: See *facilitated communication*.

FCT: See *functional communication training*.

feature matching: The process by which an AAC user's current and projected needs are matched to features of AAC symbols and devices. Because no AAC symbol set or system or device may have all of the desired features, selections that have the most desirable features for an AAC user's needs are made to achieve "goodness of fit." a.k.a., *predictive assessment*.

feedback: Information conveyed to a communicator, whether from within the communicator's body (internal/endogenous) or from the external environment or communication partner (external/exogenous), that helps the communicator monitor their communication so adjustments can be made if needed.

fetal alcohol effect: A less severe form of *fetal alcohol syndrome*.

fetal alcohol syndrome: A collection of symptoms, including developmental delay, craniofacial abnormalities, heart and other organ defects, and growth and skeletal deformities caused by the mother's excessive ingestion of alcohol during pregnancy; in its milder form, may be referred to as *fetal alcohol effect.*

fetal cytomegalovirus: A herpes group virus that can cause growth and intellectual impairment, microcephaly, brain calcification, hearing loss, and chorioretinitis (inflammation of the choroid and the retina).

fetal Dilantin (phenytoin) syndrome: A syndrome caused by maternal use of Dilantin (seizure medication), characterized by poor growth, mild cognitive impairments, unusual facies, and digit and nail myoplasia (i.e., undeveloped fingers and nails).

fifth digit syndrome: See *Coffin-Siris syndrome.*

figure: The part of a graphic symbol that depicts the important information that conveys the meaning of the symbol. See *ground.*

figure-ground: (1) The separation of perception into at least two parts, each with different attributes but influencing one another. Figure is the target of perception; ground is the contextual information (e.g., a bird [the figure] in flight seen against the sky [the ground]). (2) The tendency of certain aspects of something being perceived to stand out clearly while the rest forms a background.

file: A collection of data stored on some type of medium, such as a hard drive, floppy disk, or memory stick.

filtered activation: See *averaged activation.*

fine motor: A term that describes skillful, discrete, spatially oriented movements requiring the use of small muscle sets (e.g., speech activity or picking up a small object with the fingers).

Finger Foniks: An archaic, dedicated speech-generating device that was operated by direct selection, consisting of 36 keys, each producing an American English phoneme or phoneme pair. The device featured an optimized keyboard layout in an attempt to approach the normal rate of conversation.

fingerspelling: The use of a manual alphabet to communicate. Letters are formed by hand configurations and are produced sequentially to spell words. See also *dactylology.*

firmware: Software that is stored permanently in read-only memory.

Fitts's law: A model of human movement that predicts the time required to rapidly move from a starting position to a target as a function of the distance to, and the size of, the target.

Fitzgerald Key: Originally designed for teaching language to individuals with hearing impairments and subsequently adapted for AAC, a strategy in which symbols on a communication board are arranged from left to right in subject-verb-object order.

fixed display: A display in which the symbols or items on the board or overlay remain in a particular location, as opposed to *dynamic display.*

fixed interval reinforcement: A schedule of reinforcement in which reinforcement is delivered after a specified, consistent amount of time.

fixed ratio reinforcement: A schedule of reinforcement in which reinforcement is delivered only after a consistent number of correct responses is demonstrated.

flaccid: (1) Muscles that are hypotonic, soft, and weak. (2) A type of dysarthria seen in cerebral palsy and other neuromuscular disorders, caused by damage to the lower motor neuron system and characterized by hypernasality, nasal air emission, breathiness, and imprecise consonant production.

flashing light cue: See *constant light cue.*

Flexcom: An archaic, adjustable-speed scanning communication aid that featured remote activation via an infrared transmitter. Pictures, letters, or symbols could be displayed on removable overlays having 48, 24, or 16 positions. With additional interfaces, computer and printer output were available, along with environmental control.

flexion: Bending a joint, thereby reducing the joint angle.

floppy disk: A medium of storage for data created by computer systems.

floppy infant: A condition that occurs within the first 2 years of life, characterized by decreased muscle tone (hypotonia) with motor delay, possibly leading to a variety of cognitive or neuromotor disorders.

FMT: Common abbreviation for *functional muscle test.*

fontanel: The "soft spot" on an infant's head that usually disappears within the first year and a half of life.

force: (1) The intensity of effect. (2) The strength or power exerted on an object (i.e., pressure). See *activation force.*

format: The division of physical space on a disk into sectors and tracks so data can be stored.

fragile X syndrome: A sex-linked hereditary disorder characterized by intellectual impairment, large ears, abnormally large testicles (macroorchidism), prominent jaw, delayed motor and speech development, and in some cases, autism spectrum disorder.

free, appropriate public education: A mandate of the Education for All Handicapped Children Act of 1975 (PL 94-142), referring to the provision of the most appropriate and effective education for an individual with a disability. Free, appropriate public education typically involves special education and related services provided at public expense under public supervision that meet the standards of the state education agency and Individuals with Disabilities Education Act of 1990 (PL 101-476).

free morpheme: See *unbound morpheme.*

French Sign Language: The natural sign language used by the Deaf community in France.

frequency-of-use scanning: A scanning method that uses statistics and frequency counts to determine which items are most often accessed by the user, so that those items are arranged in the most accessible area of the display.

fringe vocabulary: Words or messages that are individualized according to an AAC user's environments, interests, and needs; as opposed to *core vocabulary*.

FSL: See *French Sign Language*.

FTC: Common medical abbreviation for family team conference.

full inclusion: The inclusion of an individual with a disability into all aspects of general educational programming.

full weight-bearing: The legs are able to bear 100% of the individual's weight. The individual has the ability to fully ambulate.

functional: Being relevant and directly applicable to an individual's daily life.

functional analysis: The experimental manipulation of an individual's environment to determine the function(s) of a variety of behaviors, including problem behavior.

functional assessment: The full range of strategies and procedures used (1) to develop and test hypotheses regarding antecedents and consequences that control behaviors, including problem behavior or (2) to determine an individual's abilities in real life situations.

functional behavioral assessment: The systematic collection and analysis of data pertaining to a student's behavior. The results of the analysis of the data are used to develop the student's behavioral intervention plan.

functional communication: Communication that allows an individual to express basic needs and desires, transfer information, establish social closeness, and demonstrate social etiquette. Individuals who fail to develop functional communication are typically limited in their independence and may exhibit learned helplessness.

functional communication training (FCT): A proactive approach for reducing challenging behaviors by teaching a more appropriate form of communication using communication-based interventions to replace challenging behavior with socially mediated consequences that serve the same function.

functional equivalence: The relationship of an alternative behavior to a problem behavior. The goal is to replace a problem behavior with a more acceptable behavior that serves the same purpose and provides the same reinforcement for the individual.

functional gain: Improvement that can be directly attributed to the addition of a new approach or device (e.g., improvement in expressive communication resulting from adding technology to an individual's AAC system).

functional muscle test: Assessment of muscle-specific strength and flexibility in persons who have neuromuscular imbalances, for the purpose of designing intervention to address and either eliminate or compensate for the imbalances.

functional outcome measures: A valid and reliable tool that helps evaluate the effectiveness of a treatment or assessment.

functional skills of communication: Communication skills that are necessary for the initiation and maintenance of daily interactions within the natural environment.

functionality of communication: The level of an individual's communication and how well it fits their role in everyday life. An individual's functionality of communication is measured by how demanding their communicative role is in the environment.

funded mandates: Federal or state legislation that mandates specific functions, services, or activities for which funds are also provided. See also *unfunded mandates*.

funding: The provision of financial support for an item or activity (e.g., funding the purchase of an AAC device and services).

funding coordinator: The member of the service delivery team whose responsibility is to guide efforts at seeking and obtaining funding.

FWB: Common medical abbreviation for *full weight-bearing*.

galactosemia: Galactose intolerance of hereditary etiology, characterized by enlargement of the liver (hepatomegaly) and spleen (splenomegaly) and failure to thrive.

gas discharge display: See *plasma display*.

Gates-MacGinitie Reading Test: A standardized reading test that uses a multiple-choice format for persons in early elementary school through college.

Gateway: see *Gateway to Language Learning*. Not to be confused with the computer company.

Gateway to Language Learning: A software program used with Dynamite and Dynavox software that organizes and facilitates the retrieval of vocabulary from various pages and levels.

GB: See *gigabyte*.

GBS: See *Guillain-Barré syndrome*.

g-byte: See *gigabyte*.

gbyte: See *gigabyte*.

generalization: The transfer of learned behaviors to novel people, settings, or stimuli.

Generalized Response: Total Assistance: Level II of the *Rancho Los Amigos Levels of Cognitive Functioning Scale-Revised*, characterized in part by generalized reflex responses to painful stimuli, response to repeated auditory stimuli by increasing or decreasing activity, response to external stimuli with gross body movement or nonpurposeful vocalizations, and significantly delayed responses.

generally understood gestures: A set of gestures used with and by persons with severe intellectual disabilities.

generation effect: Active involvement in the construction of learning content that appears to facilitate retrieval of information from long-term memory.

genetic counseling: A process whereby family members are presented with the ramifications associated with the presence of a genetic disorder in the family and the risk of reoccurrence of the disorder in future offspring.

genetics: The study of heredity.

geriatric adults: Persons of advanced age, generally considered to be in the age range of 65 years and older.

German measles: See *rubella.*

gestalt processing: An inflexible, holistic mode of information processing in which stimuli are examined in their entirety rather than in terms of their component parts.

Gestuno: A set of manual signs selected by a committee of the World Federation of the Deaf to facilitate communication among users of different sign languages.

gestural systems: Any collection of gestures that can mimic the language of the general community (e.g., gestural Morse code can be used to create the letters of the alphabet to spell an unlimited number of words; any two reliable gestures can be used to represent the dits and dahs of Morse code).

gesture: A body movement or series of coordinated body movements that represent an object, idea, or action without having the linguistic constraints of more formal gestural systems, such as manual sign. Gestures play an important role in early pre-linguistic communication and the transition to linguistic communication.

gesture dictionary: A personalized inventory of the gestures used by an individual for receptive and expressive communication.

GHz: See *gigahertz.*

gigabyte: One billion bytes (1,073,741,824 bytes), or 1,000 megabytes. See *megabyte.*

gigahertz: A unit of measure for frequency, equal to one billion Hertz, or one billion vibrations per second.

glaucoma: An eye disease characterized by increased pressure within the eyeball, resulting in blindness if not treated.

global aphasia: A severe form of aphasia that results in extensive impairment in all areas of speech and language (e.g., naming, comprehension, repetition, reading, writing).

gloss: (1) The printed word that may accompany a graphic symbol to indicate its meaning. (2) The oral-language word equivalent of a manual sign or gesture.

glossectomy: Surgical removal of all or part of the tongue, usually as a result of cancer.

glottochronology: See *numerical linguistics.*

grammar: The structure of a language. The grammar of any language consists of a limited set of basic elements (phonemes) and rules that govern the creation of meaningful combinations (words) and strings (sentences). A central part of grammar is the lexicon.

grapheme: An individual letter of the alphabet.

grapheme-phoneme correspondence: The relationship between an alphabetic letter (grapheme) and the sound or sounds that the letter represents (phoneme).

graphic: A term used to describe visual displays (e.g., drawings, logographs, paintings, photographs, printed words, or other markings).

graphic complexity: The intricateness of graphic symbols. Complexity may be a function of the number of strokes required to create a symbol (i.e., the more strokes required, the more complex the symbol) or the number of semantic elements that are used in a graphic symbol to represent the referent (i.e., the more semantic elements used, the more complex the symbol).

graphic representation of manual signs: Graphic depictions of how manual signs are produced. These include simple illustrations in sign dictionaries that show how to produce manual signs, sign-linked symbols in Sigsymbols, static representation systems, such as HANDS, SignWriting, and WorldSign, and synthetic or animated manual signs.

graphic symbol: A visual symbol that represents a referent to convey meaning (e.g., Blissymbol, line drawing, photograph, Sigsymbol).

graphic tablet: A computer input device with a touch sensitive surface that accepts drawing.

graphic user interface: A computer operating system that depicts information in graphic form on the screen, thereby allowing the user to perform tasks by manipulating pictures representing programs, files, etc.

graphophonic elements: The graphemes (letters) used in traditional orthography and the grapheme-phoneme correspondences they represent.

gross motor development: Movement and control of large muscles or muscle groups for activities, such as rolling, crawling, walking, throwing, and balance.

ground: The contextual information of a graphic symbol that may enhance its meaning. However, if there is poor figure-ground discrimination, then the ground may interfere in an individual's ability to interpret the meaning of the symbol. See *figure.*

group experimental designs: The range of experimental designs that demonstrates the effects of variables on groups of subjects or participants, with generalization to larger populations based upon the subject sample chosen.

group item scanning: See *block/group scanning.*

GUI: See *graphic user interface.*

guided interaction: A program that emphasizes the development of perception, interaction, and language moved to conversation through flexible activities.

Guillain-Barré: See *Guillain-Barré syndrome.*

Guillain-Barré syndrome : A rare, acute neurological disorder of unknown etiology, usually occurring after certain viral infections or vaccinations, and characterized by partial paralysis of several muscle groups (in some cases, those muscles responsible for speech production); a.k.a., *Guillain-Barré.*

habilitation: (1) The process of providing services and education to improve an individual's total range of functioning (e.g., educational, recreational, and vocational skills) throughout their life. (2) The mainstreaming of individuals with disabilities into all facets of community life by integrating the interactive patterns and lifestyles of individuals with and without disabilities.

hand alphabet: Unaided symbols that consist of hand configurations representing the letters of the alphabet and numbers. Several hand alphabets are in use throughout the world. These alphabets are usually analogs of their corresponding spoken language; a.k.a., *manual alphabet.*

hand configuration: See *handshape.*

hand-cued speech: A general term used to denote any unaided system that provides manual-visual cues for the interpretation of speech by a person with a profound hearing impairment. Typically, the various speech sounds are represented by different hand configurations and locations of production to make speech more visual.

hand-cued systems: See *hand-cued speech.*

handicap: The impact of a disability on an individual's role in society. The term should be avoided for describing a person unless the author intends to convey that there is a negative impact on that person's role in society.

Handivoice 130: An archaic, dedicated direct-selection speech-generating device that enabled the user to retrieve and combine single words, phrases, single letters or numbers, and sounds. See also *VOIS 130.*

hand posturing: Abnormal and sometimes painful positioning of the hands due to dystonia (involuntary muscle contractions), seen often in persons with damage to the basal ganglia.

handshape: One of the basic parameters of manual signs, along with designation, location, and movement. A manual sign system or sign language typically uses a limited set of between 25 and 50 handshapes; a.k.a., *hand configuration.*

haptic: The use of the sense of touch for perception via active exploration (as opposed to tactile, which is passive).

hard copy: Paper copy or output of an electric file or image.

hard disk: A device permanently mounted within a computer's central processing unit that stores large amounts of information that can be retrieved quickly.

hardware: The tangible or physical parts of a computer that the user can see and touch (e.g., the computer central processing unit, monitor, keyboard, and mouse; printer; external drives; scanner; speakers).

Hawaii Early Learning Profile: A developmental assessment tool for children from birth to 3 years of age that evaluates the areas of cognition, language, motor skills, social skills, and self-help skills.

HCPC: See *Health Care Financing Administration Common Procedure Coding System.*

head injury: Any injury to the skull or brain as a result of either a penetrating head wound (e.g., a gunshot) or a closed head injury.

head lag: An inability of the head to respond immediately with the trunk when a baby is pulled to a sitting position. Some degree of head lag is considered normal in children up to approximately 4 months of age.

head pointer: An adaptive device affixed to the head (e.g., with a band or helmet) to be used for direct selection; a.k.a., *head stick.*

head stick: See *head pointer.*

headlight pointer: A device that emits a focused light beam to indicate communication choices. The user directs the light beam to words, objects, or symbols to communicate.

HeadMaster Plus: An archaic device manufactured by the Prentke Romich Company that emulated a mouse to control a cursor on the screen of an Apple IIGS, Macintosh, or IBM computer. A software program called Screen Keys placed an image of the computer keyboard on the screen. The HeadMaster Plus allowed the user to input through a two step process of moving the head-mounted light beam to move the cursor on the screen and then sucking or puffing on a pneumatic switch to make the choice.

Health Care Financing Administration Common Procedure Coding System: A system of codes used by audiologists to describe hearing aid services to insurance carriers when seeking reimbursement.

Hear My Voice: Language Through AAC: A nonprofit organization that focuses on developing language through AAC. The organization has an online newsletter to which one can subscribe and scholarships aligned with its mission.

hearing impairment: A deficiency of hearing caused by a conductive, sensorineural, or mixed (conductive and sensorineural) hearing loss.

hearing threshold: The intensity level (expressed in decibels) at which an individual responds to 50% of the pure tones presented.

HELP: See *Hawaii Early Learning Profile.*

Helpmate: An archaic, lightweight assistive communication device that featured a QWERTY keyboard and a 40-character display. Words and phrases up to 250 characters could be stored in memory and recalled with a two-key sequence.

hemi: Common medical abbreviation for *hemiplegia.*

hemianopia (hemianopsia): Loss of one half of the visual field.

hemiparesis: Muscular weakness or partial paralysis confined to one side of the body. A less severe form of hemiplegia.

hemiplegia: A more severe form of paralysis that is confined to one side of the body (usually the ipsilateral arm and leg).

hertz: The unit of measure for sound frequency. Cycles per second is also used as a measure of sound frequency (defined as the number of times an object vibrates per second).

HF: See *high frequency.*

high frequency: Radio waves with frequencies between 3 and 30 MHz.

high-tech: A common abbreviation for the archaic term, *high technology.*

high technology: (1) Electronic technology that uses a computer chip or integrated circuit. (2) An electronic communication device that has speech or printed output and programming and editing capabilities. This term has been replaced by the term, *speech-generating.*

high technology communication aid: A computer-based AAC system that requires specially designed software and has printed or spoken output (and possibly both). This term is archaic and has been replaced by the term, *speech-generating device.*

highlighting: The intensifying of a selected portion of text or image (e.g., by a cursor, usually in a color that is different than the text or image being highlighted, to make it stand out).

history: An individual's chronological record of academic, developmental, employment, medical, and other experiences.

Hollerith tabulator: An early mechanical tabulator that used punched cards and was designed for processing and statistically analyzing the 1890 U.S. Census.

HOME: See *Home Observation for Measurement of the Environment.*

home-based program: Service delivery where the AAC user's natural environment is used to provide intervention services.

Home Observation for Measurement of the Environment: A checklist that is used in a child's home in order to determine whether or not the home environment is nurturing.

home row: The row of keys on a computer keyboard where the fingers are placed when they are not accessing other keys (on the standard keyboard, this row includes the letters A, S, D, F, G, H, J, K, and L).

home visit: A service delivery option where professionals provide services to the individual in their home environment; typically used with persons who have the inability to travel (i.e., because of physical impairment or lack of transportation options).

hotspot: An area of interest (e.g., a picture or photograph) on a visual scene display that is programmed with an underlying communication message. When the hotspot is activated (e.g., through touch), the message is spoken and/or displayed.

HR: Common medical abbreviation for heart rate.

HTL: See *hearing threshold.*

HTN: Common medical abbreviation for *hypertension.*

human factors: See *ergonomics.*

human factors engineering: The design and implementation of technology to assist an individual with a disability in performing the necessary responsibilities and tasks of their employment setting. See also *ergonomics.*

humoral blocks: Upper arm blocks that are attached to a wheelchair or a tray to prevent the individual's arms from retracting. This positioning places the arms in a more functional position for hand use.

Hunter syndrome: A genetic syndrome characterized by growth deficiency, coarse facies, stiff joints, and enlargement of the liver and spleen (hepatosplenomegaly).

Huntington's chorea: See *Huntington disease.*

Huntington disease: An inherited, autosomal dominant, degenerative central nervous system disorder characterized by involuntary, uncoordinated, jerky movements (chorea), dementia, and hyperkinetic dysarthria, usually striking in middle age; a.k.a., *Huntington chorea.*

Hurler syndrome: A genetic disorder characterized by growth deficiency, coarse facies, flattened nose, enlarged lips, stiff joints, enlarged liver and spleen (hepatosplenomegaly), intellectual impairment, possible hearing impairment, and cloudy corneas.

HV: Common medical abbreviation for *home visit.*

Hx: Common medical abbreviation for *history.*

hydrocephalus: A condition typically caused by a blockage in, or underdevelopment of, the ventricles of the brain, characterized by the abnormal accumulation of cerebrospinal fluid within the ventricles leading to enlargement of the head if not corrected.

hyperextension: The movement of a joint to a position of greater extension than that allowed by natural alignment.

hyperlexia: A precocious ability to recognize written words significantly above the individual's language or cognitive skill level.

hyperopia: Farsightedness.

hypertelorism: An abnormal distance between two paired organs.

hypertension: High blood pressure. See *blood pressure.*

hypertonic: Pertaining to an increase in muscle tone.

hypotheses development: Identifying possible functional relationships between a problem behavior and naturally occurring environmental events.

hypotheses testing: (1) The purpose of empirical research. (2) The testing of hypotheses developed from direct or indirect observations through a functional analysis.

hypotonic: Pertaining to a reduction of muscle tone.

Hz: See *hertz.*

IC: See *integrated circuit.*

ICD-11: See *International Classification of Diseases, Eleventh Revision.*

ICOMM: An archaic, single switch–activated scanning communication aid that featured 64 locations and 16 scanning speeds. Single characters were activated to recall factory preprogrammed phrases. Morse code input was also available. The device had an optional built-in speech synthesizer for storing custom vocabulary.

icon: A picture or symbol that represents a referent.

icon prediction: A feature of Minspeak that allows the user to retrieve stored messages more quickly and with less cognitive effort. As each Minspeak icon is selected, only the remaining icons that can be chosen next are highlighted.

iconic: A term that is used to describe symbols that readily depict referents or some easily identifiable aspect of referents (e.g., iconic symbols).

iconic encoding: A misnomer for *conceptual encoding* and *semantic encoding*.

iconicity: A term that refers to the visual relationship between a symbol (e.g., manual sign or graphic symbol) and its referent. Iconicity is frequently considered in terms of *transparency* and *translucency*. See also *opaqueness*.

ICU: Common medical abbreviation for *intensive care unit*.

IDEA: See *Individuals with Disabilities Education Act of 1990 (PL 101-476)*.

identity-first terminology: Terminology that places the impairment or disability before the individual (e.g., 'aphasic adult').

ideograph: A graphic representation that suggests the idea of the referent it represents but does not depict the referent directly. Ideographs are typically used to depict more abstract referents.

idiosyncratic: Specific to an individual (e.g., idiosyncratic gestures or signs).

idiosyncratic codes: Eye blinks, gestures, or vocalizations specific to an individual, used for the purpose of encoding words or messages; because of their idiosyncratic nature, they are not generally understood by most communication partners.

idiosyncratic gestures: Gestures developed by an individual to denote referents and meanings. These remain idiosyncratic as long as they have not become conventionalized (i.e., widely accepted and used by others).

IEP: See *Individualized Education Program*.

IFSP: See *Individualized Family Service Plan*.

IHO: See *impartial (independent) hearing officer*.

Illinois Test of Psycholinguistic Abilities: A formal, standardized test of linguistic and related abilities.

imageability: The ability of a word to elicit a visual image of the referent.

imitation: The sensorimotor scheme pertaining to the ability to copy or mimic behavior.

immittance audiometry: A battery of audiometric tests for detecting abnormalities of middle ear function.

impairment: The absence or deficiency of a specific structure or function. In most usages, the specific impairment should be identified (e.g., rather than saying that an individual has an impairment, one should state that the individual has a motor impairment).

impartial (independent) hearing officer: As applied to special education, an individual who is trained in special education law and is appointed to preside over special education hearings.

incidence: The number of new cases of a disease or disorder reported for a specific time period.

inclusion: The philosophy of educating children who have disabilities in the same setting as children who do not.

independent play: The second stage of play development in which children begin to use objects for appropriate functions.

index: A pointing sign in sign languages, typically used for pronominal reference.

indexing: The process of pointing or indicating, usually with a finger or stick.

indirect methods: In research, the use of tools other than direct observation to determine behavior, including rating scales, structured interviews, and qualitative interviews. These indirect methods are typically completed by or with partners who are familiar with the particular individual.

indirect selection: An input method that involves intermediate selection steps between indicating a choice and actually sending a keystroke or command to the computer, typically by replicating the computer's keyboard characters by using a variety of display formats (e.g., a graphic keyboard image on the screen, a textual scanning array of keyboard characters, or a menu of computer commands).

Individual Program Plan: A written document used by some agencies that provide services for adults with disabilities; a plan that specifies the client's current and future needs and ways to provide for those needs.

Individualized Education Program: A formal educational program plan designed by an Individualized Education Program team to meet the special needs of a child with a disability, as mandated by the Individuals with Disabilities Education Act of 1990 (PL 101-476).

Individualized Family Service Plan: A family-centered intervention program for children from birth through 2 years of age, as mandated by the Individuals with Disabilities Education Act of 1990 (PL 101-476).

Individuals with Disabilities Education Act of 1990 (PL 101-476): Federal legislation that modified the Education for All Handicapped Children Act of 1975 (PL 94-142), and is therefore also referred to as the Education for All Handicapped Children Act Amendments of 1990. Modifications included substituting the term *disability* for *handicapped*, adding assistive technology for individuals with disabilities, adding specific disabilities to be covered (e.g., autism spectrum disorder and brain injury), and extending services to preschoolers.

Individuals with Disabilities Education Act Amendments of 1997 (PL 105-17): Federal legislation that updated the Individuals with Disabilities Education Act of 1990. This law included appropriate accommodations for students with disabilities in state and district-wide testing, enhanced parent participation in eligibility and placement decisions, and for students 14 years of age or older, annual statements of transition service needs. Referred to as IDEA'97.

Individuals with Disabilities Education Improvement Act of 2004 (PL 108-446): Federal legislation that reauthorized the Individuals with Disabilities Education Act of 1990 and also included new requirements for personnel training, Individualized Education Programs, and research-based instruction (evidence-based practice).

infantile reflexes: See *primitive reflexes.*

informant: An individual who provides information about a topic or individual.

informational consultation: A form of consultation most closely associated with interdisciplinary service delivery, where a consultant provides information to a consultee that meets the needs of a targeted AAC user but is also broad enough that the principles may be applied to similar AAC users.

infrared rays: Light rays outside of the human visual range (and are therefore invisible to humans) that are digitally coded and typically used to activate remote-controlled devices.

Initial Teaching Alphabet: A modified orthography system originally designed in Great Britain for the purpose of making it easier for English-speaking children to learn to read English. The Initial Teaching Alphabet is introduced first, and then the child transitions to traditional orthography. The Initial Teaching Alphabet consists of 42 characters (24 standard lowercase Latin letters plus a number of special characters), each character representing a single phoneme. Some traditional orthography digraphs are represented by Initial Teaching Alphabet ligatures.

initialization: The preparation of a blank floppy disk or other storage media for use on a computer.

initiation: The spontaneous offering of interactive or communicative behavior by an individual.

inkjet printer: A nonimpact printer in which sprayed ink is used to form characters on a page.

inner language: (1) The transformation of one's experiences into verbal or nonverbal symbols for purposes of self-awareness, thinking, and adjustment. (2) Communicating with oneself. (3) A subliminal response to verbal stimuli that may or may not result in overt speech. (4) The process of verbal thought.

inner speech: Visual, auditory, and kinesthetic sensations that evoke mental images of words.

input: The transmission of data from an input device to a computer (e.g., through a keyboard, mouse, touch-sensitive screen, scanner).

input device: Any device that allows the user to input information to a computer or other electronic device (e.g., a keyboard, mouse, touch-sensitive screen, scanner).

input/output: Pertaining to the means by which information is exchanged by a computer and its peripheral devices.

inservice training: Ongoing instruction and hands-on training for service providers in education, health care, rehabilitation, and related fields for the purpose of skill development and improved care and management, typically conducted at the individual's place of employment; a form of *continuing education.*

integrate: To include someone or something into a larger whole (e.g., a mainstreamed classroom).

integrated augmentative communication device: An integrated device (including speech generation) that allows for use as a traditional computer complete with internet access and software or apps that perform tasks unrelated to the production of speech, such as environmental control, word processing, spreadsheets, music, videos, and games.

integrated circuit: An electronic circuit, usually made of silicon, in which all components are formed on a single piece of semiconductor material.

integrated environments: Settings where an individual with disabilities functions alongside peers without disabilities.

integrated objectives: Goals or objectives that target meaningful communication in natural contexts through important activities for the individual.

integrated system: Technology that encompasses more than one function (e.g., a tablet-based AAC system that also includes gaming and word processing). An integrated system also refers to the integration of assistive technology, such as mobility devices, environmental control systems, and speech-generating devices, where they share access features (e.g., eye gaze or joystick control).

integrated therapy: An approach to service delivery in which intervention centers on an individual's daily experiences as both a context and focus.

intellectual impairment: A particular state of functioning that begins in childhood and is characterized by limitations in both intelligence and adaptive skills. Intellectual impairment reflects the discrepancy between an individual's capabilities and the environmental demands that are placed upon them.

intelligibility: (1) The ability of a symbol to be recognized and understood without cues or explanations. (2) The understandability of speech (whether natural or synthetic) by persons who are unfamiliar with the speaker.

intensive care unit: A specialized acute care setting where an individual's vital functions are closely monitored.

intention tremor: Involuntary shaking or quivering that occurs during conscious, purposeful movement.

intentional communication: The expression of ideas, information, or emotional state that is planned, deliberate, and purposeful.

interactive compensatory model: A model in which skills at one level of processing can compensate for deficiencies at another level.

interdisciplinary team: In AAC, a team of individuals with expertise in widely divergent areas who share a common function or goal. The team makes decisions as a whole based upon shared information.

interdisciplinary team model: A model of team assessment and intervention in which members share information with one another to influence decision making. However, each member of the team may conduct their own assessment and intervention independently of the other team members.

interface: (1) Surfaces or devices that come together (e.g., computer devices are interfaced through the use of cables that allow the transmission of data from the output port of one computer to the input port of another). (2) The connection of the AAC user to the means of transmission and other devices (i.e., the AAC user may interface with their environment through unaided means [e.g., signs, gestures] or aided means [e.g., materials, devices]).

intermittent/variable ratio reinforcement: A schedule of reinforcement in which reinforcement is delivered after a random and unpredictable number of correct responses is given.

internal rotation: A movement that occurs when the anterior surface turns inward (e.g., turning an arm or leg inward, toward the body).

international: (1) Having global aspects or characteristics of at least being multinational in nature. (2) Symbols that are generally understood across cultures (e.g., mathematical symbols).

International Classification of Diseases, Eleventh Revision: A numerical coding system of medical conditions and procedures used for billing, research, and statistical purposes.

International Phonetic Alphabet: A modified orthography system consisting of phonetic notations devised by linguists to accurately and uniquely represent each of the wide variety of sounds (i.e., phonemes) used in spoken language. Each speech sound of a language has its own International Phonetic Alphabet character. The American English International Phonetic Alphabet system has characters for approximately 24 consonants, 14 vowels, and 5 diphthongs.

International Project on Communication Aids for the Speech Impaired: In the 1980s, a collaborative project between Canada, the United Kingdom, the United States, and Sweden in which information concerning professional and technological developments in AAC was shared.

International Sign Language: See *Gestuno*.

International Society for Augmentative and Alternative Communication: A multinational organization of professionals, AAC users, family members, and others devoted to encouraging scholarship, promoting research, and improving service delivery in the field of AAC.

interprofessional practice (IPP): An umbrella term given to a framework that describes collaboration among professionals of various disciplines with the goal of improving outcomes for clients with respect to all aspects of service delivery. Interprofessional practice is an intentional approach to collaboration. The interprofessional practice framework helps professionals learn about, from, and with colleagues from different specialties. On successful interprofessional practice teams, each member provides their professional expertise and works together on an assessment and/or treatment plan focused on the person and their family. Collaboration in interprofessional practice may be short- or long-term, depending on the goals of the collaboration.

interrupted behavior chain: A technique used to teach requesting, based on milieu teaching, which uses natural routines, or "behavior chains," as contexts for communication.

intervener: A person who works consistently, one-to-one with a learner who experiences deaf-blindness, to provide access to environmental information that is usually gained through vision and hearing, to facilitate communication development, and to promote social connectedness.

intervention: The provision of services designed to improve communication so an individual can interact more effectively and participate more fully in activities of choice, based upon a thorough assessment of the individual's strengths and limitations.

intervention planning phase: A sequence of information-gathering activities (i.e., review of records, observations and structured interactions, interviews) to determine communicative competence and to consider appropriate goals and activities.

intonation: Variations in vocal pitch and stress that influence the meaning of oral language.

intraoral speech aid: Any device that produces an electronically generated tone transmitted to the mouth of the user who then modifies the tone into speech by movements of their articulators. Typically used by laryngectomees, individuals on respirators, and patients with emphysema.

intrinsic message: The message that is inherent in a symbol that the communication partner sees; the message is inseparable from the symbol that is used to produce it.

IntroTalker: An archaic, portable, dedicated speech-generating device, intended for introductory use, that featured natural speech output and limited use of Minspeak semantic vocabulary organization. The device's standard memory allowed for 2 minutes of normal-quality or 1 minute of high-quality speech.

invented spelling: Attempts by a beginning writer to spell words when their standard spellings are unknown; the individual uses whatever knowledge of sounds or visual patterns they have to spell the words, which may or may not be the correct spellings.

inverse scanning: A message selection technique in which scanning commences upon switch activation and continues while switch closure is maintained. Upon release of the switch, scanning stops on the desired item.

invisible unaided symbols: Unaided symbols that cannot be monitored visually during production. Although speech is obviously an invisible unaided symbol, the term is more frequently used to refer to manual signs or gestures that are made outside of the visual field of the sender/producer (e.g., pointing to one's own ear).

I/O: See *input/output*.

IPA: See *International Phonetic Alphabet*.

IPCAS: See *International Project on Communication Aids for the Speech Impaired*.

IPP: See *interprofessional practice*.

IR: See *infrared rays*.

ISAAC: See *International Society for Augmentative and Alternative Communication*.

ISAAC Bulletin: The original name of the official quarterly newsletter published by ISAAC, containing scholarly articles and scientific research findings. The current name is *The Bulletin*.

ITA: See *Initial Teaching Alphabet*.

item-by-item scanning: A scanning procedure in which a cursor or communication partner moves through the items in a display one at a time, usually going from left to right and from top to bottom. The AAC user activates a switch or indicates in some manner to the communication partner when the desired item is encountered.

ITPA: See *Illinois Test of Psycholinguistic Abilities*.

jack: A piece of hardware used to complete an electrical connection. A plug of some type is typically inserted into a jack to connect switches and other electronic devices.

joint contracture: Occurs when a joint cannot be moved passively through its full range of motion. A limitation in the full range of motion of joints.

joystick: An input device that allows for directed scanning by controlling the movement of an object or cursor on a screen in several directions.

K: See *kilobyte*.

kB: See *kilobyte*.

KB: See *kilobyte*.

Ke:nx: A keyboard emulation system marketed by Don Johnston Incorporated that provides options for single-switch scanning, Morse code, alternate keyboard, and synthesized speech.

key symbols: (1) A set of graphic symbols used in functional communication that may be idiosyncratic in origin. (2) In Blissymbolics, the finite set of approximately 120 basic components that are used to create a virtually unlimited number of symbols; a.k.a., *semantic elements*.

key word signing: The manual signing of key words (e.g., nouns and verbs) as they are spoken. In Britain, the term *signs supporting English* is used.

keyboard: A peripheral device that provides a common way for an individual to communicate with the computer. The most common arrangement of keys on a keyboard is QWERTY, but a variety of layouts exists with different numbers, sizes, and shapes of keys. Key activation can be through mechanical depression, touch membrane, or touchscreen surfaces.

keyboard emulator: Any device that simulates the input functions of a keyboard (e.g., a standard mouse, trackball, IntelliKeys, Unicorn Keyboard).

keyguard: A hardware device (usually made of plastic or plexiglass) that can be placed over a standard or alternative keyboard to help prevent accidental hits while allowing for more controlled usage by individuals with physical impairments.

keypad: An alternate keyboard that is usually smaller than a standard keyboard and contains a limited number of keys, such as number or function keys.

keyword: A word that has a significantly higher frequency of occurrence in a sample of text than it does in a much larger and more general reference corpus. A word such as "teddy" may appear often in a small collection of children's books but very infrequently in a larger library. It is therefore a keyword in the children's book sample.

kHz: See *kilohertz*.

kilobyte: One thousand (1,024) bytes.

kilohertz: A unit of measure for frequency, equal to 1,000 Hertz, or 1,000 vibrations per second.

kinesics: (1) The use of facial expression, eye contact, and body movements to communicate information for the purpose of enhancing spoken language. (2) The study of the use of facial expression, eye contact, and body movements during speech.

Kleeblattshadel syndrome: See *Cloverleaf skull syndrome*.

knowledge barriers: Barriers that result from a lack of knowledge about AAC intervention and use options.

kyphosis: An increased or exaggerated forward curvature of the spine.

Landau reflex: When an infant is held in a prone position, they reflexively raise their head to a vertical position.

Landau-Kleffner syndrome: A rare seizure disorder in young children that often results in acquired aphasia.

language: An arbitrary system of symbols (e.g., manual signs, words) and rules that govern their use, used for a communicative function (e.g., expressing feelings, transferring information).

language acquisition and development: The receptive and expressive development of language (i.e., phonology, morphology, syntax, semantics, and pragmatics) that occurs throughout the entire lifespan but is primarily associated with the child's first 18 years of life.

Language Acquisition through Motor Planning (LAMP): An AAC approach designed to give individuals who are nonspeaking or who have limited verbal abilities a method of independently and spontaneously expressing themselves through use of a speech-generating device. The key components of the LAMP approach include readiness to learn, teaching in moments of joint engagement, and learning language through a unique and consistent motor plan paired with an auditory signal and a natural consequence.

language arts: Educational activities aimed at developing listening, speaking, reading, handwriting, and spelling skills.

language content: The meaning of language (semantics), as well as the rules for linking meaning with the units of language (i.e., semantic relations).

language delay: See *specific language impairment.*

language form: The sounds and sound system of a language (i.e., phonology), its units of meaning (i.e., morphology), and its grammar (i.e., syntax).

language function or use: The pragmatics of language, including the reasons for communication (e.g., requesting, commenting, protesting); topic initiation, maintenance, and termination; and repair strategies.

Language Master: A piece of electronic equipment that allows for autotutorial training. Prerecorded responses placed on cards with magnetic tape along with pictures or printed symbols serve as models of target behavior. The child then compares their responses to the models on the cards as they are fed through the device for playback.

language processing: The multidimensional process of hearing, discriminating, assigning significance to, and interpreting spoken words, phrases, clauses, sentences, and discourse.

laptray: A tray attached to a wheelchair, usually made of plexiglass, plastic, or wood.

large print display: Computer hardware or software that enlarges images on the computer monitor for persons with visual impairments.

laryngectomee: An individual whose larynx has been surgically removed, usually due to cancer.

laryngectomy: The surgical removal of all or part of the larynx.

laser printer: A nonimpact printer in which characters are formed on a page by heating dried ink that has been electrically charged on a rotating drum.

lat: Common medical abbreviation for *lateral.*

latching: A feature of some switches or controls in which activation causes them to remain in a constant state of "on" or "off" until they are activated again.

latching switch: A switch that, upon activation, locks into a "closed" or "open" position (e.g., a light switch).

late-latency response: Auditory-evoked potentials occurring between 50 and 300 msec poststimulus onset that indicate activity within the thalamus and auditory cortex.

latency: The amount of time that elapses between the introduction of a stimulus and the response to it.

lateral: To the side.

law of best fit: Select the device, system, or approach that provides a maximal match of features to the needs and characteristics of the user.

law of minimal energy: Select the device, system, or approach that requires the least amount of energy or effort on the part of the user.

law of minimal interference: Select the device, system, or approach that avoids other competing or conflicting tasks or processes (i.e., does not interfere with the user's ability to engage in other tasks or processes).

law of minimal learning: Select the device, system, or approach that requires the least amount of learning on the part of the user and communication partners.

law of parsimony: Select the simplest device, system, or approach possible.

law of practicality and use: Select the device, system, or approach that is most appropriate for the environment in which it will be used and is consistent with available resources. This law also implies conformity with all the other laws governing the selection of AAC devices, systems, or approaches (e.g., best fit, minimal energy, minimal interference, minimal learning, and parsimony).

LB: Common medical abbreviation for *lower body.*

LBW: See *low birth weight.*

LCD: See *liquid crystal display.*

LD: See *learning disability.*

l-dopa: See *levodopa.*

LE: Common medical abbreviation for lower extremity(ies).

LEA: See *local education agency.*

learned helplessness: Inactivity or passivity in a child or adult with a disability that is reinforced and entrenched due to repeated failures or lack of stimulation in interacting with people and devices.

learning disability: Any of the various cognitive, neurological, or psychological disorders that impedes a child's ability to learn, especially academic information (e.g., mathematics, reading, writing) or language skills.

least restrictive environment: (1) A legal mandate of the Education for All Handicapped Children Act of 1975 (PL 94-142) that all children with disabilities be educated with children without disabilities and that special classes, separate schooling, or removal of children from the general educational environment occurs only when the nature or severity of the disability is such that general education classes with the use of supplementary aids and services cannot be achieved satisfactorily. Children should be afforded opportunities for education, work, living, and recreation that are as near as possible to those afforded individuals without disabilities. (2) The environment in which a child is least restricted and has the greatest access to educational opportunities.

LED: See *light-emitting diode.*

lemma: In linguistics, a root or base form of a word, similar to how it would appear in a dictionary, without all its possible inflected forms. For example, the word "like" is the lemma form of "liked," "likes," and "liking."

lesion: Any change that occurs in the structure of organs or tissues as a result of injury or disease process.

letter arrays: Any arrangement or configuration of the letters of the alphabet for the purpose of using them in communication or word processing (e.g., QWERTY array, frequency-of-use array, alphabetic-order array).

letter category encoding: The systematic organization of information or messages for storage and retrieval by using letters to represent categories, for the purpose of language formulation.

letter coding/encoding: See *alphabet encoding.*

leukodystrophies: A group of rare, genetic neurological disorders that cause abnormal growth of white matter (i.e., myelinated neuronal axons) in the brain. These disorders can have an onset shortly after birth, later in childhood, or into adulthood.

level of abstraction: The amount of detail that is provided in the object or event being depicted in a symbol (i.e., the figure as opposed to the ground). The less detail that is provided in a symbol, the greater its level of abstraction, and vice versa.

levels: See *pages.*

Levels of Cognitive Functioning Scale: A scale designed for the classification of persons who have experienced traumatic brain injury. The intent is to describe cognitive and language behaviors that occur during recovery according to 10 levels: (1) No Response: Total Assistance, (2) Generalized Response: Total Assistance, (3) Localized Response: Total Assistance, (4) Confused/Agitated: Maximal Assistance, (5) Confused, Inappropriate Non-Agitated: Maximal Assistance, (6) Confused, Appropriate: Moderate Assistance, (7) Automatic, Appropriate: Minimal Assistance for Daily Living Skills, (8) Purposeful, Appropriate: Stand-By Assistance, (9) Purposeful, Appropriate: Stand-By Assistance on Request, and (10) Purposeful, Appropriate: Modified Independent; a.k.a., *Ranchos Los Amigos Levels of Cognitive Functioning Scale-Revised.*

levodopa: A drug for individuals with Parkinson's disease that replaces dopamine, a substance in the neurotransmitter system facilitating volitional movements.

lexical prediction: See *word prediction.*

lexicon: A collection of manual signs and/or vocabulary words.

lexigrams: An aided set of graphic symbols composed of combinations of nine basic design elements originally developed for language research with the chimpanzee Lana at the Yerkes Regional Primate Center in Atlanta, Georgia. See also *Yerkish.*

LF: See *low frequency.*

license: Legal status granted by a state to an individual to engage in a defined professional practice that also provides legal penalties for violations in that practice.

life history book: A book of genealogical charts, mementos, photographs, and other items, typically along with simple text, that provide information about the life of an individual who exhibits memory impairment.

light emitting diode: Electronic visual display component for a communication device that gives off light; many of them are arranged so that letters, numbers, and other characters can be formed by the patterns of LEDs that are illuminated.

light pen: An alternate computer input device (e.g., the Robin Light Pen used with the BBC Micro/Master computers).

light pointer: A device that focuses a beam of light on the surface of a communication device for the purpose of direct selection of symbols, words, or other items.

Light Talker: An archaic, portable, dedicated speech-generating device that accepted multiple-switch input (e.g., optical head pointer, joystick, Morse code, variety of scanning modes) to recall stored utterances using Express or Minspeak software. The device could be operated with 8-, 32-, or 128-location overlays. It could also be used as a keyboard emulator or to serve an environmental control function.

Lightwriter: An archaic, portable, dedicated speech-generating device that featured a direct selection standard keyboard for spontaneous use or recall of prestored common words and phrases with a limited user-programmable memory. Output included two bright fluorescent visual displays for both the user and listener; a built-in text-to-speech synthesizer and printer were optional.

limited English proficiency: Individuals who are not fluent in English, and as such, cannot communicate effectively with English-speaking caregivers.

limited use policy: A policy by most public school districts that prohibits students who use AAC devices purchased with school funds to take them home after school, or in some cases, to take them out of the school building for community-based instruction.

linear predictive coding: A method of speech output that utilizes a combination of speech digitizing and mathematical modeling to reconstruct and produce a high-quality voice. Special hardware and software are required to reconstruct and simulate the original speech signal. Linear predictive coding is often referred to as *custom-encoded speech.*

linear scanning: A message selection technique in which items are scanned one-by-one in a specific sequence (e.g., in a circular direction or by columns within rows).

linguistic characteristics: AAC symbols possessing the ability to produce or approximate the production of language.

linguistic communication: Signed, spoken, or written communication that uses linguistic symbols according to the combination rules (i.e., syntax) of a naturally developed language (e.g., sign language, spoken language).

linguistic competence: (1) Knowledge of the rules of syntax, semantics, morphology, phonology, and pragmatics necessary to produce and understand an unlimited number of grammatical utterances of a language. (2) Mastery of symbols and symbol arrangements of an AAC system, leading to the ability to use the system to accomplish linguistic exchanges.

linguistics: The study of language, including phonology, morphology, semantics, syntax, and pragmatics.

liquid crystal display: A type of flat panel display in which liquid crystals placed between two sheets of glass emit light as a result of changes in electrical charge (e.g., the screen of notebook computers).

lissencephaly: A condition in which the gyri (convolutions) are malformed or do not develop on the surface of the cerebrum, often resulting in severe intellectual impairment and hypotonia.

literal comprehension task: A task that challenges a child's ability to perform a grammatical analysis on an incoming message. The child identifies the meaning of the lexical items and then determines the syntactic relationship that exists between and among the lexical items.

literate: A term used to describe an individual who has learned to read, write, and spell.

LLC: See *logical letter coding.*

LLR: See *late-latency response.*

LMN: See *lower motor neurons.*

LOA: Common medical abbreviation for leave of absence.

LOB: Common medical abbreviation for loss of balance.

local education agency: A public agency that is authorized or required to provide free, appropriate public education for children with disabilities.

localization: The systematic use of points in space for the purpose of referencing in manual signing. It is one of the major syntactical mechanisms in sign languages.

Localized Response: Total Assistance: Level III of the *Ranchos Los Amigos Levels of Cognitive Functioning Scale-Revised,* characterized in part by withdrawing or vocalizing in response to painful stimuli, turning of the head toward or away from an auditory stimulus, tracking moving objects as they pass within the visual field, responding inconsistently to simple commands, and responding that is directly related to the type of stimulus being presented.

location: One of the basic parameters of manual signs along with handshape, movement, and designation, defined as the area on or near the signer's body where a sign is made.

LOCF: See *Levels of Cognitive Functioning Scale.*

locked-in syndrome: A rare condition of neurological etiology that is characterized by quadriplegia, visual impairment, mutism, and ventilator dependency with (nearly) intact cognitive abilities; often results from bilateral damage to the pyramidal tract in the upper pons due to occlusion of the basilar artery.

locus coeruleus: A bluish-gray nucleus found in the floor of the fourth ventricle of the brain responsible for production of the neurotransmitter norepinephrine.

logic: The inherent conformity of a symbol system to rules allowing the creation of new symbols (expansion capability) that are consistent with symbols already existing in the system. A characteristic that separates symbol sets from symbol systems.

logical letter coding: The systematic organization of information or messages for storage and retrieval based on the use of letters and letter combinations that have meaning for the user (e.g., HM could be the code for the message "Help me"); a.k.a., *salient letter encoding.*

logograph: A letter, character, or other graphic symbol that is used to represent a word.

LOLEC: See *logical letter coding.*

Lombard effect: The involuntary tendency of an individual to increase vocal loudness in the presence of a noisy environment (e.g., at a busy nightclub or music concert).

long-term goal: A goal one expects to accomplish over a relatively lengthy period of time. Long-term goals are general statements about the ultimate outcome that is expected. They are usually followed by a number of more specifically written short-term goals or objectives that break the long-term goal down into more manageable steps.

long-term memory: The relatively permanent memory of experiences, ideas, etc. that can be called up and used by the individual when needed.

longitudinal research: A research method that involves the collection of information from an individual or group across a period of time (usually a year or more). This type of research is most often observational and typically involves documentation of the acquisition of particular skills or outcomes of intervention techniques.

Lorma alphabet: The alphabet most commonly used by persons with dual sensory impairment in Poland; use of this alphabet involves drawing lines or touching points on the hands of communication partners, one to the other, to the spaces assigned to individual letters of the conventional alphabet.

Lou Gehrig's disease: See *amyotrophic lateral sclerosis.*

low birth weight: Weight at birth that is less than 2,500 grams (approximately 5.5 pounds).

low frequency: Radio waves with frequencies between 30 and 300 kHz.

low technology: Any nonelectronic or simple electronic device that does not use a computer chip or integrated circuit or have moving parts. This term is archaic and has been replaced by the term, *non–speech-generating.*

low-tech: A common abbreviation for the archaic term, *low technology.*

low-technology communication aid: Simple communication devices that do not utilize computer chips or integrated circuits, nor produce written or spoken output or have programming capabilities. This term is archaic and has been replaced by the term, *non–speech-generating device.*

low-technology device: Any device that includes no electronic components (e.g., computer chips or integrated circuits) and functions more as a passive aid. This term is archaic and has been replaced by the term, *non–speech-generating device.*

lower extremities: The legs and feet.

lower motor neurons: Nerve cells that start in the spinal cord and terminate at a skeletal muscle. The loss of lower motor neurons leads to weakness, muscle fasciculations, and muscle atrophy. See also *flaccid* and *upper motor neurons.*

LPC: See *linear predictive coding.*

LRE: See *least restrictive environment.*

LTG: See *long-term goal.*

LTM: See *long-term memory.*

luminance: Refers to the brightness of images on a computer screen.

MA: See *mental age.*

macro command: A recorded group of computer commands treated by the computer as a unit and usually executed by the function keys on the keyboard.

macrocephaly: A condition in which an individual has an abnormally large head, often associated with a variety of syndromes and often a precursor for hydrocephalus.

macroglossia: An abnormal enlargement or oversizing of the tongue.

macula: The small, highly sensitive central area of the retina of the eye.

magnetic resonance imaging: An imaging procedure that uses the magnetic resonance of atoms to provide clear images of internal parts of the body, particularly useful in diagnosing structural abnormalities of the brain.

magnification hardware: Special magnification card for the computer that replaces the existing video card.

magnification software: Computer software that allows the user to enlarge the text displayed on a computer screen and designed to run in conjunction with other applications.

mainstream: A philosophy of educating children with disabilities in a general education setting with children without disabilities.

mainstreaming: The practice of placing students with various disabilities in classes that are predominantly composed of students without disabilities.

Makaton: An instructional program that is arranged in nine stages for the purpose of teaching a preselected vocabulary of approximately 350 manual signs from British Sign Language.

malignant in MS: A severe form of multiple sclerosis marked by rapid and extensive degeneration of cognitive, cerebellar, and pyramidal systems leading to death.

Maltron keyboard: A keyboard that is designed specifically for the comfort and accuracy of physically impaired individuals; used with the BBC microcomputer.

managing facilitator: Coordinates primary areas of responsibility, such as linguistic or operational competence, and includes leading the AAC team to consensus about intervention roles, scheduling intervention activities, clarifying the roles of other facilitators, and documenting progress.

mandated funding: See *funded mandate.*

mand-model procedure: A procedure that is used for promoting expressive communication, involving a sequence of steps, including gaining the learner's attention, producing a mand (i.e., request or command), pausing to allow for a response, and modeling the correct response if necessary.

manual: Pertaining to the use of the hands (e.g., gestures and manual signs, which are produced by varying conventional or idiosyncratic handshapes and/or movements).

manual alphabet: See *hand alphabet.*

manual English: An unaided pedagogical system developed by the Washington State School for the Deaf that utilizes manual signs to code spoken English.

manual pointing: A form of direct selection involving pointing with the hand or fingers, with or without a pointing aid.

manual signs: Unaided symbols that can be applied to either a natural sign language (e.g., American Sign Language, British Sign Language) or used as a code for a spoken language (e.g., Signed English or Signing Exact English). When used as a code for a spoken language, manual signs are used simultaneously with speech, either by signing each spoken word or by signing only the key words spoken (e.g., key word signing, manually coded English, signs supporting English).

manually coded English: See *manually coded language.*

manually coded language: An unaided communication system in which manual signs are used to represent the successive elements of a spoken language. Typically, manual signs are used as labels for whole words, but they can also be used for part words, such as suffixes (e.g., ed, ing) or prefixes (e.g., a , un). Manually coded languages differ in the degree to which they represent all the elements of a spoken language. For teaching purposes, where the accurate representation of the spoken language is important, more strict systems, such as Signed English or Signing Exact English, are sometimes preferred. Conversely, for general communication purposes, key word signing is often preferred, especially with hearing individuals who have intellectual impairments.

manufacturer: A company that designs, manufactures, sells, and in most cases, provides technical support, for AAC devices or materials or assistive technology (e.g., Prentke Romich Company, Tobii Dynavox, Words+, Inc., Zygo Industries).

maple syrup urine disease: A metabolic degenerative disorder in which amino acids are broken down, causing urine to smell like maple syrup. If untreated, this disorder may lead to spasticity, arching of the back (opisthotonos), hypertonia, and intellectual impairment.

Mark I: An early version of an IBM computer that used mechanical switches controlled by punched tape.

masked facies: Diminished facial expression, giving the person an expressionless appearance; seen often in Parkinson's disease.

match-to-sample: A stimulus-equivalence technique in which the learner is given an exemplar from a class of objects or pictures along with a group of similar and dissimilar objects or pictures, then is asked to find all the other objects or pictures that have a characteristic or characteristics in common.

maximal assessment: An assessment model consisting of a thorough evaluation of an individual's abilities across cognitive, academic, perceptual, linguistic, and motor domains, for the purpose of determining which AAC system to implement.

MB: See *megabyte.*

MBD: See *minimal brain damage/dysfunction.*

MBS: Common medical abbreviation for *modified barium swallow.*

MCE: Abbreviation for *manually coded English.* See *manually coded language.*

MD: See *muscular dystrophy.*

means-ends relationships: A sensorimotor scheme involving the understanding that problem solving has two components: a problem-solving process (i.e., means) and a solution or problem-solving goal (i.e., ends).

means to represent: One of the transmission processes of the AAC model proposed by Lloyd and colleagues (1990) that refers to the symbols (aided and unaided) used to encode a message for communication.

means to select: One of the transmission processes of the AAC model proposed by Lloyd and colleagues (1990) that refers to the manner in which the user makes symbol choices. The means to select can be either aided (e.g., direct selection with a head pointer) or unaided (e.g., direct selection with a finger).

means to transmit: One of the transmission processes of the AAC model proposed by Lloyd and colleagues (1990) that refers to the manner in which a user transmits a message. The means to transmit can be either aided (e.g., a communication board) or unaided (e.g., direct transmission through body parts).

measured intelligence: The demonstration of current intellectual functioning through use of an intelligence test.

Medicaid: A federal health program in the United States for individuals who qualify on the basis of financial hardship.

Medicaid waiver: A source of medical funding in the United States that varies from state to state. For example, in several states, the individual must be Medicaid-eligible (criteria for eligibility are usually waived when children are under 18 years of age) and at risk for institutionalization. The following individuals are typically eligible: adults who are aged, children who are medically fragile, individuals with autism, and persons with developmental disabilities.

medical decision making: The process of making decisions about what medical interventions should be undertaken.

Medicare: A federal health program in the United States for persons 65 years of age and older.

medium frequency: Radio waves with frequencies between 300 kHz and 3 MHz.

med-speak: An inappropriate speech-generating device medical need limitation advanced by some funding sources. Med-speak misstates the "purpose" or "medical purpose" of speech as being focused on the content of speech produced, as well as the role of the communication partner as a health care provider (i.e., that the medical need for a speech-generating device is to enable clients to produce "medically necessary communication" or "to communicate medical needs," or that speech-generating devices are medically necessary for clients unable to "communicate their basic needs through oral speech or manual sign language.") Med-speak inappropriately focuses on communication of medically related words, phrases, and messages to physicians and other care providers. Med-speak is inappropriate because it ignores the basis for stating clients have a medical need for speech-language pathology treatment, (i.e., that they are unable to meet *all* daily communication needs using speech or other natural communication methods). No speech-language pathology treatment method is focused exclusively on the production of messages on a specific topic or to specific communication partners.

meg: See *megabyte*.

megabyte: One million bytes (1,048,576 bytes).

megahertz: A unit of measure for frequency; one megahertz is equal to one million Hertz, or one million vibrations per second.

melodic intonation therapy: An approach to speech and language therapy for aphasic individuals, where speech is paired with simple melodic patterns, similarly to singing.

membrane board: A hard contact keyboard in which each key is housed in a foam rubber dome that, when pressed, completes an electrical circuit to activate the controller chip.

membrane keyboard: A keyboard that is typically flat and programmable with numerous pressure sensitive switches located under a soft surface.

membrane keys: An input device with a flat, continuous surface, having individual switches that are activated by pressure.

memorabilia box: A box filled with personal items that remind the user of personal events, to encourage meaningful conversation, and to serve as a memory aid. The box is used to assist in focusing the attention of the user, directing conversations, and reducing frustrating behavior.

memory: (1) A human's capacity for storing and retrieving information. (2) The amount of data that can be stored, either in random access memory or on a floppy or hard drive.

memory-based encoding: The process of language formulation in which the storage and retrieval of words, phrases, or other items are committed to memory (as opposed to a chart based system).

memory binder: A 3-ring book with pages containing photographs, pictures, and mementos to assist an individual with diminished memory; the pages can be removed and inserted depending on the context or environment.

Memowriter: An archaic, portable communication device that featured a typewriter keyboard, calculator, and printer. Up to 800 characters could be stored in memory and recalled using three-key sequences.

meningitis: An inflammation or infection of the meninges, the layers of tissue that cover the brain and spinal cord.

mental age: An age-equivalent score usually obtained by formal evaluation, frequently compared to chronological age to indicate an individual's level of intellectual functioning.

mental handicap: A condition of arrested or incomplete development of the mind that is characterized by below-normal intelligence.

mental retardation: As defined by the American Association on Intellectual and Developmental Disabilities, cognitive deficits that occur during the developmental period. More specifically, the individual must score at least two standard deviations below the mean for their age group on a standardized intelligence test and show significant impairment in adaptive behavior. The term *intellectual impairment* is typically used instead, as this term has negative connotations.

menu: A list of options, usually on a computer screen, from which the user can make choices.

message: A meaningful, purposeful attempt to communicate (e.g., expressing an opinion, making a request).

message banking: The electronic storage of recorded whole phrases, sentences and/or messages early in the progression of a disease (e.g., amyotrophic lateral sclerosis) to be used later in the disease process or as a vocal legacy for family members upon the individual's demise.

message prediction: A message retrieval strategy that allows the user to retrieve messages more quickly and with less effort; as the first and subsequent symbols are chosen, only the remaining possible choices light up or are otherwise presented to the user.

message retrieval: The process by which entire messages can be retrieved in response to a short code.

metalinguistic ability: The ability of an individual to consciously reflect on the form and functions of language separate from its use in context; metalinguistic abilities are presumed to develop in tandem with language itself.

methicillin-resistant staphylococcus aureus: A highly infectious bacterial infection of the skin that is resistant to the antibiotic methicillin at its variants.

method: (1) An orderly or systematic way of doing something. (2) A predetermined procedure.

MF: See *medium frequency*.

MHz: See *megahertz*.

MI: See *measured intelligence*.

microcephaly: A condition in which an individual has an abnormally small head; often associated with intellectual impairment, learning disabilities, or language disorders.

microcultures: Social organizations that result from associations of individuals with common characteristics, such as age, education, gender, health, occupation, and socioeconomic status.

microglossia: A condition in which the tongue is abnormally small or undersized.

micromike: A voice input device for the BBC Micro/Master computer series.

microscribe: A portable word processor featuring a QWERTY keyboard and optional speech output. Up to 10 messages can be stored for retrieval for communication along with an 8,000-character text memory.

microswitch: A small switch, usually used to control a computer, environmental control system, or power wheelchair, that has been adapted so that less pressure than normal is required to activate it.

microwriter: A portable communication device that utilizes combinations of six keys to produce alphabet letters and store text. It can be linked to a speech synthesizer, printer, or television.

middle-latency response: Auditory-evoked potentials occurring during the first 50 msec poststimulus onset, which indicate activity within or in the vicinity of the auditory cortex.

milieu: Referring to teaching that occurs in meaningful and relevant contexts or environments.

mime: An elaborate form of gesturing where the user typically assumes a role and enacts sequences of gestures to communicate a message.

mini keyboard: A small keyboard in which the keys are arranged closely together so they can be activated by individuals with a limited range of motion.

mini rocker lever: A smaller version of the dual switch, in which a plate sets upon a fulcrum so that it can be rocked back and forth.

mini talking card reader: An archaic hand-held speech-generating device that recorded and played back strips of audio tape attached to cards. Two seconds of sound could be recorded and played back on each inch of tape.

miniature objects: Smaller versions of larger objects (e.g., pieces of doll house furniture) used by some individuals with severe intellectual impairments to represent the larger object. The miniatures are used because of their portability and are typically stored in a calendar box, display box, or communication vest with transparent pockets. In some instances, miniature objects are used to represent concepts that are related to the object (e.g., a miniature comb used to represent the concept of self-care, including washing the face, shaving, brushing teeth).

Miniboard: A pictorial or graphic symbol display that can be used as an overlay on electronic devices or as a stand-alone non–speech-generating device.

minimal brain damage/dysfunction: A less severe form of brain injury, characterized by any of the following symptoms: short attention span, distractibility, impulsivity, hyperactivity, emotional lability, motor incoordination, visual-perceptual motor disturbance, and language disorder.

minimal pair: Two lexical items (e.g., words, manual signs, pictures) that differ only in one of their constituting elements (e.g., the words "cave" and "gave" differ only in their initial sound; the manual signs for "good" and "bad" differ only in the movement of the hand during their production).

minor dysmorphic features: Superficial malformations of the body that are usually considered to be normal variants or familial traits; the presence of several of these features may contribute to an overall appearance that is part of a specific syndrome.

Minspeak: A system for encoding and organizing messages for storage and retrieval based on the use of pictures (i.e., icons) that have multiple meanings.

mismatched negativity: A negative wave from the auditory-evoked potential, occurring approximately 150 to 275 msec poststimulus onset that indicates the patient's ability to discriminate one signal from preceding signals without directly attending to the auditory stimulus. The clinical applications of mismatched negativity are yet unknown due to a lack of research.

MIT: See *melodic intonation therapy*.

mixed aphasia: A type of aphasia in which sensory and motor abilities are adversely affected.

mixed cerebral palsy: A term used to describe an individual with more than one type of cerebral palsy (e.g., both athetoid and spastic).

mixed hearing impairment: A hearing loss that has both conductive and sensorineural components. With intervention, the conductive component can be resolved, but the sensorineural component is permanent.

MLR: See *middle-latency response*.

MMN: See *mismatched negativity*.

mobility: An individual's ability to move about safely and effectively within the environment.

modality: The particular channel through which information is transmitted or received.

mode: A particular manner of communication (e.g., oral mode, manual motor mode, ocular motor mode).

model: (1) A graphic representation of a structured theory or principle designed to organize hypotheses and knowledge. Some taxonomies serve as models. (2) A target behavior to be imitated.

modeling: Presenting a target behavior for an individual to imitate.

modem: Short for modulator/demodulator, a hardware device that allows computers to communicate with each other. Modems operate at different speeds.

modification: A process which changes the prescribed curriculum to meet a student's special educational needs. Modified courses do not provide the same credit as a prescribed course. Details of the modified course must be included in the student's file and the transcript should indicate that the course has been modified.

modified barium swallow: An x-ray procedure that obtains views of swallowing function that are then recorded on videotape. The modified barium swallow is useful in determining the presence or absence of aspiration of material into the airway and the movement of material into and through the upper portion of the esophagus. Small amounts of flavored barium (a radioactive material) are mixed with foods differing in texture and thickness and then swallowed. An x-ray image is then captured of the swallowing process.

modified orthography: Orthography that has been accentuated or enhanced so that a word bears some resemblance to its referent (e.g., drawing icicles on the word ice).

modulator/demodulator: See *modem.*

moisture guard: A soft, plastic cover molded to the shape of a keyboard or device to protect it from moisture.

molded seats: See *custom contoured seats.*

molding: See *physical guidance.*

momentary light cue: If an AAC user is aware that a communicative opportunity has arisen, is visually scanning an overlay but does not call forth a message after a brief period, the clinician or educator shines a light momentarily on a target symbol(s) as a cue to the user.

momentary switch: A switch that opens or closes only when it is activated.

monitor: A display device that receives video signals by direct connection to a computer or AAC device. A wide variety of technology is available, including cathode ray tube, liquid crystal display, and plasma.

monoplegia: Complete paralysis of a single limb, muscle, or muscle group.

morphology: A branch of linguistics that examines the way in which words can change based on how they are used in relation to other words in a sentence. Adding "s" to a regular noun to make it plural is an example of morphology, as is altering the vowel in "run" to "ran" to mark a change in tense from present to past.

Morse code: An international system that represents the letters of the alphabet and other characters via a series of dits and dahs. Morse code can be input through switches to communication devices or computers and output as letters, punctuation, and numbers.

Morse code equalizer: An archaic, dedicated speech-generating device and word processor that was accessed by single or dual switch Morse code inputs appropriate for visually impaired users. User strategies included abbreviation expansion and Instant Speech.

mother board: A large circuit board, housed in the central processing unit, into which all other computer components are plugged.

motor access: The ways in which an individual will physically approach and use an AAC system.

motor control: The voluntary initiation and execution of movement.

motor development: The typical sequence of gross and fine motor skills a child develops, such as holding the head up, sitting up, crawling, walking, jumping, and writing, to name a few.

motor encoding: A storage and retrieval organization scheme based on motor patterns.

motor learning: The development of an understanding of the consequences of motor activity, including interface control.

motor performance: The ability to perform a motor task. Having the ability to carryover between one movement pattern and other functional movement patterns. Components of motor performance include (a) timing and force of muscle activation, (b) initiation, sustained holding of contraction, and/or termination of movement, (c) speed of movement, and (d) patterns of movement. The appropriate and efficient control of motor processes and the movements of the body in such functions as dancing, jumping, running, and walking.

mounting: The securing or attachment of a switch, control, or other device so that a user may gain access to it to operate technology.

mouse: An input device that allows selection of items on the screen. The pointer or cursor on the screen moves in accordance with the mouse as it is dragged across a surface.

mouse button: The button(s) on top of the mouse. The user presses the mouse button to choose commands from menus or to move items around on the screen.

mouse emulator: Any device that simulates the input functions of the standard mouse (e.g., Headmouse).

Mouth-Hand System: See *Danish Mouth Hand System.*

mouthstick: An adaptive device (i.e., stick) that is held in the mouth and used to point to a desired object, picture, or word from an array of choices.

movement: One of the basic parameters of manual signs along with handshape, location, and designation.

movement-based approach: A systematic approach developed Van Dijk (1966) for individuals with dual sensory impairments. It includes six components: (1) nurturance, (2) resonance, (3) coactive movement, (4) nonrepresentational reference, (5) deferred imitation, and (6) natural gestures.

MR: See *mental retardation.*

MRI: See *magnetic resonance imaging.*

MRSA: See *methicillin-resistant staphylococcus aureus.*

MS: See *multiple sclerosis.*

MS-DOS: A disk-operating system made by Microsoft Corporation, it was the dominant operating system for PC-compatible computers during the 1980s. It was gradually replaced on consumer desktop computers with various generations of the Windows operating system. See also *disk-operating system*.

MSUD: See *maple syrup urine disease*.

multicultural: Simultaneously belonging to two or more cultural groups.

multidimensional scanning: See *block/group scanning*.

multidisciplinary team model: One of several models for team assessment and intervention in which members of different professions or disciplines function relatively independently of one another.

multihandicapped: Having a physical or sensory disability plus one or more additional disabilities that make education in the regular classroom difficult; because of this, special services usually are required.

multimodal: The use of more than one mode, channel, or form (e.g., auditory, visual, tactile).

multimodal approach: An intervention approach that uses more than one mode of communication (e.g., concurrent use of residual speech, gestures, manual signs, graphic symbols).

multimodal communication: The use of more than one mode, channel, or form for the purpose of communication (e.g., concurrent use of residual speech, gestures, manual signs, graphic symbols).

multiple primary interactants: Caregivers, teachers, public school paraprofessionals, nursing home staff, job coaches, etc., who are actively involved in AAC service delivery. The interactants must have a working knowledge of the individual's AAC system (i.e., non–speech-generating and speech-generating technology).

multiple sclerosis: A disease of the central or peripheral nervous system characterized by degeneration of the fatty sheaths (i.e., myelin) surrounding the nerve fibers resulting in a variety of symptoms, such as double vision, loss or reduction of sensation, tingling in the extremities, dizziness, and dysarthria. Multiple sclerosis occurs more often in young adults and is characterized by cycles of remission and relapse.

multiple-switch scanning: Scanning in which the user utilizes two or more switches.

muscle imbalance: Occurs when opposing muscles provide different directions of tension due to tightness and/or weakness. The strength or size of muscle on one side is not symmetrical to the strength or size of muscle on the other side of the body.

muscle stiffness: Abnormal muscle contraction or lack of extensibility, often caused by spasticity or simultaneous contraction of muscles on both sides of a joint.

muscle tone: The natural state of tension within muscles. Muscles are always in a slight state of tension.

muscle weakness: A reduced ability to create and apply force or strength, usually due to a neuromuscular disease or disorder.

muscular dystrophy: A progressive neuromotor disease characterized by weakness and wasting away of muscle tissue (atrophy).

musculoskeletal: Pertaining to the muscles and skeleton, and the relationship between them.

mvmt: Common medical abbreviation for *movement*.

myelin sheath: A sheath of fatty tissue that surrounds and insulates the axons of nerve cells; plays a role in neural transmission.

myelomeningocele: A condition seen in spina bifida where the spinal cord and its covering protrude from the infant's back.

myoclonus: Sudden, brief involuntary twitching or jerking of a muscle or groups of muscles. It is not considered a disease per se but rather a clinical manifestation of another disease or disorder.

myopia: Nearsightedness.

nasogastric tube: A short-term feeding tube that is passed through the nose, down the back of the throat and esophagus, and into the stomach.

National Institute on Disability, Independent Living, and Rehabilitation Research: A federal agency of the U.S. government housed within the Office of Special Education and Rehabilitative Services of the U.S. Department of Education. National Institute on Disability, Independent Living, and Rehabilitation Research funds Tech Act projects, Rehabilitation Engineering Research Centers, and other projects related to AAC and assistive technology.

National Institute on the Education of At-Risk Students (At-Risk Institute): One of five institutes created by the Educational Research, Development, Dissemination and Improvement Act of 1994, located within the Office of Educational Research and Improvement within the United States Department of Education. The institute supports a wide range of research and development activities designed to improve the education of students at risk for educational failure due to limited English proficiency, poverty, race, geographic location, or economic disadvantage.

native language: (1) The language that is normally used by an individual in their home. (2) For an individual who is deaf or hard of hearing or visually impaired or with no ability to use written language, the mode of communication that is normally used by the individual (e.g., sign language, Braille, or oral communication).

natural contexts: The settings and activities in which an individual would normally function (e.g., home, work, community) if not engaged in an intervention program.

natural contingency: The natural consequence that happens in the environment without an individual controlling the consequence of the behavior; naturally occurring consequence of behavior occurring in everyday situations.

natural gestures: One of six components of Van Dijk's (1966) Movement Based Approach that encourages the use of "self-developed" gestures that are iconic to the individual.

natural language: Any language that has evolved over time from the social interaction between human beings (i.e., has not been artificially invented).

natural language acquisition: A systematic way of analyzing typical language development in relation to communicative intents that provides a framework of intervention that follows typical language development and allows for spontaneous self-generated grammar.

natural language teaching: A method of language instruction in which a child's voluntary engagement with an object is used for the purpose of object labeling. Any clear verbal response by the child is reinforced and shaped. Reinforcement comes in the form of praise or the continued opportunity to play with the target object.

natural speech: The use of the oral motor mechanism (i.e., lips, tongue, cheeks) to produce spoken words to request wants or needs during conversational exchanges.

navigation ring: A D-shaped layout on a visual screen display where thumbnails of other available visual scenes surround the currently active visual screen display.

NDT: See *neurodevelopmental therapy.*

neck collar: A head support for an individual in a wheelchair that keeps the head centered in midline and prevents it from falling too far back or to the side. The head should be positioned so the face is perpendicular to the floor and is in midline. This positioning is critical for the functions of breathing, vision, feeding, and attention.

neck dissection: A surgical procedure by which lymphatic tissue is removed from the neck; may be performed along with a laryngectomy.

needs assessment: An assessment of the communication needs of an AAC user. Once a specific list of mandatory or desirable needs is generated, AAC technologies that can support these needs are sought.

negative reinforcement: The removal of an aversive or undesirable consequence that results in an increase in desired behavior.

neonatal intensive care unit: A facility within a hospital where life-threatening perinatal problems are diagnosed and treated.

network: (1) A group of computers linked together so their users can share information or peripheral devices. (2) A group of professionals, agencies, or other entities that shares a common interest, goal, or service.

neurodevelopmental therapy: Intervention in which normal developmental stages serve as the underlying principle or theory; the basis for practice in physical and occupational therapy.

neurogenic degenerative diseases: Diseases having a neurological etiology that cause progressive deterioration in functioning as they progress.

neuromotor system: The relationship between the nervous system and movement that entails the transmission of the nerves or nerve impulses to muscles to create movement.

neuromuscular: Pertaining to the nerves and muscles and the relationship between them.

neuromusculoskeletal: Pertaining to the nerves, muscles, and skeleton and the relationship among them.

neurotransmitter: Any substance that plays a role in the transmission of nerve impulses between two neurons or between a nerve and a muscle (e.g., acetycholine, dopamine).

NG tube: See *nasogastric tube.*

NICU: See *neonatal intensive care unit.*

NIDILRR: See *National Institute on Disability, Independent Living, and Rehabilitation Research.*

NLA: See *natural language acquisition.*

No Response: Total Assistance: Level I of the *Ranchos Los Amigos Levels of Cognitive Functioning Scale-Revised,* characterized by a complete absence of an observable change in behavior when presented with auditory, visual, tactile, proprioceptive, vestibular, or painful stimuli.

noncontact signs: Manual signs in which the hands do not make contact with each other or with any other body part during production.

nondedicated AAC system: A device that is not specifically designed for communication that can be adapted to function as an AAC device (e.g., a computer).

nondedicated communication aid: A system consisting of a standard microcomputer that has been adapted for use as an AAC aid by adding special software, synthetic speech, or other peripherals.

nondedicated communication device: A computer-based communication device or system, not limited in its function to just communication; the computer can also perform a number of work functions, such as database, spreadsheet, or statistical operations, and can switch back and forth between these operations and the communication function.

nonelectronic: A term used to describe assistive technology that does not rely on electronic components, such as transistors, vacuum tubes, integrated circuits, or computer chips

nonintentional act: Any behavior that is performed without an intent, plan, or purpose.

nonintentional communication: The interpretation of nonintentional acts as a communicative message.

non-linguistic communication: The use of vocal, graphic, or gestural symbols for the purpose of communication but are not part of a linguistic system, such as speech or a natural sign language (e.g., vocalizations that express pleasure, discomfort, or pain; simple line drawings; basic gestures).

nonliterate: A term that is used to describe an individual who has had the time and opportunity to learn to read or write but has not yet accomplished the skill.

nonmanual component: A significant element of manual signs that is not expressed by configurations or movements of the hands or arms (e.g., facial or bodily expressive elements used in a systematic way, such as raising the eyebrows to mark a question).

nonoral: (1) Literally, without speech, voice, or oral production. (2) A term that was used in the past to describe AAC.

nonrelational words: Words that have tangible referents in the real world (e.g., chair, dog, shirt).

nonrepresentational reference: One of the six components of Van Dijk's (1966) Movement Based Approach. This component is based on the principle of "learning through doing" by teaching the individual to identify three- and then two-dimensional representations of body parts for the purpose of developing body image, pointing skills, and independence.

nonspeech: (1) Literally, without spoken words. (2) A term that was used in the past to describe AAC.

non–speech-generating: Any process, device, or system that does not include natural or synthetic speech.

non–speech-generating device: A device or instrument that does not produce natural or synthetic speech.

nonsymbolic: Eye gaze, gestures, facial expressions, body movements, vocal sounds, and other expressions that enhance communication but are not considered part of symbolic communication systems.

nonverbal: (1) An ambiguous term that technically means without language. It is generally used to describe evaluation tools that purport to measure the *nonverbal* intelligence of individuals who have difficulty comprehending or producing spoken language, through the use of spatial and motor tasks with gestural instructions. (2) Used sometimes to describe individuals with little or no functional speech. However, the term should only be used to describe communication and should not be used to describe individuals with little or no functional speech.

nonverbal cognition: Cognitive functions and skills that are not language-based (e.g., attention, flexibility).

nonvocal: See *nonoral*.

nonvocal communication: Communication that bypasses the acoustic mode (e.g., writing, signing, or pointing to graphic symbols without vocalization).

non–weight-bearing: The legs cannot support the weight of the individual, so walking distances or climbing stairs is virtually impossible. The individual may be able to transfer short distances by hopping.

Noonan syndrome: A syndrome occurring in both males and females, without chromosomal abnormality, with characteristics similar to Turner's syndrome, such as short stature, webbed neck, low posterior hairline, a shieldlike chest, lateral deviation of the forearm, and abnormalities of the earlobes.

norm-referenced test: Any commercially prepared test that can be administered to large groups of individuals and used for the purpose of comparing the performance of the individual being tested to similar individuals making up the normative sample.

number encoding: See *numeric encoding*.

numeric encoding: The systematic organization of information or messages for storage and retrieval using numbers and number combinations for the purpose of language formulation; a.k.a., *number encoding*.

numerical linguistics: A method of analysis in historical linguistics that attempts to determine the evolutionary relationships among various human languages. It accomplishes this by comparing lists of supposedly core (or basic) words between languages and finding relationships by determining the percentage of cognates between them; a.k.a., *glottochronology*.

nursing home: See *skilled nursing facility*.

Nurturance: One of six components of Van Dijk's (1966) Movement Based Approach. The goal is to develop a warm, positive relationship between the individual with a disability and the facilitator, to promote an interest in communication interactions, and to enhance the individual's willingness to participate in social exchanges.

NWB: Common medical abbreviation for *non–weight-bearing*.

nystagmus: Involuntary, rapid movements of the eye.

O & M: See *orientation and mobility* and *orientation and mobility specialist*.

OAE(s): See *otoacoustic emissions*.

Oakland Picture Dictionary: A dictionary of nearly 600 clear, realistic drawings. The symbols are black and white and according to the author are appropriate for persons of all ages.

object: A physical item used for symbolic representation (e.g., real objects, parts of objects, or miniature objects). See *tangible symbols*.

object concept: The sensorimotor scheme pertaining to the ability to apply appropriate behaviors to act on objects, as influenced by the objects' perceptual properties.

object permanence: The sensorimotor scheme pertaining to a knowledge that objects still exist when they are not perceptible.

OCB: See *olivocochlear bundle*.

occupational therapist: A professional who is qualified to work with individuals with disabilities to establish or re-establish life functions (e.g., fine motor function, wheelchair transfers, mobility). An occupational therapist who has earned their credentials is referred to as an occupational therapist, registered. Assistants who have special training but not to the degree of an occupational therapist are referred to as *occupational therapist aides.*

occupational therapy: The rehabilitation discipline in which purposeful activities are employed as a basis for improving muscular control. Physical and mental recovery is the primary objective, with a secondary objective being helping the individual acquire a job or self-help skills.

OCR: See *optical character recognition.*

ocular mobility: Coordinated functioning of the eye muscles that enables the eyes to move together smoothly in all directions.

Office of Special Education and Rehabilitative Services: An office of the U.S. Department of Education that supports programs that assist in educating children with special needs, provides for the rehabilitation of youth and adults with disabilities, and supports research to improve the lives of individuals with disabilities. Its organizational structure includes three entities: National Institute of Disability, Independent Living, and Rehabilitation Research, Rehabilitation Services Administration, and Office of Special Education Programs.

Office of Special Education Programs: An office within the Office of Special Education and Rehabilitative Services of the U.S. Department of Education dedicated to improving the lives of infants, toddlers, children, and youth with disabilities ages birth through 21 years by providing leadership and financial support to assist states and local districts.

OHCs: See *outer hair cells.*

olivocochlear bundle: A group of efferent (i.e., descending) or motor neural pathways connecting the superior olivary complex with the cochlea that assists in the detection and processing of auditory stimuli in the presence of noise; a.k.a., *Rasmussen's bundle.*

OM: See *otitis media.*

OME: See *otitis media with effusion.*

onset: Any consonants that precede the vowel in a syllable. See *onset-rime.*

onset-rime: The components of a syllable; any consonants that precede the vowel in a syllable are referred to as the onset, and the vowel and any successive consonants in the syllable are called the rime.

onsite facilitator: Similar to an e-helper, this person is onsite with the person who uses AAC during a telepractice session and facilitates the session. They may or may not be the e-helper. The facilitator provides support so a session runs smoothly and may help co-construct an AAC user's message to the clinician.

OOB: Common medical abbreviation for *out of bed.*

opaque: A term used to describe a symbol that has little to no visual relationship to its referent.

opaque symbol: Any symbol (whether aided or unaided) that bears very little visual resemblance, if any, to its referent. The creation of opaque symbols tends to be arbitrary, and therefore, the meaning of these symbols must be learned.

opaqueness: A term used to describe the absence of iconicity due to symbols that have little to no visual resemblance to their referents. See also *iconicity, transparency,* and *translucency.*

open reduction internal fixation: A surgical technique to repair a bone fracture; it involves opening the body part that houses the fractured bone and then using plates or screws to repair the fracture so it will heal.

operational competence: The ability to effectively, efficiently, and independently operate an AAC system.

opportunity barriers: Barriers imposed by other persons or by obstacles in the AAC user's environment that impede their ability to use AAC (e.g., policies, attitudes, lack of knowledge, and lack of communication opportunities).

opportunity strand: A principle that states that once access issues have been resolved, the person with a disability must be allowed the opportunity to participate.

opsoclonus-myoclonus syndrome: A rare neurological disorder in which the sufferer exhibits an unsteady, trembling gait; intermittent shock-like spasms of the muscles; and irregular, rapid eye movements.

optical character recognition: A process by which visual information (e.g., print) is digitized for computer storage and retrieval.

optical headpointer: Used with some electronic communication devices, a head-mounted optical interface that is used to select keys or symbols on a device by activating built-in light-emitting diodes.

optical input: The transmission of visual data into a computer (e.g., a scanner).

optical pointer: Any device that focuses a beam of nonvisible (i.e., infrared) light or other energy (e.g., sonar) on the surface of a communication system to activate it.

optical scanning: The process of using an optical device to scan visual information (e.g., words, graphic symbols) into a computer.

oral: Pertaining to or surrounding the mouth; performed by the mouth (e.g., speech).

oral motor function: Motor and sensory function of the structures of the oral cavity and pharynx related to the process of swallowing up to the point that food enters the esophagus.

orientation: A parameter of manual signs related to the direction the palms and fingers are facing (e.g., to the front, to the left, upward) during sign production; often considered to be a minor parameter of manual signs because it gives additional information about the handshape parameter.

orientation and mobility: Pertaining to the provision of assistive technology and services to persons who are blind or have low vision to allow them to function within their environments.

orientation and mobility specialist: A professional who assists individuals with low vision to acquire mobility skills.

orientation of display: The spatial position of a display in relation to the floor.

ORIF: Common medical abbreviation for *open reduction internal fixation.*

oromotor dysfunction: Exhibiting difficulty in the planning, coordination, or execution of motor activity related to the lips, tongue, cheeks, and pharynx.

Orovox: An archaic, programmable speech synthesizer that could recall up to 250 phrases with a single key. It could also be interfaced to a computer and printer.

orthography: Written language. See *traditional orthography.*

orthopedic: (1) Generally referring to the bones, joints, and muscles. (2) In describing surgery, to straighten, restore, or preserve muscles, bones, or joints to correct body deformities.

orthosis: An external orthopedic appliance that prevents or assists the movement of the spine or limbs.

orthotics: Devices or equipment that support weak or ineffective joints or muscles (e.g., braces, shoe inserts, splints).

OSEP: See *Office of Special Education Programs.*

OSERS: See *Office of Special Education and Rehabilitative Services.*

osteogenesis imperfecta: A group of hereditary disorders affecting connective tissue, resulting in fragile bones. Although individuals who have the disorder do not experience concomitant intellectual or language impairments, they may require alternative access for written communication due to writing difficulties that occur as a result of frequent fractures; a.k.a., *brittle bone disease.*

OT: See *occupational therapist.*

OTA: Common medical abbreviation for *occupational therapist aide.* See *occupational therapist.*

otitis media: An inflammation of the middle ear, usually caused by malfunction of the Eustachian tube leading to poor ventilation of the middle ear cavity. As the disorder progresses, negative pressure (in relation to atmospheric pressure) builds in the middle ear cavity, causing the mucous membrane lining to secrete fluid that fills the middle ear space. At this point, the individual has *otitis media with effusion.*

otitis media with effusion: See *otitis media.*

otoacoustic emissions: Low-level, inaudible sounds produced by the cochlea's outer hair cells as they respond to a sound presented to a stimulus ear. A tiny microphone is placed within the external ear canal to pick up the sounds. Otoacoustic emissions can be used as a general measure of the integrity of the cochlea and auditory neural pathway and are often used during infant hearing screenings.

OTR: Common medical abbreviation for *occupational therapist, registered.* See *occupational therapist.*

outer hair cells: Sensory receptor cells within the organ of Corti that activate the cochlear neurons of cranial nerve VIII when stimulated by fluid displacement within the cochlea.

output: (1) The transmission of data from a computer to devices, such as monitors and printers. (2) The products of aided speech-generating devices, including voice output and print.

overflow: A generalized increase in muscle tone that occurs when an individual engages in considerable physical effort.

overlay: A sheet of paper, plastic, or other material, usually removable, on which pictures, symbols, and messages are mounted on a communication board or device.

PA: See *prior authorization.*

PAC: See *personal aid for communication.*

PACA: See *Portable Anticipatory Communication Aid.*

PACE: See *Promoting Aphasics' Communicative Effectiveness Therapy.*

paddle: An input device used for moving objects around a monitor screen, usually when playing arcade games.

pages: In some electronic communication devices with dynamic display capability, the vocabulary is stored on a series of virtual pages or levels. When a symbol is activated, it may lead to further vocabulary on a different page. The new page automatically displays itself on the screen and remains there until activation of a symbol leads to vocabulary on a different page.

Paget Gorman Sign System: An entirely pedagogical sign system designed in Britain to represent the English language.

PalmPilot: One of the more popular *personal digital assistants* manufactured by Palm, Inc.

palm writing: Spelling out messages by using the index finger to draw the letters of the alphabet in the palm of the message receiver's hand.

paralanguage/paralinguistics: Features that are not part of the language but are important in the comprehension and expression of the language (e.g., body postures, facial expressions, hand gestures, stress, intonation, volume, and phrasing).

parallel play: The third stage of play development in which children play in proximity to each other but still remain independent of each other.

parallel port: A computer port that allows the transmission of data eight bits at a time, a transmission speed that is much faster than for serial ports. See also *port* and *serial port*.

parallel training: A training method where a new set of complex skills is introduced at the same time the learner is mastering an easier set of skills.

parallel transmission: A method of sending data between a computer and a peripheral device through a parallel port, usually eight bits at a time along separate wires.

paralysis: A loss or impairment of muscle power, function, or sensation (anaesthesia) due to lesions of the neural or muscular system.

paraplegia: Paralysis of both legs and generally the lower trunk.

paresis: Partial paralysis.

Parkinson's disease: A neurological disease that usually results from arteriosclerotic changes in the basal ganglia and characterized by rhythmic tremors of the limbs, slowness and stiffness of voluntary movement, rigid facial expression, and stooped posture.

partial weight-bearing: The ability to bear between 20% and 50% of the body's weight with the legs. The individual may be able to ambulate for short distances but may not be able to climb stairs.

participation model: An assessment and intervention model based on functional participation of an AAC user as compared to able-bodied peers of the same chronological age.

partner-assisted scanning: A message selection technique in which an assistant or aide scans items for the AAC user through spoken, tactile, or visual means.

PAS: See *personal amplification system*.

passive matrix screen: A laptop computer monitor that uses less expensive technology, resulting in a graphic image that is of poor quality, with fewer available colors, poor color depth and contrast, and ghosting when images on the monitor change.

passive range of motion: Range of movement of a joint when the joint is manipulated by another person (e.g., a doctor) without any active participation by patient.

Patau syndrome: Also known as Trisomy 13; Patau syndrome is a serious genetic disorder associated with a third copy of chromosome 13 in some or all cells of the body. Individuals born with this condition experience a variety of severe medical conditions; only approximately 10% of infants survive to reach 1 year of age.

patient care conference: A meeting of members of the health care team, the patient, and their family where discussions are held to discuss specific issues and reach consensus on decisions about the patient's treatment plan.

Patient Initiated Light Operated Telecontrol: A pointer controlled by movements of the head, providing access opportunities for individuals who are not able to make selections with other body parts.

Patient Operated Selector Mechanism: One of the earliest assistive technology devices; a special typewriter control involving scanning and selection through the activation of a switch.

patient-provider communication: Communication between patients and their care providers.

pause time: The time during which a communication partner pauses without giving additional prompts in anticipation of a response. See *time delay*.

PCA: Common medical abbreviation for *personal care attendant*.

PCC: Common medical abbreviation for *patient care conference*.

PCS: See *Picture Communication Symbols*.

PD: See *Parkinson's disease*.

PDA: See *personal digital assistant*.

PDD: See *pervasive developmental disorders*.

Peabody Individual Achievement Test: A multiple-choice assessment of academic skills, such as spelling, reading, and math.

Peabody Picture Vocabulary Test-Revised: A norm-referenced receptive vocabulary test with a multiple-choice response format.

PECS: See *Picture Exchange Communication System*.

pectoral flap: A reconstructive procedure where tissue with its blood supply from the pectoral region is positioned to fill a defect resulting from trauma to the neck or surgery for oropharyngeal cancer.

peculiar facies: Unusual facial features typically seen in persons exhibiting certain syndromes affecting the craniofacial structures.

pedagogical sign system: See *artificial sign system*.

pedagogical signs: Any set of manual signs used to provide an easy transition to written English or to speech; related to manually coded English. See also *Paget Gorman Sign System*, *Signing Exact English*, and *Signed English*.

peer tutoring: A method that is used to integrate students with handicaps in regular classrooms, based on the notion that students can effectively tutor one another. The role of learner or teacher may be assigned to either the student with a disability or a peer without a disability.

pelvic obliquity: A condition in which one side of the pelvis is higher than the other.

pelvic rotation: A condition in which one side of the pelvis is more forward than the other side.

pelvic tilt: An incline of the pelvic girdle in a forward or backward alignment.

perceptual distinctness: The degree to which symbols can be easily discriminated from each other or are perceived as appearing distinctly different.

perinatal: The period immediately before, during, and after birth.

peripheral device: A piece of hardware that is physically separate from the computer (e.g., monitors, external disk drives, printers, scanners).

Perkins Brailler: A machine that produces Braille, having six keys and a space bar for production of letters and other characters.

perlocutionary behaviors: Behaviors that are not intentional but may be interpreted as intentional by the listener (e.g., a listener may conclude that an infant cries to express hunger).

perseverative speech: Speech seen in some individuals with autism, intellectual impairment, or developmental disabilities that is characterized by continuous repetitions of the same utterances. See also *unconventional verbal behavior*.

person-first terminology: Terminology that places the individual before the impairment or disability (e.g., "children with autism spectrum disorder.")

personal aid for communication: A simple, archaic communication device that featured switch activation of an array of lights to designate pictures, symbols, or words placed on an overlay. The standard personal aid for communication contained up to eight lights.

personal amplification system: A hardware amplification system consisting of a body worn amplifier and headphones for an individual with hearing impairment.

personal care attendant: A person who performs personal care duties or services for a person with a disability (e.g., assisting with activities of daily living, monitoring vital signs, transporting and escorting, assisting with household maintenance, and retrieving desired items).

personal digital assistant: An electronic personal organizer that may have any number of the following capabilities: (a) basic calendar, (b) address book, (c) task organizer, (d) wireless connection to the internet, (e) MP3 player, (f) digital photography, (g) global positioning, and (h) mobile phone.

personal speech amplifier: A portable amplification device featuring an over-the-ear microphone and an amplifier that can be attached to a pocket or belt, allowing the user freedom of movement.

pervasive developmental disorders: Several disorders that involve problems in the domains of social-emotional and communicative development. The most common of all pervasive developmental disorders is autism.

PET: See *positron emission tomography*.

PGSS: See *Paget Gorman Sign System*.

phenotype: The interaction of genetics with the environment, giving way to the physical characteristics of an individual, including morphology, biochemistry, and physiology.

phenylketonuria: A metabolic disorder in which there is an increase in the level of the amino acid phenylalanine in the blood. Untreated phenylketonuria is associated with intellectual impairment, microcephaly, seizures, athetosis, hand posturing, and behavioral stereotypies.

phoneme: A speech sound, such as a consonant, vowel, or diphthong.

phoneme analysis: The operation of analyzing a spoken syllable or word into individual phonemes; a.k.a., *phoneme segmenting*.

phoneme blending: The operation of producing a complete syllable or word upon hearing the spoken individual phonemes; a.k.a., *phoneme synthesis*.

phoneme segmenting: See *phoneme analysis*.

phoneme synthesis: See *phoneme blending*.

phonemics: (1) The study of the phonological segments of speech sounds. (2) Of or relating to the smallest category of speech sound or the smallest unit of sound that distinguishes one word from another.

phonetically balanced words: Monosyllabic words used as stimuli for assessing speech recognition threshold in speech audiometry.

phonetics: (1) The study of the description and classification of speech sounds. (2) Of or relating to the actual or variant production of a phoneme (e.g., aspirated vs. unaspirated /p/).

phonics: (1) Of or relating to the sounds of speech. (2) A method of teaching reading by demonstrating the relationship of letters to sounds.

phonological awareness: A skill thought to be necessary for the development of reading ability, the ability to consciously reflect on the sound system of a language, to manipulate phonemic structure, and to recognize similarities and differences in phonemic properties.

phonological store: A component of short-term or working memory thought to mediate spoken and written information in phonological or verbal form.

phonology: The study of the sound system of a language, including the speech sounds (or segments), suprasegmentals (e.g., stress, intonation, tempo), syllables, and phonotactics.

phonotactics: Rules that govern the allowable combinations of speech sounds in a given language (e.g., no word in the English language begins with the "ng" sound).

photoreceptors: Sensory nerve endings, cells, or groups of cells specialized to sense or receive light.

Phototonic wand: An input device for the BBC microcomputer that consists of a head-mounted light beam for producing graphics, text, and music utilizing special computer software.

phrenic nerve pacer: For individuals with paralysis of the diaphragm due to a spinal cord lesion above the nuclei of the phrenic nerves, a device that stimulates the phrenic nerves to contract the diaphragm.

physical attributes: See *physical characteristics.*

physical characteristics: Also known as physical attributes, they are components of aided AAC symbols referring to the physical nature of the symbols. There are four physical characteristics of aided symbols: two-dimensional, three-dimensional, animated, and acoustic.

physical effort: The amount or degree of physical activity (i.e., calories of energy expended) that is required to perform a response.

physical guidance: Providing physical assistance to move an individual through desired motor behaviors; a.k.a., *molding.*

physical therapist: A professional who is qualified to work with individuals who have muscular or neurological impairment to restore gross motor functions. A physical therapist who has earned their credentials is referred to as a *physical therapist, registered.* Assistants who have special training but not to the degree of a physical therapist are referred to as *physical therapy assistants.*

physical therapy: The rehabilitative discipline that is concerned with the use of massage, exercise, water, light, heat, and certain forms of electricity (all of which are mechanical rather than medical in nature) in the treatment of persons with disabilities. A physical therapist may also develop and recommend appropriate adaptive positioning for persons with physical impairments.

physically handicapped: A term used to describe disabling conditions that involve motor dysfunction or chronic health problems that interfere with education, development, or adjustment (sensory impairments, such as vision or hearing, are usually excluded).

PIAT: See *Peabody Individual Achievement Test.*

PIC: See *Pictogram Ideogram Communication.*

pica: An abnormal craving or appetite for nonfood items, such as dirt or paint chips.

PICSYMS: A graphic symbol system developed by Faith Carlson and consisting of pictographs and ideographs.

pictogram: See *pictograph.*

Pictogram Ideogram Communication: A graphic symbol set that features white symbols on a black background. Renamed *Pictogram Symbols.*

Pictogram Symbols: See *Pictogram Ideogram Communication.*

pictograph: A symbol that depicts a concrete or abstract referent easily represented by simple pictures or line drawings; a.k.a., *pictogram.*

Picture Communication Symbols: A large set of graphic symbols composed primarily of simple line drawings with words printed above them. One of the most commonly used symbol sets in the United States.

Picture Exchange Communication System: An alternative language system developed for use with children with autism. Picture Exchange Communication System integrates principles from applied behavior analysis and speech-language pathology to encourage functional communication skills. Generally, the learner uses a picture symbol or line drawing in combination with a Fitzgerald key to visually express messages to their communication partner. The system consists of six phases: (1) the physical exchange, (2) expanding spontaneity, (3) picture discrimination, (4) sentence structure, (5) responding to "What do you want?," and (6) responsive and spontaneous commenting.

picture schedule system: A vertical or horizontal display of each day's activities with each activity being represented by a separate card fastened to the schedule by a paper clip or Velcro.

Pierre Robin sequence/syndrome: A genetic syndrome characterized by a small jaw (mandibular hypoplasia), cleft soft palate, and forward displacement of the tongue (glossoptosis) resulting in a "shrew" facies. Upper airway obstruction and early failure to thrive are the primary and immediate medical concerns associated with the disorder.

piezoelectric crystal switch: A switch that has a crystal that generates a voltage when it is activated by eye movements.

pillow switch: A type of pneumatic switch that is activated when pressure is applied to an air-filled pillow or cushion that houses the switch.

PILOT: See *Patient Initiated Light Operated Telecontrol.*

pixel: A tiny dot of light representing bits of graphic information on a computer screen. The greater the number of pixels, the better the screen resolution.

PKU: See *phenylketonuria.*

PL: In the United States, *Public Law.*

PL 74-271: See *Social Security Act of 1935.*

PL 91-230: See *Elementary and Secondary Education Act Amendments of 1969 (PL 91-230).*

PL 91-517: See *Developmental Disabilities Services and Facilities Construction Amendments of 1970.*

PL 93-112: See *Rehabilitation Act of 1973.*

PL 93-380: See *Education Amendments of 1974.*

PL 94-103: See *Developmental Disabilities Assistance and Bill of Rights Act Amendments of 1975.*

PL 94-142: See *Education for All Handicapped Children Act of 1975.*

PL 98-199: See *Education for All Handicapped Children Act Amendments of 1983.*

PL 99-457: See *Education for All Handicapped Children Act Amendments of 1986.*

PL 100-146: See *Developmental Disabilities Assistance and Bill of Rights Act Amendments of 1987.*

PL 100-407: See *Technology-Related Assistance for Individuals with Disabilities Act of 1988.*

PL 101-336: See *Americans with Disabilities Act of 1990*.

PL 101-476: See *Individuals with Disabilities Education Act of 1990*.

PL 101-496: See *Developmental Disabilities Assistance and Bill of Rights Act Amendments of 1990*.

PL 105-17: See *Individuals with Disabilities Education Act Amendments of 1997*.

PL 106-170: See *Ticket to Work and Work Incentives Improvement Act of 1999*.

PL 108-446: See *Individuals with Disabilities Education Improvement Act of 2004*.

planar seats: Chairs and other seats with flat or nearly flat surfaces.

plantar flexion: Bending the foot downward in the direction of the sole.

plasma display: Flat-screen technology that uses tiny cells lined with phosphor that are full of inert ionized gas (typically a mix of xenon and neon). Each pixel consists of three cells (one cell has red phosphor, one green, one blue). The cells are sandwiched between two panels, and a cell is selected by charging the appropriate panel electrodes. A charge causes the gas in the cell to emit ultraviolet light, which in turn causes the phosphor to emit color. The amount of charge determines the intensity, and the combination of the different intensities of red, green, and blue produce all the required colors; a.k.a., *gas discharge display*.

play: An activity that is done for its own intrinsic value rather than as a means to achieve any specific end. Play is spontaneous and voluntary, undertaken by choice and done for fun.

play audiometry: Hearing assessment procedure in which responses are made through play (e.g., a young child may be instructed to drop a block in a box after hearing a pure tone stimulus).

plug: Hardware used to complete electrical connections. Switches typically have plugs that are inserted into a jack within a device to allow the switch user to access the device.

PND: See *progressive neurological disease*.

pneumatic switch: Any switch that is activated by air pressure, either negative (e.g., a sip) or positive (e.g., a puff), or both.

PODD: See *Pragmatic Organized Dynamic Display*.

pointing: (1) The indexing of objects, persons, or events in the immediate environment. Pointing is typically done with an extended index finger but can also be accomplished through other body parts or movements. (2) An unaided method of direct selection. (3) An index used in sign languages for pronominal reference.

policy barriers: Barriers that are the result of legislation, regulations, and administrative policies that limit the full participation of AAC users (e.g., school policies that segregate AAC users from their peers without disabilities or that limit the use of communication devices purchased with school funding to classroom use only).

polysemic symbols: Pictographic symbols having multiple meanings that are used as a code to recall prestored phrases and sentences (e.g., the Minspeak semantic encoding approach).

pop-up: A page or banner that appears on a computer screen, superimposed over the original page that was being displayed.

port: A receptacle on the back of the central processing unit of a computer that permits the interfacing of an input or output device. There are two types of ports: *serial* and *parallel*.

Portable Anticipatory Communication Aid: Special computer software adapted to a laptop computer to increase the rate of single switch input for spelling by continually using predictive routines to rank all the user's selections according to frequency of use. Portable Anticipatory Communication Aid could be accessed by row-column scanning and featured a built-in printer, microcassette storage unit, and optional voice output.

Portable Pocket Typewriter/Computer: An archaic communication aid that used a QWERTY keyboard and featured an 11-character display and a built-in printer with adding machine-type paper. A limited number of phrases could be stored in memory and retrieved.

Portable Voice II: An archaic portable speech-generating device that featured an Espon HX-20 computer with speech synthesizer and commanded by an expanded keyboard or through switch activation (with Morse code). Stored phrases and sentences could be recalled using an abbreviation expansion code or with any symbol system attached to the expanded keyboard.

portability: A selection consideration that refers to the ease or difficulty that an AAC user experiences in transporting symbols or communication devices from environment to environment.

position statements: Official statements from the American Speech-Language-Hearing Association that specify policy and stance on a matter that is important not only to the membership but also to outside agencies or groups.

positioning: Placing and maintaining a person in a sitting, side-lying, standing, prone, or other postural alignment.

positive behavior supports: Positive (i.e., nonpunitive) strategies that increase appropriate or desired behavior, such as visual schedules, behavior maps, social stories, and token boards.

positive reinforcement: The consequence that adds something (i.e., a reinforcer such as events, objects, or sensory stimuli). Positive reinforcement increases the likelihood of a behavior.

positive support reflex: When holding a baby under the arms, supporting the head, and allowing the feet to bounce on a flat surface, the baby will extend (straighten) their legs for about 20 to 30 seconds to support themselves, before they flex their legs again and go to a sitting position. This reflex usually disappears by 2 to 4 months, until it becomes a more mature reflex in which there is a sustained extension of the legs and support of the body by about 6 months.

positron emission tomography: Imaging technique that utilizes radioactive chemical compounds to study the metabolism of an organ, most commonly the brain.

POSM: See *Patient Operated Selector Mechanism.*

POSSUM: See *Patient Operated Selector Mechanism.*

posterior: Behind.

post-traumatic amnesia: A disturbance of memory that occurs after a traumatic brain injury. There are two types of post-traumatic amnesia: (1) retrograde amnesia, a partial or total loss of the ability to recall events that occurred immediately prior to the brain injury; (2) anterograde amnesia, a reduced ability to form new memory after a brain injury, often accompanied by decreased attention and inaccurate perception.

postural control: The regulation of the body's spatial position for stability and orientation.

postural stability: An automatic function that involves control of the body's position in space to obtain stability and orientation. Stability is achieved, maintained, or regained when the position of the body is over its base of support (i.e., center of body mass) to prevent falling during static or dynamic activities. Orientation is attained when the body parts are aligned for the task being accomplished.

potential communicative act: Any behavior produced by an individual that a communication partner interprets as holding meaning, including changes in respiration, body movement, stereotypy, vocalization, eye gaze, facial expression, and/or challenging behavior, as well as words and AAC symbols; may be intentional or nonintentional.

powered mobility: Devices (e.g., wheelchairs, scooters, and other devices) that use electrical or other power sources under the user's control to propel them.

PowerPad: A high quality, lithium-ion battery pack used in personal computers and other electronic equipment. It has a relatively short charging time and has a life of approximately 24 hours.

PPP: See *preferred practice patterns.*

PPVT-R: See *Peabody Picture Vocabulary Test-Revised.*

practice barriers: Barriers that result from the precedents, procedures, and common practices within a school or other environment that are not actual policies or laws but are assumed to be; the net effect is the limiting of full participation of AAC users.

practice guidelines: A recommended set of procedures for a specific area of practice, based on research findings and best practice, that details the knowledge, skills, or competencies needed to perform the procedures effectively.

Pragmatic Organized Dynamic Display (PODD): A system of organizing and selecting words or symbol vocabulary on a non–speech-generating or speech-generating AAC system. PODD includes symbols for navigation, colored page tabs that match page numbers on symbols displayed on the first page, and symbols for specific operational commands, such as "Turn the page," or "Go to page____."

pragmatics: The use of language in communicative contexts. It is more concerned with how a message is communicated than its content.

predictive assessment: A focused assessment process that evaluates the skills necessary for developing an AAC prescription by matching the skills of the person with a disability to the features of a given AAC system; a.k.a., *feature matching process.*

predictive profiling: A type of criteria based profiling in which an individual's abilities are judged against a set of standards considered essential to a skill area. A prognosis or prediction is made about the individual's potential for the development of certain skills based upon the findings.

predictive scanning: A scanning method in which only the potential symbol choices are included in the scan (e.g., on some devices, blank keys are excluded from scanning). More sophisticated predictive scanning will only include symbols that are predicted based on previous selection patterns.

preferred practice patterns: Statements that define universally applicable characteristics of activities that are directed toward individual patients or clients and also address structural requisites of the practice, processes to be carried out, and expected outcomes.

prehension: Reaching toward something, shaping the hand in anticipation, and closing the fingers to grasp or take hold.

preliterate: A descriptive term for an individual who has not yet learned to read, write, and spell but appears to have the cognitive skills to do so if given the opportunity.

Premack-type symbols: Uniquely shaped and color-coded plastic or masonite shapes, each representing a word, based on Premack's work with chimpanzees. The shapes were arbitrarily assigned meanings to control for effects of iconicity.

presbyopia: The gradual decrease in visual acuity due to the aging process.

preschool: (1) The birth-to-5-years age group. (2) Demonstrating skills associated with the birth-to-5-years age level.

preset scanning: Process in which the scanning indicator moves in a predetermined, predictable pattern controlled by the electronic scanning device. Patterns of scanning may be either linear, circular, row-column, or block.

prestored message: Words, phrases, and sentences that are preprogrammed into a computer or AAC device for later playback.

presymbolic: Basic communicative functions that are learned early in child development consisting of two stages: (1) perlocutionary stage (occurring around the age of 8 months and characterized by the caregiver assigning meaning to the child's behaviors), (2) illocutionary stage (beginning at around 8 to 9 months, the child begins to use signals to deliberately communicate to regulate the behavior of others, to establish joint attention, or to engage in social interaction).

prevalence: The total number of cases of a disease or disorder reported for a given time period.

primitive reflexes: Automatic responses that produce change in muscle tone and movement of the limbs. These reflexes are typically present in newborns; however, in individuals with brain damage, they may persist into adult life (e.g., the asymmetrical and symmetrical tonic neck reflexes). a.k.a., *infantile reflexes.*

print-on-palm: A tactile communication method; a sighted partner uses their index finger to print block letters on the palm (or arm or wrist) of a person who is deaf-blind and familiar with conventional orthographic spelling.

prior authorization: An agreement by Medicaid and many insurance companies to fund certain medical procedures; however, it does not set a specific dollar amount for the funding. In the case of Medicaid, the prior authorization must be submitted along with an evaluation report and prescription letter.

private practice and contractual services: Professionals who own and operate their own business provide both direct and indirect services and can be contracted either by individuals or agencies (e.g., group homes, skilled nursing facilities, and school programs).

prn: Common medical abbreviation for *as needed.*

problem behavior: Any behavior that is detrimental to the educational or communicative process (e.g., aggression, autistic leading, disruption, self injurious behavior, tantrums, and unconventional verbal behavior).

production-based techniques: Message transmission techniques in which the individual actually produces the symbols used for communication. Most production-based techniques are the same as those used by unimpaired individuals (e.g., gesturing, writing).

professional-family fit: The degree to which a professional's recommendations match a family's ability to follow through with them. The fit should improve over time as each individual involved becomes more skilled in using feedback from others.

professional preparation: The training of individuals to become professional clinicians or educators (e.g., occupational therapists, physical therapists, speech-language pathologists, regular educators, special educators), taking place in the higher education environment, typically in programs that are accredited by professional regulatory bodies.

prognosis: A prediction of the probable course of an individual's disease or chances of recovery, based upon such variables as the extent and severity of the disorder, the patient's response to intervention, the patient's motivation, and environmental supports.

progressive neurological disease: Diseases affecting the central or peripheral nervous system whose symptoms worsen over time (e.g., amyotrophic lateral sclerosis, Huntington's disease, multiple sclerosis, and Parkinson's disease).

progressive supranuclear palsy: A sporadic degenerative condition characterized primarily by an inability to aim the eyes properly. As the disease progresses, there may be postural impairment, general motor decline, and mild dementia.

projectability: A selection consideration that refers to the degree to which a message can be transmitted over a distance using symbols or a communication device.

PROM: Common medical abbreviation for *passive range of motion.*

Promoting Aphasics' Communicative Effectiveness Therapy: An intervention approach for aphasic individuals developed by Davis (1980) that uses pictures and focuses on the development of meaningful communication interaction (e.g., face-to-face conversations).

PROMPT: See *Prompts for Restructuring Oral Muscular Phonetic Targets.*

prompting: Additional assistance provided before, during, or after a communication strategy. Typically, a prompting hierarchy may include least-to-most intrusive prompts or most-to-least intrusive prompts. A least-to-most approach is usually recommended to facilitate fading and independence.

prompts: The stimuli and other forms of assistance given to help an individual produce a desired response or behavior. Prompts may be partial or full. They may be verbal (spoken, signed, written), gestural, physical, and/or visual.

Prompts for Restructuring Oral Muscular Phonetic Targets: A technique with four levels of prompting (parameter, syllable, complex, and surface) that supports the broader, holistic philosophy that addresses the transition of motor speech development to conversation. Used with children who have phonological impairment, developmental and acquired dysarthria and apraxia, hearing impairment, autism spectrum disorders, and fluency disorders.

pronation: Turning downward or outward.

prone: Lying face down (on the stomach).

pronominal reference: Referring to someone or something by using a pronoun.

proprioception: Unconscious, endogenous sensory feedback that occurs during movement to keep the nervous system appraised of body status.

proprioceptive system: The sensory system that provides a sense of body awareness and detects/controls force and pressure; the internal sense that informs a person what their body is doing and where their body is in space.

prosody: (1) Variations in pitch, loudness, rhythm, rate, and stress patterns of speech that contribute to meaning. (2) The analysis and study of speech and verse.

prosthesis: An artificial device, often mechanical or electrical, used to replace a missing part or assist a defective part of the body (e.g., electrolarynx, eyeglasses, hearing aid, speech-generating device).

prosthetic device: There is no uniform definition of prosthetic devices across funding programs. Medicare defines prosthetic devices as "devices that replace all or part of an internal body organ, … and replacement of such devices and supplies." This definition is supplemented by the following: Prosthetic devices are "devices that replace all or part of an internal body organ or replace all or part of the function of a permanently inoperative or malfunctioning internal body organ." Federal Medicaid regulations define prosthetic devices as "replacement, corrective, or supportive devices prescribed by a physician or other licensed practitioner of the hearing arts within the scope of [their] practice as defined by state law to artificially replace a missing portion of the body; prevent or correct physical deformity or malfunction; or support a weak or deformed portion of the body."

protoreading: Reading-like behavior in which children turn the pages of a book and engage in oral storytelling.

proxemics: (1) The study of variations in posture, distance, and tactile contact in human communication that may be culture-specific and can be analyzed in terms of gender, age, intimacy, social role, and other such factors. (2) Awareness of four areas of interpersonal territory: intimate, social, personal, and public.

proximal: Situated nearest to the center of the body. Opposite of *distal*.

p-switch: See *piezoelectric crystal switch*.

PSP: See *progressive supranuclear palsy*.

psycholinguistics: (1) A discipline that integrates the disciplines of psychology and linguistics to study human behavior and culture and their relationship to human language function. (2) The study of the relationship between grammatical and psychological complexity that attempts to distinguish between what people know about their language and how they use it.

psychometric: Pertaining to the measurement of psychological variables, such as intelligence, aptitude, and emotional disturbance.

pt: Common medical abbreviation for *patient*.

PT: See *physical therapist*.

PTA: Common medical abbreviation for *physical therapy assistant* (see *physical therapist*), *post-traumatic amnesia*, or *prior to admission*.

ptosis: An involuntary drooping of the upper eyelid.

PTR: Common medical abbreviation for *physical therapist, registered*. See *physical therapist*.

Purposeful, Appropriate: Modified Independent: Level X (the highest level) of the *Rancho Los Amigos Levels of Cognitive Functioning Scale-Revised*, characterized in part by the ability to handle multiple tasks simultaneously with periodic breaks, ability to independently initiate and carry out steps to complete a task with additional time or compensatory strategies, ability to independently think about the consequences of decisions or actions with additional time or compensatory strategies, ability to recognize the needs and feelings of others and automatically respond in an appropriate manner, and social interaction that is consistently appropriate.

Purposeful, Appropriate: Stand-By Assistance: Level VIII of the *Rancho Los Amigos Levels of Cognitive Functioning Scale-Revised*, characterized in part by consistent orientation to person, place, and time, ability to attend to and complete familiar tasks for one hour in a distracting environment, ability to recall and integrate past and current events, ability to think about consequences of decisions or actions with minimal assistance, over- or underestimation of their own abilities, ability to acknowledge and respond to other people's needs and feelings with minimal assistance, and ability to recognize and acknowledge inappropriate social interaction while it is occurring and to take corrective action with minimal assistance.

Purposeful, Appropriate: Stand-By Assistance on Request: Level IX of the Rancho Los Amigos Levels of Cognitive Functioning Scale-Revised, characterized in part by an ability to shift back and forth between tasks and to complete them accurately for at least two consecutive hours, ability to initiate and carry out steps to complete a familiar task on request with assistance, ability to think about the consequences of decisions or actions on request with assistance, accurate estimation of abilities but requiring stand-by assistance to adjust to task demands, ability to acknowledge other people's needs and feelings and to respond appropriately with stand-by assistance, and ability to monitor the appropriateness of social interactions with stand-by assistance.

PWB: Common medical abbreviation for *partial weight-bearing*.

PWUAAC: Person who uses augmentative and alternative communication.

pyramidal: A term that refers to the primary motor nerve tracts that cross over at the pyramids of the medulla.

QED Scribe: An archaic, portable communication aid that featured a liquid crystal display and paper printout via a built-in printer. Messages could be typed on an alphanumeric membrane keyboard for immediate printout or storage of up to 26 messages.

quadriplegia: Paralysis of all four body extremities (i.e., both arms and both legs).

qualitative research: Descriptive research that relies primarily upon observations of persons, behaviors, or events and uses descriptions, categories, and words more than numbers or statistics; includes case studies, interviews and questionnaires, and surveys, to name a few.

questionnaire: A type of qualitative research that seeks to determine opinions, attitudes, or behaviors of a selected group of people. The typical questionnaire is mailed to the respondents and consists of a section that requests demographic information and a section that is designed to probe the opinions, attitudes, or behaviors of the respondents.

Quicktalk: An archaic, computer-based system for prestoring predictable or often-used messages.

Quinkey keyboard: An alternative one-handed keyboard for the BBC microcomputer operated by activating various key combinations to produce different characters.

QWERTY keyboard: The standard computer (and typewriter) keyboard that has four main rows of keys (the first row houses the numerals 1 through 0; the second row starts with the letters Q, W, E, R, T, and Y; the third or "home" row starts with the letters A, S, D, F, and G; and the fourth row starts with the letters Z, X, C, V, and B).

radio frequency: Signals transmitted through the air that are within the same general range as radio broadcasts (e.g., 300 kHz to 3 MHz for AM, 30 to 300 MHz for FM, and 300 to 3,000 MHz for UHF).

RAM: See *random access memory*.

Ranchos Los Amigos Levels of Cognitive Functioning Scale: See *Levels of Cognitive Functioning Scale*.

Ranchos Los Amigos Levels of Cognitive Functioning Scale-Revised: See *Levels of Cognitive Functioning Scale*.

random access memory: The temporary or working memory in the computer that is accessed by the central processing unit. Information in this memory is lost when the computer is turned off.

random activity or movement: Movement that occurs without purpose (i.e., is not goal-directed or elicited by specific situational cues).

range of motion: The maximal distance across which an individual can move a body part.

raphe nuclei neurons: Neural cells located along the midline of the medulla, connected to neural fibers that generate the neurotransmitters serotonin, noradrenaline, and dopamine.

Rasmussen's bundle: See *olivocochlear bundle*.

rate: The speed at which communication takes place. The rate of natural speech production (approximately 175 words per minute) is the standard by which the various forms of AAC are compared.

rate enhancement strategy: Any technique that improves the rate of production of AAC or written communication (e.g., abbreviation expansion, word prediction).

Raven's Progressive Matrices Test: A test of nonverbal intelligence that uses a multiple-choice response format.

RDS: See *respiratory distress syndrome in infants*.

reaction time: The time that elapses from the onset of a stimulus to a response.

reactive behaviors: Behaviors that are unintentional and largely involuntary (e.g., movements, crying, and gurgling). The learner has little awareness or understanding of the social bases or context in which the behaviors are elicited.

reading: The literacy process in which an individual demonstrates an ability to comprehend the written or printed word.

reading readiness: See *emergent literacy*.

reading recognition: Reading words by graphic presentation only (e.g., recognizing that the "golden arches" means McDonald's).

read-only memory: The permanent memory of a computer. Data in read-only memory can only be read, not modified, and is not lost when the computer is turned off.

real objects: Life-sized tangible objects that are used by some individuals with intellectual impairments to communicate. These objects may be used to represent themselves or to represent concepts that are related in some way to the object (e.g., a pair of glasses can be used to represent themselves or can be used by the individual to signal a desire for reading time).

RealVoice with Epson HX-20: An archaic, portable, dedicated speech-generating device (originally called SpeechPAC) that featured a standard keyboard, built-in printer, liquid crystal display, and a microcassette drive. It used an abbreviation expansion program to recall prestored messages. Switches could also be used to scan the alphabet on the display. Morse code or an expanded keyboard could also be used.

rebus: (1) Latin word for *thing*. (2) A representation of syllables or words by pictures with names that sound the same as the intended syllables or words. See *basic rebus* and *expanded rebus*.

rebus symbols: (1) Originally designed as an alternate method for teaching reading to language delayed or mildly intellectually impaired children (e.g., the *Peabody Rebus Reading Program*, a programmed approach to reading readiness and beginning reading). (2) Predominantly pictographic symbols (i.e., line drawings) that represent whole words or parts of words. Rebuses can have phonological, morphological, or semantic significance. A rebus may consist of a single symbol, several symbols, or a combination of letters of the alphabet and symbols.

recasting: Paraphrasing an individual's utterance by expanding, reordering, or omitting lexical structural information.

receiver: The person in a communication dyad who receives the message.

receptive communication: The process of receiving and understanding a message.

receptive language: An individual's ability to understand language.

receptive vocabulary: Words and messages that are received and understood by a listener.

reciprocal interaction: The mutual exchanges between two people as they alternate between sending and receiving messages.

reciprocity: (1) The give and take nature of communication exchanges and bidirectional influences of communicators on each other. (2) An agreement between states to accept an applicant's professional credentials although there may be differences between the states in terms of the criteria required for credentialing.

recline: The position of a chair when the back is lowered or raised, thereby altering the seat-to-back angle.

referent: An object, person, place, abstract idea, or other entity that is represented by a symbol.

reflex: An automatic, involuntary movement in response to an external stimulus.

regional AAC center: A center that is set up to conduct AAC evaluations and make recommendations for interventions or equipment. Staff members are well trained and experienced in the area of AAC and the center is well equipped. Referral can be made by the potential AAC users or family or by other professionals (e.g., educational, medical, social services, vocational).

regulators: Nonverbal behaviors that serve to maintain and regulate conversational speaking and listening between two or more people.

Rehabilitation Act of 1973 (PL 93-112): Federal legislation that mandated civil rights protection for persons with disabilities (Section 504) and established rehabilitation programs and services.

rehabilitation center: A center where several levels of care, including AAC assessment and intervention, may be provided.

rehabilitation engineer: A professional who specializes in designing, adapting, or constructing equipment for individuals with disabilities.

Rehabilitation Engineering and Assistive Technology Society of North America: (Formerly known as the Rehabilitation Engineering Society of North America). An interdisciplinary organization interested in issues related to assistive technology and includes such areas as audiology, occupational therapy, orthotics, physical therapy, prosthetics, rehabilitation engineering, special education, and speech language pathology. It is organized with professional specialty groups that are discipline-specific and a large number of relevant special interest groups, including AAC, computer applications, and special education.

reinforcement: Within the antecedent-behavior-consequence model, reinforcement is a consequence that immediately follows a behavior that then leads to the likelihood that the behavior will increase.

rejection signal: A communication from an individual to briefly stop or terminate a routine or to explore alternative routines (e.g., a vocalization with an angry tone).

relapse/remitting with chronic progression: A stage of multiple sclerosis marked by gradual deterioration of capabilities over time with periods of remission.

relapsing and remitting: A virtual full recovery between relapses of multiple sclerosis.

related services: Services determined by the case conference committee to be necessary in order for a student to benefit from special education, including but not limited to audiological services, counseling, early identification and assessment, medical services for evaluation, occupational therapy, orientation and mobility services, parent counseling and training, physical therapy, psychological services, recreation, rehabilitation counseling, school health services, social work services in schools, speech-language pathology, and transportation.

relational words: Words that do not have a real-world referent (e.g., in/out, hot/cold). Typically includes adjectives, adverbs, conjunctions, and prepositions.

reliability: The extent to which performance on an evaluation or test is consistent across items (i.e., internal consistency), forms (i.e., alternate reliability), and time (i.e., test-retest reliability).

remnant book: A topic setting approach that provides a way for a beginning symbol user with limited verbal output to tell people about past events, such as those that occurred during the day at school or at home.

remnant page: A sheet of card stock or paper with attached remnants of events (e.g., concert stubs), places (e.g., admission ticket to a museum), or occasions (e.g., confetti from a New Year's celebration) to serve as memory aids during conversation with a person who has impaired memory.

repetition of response: See *response repetition.*

repetition rate: See *response repetition.*

repetitive strain injury: Soft tissue damage that results from continuous, prolonged movement over time; a.k.a., *repetitive stress syndrome.*

repetitive stress syndrome: See *repetitive strain injury.*

representational gesture: A natural gesture used to establish reference (i.e., to an object, action, person, location), which carries some specific semantic value; includes both iconic and conventional gesture types.

representational range: A selection consideration referring to the breadth of thought that symbols allow the user to express. A wide representational range implies that the user can express both concrete and abstract thoughts.

representational thinking skill: Cognitive ability to hold information in mind when the referent is not present in the here and now; the ability to comprehend that one thing stands for or refers to something else; integrally involved in the ability to communicate symbolically.

representativeness: A term tied to Paivio's Dual Coding Model, defined as the visual relationship between a symbol and its referent. Although representativeness is essentially the same concept as translucency, the term is used more often in the psychological literature, while translucency is most frequently used in the AAC literature. See *iconicity* and *translucency.*

reproducibility: A selection consideration that refers to how easy or difficult symbols are to duplicate or create, either by hand or photocopying.

required specificity of the means to represent: The minimal amount or degree of specificity necessary in a symbol to convey meaning. As a guiding principle, symbols should be sufficiently generic to allow the user to communicate in a large range of contexts while being sufficiently specific to minimize the communicative burden on the partner.

Rescue Speech System: An archaic, dedicated speech-generating device that featured a standard computer (Laser 128), monitor, printer, environmental controller and module, cart, SynPhonix synthesizer, switches, and speech and writing software.

residual natural speech: Limited speech or vocal ability that can be integrated into an individual's AAC system.

RESNA: See *Rehabilitation Engineering and Assistive Technology Society of North America.*

resolution: (1) The detail and clarity of an image on a visual or graphics display. (2) Reduction to a simpler form.

resolution of motion: The minimal (refined) movement an individual can reliably and accurately execute.

resonance activities: One of the six components of Van Dijk's (1996) Movement Based Approach that includes rhythmic movements that the individual and the facilitator perform while in direct physical contact. These movements are designed to shift the individual's attention from self to the external world of people and objects (e.g., hand-on-hand prompt to assist the individual to wipe a tabletop with a sponge).

respirator: See *ventilator.*

respirator-dependent: Describes an individual who cannot breathe without the aid of a respirator (ventilator).

respiratory distress syndrome in infants: A disorder seen in newborn infants that is characterized by difficulty in breathing (dyspnea) and a blue color (cyanosis). Long-term effects can include chronic lung disease and neurological and developmental impairments.

response efficiency: The efficiency of an alternative behavior in relation to the problem behavior. Three variables affect the efficiency of response: physical effort, schedule of reinforcement, and time delay. An alternative behavior must be more efficient than the problem behavior for it to replace the problem behavior.

response generalization: The tendency of an individual to respond to stimuli that are similar to a previously conditioned stimulus.

response repetition: The average number of responses that can be made during a specified time period.

response repetition rate: See *response repetition.*

retinitis pigmentosa: A hereditary degenerative disease of the retina, characterized by night blindness, pigmentary changes within the retina, and eventual loss of vision. See also *Usher's syndrome.*

retinopathy: Pathological changes in the retina, usually associated with systemic disease.

retinopathy of prematurity: An eye disease most often found in premature infants that often results in blindness.

RF: See *radio frequency.*

RGB (red, green, blue) monitor: An early color monitor that allowed display of three colors: red, green, and blue.

rhyme: The result when the rimes of syllables from two words sound the same.

Rifton Activity Chair: An assistive chair specifically designed to promote an upright, seated posture for functional activities at home, school, or therapy.

rime: The vowel and any subsequent consonants in a syllable. See *onset-rime.*

role extension: Refers to an increase in a professional's knowledge of other professional disciplines and the incorporation of this knowledge into their own discipline.

role release: The sharing of information and function across members of a transdisciplinary team. Role release grows out of continuous staff development.

ROM: See *read-only memory* or *range of motion.*

ROP: See *retinopathy of prematurity.*

rotation: Movement that turns a body part on its own axis (e.g., turning of the head).

routines: Activities that are designed to provide scaffolding to assist in overcoming receptive language difficulties.

row-column scanning: A message selection technique in which selections are offered by scanning down row-by-row until the user interrupts the scan. Selections are then offered by scanning item-by-item (i.e., across the columns) in the selected row.

RR: Common medical abbreviation for *respiratory rate.*

RSI: See *repetitive strain injury.*

rubella: A disease that, when contracted during the first trimester of pregnancy, may cause severe, multiple abnormalities in the infant, such as hearing impairment, visual impairment, and developmental delay; a.k.a., *German measles.*

rumination: The process of regurgitating partially digested food and rechewing it before swallowing it or spitting it out.

rural service delivery: A service delivery model that offers creative solutions for providing AAC services to persons who live in rural areas, where long distances, rugged terrain, and adverse weather conditions may prove to be problematic.

sacral setting: A sitting position in which the lower back is rounded, and the upper trunk is usually flexed due to the pelvis being tilted posteriorly.

salient letter encoding: See *logical letter coding.*

sanction: A public acknowledgment of wrongdoing, often published in professional journals. The person receiving the sanction may be expelled from membership or lose credentials in the professional organization, but there is no legal punishment (e.g., imprisonment).

Say-It-All II: A portable, dedicated speech-generating device that features unlimited vocabulary and a large print display and can be connected to several printers and computers.

Say-It-All II Plus: A portable, dedicated speech-generating device similar to the Say-It-All II with the capability of storing and recalling phrases.

Say-It-Simply Plus: A portable, dedicated speech-generating device that features storage of words and phrases under different size response areas on several levels, accessed via direct selection.

scaffolding: Involves the caregiver's efforts to adjust the environment in order to permit participation in a communication event of which the child would not otherwise be capable.

scan mode: The manner in which a switch interface operates in conjunction with the scanning device to achieve the scanning process.

Scan Wolf: An archaic, portable, dedicated speech-generating device that featured a 500-word user-specified vocabulary, preprogrammed by the manufacturer before purchase. It used two scanning modes with single-switch access to select multiple levels via a 6 x 6 light emitting diode array.

scanner: An input device that reads text and pictures, then stores them in digital form within the computer. Special software called *optical character recognition* allows interpretation of the character configurations for handwritten and printed text.

scanning: (1) A message selection technique in which symbols, words, or other entities are presented in some kind of order for the AAC user to indicate choice (e.g., automatic scanning, partner assisted scanning, row-column scanning, block/group scanning, circular scanning, auditory scanning, multidirectional scanning). (2) The process an individual goes through as they read or locate words, symbols, or other visual information.

scanning pattern: The visual layout of pictures, symbols, or text and the manner in which the scanning indicator moves across patterns (e.g., linear, circular, row-column).

scanning speech: An abnormal pattern of speech production in which words are produced in a measured or scanned manner (e.g., pausing after each syllable and pronouncing the syllables slowly).

scanning technique: The method by which an individual uses a switch to select a communication symbol (e.g., step scanning, automatic scanning, and directed scanning).

schedule of reinforcement: The precise rules that are used to present reinforcers following a specified operant behavior. These rules are defined in terms of the time or the number of responses that are required in order to present a reinforcer (e.g., ratio schedule, interval schedule, fixed schedule, variable schedule).

school-based programs: School-based programs in which a full range of AAC services are provided to preschool and school-aged children. Services may be provided from the individual school system, a consortium, or a cooperative.

scientific antecedents: The scientific base developed when special education and rehabilitation programs began to apply the principles of operant technology in their teaching programs, representing a partnership between behavior analysis and the teaching of pragmatics, semantics, and syntax related to AAC.

scoliosis: Sideways (i.e., lateral) deviation of the spine with or without rotation or deformity of the vertebrae.

scope of practice statement: A list of professional activities that defines the range of services that are offered within speech-language pathology or another profession.

screen: The part of the computer monitor where information is displayed.

screening: A relatively quick and shortened evaluation process where individuals are sorted into two groups: those who need follow up (i.e., evaluation) and those who do not.

Screenreader: Software that works in conjunction with other applications to convert text on the computer screen to speech output.

scripting: The process of analyzing an activity into small steps and then recording the words and expressions needed to participate in the activity.

SEA: See *state education agency.*

search light cue: A cue given by the clinician or educator to the AAC user that a communicative opportunity is at hand. The cue consists of the clinician or educator scanning a light across all or a portion of the user's symbol overlay.

seat elevators: Components used to lower or raise a seat. Seat elevators have several medical benefits, including assisting with safe transfers, increasing reach, and increased psychological benefits.

seating: Devices and their components that are used to assist people in maintaining a sitting position. Seating can involve ordinary seats (e.g., office chairs and couches) or specialized seats designed for individuals with disabilities (e.g., Rifton Activity Chair).

seating system: Composed of the primary support surface (seats and backs) and secondary supports (e.g., lateral trunk supports, head supports, pelvic-positioning belts) designed to accommodate and support a fixed posture while in a wheelchair.

SEE-I: See *Seeing Essential English*.

SEE-II: See *Signing Exact English*.

Seeing Essential English: A pedagogical sign system that uses modifications of American sign language to resemble English. English words are represented by the traditional American sign plus affixes. Complete English syntax is emphasized (e.g., verb tense is clearly indicated, and irregular verb forms have signed representation).

segmentation: Analyzing larger linguistic or phonological information into smaller components (e.g., separating the individual sounds /k/, /æ/, and /t/ from the word "cat"; analyzing the word "running" into its root word "run" and the present progressive morpheme *-ing*).

seizure: Abnormal electrical activity in the central nervous system that may be characterized by a loss of consciousness, involuntary motor movements, or language disturbances. A seizure disorder may also be referred to as *epilepsy*.

selection-based techniques: Message transmission techniques in which the AAC user directly selects or otherwise indicates the desired symbols from a preformed set rather than actually produce the symbols physically.

selection considerations: Empirically tested or clinically conceived variables that allow educators or clinicians to make sound decisions regarding the selection of appropriate symbols or communication devices for individuals with severe communication disabilities.

selection technique: The means by which a user selects items that will in turn create or retrieve messages for communication.

selective integration: Inclusion of a student with a disability into the regular classroom only during special classroom activities while remedial instruction occurs for other curricular activities. Intervention may be provided during nonacademic classroom activities.

self-injurious behavior: Behavior that causes injury to self (e.g., headbanging, pica, rumination, self-biting, self-slapping, vomiting).

self-stimulating behavior: See *stereotypic behavior*.

semantic compaction: The encoding system used with Minspeak in which each symbol or icon can have many associated meanings. See *Minspeak*.

semantic elements: See *key symbols*.

semantic encoding: The systematic organization of information or messages for storage and retrieval according to an individual's association of meanings with symbols for the purpose of language formulation (e.g., Minspeak).

semantics: The study or science of meaning in language.

Semi-Independent Living Program: A program used by some agencies that provides services for adults with disabilities, where the person with a disability lives in their own private facility but receives daily living support from a paid assistant.

semiotics: The scientific study of the properties of natural and artificial signaling systems. Originally, it referred to the philosophical study of sign and symbol systems in general.

semiphonetic spelling: Spelling in which some aspect of the sound a letter makes is incorporated; the phonetic information may derive from the name of the letter rather than the phoneme it represents (e.g., "you are" may be written "U R").

sender: The person in a communication dyad who sends a message.

sensorineural hearing impairment: A permanent hearing loss caused by damage to the inner ear structures, such as the cochlea or auditory nerve.

sensory-consequences-motivated problem behavior: See *automatic-reinforcement-motivated problem behavior*.

sensory defensiveness: (1) A reluctance or inability of some technology users to tolerate contact of their skin or other body parts with switches, controls, or other surfaces. (2) The inability or reluctance of an individual to tolerate being touched by another person; a.k.a., *tactile defensiveness*.

sensory integration: A form of occupational therapy in which special exercises are used to strengthen the child's senses of touch, balance, and proprioception, typically conducted with persons with movement disorders or severe over- or under-sensitivity to sensory input.

sensory system: This system consists of sensory receptors, neural pathways, and parts of the brain involved in sensory perception. These systems include vision, hearing, somatic sensation (i.e., touch), taste, and olfaction (i.e., smell).

serial port: A computer port that allows the transmission of data one bit at a time. See also *port* and *parallel port*.

serial transmission: A method of sending data between a computer and a peripheral device, one bit at a time along a single wire. Serial transmission is much slower than parallel transmission and is often used with printers and modems.

service delivery: A general term that denotes the manner in which assessment, intervention, and other services are provided to persons with disabilities.

set: A collection or finite number of symbols with no rules or logic governing expansion.

severe aphasia: A neurological disorder that results in extensive impairment in at least one area of speech or language.

severe disabilities: Individuals of all ages who require extensive ongoing support in more than one major life activity in order to participate in integrated community settings and to enjoy a quality of life that is available to citizens with no or fewer disabilities.

severe-profound hearing impairment: A sensorineural hearing loss in the better ear of 70 dB HL or greater at a frequency of 1,000 Hz. Persons with a hearing impairment of this magnitude may be classified as "hard of hearing." See also *sensorineural hearing impairment.*

severity: The degree or magnitude of an impairment (e.g., mild, moderate, severe, profound).

SGD: See *speech-generating device.*

shadow light cueing: A technique in which the educator or clinician provides light cues on the user's symbol overlay in an attempt to promote communication.

shaping: A training technique based on behaviorism, which initially accepts a response that only grossly approximates the desired response. Gradually, an individual must produce more and more accurate responses until the desired response is produced. See also *successive approximation.*

Sharp Expanded Keyboard Memowriter: A Sharp Memowriter with an expanded keyboard.

Sharp Memowriter: A "family" of archaic dedicated communication devices that featured letter-by-letter spelling, limited message retrieval, and calculation. Output appeared on a built-in display and a printer.

shear: Occurs when opposing forces take place in a parallel direction to each other. Shear forces often result in shear strain. In a wheelchair, the client may experience increased force between their back and the seat-back surface that can lead to tears in the skin that in turn can lead to pressure ulcers.

sheltered workshop: A segregated vocational placement for individuals with disabilities where they receive training and support in learning job skills that will then potentially make them marketable for work in a community-based setting.

SHF: See *super high frequency.*

short-term goal: A smaller step in a series of steps that are performed to master a more complex target behavior; the target behavior may be worded generally in the form of a long-term goal, which is then broken down into smaller, more manageable steps. Each of these manageable steps is operationally defined as a STG. See also *long-term goal.*

short-term memory: A system for storing and managing information required to carry out complex cognitive tasks, such as learning, reasoning, and comprehension. Short-term memory is involved in the selection, initiation, and termination of information-processing functions, such as encoding, storing, and retrieving data. a.k.a., *working memory.*

SIB: See *self-injurious behavior.*

Siglish: See *Signed English.*

sign language: The visual language used by many deaf individuals (e.g., American Sign Language, British Sign Language). It is not a universal language and is different from the spoken language of the corresponding hearing community. Sign language most probably evolved quickly (within one single generation of users) from an iconic gestural level through conventionalization to a linguistic level with decreased iconicity. The term "sign language" should not be used if one is referring to the simultaneous use of both speech and manual signs.

sign languages other than American Sign Language and British Sign Language: For many of the oral languages of the world, there is a corresponding sign language used by the Deaf community (e.g., Chinese Sign Language; German Sign Language; Korean Sign Language). See also *sign language.*

sign space: Refers to an imaginary physical space in which manual signs are produced; this space is generally from the forehead to waist vertically, and outer aspect of one arm to the other horizontally.

sign system: A collection of manual signs that does not constitute a language but uses signs to represent words and morphological endings and uses the grammar of spoken language.

signal channel: See *transmission environment.*

signed English: See *manually coded language.*

Signed English: A system that utilizes manual signs to code spoken English, which shares some of the characteristics of both English and American Sign Language, with the grammar of each language being reduced.

Signing Exact English: A pedagogical sign system based on American Sign Language that utilizes manual signs to code spoken English. The manual signs are used in exact English word order, with some additional signs for conventions (e.g., present progressive, past tense).

signing key words: A process used in simultaneous communication where the individual signs the keys words that are being spoken (i.e., typically the nouns, verbs, and other important words). See also *key word signing.*

sign-linked graphic symbols: Symbols that illustrate how a manual sign is produced or that realistically or schematically depict some aspect of manual sign production (e.g., some Sigsymbols).

sign-linked symbols: See *sign-linked graphic symbols*.

signs supporting English: British term for *key word signing*.

Sigsymbols: A graphic symbol system of pictographs, ideographs, and sign linked symbols that is composed primarily of graphic representations of manual signs from British or American Sign Language.

SILP: See *Semi-Independent Living Program*.

simple rebus: See *basic rebus*.

simultaneous communication: The simultaneous use of two modes of communication. Typically, a manually coded language (e.g., Signed English) is used at the same time as spoken language. The manual signs and spoken words parallel each other synchronously.

simultaneous method: The use of simultaneous communication, often manual signing and speaking.

sincere message or information message: The principle that the communication partner should ask questions of the patient because they truly want to know the answer.

single letter prediction: A probability-based strategy to enhance the rate of communication, based on the probability of another letter occurring after a certain letter or combination of letters (e.g., for the letter combination of "in" in the English language, there is a higher probability of "g" following than "q").

single-service provider model: A form of multidisciplinary team service delivery in which a single professional provides services in a particular area of need.

single-subject research: A research approach in which participants serve as their own controls, with controlled introduction of treatment following a baseline (no treatment) phase; and may involve replication of treatment effects across additional participants. See *case study*.

sip-and-puff switch: A pneumatic switch that is held in the mouth during use and is controlled by the amount of air that is sucked in or puffed out. Sipping activates one switch and puffing activates a second switch.

situational teaching: A nonstructured, naturalistic teaching strategy that takes advantage of daily activities to teach skills.

size: A quantitative amount proportionally measured.

skeletal deformities: Abnormalities of the skeletal system that gives the body its basic framework, structure, protection, and movement. This may include scoliosis (i.e., sideways bending of the spine, which is usually combined with rotation of the vertebrae), kyphosis (i.e., forward bending of the spine), and hip dislocation (i.e., the hip joint separates, with the ball on the top of the femur coming out of the socket of the pelvis).

skill: (1) A high level or degree of ability or proficiency, usually developed over time through training and practice. (2) An activity that requires expertise for competent performance.

skill barriers: Barriers that are related to the limits of the technical and communication knowledge and skill of those responsible for the AAC assessment and intervention plan. In other words, skill barriers refer to the skill of the individuals who assist AAC users and not to the AAC users themselves.

skilled nursing facility: A residential living facility that provides long-term care for individuals with medical needs or disabilities; a.k.a., *nursing home*.

SLD: See *specific learning disability*.

SLI: See *specific language impairment*.

sling seat: The sagging, vinyl seat often found on a wheelchair. This type of seat encourages asymmetrical posture and does not provide sufficient stability.

SLP: See *speech-language pathologist*.

Small Talk: An archaic, portable speech-generating device that featured a liquid crystal display, a built-in printer, word processing (WordTalk), and calculator (CalcTalk) with a standard keyboard. Up to six pages of text could be stored on a microcassette. The device could be connected to printers and computers.

Smooth Talker Speech Update for Light Talker and Touch Talker: A more natural sounding, intelligible synthesized speech provided as an option to the speech output of the Light Talker and Touch Talker.

SNF: See *skilled nursing facility*.

SOB: Common medical abbreviation for *shortness of breath*.

SOC: See *superior olivary complex*.

social attention motivated problem behavior: Problem behavior used to elicit or request attention that has been reinforced by obtaining social attention.

social cognition: The various psychological processes that enable a person to engage as a functional member of a social group (e.g., perception and understanding of social cues, decision-making within the social context).

social competence: The ability to appropriately use the pragmatic aspects of communication such as when to talk and what to talk about.

social haptic: Communication between people that relies on touch messages (i.e., "haptices") in a social context. With individuals who experience dual sensory impairment, social haptic communication most frequently involves the presentation of messages on the back of the person with dual sensory impairment, primarily to enhance information regarding emotion, facial expression, and/or the physical environment.

Social Security Act of 1935 (PL 74-271): Federal legislation that ensured basic retirement income for all individuals who had worked for a designated minimal number of quarters (i.e., quarter-year periods). The act was amended to provide income for children of deceased individuals and individuals who became unable to work.

social worker: A professional who coordinates and dispenses information, therapy, and related services to individuals with disability, illness, trauma, and other impairments.

sociolinguistics: The study of linguistic behavior as influenced by social and cultural factors.

soft neurological sign: A neurological finding that cannot be interpreted as physiological or pathological without taking into account the individual's age.

software: Programs that include commands written in computer language (e.g., DOS, BASIC) that instruct the computer to perform specific functions (e.g., word processing, databasing, statistics). The programs are typically purchased on separate floppy disks or CD-ROMs that are installed on the computer's hard drive, or downloaded from internet web sites.

Sonas: Calm music from Ireland that is used with individuals who have Alzheimer's disease.

Sonoma Voice: An archaic, portable, dedicated speech-generating device that featured 16 one-and one-half inch phrase keys to access up to 256 phrases on 16 levels. Phrases were preprogrammed by the manufacturer according to user specifications.

s/p: Common medical abbreviation for *status post*.

spastic cerebral palsy: A congenital or early acquired motor impairment characterized by muscular incoordination resulting from muscle spasms, hypertonicity, and contractions of opposing muscle groups.

spasticity: A condition usually associated with stroke or spinal cord disease whereby stretch reflexes are exaggerated and may even occur spontaneously, producing involuntary muscle contractions.

spatial information: Concrete, permanent, and predictable units of meaning, presented holistically and resulting in a more stable time relationship for processing (i.e., line drawings, pictures).

spatial relationships: The sensorimotor scheme having to do with an ability to understand the three-dimensionality of objects.

special education: Education for children designated as having a disability, with varying degrees of direct and support services provided.

special educator: A professional who works with children who have a variety of special needs related to cognitive, motor, psychological, or sensory impairments.

Special Friend: An archaic, portable, dedicated speech-generating device that featured a typewriter-style membrane keyboard to recall preprogrammed and user-programmed phrases and sentences. It could also produce music.

specific language impairment: A primary language disorder thought to be an impairment of language expression, comprehension, or both, and is characterized by uneven language development, poor auditory processing skills, short auditory memory, disordered temporal sequencing, and repetition of auditory patterns; a.k.a., *developmental aphasia* or *dysphasia*, *developmental language disorder*, and *language delay*.

specific learning disability: A disorder in which there is a severe discrepancy between a child's intellectual ability and their academic performance in one or more of the basic psychological processes involved in comprehending or using language (spoken or written), including the ability to listen, perform mathematic calculations, read, speak, spell, think, or write.

specific need communicator: In AAC intervention, one of the five categories of persons with aphasia described by Garrett and Beukelman (1992); individuals with mild to moderate aphasia who generally have the ability to communicate through simple syntactic constructions and gestures, so communication support is provided only in specific situations.

speech: The human or electronic production of spoken language. Speech is considered to be vocal, although not all vocalizations are speech. It is the standard by which all other modes of communication are compared in terms of rate and efficiency.

speech digitizer: A device that allows digitally recorded speech to be converted into electronic patterns that can then be stored in computer memory.

speech-generating: The process of producing natural or synthetic speech.

speech-generating device: An assistive communication device that provides synthesized or digitized speech, or both. This term is currently being used in the literature more often than *voice output communication aid*.

speech impairment: An impairment in the production of speech due to the absence or deficiency of a specific structure or physiological function.

speech-language pathologist: A professional who is qualified to work with individuals who have a variety of communication disorders (e.g., aphasia, articulation and phonological disorders, communication disorders of neuromotor etiology, fluency disorders, receptive and expressive language disorders, swallowing disorders, voice and resonance disorders).

speech-language pathology: The professional discipline concerned with disorders of speech, language, and swallowing. Speech disorders include impairments of articulation, fluency, and voice. Language disorders include impairments in the comprehension or production of language, whether oral or written.

speech-linked graphic symbols: Graphic symbols that have a correspondence to spoken symbols (i.e., speech). For example, in traditional orthography or writing, the phonemes in speech correspond to the letters (graphemes) or combination of letters. In English traditional orthography, there is not a one-to-one correspondence of phoneme to grapheme. In some modified orthographies, such as the International Phonetic Alphabet or the Initial Teaching Alphabet, there is a one-to-one correspondence of phoneme to grapheme.

speech output software: Software that translates standard text into a special code that can be converted and spoken by a speech synthesizer.

speech pathologist: See *speech-language pathologist*.

speech pathology: See *speech-language pathology*.

speech reception threshold: The level at which an individual can correctly identify at least 50% of spoken spondaic words (e.g., baseball, cupcake). See *spondaic word*.

speech recognition: The process by which a computer accepts commands that are inputted though the user's speech or voice. Speech recognition software matches the user's voice to prestored, digitally recorded patterns; if a match occurs, the software accepts the command. a.k.a., *voice recognition*.

speech supplementation: The process of enhancing speech intelligibility through the use of an aid or device (e.g., using an alphabet board where the speaker points at the first letter of each word spoken; this slows the rate of speech and increases intelligibility).

speech synthesis: Computer generation of speech by phonetic and mathematical rules and algorithms for the parameters of the speech signal. It is highly flexible and can use text-to-speech synthesis to produce virtually any typed message. There is a wide range of quality depending on the rules/algorithms stored in the computer memory. In general, the intelligibility of synthesized speech is not as good as digitized speech. a.k.a., *synthesized speech*.

speech synthesizer: An electronic device that converts text into artificial speech. The device may be connected to a computer or exist as an internal chip, circuit card, or software.

speech therapist: See *speech-language pathologist*.

speech therapy: See *speech-language pathology*.

SpeechAid: An archaic, portable speech-generating device that featured 80 preprogrammed commonly used phrases (two-keystroke recall), storage of custom vocabulary (single keystroke recall), and immediate speech output of typed words or phrases. The device could also speak musical tones in a five-octave range.

SpeechPAC/Epson: An archaic, portable, dedicated speech-generating device that featured a standard keyboard, built-in printer, liquid crystal display, and microcassette drive. The device used an abbreviation expansion program to recall prestored messages. Switches could be used to scan the alphabet on the display. Morse code or an expanded keyboard could also be used.

SpeechPAC/Epson with Photo Board and Light Pointer: An archaic, portable, dedicated speech-generating device that was activated by a Light Pointer and featured logical letter coding and an expansion program for recall of messages of up to 250 characters. The user could store programs on 15 different levels with additional programs available on microcassette.

SpeechPAC/Epson with Unicorn Board: An archaic, portable, dedicated speech-generating device that had the same features as the SpeechPAC/Epson but with an expanded keyboard. The Unicorn Keyboard could be sectioned up to 128 squares for use with the alphabet or with small or large pictures. Up to 15 different programs could be stored with additional programs available on microcassette.

SpeechPAC/ScanPAC/Epson: An archaic, portable, dedicated speech-generating device based on the SpeechPAC system and operated by switches and joysticks with a user-adjustable scanning rate. Programs could be stored on 15 different levels.

SpeechPad: An archaic, portable, dedicated speech-generating device that was built into the PowerPad (a 12 x 12 membrane surface) that could store and recall words and phrases under different size squares and levels. Programming could be done using the device itself or with an Apple II computer and then transferred to the SpeechPad.

SpeechVive: A wearable prosthetic device similar to a hearing aid that introduces noise into the ear, thereby creating the Lombard effect, which causes the wearer to increase their vocal precision and loudness; designed to assist persons with Parkinson's disease to increase their vocal intensity and improve their intelligibility.

speed: The rapidity or rate of movement.

Speller Teller Communicator: An archaic, dedicated, scanning communication aid that featured letters, numbers, and symbols on a clock-like panel. Two switches rotated a pointer clockwise or counterclockwise around the panel.

spelling: The literacy process that involves an individual's ability to form words with letters in an accepted order.

spina bifida: A congenital abnormality of the spine in which the spine fails to close completely. Children with spina bifida will have paralysis below the spinal opening and may have bladder, orthopedic, language, and learning difficulties. See also *myelomeningocele*.

spinal amyotrophic lateral sclerosis: A form of amyotrophic lateral sclerosis that refers to predominant involvement of the spine. These individuals may exhibit normal to mildly dysarthric speech for a considerable period of time, even as they experience extensive motor impairments in their trunk and limbs. For these individuals, the need for an augmented writing system often precedes the need for a conversational system.

spinal cord injury: Damage to the spinal cord that results in a loss of function, such as mobility or feeling, typically caused by trauma (e.g., car accident, gunshot, falls) or disease (e.g., polio, spina bifida, Friedreich's ataxia). Loss of functioning is not restricted to a severed spinal cord; the spinal cord can remain intact and there may still be a loss of function.

spinal cord lesion: An injury to, or growth on, the spinal cord.

spintronics: Technology that uses electrons to represent binary (0 or 1) data.

Splink: A shortening of "speech link," it is a system comprised of a small electronic word board that has 950 basic words, letters, numerals, common phrases, and various prefixes and suffixes plus instructions. The system can fit on the patient's knee and can transmit a signal by infrared light to a microprocessor box plugged into the aerial socket of an ordinary TV set. Thus, images can appear on the screen. There are no wires, but the patient must keep within 12 to 15 feet of the television set. Two or more word boards can be used with a single microprocessor so that Splink can be used with groups.

spoken: Information presented through the oral modality, typically where verbal or nonverbal information is conveyed through an acoustic signal.

spondaic word: A two-syllable word in which each syllable has equal stress (e.g., airplane, baseball, cowboy, cupcake); a.k.a., *spondee*.

spondee: See *spondaic word*.

spreadsheet: An organized display of data by rows and columns, typically used by accountants and statisticians. Computer spreadsheet programs (e.g., Microsoft Excel) allow for the organization of alphabetic and numeric data and the use of predetermined formulas to enable instantaneous, automatic calculation of data as it is entered.

SRT: See *speech reception threshold*.

SSI: See *supplemental security income*.

SSL: See *Swedish Sign Language*.

state education agency: The government agency that is responsible for monitoring and enforcing all policies related to education.

static: A term used to describe symbols in which movement or change is not necessary to understand meaning (e.g., most aided symbols).

static display: Communication aids or computer displays that never change or vary.

statistical significance: Used in statistical analysis of data, it is the probability that an observed or measured behavior or phenomenon did not occur by chance; usually expressed by an alpha level (e.g., .05, .01, .001). An alpha level of .01 means there is a 1% probability an observation or measurement occurred by chance.

statistics—nonparametric: Statistical tests of significance that are used with nominal or ordinal data. No assumption is made as to whether the data conform to a normal distribution. The data cannot be added, subtracted, multiplied, or divided.

statistics—parametric: Statistical tests of significance that are used with interval and ratio data. The data meet the assumption of a normal distribution and can be manipulated mathematically. As a group, parametric statistics are more powerful than nonparametric statistics.

status post: A term meaning after an event has occurred.

Steeper Communication Teaching Aid: An archaic, portable, dedicated communication aid that was designed for individuals who are very young or have severe disabilities and featured a switch-operated light scanning system where the entire cell is lit (16 cells total). It could also be set up horizontally for holding small objects.

step-linear scanning: A manual scanning method in which a cursor is moved through an array one item at a time until the user's choice is encountered. The user typically pushes a switch to begin the scanning process and then presses and releases the switch to move the cursor through the array and to the desired item. Because this method requires repeated switch activations, it can be fatiguing on the user.

step scanning: See *step-linear scanning*.

stereotypic behavior: Repetitive behavior (e.g., incessant rocking back and forth, repetitively moving fingers in front of eyes, flapping hands in the air) seen often in persons with developmental disabilities, especially autism; a.k.a., *self-stimulating behavior*.

stereotypic movement: Limited variety of movement options that results in the use of the same or similar patterns of movement to accomplish different motor tasks.

STG: See *short-term goal*.

sticky key: Memory-resident utility software that provides keyboard assistance. Sticky key features allow head-stick users and single-finger typists to simultaneously depress two or more keys. A single keystroke can then be used to capitalize letters or to enter multiple control key sequences.

stimulus equivalence: A type of learning in which stimuli become equivalent even though the individual has never observed a relation between them; may be involved in learning how to read and manipulate symbols.

stimulus generalization: The ability to transfer learning of stimuli in the clinical or educational setting to novel stimuli outside these environments.

stimulus shaping: The process of gradually adding items to an array to increase discriminative demands on the learner.

STM: See *short-term memory.*

STNR: See *symmetrical tonic neck reflex.*

strabismus: An oculomotor impairment that prevents an individual from maintaining proper eye position, caused by weak eye muscles or cranial nerve damage. The eyes stray from the binocular fixation position in a converging (internal strabismus, or "crosseyed") or diverging (external strabismus) manner.

strategic competence: The ability to use compensatory strategies to communicate effectively within the restrictions imposed by the AAC system.

strategy: (1) A plan of action. (2) A process that involves the implementation of assessment and intervention.

strength: Muscular force that produces movement or stability in a joint.

stroke: See *cerebrovascular accident.*

strokes: A measure that may be an indicator of the complexity of graphic symbols, it is the number of lines that must be drawn to produce a symbol. Any lifting of the pen or change in angle constitutes a new stroke. See also *complexity.*

structure barriers: Barriers that might limit opportunities for an AAC user (e.g., inappropriately designed workstations that do not accommodate wheelchairs; extremely noisy environments that prevent effective communication with speech-generating devices).

structured guidance: Teaching techniques provided by a skilled partner that allow performance of language and cognitive levels a child would not otherwise be capable of reaching.

structured teaching: Teaching that uses specific activities devised for teaching targeted skills; in intervention, time is set aside to address certain domains (e.g., a 30-minute block of therapy may be designated as language use time).

subASIS bar: A rigid padded bar secured below the anterior superior iliac spine used to maintain the position of the pelvis in the seated position.

subclinical aphasia: Linguistic processing deficits found during assessment that are not demonstrated by clinical manifestation of linguistic impairment.

subordinate level: In taxonomies, levels of lower classification below the superordinate level (e.g., in the symbol taxonomy described by Lloyd and Fuller [1986] and Fuller and colleagues [1992], static/dynamic, iconic/opaque, and set/system are all subordinate levels of symbol classification under the main classification of aided/unaided).

substantia nigra: A nucleus in the midbrain composed of deeply pigmented nerve cells (due to the presence of neuromelanin) that produces the neurotransmitter dopamine and is thought to be related to certain aspects of movement and attention.

successive approximation: Associated with shaping, a complex behavior is broken down into smaller steps, each one more closely resembling the target behavior. The individual's gross behaviors are shaped gradually until the target behavior is mastered. Each successively more complex step along the way is a successive approximation. See also *shaping.*

sundowing: A behavioral phenomenon exhibited by persons with Alzheimer's disease characterized by greater confusion, restlessness, and insecurity demonstrated late in the day, especially after dark.

super high frequency: Radio waves with frequencies between 2.9 GHz and 30 GHz.

superior olivary complex: A group of small nuclei within the medulla located dorsal to the inferior olivary nuclei that is part of the auditory pathway.

superordinate level: In a taxonomy, the highest level of classification. For example, in the symbol taxonomy proposed by Lloyd and Fuller (1986) and Fuller and colleagues (1992), the aided/unaided dichotomy is the superordinate level of classification.

supination: Turning upward.

supine: Lying face up (on the back).

supplemental security income: In the United States, the section of the Social Security system in which Medicaid exists. Criteria for eligibility vary from state to state, but generally, an individual must meet the following criteria: (a) inability to be gainfully employed, (b) medically diagnosed with physical or mental impairment that has or is expected to last for 12 months or result in death, (c) have little or no income, and (d) have countable resources less than $2,000.

supplemented speech: A strategy used with dysarthric speakers to improve their intelligibility, consisting of the use of an alphabet board or other AAC device to allow the speaker to indicate the first letter of each word as they say them. Those receiving the message are then able to narrow down the range of possibilities, and intelligibility is increased while still allowing for natural speech.

supported employment: Human, technological, and other supports that are provided to a person with a disability in an effort to achieve competitive employment in a community setting.

suprasegmentals: The prosodic features of language, including stress, intonation, duration, and juncture (i.e., the use of pausing). The suprasegmentals are transmitted along with the speech sounds in connected speech and provide additional cues as to the speaker's intended meaning.

Swedish Sign Language: The natural sign language used by the Deaf community in Sweden. See also *manual signs* and *sign language.*

switch: A component of an AAC system that serves to interface the user with a communication device by allowing the user to make selections via scanning.

switch control: The ability of the user to effectively use a switch. There are five components to assess for switch control: (1) wait—waiting for the appropriate time to activate, (2) activation—closing of the switch, (3) holding—maintaining contact with the switch to hold it closed or activated, (4) release—lifting the contact with the switch to open it and stop activation, and (5) reactivation—closing or activating the switch again, which would require going through the previous steps.

switch latch timer: A piece of equipment that allows the user to use a switch to turn a device on and off or to turn on a device for a specific length of time.

switch mounting system: A custom-made or commercial adaptation designed to hold single switches in place.

switch toys: Battery- or radio-operated toys that have been adapted for single-switch use.

symbol: (1) Something used to stand for or represent another thing or concept (e.g., real object, picture, line drawing, word). (2) In communication, anything used to represent thought (e.g., acoustic symbols via speech, letters of the alphabet via writing). AAC symbols can be acoustic, graphic, manual, or tactile. A symbol may be classified as aided or unaided, static or dynamic, and iconic or opaque. Symbols may also be taxonomically grouped as sets or systems. In some countries (e.g., United Kingdom) the use of the word symbol is limited to only graphic symbols.

symbol collection: (1) A combination of symbol sets and systems that facilitates multimodal communication. (2) In the AAC symbol quaternary continuum, a corpus of symbols with no rules for expansion beyond the original corpus.

symbol complexity: See *complexity.*

symbol corpus: A general term used to describe a collection or group of symbols.

symbol set: (1) A defined number (i.e., closed set) of symbols. A set can be expanded (e.g., by using the symbols in conjunction with traditional orthography), but it does not have clearly defined rules or logic for expansion. (2) The second lowest point along the AAC symbol quaternary continuum; it has poor to fair internal logic, resulting in limited expansion capability and limited increase in vocabulary size; the net effect is a limited representational range and very little correspondence to the oral and written language of the community.

symbol system: Symbols designed to work together for maximum communication. It is a set or collection of symbols that includes generative rules or logic for the development of additional symbols beyond the original set.

symbolic: Pertaining to the use of symbols to represent elements, relations, or qualities (e.g., written words, spoken words, sign language, Blissymbolics, Braille).

symbolic load: The extent to which a gesture is an arbitrary symbol for the concept it conveys.

symbolic play: The final stage of play development in which children begin to participate in make-believe and pretending.

symbolization: The representation of ideas or tangible objects with symbols.

symmetrical: A characteristic of gestures or manual signs where both hands perform mirror image movement patterns. Symmetrical gestures and manual signs are generally easier to learn than asymmetrical patterns in young children and individuals with intellectual or developmental disabilities.

symmetrical tonic neck reflex: A postural reflex often seen in children with cerebral palsy. When the neck is extended, the arms extend and the hips flex. When the neck is flexed, the arms flex and the hips extend.

synchronous: Services conducted with real-time audio and/or video connection to create an experience similar to that achieved in an in-person traditional encounter. Synchronous services may include, for example, connecting a client or a group of clients with a clinician, or they may include consultation between a clinician and a specialist. Telehealth visits, virtual check-ins, e-visits, or virtual consultations are examples of synchronous services.

syndactyly: A physical characteristic seen in a number of syndromes where there is webbing or fusion of the fingers or toes.

syndrome: A term that is used to denote the appearance of multiple signs and symptoms, which collectively result in the clinical presentation of a disease or disorder.

syntax: The structural or grammatical aspects of a language.

syntax morphology: The syntax of a language and the rules that exist for the modification of words to reflect grammatical changes that occur in generating various sentence types (e.g., morphological changes that occur to a verb when the sentence changes from present progressive to past tense).

synthesized speech: Speech that is artificially produced (i.e., by electronic means) rather than by the human vocal tract. See *speech synthesis.*

synthesized speech output: Prerecorded verbal information that is produced by an electronic device when symbols are selected by the user to activate and create messages.

system: (1) An integrated group of components that work as a unit or whole. (2) As related to symbols, having generative rules or logic for expansion beyond the original collection. (3) In the broader context of AAC, the use of a variety of means to represent, means to select, and means to transmit messages.

system efficiency: A selection consideration related to the relationship between symbols or activations and the number of messages they convey. The fewer the number of symbols or activations required to generate the most messages, the higher the system efficiency.

systems approach: A holistic approach to AAC assessment and intervention for persons who exhibit degenerative, progressive neurological disorders.

systems consultation: A consultation model associated with interdisciplinary service delivery. A consultant provides assessment, prescribes intervention, and evaluates intervention effectiveness as a consultee carries out programs. Set procedures of consultant follow up should exist.

T+A+C: A speech-generating device constructed or comprised of an off-the-shelf <u>T</u>ablet computer, plus (+) a speech-generating <u>A</u>pp, plus (+) a protective <u>C</u>ase.

tactile: The use of the sense of touch to perceive (e.g., a texture) via passive stimulation of the skin (as opposed to *haptic*, which is active).

tactile defensiveness: See *sensory defensiveness*.

tactile fingerspelling: A manual form of the alphabet; this is one tactile communication mode utilized by individuals who experience dual sensory impairment. The communication partner spells words using tactile signs and the person with dual sensory impairment places their hands over the hands of the partner to decipher the fingerspelling.

tactile symbols: Symbols that have discernible differences in their tactile qualities, typically used with individuals with visual or dual sensory impairments.

Tadoma method: A vibrotactile method in which the user places a hand on the speaker's jaw and lips to perceive breath from the nose, movements of the lips, and vibrations from the throat. This method gives the user cues as to what is being spoken by allowing the user to feel the speaker's speech production.

Talker II: An archaic, portable, dedicated speech-generating device that featured a text-to-speech mode and unlimited user-programmable levels for storage and recall. An overlay kit with different-sized target areas and a keyguard were also available.

Talking Brooch: An early assistive communication device with a liquid crystal display that could be worn on clothing.

Talking Mats: A pre-linguistic symbol set designed by AAC practitioners in the United Kingdom, used to support the communication of persons with Alzheimer's disease, aphasia, dementia, Huntington's disease, and other neurological and neurodegenerative disorders.

tangible consequences: Tangible items (e.g., toys, food, activities) that have become positively reinforcing for an individual.

tangible consequences motivated problem behavior: Problem behavior that is positively reinforced by the individual obtaining or maintaining access to tangible items (e.g., toys, food, activities).

tangible reinforcement operant conditioning audiometry (TROCA): A form of audiometric pure tone testing that involves providing the child with an edible reinforcer each time they respond appropriately to the sound stimuli presented.

tangible symbols: An aided set of objects, parts of objects, miniature objects, or textures that may be accessed by tactile or haptic means.

tantrum: A problem behavior that involves prolonged screaming, crying, or acting out.

task analysis: A strategy in which complex activities are broken down into a series of smaller steps that are arranged in the proper sequence.

taxonomy: The classification of organisms, events, or phenomena in an ordered system that indicates natural relationships.

TBI: See *traumatic brain injury*.

TC: See *total communication* and *total communication approach*.

TDWB: Common medical abbreviation for *touch down weight-bearing*.

TEACCH: See *Treatment and Education of Autistic and Related Communication Handicapped Children*.

teacher of record: The single special education teacher to whom a student with a disability is assigned; the individual must be appropriately licensed or trained to work with students with special needs.

Tech Act: See *Technology Related Assistance for Individuals With Disabilities Act of 1988 (PL 100-407)*.

technique: An approach or method of performance used in service delivery.

technology: (1) The application of science to industrial use. (2) The science of mechanical and industrial arts. (3) A term that refers to devices used to perform industrial, mechanical, and other functions (e.g., use of orthotics and prostheses, such as assistive technology and communication devices in AAC).

Technology-Related Assistance for Individuals With Disabilities Act of 1988 (P.L. 100-407): Federal legislation that encouraged states to develop programs for increasing awareness, training, and availability of technology for individuals with disabilities. This act was extended and further updated in 1994 by P.L. 103-218.

technology selection: The process of matching the strengths and needs of people who use or could benefit from AAC to the features of technology. This is considered a subset of the feature-matching process.

technophobia: Fear, dislike, or avoidance of new technology. The adoption of new technology may be disrupted or delayed when the end user and/or significant others display a sense of technophobia.

tele-AAC: AAC services provided via telepractice rather than in person. This may include assessment for AAC, intervention for AAC, consultation for AAC, and training of team and family members to implement AAC.

telepractice: Delivery of services using telecommunication and internet technology to remotely connect clinicians to clients, other health care providers, and/or educational professionals for screening, assessment, intervention, consultation, and/or education. Telepractice is an appropriate model of service delivery for audiologists and speech-language pathologists and may be the primary mode of service delivery or may supplement in-person services (known as hybrid service delivery).

temporal information: Abstract units of meaning that are presented sequentially, resulting in processing of information that is transient in nature and fades over time (i.e., spoken language).

teratogen: Any chemical or physical agent that causes or increases the incidence of congenital malformations; these intrauterine toxins generally have their greatest impact early in pregnancy.

terminate-and-stay-resident: A computer software program that resides in random access memory and remains active in the background while other applications run in the foreground.

text-to-speech synthesis: The creation of artificial speech by typing letters on a keyboard (or emulator) in which the retrieval and arrangement of stored phonemes is accomplished according to a prescribed set of phonetic and mathematical rules and algorithms.

textured symbols: A specific type of tangible symbol which uses different textures to represent various referents. See also *tangible symbols*.

The Arc: See *Arc of the United States, The.*

The Joint Commission: An organization that accredits hospitals in the United States.

Therapy Material BUILLD: Bringing Unity into Language and Learning Development; a product of the Prentke Romich Company that assists educators or clinicians in using the Unity program with their children. See also *Unity.*

thermal printer: An early type of printer that used heat sensitive paper that accepted a liquid ink spray.

THR: Common medical abbreviation for *total hip replacement.*

three-dimensional symbols: Aided AAC symbols having the dimensions of height, width, and depth; these include objects and some tangible and textured symbols.

three-point eye referencing: A skill used by an AAC user when using an eye-gaze system. The user initiates communication by establishing eye contact with their communication partner, then eye gazes to the chosen symbol, and finally re-establishes eye contact with the partner to complete the communication process.

Ticket to Work and Work Incentives Improvement Act of 1999 (PL 106-170): Federal legislation that amended Title XIX (Medicaid) of the Social Security Act and created Medicare coverage in order to provide Medicaid/Medicare for individuals with disabilities who are in the workforce. In essence, this law allows individuals with disabilities to be employed without losing government-sponsored medical benefits.

tilt in space: A feature of a seat that permits it to be tipped back, upright, or forward without altering the seat-to-back angle.

tilt, recline, and elevating leg rests: The most common medically necessary positioning features available on almost all manual and power wheelchairs. Tilt is the ability to rotate a specific seating system around a fixed axis. Recline is the ability change the position of the seat-to-back angle. Elevating leg rests allow a client to change the leg and footrest angle relative to the seat to flex or extend the lower extremities at the knee.

time delay: (1) The time during which a communication partner waits for an initiation or response from an AAC user without providing additional prompts; a.k.a., *pause time.* (2) A teaching strategy that involves pairing a known stimulus that has meaning for an individual with a new stimulus. The new stimulus is presented prior to the old one, and the time span is gradually increased until the individual responds to the new stimulus. (3) The time between the presentation of the discriminative stimulus for a target response and delivery of the reinforcer for that response.

timed activation: Switch activation that is set for a specified time.

Timothy Communications Package: An archaic microcomputer-based communication aid that featured both printed and synthetic speech output operated by scanning with a single switch or with up to five switches. Additional programs were included in the package for adding and storing phrases, message composition, and a switch evaluation program.

TO: See *traditional orthography.*

toe touch weight-bearing: A term used interchangeably with *touch down weight-bearing.*

Tokyo Artificial Larynx: A pneumatic artificial larynx that consists of a trumpet-like mouthpiece, a metal cavity containing a tightly stretched rubber strip, and a rubber or plastic tube that is inserted into the mouth. The mouthpiece is placed directly on the stoma and expired pulmonary air passes through the mouthpiece and into the metal cavity, causing the rubber strip to vibrate. The resulting sound is then passed into the oral cavity through the tube and speech is produced by the movement of the articulators. Also known as the *Tokyo Reed.*

Tokyo Reed: See *Tokyo Artificial Larynx.*

tongue switch: A dual switch that can be activated not only by minimal movement of the tongue but by the nose, chin, or finger as well.

tonic neck reflex: A primitive or infantile reflex seen in very young children; when the head is turned to one side, the arm behind the head bends with the hand close to the back of the head, while the arm in front of the face is stretched out. If you turn the head the opposite direction, the arms change accordingly. See also *primitive reflexes.*

top down strategy: A cognitive style of information processing (linguistic or non-linguistic) in which an individual starts with a contextual or global concept and relationship of elements and then proceeds to more basic low level structures and elements. This strategy is generally predictive and sets forward hypotheses.

topic board: A display on a communication board that designates which topic the speaker has chosen. It is similar to an alphabet board because it provides the listener with a cue, in this case the cue references the topic.

topic identification: An AAC technique that may be used if a person's speech is marginally intelligible; their message can often be understood if the communication partner is made aware of the semantic context of the topic.

topic setter cards: Cards or notes with simple drawings or symbols that pertain to the child's interests, used in conjunction with collections, remnant books, or other topic-setting techniques.

topic supplementation: Similar to the use of an alphabet board for speech supplementation, a non–speech-generating display consisting of a list or lists of topics to which an individual with a memory deficit can refer to initiate and maintain a conversation.

topographical dissimilarity: The minimal differences between manual signs in terms of their handshapes, locations, or movements; a physical characteristic of manual signing that distinguishes the shared features between symbols. See *minimal pair.*

topographical similarity: Occurs when manual signs share two of the three parameters of handshape, location, and movement. They may be thought of as minimal pairs for unaided symbols.

TORCH: An acronym for toxoplasmosis, other infection, rubella, cytomegalovirus, herpes. These five diseases are grouped together because they can cause a cluster of symptomatic birth defects in newborns. The symptoms of TORCH include a small head in proportion to the length of the mother's pregnancy at the time of delivery, an enlarged liver or spleen, a low level of platelets in the blood, a skin rash, central nervous system involvement, and jaundice.

total communication: A philosophy developed in the 1960s in the field of deafness stressing the importance of communication and language development regardless of the modes or methods. It embraced the use of the most appropriate communication modes or methods for the individual. Although it was originally developed as a philosophy, some refer to it as a communication method.

total communication approach: An intervention approach that emphasizes language and communication development without regard to sensory system or communication modes. It usually implies the pairing of speech and manual sign.

TouCan Communicator: An archaic, portable communication device that was operated by two switches that could be accessed by hand, foot, or chin. It featured two 80-character displays (one facing the message sender and the other the receiver), message storage and retrieval, and optional microcomputer, printer, and speech synthesizer access.

touch cue: A consistent tactile cue given as additional information to spoken words before each step in a routine (e.g., touching the waist before unbuckling a seat belt for transfer). See also *verbal cue.*

touch down weight-bearing: Allowing the weight of the leg to rest on the floor as an individual steps, accounting for up to 20% of body weight. This procedure relaxes the hip muscles and reduces the stresses through the hip. This is very hard work if done properly, and the arms must be strong enough to support most of the individual's weight.

touch membrane keyboard: A keyboard that consists of two electrically conductive flat surfaces separated by nonconductive spacers. Lightly touching the keyboard presses the two surfaces together, which sends an electronic signal to the AAC system.

touch screen: A transparent device or interface that can be attached to a computer monitor that allows input by touching areas on the screen.

touch tablet: An input device that senses the position of a finger or stylus on a flat, touch-sensitive surface. Touch tablets can be used to control cursor movements, act as an alternative keyboard, or replace a mouse or a joystick.

Touch Talker: An archaic, portable, dedicated speech-generating device that featured 8-, 32-, or 128-selection overlays to recall stored vocabulary using Express or Minspeak software for symbols and message retrieval meaningful to the user. The device could also be used as an alternate keyboard or to operate environmental control.

TPBA: See *transdisciplinary play-based assessment.*

TR: Common medical abbreviation for *therapeutic recreation.*

tracheostomy tube: A tube placed through a stoma (a surgically created opening in the anterior neck) and into the trachea to keep the airway to the lungs open following neck surgery.

tracheotomy: A surgical procedure involving cutting into the trachea through the outer skin of the neck to alleviate breathing difficulties. The opening may be temporary or permanent.

trackball: An input device containing a visible ball or sphere mounted into a stationary container. The device functions similarly to an upside-down mouse by moving the cursor on screen as the ball is moved or rotated by the user's hand.

trackpad: An input device that allows selection of items on a computer screen. The pointer or cursor on the screen moves in accordance with the movement of a finger along a touch sensitive pad.

traditional orthography: An aided system of alphabet letters (or characters) that are used to encode the language of the community in written form (e.g., the 26 letters of the English alphabet).

transceiver: A hardware device that is capable of transmitting and receiving information.

transdisciplinary approach: A team approach to assessment and treatment where a professional not only performs their own duties but also acquires knowledge of related disciplines, incorporating that knowledge into their own practice. Thus, although several disciplines may be involved in the provision of services, one professional on the team assumes primary responsibility for direct client contact.

transdisciplinary play-based assessment: Typically used with children functioning developmentally between 6 months and 6 years of age, TPBA consists of a set of criterion-referenced informal assessment scales where a videotaped play interaction session is scored by multiple professionals who observe four domains: (1) cognitive, (2) social-emotional, (3) communication and language, and (4) sensorimotor.

transdisciplinary team model: One of several models for team assessment and intervention in which members jointly engage in decision making. Transdisciplinary teams are based on maximum collaboration and interaction among team members who are expected to cross boundaries and release roles to share knowledge and responsibility.

transition planning: A planning process implemented by the early intervention service coordinator that considers the transition from early intervention to early childhood services prior to a child's third birthday so the child will be able to adapt to new services with little difficulty.

transition services: The process or delivery of services that involves assisting individuals to smoothly pass from one environment or situation to another (e.g., from home to school, school to school, school to work).

translucency: An aspect of iconicity in which the visual relationship between a symbol and its referent or meaning is not readily understood (i.e., guessable) but the relationship generally becomes recognized or understood when symbol and referent appear together. In the psychology discipline, this term is referred to as *representativeness*. See also *iconicity*, *opaqueness*, and *transparency*.

translucent: A term used to describe symbols that are not readily understood (i.e., guessable) without knowing the referents.

transmission: The sending of a message to a communication partner. In AAC, transmission can be accomplished through a variety of means (e.g., visual, gestural, voice, print).

transmission environment: A component of the AAC model proposed by Lloyd and colleagues (1990) that describes the media in which communication symbols are sent and received (e.g., air, light waves, vibration); a.k.a., *signal channel* or *transmission/signal channel*.

transmission processes: A component of the AAC model proposed by Lloyd and colleagues (1990); refers to the means of communicating a message using AAC, including the means to represent (i.e., symbols), the means to select symbols, and the means to transmit symbols.

transmission/signal channel: See *transmission environment*.

transmission techniques: The manner in which an AAC user transmits a message. A transmission technique can be either aided (e.g., communication boards, pen and paper, speech-generating devices) or unaided (i.e., direct transmission using various parts of the body).

transparency: An aspect of iconicity in which the visual relationship between a symbol and its referent or meaning is readily understood (i.e., guessable) even when the referent is not present. See also *iconicity*, *opaqueness*, and *translucency*.

transparent: A term used to describe symbols that are readily understood (i.e., guessable) because of their visual relationship to their referents.

traumatic brain injury: Physical damage to the brain or nervous system caused by bruises, lacerations, penetrations, or shearing as a result of any number of sudden physical, violent injuries. An injury that does not involve penetration or laceration may be called a closed head injury.

Treacher Collins syndrome: A variable genetic syndrome involving several atypical features, including undergrowth of the midface with flattened or depressed cheekbones, antimongoloid slant, absence of the lower eyelashes, a large fishlike mouth, a receding chin, and malformations of the external ear. Intellectual impairment is present in only 5% of cases, but learning disabilities occur in almost 50% of cases.

Treatment and Education of Autistic and Related Communication Handicapped Children: A program developed in North Carolina that provides a wide range of services to persons with autism and their families, including diagnosis and assessment, individualized treatment programs, special education, social skills training, vocational training, school consultations, parent training and counseling, and the facilitation of parent group activities. The primary aim of the program is to help to prepare people with autism to live or work more effectively at home, at school, and in the community. Special emphasis is placed on helping people with autism and their families to live together more effectively by reducing or eliminating the behaviors that are associated with autism. Also known as *TEACCH.*

trial: A systematic examination of performance, quality, or goodness of fit.

Trine system: An archaic, three-function communication aid developed at the Trace Center (Madison, Wisconsin) that featured a portable electronic notebook, a communication aid with printed or synthesized speech output, and computer control. It was based on the Epson HX-20 portable computer with a standard keyboard, liquid crystal display, built-in printer, and microcassette storage unit. The QuicKey abbreviation expansion program was included for message storage and retrieval.

triplegia: (1) Paralysis of an upper and lower extremity on one side of the body in addition to the face. (2) Paralysis of both extremities on one side of the body and one extremity on the opposite side.

TROCA: See *tangible reinforcement operant conditioning audiometry.*

TSR: See *terminate-and-stay-resident.*

TTWB: Common medical abbreviation for *toe touch weight-bearing.*

two-dimensional symbols: Aided AAC symbols having the dimensions of height and width; these include but are not limited to pictures, line drawings, and alphabet-based symbols drawn or typed on a medium such as paper.

TWWIIA: See *Ticket to Work and Work Incentives Improvement Act of 1999 (PL 106-170).*

tx: Common medical abbreviation for *treatment.*

tx fdg: Common medical abbreviation for *therapeutic feeding.*

tympanogram: The graphic output of tympanometry (one of three immittance audiometry tests) that depicts the mobility of the tympanic membrane (eardrum) to variations in air pressure. A "flat" tympanogram indicates that the tympanic membrane is not as mobile as it should be, indicating some kind of pathology (e.g., otitis media with effusion, perforated eardrum, tumor in the middle ear cavity).

type-one structure: Defined by Lindblom (1990) as animal communication that has no dual structure. Their signals are gestalts, communicating by means of holistic patterns.

type-one symbols: A class of symbols in which the symbol representation relates to the visual appearance of the referent.

type-two structure: Defined by Lindblom (1990) as human language, characterized by combinatorial use of discrete units at two levels of structure—the phonological level and the syntactic level. This structure results in an unlimited number of messages that language can convey.

type-two symbols: Class of symbols in which the symbol relates to domains other than visual appearance (e.g., phonological or semantic domains). These symbols portray meaning by the sequencing of their components and the logic or rules by which these components are ordered both on an intrasymbolic and an intersymbolic level.

typology: The classification of things according to their characteristics. See also *taxonomy.*

UB: Common medical abbreviation for *upper body.*

UbD: See *Understanding by Design.*

UE: Common medical abbreviation for *upper extremity(ies).*

UFAS: See *Uniform Federal Accessibility Standards.*

UHF: See *ultra high frequency.*

ultra high frequency: Radio waves with frequencies between 328.6 MHz and 2.9 GHz.

UMN: See *upper motor neurons.*

unaided: A term used to refer to communication symbols, approaches, strategies, or techniques in which only the body or parts of the body are used to represent, select, or transmit information.

unaided approach: The use of unaided symbols and techniques to accomplish effective communication.

unaided communication: Communication using unaided symbols and only parts of the body without any aids or devices (e.g., facial expressions, gestures, manual signs, natural speech).

unaided communication technique: A technique that does not require a physical aid for transmission (e.g., gesture, manual sign, facial expression, natural speech).

unaided symbols: AAC symbols selected and transmitted through parts of the body, thereby requiring no external aid or device (e.g., gestures, manual signs, pantomime).

unbound morpheme: A meaningful unit of language that can stand alone as a word (e.g., dog, house, car, him, sad). Bound morphemes can be affixed to unbound morphemes to change their meaning (e.g., "un-" affixed to "happy" results in "unhappy"; "-ing" affixed to "walk" results in "walking"). a.k.a., *free morpheme.*

unconventional verbal behavior: Verbal behavior not typically used for effective communication (e.g., *echolalia, perseverative speech,* incessant questioning).

Understanding by Design (UbD): An educational approach and planning process in which the educational target is identified and an approach for reaching it is created that allows access to the goal from a variety of perspectives and approaches to accommodate all learners.

unfunded mandate: Federal or state legislation requiring specific functions, services, or activities for which no funds are provided. See *funded mandates.*

Unicorn Keyboard: An expanded membrane keyboard consisting of pressure-sensitive cells that allows a variety of configurations to meet a user's needs (e.g., size, location, pressure, delay time). It can be used with a variety of computers interfaced through a device, such as an Adaptive Firmware Card or Ke:nx.

unidisciplinary model: One of several models for assessment and intervention in which only one discipline is involved.

Uniform Federal Accessibility Standards: Standards issued in 1984 as construction guidelines for accessibility to federal buildings and facilities. In 1991, they replaced ANSI standards because Uniform Federal Accessibility Standards covered both private and public facilities. In 2006, the Uniform Federal Accessibility Standards were replaced by the Americans with Disabilities Act of 1990 and the Architectural Barriers Act of 1968 *Accessibility Guidelines for Buildings and Facilities.*

unilateral: Referring to one side of the body (e.g., unilateral hearing loss).

United States Architectural and Transportation Barriers Compliance Board: A board whose primary responsibility is to ensure compliance with the standards prescribed by the Architectural Barriers Act of 1968, which mandated that certain buildings financed with federal funds be constructed to be accessible to persons with physical disabilities.

United States Department of Justice: Headed by the Attorney General of the United States, the U.S. Department of Justice is responsible for enforcing the law and defending the interests of the United States according to the law and ensuring fair and impartial administration of justice for all Americans, including persons with disabilities.

United States Society for Augmentative and Alternative Communication: A national chapter of the *International Society for Augmentative and Alternative Communication.* United States Society for Augmentative and Alternative Communication is an interdisciplinary society for the advancement of research and service delivery of AAC in the United States.

Unity: A software program developed by the Prentke Romich Company to assist educators or clinicians in developing vocabulary and other support materials for use with individuals using Prentke Romich Company devices.

universal cuff: An assistive device that allows an individual with limited hand function to access a keyboard with greater effectiveness.

upper extremities: The arms and hands.

upper motor neurons: Neurons that start in the motor cortex of the brain and terminate within the medulla or spinal cord. Damage to upper motor neurons can result in spasticity and exaggerated reflexes. See also *lower motor neurons* and *spasticity.*

USATBCB: See *United States Architectural and Transportation Barriers Compliance Board.*

USDOJ: See *United States Department of Justice.*

user interface: Any device that is used by an individual to access a communication aid or computer (e.g., switches, touch panels, joysticks, lightbeams and sensors, or other means). To interface an individual means to find the anatomical site and control mechanism or technique that the individual can use most effectively to operate an aid or device.

user preference: The concept that AAC users can choose how and what they want to communicate with their choice of AAC device or AAC strategy.

Usher's syndrome: A genetic condition of dual sensory impairment characterized by hearing loss at birth and progressive visual loss from *retinitis pigmentosa* beginning by age 10 years; it accounts for more than half of the cases of dual sensory impairment in the United States.

USSAAC: See *United States Society for Augmentative and Alternative Communication.*

vacuum tube: The earliest type of electronic switch consisting of a glass tube housing electric circuitry in a vacuum. By heating a wire (cathode plate), electrons are accelerated in movement through a vacuum to a positively charged plate (anode). This speeding up of electrons is the process that was used in early amplifiers. Vacuum tubes were replaced by transistors.

variable depth techniques: Techniques that require shorter selection times for some items and longer selection times for others; all scanning techniques are variable depth techniques. Morse code is an example of a variable depth encoding technique.

ventilator: A mechanical device that provides oxygen and supports breathing for a person who cannot breathe independently; a.k.a., *respirator.*

ventral pontine syndrome: An acquired condition due to damage to the pons, characterized by general weakness of the upper and lower extremities, lateral gaze weakness, and possible weakness of the facial muscles; intellectual impairment is not a characteristic of the disorder.

verbal: A term that technically means the use of words (implying linguistic or language ability). It is occasionally used to mean "with speech."

verbal cue: A general spoken description that accompanies the touch cue (e.g., "It's time to get out of your wheelchair" while taking the individual by the arm to assist). See also *touch cue.*

verbal stereotypy: See *perseverative speech.*

VersaScan: An archaic scanning communication aid featuring 2 to 16 lamps in a circular array operated by a single switch. Pictures, symbols, words, or letters could be placed on the overlay. Optional remote lamps were available for scanning a larger area.

versatility: The ability to perform in a variety of ways for different purposes (e.g., a hand has more ways of moving and can be used for more purposes than a foot or an eye).

very high frequency: Radio waves with frequencies between 30 MHz and 328.6 MHz.

very low birth weight: Weight at birth that is below 1,500 grams (approximately 3.3 pounds).

very low frequency: Radio waves with frequencies between 10 kHz and 30 kHz.

vestibular system: Part of the inner ear; in human beings, this system is a collection of structures, primarily the semicircular canals, that provide primary input to a person's sense of balance, awareness of one's orientation in space, and coordination of movement with balance.

VGA: See *video graphics adapter*.

VHF: See *very high frequency*.

vibrotactile codes: Any coding system in which a person who is deaf interprets sounds through their sense of touch (i.e., through movements or vibrations). See also *Tadoma method*.

VIC: See *visual input communication system*.

video graphics adapter: High-quality color monitor, allowing display of 256 colors with pixel resolution of 640 x 480 dots per inch or better.

violation of expectation: A disturbing event or conflict that interferes with a previously established mental state that instilled within the individual a firm belief or feeling of confidence; often seen when an individual is informed they have a progressive degenerative neurological disorder, such as amyotrophic lateral sclerosis or Parkinson's disease.

visible unaided symbol: An unaided symbol that can be visually monitored by the user during production. Most gestures and manual signs are at least partially visible to the signer.

visual acuity: The clarity of vision that allows an individual to discriminate details through the sense of sight. Normal visual acuity is general accepted as 20/20 (i.e., the individual can see at 20 feet what a typical person can see).

visual attention: The perceptual process of receiving neural signals in the visual cortex and directing those signals toward higher cognitive centers in the brain to make meaning of visual information, incorporating visual memory and pattern recognition.

Visual Communication System: See *visual input communication system*.

visual disability: Functional limitations that may result from a visual impairment and how the impairment affects the individual's lifestyle.

visual discrimination: The ability to detect specific features of an object to recognize, match, duplicate, and categorize it.

visual field: Refers to the area in which objects are visible to the eye without a shift in gaze. This normally extends in an arc of 150 degrees from right to left and 120 degrees up and down.

visual impairment: Any impairment in the ability to perceive or process visual information due to the absence or deficiency of a specific structure or physiological function.

visual input communication system: A system of visual symbols that has been used in intervention with individuals with severe and global aphasia with some success.

visual-motor: The performance of a motor task or function in response to visual input.

visual motor encoding: A storage and retrieval organization system based on visual representations that relate to motor components of manual signs or gestures that represent meaning.

visual perception: One of the senses, consisting of the ability to detect light (i.e., color and intensity) and interpret it as sight or vision.

visual pursuit: See *visual tracking*.

visual reinforcement audiometry: A method of assessing for auditory acuity in which a loud tone is presented (usually in a sound treated booth) followed by some type of visual reinforcement (e.g., activation of a light or video display or movement of a mechanical toy). The audiologist notes when the individual looks toward a reinforcer in anticipation that it will be activated.

visual scanning: A message selection technique in which symbols are presented to the user through the visual modality.

visual scene display (VSD): A message communicated through pictures or photos of common scenes for the user. The user will click on images in the scene (referred to as "hotspots") to communicate a message that has been preprogrammed. Visual scene displays are composed of those people, events, and activities that encompass the everyday milieu of the user.

visual-spatial store: A component of short-term or working memory thought to mediate visual information and spatial relationships between and among visual stimuli.

visual tracking: Smooth eye movements that involve following or tracking a moving target.

visually impaired (handicapped): In the field of education, defined as children whose visual impairment is such that special provisions are necessary for their successful participation in the learning process.

vital signs: Signs used by medical professionals as a general gauge of a person's health status (e.g., heart rate, blood pressure, and respiratory rate).

VLBW: See *very low birth weight*.

VLF: See *very low frequency*.

VOCA: An abbreviation for *voice output communication aid.* See *speech-generating device.*

vocabulary masking: Allows the practitioner to show only a subset of vocabulary items (depending upon client abilities and characteristics), and therefore, provides the opportunity to teach targeted words while minimizing distractions.

vocabulary selection: The process of choosing referents and their representations (e.g., spoken or written words, graphic symbols, gestures, manual signs) for the purpose of communication.

Vocaid: An archaic, portable, dedicated speech-generating device that featured a 36-key direct selection keyboard and four levels of preprogrammed vocabulary. A total of 140 words, letters, and numbers were provided.

vocal: Pertaining to voice or the oral production of sounds that may or may not be speech sounds (e.g., cries, moans, sighs).

vocalization: An utterance viewed only as a sound (i.e., produced by vocal cord vibration) without reference to its linguistic structure.

vocational rehabilitation: (1) The retraining of individuals who have injuries or disabilities so they can return to work. (2) A federally funded program enacted under the Rehabilitation Act Amendments of 1992 (P.L. 102-569) that provides vocational placement, training, and support for individuals with disabilities.

voice banking: A process that allows individuals to create a synthesized version of their natural speaking voice to be used in a speech-generating device at a time that the individual loses the ability to produce intelligible, natural speech.

voice input: The use of voice to activate a computer in place of the standard keyboard or other means of input. See also *speech recognition.*

voice onset time: The amount of time that elapses between the release of a plosive sound and the beginning of vocal fold vibration, measured in milliseconds. There are three types of voice onset time: (1) zero voice onset time, where onset of vocal fold vibration is simultaneous with plosive release; (2) positive voice onset time, where there is a delay in the onset of vocal fold vibration after plosive release; and (3) negative voice onset time, where the onset of vocal fold vibration precedes plosive release.

voice output communication aid: See *speech-generating device.*

voice recognition: See *speech recognition.*

voice recognition system: A computer access system designed to be used as the input device. See also *voice input* and *speech recognition.*

voice synthesis: See *speech synthesis.*

VOIS 130: An archaic, portable, dedicated speech-generating device that featured a 128-square touch sensitive keyboard containing four preprogrammed levels accessible by a single master overlay. A fifth level was available with 118 user-programmable locations.

VOIS 135: An archaic, portable, dedicated speech-generating device that featured a 128-square touch sensitive keyboard containing one preprogrammed level and four separate user-programmable levels (a total of 114 user locations).

VOIS 136: An archaic, portable, dedicated speech-generating device that featured over 21,000 user-programmable entries on multiple levels, recalled by a direct selection membrane keyboard that could be configured into three-fourth–inch squares, multiple squares, or the entire keyboard.

VOIS 140: An archaic, portable, dedicated speech-generating device that featured a three-digit encoding system to recall 980 preprogrammed words, letter, phrases, numbers, and phonemes using the numerals 0 through 9. The device had an additional user-programmable memory for 100 entries.

VOIS 150: An archaic, portable, dedicated speech-generating device that was similar to the VOIS 140, but was accessible by any single switch or joystick. The device featured a special tone system for individuals with visual impairments, as well as row-column or directed scanning.

VOIS 160: An archaic, portable, dedicated speech-generating device that featured text-to-speech synthesis (male or female voices) with vocabulary storage for up to 50,000 entries on seven levels. Text was also shown on a two-line liquid crystal display. User-created vocabulary could be saved or special vocabulary loaded via computer.

VOT: See *voice onset time.*

VR: See *vocational rehabilitation.*

VRA: See *visual reinforcement audiometry.*

VS: Common medical abbreviation for *vital signs.*

VSD: See *visual scene display.*

Waardenburg syndrome: A genetic syndrome characterized by pigmentary disturbances, different-colored, widely-spaced eyes, white patches on the skin, and sensorineural hearing loss. Severe congenital bilateral hearing loss is present in 25% to 50% of cases.

WAIS: See *Wechsler Adult Intelligence Scale.*

WB: Common medical abbreviation for *weight-bearing.*

WBAT: Common medical abbreviation for *weight-bearing as tolerated.*

W/C: Common medical abbreviation for *wheelchair.*

Web 2.0: A general term used to denote the second generation of the web's development. It is an information and computing platform as opposed to a storehouse for content.

Wechsler Adult Intelligence Scale: An individually administered intelligence test battery that includes 11 subtests. Three IQ scores can be determined: verbal IQ, performance IQ, and full-scale IQ.

weight-bearing: A range of abilities in which an individual is able to bear their body weight upon the legs (which stresses the hip joints); in order of greatest to least: *full weight-bearing, weight-bearing as tolerated, partial weight-bearing, touch down weight-bearing,* and *non–weight-bearing.*

weight-bearing as tolerated: An individual bears as much weight on their legs as they feel able to do; approximately 50% to 100% of the individual's body weight.

Wernicke's aphasia: A type of aphasia caused by cortical lesions in the posterior portion of the left first temporal gyrus, characterized by a loss of comprehension of spoken language, loss of ability to read (silently) and write, and a distortion of articulate speech. However, hearing tends to remain intact. The individual may speak fluently with a natural language rhythm, but the result has neither understandable meaning nor syntax. Despite the loss of comprehension, word memory is preserved and words are often chosen correctly. Secondary impairments may include alexia, agraphia, and acalculia.

WFL: Common medical abbreviation for *within functional limits.*

wheelchair: A manually operated or power-driven seating device designed primarily for use by an individual with a mobility disability for the main purpose of indoor, or both indoor and outdoor, locomotion.

wheelchair mounting systems: Custom-made or commercial adaptations designed to support the AAC device at the correct height and viewing angle.

whole language: A theory that incorporates teaching strategies and experiences to promote learning to read, write, speak, and listen in more natural language situations. A whole language approach is more informal, transactional, and follows a psychosociolinguistic approach.

Wide Range Achievement Test: A standardized test that measures a variety of academic performance areas.

WiFi: See *wireless fidelity.*

WIIA: Abbreviation for *Work Incentives Improvement Act.* See *Ticket to Work and Work Incentives Improvement Act of 1999 (P.L. 106-170).*

wireless fidelity: A general term used to denote wireless technology in the IEEE 802.11 specification. Simply put, WiFi allows a laptop computer user to access the internet without being hardwired. WiFi is similar but not synonymous with Bluetooth technology.

within normal limits: Anatomical structures, physiological functions, or performance that are observed in typically developing or typically developed individuals (e.g., in auditory testing, this abbreviation means that auditory thresholds are indicative of normal hearing).

WNL: See *within normal limits.*

wobble switch: A single switch that is activated by gross movements in any direction.

Wolf: An archaic, portable, dedicated speech-generating device that originally featured a 500-word user-specified vocabulary (programmed by the manufacturer) but was expanded to include an 800-word user-programmable memory. Words and phrases were recalled by direct selection on a touch pad grid with varying sized selection areas.

word completion: See *word prediction.*

word prediction: (1) An encoded retrieval system that facilitates and increases word retrieval by selecting high-frequency words based on the initial letter selected. (2) Software that minimizes keystrokes by presenting the user with a menu of numbered or lettered choices based on input letters; it may be organized by frequency of use or user's conceptual pattern. a.k.a., *lexical prediction.*

word processing: (1) The process of selecting and arranging the order and display of letters to form words and sentences. (2) Computer programs that enable the user to input letters to form words and sentences in a manner similar to a typewriter, except that changes in text can be made immediately and on an ongoing basis (e.g., deleting, editing, inserting, merging, saving).

working memory: See *short-term memory.*

WRAT: See *Wide Range Achievement Test.*

writing aid: Any device or instrument that assists an individual with motor impairments in writing words or drawing.

writing skills: The literacy process where an individual demonstrates the ability to spell and write words correctly, following all the conventions of their language (e.g., syntax, morphology, semantics).

written choice conversation: A technique in which a person answers open-ended questions by pointing to written choices generated by communication partners. Partners provide a short list of appropriate responses to their questions and say the written choices as the person points to the word representing their response or choice.

Yerkish: An opaque graphic communication system originally created at the Yerkes Primate Laboratory (Atlanta, Georgia) to teach a chimpanzee to communicate. The system utilizes a large symbol board that is touched to translate into commands. The system more recently has been tried with persons with intellectual impairment with some success. See also *lexigrams.*

yes/no headshakes: A means of communication in which the user responds to questions by their communication partner with yes or no gestures. The yes and no gestures can be the common head nod and head shake or any two consistent, reliable gestures, movements, or vocalizations.

yes/no verbal scanning: A scanning method in which the communication partner or aide points to all possible choices as the user responds yes or no to each selection.

zero reject principle: The principle that states that all children are eligible to participate in the educational process without having to meet any specified criteria.

Zika syndrome: A congenital condition, it is a group of birth defects associated with infection of the mother from the Zika virus transmitted primarily by Aedes mosquitoes. Birth defects may include microcephaly, brain atrophy and asymmetry, absent brain structures, hydrocephalus, damage to the back of the eye, hearing loss, cerebral palsy, low birth weight, problems with the limbs or joints, hypertonia, and excessive skin on the scalp. Zika syndrome has also been associated with Guillain-Barré syndrome.

zone of proximal development: Based on the work of Vygotsky (1978), it involves the difference between a child's actual level of development as determined by independent performance and the child's potential level of development accomplished through collaborative interaction with a more skilled partner.

ZYGO Model 100 Communication System/Keyboard Emulator: An archaic, portable, 100-light row-column scanning communication aid that could also function as a keyboard emulator for the Apple II+ and IIe computers. Overlays with custom vocabulary could be attached.

ZYGO Model 16C: An archaic 16-position scanning communication aid featuring single or dual switch input. Overlays could be attached to the panel so that 2 to 16 lighted positions could be used.

ZYGO Notebook: An archaic portable communication and writing aid featuring liquid crystal display and optional printed output to an external printer. It has a standard typewriter keyboard, text memory, and an abbreviation expansion program (called Abex).

ZYGO Parrot: An archaic small, dedicated speech-generating device featuring natural speech output for 16 messages by direct selection of one-half-inch squares. The Parrot-JK model is switch-activated.

ZYGO scanWRITER: An archaic portable, dedicated speech-generating device that uses row-column or directed scanning to retrieve single letters or entire words or phrases for printed output. It can also function as a notetaker, calculator, and keyboard emulator. Optional modules include speech output and a remote system for addressing computers without a cable connection.

ZYGO Secretary: An archaic portable, dedicated speech-generating device that combines the characteristics of the ZYGO QUE Scribe, which utilizes input on a standard typewriter keyboard for print and liquid crystal display, and the ZYGO Parrot, which utilizes prerecorded natural speech for a small number of messages.

ZYGO Talking Notebook II: An archaic portable, dedicated speech-generating device that features a lap style personal computer with a liquid crystal display screen. Special software allows for single pointer access, file storage, talking scratchpad, math scratchpad, and perpetual calendar/clock.

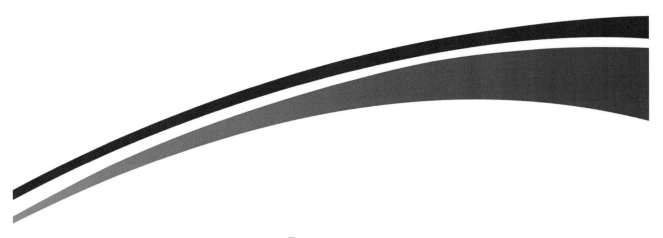

REFERENCES

AAC Institute. (2001). *Performance report tool [computer software]*. AAC Institute.

AAC Institute. (2015). *Language sample collection in AAC*. Retrieved from https://aacinstitute.org/language-sample-collection-in-aac/

Abbott, M. A., & McBride, D. (2014). AAC decision-making and mobile technology: Points to ponder. *Perspectives on Augmentative and Alternative Communication, 23*, 104-111.

Abedi, J. (2010). Research and recommendations for formative assessment with English language learners. In H. Andrade & G. J. Cizek (Eds.), *Handbook of formative assessment* (pp. 181-197). Routledge.

Acredolo, L., & Goodywn, S. (1988). Symbolic gesturing in normal infants. *Child Development, 59*, 450-466.

Adams, M. J. (1990). *Beginning to read: Thinking and learning about print*. The MIT Press.

Adamson, L. B., Romski, M. A, Deffebach, K., & Sevcik, R. A. (1992). Symbol vocabulary and the focus of conversations: Augmenting language development for youth with mental retardation. *Journal of Speech and Hearing Research, 35*, 1333-1343.

Adelman, R., Tmanova, L., Delgado, D., Dion, S., & Lachs, M. (2014). Caregiver burden: A clinical review. *Journal of the American Medical Association, 311*(10), 1052-1059.

Adult Hearing Screening. (n.d.). Retrieved from https://www.asha.org/PRPSpecificTopic.aspx?folderid=8589942721&section=Key_Issues

Aftonomos, L., Appelbaum, J., & Steele, R. (1999). Improving outcomes for persons with aphasia in advanced community-based treatment programs. *Stroke: A Journal of Cerebral Circulation, 30*(7), 1370-1379.

Aftonomos, L., Steele, R., & Wertz, R. (1997). Promoting recovery in chronic aphasia with an interactive technology. *Archives of Physical Medicine and Rehabilitation, 78*(8), 841-846.

Ahlgren, I., Bergman, B., & Brennan, M. (Eds.). (1994). *Papers from the Fifth International Symposium on Sign Language Research. Volume I: Perspectives on sign language structure. Volume II: Perspectives on sign language use*. International Sign Linguistics Association and Deaf Studies Research Unit, University of Durham.

Ahmed, M. A., Zaidan, B. B., Zaidan, A. A., Salih, M. M., & Lakulu, M. M. B. (2018). A review on systems-based sensory gloves for sign language recognition state of the art between 2007 and 2017. *Sensors, 18*(7), 2208.

Alant, E. (2017a). *Augmentative and alternative communication: Engagement and participation*. Plural Publishing.

Alant, E. (2017b). Engagement, participation, and people with severe dementia. In E. Alant, *Augmentative and alternative communication: Engagement and participation* (pp. 227-249). Plural Publishing.

Alant, E., Bornman, J., & Lloyd, L. L. (2006). Issues in AAC research: How much do we really understand? *Disability and Rehabilitation, 28*(3), 143-150.

Alant, E., Champion, A., & Peabody, E. C. (2013). Exploring interagency collaboration in AAC intervention. *Communication Disorders Quarterly, 34*(3), 172-183.

Alant, E., Geyer, S., & Verde, M. (2015). Developing empathetic skills among teachers and learners in high schools in Tshwane: An intergenerational approach involving people with dementia. *Perspectives in Education, 33*(3), 141-158.

Alegria, J., Leybaert, J., Charlier, B., & Hage, C. (1992). On the origin of phonological representations in the deaf: Listening to the lips and the hands. In J. Morais (Ed.), *Analytic Approaches to Human Cognition* (pp. 107-132). North Holland.

Alexander, P. K. (1990). The effects of brain damage on visual functioning in children. *Journal of Visual Impairment and Blindness, 84*, 372-376.

Allgood, M. H., Heller, K. W., Easterbrooks, S. R., & Fredrick, L. D. (2009). Use of picture dictionaries to promote functional communication in students with deafness and intellectual disabilities. *Communication Disorders Quarterly, 31*(1), 53-64.

Alnfiai, M., & Sampali, S. (2017). Social and communication apps for the deaf and hearing impaired. *International Conference on Computer and Applications*, 120-126. Retrieved August 26, 2018, from http://ieeexplore.ieee.org/document/8079756/

Alpiner, J. G., & McCarthy, P. A. (Eds.). (2000). *Rehabilitative audiology: Children and adults* (3rd ed.). Lippincott Williams & Wilkins.

Alter, P. J., Conroy, M. A., Mancil, G. R., & Haydon, T. (2008). A comparison of functional behavior assessment methodologies with young children: Descriptive methods and functional analysis. *Journal of Behavioral Education, 17*, 200-219.

Altmann, L., & Troche, M. (2011). High-level language production in Parkinson's disease: A review. *Parkinson's Disease, 2011*, 12.

Alzheimer's Association. (2018). 2018 Alzheimer's disease facts and figures. *Alzheimer's and Dementia, 14*(3), 367-429.

Amatya, P., Sergieieva, K., & Meixner, G. (2018). Translation of sign language into text using Kinect for Windows v2. *The Eleventh International Conference on Advances in Computer-Human Interactions* (pp. 19-26). Retrieved January 22, 2019, from https://www.thinkmind.org/download.php?articleid=achi_2018_2_10_20002

Fuller, D. R., & Lloyd, L. L. *Principles and Practices in Augmentative and Alternative Communication* (pp. 579-623).
© 2023 Taylor & Francis Group.

Amend, S. (1987). *Research report regarding visual phonics to the Sertoma Foundation*. International Communication Learning Institute.

American Association of the Deaf-Blind. (2009). Frequently asked questions about deaf-blindness. Retrieved May 3, 2019, from http://www.aadb.org/FAQ/faq_DeafBlindness.html#count

American Hospital Association. (2017). Fast facts on U.S. hospitals. Retrieved from http://www.aha.org/research/rc/stat-studies/fast-facts.shtml

American Psychiatric Association. (2013). *Diagnostic and statistical manual of mental disorders* (5th ed.). American Psychiatric Publishing.

American Speech-Language-Hearing Association. (1991). Report: Augmentative and alternative communication. *ASHA, 33*(Suppl. 5), 9-12.

American Speech-Language-Hearing Association. (1992). Guidelines for meeting the communication needs of persons with severe disabilities. *National Student Speech Language Hearing Association Journal, 19*, 41-48.

American Speech-Language-Hearing Association. (2004a). *Preferred practice patterns for the profession of speech-language pathology*. Retrieved from www.asha.org/policy

American Speech-Language-Hearing Association. (2004b). *Roles and responsibilities of speech-language pathologists with respect to augmentative and alternative communication: Technical report*. Retrieved from http://www.asha.org/policy/TR2004-00262/

American Speech-Language-Hearing Association. (2005). *Evidence-based practice in communication disorders* [Position Statement]. Retrieved from www.asha.org/policy

American Speech-Language-Hearing Association. (2015). *Highlights and trends: Member and affiliate counts, Year-end 2015*. Retrieved from https://www.asha.org/uploadedFiles/2016-Member-Counts.pdf

American Speech-Language-Hearing Association. (2016a). *Augmentative and alternative communication* (AAC). Retrieved from http://www.asha.org/public/speech/disorders/AAC

American Speech-Language-Hearing Association. (2016b). *Code of ethics* [Ethics]. Retrieved from www.asha.org/policy/

American Speech-Language-Hearing Association. (2016c). *Scope of practice in speech-language-pathology* [Scope of Practice]. Retrieved from www.asha.org/policy/

American Speech-Language-Hearing Association. (2017). *Practice portal and professional issues in augmentative and alternative communication*. Retrieved from https://www.asha.org/Practice-Portal/Professional-Issues/Augmentative-and-Alternative-Communication/

American Speech-Language-Hearing Association. (2018a). *Augmentative and alternative communication*. Retrieved from https://www.asha.org/NJC/AAC/

American Speech-Language-Hearing Association. (2018b). *Facilitated communication* [Position statement]. Retrieved from www.asha.org/policy/PS2018-00352/

American Speech-Language-Hearing Association. (2018c). *Rapid prompting method* [Position statement]. Retrieved from www.asha.org/policy/

American Speech-Language-Hearing Association. (n.d.a). Retrieved from https://www.asha.org/SLP/Cautions-Against-Use-of-FC-and-RPM-Widely-Shared/

American Speech-Language-Hearing Association. (n.d.b). *Augmentative and alternative communication*. Retrieved from https://www.asha.org/njc/aac/

American Speech-Language-Hearing Association. (n.d.c). *Augmentative and alternative communication decisions*. Retrieved from https://www.asha.org/public/speech/disorders/communicationdecisions/

American Speech-Language-Hearing Association. (n.d.d). *Definition of communication and appropriate targets*. Retrieved from https://www.asha.org/NJC/Definition-of-Communication-and-Appropriate-Targets/

American Speech-Language-Hearing Association. (n.d.e). *Hearing screening*. Retrieved from https://www.asha.org/PRPSpecificTopic.aspx?folderid=8589942721&section=Key_Issues

American Speech-Language-Hearing Association. (n.d.f). *Introduction to evidence-based practice*. Retrieved from https://www.asha.org/Research/EBP/Introduction-to-Evidence-Based-Practice/

American Speech-Language-Hearing Association. (n.d.g). *Medicare coverage policy on SGDs*. Retrieved from https://www.asha.org/practice/reimbursement/medicare/sgd_policy/

American Speech-Language-Hearing Association. (n.d.h). *Practice portal: AAC*. Retrieved from https://www.asha.org/

American Speech-Language-Hearing Association. (n.d.i). *About the American Speech-Language-Hearing Association*. Retrieved from https://www.asha.org/about

American Speech-Language-Hearing Association. (n.d.j). *Practice portal: Telepractice*. Retrieved from https://www.asha.org/Practice-Portal/Professional-Issues/Telepractice/

Americans with Disabilities Act Amendments Act. (2008). P.L. 110-325. Retrieved from https://www.eeoc.gov/statutes/ada-amendments-act-2008

Anderberg, P., & Jönsson, B. (2005). Being there. *Disability and Society, 20*(7), 719-733.

Andersen, P. M, & Al-Chalabi, A. (2011). Clinical genetics of amyotrophic lateral sclerosis: What do we really know? *Nature Reviews Neurology, 7*, 603-615.

Andersen, P. M., Nilsson, P., Keränen, M. L., Forsgren, L., Hägglund, J., Karlsborg, M., Ronnevi, L. O., Gredal, O., & Marklund, S. L. (1997). Phenotypic heterogeneity in motor neuron disease patients with CuZn-superoxide dismutase mutations in Scandinavia. *Brain: A Journal of Neurology, 120*(10), 1723-1737.

Anderson, K., Boisvert, M. K., Doneski-Nicol, J., Gutmann, M. L., Hall, N. C., Morelock, C., Steele, R., & Cohn, E. R. (2012). Tele-AAC resolution. *International Journal of Telerehabilitation, 4*(2), 79-82.

Anderson, N. B., & Shames, G. H. (2013). *Human communication disorders: An introduction* (8th ed.). Allyn and Bacon.

Anderson, S. B. (1998). *We are not alone: Fountain House and the development of clubhouse culture*. Fountain House.

Anthony, D. (1974). *The seeing essential English manual*. The University of Northern Colorado.

Apel, K., Henbest, V. S., & Petscher, Y. (2022). Morphological awareness performance profiles of first- through sixth-grade students. *Journal of Speech, Language, and Hearing Research, 65*(3), 1070-1086.

Aram, D. M., Ekelman, B. L., & Nation, J. E. (1984). Preschoolers with language disorders: Ten years later. *Journal of Speech and Hearing Research, 27*, 232-244.

Arlinger, S. (2003). Negative consequences of uncorrected hearing loss—A review. *International Journal of Audiology, 42*(2), 17-20.

Armstrong, D. F. (2014). *The history of Gallaudet University: 150 years of a deaf American institution*. Gallaudet University Press.

Arthur-Kelly, M., Sigafoos, J., Green, V., Mathisen, B., & Arthur-Kelly, R. (2009). Issues in the use of visual supports to promote communication in individuals with autism spectrum disorder. *Disability and Rehabilitation, 31*(18), 1474-1486.

Artiles, A. J. (2011). Toward an interdisciplinary understanding of educational equity and difference: The case of the racialization of ability. *Educational Researcher, 40*(9), 431-445.

Artiles, A. J., Kozleski, E. B., Trent, S. C., Osher, D., & Ortiz, A. (2010). Justifying and explaining disproportionality, 1968-2008: A critique of underlying views of culture. *Exceptional Children, 76*(3), 279-299.

Arva, J., Paleg, G., Lange, M., Lieberman, J., Schmeler, M., Dicianno, B., & Rosen, L. (2009). RESNA position on the application of wheelchair standing devices. *Assistive Technology, 21*(2), 161-168.

Arva, J., Schmeler, M. R., Lange, M. L., Lipka, D. D., & Rosen, L. (2009). RESNA Position on the application of seat-elevating devices for wheelchair users. *Assistive Technology, 21*(2), 69-72.

ASHA Leader Live. (2019). *ASHA-endorsed telehealth legislation introduced in House, Senate*. Retrieved from https://blog.asha.org/2019/11/01/asha-endorsed-telehealth-legislation-introduced-in-house-senate/

Assistive Technology Act of 1998, PL No. 105-394, 29 U.S.C. 3001 (1998).

Assistive Technology Act of 2004, PL No. 108-364, 29 U.S.C. 3002 (2004).

Assistive Technology Guide. (2016). *AT guide: Assistive technology guide*. Retrieved from http://www.assistivetechnologyguide.co.uk/guides/

Atcherson, S. R., Franklin, C. A., & Smith-Olinde, L. (2015). *Hearing assistive and access technology*. Plural Publishing.

Atkinson, J. (1989). New test of vision screening and assessment in infants and young children. In J. H. French, S. Harel, & P. Casaer (Eds.), *Child neurology and developmental disabilities*. Review, 25, 57-66.

Atkinson, R. C., & Shiffrin, R. M. (1968). Human memory: A proposed system and its control processes. In K. W. Spence & J. T. Spence (Eds.), *The psychology of learning and motivation* (Vol. 2, pp. 89-195). Academic Press.

Autism Speaks. (2014). *Community based functional skills assessment for transition aged youth with autism spectrum disorder*. Virginia Commonwealth University Rehabilitation Research and Training Center. Retrieved from http://www.vcuautismcenter.org/documents/finalcommunityassessment711141.pdf

Axline, V. M. (1964). *Dibs in search of self*. Prestwick House, Inc.

Ayers, J. (2005). *Sensory integration and the child: Understanding hidden sensory challenges* (2nd ed.). Western Psychological Service.

Azzam, D., & Ronquillo, Y. (2022). Snellen chart. In *StatPearls* [Internet]. StatPearls Publishing.

Baddeley, A. D., & Hitch, G. J. (1974). Working memory. In G. A. Bower (Ed.)., *The psychology of learning and motivation: Advances in research and theory* (pp. 47-89). Academic Press.

Baddeley, A. D., Thomson, N., & Buchanan, M. (1975). Word length and the structure of short-term memory. *Journal of Verbal Learning and Verbal Behavior, 14*, 575-589.

Baer, D. M., Wolf, M. M., & Risley, T. R. (1968). Some current dimensions of applied behavior analysis. *Journal of Applied Behavior Analysis, 1*(1), 91.

Bailey, B. R., & Head, D. N. (1993). Providing O & M services to children and youth with severe multiple disabilities. *Review, 25*, 57-66.

Bailey, R., Parette, H. P., Stoner, J. B., Angell, M. E., & Carroll, K. (2006). Family members' perceptions of augmentative and alternative communication device use. *Language, Speech, and Hearing Services in Schools, 37*, 50-60.

Baio, J., Wiggins, L., Christensen, D. L., Maenner, M. J., Daniels, J., Warren, Z., Kurzius-Spencer, M., Zahorodny, W., Rosenberg, C. R., White, T., Durkin, M. S., Imm, P., Nikolaou, L., Yeargin-Allsopp, M., Lee, L., Harrington, R., Lopez, M., Fitzgerald, R. T., Hewitt, A., … Dowling, N. F. (2018). Prevalence of autism spectrum disorder among children aged 8 years—Autism and developmental disabilities monitoring network, 11 sites, United States, 2014. *Morbidity and Mortality Weekly Report Surveillance Summaries, 67*(6), 1-23.

Baker, B. (1982). Minspeak: A semantic compaction system that makes self-expression easier for communicatively disabled individuals. *Byte, 7*(9), 186-202.

Baker, B. (1987, June). *Semantic compaction for sub-sentence vocabulary units compared to other encoding and prediction systems*. RESNA '87, Meeting the Challenge: Tenth Annual Conference on Rehabilitation Engineering.

Baker, L., & Cantwell, D. P. (1982). Developmental, social, and behavioral characteristics of speech and language disordered children. *Child Psychiatry and Human Development, 12*, 195-206.

Baker, N. D., & Nelson, K. E. (1984). Recasting and related conversational techniques for triggering syntactic advances by young children. *First Language, 5*, 3-22.

Balandin, S. (1995). The topics and vocabulary of meal break conversations. Unpublished doctoral dissertation, Macquarie University.

Balandin, S. (2002). Message from the president. *The ISAAC Bulletin, 67*, 2.

Balandin, S., Hemsley, B., Sigafoos, J., & Green, V. (2007). Communicating with nurses: The experiences of 10 adults with cerebral palsy and complex communication needs. *Applied Nursing Research, 20*(2), 56-62.

Balandin, S., & Iacono, T. (1998a). A few well-chosen words. *Augmentative and Alternative Communication, 14*, 147-161.

Balandin, S., & Iacono, T. (1998b). Topics of meal-break conversations. *Augmentative and Alternative Communication, 14*, 131-146.

Balandin, S., & Iacono, T. (1999). Crews, wusses, and whoppas: Core and fringe vocabularies of Australian meal-break conversations in the workplace. *Augmentative and Alternative Communication, 15*, 95-109.

Balandin, S., & Morgan, J. (2001). Preparing for the future: Aging and alternative and augmentative communication. *Augmentative and Alternative Communication, 17*(2), 99-108.

Ball, L. J., Chavez, S., Perez, G., Bharucha-Goebel, D., Smart, K., Kundrat, K., Carruthers, L., Brady, C., Leach, M., & Evans, S. (2018, March). *Functional communication of children with spinal muscular atrophy type 1*. Muscular Dystrophy Association 2018 Clinical Conference. Proceedings at www.mdausa.org

Ball, L., Beukelman, D. R., & Pattee, G. (2004a). Augmentative and alternative communication acceptance by persons with amyotrophic lateral sclerosis. *Augmentative and Alternative Communication, 20*, 113-123.

Ball, L., Beukelman, D. R., & Pattee, G. (2004b). Communication effectiveness of individuals with amyotrophic lateral sclerosis. *Journal of Communication Disorders, 37*, 197-215.

Ball, L., Nordness, A., Fager, S., Kersch, K., Mohr, B., & Pattee, G. (2010). Eye-gaze access to AAC technology for people with amyotrophic lateral sclerosis. *Journal of Medical Speech-Language Pathology, 18*(3), 11-23.

Banajee, M., Dicarlo, C., & Buras Stricklin, S. (2003). Core vocabulary determination for toddlers. *Augmentative and Alternative Communication, 19*(2), 67-73.

Bane, M. C, & Birch, E. E. (1992). Forced-choice preferential looking and visual evoked potential acuities of visually impaired children. *Journal of Visual Impairment and Blindness, 86*, 21-24.

Banks, J. A. (Ed.). (2009). *The Routledge international companion to multicultural education*. Routledge.

Bannatyne, A. (1968). *Psycholinguistic color system. A reading, writing, spelling, and language program*. Learning Systems Press.

Baranek, G. T. (1999). *Sensory processing assessment for young children (SPA)*. Unpublished manuscript, University of North Carolina at Chapel Hill.

Baranek, G. T., Boyd, B. A., Poe, M. D., David, F. J., & Watson, L. R. (2007). Hyperresponsive sensory patterns in young children with autism, developmental delay, and typical development. *American Journal on Mental Retardation, 112*(4), 233-245.

Barker, R. M., Saunders, K. J., & Brady, N. C. (2012). Reading instruction for children who use AAC: Considerations in the pursuit of generalizable results. *Augmentative and Alternative Communication, 28*(3), 160-170.

Barron, R. W., Golden, J. O., Seldon, D. M., Tait, C. R., Marmurek, H. H. C., & Haines, L. P. (1992). Teaching prereading skills with a talking computer. *Reading and Writing: An Interdisciplinary Journal, 4*, 179-204.

Bartlett, G., Blais, R., Tamblyn, R., Clermont, R. J., & MacGibbon, B. (2008). Impact of patient communication problems on the risk of preventable adverse events in acute care settings. *Canadian Medical Association Journal, 178*(2), 1555-1562.

Bashinski, S. M. (2011a). Assessment of prelinguistic communication of individuals with CHARGE. In T. S. Hartshorne, M. Hefner, S. Davenport, & J. W. Thelin (Eds.), *CHARGE syndrome* (pp. 275-293). Plural Publishing.

Bashinski, S. M. (2011b). *Introduction to the etiologies and characteristics associated with learners who have deaf-blindness: Part II*. One in a series of 12 web-based professional development modules re: deaf-blindness, Kansas State Deaf-Blind Project.

Bashinski, S. M. (2012). *Gestural development*. One in a series of 12 web-based professional development modules re: deaf-blindness, Kansas State Deaf-Blind Project.

Bashinski, S. M. (2013a). *Interactions with objects: Important considerations for learners with deaf-blindness*. One in a series of 12 web-based professional development modules re: deaf-blindness, Kansas State Deaf-Blind Project.

Bashinski, S. M. (2013b). *Interactions with touch: Important considerations for learners with deaf-blindness*. One in a series of 12 web-based professional development modules re: deaf-blindness, Kansas State Deaf-Blind Project.

Bashinski, S. M. (2014a). *Calendar systems: Important considerations for learners with deaf-blindness*. One in a series of 12 web-based professional development modules re: deaf-blindness, Kansas State Deaf-Blind Project.

Bashinski, S. M. (2014b). *Intentionality*. One in a series of 12 web-based professional development modules re: deaf-blindness. Kansas State Deaf-Blind Project.

Bashinski, S. M. (2014c). *Symbolization*. One in a series of 12 web-based professional development modules re: deaf-blindness. Kansas State Deaf-Blind Project.

Bashinski, S. M. (2015a). Communication programming for learners with CHARGE syndrome: Augmenting comprehension and expression. *Perspectives on Augmentative and Alternative Communication, 24*(3), 86-93.

Bashinski, S. M. (2015b). Receptive and expressive dictionaries for students who do not use symbols. *Word of Mouth, 26*(4), 13-16.

Bashinski, S. M. (2018). *Laying the foundation for communication exchange: Critical points of understanding*. National Center on Deaf-Blindness.

Bashinski, S. M. (2021). Prelinguistic communication. In T. S. Hartshorne, M. A. Hefner, & K. D. Blake (Eds.), *CHARGE syndrome* (2nd ed., pp. 353-390). Plural Publishing.

Bashinski, S. M., Braddock, B. A., Neal, C. A., & Heithaus, J. (2017, July). *Families' perspectives: Types and purposes of communication used by their children with CHARGE syndrome*. Paper presented at the 13th International CHARGE Syndrome Conference.

Bashinski, S. M., & Bruce, S. M. (2018, April). *Implementing the tri-focus framework strategies through interprofessional collaborative practice*. Paper presented at the Deaf-blind International Network of the Americas Conference.

Basil, C., & Ruiz, R. (1985). *Sistemas de communicacion no vocal. Para niños con disminuciones fisicas (Nonvocal communication systems for children with physical handicaps)*. Los Libros de Fundesco.

Bastawrous, M. (2013). Caregiver burden—A critical discussion. *International Journal of Nursing Studies, 50*, 431-441.

Bates, E. (1976). *Language and context: The acquisition of pragmatics*. Academic Press.

Bates, E. (1999). Plasticity, localization and language development. In S. H. Broman & J. M. Fletcher (Eds.), *The changing nervous system: Neurobehavioral consequences of early brain disorders* (pp. 214-253). Oxford University Press.

Bates, E., Benigni, L., Bretheron, I., Camaioni, L., & Volterra, V. (1979). *The emergence of symbols: Cognition and communication in infancy*. Academic Press.

Bates, K., & Macleod, K. (2017). Assessing communication for children with movement disorders: A practical approach. *Pediatrics and Child Health, 27*(10), 465-469.

Batorowicz, B., & Shepherd, T. A. (2011). Teamwork in AAC: Examining clinical perceptions. *Augmentative and Alternative Communication, 27*(1), 16-25.

Batshaw, M. L., & Perret, Y. M. (1992). *Children with handicaps: A medical primer* (3rd ed.). Paul H. Brookes Publishing Co.

Batstone, S., & Harris, G. (1990). *Questions regarding the functional vision of people with multiple disabilities with reference to communication needs*. Arbitrus Society for Children.

Battle, D. (2012). *Communication disorders in multicultural and international populations* (4th ed.). Elsevier Mosby.

Bauby, J. D. (1997). *The diving bell and the butterfly*. Vintage Books.

Bauer, S. E., Schumacher, J. R., Hall, A., Marlow, N. M., Friedel, C., Scheer, D., & Redmon, S. (2016). Disability and physical and communication-related barriers to health care related services among Florida residents: A brief report. *Disability and Health Journal, 9*(3), 552-556.

Baxter, S., Enderby, P., Evans, P., & Judge, S. (2012). Barriers and facilitators to the use of high-technology augmentative and alternative communication devices: A systematic review and qualitative synthesis. *International Journal of Language and Communication Disorders, 47*(2), 115-129.

Bayldon, H., Clendon, S. & Doell, E. (2021). Shared storybook intervention for children with complex physical, cognitive and sensory needs who use partner-assisted scanning. *International Journal of Disability, Development and Education* [Online First]. https://doi.org/10.1080/1034912X.2021.1913719

Bayles, K., Tomoeda, C., Cruz, R., & Mahendra, N. (2000). Communication abilities of individuals with late-stage Alzheimer disease. *Alzheimer Disease and Associated Disorders, 14*(3), 176-181.

Baylor, C., Yorkston, K., Eadie, T., Kim, J., Chung, H., & Amtmann, D. (2013). The Communication Participation Item Bank (CPIB): Item bank calibration and development of a disorder-generic short form. *Journal of Speech, Language, and Hearing Research, 56*, 1190-1208.

Bean, A., Cargill, L. P., & Lyle, S. (2019). Framework for selecting vocabulary for preliterate children who use augmentative and alternative communication. *American Journal of Speech-Language Pathology, 28*, 1000-1009.

Bear, M. F., Connors, B. W., & Paradiso, M. A. (2015). *Neuroscience: Exploring the brain* (4th ed.). Wolters Kluwer.

Beavers, G. A., Iwata, B. A., & Lerman, D. C. (2013). Thirty years of research on the functional analysis of problem behavior. *Journal of Applied Behavior Analysis, 46*, 1-21.

Beck, A. R., Stoner, J. B., Bock, S. J., & Parton, T. (2008). Comparison of PECS and the use of VOCA: A replication. *Education and Training in Developmental Disabilities, 43*, 198-216.

Bedore, L. M., Peña, E. D., García, M., & Cortez, C. (2005). Conceptual versus monolingual scoring: When does it make a difference? *Language, Speech, and Hearing Services in Schools, 36*(3), 188-200.

Beeldman, E., Raaphorst, J., Klein Twennaar, M., de Visser, M., Schmand, B. A., & de Haan, R. J. (2016). The cognitive profile of ALS: A systematic review and meta-analysis update. *Journal of Neurology Neurosurgery and Psychiatry, 87*, 611-619.

Beevers, R., & Hallinan, P. (1990). Talking word processors and text editing for visually impaired children: A pilot case study. *Journal of Visual Impairment and Blindness, 84*, 552-555.

Beginnings Board of Directors. (2007). *BEGINNINGS for parents of children who are deaf or hard of hearing*. Author.

Bellaire, K., Georges, J., & Thompson, C. (1989, June). *Establishing functional communication board use for nonverbal aphasic subjects*. Paper presented at the Clinical Aphasiology Conference.

Bellaire, K. J., Georges, J. B., & Thompson, C. K. (1991). Establishing functional communication board use for nonverbal aphasic subjects. *Clinical Aphasiology, 19*, 219-227.

Bellugi, L., & Klima, E. (1976). Two faces of sign: Iconic and abstract. In S. R., Hamad (Ed.), *Origins and evolution of language and speech* (Vol. 280, pp. 514-538). Annals of the New York Academy of Sciences.

Bennet, T. L. (1992). *The neuropsychology of epilepsy*. Plenum Press.

Benson-Goldberg, S., Geist, L., & Erickson, K. (2022). Expressive communication over time: A longitudinal analysis of the Project Core Implementation Model. *Communication Disorders Quarterly* [Online First]. https://doi.org/10.1177/15257401221120790

Bentz, C., & Kiela, D. (2014). Zipf's Law across languages of the world: Towards a quantitative measure of lexical diversity. In E. A. Cartmill, S. Roberts, H. Lyn, & H. Cornish (Eds.), *The evolution of language: Proceedings of the 10th international conference* (pp. 385-386). World Scientific.

Bergbom-Engberg, I., & Haljamae, H. (1993). The communication process with ventilator patients in the ICU as perceived by the nursing staff. *Intensive and Critical Care Nursing, 9,* 40-47.

Berger, K. (1968). The most common words used in conversations. *Journal of Communication Disorders, 1*(3), 201-214.

Berko, R. M., Wolvin, A. D., & Wolvin, D. R. (1977). *Communicating: A social and career focus.* Houghton.

Bertsch, S., Pesta, B. J., Wiscott, R., & McDaniel, M. A. (2007). The generation effect: A meta-analytic review. *Memory and Cognition, 35,* 201-210.

Bess, F. H., & Humes, L. E. (2008). *Audiology: The fundamentals* (4th ed). Wolters Kluwer.

Betancourt, J. R., Renfrew, M. R., Green, A. R., Lopez, L., & Wasserman, M. (2012, September). *Improving patient safety systems for patients with limited English proficiency: A guide for hospitals.* Agency for Health Care Research and Quality, AHRQ Publication No. 12-0041.

Beukelman, D. R., & Ball, L. (2002). Improving AAC use for persons with acquired neurogenic disorders: Understanding human and engineering factors. *Assistive Technology, 14*(1), 33-44.

Beukelman, D. R., Ball, L. J., & Fager, S. (2008). An AAC personnel framework: Adults with acquired complex communication needs. *Augmentative and Alternative Communication, 24*(3), 255-267.

Beukelman, D. R., & Cumley, G. (1992). Models and objectives for personnel preparation in the augmentative and alternative communication field. *Resource Papers of the Augmentative and Alternative Communication Intervention, Consensus Validation Conference of the National Institute on Disability and Rehabilitation Research,* 9-22.

Beukelman, D. R., Fager, S., Ball, L., & Dietz, A. (2007). AAC for adults with acquired neurological conditions: A review. *Augmentative and Alternative Communication, 23*(3), 230-242.

Beukelman, D.R, Fager, S., & Nordness, A. (2011). *Communication support for people with ALS.* Neurology Research International, Volume 2011, Article ID 714693.

Beukelman, D. R., & Garrett, K. (1988). Augmentative and alternative communication for adults with acquired severe communication disorders. *Augmentative and Alternative Communication, 4,* 104-121.

Beukelman, D. R., Garrett, K., & Yorkston, K. (2007). *Augmentative communication strategies for adults with acute or chronic medical conditions.* Paul H. Brookes Publishing Co.

Beukelman, D. R., Hux, K., Dietz, A., McKelvey, M., & Weissling, K. (2015). Using visual scene displays as communication support options for people with chronic, severe aphasia: A summary of the AAC research and future research directions. *Augmentative and Alternative Communication, 31*(3), 234-245.

Beukelman, D. R., Jones, R., & Rowan, M. (1989). Frequency of word usage by nondisabled peers in integrated preschool classrooms. *Augmentative and Alternative Communication, 5,* 243-248.

Beukelman, D. R., & Light, J. (2020). *Augmentative and alternative communication: Supporting children and adults with complex communication needs* (5th ed.). Paul H. Brookes Publishing Co.

Beukelman, D. R., McGinnis, J., & Morrow, D. (1991). Vocabulary selection in augmentative and alternative communication. *Augmentative and Alternative Communication, 7,* 171-185.

Beukelman, D. R., & Mirenda, P. (1992). *Augmentative and alternative communication: Management of severe communication disorders in children and adults.* Paul H. Brookes Publishing Co.

Beukelman, D. R., & Mirenda, P. (1998). *Augmentative and alternative communication: Management of severe communication disorders in children and adults* (2nd ed.). Paul H. Brookes Publishing Co.

Beukelman, D. R., & Mirenda, P. (2005). *Augmentative and alternative communication: Supporting children and adults with complex communication needs* (3rd ed.). Paul H. Brookes Publishing Co.

Beukelman, D. R., & Mirenda, P. (2013). *Augmentative and alternative communication: Supporting children and adults with complex communication needs* (4th ed.). Paul H. Brookes Publishing Co.

Beukelman, D. R., & Nordness, A. (2015). Inpatient and outpatient rehabilitation. In S. W. Blackstone, D. R. Beukelman, & K. M. Yorkston (Eds.), *Patient provider communication: Roles for SLPs and other health care professionals* (pp. 225-256). Plural Publishing.

Beukelman, D. R., & Ray, P. (2010). Communication supports in pediatric rehabilitation. *Journal of Pediatric Rehabilitation Medicine, 3*(4), 279-288.

Beukelman, D. R., & Yorkston, K. M. (1977). A communication system for the severely dysarthric speaker with an intact language system. *Journal of Speech and Hearing Disorders, 42,* 265-270.

Beukelman, D. R., Yorkston, K. M., & Dowden, P. (1985). *Communication augmentation: A casebook of clinical management.* Pro-Ed.

Beukelman, D. R., Yorkston, K. M., Poblete, M., & Naranjo, C. (1984). Frequency of word occurrence in communication samples produced by adult communication aid users. *Journal of Speech and Hearing Disorders, 49,* 360-367.

Bhatnagar, S. C. (2017). *Neuroscience for the study of communicative disorders* (5th ed.). Wolters Kluwer.

Bigge, J. L. (1982). *Teaching individuals with multiple disabilities* (2nd ed.). Charles E. Merrill.

Biggs, E. E., Carter, E. W., Bumble, J. L., Barnes, K., & Mazur, E. L. (2018). Enhancing peer network interventions for students with complex communication needs. *Exceptional Children, 85*(1), 66-85.

Bijou, S. W., Peterson, R. F., & Ault, M. H. (1968). A method to integrate descriptive and experimental field studies at the level of data and empirical concepts. *Journal of Applied Behavior Analysis, 1,* 175-191.

Biklen, D., Morton, M., Gold, D., Berrigan, C., & Swaminathan, S. (1992). Facilitated communication: Implications for individuals with autism. *Topics in Language Disorders, 12*(4), 1-28.

Binger, C. (2008). Grammatical morpheme intervention issues for students who use AAC. *Perspectives on Augmentative and Alternative Communication, 17,* 62-68.

Binger, C., Ball, L., Dietz, A., Kent-Walsh, J., Lasker, J., Lund, S., McKelvey, M., & Quach, W. (2012). Personnel roles in the AAC assessment process. *Augmentative and Alternative Communication, 28*(4), 278-288.

Binger, C., Kent-Walsh, J., Berens, J., Del Campo, S., & Rivera, D. (2008). Teaching Latino parents to support the multi-symbol message productions of their children who require AAC. *Augmentative and Alternative Communication, 24*(4), 323-338.

Binger, C., Kent-Walsh, J., Ewing, C., & Taylor, S. (2010). Teaching educational assistants to facilitate the multisymbol message productions of young students who require augmentative and alternative communication. *American Journal of Speech-Language Pathology, 19,* 108-120.

Binger, C., & Light, J. (2007). The effect of aided AAC modeling on the expression of multi-symbol messages by preschoolers who use AAC. *Augmentative and Alternative Communication, 23*(1), 30-43.

Binger, C., Maguire-Marshall, M., & Kent-Walsh, J. (2011). Using aided AAC models, recasts, and contrastive targets to teach grammatical morphemes to children who use AAC. *Journal of Speech, Language, and Hearing Research, 54,* 160-176.

Birch, E. E., & Bane, M. C. (1991). Forced-choice preferential looking acuity of children with cortical visual impairment. *Developmental Medicine and Child Neurology, 33,* 722-729.

Bird, F., Dores, P. A., Moniz, D., & Robinson, J. (1989). Reducing severe aggressive and self-injurious behaviors with functional communication training: Direct, collateral and generalized results. *American Journal on Mental Retardation, 94,* 37-48.

Bishop, K., Rankin, J., & Mirenda, P. (1994). Impact of graphic symbol use on reading acquisition. *Augmentative and Alternative Communication, 10,* 113-125.

Bishop, V. (1988). Making choices in functional vision evaluation: "Hoodles, needles, and haystacks." *Journal of Visual Impairment and Blindness, 82,* 94-99.

Blachman, B. A. (1991). Early intervention for children's reading problems: Clinical applications of the research in phonological awareness. *Topics in Language Disorders, 12*(1), 51-65.

Black, R., Waller, A., Turner, R., & Reiter, E. (2012). Supporting personal narratives for children with complex communication needs. *ACM Transactions on Computer-Human Interaction, 19*(2), 15.

Blackstone, S. W. (1999). Communication partners. *Augmentative Communication News, 12*(February), 1-16.

Blackstone, S. W. (2005). Vision and AAC. *Augmentative Communication Newsletter,* (4). Retrieved from www.augcominc.com/newsletters/index.cfm/newsletter_34.pd

Blackstone, S. W., Beukelman, D. R., & Yorkston, K. M. (2015). *Patient-provider communication: Roles for speech-language pathologists and other health care professionals.* Plural Publishing.

Blackstone, S. W., & Hunt-Berg, M. (2003). *Social networks: A communication inventory for individuals with complex communication needs and their communication partners.* Augmentative Communication Inc.

Blackstone, S. W., & Hunt-Berg, M. (2012). *Social networks: A communication inventory for individuals with complex communication needs and their communication partners* [assessment instrument]. Attainment Company.

Blackstone, S. W., Luo, F., Canchola, J., Wilkinson, K. M., & Roman-Lantzy, C. (2021). Children with cortical visual impairment and complex communication needs: Identifying gaps between needs and current practice. *Language, Speech, and Hearing Services in Schools, 52*(2), 612-629.

Blackstone, S. W., Williams, M., & Wilkins, D. (2007). Key principles underlying research and practice in AAC. *Augmentative and Alternative Communication, 23*(3), 191-203.

Blaha, R. (2001). *Calendars for students with multiple impairments including deafblindness.* Texas School for the Blind and Visually Impaired.

Blaikie, A. (2014). *Visual field confrontation.* Retrieved from https://optic-disc.org/visual-fields-examination

Blaiser, K. M., & Culbertson, D. S. (2013). Language and speech of the deaf and hard-of-hearing. In R. L. Schow & M. A. Nerbonne (Eds.), *Introduction to audiologic rehabilitation* (6th ed., pp. 211-238). Pearson.

Blake Huer, M. (1997). Culturally inclusive assessments for children using augmentative and alternative communication (AAC). *Journal of Children's Communication Development, 19*(1), 23-34.

Blake, D. J., & Bodine, C. (2002). An overview of assistive technology for persons with multiple sclerosis. *Journal of Rehabilitation Research and Development, 39*(2), 299-312.

Blieszner, R., Roberto, K., Wilcox, K., Barham, E., & Winston, B. (2007). Dimensions of ambiguous loss in couples coping with mild cognitive impairment. *Family Relations, 56*(April), 196-209.

Blishack, D. M. (1993, April). *AAC assessment.* Presentation at Howard University.

Blischak, D. M. (1994). Phonological awareness: Implications for individuals with little or no functional speech. *Augmentative and Alternative Communication, 10,* 245-254.

Blischak, D. M. (1995). Thomas the writer: Case study of a child with severe physical, speech, and visual impairments. *Language, Speech, and Hearing Services in Schools, 26,* 11-20.

Blischak, D. M. (2003). Use of speech-generating devices in support of natural speech. *Augmentative and Alternative Communication, 19,* 29-35.

Blischak, D. M., & Lloyd, L. L. (1996). Multimodal augmentative and alternative communication. *Augmentative and Alternative Communication, 12,* 37-46.

Blischak, D. M., & McDaniel, M. A. (1995). Effects of picture size and placement on memory for written words. *Journal of Speech and Hearing Research, 38,* 1-7.

Bliss, C. K. (1949). *Semantography.* Semantography Publications.

Bliss, C. K. (1965). *Semantography* (2nd ed.). Semantography Publications.

Bloomberg, K. (1984). *The comparative translucency of initial lexical items represented by five graphic symbol systems.* Unpublished master's thesis, Purdue University.

Bloomberg, K., Karlan, G. R., & Lloyd, L. L. (1990). The comparative translucency of initial lexical items represented by five graphic symbol systems. *Journal of Speech and Hearing Research, 33,* 717-725.

Bloomberg, K., West, D., Johnson, H., & Iacono, T. (2009). *Triple C manual and checklists, revised.* Victoria: SCOPE.

Blyden, A. E. (1989). Survival word acquisition in mentally retarded adolescents with multihandicaps: Effects of color-revised stimulus materials. *Journal of Special Education, 22,* 493-501.

Boenisch, J., & Sachse, S. K. (2007). Sprachförderung von Anfang an. *Unterstützte Kommunikation, 3,* 12-20.

Boenisch, J., & Soto, G. (2015). The oral core vocabulary of typically developing English-speaking school-aged children: Implications for AAC practice. *Augmentative and Alternative Communication, 31,* 77-84.

Boesch, M. C., Wendt, O., Subramanian, A., & Hsu, N. (2013). Comparative efficacy of the Picture Exchange Communication System (PECS) versus a speech-generating device: Effects on requesting skills. *Research in Autism Spectrum Disorders, 7,* 480-493.

Boisvert, M., Hall, N., Andrianopoulos, M., & Chaclas, J. (2012). The multi-faceted implementation of telepractice to service individuals with autism. *International Journal of Telerehabilitation, 4*(2), 11-24.

Bondy, A. S., & Frost, L. A. (1994). The Picture Exchange Communication System. *Focus on Autistic Behavior, 9*(3), 1-19.

Bonilla-Silva, E. (2009). *Racism without racists: Colorblind racism and the persistence of inequality in America.* Rowman & Littlefield.

Bonvillian, J. D., & Miller, A. J. (1995). Everything old is new again: Observations from the nineteenth century about sign communication training with mentally retarded children. *Sign Language Studies, 88*(1), 245-254.

Bonvillian, J. D., & Nelson, K. (1978). Development of sign language in autistic children and other language-handicapped individuals. In P. Siple (Ed.), *Understanding language through sign language research* (pp. 187-209). Academic Press.

Bonvillian, J. D., & Siedlecki, T. (1996). Young children's acquisition of the location aspect of American Sign Language signs: Parental report findings. *Journal of Communication Disorders, 29,* 13-35.

Bopp, K. D., Brown, K. E., & Mirenda, P. (2004). Speech-language pathologists' roles in the delivery of positive behavior support for individuals with developmental disabilities. *American Journal of Speech-Language Pathology, 13,* 5-19.

Bora, E., Velakoulis, D., & Walterfang, M. (2016). Social cognition in Huntington's disease: A meta-analysis. *Behavioral Brain Research, 297,* 131-140.

Borden, P.A., Berliss, J., & Vanderheiden, G. (1993). *Trace resource book: Assistive technologies for communication, control, and computer access* (1993-1994 ed.). Trace Resource and Development Center.

Borgestig, M., Sandqvist, J., Ahlsten, G., Falkmer, T., & Hemmingsson, H. (2017). Gaze-based assistive technology in daily activities in children with severe physical impairments: An intervention study. *Developmental Neurorehabilitation, 20*(3), 129-141.

Bornman, J. (2011). Low technology. In O. Wendt, R. W. Quist, & L. L. Lloyd (Eds.), *Assistive technology: Principles and applications for communication disorders and special education.* Emerald Press.

Bornman, J., Bryen, D. N., Moolman, E., & Morris, J. (2016). Use of consumer wireless devices by South Africans with severe communication disability. *African Journal of Disability, 5*(1), 1-9.

Bornstein, H. (1990). *Manual communication: Implications for education.* Gallaudet University Press.

Bornstein, H., & Jordan, I. K. (1984). *Functional signs: A new approach from simple to complex.* University Park Press.

Bornstein, H., & Saulnier, K. L. (1984). *Signed English: A basic guide.* Crown Publishers.

Boss, P. (1999). *Ambiguous loss: Learning to live with unresolved grief.* Harvard University Press.

Boss, P. (2010). The trauma and complicated grief of ambiguous loss. *Pastoral Psychology, 59,* 137-145.

Boss, P., & Couden, B. A. (2002). Ambiguous loss from chronic physical illness: Clinical interventions with individuals, couples, and families. *Journal of Clinical Psychology, 58,* 1351-1360.

Boulton, A. (2010). Data-driven learning: Taking the computer out of the equation. *Language Learning, 60,* 534-572.

Boulton, A. (2015). Applying data-driven learning to the web. In A. Lenko-Szymanska & A. Boulton (Eds.), *Multiple affordances of language corpora for data-driven learning* (pp. 267-295). John Benjamins.

Boulton, A., & Vyatkina, N. (2021). Thirty years of data-driven learning: Taking stock and charting new directions over time. *Language Learning & Technology, 25*(3), 66-89.

Bourgeois, M. S. (1992). Evaluating memory wallets in conversation with persons with dementia. *Journal of Speech and Hearing Research, 35*(6), 1344-1357.

Bourgeois, M. S. (1993). Effects of memory aids on the dyadic conversations of individuals with dementia. *Journal of Applied Behavior Analysis, 26*(1), 77-87.

Bourgeois, M. S. (1994). Teaching caregivers to use memory aids with patients with dementia. *Seminars in Speech and Language, 15,* 291-305.

Bourgeois, M. S. (2014). *Memory and communication aids for people with dementia.* Health Professions Press.

Bourgeois, M. S., Dijkstra, K., Burgio, L., & Allen-Burge, R. (2001). Memory aids as an augmentative and alternative communication strategy for nursing home residents with dementia. *Augmentative and Alternative Communication, 17*(3), 196-210.

Bowen, C. (2011). Brown's stages of syntactic and morphological development. Retrieved from www.speech-language-therapy.com/index.php?option=com_content&view=article&id=33

Bower, G. H., Clark, M. C., Lesgold, A. M., & Winzenz, D. (1969). Hierarchical retrieval schemes in recall of categorized word lists. *Journal of Verbal Learning and Verbal Behavior, 8,* 323-343.

Bowers, P., & Kirby, J. (2010). Effects of morphological instruction on vocabulary acquisition. *Reading and Writing, 23,* 515-537.

Boyd, L. H., Boyd, W. L., & Vanderheiden, G. C. (1990). The graphical user interface: Crisis, danger, and opportunity. *Journal of Visual Impairment and Blindness, 84,* 496-502.

Boyes-Braem, P. (1973). *A study of the acquisition of the DEZ in American Sign Language.* Unpublished paper, Salk Institute.

Braddock, B. (2015). Support organization for Trisomy 18, 13, and related disorders (SOFT) promotes interprofessional collaboration. *Perspectives on Augmentative and Alternative Communication, 24*(3), 63-66.

Braddock, B., McDaniel, J., Spragge, S., Loncke, F., Braddock, S., & Carey, J. C. (2012). Communication ability in persons with trisomy 18 and trisomy 13. *Augmentative and Alternative Communication, 28,* 266-277.

Brady, N. C., & Bashinski, S. M. (2008). Increasing communication in children with concurrent vision and hearing loss. *Research and Practice for Persons with Severe Disabilities, 33*(1-2), 59-70.

Brady, N. C., Bruce, S., Goldman, A., Erickson, K., Mineo, B., Ogletree, B. T., Paul, D., Romski, M. A., Sevcik, R., Siegel, E., Schoonover, J., Snell, M., Sylvester, L., & Wilkinson, K. (2016). Communication services and supports for individuals with severe disabilities: Guidance for assessment and intervention. *American Journal on Intellectual and Developmental Disabilities, 121*(2), 121-138.

Brady, N. C., Marquis, J., Fleming, K., & McLean, L. (2004). Prelinguistic predictors of language growth in children with developmental disabilities. *Journal of Speech, Language, and Hearing Research, 47,* 663-677.

Branson, D., & Demchak, M. (2009). The use of augmentative and alternative communication methods with infants and toddlers with disabilities: A research review. *Augmentative and Alternative Communication, 25,* 274-286.

Brennan, A., Worrall, L., & McKenna, K. (2005). The relationship between specific features of aphasia-friendly written material and comprehension of written material for people with aphasia. *Aphasiology, 19,* 693-711.

Brezina, V., & Gablasova, D. (2013). Is there a core general vocabulary? Introducing the new general service list. *Applied Linguistics, 36,* 1-22.

Bridges, S.J. (2004). Multicultural issues in augmentative and alternative communication and language. *Topics in Language Disorders, 24*(1), 62-75.

Briggs, T. R. (1983). *An investigation of the efficiency and effectiveness of three nonvocal communication systems with severely handicapped students.* Unpublished doctoral dissertation, Georgia State University.

Brock, K., Koul, R., Corwin, M., & Schlosser, R. (2017). A comparison of visual scene and grid displays for people with chronic aphasia: A pilot study to improve communication using AAC. *Aphasiology, 31*(11), 1282-1306.

Brock, K., & Thomas, E. (2021). The effectiveness of aided AAC modeling on Belizean children: A case study. *Perspective of the ASHA Special Interest Groups, 6,* 1182-1197.

Bronfenbrenner, U. (1979). *The ecology of human development: Experiments by nature and design.* Harvard University Press.

Brown, F. E., McDonnell, J. J., & Snell, M. E. (2020). *Instruction of students with severe disabilities: Meeting the needs of children and youth with intellectual disabilities, multiple disabilities, and autism spectrum disorders* (9th ed.). Pearson.

Brown, K. E., & Mirenda, P. (2006). Contingency mapping: Use of a novel visual support strategy as an adjunct to functional equivalence training. *Journal of Positive Behavior Interventions, 8,* 156-163.

Brown, R. (1973). *A first language: The early stages.* Harvard University Press.

Brown, R. (1977). Why are signed languages easier to learn than spoken languages? In W. C. Stokoe (Ed.), *National symposium on sign language research and teaching* (pp. 9-24). National Association of the Deaf.

Brown, R. (1978). Why are signed languages easier to learn than spoken languages?—Part two. *Bulletin of the American Academy of Arts and Sciences, 32*(3), 25-44.

Brownlee, A., & Bruening, L. (2012). Methods of communication at end of life for the person with ALS (PALS). *Topics in Language Disorders, 32,* 171-188.

Bruce, S. M. (2005). The application of Werner and Kaplan's "distancing" to children who are deaf-blind. *Journal of Visual Impairment and Blindness, 99,* 464–477.

Bruce, S. M., & Bashinski, S. M. (2017). The tri-focus framework and interprofessional collaborative practice in severe disabilities. *American Journal of Speech-Language Pathology, 26,* 162-180.

Bruce, S. M., Bashinski, S. M., Covelli, A. J., Bernstein, V., Zatta, M. C., & Briggs, S. (2018). Positive behavior supports for individuals who are deafbind with CHARGE syndrome. *Journal of Visual Impairment and Blindness, 112,* 497-508.

Bruce, S. M., Brum, C., & Nannemann, A. (2015). Communication programming implications for individuals with genetic causes of severe disability and visual impairment. *Perspectives on Augmentative and Alternative Communication, 24*(3), 94-105.

Bruce, S. M., Janssen, M. J., & Bashinski, S. M. (2016). Individualizing and personalizing communication and literacy instruction for children who are deafblind. *Journal of Deafblind Studies on Communication, 2*(1), 73-87.

Bruce, S. M., Randall, A., & Birge, B. (2008). Colby's growth to language and literacy: The achievements of a child who is congenitally deafblind. *TEACHING Exceptional Children Plus, 5*(2), Article 6. Retrieved [date] from https://eric.ed.gov/?id=EJ967739

Bruce, S. M., Trief, E., & Cascella, P. W. (2011). Teachers' and speech-language pathologists' perceptions of a tangible symbols intervention: Efficacy, generalization, and recommendations. *Augmentative and Alternative Communication, 27*, 172-182.

Bruno, J. (2017). *The test of aided-communication symbol performance: An AAC assessment tool.* Communication Technology Resources.

Bruno, J., & Trembath, D. (2006). Use of aided language stimulation to improve syntactic performance during a weeklong intervention program. *Augmentative and Alternative Communication, 22*(4), 300-313.

Bryen, D. N., Bornman, J., Morris, J., Moolman, E., & Sweatman, F. M. (2017). Use of mobile technology by adults who use AAC: Voices from two countries. *Assistive Technology Outcomes and Benefits, 11*, 66-81.

Buie, A. (2013). *Behavior mapping: A visual strategy for teaching appropriate behavior to individuals with autism spectrum and related disorders.* AAPC.

Bulwer, J. B. (1644). *The natural language of the hand.* R. Whitaker.

Burd, L., Hammes, K., Bornhoeft, D., & Fisher, W. (1988). A North Dakota prevalence study of nonverbal school-age children. *Language, Speech, and Hearing Services in Schools, 19*, 371-383.

Burkhart, L., & Porter, G. (2006). Partner-assisted communication strategies for students who face multiple challenges. Retrieved from http://www.lburkhart.com/handouts.htm

Burns, C., Ward, E., Hill, A., Phillips, N., & Porter, L. (2016). Conducting real-time videofluoroscopic swallow study via telepractice: A preliminary feasibility and reliability study. *Dysphagia, 31*, 473-483.

Burroughs, J., Albritton, E., Eaton, B., & Montague, J. (1990). A comparative study of language delayed preschool children's ability to recall symbols from two symbol systems. *Augmentative and Alternative Communication, 6*, 202-206.

Byers, V. W., & Bristow, D. C. (1990). Audiologic evaluation of nonspeaking, physically challenged populations. *Ear and Hearing, 11*, 382-386.

Caesar, L. G., & Kohler, P. D. (2007). The state of school-based bilingual assessment: Actual practice versus recommended guidelines. *Language, Speech, and Hearing Services in Schools, 38*, 190-200.

Calculator, S. N. (2002). Use of enhanced natural gestures to foster interactions between children with Angelman syndrome and their parents. *American Journal of Speech-Language Pathology, 11*, 3340-3355.

Calculator, S. N. (2009). Augmentative and alternative communication (AAC) and inclusive education for students with the most severe disabilities. *International Journal of Inclusive Education, 13*(1), 93-113.

Calculator, S. N. (2015). AAC considerations for individuals with Angelman syndrome. *Perspectives on Augmentative and Alternative Communication, 24*(3), 106-113.

Calculator, S. N., & Diaz-Caneja Sela, P. (2014). Overview of the enhanced natural gestures instructional approach and illustration of its use with three students with Angelman syndrome. *Journal of Applied Research in Intellectual Disabilities, 28*, 145-158.

Campbell, A., & Lloyd, L. L. (1986, May). *Graphic symbols and symbol systems: What research and clinical practice tell us.* Paper presented at the Conference of the American Association on Mental Deficiency.

Campbell, R., Dodd, B., & Burnham, D. (Eds.). (1998). *Hearing by eye II: Advances in the psychology of speechreading and auditory-visual speech.* Psychology Press.

Canale, M. (1983). From communicative competence to communicative language pedagogy. In J. C. Richards & R. W. Schmidt (Eds.), *Language and communication* (pp. 2-27). Longman.

Cannella-Malone, H. I., DeBar, R. M., & Sigafoos, J. (2009). An examination of preference for augmentative and alternative communication devices with two boys with significant intellectual disabilities. *Augmentative and Alternative Communication, 25*, 262-273.

Cantrell, R. J., Fusaro, J. A., & Dougherty, E. A. (2000). Exploring the effectiveness of journal writing on learning social studies: A comparative study. *Reading Psychology, 21*(1), 1-11.

Cantwell, D. P., Baker, L., & Mattison, R. E. (1980). Psychiatric disorders in children with speech and language retardation. *Archives of General Psychiatry, 37*, 423-426.

Carlson, F. (1981). A format for selecting vocabulary for the nonspeaking child. *Language, Speech, and Hearing Services in Schools, 12*, 240-245.

Carlson, F. (1985). *PICSYMS categorical dictionary.* Baggeboda Press.

Carlson, F., & James, C. A. (1980). *PICSYMS symbol system.* Unpublished paper, Meyer Children's Rehabilitation Institute of the University of Nebraska Medical Center.

Carlson, F., & Kovarik, A. M. (1985, November). *Developmental comprehension of PICSYMS, an augmentative communication symbol system.* Paper presented at the Annual Convention of the American Speech-Language-Hearing Association.

Caron, J. G. (2015). "We bought an iPad": Considering family priorities, needs, and preferences as an AAC support provider. *Perspectives on Augmentative and Alternative Communication, 24*, 5-11.

Caron, J. G., Costello, J., & Shane, H. (2014, July). *Mobile devices and app selection: Who's driving the decision process?* Mini-seminar presented at the 2014 Biennial Meeting of the International Society for Augmentative and Alternative Communication.

Caron, J. G., Light, J., & Drager, K. (2016). Operational demands of AAC mobile technology applications on programming vocabulary and engagement during professional and child interactions. *Augmentative and Alternative Communication, 32*(1), 12-24.

Caron, J. G., Light, J., & McNaughton, D. (2020). Effects of an AAC app with transition to literacy features on single-word reading of individuals with complex communication needs. *Research and Practice for Persons with Severe Disabilities, 45*(2), 115-131.

Carr, E. G. (1988). Functional equivalence as a means of response generalization. In R. H. Homer, G. Dunlap, & R. L. Koegel (Eds.), *Generalization and maintenance: Life style changes in applied settings* (pp. 221-241). Paul H. Brookes Publishing Co.

Carr, E. G., Binkoff, J., Kologinsky, E., & Eddy, M. (1978). Acquisition of sign language by autistic children: I. Expressive labeling. *Journal of Applied Behavior Analysis, 11*, 459-501.

Carr, E. G., & Durand, V. M. (1985a). Reducing behavior problems through functional communication training. *Journal of Applied Behavior Analysis, 18*, 111-126.

Carr, E. G., & Durand, V. M. (1985b). The social-communicative basis of severe behavior problems in children. In S. Reiss & R. R. Bootzin (Eds.), *Theoretical issues in behavior therapy* (pp. 219-254). Academic Press.

Carr, E. G., Levin, L., McConnachie, G., Carlson, J. I., Kemp, D. C. , & Smith, C. E. (1994). *Communication-based intervention for problem behavior: A user's guide for producing positive change.* Paul H. Brookes Publishing Co.

Carter, C. K., & Hartley C. (2021). Are children with autism more likely to retain object names when learning from color photographs or black-and-white cartoons? *Journal of Autism and Developmental Disorders, 51*(9), 3050-3062.

Caselli, M. C., Rinaldi, P., Stefanini, S., & Volterra, V. (2012). Early action and gesture "vocabulary" and its relation with word comprehension and production. *Child Development, 83*, 526-542.

Cason, J., & Cohn, E. (2014). Telepractice: An overview and best practices. *Perspectives on Augmentative and Alternative Communication, 23*(1), 4-17.

Catania, A. C., Harnad, S. R., & Skinner, B. F. (1988). *The selection of behavior: The operant behaviorism of B. F. Skinner: Comments and consequences.* Cambridge University Press.

Caulfield, M. B., Fischel, J., DeBarshye, B. D., & Whitehurst, G. J. (1989). Behavioral correlates of developmental expressive language disorders. *Journal of Abnormal Child Psychology, 17*, 187-201.

Caves, K., Shane, H. C., & DeRuyter, F. (2002). Connecting AAC devices to the world of information technology. *Assistive Technology, 14*(1), 81-89.

Centers for Disease Control and Prevention. (2018). Cytomegalovirus (CMV) and congenital CMV infection. Retrieved from https://www.cdc.gov/cmv/congenital-infection.html

Centers for Medicare and Medicaid Services. (2014). Speech-generating devices. Retrieved from https://www.cms.gov/medicare-coverage-database/details/medicare-coverage-document-details.aspx?MCDId=26#Top

Cereda, A., & Carey, J. C. (2012). The trisomy 18 syndrome. *Orphanet Journal of Rare Diseases, 7*(81), 1-14.

Chairdex. (n.d.). Types of wheelchairs. Retrieved from http://www.chairdex.com/types.htm

Chalifoux, L. M. (1991). Macular degeneration: An overview. *Journal of Visual Impairment and Blindness, 85,* 249-252.

Chall, J. S. (1983). *Stages of reading development.* McGraw-Hill.

Chandler, D. (2002). *Semiotics: The basics.* Routledge.

Chang, M. Y., & Borchert, M. S. (2020). Advances in the evaluation and management of cortical/cerebral visual impairment in children. *Survey of Ophthalmology, 65*(6), 708-724.

Chao, T. K., Hu, J., & Pringsheim, T. (2017). Risk factors for the onset and progression of Huntington disease. *Neurotoxicology, 61,* 79-99.

Chapin, S. E., McNaughton, D., Light, J. C., McCoy, A., & Caron, J. (2018, July). *Effects of video visual scene display technology on the symbolic communicative turns taken by preschoolers with ASD during a shared activity.* Paper presented at the Annual Conference of the Rehabilitation Engineering and Assistive Technology Society of North America (RESNA).

Chapman, B. L. M. (1982). Computer assisted teaching of communication to handicapped users project. In *Research unit handbook.* Research Unit, School of Education, University of Bristol, England.

Chapman, R., & Miller, J. (1980). Analyzing language and communication in the child. In R. L. Schiefelbusch (Ed.), *Nonspeech language and communication: Acquisition and intervention* (pp. 159-196). University Park Press.

CHARGE Syndrome Foundation. (2019). Overview. Retrieved from https://www.chargesyndrome.org/about-charge/overview/

CHARGE Syndrome Foundation. (2022). CHARGE syndrome fact sheet. Retrieved from https://www.chargesyndrome.org/wp-content/uploads/2016/03/4-Fact-Sheet.pdf

Chaudhuri, A., & Behan, P. (2004). Fatigue in neurological disorders. *Lancet Neurology, 363,* 978-988.

Chaudhuri, K., Healy, D., & Schapira, A. (2006). Non-motor symptoms of Parkinson's disease: Diagnosis and management. *Lancet Neurology, 5,* 235-245.

Chaves, T., & Solar, J. (1974). Pedro Ponce de Leon: First teacher of the deaf. *Sign Language Studies, 5,* 48-63.

Chazin, K. T., & Ledford, J. R. (2016). Multiple stimulus without replacement (MSWO) preference assessment. In *Evidence-based instructional practices for young children with autism and other disabilities.* Retrieved from https://ebip.vkcsites.org/multiple-stimulus-without-replacement/

Checchetto, A., Geraci, C., Cecchetto, C., & Zucchi, S. (2018). The language instinct in extreme circumstances: The transition to tactile Italian Sign Language (LISt) by Deafblind signers. *Glossa: A Journal of General Linguistics, 3*(1), 1-28.

Chen, D., & Downing, J. E. (2006). *Tactile strategies for children who have visual impairments and multiple disabilities: Promoting communication and learning skills.* AFB Press.

Chen, D., Downing, J. E., Minor, L., & Rodriguez-Gil, G. (2005a). Successful adaptations for learning to use touch effectively: Interaction with children who are deaf-blind or visually impaired and have additional disabilities. California State University, Department of Special Education. Retrieved from http://projectsalute.net

Chen, D., Downing, J. E., Minor, L., & Rodriguez-Gil, G. (2005b). Successful adaptations for learning to use touch effectively: Interaction with children who are deaf-blind or visually impaired and have additional disabilities: Object cue. California State University, Department of Special Education. Retrieved from http://www.projectsalute.net/Learned/Learnedhtml/ObjectCue.html

Chen, D., Downing, J. E., Minor, L., & Rodriguez-Gil, G. (2005c). Successful adaptations for learning to use touch effectively: Interaction with children who are deaf-blind or visually impaired and have additional disabilities: Tangible symbols. California State University, Department of Special Education. Retrieved from http://www.projectsalute.net/Learned/Learnedhtml/TangibleSymbols.html

Chen, D., Downing, J. E., Minor, L., & Rodriguez-Gil, G. (2005d). Successful adaptations for learning to use touch effectively: Interaction with children who are deaf-blind or visually impaired and have additional disabilities: Touch cue. California State University, Department of Special Education. Retrieved from http://www.projectsalute.net/Learned/Learnedhtml/TouchCue.html

Chen, D., & Smith, J. (1992). Developing orientation and mobility skills in students who are multihandicapped and visually impaired. *Review, 24,* 133-139.

Cheok, M. J., Omar, Z., & Jaward, M. H. (2017). A review of hand gesture and sign language recognition techniques. *International Journal of Machine Learning and Cybernetics, 10*(1), 131-153.

Cherney, L., & van Vuuren, S. (2012). Telerehabilitation, virtual therapists, and acquired neurologic speech and language disorders. *Seminars in Speech and Language, 33*(3), 243-257.

Chiaravalloti, N., & DeLuca, J. (2008). Cognitive impairment in multiple sclerosis. *Lancet Neurology, 7,* 1139-1151.

Childes, J. M., Palmer, A. D., Fried-Oken, M., & Graville, D. J. (2017). The use of technology for phone and face-to-face communication after total laryngectomy. *American Journal of Speech-Language Pathology, 26,* 99-112.

Childhood Hearing Screening. (n.d.). Retrieved from https://www.asha.org/PRPSpecificTopic.aspx?folderid=8589935406&section=Key_Issues

Chiò, A., Vignola, A., Mastro, E., Dei Giudici, A., Iazzolino, B., Calvo, A., Moglia, C., & Montuschi, A. (2010). Neurobehavioral symptoms in ALS are negatively related to caregivers' burden and quality of life. *European Journal of Neurology, 17,* 1298-1303.

Chiou, H., & Kennedy, M. (2009). Switching in adults with aphasia. *Aphasiology, 23*(7), 1065-1075.

Cho Lieu, J. E. (2004). Speech-language and educational consequences of unilateral hearing loss in children. *Archives of Otolaryngology-Head and Neck Surgery, 130*(5), 524-530.

Chomsky, N. (1965). *Aspects of the theory of syntax.* MIT Press.

Christensen, D. L., Van Naarden Braun, K., Baio, J., Bilder, D., Charles, J., Constantino, J. N., Daniels, J., Durkin, M. S., Fitzgerald, R. T., Kurzius-Spencer, M., Lee, L., Pettygrove, S., Robinson, C., Schulz, E., Wells, C., Wingate, M. S., Zahorodny, W., & Yeargin-Allsopp, M. (2018). Prevalence and characteristics of autism spectrum disorder among children aged 8 years—Autism and developmental disabilities monitoring network, 11 sites, United States, 2012. *Morbidity and Mortality Weekly Report Surveillance Summaries, 65*(13), 1.

Chujo, K., Oghigian, K., Anthony, L., & Yokota, K. (2013). Teaching remedial grammar through data-driven learning using AntPConc. *Taiwan International ESP Journal, 5*(2), 65-89.

Chung, Y., Carter, E. W., & Sisco, L. G. (2012). Social interactions of students with disabilities who use augmentative and alternative communication in inclusive classrooms. *American Journal on Intellectual and Developmental Disabilities, 117*(5), 349-367.

Chung, Y., & Stoner, J. B. (2016). A meta-synthesis of team members' voices: What we need and what we do to support students who use AAC. *Perspectives on Augmentative and Alternative Communication, 32,* 175-186.

Church, G., & Glennen, S. (1992). *The handbook of assistive technology.* Singular Publishing Group.

Churchman, C. W., & Churchman, C. W. (1968). *The systems approach* (Vol. 1, p. 984). Dell.

City Ergonomics. (2018). DXT ergonomic wireless mouse 2. Retrieved from http://www.ergocanada.com/detailed_specification_pages/city_ergonomics_dxt_ergonomic_wireless_mouse_2.html

Clark, C. R. (1977). *Research report #107: A comparative study of young children's ease of learning words represented in the graphic systems of Rebus, Bliss, Carrier-Peak, and traditional orthography.* Unpublished manuscript, Research, Development and Demonstration Center in Education of Handicapped Children.

Clark, C. R. (1981). Learning words using traditional orthography and the symbols of Rebus, Bliss, and Carrier. *Journal of Speech and Hearing Disorders, 46,* 191-196.

Clark, C. R. (1984). A close look at the standard rebus system and Blissymbolics. *Journal of the Association for Persons with Severe Handicaps, 9,* 37-48.

Clark, C. R., Davies, C. O. & Woodcock, R. W. (1974). *Standard rebus glossary.* American Guidance Service.

Clark, C. R., & Woodcock, R. W. (1976). Graphic systems of communication. In L. L. Lloyd (Ed.), *Communication assessment and intervention strategies* (pp. 549-605). University Park Press.

Clarke, V. (2016). Is AAC feature matching still relevant? Retrieved from http://praacticalaac.org/praactical/aac-assessment-corner-by-vicki-clarke-is-aac-feature-matching-still-relevant/

Classen, D. C., Resar, R., Griffin, F., Federico, F., Frankel, T., Kimmel, N., Whittington, J. C., Frankel, A., Seger, A., James, B. C. (2011). "Global Trigger Tool" shows that adverse events in hospitals may be ten times greater than previously measured. *Health Affairs, 30*(4), 581-589.

Clay, M. M. (1991). *Becoming literate.* Heinemann Educational Books Limited.

Cleave, P. L., & Fey, M. E. (1997). Two approaches to the facilitation of grammar in children with language impairments: Rationale and description. *American Journal of Speech-Language Pathology, 6*(1), 22-32.

Clendon, S. A., & Erickson, K. A. (2008). The vocabulary of beginning writers: Implications for children with complex communication needs. *Augmentative and Alternative Communication, 24,* 281-293.

Clendon, S. A., Sturm, J. M., & Cali, K. S. (2003, November). *The vocabularies of beginning writers: Implications for students who use AAC.* Paper presented at the American Speech-Language-Hearing Association Convention.

Clendon, S. A., Sturm, J. M., & Cali, K. S. (2013). Vocabulary use across genres: Implications for students with complex communication needs. *Language, Speech, and Hearing Services in Schools, 44,* 61-72.

Cline, D., Hofstetter, H. W., & Griffin, J. (1997). *Dictionary of visual science* (4th ed.). Butterworth-Heinemann.

Coelho, C. A. (2007). Management of discourse deficits following traumatic brain injury: Progress, caveats, and needs. *Seminars in Speech and Language, 28,* 122-135.

Cohen, A. L., Rivara, F., Marcuse, E. K., McPhillips, H., & Davis, R. (2005). Are language barriers associated with serious medical events in hospitalized pediatric patients? *Pediatrics, 116*(3), 575-579.

Cohen, E. T., Allgood, M., Heller, K. W., & Castelle, M. (2001). Use of picture dictionaries to promote written communication by students with hearing and cognitive impairments. *Augmentative and Alternative Communication, 17*(4), 245-254.

Cohen, K. J., & Light, J. C. (2000). Use of electronic communication to develop mentor-protégé relationships between adolescent and adult AAC users: Pilot study. *Augmentative and Alternative Communication, 16*(4), 227-238.

Cohut, M. (2018). Hugs and kisses: The health impact of affective touch. *MedicalNewsToday.* Retrieved from https://www.medicalnewstoday.com/articles/323143.php

Cole, E. B., & Flexer, C. (2016). *Children with hearing loss: Developing listening and talking- Birth to six* (3rd ed.). Plural Publishing.

Coleman, C. I., & Meyers, L. (1991). Computer recognition of the speech of adults with cerebral palsy and dysarthria. *Augmentative and Alternative Communication, 7,* 34-43.

Collaboration and Teaming. (n.d.). Retrieved from https://www.asha.org/Practice-Portal/Clinical-Topics/Intellectual-Disability/Collaboration-and-Teaming/

Committee on Children with Disabilities. (1992). Pediatrician's role in the development and implementation of an individual education plan (IEP) and/or an individual family service plan (IFSP). *Pediatrics, 89*(2), 340-342.

Conlon, C., & McNeil, M. (1991). The efficacy of treatment for two globally aphasic adults using visual action therapy. In T. Prescott (Ed.), *Clinical aphasiology* (Vol. 19, pp. 185-195). Pro-Ed.

Constantinescu, G. A., Theodoros, D. G., Russell, T. G., Ward, E. C., Wilson, S. J., & Wootton, R. (2010). Home-based speech treatment for Parkinson's disease delivered remotely: A case report. *Journal of Telemedicine and Telecare, 16,* 100-104.

Cook, A. M. (2011). It's not about the technology, or is it? Realizing AAC through hard and soft technologies. *Perspectives on Augmentative and Alternative Communication, 20,* 64-68.

Cook, A. M., & Hussey, S. M. (1995). *Assistive technologies: Principles and practice.* Mosby Elsevier.

Cook, A. M, & Polgar, J. M. (2015). *Cook and Hussey's assistive technologies: Principles and practice* (4th ed.). Elsevier Health Sciences.

Cooper, J. O., Heron, T. E., & Herward W. L. (2007). *Applied behavior analysis* (2nd ed.). Pearson.

Cooper, R., & Fuller, D. R. (1994). *Differences in preschool children's learning of black-on-white versus white-on-black graphic symbols.* Unpublished manuscript, University of Arkansas at Little Rock/University of Arkansas for Medical Sciences.

Copeland, K. (1974). *Aids for the severely handicapped.* Grune & Stratton.

Cornett, R. O. (1967). Cued speech. *American Annals of the Deaf, 112,* 3-13.

Corrington, R. S. (1993). *An introduction to C.S. Peirce philosopher, semiotician, and ecstatic naturalist.* Rowman & Littlefield.

Corwin, M., & Koul, R. K. (2003). Efficacy of AAC intervention in individuals with chronic severe aphasia: An evidence-based practice process illustration. *Perspectives on Augmentative and Alternative Communication, 12*(4), 11-15.

Costello, J. M. (2000). AAC intervention in the intensive care unit: The Children's Hospital Boston model. *Augmentative and Alternative Communication, 16*(3), 137-153.

Costello, J. M. (Producer). (2014). *Boston Children's Hospital message banking examples from people with ALS.* Boston Children's Hospital.

Costello, J. M., Patak, L., & Pritchard, J. (2010). Communication vulnerable patients in the pediatric ICU: Enhancing care through augmentative and alternative communication. *Journal of Pediatric Rehabilitation Medicine, 3*(4), 289-301.

Costello, J. M., Santiago, R. M., & Blackstone, S. W. (2015). Pediatric acute and intensive care in hospitals. In S. Blackstone, D.R. Beukelman, & K. Yorkston (Eds.), *Patient provider communication in health care settings: Roles for speech-language pathologists and other professionals.* Plural Publishing.

Costello, J. M., & Shane, H. C. (1994, November). *Augmentative communication assessment and the feature matching process.* Presentation at the Annual Convention of the American Speech-Language-Hearing Association.

Costigan, F. A., & Light, J. (2010a). A review of preservice training in augmentative and alternative communication for speech-language pathologists, special education teachers, and occupational therapists. *Assistive Technology, 22,* 210-212.

Costigan, F. A., & Light, J. (2010b). Effect of seated position on upper-extremity access to augmentative communication for children with cerebral palsy: Preliminary investigation. *The American Journal of Occupational Therapy, 64*(4), 596-604.

Cotter, J., Firth, J., Enzinger, C., Kontopantelis, E., Yung, A. R., Elliott, R., & Drake, R. J. (2016). Social cognition in multiple sclerosis: A systematic review and meta-analysis. *Neurology, 87,* 1727-1736.

Council for Exceptional Children (CEC). (2015). *What every special educator must know: Professional ethics and standards.* Author.

Cowan, R. J. & Allen, K. D. (2007). Using naturalistic procedures to enhance learning in individuals with autism: A focus on generalized teaching within the school setting. *Psychology in the Schools, 44,* 701-715.

Coyle, J. (2012). Tele-dysphagia management: An opportunity for prevention, cost-savings and advanced training. *International Journal of Telerehabilitation, 4*(1), 37-40.

Craddock, D., O'Halloran, C., Borthwick, A., & McPherson, K. (2006). Interprofessional education in health and social care: Fashion or informed practice? *Learning in Health and Social Care, 5,* 220-242.

Crais, E. R., Douglas, D., & Campbell, C. (2004). The intersection of the development of gestures and intentionality. *Journal of Speech, Language, and Hearing Research, 47,* 678-694.

Crais, E. R., Watson, L. R., & Baranek, G. T. (2009). Use of gesture development in profiling children's prelinguistic communication skills. *American Journal of Speech-Language Pathology, 18,* 95-108.

Creech, R. (1992). *Reflections from a unicorn.* R.C. Publishing.

Creer, S., Cunningham, S., Green, P., & Yamagishi, J. (2013). Building personalized synthetic voices for individuals with severe speech impairment. *Computer Speech and Language, 27,* 1178-1193.

Creer, S., Enderby, P. Judge, S., & John, A. (2016). Prevalence of people who could benefit from augmentative and alternative communication (AAC) in the UK: Determining the need. *International Journal of Communication Disorders, 51*(6), 639-653.

Cregan, A. (1982). *Sigsymbol dictionary.* Author.

Cregan, A. (1993). Sigsymbol system in a multimodal approach to speech elicitation: Classroom project involving an adolescent with severe mental retardation. *Augmentative and Alternative Communication, 9,* 146-160.

Cregan, A., & Lloyd, L. L. (1990). *Sigsymbols: American edition.* Don Johnston Developmental Equipment, Inc.

Crema, C. (2009). Augmentative and alternative communication in the geriatric population: A review of literature. *Perspectives on Gerontology, 14*(2), 42-46.

Cress, C., Arens, K. B., & Zajicek, A. K. (2007). Comparison of engagement patterns of young children with developmental disabilities between structured and free play. *Education and Training in Developmental Disabilities, 42,* 152-164.

Cress, C., & French, G. J. (1994). The relationship between cognitive load measurements and estimates of computer input control skills. *Assistive Technology, 6,* 54-66.

Cress, C., & Goltz, C. (1989). Cognitive factors affecting accessibility of computers and electronic devices. In *Proceedings of the 12th annual RESNA conference* (pp. 25-26). RESNA.

Cress, C., & Marvin, C. (2003). Common questions about AAC services in early intervention. *Augmentative and Alternative Communication, 19,* 254-272.

Cress, P. J., Spellman, C. R., DeBriere, T. J., Sizemore, A. C., Northam, J. K., & Johnson, J. L. (1981). Vision screening for persons with severe handicaps. *Journal of the Association for the Severely Handicapped, 6,* 41-50.

Crestani, C. A. M., Clendon, S. A., & Hemsley, B. (2010). Words needed for sharing a story: Implications for vocabulary selection in augmentative and alternative communication. *Journal of Intellectual and Developmental Disability, 35,* 268-278.

Cross, R. T. (2010). Developing evidence-based clinical resources. In H. Roddam & J. Skeat (Eds.), *Embedding evidence-based practice in speech and language therapy* (pp. 114-121). John Wiley & Sons, Ltd.

Cross, R. T. (2015, July). *Using corpora in the field of augmentative and alternative communication (AAC) to provide visual representations of vocabulary use by non-speaking individuals.* Paper presented at the 8th International Corpus Linguistics Conference, Lancaster University.

Cross, R. T., Baker, B. R., Klotz, L. S, & Badman, A. L. (1997). Static and dynamic keyboards: Semantic compaction in both worlds. Proceedings of the 18th Annual Southeast Augmentative Communication Conference (pp. 9-17). SEAC Publications.

Crossley, R., & Remington-Gurney, J. (1992). Getting the words out: Facilitated communication training. *Topics in Language Disorders, 12*(4), 29-45.

Culbertson, D. S. (2007). Language and speech of the deaf and hard-of-hearing. In R. L. Schow & M. A. Nerbonne (Eds.), *Introduction to audiologic rehabilitation* (5th ed.). Pearson.

Cunningham, L. L., & Tucci, D. L. (2017). Hearing loss in adults. *The New England Journal of Medicine, 377,* 2465-2473.

Cutson, T. M., & Bongiorni, D. R. (1996). Rehabilitation of the older lower limb amputee: A brief review. *Journal of the American Geriatrics Society, 44*(11), 1388-1393.

da Costa Monsanto, R., Bittencourt, A. G., Neto, N. J. B., Beilke, S. C. A., de Lima, N. F. G., Lorenzetti, F. T. M., & Salomone, R. (2014). Auditory brainstem implants in children: Results based on a review of the literature. *Journal of International Advanced Otology, 10*(3), 284-290.

Dammeyer, J. (2012). Development and characteristics of children with Usher syndrome and CHARGE syndrome. *International Journal of Pediatric Otorhinolaryngology, 76,* 1292-1296.

Dandashi, A., Karkar, A. G., Saad. S., Barhoumi. Z., Al-Jaam, J. & El Saddik, A. (2015). Enhancing the cognitive and learning skills of children with intellectual disability through physical activity and edutainment games. *International Journal of Distributed Sensor Networks, 2015,* Article ID 165165.

Daniloff, J., & Vergara, D. (1984). Comparison between the motoric constraints for Amer-Ind and ASL sign formation. *Journal of Speech and Hearing Research, 27,* 76-88.

Dara, C., Monetta, L., & Pell, M. D. (2008). Vocal emotion processing in Parkinson's disease: Reduced sensitivity to negative emotions. *Brain Research, 1188,* 100-111.

Daumuller, M., Bogenhausen, K., & Goldenberg, G. (2010). Therapy to improve gestural expression in aphasia: A controlled clinical trial. *Clinical Rehabilitation, 24,* 55-65.

Davidson, K., & Hettenhausen, A. (2016). *Using automated data logging to track progress and plan intervention: A case study.* Paper presented at the 2016 ISAAC Biennial Conference.

Davies, M. (2008). The corpus of contemporary American English: 425 million words, 1990-present. Available from Brigham Young University, The Corpus of Contemporary America English. Retrieved from http://corpus.byu.edu/coca

Davies, M. (2013a). Corpus of global web-based English: 1.9 billion words from speakers in 20 countries (GloWbE). Retrieved from https://corpus.byu.edu/glowbe/

Davies, M. (2013b). Corpus of news on the web (NOW): 3+ billion words from 20 countries, updated every day. Retrived from https://english-corpora.org/now

Davies, M. (2016). Corpus of newspapers on the web: 2.8+ billion words from speakers in 20 countries. Retrieved from http://corpus.byu.edu/now/

Davies, M. (2018). English-corpora.org. Retrieved from https://www.english-corpora.org/

Davis, P., Lay-Yee, R., Briant, R., Ali, W., Scott, A., & Schug, S. (2002). Adverse events in New Zealand public hospitals I: Occurrence and impact. *New Zealand Medical Journal, 115*(1167), 1-9.

Davis, T. N., Barnard-Brak, L., Dacus, S., & Pond, A. (2010). Aided AAC systems among individuals with hearing loss and disabilities. *Journal of Developmental and Physical Disabilities, 22*(3), 241-256.

Dawson, G., Rogers, S., Munson, J., Smith, M., Winter, J., Greenson, J., Donaldson, A., & Varley, J. (2010). Randomized, controlled trial of an intervention for toddlers with autism: The Early Start Denver Model. *Pediatrics, 125*(1), e17-e23.

Day, R. M., Johnson, W. L., & Schussler, N. G. (1986). Determining the communicative properties of self-injury: Research, assessment, and treatment implications. In K. D. Gadow (Ed), *Advances in learning and behavioral disabilities* (Vol. 5, pp. 117-139). JAI Press.

de Andrade Figueiredo, M. Z., Chiari, B. M., & de Goulart, B. N. G. (2013). Communication in deafblind adults with Usher syndrome: Retrospective observational study. *CoDAS, 25,* 319-324.

Deckers, S. R. J. M., Van Zaalen, Y., van Balkom, H., & Verhoeven, L. (2017). Core vocabulary of young children with Down syndrome. *Augmentative and Alternative Communication, 33,* 77-86.

de Lamo White, C., & Jin, L. (2011). Evaluation of speech and language assessment approaches with bilingual children. *International Journal of Language and Communication Disorders, 46*(6), 613-627.

Desrochers, M., & Fallon M. (2014). *Instruction in functional assessment.* SUNY Textbooks.

de Valenzuela, J. S., Bird, E. K. R., Parkington, K., Mirenda, P., Cain, K., MacLeod, A. A., & Segers, E. (2016). Access to opportunities for bilingualism for individuals with developmental disabilities: Key informant interviews. *Journal of Communication Disorders, 63,* 32-46.

de Vries, E. N., Ramrattan, M. A., Smorenburg, S. M., Gouma, D. J., & Boermeestert, M. A. (2008). The incidence and nature of in-hospital adverse events: A systematic review. *Quality and Safety in Health Care, 17,* 216-223.

DeCarlo, J., Bean, A., Lyle, S., & Paden Miller Cargill, L. (2019). The relationship between operational competency, buy-in, and augmentative and alternative communication use in school-age children with autism. *American Journal of Speech-Language Pathology, 28*(2), 469-484.

Dekker, R., & Koole, F. D (1992). Visually impaired children's visual characteristics and intelligence. *Developmental Medicine and Child Neurology, 34,* 123-133.

DeKlerk, H. M., Dada, S., & Alant, E. (2014). Children's identification of graphic symbols representing four basic emotions: Comparison of Afrikaans-speaking and Sepedi-speaking children. *Journal of Communication Disorders, 52,* 1-15.

Demasco, P. (1994). Human factors consideration in the design of language interfaces in AAC. *Assistive Technology, 6,* 10-25.

Dennis, R., Reichle, J., Williams, W., & Vogelsberg, R. T. (1982). Motor factors influencing the selection of vocabulary for sign production programs. *Journal of the Association for the Severely Handicapped, 7,* 20-32.

DeRuyter, F., McNaughton, D., Caves, K., Bryen, D. N., & Williams, M. B. (2007). Enhancing AAC connections with the world. *Augmentative and Alternative Communication, 23*(3), 258-270.

Devereux, K., & van Oosterom, J. (1984). *Learning with rebuses.* National Council for Special Education (Developing Horizons in Special Education Series, No. 8).

Dicianno, B. E., Lieberman, J., Schmeler, M. R., Schuler, A. E., Cooper, R., Lange, M., & Jan, Y. (2015). RESNA position on the application of tilt, recline and elevating legrests for wheelchair literature update. *Assistive Technology, 21*(1), 13-22.

Di Filippo, M., Portaccio, E., Mancini, A., & Calabresi, P. (2018). Multiple sclerosis and cognition: Synaptic failure and network dysfunction. *Nature Reviews Neuroscience, 19*(October), 599-609.

Diehl, S., & de Riesthal, M. (2019). Augmentative and alternative communication use by individuals with Huntington's disease: Benefits and challenges of implementation. *Perspectives of the ASHA Special Interest Groups, 4*(June), 456-463.

Diemart, R. (2018, February 16). 32 million American adults can't read: Why literacy is the key to growth. *One Young World.* Retrieved from https://medium.com/@OneYoungWorld_/32-million-american-adults-cant-read-why-literacy-is-the-key-to-growth-818996739523

Dietz, A., McKelvey, M., & Beukelman, D. R. (2006). Visual scene displays (VSD): New AAC interface for persons with aphasia. *Perspectives on Augmentative and Alternative Communication, 15*(1), 13-17.

Dietz, A., Quach, W., Lund, S. K., & McKelvey, M. (2012). AAC assessment and clinical-decision making: The impact of experience. *Augmentative and Alternative Communication, 28*(3), 148-159.

Dietz, A., Thiessen, A., Griffith, J., Peterson, A., Sawyer, E., & McKelvey, M. (2013). The renegotiation of social roles in chronic aphasia: Finding a voice through AAC. *Aphasiology, 27*(3), 309-325.

Dietz, A., Vannest, J., Maloney, T., Altaye, M., Holland, S., & Szaflarski, J. P. (2018). The feasibility of improving discourse in people with aphasia through AAC: Clinical and functional MRI correlates. *Aphasiology, 32*(6), 693-719.

Dietz, A., Weissling, S. E., Griffith, J., & McKelvey, M. L. (2013). Personalizing AAC for people with aphasia: The role of text and pictures. *Special Education and Communication Disorders Faculty Publications, 154,* 1-12.

Ding, D., Leister, E., Cooper, R. A., Cooper, R., Kelleher, A., Fitzgerald, S. G., & Boninger, M. L. (2008). Usage of tilt-in-space, recline, and elevation seating functions in natural environment of wheelchair users. *Journal of Rehabilitation Research and Development, 45*(7), 973-984.

Disabled World. (2017). Wheelchairs: Information and reviews. Retrieved from https://www.disabled-world.com/assistivedevices/mobility/wheelchairs/

Dixon, H. N. (1890). *Simplification of the letters of the alphabet and methods of teaching deaf-mutes to speak* (J. P. Bonet, Trans.). Harrogate: Farrar. (Original work published 1620.)

Dixon, L. S. (1981). A functional analysis of photo-object matching skills of severely retarded adolescents. *Journal of Applied Behavior Analysis, 14,* 465-478.

Dodd, J. L., & Gorey, M. (2013). AAC intervention as an immersion model. *Communication Disorders Quarterly, 35,* 103-107.

Doherty, J. E. (1985). The effects of sign characteristics on sign acquisition and retention: An integrative review of the literature. *Augmentative and Alternative Communication, 1,* 108-121.

Doherty, J. E. (1986). The effects of translucency and hand-shape difficulty on sign acquisition by preschool children. (Doctoral dissertation, Purdue University, 1985). *Dissertation Abstracts International, 46,* 3317A.

Doherty, J. E., Daniloff, J., & Lloyd, L. L. (1985). The effect of categorical representation on Amer-Ind transparency. *Augmentative and Alternative Communication, 1,* 10-16.

Dominowska, E. (2002). *A communication aid with context-aware vocabulary prediction.* Unpublished Master's in Engineering Dissertation, Massachusetts Institute of Technology.

Donnellan, A. M., Mirenda, P., Mesaros, R. A., & Fassbender, L. L. (1984). Analyzing the communicative functions of aberrant behavior. *Journal of the Association for Persons with Severe Handicaps, 9,* 201-212.

Dorn, L. J., & Soffos, C. (2001). *Shaping literate minds: Developing self-regulated learners.* Stenhouse.

Doss, L. S., & Reichle, J. (1989). Establishing communicative alternatives to the emission of socially motivated excess behavior: A review. *Journal of the Association for Persons with Severe Handicaps, 14,* 101-112.

Doss, L. S., & Reichle, J. (1991). Replacing excess behavior with an initial communicative repertoire. In J. Reichle, J. York, & J. Sigafoos (Eds.), *Implementing augmentative and alternative communication: Strategies for learners with severe disabilities* (pp. 215-237). Paul H. Brookes Publishing Co.

Douglas, S., Light, J., & McNaughton, D. (2012). Teaching paraeducators to support the communication of young children with complex communication needs. *Topics in Early Childhood Education, 33,* 91-101.

Dowden, P. A. (1997). Augmentative and alternative communication decision making for children with severely unintelligible speech. *Augmentative and Alternative Communication, 13,* 48-58.

Dowden, P. A. (2016). University of Washington augmentative and alternative communication. Retrieved from https://depts.washington.edu/augcomm

Downey, D., & Happ, M. B. (2013). The need for nurse training to promote improved patient-provider communication for patients with complex communication needs. *Perspectives on Augmentative and Alternative Communication, 22*(2), 112-119.

Downing, J. E. (1963). *The Downing readers.* Initial Teaching Publication.

Downing, J. E. (1970). Cautionary comments on some American i.t.a. reports. *Educational Research, 13,* 70-72.

Downing, J. E. (2005). *Teaching communication skills to students with severe disabilities* (2nd ed.). Paul H. Brookes Publishing Co.

Downing, J. E., & Eichinger, J. (1990). Instructional strategies for learners with dual sensory impairments in integrated settings. *Journal of the Association for Persons with Severe Handicaps, 15,* 98-105.

Downing, J. E., Hanreddy, A., & Peckham-Hardin, K. (2015). *Teaching communication skills to students with severe disabilities* (3rd ed.). Paul H. Brookes Publishing Co.

Downing, J. E., & Jones, B. (1966). Some problems of evaluating i.t.a.: A second experiment. *Educational Research, 8,* 100-114.

Draffan, E. A., Kadous, A., Idris, A., Banes, D., Zeinoun, N., Wald, M., & Halabi, N. (2015). A participatory research approach to develop an Arabic symbol dictionary. *Studies in Health Technology and Informatics, 217,* 796-804.

Draffan, E. A., Wald, M., Halabi, N., Sabia, O., Zaghouani, W., Kadous, A., … Banes, D. (2015, September). *Generating acceptable Arabic core vocabularies and symbols for AAC users.* Paper presented at the 6th Workshop on Speech and Language Processing for Assistive Technologies. Retrieved from http://eprints.soton.ac.uk/384316/

Drager, K. D., & Light, J. C. (2006). Designing dynamic display AAC systems for young children with complex communication needs. *Perspectives on Augmentative and Alternative Communication, 15*(1), 3-7.

Drager, K. D. R., Light, J., Currall, J., Muttiah, N., Smith, V., Kreis, D., Nilam-Hall, A., Parratt, D., Schuessler, K., Shermetta, K., & Wiscount, J. (2017). AAC technologies with visual scene displays and "just in time" programming and symbolic communication turns expressed by students with severe disability. *Journal of Intellectual and Developmental Disability, 44,* 1-16.

Drager, K. D., Light, J. C., Curran Speltz, J., Fallon, K. A., & Jeffries, L. Z. (2003). The performance of typically developing 2 ½-year-olds on dynamic display AAC technologies with different system layouts and language organizations. *Journal of Speech, Language, and Hearing Research, 46*(2), 298-312.

Drager, K. D., Light, J. C., & Finke, E. (2009). Using AAC technologies to build social interaction with young children with autism spectrum disorders. In P. Mirenda & T. Iacono (Eds.), *Autism spectrum disorders and AAC* (pp. 247-278). Paul H. Brookes Publishing Co.

Drager, K. D., Light, J. C., & McNaughton, D. (2010). Effects of AAC interventions on communication and language for young children with complex communication needs. *Journal of Pediatric Rehabilitation Medicine, 3*(4), 303-310.

Du, Y., Boyd, L., & Ibrahim, S. (2018). From behavioral and communication intervention to interaction design: User perspectives from clinicians. In *Proceedings of the 20th International ACM SIGACCESS Conference on Computers and Accessibility* (pp. 198-202). ACM.

Dubois, B., & Pillon, B. (1997). Cognitive deficits in Parkinson's disease. *Journal of Neurology, 244,* 2-8.

Duchastel de Montrouge, C. (2014). [Review of the book Disability and new media by K. Ellis and M. Kent]. *Canadian Journal of Disability Studies, 3*(2), 135-141.

Duffy, J. R. (2005). *Motor speech disorders: Substrates, differential diagnosis, and management.* Mosby.

Duffy, J. R. (2013). *Motor speech disorders: Substrates, differential diagnosis, and management* (3rd ed.). Elsevier Mosby.

Duffy, L. (1977). *An innovative approach to the development of communication skills for severely speech handicapped cerebral palsied children.* Unpublished master's thesis, University of Nevada, Las Vegas.

Duker, P. C., & Remington, B. (1991). Manual sign-based communication for individuals with severe or profound mental handicap. In B. Remington (Ed.), *The challenge of severe mental handicap: A behavior analytic approach* (pp. 167-187). John Wiley.

Dukhovny, E., & Kelly, E. B. (2015). Practical resources for provision of services to culturally and linguistically diverse users of AAC. *Perspectives on Communication Disorders and Sciences in Culturally and Linguistically Diverse Populations, 22*(1), 25-39.

Dukhovny, E., & Thistle, J. J. (2017). An exploration of motor learning concepts relevant to use of speech-generating devices. *Assistive Technology, 31*(3), 126-132.

Duncan, J. L., & Silverman, F. H. (1977). Impacts of learning American Indian Sign Language on mentally retarded children: A preliminary report. *Perceptual and Motor Skills, 44,* 1138.

Dunlap, G., Sailor, W., Horner R. H., & Sugai, G. (2009). Overview and history of positive behavior support. In W. Sailor, G. Dunlap, G. Sugai, & R. Horner (Eds.), *Handbook of positive behavior supports* (pp. 3-16). Springer.

Dunlap, G., Strain, P. S., Fox, L., Carta, J. J., Conroy, M., Smith, B. J., Kern, L., Hemmeter, M. L., Timm, M. A., McCart, A., Sailor, W., Markey, U., Markey, D. J., Lardieri, S., & Sowell, C. (2006). Prevention and intervention with young children's challenging behavior: Perspectives regarding current knowledge. *Behavioral Disorders, 32,* 29-45.

Dunn, M. L. (1982). *Pre-sign language motor skills: Skill starters for motor development.* Communication Skill Builders.

Dunst, C., & Lowe, L. W. (1986). From reflex to symbol: Describing, explaining, and fostering communicative competence. *Augmentative and Alternative Communication, 2*(1), 11-18.

Durand, V. M. (1990). *Severe behavior problems. A functional communication training approach.* Guilford Press.

Durand, V. M. (1993). Functional communication training using assistive devices. Effects on challenging behavior and affect. *Augmentative and Alternative Communication, 9,* 168-176.

Durand, V. M. (2012). Functional communication training: Treating challenging behavior. In P. A. Prelock & R. J. McCauley (Eds.), *Treatment of autism spectrum disorders: Evidence-based intervention strategies for communication and social interaction* (pp. 107-138). Paul H. Brookes Publishing Co.

Durand, V. M., & Berotti, D. (1991). Treating behavior problems with communication. *ASHA, 33,* 37-39.

Durand, V. M., Berotti, D., & Weiner, J. (1993). Functional communication training: Factors affecting effectiveness, generalization, and maintenance. In J. Reichle & D. P. Wacker (Eds.), *Communicative alternatives to challenging behavior: Integrating functional assessment and intervention strategies* (pp. 317-340). Paul H. Brookes Publishing Co.

Durand, V. M., & Carr, E. G. (1991). Functional communication training to reduce challenging behavior: Maintenance and application in new settings. *Journal of Applied Behavior Analysis, 24,* 251-264.

Durand, V. M., & Crimmins, D. B. (1992). *The Motivation Assessment Scale (MAS) administration guide.* Moinaco & Associates.

Durand, V. M., & Merges, E. (2001). Functional communication training: A contemporary behavior analytic intervention for problem behaviors. *Focus on Autism and Other Developmental Disabilities, 16,* 110-119.

Dybwad, G., & Bersani, H. A. (Eds.). (1996). *New voices: Self-advocacy by people with disabilities.* Brookline Books.

Dye, R., Alm, N., Arnott, J. L., Harper, G., & Morrison, A. I. (1998). A script-based AAC system for transactional interaction. *Natural Language Engineering, 4*(1), 57-71.

Ecklund, S., & Reichle, J. (1987). A comparison of normal children's ability to recall symbols from two logographic systems. *Language, Speech, and Hearing Services in Schools, 18,* 34-40.

Edman, P. (1991). Relief Bliss: A low tech technique. *Communicating Together, 9,* 21-22.

Edrisinha, C. D. (2014). Tangible symbols as an AAC option for individuals with developmental disabilities: A systematic review of intervention studies. *Augmentative and Alternative Communication, 30*(1), 28-39.

Edwards, A., Theodoros, D., & Davidson, B. (2018). Group therapy for maintenance of speech in Parkinson's disease following LSVT LOUD: A pilot study. *Speech, Language and Hearing, 21*(2), 105-116.

Eide, A. H., & Øderud, T. (2009). Assistive technology in low-income countries. In M. MacLachlan & L. Swartz (Eds.), *Disability and international development: Towards inclusive global health.* Springer.

Elliott, J. (2003). Dynamic assessment in educational settings: Realizing potential. *Educational Review, 55,* 15-32.

Elliott, L. L., & Katz, D. R. (1980). *Northwestern University children's perception of speech (NU-CHIPS).* Auditec of St. Louis.

Ellis, N. (1991). Spelling and sound in learning to read. In M. Snowling & M. Thomson (Eds.), *Dyslexia: Integrating theory and practice* (pp. 80-94). Whurr Publishers Ltd.

Ellis, N. (1993). *Reading, writing and dyslexia: A cognitive analysis* (2nd ed.). Lawrence Erlbaum Associates.

Ellsperman, S. E., Nairn, E. M., & Stucken, E. Z. (2021). Review of bone conduction hearing devices. *Audiology Research, 11*(2), 207-219.

Emerson, E. (2001). *Challenging behaviour: Analysis and intervention in people with learning disabilities* (2nd ed.). Cambridge University Press.

Emmorey, K., Korpics, F., & Petronio, K. (2009). The use of visual feedback during signing: Evidence from signers with impaired vision. *Journal of Deaf Studies and Deaf Education, 14,* 99-104.

Erhardt, R. P. (1987). Visual function in the student with multiple handicaps: An integrative transdisciplinary model for assessment and intervention. *Education of the Visually Impaired, 19,* 87-98.

Erhardt, R. P. (1990). *Developmental visual dysfunction.* Therapy Skill Builders.

Erickson, K., & Clendon, S. (2009). Addressing the literacy demands of the curriculum for beginning readers and writers. In G. Soto & C. Zangari (Eds.), *Practically speaking: Language, literacy, and academic development for students with AAC needs* (pp. 195-215). Paul H. Brookes Publishing Co.

Erickson, K. A., & Geist, L. A. (2016). The profiles of students with significant cognitive disabilities and complex communication needs. *Augmentative and Alternative Communication, 32,* 1-11.

Erickson, K. A., & Koppenhaver, D. A. (2007). *Children with disabilities: Reading and writing the Four Blocks way.* Carson-Dellosa.

Erickson, K. A., & Koppenhaver, D. A. (2020). *Comprehensive literacy for all: Teaching students with significant disabilities to read and write.* Paul H. Brookes Publishing Co.

Erickson, W., Lee, C., & von Schrader, S. (2017). Disability statistics from the American community survey (ACS). *Cornell University.* Retrieved from www.disabilitystatistics.org

ESL Lounge. (2020). 50 most common irregular verbs. Retrieved from http://www.esl-lounge.com/reference/grammar-reference-most-common-irregular-verb-list.php

Evans, M. (2017). Empowering people experiencing Usher syndrome as participants in research. *British Journal of Social Work, 47,* 2328-2345.

Evidence Based Practice (EBP). (n.d.) Retrieved from https://www.asha.org/Research/EBP/Evidence-Based-Practice

Fadiman, A. (1997). *The spirit catches you and you fall down: A Hmong child, her American doctors and the collision of two cultures.* Farrar, Straus, & Giroux.

Fager, S. K., Bardach, L., Russell, S., & Higginbotham, J. (2012). Access to augmentative and alternative communication: New technologies and clinical decision-making. *Journal of Pediatric Rehabilitation Medicine, 5,* 53-61.

Fager, S. K., Beukelman, D. R., Fried-Oken, M., Jakobs, T., & Baker, J. (2011). Access interface strategies. *Assistive Technology, 24*(1), 25-33.

Fager, S. K., Fried-Oken, M., Jakobs, T., & Beukelman, D. R. (2019). New and emerging access technologies for adults with complex communication needs and severe motor impairments: State of the science. *Augmentative and Alternative Communication, 35*(1), 13-25.

Fairbanks, G. (1954). Systematic research in experimental phonetics: 1. A theory of the speech mechanism as a servomechanism. *Journal of Speech and Hearing Disorders, 19,* 133-139.

Falck, K. (2001). *The practical application of Pictograms.* Swedish Institute for Special Needs Education.

Falkman, K., Dahlgren-Sandberg, A., & Hjelmquist, E. (2002). Preferred communication modes: Prelinguistic and linguistic communication in non-speaking preschool children with cerebral palsy. *International Journal of Language and Communication Disorders, 37,* 59-68.

Fallon, K. A., Light, J. C., & Paige, T. K. (2001). Enhancing vocabulary selection for preschoolers who require augmentative and alternative communication (AAC). *American Journal of Speech-Language Pathology, 10,* 81-94.

Fanelli, D. (2012). Negative results are disappearing from most disciplines and countries. *Scientometrics, 90,* 891-904.

Fannin, D. K. (2016). The intersection of culture and ICF-CY personal and environmental factors for alternative and augmentative communication. *Perspectives of the ASHA Special Interest Groups SIG 12, 1*(12), 63-82.

Farrall, J. (2013). AAC apps lists. Retrieved from http://www.janefarrall.com/aac-apps-lists/

Faurot, K., Dellinger, D., Eatough, A., & Parkhurst, S. J. (2000). *The identity of Mexican sign as a language.* Summer Institute of Linguistics International Publications. Retrieved from https://www.sil.org/resources/publications/entry/9069

Feinstein, A., Freeman, J., & Lo, A. (2015). Treatment of progressive multiple sclerosis: What works, what does not, and what is needed. *Lancet Neurology, 14,* 194-207.

Felce, D., & Kerr, M. (2013). Investigating low adaptive behaviour and presence of the triad of impairments characteristic of autistic spectrum disorder as indicators of risk for challenging behaviour among adults with intellectual disabilities. *Journal of Intellectual Disability Research, 57*(2), 128-138.

Feldman, R. (2003). Infant–mother and infant–father synchrony: The co-regulation of positive arousal. *Infant Mental Health Journal: Official Publication of the World Association for Infant Mental Health, 24*(1), 1-23.

Ferm, U., Wallfur, P.E., Gelfgren, E., & Hartelius, L. (2012). Communication between Huntington's disease patients, their support persons and the dental hygienist using Talking Mats. In N. E. Tunali (Ed.), *Huntington's disease: Core concepts and current advances* (Ch. 23, pp. 531-555). InTech.

Ferm, U., Sahlin, A., Sundin, L., & Hartelius, L. (2010). Using Talking Mats to support communication in persons with Huntington's disease. *International Journal of Language and Communication Disorders, 5,* 523-536.

Fey, M., Warren, S., Brady, N., Finestack, L., Bredin-Oja, S., & Fairchild, M. (2006). Early effects of prelinguistic milieu teaching and responsivity education for children with developmental delays and their parents. *Journal of Speech, Language and Hearing Research, 49,* 526-547.

FIRST WORDS Project. (2014). 16 gestures by 16 months. Florida State University. Retrieved from http://firstwordsproject.com/

Fischer, S., Metz, D., Brown, P., & Caccamise, F. (1991). The effects of bimodal communication on the intelligibility of sign and speech. In P. Siple & S. Fischer (Eds.), *Theoretical issues in sign language research. Volume 2: Psychology* (pp. 135-147). University of Chicago Press.

Fisher, W., Piazza, C., Cataldo, M., Harrell, R., Jefferson, G., & Conner, R. (1993). Functional communication training with and without extinction and punishment. *Journal of Applied Behavior Analysis, 26,* 23-36.

Fishman, C. E., & Nickerson, A. B. (2015). Motivations for involvement: A preliminary investigation of parents of students with disabilities. *Journal of Child and Family Studies, 24,* 523-535.

Fishman, I. (2011). Guidelines for teaching speech-language pathologists about the AAC assessment process. *Perspectives on Augmentative and Alternative Communication, 20*(3), 82-86.

Flanagan, J. L. (1972). Speech synthesis. In *Speech Analysis, Synthesis, and Perception* (2nd ed., Ch. 6, pp. 204-276). Springer Verlag.

Flener, B., & Nygard, J. (2015). *TactileTalk guidebook: Strategies for functional communication and literacy.* Attainment Company.

Flexer, C. (1999). *Facilitating hearing and listening in young children* (2nd ed.). Singular Publishing.

Flodin, M. (2004). *SIGNING illustrated: The complete learning guide.* The Penguin Group.

Flowerdew, L. (2009). Applying corpus linguistics to pedagogy: A critical evaluation. *International Journal of Corpus Linguistics, 14,* 393-417.

Foley, A., & Ferri, A. (2012). Technology for people, not disabilities: Ensuring access and inclusion. *Journal of Research in Special Educational Needs, 12,* 192-200.

Foley, B. E. (1993). The development of literacy in individuals with severe congenital speech and motor impairments. *Topics in Language Disorders, 13*(2), 16-32.

Fonner, K., & Marfilius, S. (2011). Sorting through AAC apps. Retrieved from http://www.spectronics.com.au/conference/2012/pdfs/handouts/kelly-fonner/Sorting%20AAC%20aaps%20OCT302011.pdf

Forsberg, K., Graffmo, K., Pakkenberg, B., Weber, M., Nielsen, M., Marklund, S., Brännström, T., & Andersen, P. M. (2019). Misfolded SOD1 inclusions in patients with mutations in C9orf72 and other ALS/FTD-associated genes. *Journal of Neurology Neurosurgery and Psychiatry, 90,* 861-869.

Fountas, I. C., & Pinnell, G. S. (1996). *Guided reading: Good first teaching for all children.* Heinemann.

Fox, C., Ramig, L., Ciucci, M., Sapir, S., McFarland, D., & Farley, B. (2006). The science and practice of LSVT/LOUD: Neural plasticity-principled approach to treating individuals with Parkinson's. *Seminars in Speech and Language, 27*(4), 283-299.

Fox, L., & Fried-Oken, M. (1996). AAC aphasiology: Partnership for future research. *Augmentative and Alternative Communication, 12*(4), 257-271.

Francis, W. N., Kucera, H., & Mackie, A. W. (1982). *Frequency analysis of English usage: Lexicon and grammar.* Houghton Mifflin.

Frank, R. G., & Glied, S. (2006). *Better but not well: Mental health policy in the U.S. since 1950.* Johns Hopkins University Press.

Frankel, T., Penn, C., & Ormond-Brown, D. (2007). Executive dysfunction as an explanatory basis for conversation symptoms in aphasia: A pilot study. *Aphasiology, 21*(6-8), 1-15.

Frankoff, D. (2010). *Exploring legal consciousness: Experiences of families seeking funding for assistive technologies for children with disabilities.* Available from ProQuest Dissertations and Theses Global: The Humanities and Social Sciences Collection Database.

Frankoff, D., & Hatfield, B. (2011). Augmentative and alternative communication in daily practice: Strategies and tools for management of severe communication disorders. *Topics in Stroke Rehabilitation, 18*(2), 112-119.

Franzone, E. (2009). *Implementation checklist for functional communication training (FCT).* The National Professional Development Center on Autism Spectrum Disorders, Waisman Center, University of Wisconsin.

Frederick, A. A., Kingdom, F. A. A., & Prins, N. (2016). *Psychophysics: A practical introduction* (2nd ed.). Academic Press.

Frederiksen, J. R., & Collins, A. (1989). A systems approach to educational testing. *Educational Researcher, 18*(9), 27-32.

Friederich, A., Bernd, T., & De Witte, L. (2010). Methods for the selection of assistive technology in neurological rehabilitation practice. *Scandinavian Journal of Occupational Therapy, 17*(4), 308-318.

Fried-Oken, M. (1992). The AAC assessment cube for adults with severe communication disabilities. *Communication Outlook, 14*(1), 14-18.

Fried-Oken, M. (2001). Been there, done that: A very personal introduction to the special issue on augmentative and alternative communication and acquired disorders. *Augmentative and Alternative Communication, 17,* 138-140.

Fried-Oken, M., Beukelman, D. R., & Hux, K. (2012). Current and future AAC research considerations for adults with acquired cognitive and communication impairments. *Assistive Technology, 24*(1), 56-66.

Fried-Oken, M., Mooney, A., & Peters, B. (2015). Supporting communication for patients with neurodegenerative disease. *Neurological Rehabilitation, 37,* 69-87.

Fried-Oken, M., Mooney, A., Peters, B., & Oken, B. (2015). A clinical screening protocol for the RSVP keyboard brain-computer interface. *Disability and Rehabilitation: Assistive Technology, 10*(1), 11-18.

Fried-Oken, M., & More, L. (1992). An initial vocabulary for nonspeaking preschool children based on developmental and environmental language sources. *Augmentative and Alternative Communication, 8,* 41-56.

Fried-Oken, M., Rowland, C., Daniels, D., Dixon, M., Fuller, B., Mills, C., Noethe, G., Small, J., Still, K., & Oken, B. (2012). AAC to support conversation in persons with moderate Alzheimer's disease. *Augmentative and Alternative Communication, 28*(4), 219-231.

Fristoe, M. (1975). *Language intervention systems for the retarded.* Lurleen B. Wallace Developmental Center.

Fristoe, M., & Lloyd, L. L. (1979a). Nonspeech communication. In N. R. Ellis (Ed.), *Handbook of mental deficiency: Psychological theory and research* (2nd ed., pp. 401-430). Lawrence Erlbaum Associates.

Fristoe, M., & Lloyd, L. L. (1979b). Signs used in manual communication training with persons having severe communication impairment. *AAESPH Review, 4,* 364-373.

Fristoe, M., & Lloyd, L. L. (1980). Planning an initial expressive sign lexicon for persons with severe communication impairment. *Journal of Speech and Hearing Disorders, 45*(2), 170-180.

Frost, L., & Bondy, A. (2002). *PECS: The Picture Exchange Communication System training manual.* Pyramid Educational Products, Inc.

Frost, L., & Silverman-McGowan, J. (2014). Strategies for transitioning from PECS to SGD, part 2: Maintaining communication competency. *Perspectives on Augmentative and Alternative Communication, 21*(1), 3-10.

Fry, E. (1964). A diacritical marking system to aid beginning reading instruction. *Elementary Engineering, 41,* 526-529.

Fuchs, L., & Fuchs, D. (1984). Teaching beginning reading skills: A unique approach. *Teaching Exceptional Children, 17,* 48-53.

Fuchs, S., Johnston, M., Hale, K. S., & Axelsson, P. (2008). Results from pilot testing a system for tactile reception of advanced patterns (STRAP). *Proceedings of the Human Factors and Ergonomics Society Annual Meeting, 52*(18), 1302-1306.

Fujisawa, K., Inoue, T., Yamana, Y., & Hayashi, H. (2011). The effect of animation on learning action symbols by individuals with intellectual disabilities. *Augmentative and Alternative Communication, 27*(1), 53-60.

Fuller, D. R. (1988). *Effects of translucency and complexity on the associative learning of Blissymbols by cognitively normal children and adults.* (Doctoral dissertation, Purdue University, 1987). *Dissertation Abstracts International, 49,* 710B.

Fuller, D. R. (1997). Initial study into the effects of translucency and complexity on the learning of Blissymbols by children and adults with normal cognitive abilities. *Augmentative and Alternative Communication, 13*(1), 30-39.

Fuller, D. R. (2019a, November). *AAC terminology issues, part I: Describing persons who rely on AAC to communicate.* Poster session presented at the Annual Convention of the American Speech-Language-Hearing Association.

Fuller, D. R. (2019b, November). *AAC terminology issues, part III: Revisiting terminology for communication technology.* Poster session presented at the Annual Convention of the American Speech-Language-Hearing Association.

Fuller, D. R., & Lloyd, L. L. (1987). A study of physical and semantic characteristics of a graphic symbol system as predictors of perceived complexity. *Augmentative and Alternative Communication, 3,* 26-35.

Fuller, D. R., & Lloyd, L. L. (1991). Toward a common usage of iconicity terminology. *Augmentative and Alternative Communication, 7,* 215-220.

Fuller, D. R., & Lloyd, L. L. (1997a). AAC model and taxonomy. In L. L. Lloyd, D. R. Fuller, & H. H. Arvidson (Eds.), *Augmentative and alternative communication: A handbook of principles and practices* (pp. 27-37). Allyn & Bacon.

Fuller, D. R., & Lloyd, L. L. (1997b). Symbol selection. In L. L. Lloyd, D. R. Fuller, & H. H. Arvidson (Eds.), *Augmentative and alternative communication: A handbook of principles and practices* (pp. 214-225). Allyn & Bacon.

Fuller, D. R., Lloyd, L. L., & Schlosser, R. W. (1991, October). *Symbol selection considerations: An integrative review.* Paper presented at the 1991 Think Tank Symposium, Purdue University.

Fuller, D. R., Lloyd, L. L., & Schlosser, R. W. (1992). Further development of an augmentative and alternative communication symbol taxonomy. *Augmentative and Alternative Communication, 8,* 67-74.

Fuller, D. R., Lloyd, L. L., & Schlosser, R. W. (1997). *What do we know about graphic AAC symbols, and what do we still need to know about them? Theoretical and methodological issues in augmentative and alternative communication.* Proceedings of the fourth ISAAC research symposium, Vancouver, Canada, August 11-12, 1996. Malardalen University Press.

Fuller, D. R., Lloyd, L. L., & Stratton, M. (1997). Aided AAC symbols. In L. L. Lloyd, D. R. Fuller, & H. H. Arvidson (Eds.), *Augmentative and alternative communication: A handbook of principles and practices* (pp. 48-79). Allyn & Bacon.

Fuller, D. R., & Pampoulou, E. (2022). Opinion: Revisiting the means to select and transmit of the AAC model. *Journal of Enabling Technologies, 16*(1), 28-37.

Fuller, D. R., Schlosser, R. W., & Lloyd, L. L. (1994). *Aided symbol selection considerations. An integrative review.* Unpublished manuscript, University of Arkansas at Little Rock.

Fuller, D. R., & Stratton, M. M. (1991). Representativeness versus translucency: Different theoretical backgrounds, but are they really different concepts? A position paper. *Augmentative and Alternative Communication, 7,* 51-58.

Gaebler-Spira, D., & Girolami, G. L. (2013). The framework of movement and implications for clinical practice. Retrieved from https://www.aacpdm.org/UserFiles/file/IC37.pdf

Galda, L., Cullinan, B., & Strickland, D. (1993). *Language, literacy and the child.* Harcourt Brace Jovanovich College Publishers.

Galyas, K., Fant, G., & Hunnicut, S. (1993). *Voice output communication aids.* Handikappinsti-tutet.

Gambier, Y., & Gottlieb, H. (Eds.). (2001). *(Multi) media translation: Concepts, practices, and research* (Vol. 34). John Benjamins Publishing.

Gans, D., & Gans, K. D. (1993). Development of a hearing test protocol for profoundly involved multi-handicapped children. *Ear and Hearing, 14*(2), 128-140.

Ganz, J. B., Earles-Vollrath, T. L., Heath, A. K., Parker, R. I., Rispoli, M., & Duran, J. B. (2012). A meta-analysis of single case research studies on aided augmentative and alternative communication systems with individuals with autism spectrum disorders. *Journal of Autism and Developmental Disorders, 42,* 60-74.

Ganz, J. B., Hong, E. R., Gilliland, W., Marin, K., & Svenkerud, N. (2015). Comparison between visual scene displays and exchange based communication in augmentative and alternative communication for children with ASD. *Research in Autism Spectrum Disorders, 11,* 27-41.

Gardner, W. H. (1962). The whistle technique in esophageal speech. *Journal of Speech and Hearing Disorders, 27,* 187-188.

Garg, H., Bush, S., & Gappmaier, E. (2016). Associations between fatigue and disability, functional mobility, depression, and quality of life in people with multiple sclerosis. *International Journal of Multiple Sclerosis Care, 18,* 71-77.

Garrett, K. L., Beukelman, D. R., & Low-Morrow, D. (1989). A comprehensive augmentative communication system for an adult with Broca's aphasia. *Augmentative and Alternative Communication, 5*(1), 55-61.

Garrett, K. L., & Huth, C. (2002). The impact of graphic contextual information and instruction on the conversational behaviors of a person with severe aphasia. *Aphasiology, 16*(4-6), 523-536.

Garrett, K. L., & Lasker, J. P. (2004). Multimodal communication screening task for persons with aphasia. Retrieved from http://cehs.unl.edu/aac/aphasia-assessment-materials/

Garrett, K. L., & Lasker, J. (2005). *The Multimodal Communication Screening Test for Persons with Aphasia (MCST-A).* Retrieved from https://cehs.unl.edu/aac/aphasia-assessment-materials/

Garrett, K. L., & Lasker, J. P. (2007). AAC and severe aphasia - Enhancing communication across the continuum of recovery. *Perspectives on Neurophysiology and Neurogenic Speech and Language Disorders, 17*(3), 6-15.

Garrett, K. L, Lasker, J. P., Beukelman, D. R., & Mirenda, P. (2013). Adults with severe aphasia and apraxia of speech. In D. R. Beukelman & P. Mirenda (Eds.), *Augmentative and alternative communication: Supporting children and adults with complex communication needs* (4th ed., pp. 405-446). Brookes Publishing.

Garrett, S. (1986). A case study in tactile Blissymbols. *Communicating Together, 4,* 16.

Gately, G. (1971). A technique for teaching the laryngectomized to trap air for the production of esophageal speech. *Journal of Speech and Hearing Disorders, 36,* 484-485.

Gdowski, B. S., Sanger, D. D., & Decker, T. N. (1986). Otitis media effect on a child's learning. *Academic Therapy, 21,* 283-289.

Geist, L., Erickson, K., Greer, C., & Hatch, P. (2021). Initial evaluation of the Project Core Implementation Model. *Assistive Technology Outcomes and Benefits, 15,* 29-47.

Geist, L., Erickson, K., Hatch, P., Dorney, K., & Benson-Goldberg, S. (2018, November). *Implementation of classroom-based core vocabulary instruction for beginning communicators with significant disabilities: Year three results.* Paper presented at the Annual Convention of the American Speech-Language-Hearing Association.

Gellhaus, M. M., & Olson, M. R. (1993). Using color and contrast to modify the educational environment of visually impaired students with multiple disabilities. *Journal of Visual Impairment and Blindness, 87,* 19-20.

Genetics Home Reference. (2017). Usher syndrome. Retrieved from https://ghr.nlm.nih.gov/condition/usher-syndrome#statistics

Gentry, J. R. (2007). *Breakthrough in beginning reading and writing: The evidence-based approach to pinpointing students' needs and delivering targeted instruction.* Scholastic.

Georgia Project for Assistive Technology (GPAT). (n.d.). Augmentative Evaluation Communication Summary. [Assessment]. Retrieved from https://www.gadoe.org/Curriculum-Instruction-and-Assessment/Special-Education-Services/Documents/GPAT%20AAC_Evaluation_Protocol.pdf

Gerard, J. M., Thill, M. P., Chantrain, G., Gersdorff, M., & Deggouj, N. (2012). Esteem 2 middle ear implant: Our experience. *Audiology Neurotology, 22,* 267-274.

Gerber, D. A. (2003). Disabled veterans, the state, and the experience of disability in Western societies, 1914-1950. *Journal of Social History, 36*(4), 899-916.

Gerber, S., & Kraat, A. (1992). Use of a developmental model of language acquisition: Applications to children using AAC systems. *Augmentative and Alternative Communication, 8*(1), 19-32.

Geruschat, D. R. (1992). Using the acuity card procedure to assess visual acuity in children with severe and multiple impairments. *Journal of Visual Impairment and Blindness, 86,* 25-27.

Gevarter, C., O'Reilly, M. F., Kuhn, M., Watkins, L., Ferguson, R., Sammarco, N., Rojeski, L., & Sigafoos, J. (2016). Assessing the acquisition of requesting a variety of preferred items using different speech generating device formats for children with autism spectrum disorder. *Assistive Technology, 1,* 1-8.

Gevarter, C., O'Reilly, M. F., Rojeski, L., Sammarco, N., Lang, R., Lancioni, G. E., & Sigafoos, J. (2013). Comparing communication systems for individuals with developmental disabilities: A review of single-case research studies. *Research in Developmental Disabilities, 34*(12), 4415-4432.

Gevarter, C., O'Reilly, M. F., Rojeski, L., Sammarco, N., Sigafoos, J., Lancioni, G. E., & Lang, R. (2014). Comparing acquisition of AAC-based mands in three young children with autism spectrum disorder using iPad applications with different display and design elements. *Journal of Autism and Developmental Disorders, 44*(10), 2464-2474.

Gillam, R. B., & Johnston, J. R. (1992). Spoken and written relationships in language/learning impaired and normally achieving school-age children. *Journal of Speech and Hearing Research, 35*, 1303-1315.

Glennen, S. L., & DeCoste, D. C. (1997). *Handbook of augmentative and alternative communication.* Singular Publishing Group.

Glosser, G., Wiener, M., & Kaplan, E. (1986). Communicative gestures in aphasia. *Brain and Language, 27,* 345-359.

Godsil, R., Tropp, L. R., Goff, P. A., & Powell, J. A. (2014). The science of equality, volume 1: Addressing implicit bias, racial anxiety, and stereotype threat in education and health care. Retrieved from https://perception.org

Goh, S. K. Y., Tham, E. K. H., Magiati, I., Sim, L., Sanmugam, S., Qiu, A., Daniel, M. L., Broekman, B. F. P., & Rifkin-Graboi, A. (2017). Analysis of item-level bias in the Bayley-III Language Subscales: The validity and utility of standardized language assessment in a multilingual setting. *Journal of Speech, Language, and Hearing Research, 60*(9), 2663-2671.

Goldberg, H. R., & Fenton, J. (1960). *Aphonic communication for those with cerebral palsy: Guide for the development and use of communication boards.* United Cerebral Palsy of New York State.

Goldman, R., & Lynch, M. (1971). *Goldman-Lynch sounds and symbols developmental kit.* American Guidance Service.

Golinker, L. (1992). Funding assistive technology. *Rehabilitation Management, 5,* 129-133.

Golinker, L. (2019). AAC from a broad perspective. Based on an email discussion of technology taxonomies, February 14, 2019.

Gona, J. K., Newton, C. R., Hartley, S., & Bunning, K. (2014). A home-based intervention using augmentative and alternative communication (AAC) techniques in rural Kenya: What are the caregivers' experiences? *Child: Care, Health and Development, 40*(1), 29-41.

Good, J. E., Lance, D. M., & Rainey, J. (2015). The effects of morphological awareness training on reading, spelling, and vocabulary skills. *Communication Disorders Quarterly, 36*(3), 142-151.

Goodenough-Trepagnier, C. (1981, June). *Representation of language for nonvocal communication.* Paper presented at the AACP&T-NEMC meeting on Advances in Technical Aids for Children with Physical Disabilities, Tufts University.

Goodenough-Trepagnier, C. (1994). Design goals for augmentative communication. *Assistive Technology, 6,* 3-9.

Goodenough-Trepagnier, C., & Prather, P. (1981). Communication systems for the nonvocal based on frequent phoneme sequences. *Journal of Speech and Hearing Research, 24,* 322-329.

Goodenough-Trepagnier, C., Tarry, E., & Prather, P. (1982). Derivation of an efficient nonvocal commumcation system. *Human Factors, 24,* 163-172.

Goodwin, A. P., Lipsky, M., & Ahn, S. (2012). Word detectives: Using units of meaning to support literacy. *The Reading Teacher, 65,* 461-470.

Goodwin, A. P., & Ahn, S. (2010). A meta-analysis of morphological interventions: Effects on literacy achievement of children with literacy difficulties. *Annals of Dyslexia, 60,* 183-208.

Goossens', C. A. (1984). The relative iconicity and learnability of verb referents differentially represented as manual signs, Blissymbolics, and rebus symbols. An investigation with moderately retarded individuals, (Doctoral dissertation, Purdue University, 1983). *Dissertation Abstracts International, 45,* 809A.

Goossens', C. A. (1989). Aided communication intervention before assessment: A case study of a child with cerebral palsy. *Augmentative and Alternative Communication, 5,* 14-26.

Goossens', C. A., & Crain, S. (1986). *Augmentative communication: Intervention resource.* Don Johnston Incorporated.

Goossens', C. A., Crain, S., & Elder, P. (1992). *Engineering the preschool environment for interactive, symbolic communication.* SEAC Publications.

Gosnell, J., Costello, J., & Shane, H. (2011). Using a clinical approach to answer "What communication apps should we use?" *Perspectives on Augmentative and Alternative Communication, 20,* 87-96.

Goswami, U. (1994). Reading by analogy: Theoretical and practical perspectives. In C. Hulme & M. Snowling (Eds.), *Reading development and dyslexia* (pp. 18-30). Whurr Publishers Limited.

Grandin, T. (2006). *Thinking in pictures, expanded edition: My life with autism.* Vintage Books.

Granlund, M., Björck-Åkesson, E., Wilder, J., & Ylvén, R. (2008). AAC interventions for children in a family environment: Implementing evidence in practice. *Augmentative and Alternative Communication, 24*(3), 207-219.

Gray, H., & Tickle-Degnen, L. (2010). A meta-analysis of performance on emotion recognition tasks in Parkinson's disease. *Neuropsychology, 24*(2), 176-191.

Graziano, M., & Gullberg, M. (2018). When speech stops, gesture stops: Evidence from developmental and crosslinguistic comparisons. *Frontiers in Psychology, 9,* 1-17.

Gregory, M. K., DeLeon, I. G., & Richman, D. M. (2009). The influence of matching and motor-imitation abilities on rapid acquisition of manual signs and exchange-based communicative responses. *Journal of Applied Behavior Analysis, 42,* 399-404.

Grether, S. M. (2015). AAC supports for individuals with Rett syndrome across the lifespan. *Perspectives on Augmentative and Alternative Communication, 24*(3), 74-85.

Griffith, P. L. (1979). *The influence of iconicity and phonological similarity on sign learning in mentally retarded persons.* Unpublished doctoral dissertation, Kent State University.

Griffith, P. L., & Robinson, J. H. (1980). Influence of iconicity and phonological similarity on sign learning by mentally retarded children. *American Journal of Mental Deficiency, 85,* 291-298.

Groba, B., Nieto-Riveiro, L., Canosa, N., Concheiro-Moscoso, P., Miranda-Duro, M., & Pereira, J. (2021). Stakeholder perspectives to support graphical user interface design for children with autism spectrum disorder: A qualitative study. *International Journal of Environmental Research and Public Health, 18*(9), 4631.

Grove, N. (2010). *The big book of storysharing.* SENJIT, Institute of Education, University of London.

Grove, N. (2018, September). Sign language and AAC: From yesterday to tomorrow. Tribute to John Bonvillian presented at the 2018 Clinical AAC Research Conference.

Grove, N., & Walker, M. (1990). The Makaton vocabulary: Using manual signs and graphic symbols to develop interpersonal communication. *Augmentative and Alternative Communication, 6,* 15-28.

Guo, Y., Roehrig, A. D., & Williams, R. S. (2011). The relation of morphological awareness and syntactic awareness to adults' reading comprehension: Is vocabulary knowledge a mediating variable? *Journal of Literacy Research, 43,* 159-183.

Gurgel, R. K., & Shelton, C. (2013). The SoundBite hearing system: Patient-assessed safety and benefit study. *The Laryngoscope, 123*(11), 2807-2812.

Gustason, G. (1990). Signing Exact English. In H. Bornstein (Ed.), *Manual communication: Implications for education* (pp. 108-127). Gallaudet University Press.

Gustason, G., Pfetzing, D., & Zawolkow, E. (1980). *Signing Exact English.* Modern Signs Press.

Gutierrez-Clellen, V. F., & Peña, E. (2001). Dynamic assessment of diverse children: A tutorial. *Language, Speech, and Hearing Services in Schools, 32,* 212-224.

Gutmann, M. (2016). Use of simulation with standardized patients in AAC pre-service training: Potentiating practical learning. *Perspectives on Augmentative and Alternative Communication, 1,* 38-44.

Gutmann, M., & Gryfe, P. (1996, August). *The communication continuum in ALS: Critical paths and client preferences.* Paper presented at the Seventh Biennial conference of the International Society for Augmentative and Alternative Communication (ISAAC).

Gutman, S. (2017). *Quick reference neuroscience for rehabilitation professionals: The essential neurologic principles underlying rehabilitation practice.* SLACK Incorporated.

Gutman, S., & Schonfeld, A. (2009). *Screening adult neurologic populations* (2nd ed.). AOTA Press.

Hadley, P. A., Rispoli, M., & Hsu, N. (2016). Toddlers' verb lexicon diversity and grammatical outcomes. *Language, Speech, and Hearing Services in Schools, 47*, 44-58.

Hagood, L. (1992). *A standard tactile symbol system: Graphic language for individuals who are blind and unable to read braille.* Texas School for the Blind and Visually Impaired Outreach Programs. Retrieved from https://www.tsbvi.edu/tagged-resources/203-resources/1315-standard-tactile-symbol-system

Hall, A., Orel-Bixler, D., & Haegerstrom-Portnoy, G. (1991). Special visual assessment techniques for multiple handicapped persons. *Journal of Visual Impairment and Blindness, 85*, 23-29.

Hall, J. W. (2014). *Introduction to audiology today.* Pearson.

Hall, N., & Boisvert, M. (2014). Clinical aspects related to tele-AAC: A technical report. *Perspectives on Augmentative and Alternative Communication, 23*, 18-31.

Hall, N., Boisvert, M., & Steele, R. (2013). Telepractice in the assessment and treatment of individuals with aphasia: A systematic review. *International Journal of Telerehabilitation, 5*(1), 27-38.

Hall, N., Jeungling-Sudkamp, J., Gutmann, M., & Cohn, E. (2019). *Tele-AAC: Augmentative and alternative communication through telepractice.* Plural Publishing.

Hallberg, L., Mellgren, E., Hartelius, L., & Ferm, U. (2013). Talking Mats in a discussion group for people with Huntington's disease. *Disability and Rehabilitation: Assistive Technology, 8*(1), 67-76.

Halloran, C., & Halloran, J. (2013). *LAMP: Language acquisition through motor planning.* The Center for AAC and Autism.

Hamilton, A., Ferm, U., Heemskerk, A. -W., Twiston-Davis, R., Matheson, K. Y., Simpson, S. A., & Rae, D. (2012). Management of speech, language and communication difficulties in Huntington's disease. *Neurodegenerative Disease Management, 2*(1), 67-77.

Hanke, T. (2004). HamNoSys - Representing sign language data in language resources and language processing contexts. LREC 2004 Workshop proceedings: Representation and processing of sign languages (pp. 1-6). Retrieved from https://www.sign-lang.uni-hamburg.de/dgs-korpus/files/inhalt_pdf/HankeLRECSLP2004_05.pdf

Hanson, E. K. (2007). Documentation in AAC using goal attainment scaling. *Perspectives on Augmentative and Alternative Communication, 16*(4), 6-9.

Hanson, E. K., Beukelman, D. R., & Yorkston, K. M. (2013). Communication support through multimodal supplementation: A scoping review. *Augmentative and Alternative Communication, 29*(4), 310-321.

Hanson, E. K., Yorkston, K. M., & Beukelman, D. R. (2004). Speech supplementation techniques for dysarthria: A systematic review. *Journal of Medical Speech-Language Pathology, 12*(2), ix-xxix.

Hanson, E. K., Yorkston, K. M., & Britton, D. (2011). Dysarthria in amyotrophic lateral sclerosis: A systematic review of characteristics, speech treatment, and augmentative and alternative communication options. *Journal of Medical Speech-Language Pathology, 19*, 12-30.

Harbo, H., Gold, R., & Tintore, M. (2013). Sex and gender issues in multiple sclerosis. *Therapeutic Advances in Neurological Disorders, 6*(4), 237-248.

Hardy, J. C. (1983). *Cerebral palsy.* Prentice Hall.

Harmon, A. C., Schlosser, R. W., Gygi, B., Shane, H. C., Kong, Y. Y., Book, L., Macduff, K., & Hearn, E. (2014). Effects of environmental sounds on the guessability of animated graphic symbols. *Augmentative and Alternative Communication, 30*(4), 298-313.

Harrison, M. (2017). Facilitating communication in infants and toddlers with hearing loss. In A. M. Harpe & R. Seewald (Eds.), *Comprehensive handbook of pediatric audiology* (2nd ed., pp. 829-848). Plural Publishing.

Harry, B. (2008). Collaboration with culturally and linguistically diverse families: Ideal versus reality. *Exceptional Children, 74*(3), 372-388.

Harry, B., Allen, N., & McLaughlin, M. (1995). Communication versus compliance: African-American parents' involvement in special education. *Exceptional Children, 61*(4), 364-377.

Hartelius, L., Carlstedt, A., Ytterberg, M., Lillvik, M., & Laasko, K. (2003). Speech disorders in mild and moderate Huntington's disease: Results of dysarthria assessment of 19 individuals. *Journal of Medical Speech-Language Pathology, 11*(1), 1-14.

Hartelius, L., Jonsson, M., Rickeberg, A., & Laasko, K. (2010). Communication and Huntington's disease: Qualitative interviews and focus groups with persons with Huntington's disease, family members, and carers. *International Journal of Language and Communication Disorders, 45*(3), 381-393.

Hartshorne, T. S., Hefner, M. A., & Blake, K. D. (Eds.). (2021). *CHARGE syndrome* (2nd ed.). Plural Publishing.

Hartshorne, T. S., Hefner, M. A., Davenport, S. L. H., & Thelin, J. W. (2011b). Introduction. In T. S. Hartshorne, M. A. Hefner, S. L. H. Davenport, & J. W. Thelin (Eds.), *CHARGE syndrome* (pp. xi-xv). Plural Publishing.

Hawley, M., Cunningham, S., Cardinaux, F., Coy, A., O'Neill, P., Seghal, S., & Enderby, P. (2007, October). *Challenges in developing a voice input voice output communication aid for people with severe dysarthria.* AAATE 2007: 9th European Conference for the Advancement of Assistive Technology in Europe.

Hayes, A. W. (Ed.). (1985). *Toxicology of the eye, ear, and other special senses.* Raven Press.

Hazamy, A. (2009). *Influence of pictures on word recognition.* Electronic Theses and Dissertations, Graduate Studies, Jack N. Averitt College of Graduation Studies, Georgia Southern University.

Hazenkamp, J., & Huebner, K. M (1989). *Program planning and evaluation for blind and visually impaired students.* American Foundation for the Blind.

Heath, A. K., Ganz, J. B., Parker, R., Burke, M., & Ninci, J. (2015). A meta-analytic review of functional communication training across mode of communication, age, and disability. *Review Journal of Autism and Developmental Disorders, 2*(2), 155-166.

Hecht, M., Hillemacher, T., Gräsel, E., Tigges, S., Winterholler, M., Heuss, D., Hilz, M. J., & Neundörfer, B. (2002). Subjective experience and coping in ALS. *Amyotrophic Lateral Sclerosis and Other Motor Neuron Disorders, 3*(4), 225-231.

Hefner, M. (1999). Diagnosis, genetics and prenatal diagnosis in CHARGE. *The CHARGE Syndrome Foundation.* Retrieved from https://www.chargesyndrome.org/wp-content/uploads/2016/05/Diagnosis-Genetics-and-Prenatal-Diagnosis.pdf

Heilmann, J., Nockerts, A., & Miller, J. (2010). Language samples: Does the length of the transcript matter? *Language, Speech, and Hearing Services in Schools, 41*, 393-404.

Heller, M. A., Calcaterra, J. A., Burson, L. L., & Tyler, L. A. (1996). Tactual picture identification by blind and sighted people: Effects of providing categorical information. *Perception and Psychophysics, 58*, 310-332.

Helling, C. R., & Minga, J. (2014). Developing an effective framework for the augmentative and alternative communication evaluation process. *Perspectives on Augmentative and Alternative Communication, 23*, 91-98.

Hemphill, L., & Tivnan, T. (2008). The importance of early vocabulary for literacy achievement in high-poverty schools. *Journal of Education for Students Placed at Risk, 13*, 426-451.

Hemsley, B., Balandin, S., Palmer, S., & Dann, S. (2017). A call for innovative social media research in the field of augmentative and alternative communication. *Augmentative and Alternative Communication, 33*(1), 14-22.

Hemsley, B., Balandin, S., Sigafoos, J., Forbes, R., Taylor, C., Green, V., & Parmenter, T. (2001). Nursing the patient with severe communication impairment. *Journal of Advanced Nursing, 35*, 827-835.

Hemsley, B., Balandin, S., & Togher, L. (2007). Narrative analysis of the hospital experience for older parents of people who cannot speak. *Journal of Aging Studies, 21*, 239-254.

Hemsley, B., Balandin, S., & Worrall, L. (2011). The 'Big 5' and beyond: Nurses, paid careers, and adults with developmental disability discuss communication needs in hospital. *Applied Nursing Research, 24*(1), e51-e58.

Hemsley, B., & Murray, J. (2015). Distance and proximity: Research on social media connections in the field of communication disability. *Disability Rehabilitation, 37*(17), 1509-1510.

Hern, S., Lammers, J., & Fuller, D. R. (1994). *The effects of translucency, complexity, and other variables on the acquisition of Blissymbols by institutionalized individuals with mental retardation.* Unpublished manuscript, University of Arkansas at Little Rock/University of Arkansas for Medical Sciences.

Hershberger, D. (2011). Mobile technology and AAC apps from an AAC developer's perspective. *Perspectives on Augmentative and Alternative Communication, 20*(1), 28-33.

Hetzroni, O. (2004). AAC and literacy. *Disability and Rehabilitation, 26*(21), 1305-1312.

Hetzroni, O., & Harris, O. (1996). Cultural aspects in the development of AAC users. *Augmentative and Alternative Communication, 12*(1), 52-58.

Higdon, C. W., & Hill, K. (2015). Five SGD funding rules of commitment. *Perspectives on Augmentative and Alternative Communication, 24*, 129-134.

Higginbotham, D. J. (1992). Evaluation of keystroke savings across five assistive communication technologies. *Augmentative and Alternative Communication, 8*(4), 258-272.

Higginbotham, D. J., Lesher, G. W., Moulton, B. J., & Roark, B. (2012). The application of natural language processing to augmentative and alternative communication. *Assistive Technology, 24*(1), 14-24.

Higginbotham, D.J., Shane, H., Russell, S., & Caves, K. (2007). Access to AAC: Present, past, and future. *Augmentative and Alternative Communication, 23*(3), 243-257.

Hill, K. (2001). The development of a model for automated performance measurement and the establishment of performance indices for augmented communicators under two sampling conditions. *Dissertation Abstracts International, 62*(05), 2293.

Hill, K. (2004). Augmentative and alternative communication and language: Evidence-based practice and language activity monitoring. *Topics in Language Disorders, 24*, 18-30.

Hill, K., & Romich, B. (2002). A rate index for augmentative and alternative communication. *Journal of Speech Technology, 5*, 57-64.

Hillier, S., Immink, M., & Thewlis, D. (2015). Assessing proprioception: A systematic review of possibilities. *Neurorehabilitation Neural Repair, 29*(10), 933-949.

Hjelmquist, E., Sandberg, A. D., & Hedelin, L. (1994). Linguistics, AAC, and metalinguistics in communicatively handicapped adolescents. *Augmentative and Alternative Communication, 10*, 169-183.

Ho, K., Weiss, S., Garrett, K., & Lloyd, L. (2005). The effect of remnant and pictographic books on the communicative interaction of individuals with global aphasia. *Augmentative and Alternative Communication, 21*(3), 218-232.

Hoffman, J. M., Yorkston, K. M., Shumway-Cook, A., Ciol, M. A., Dudgeon, B. J., & Chan L. (2005). Effect of communication disability on satisfaction with health care: A survey of Medicare beneficiaries. *American Journal of Speech-Language Pathology, 14*(3), 221-228.

Hofstede, G. (2011). Dimensionalizing cultures: The Hofstede Model in context. *Online Readings in Psychology and Culture, 2*, 8.

Hofstetter, H. W. (1991). Efficacy of low vision services for visually impaired children. *Journal of Visual Impairment and Blindness, 85*, 20-22.

Holland, A. L., & Beeson, P. (1993). Finding a new sense of self: What the clinician can do to help. *Aphasiology, 7*(6), 581-584.

Holland, A. L., & Nelson, R. L. (2014). *Counseling in communication disorders: A wellness perspective.* Plural Publishing.

Holland, A. L., Weinberg, P., & Dittelman, J. (2012). How to use apps clinically in the treatment for aphasia. *Seminars in Speech and Language, 33*, 223-233.

Holstrum, W. J., Biernath, K., McKay, S., & Ross, D. S. (2009). Mild and unilateral hearing loss. *Infants and Young Children, 22*(3), 177-187.

Holvoet, J. F., & Helmstetter, E. (1989). *Medical problems of students with special needs: A guide for educators.* College-Hill Press.

Holyfield, C., Caron, J., Drager, K. D., & Light, J. C. (2019). Effect of mobile technology featuring visual scene displays and just-in-time programming on communication turns by preadolescent and adolescent beginning communicators. *International Journal of Speech-Language Pathology, 21*(2), 201-211.

Holyfield, C., Drager, K., Kremkow, J., & Light, J. (2017). Systematic review of AAC intervention research for adolescents and adults with autism spectrum disorder. *Augmentative and Alternative Communication, 33*, 201-212.

Holyfield, C., Pope, L., Light, J. C., McNaughton, D., & Drager, K. D. (2016, November). *Visual scene displays (VSDs) with dynamic text: Supporting early reading in adults with intellectual disabilities (ID).* Presentation at the American Speech-Language Hearing Association Convention.

Honsinger, M. (1989). Midcourse intervention in multiple sclerosis: An inpatient model. *Augmentative and Alternative Communication, 5*, 71-73.

HonuIntervention. (2017). Function-based intervention (PDF). Retrieved from https://72aa752c-61fb-4cc4-a8c1-828003da22ee.filesusr.com/ugd/6ce87f_2fa2989c391e4b2a88977680ee7e9868.pdf

Hoogeveen, F. R., Smeets, P. M., & Lancioni, G. E. (1989). Teaching moderately mentally retarded children basic reading skills. *Research in Developmental Disabilities, 10*, 1-18.

Hooper, J., & Lloyd, L. L. (1986). *An investigation of the effect of element explanation on the ability of preschool children to learn Blissymbols.* Unpublished manuscript, Purdue University.

Hopper, T. (2001). Indirect interventions to facilitate communication in Alzheimer's disease. *Seminars in Speech and Language, 22*(4), 305-315.

Hopper, T., Douglas, N., & Khayum, B. (2015). Direct and indirect interventions for cognitive-communication disorders of dementia. *Perspectives on Neurophysiology and Neurogenic Speech and Language Disorders, 25*, 142-157.

Horner, R. H. (1994). Functional assessment: Contributions and future directions. *Journal of Applied Behavior Analysis, 27*, 401-404.

Horner, R. H., & Day, H. M. (1991). The effects of response efficiency on functionally equivalent competing behaviors. *Journal of Applied Behavior Analysis, 24*, 719-732.

Horner, R. H., Sprague, J. R., O'Brien, M., & Heathfield, L. (1990). The role of response efficiency in the reduction of problem behaviors through functional equivalence training: A case study. *Journal of the Association for Persons with Severe Handicaps, 15*, 91-97.

Hornero, G., Conde, D., Quílez, M., Domingo, S., Rodríguez, M. P., Romero, B., & Casas, O. (2015). A wireless augmentative and alternative communication system for people with speech disabilities. *IEEE Access, 3*, 1288-1297.

Hourcade, J., Everhart Pilotte, T., West, E., & Parette, P. (2004). A history of augmentative and alternative communication for individuals with severe and profound disabilities. *Focus on Autism and Other Developmental Disabilities, 19*(4), 235-244.

Howard, D., & Hatfield, F. M. (2018). *Aphasia therapy: Historical and contemporary issues.* Routledge.

H. R. 2903. (2021). Creating opportunities now for necessary and effective care technologies (CONNECT) for health act of 2021. Retrieved from https://www.govtrack.us/congress/bills/117/hr2903

Hudson, R. (1994). About 37% of word-tokens are nouns. *Language, 70*(2), 331-339.

Huer, M. B. (1999). Augmentative and alternative communication: Changing demographic patterns. *Perspectives on Communication Disorders and Sciences in Culturally and Linguistically Diverse Populations, 5*(1), 2-3.

Huer, M. B. (2000). Examining perceptions of graphic symbols across cultures: Preliminary study of the impact of culture/ethnicity. *Augmentative and Alternative Communication, 16*(3), 180-185.

Huer, M. B., & Lloyd, L. L. (1988a). Parents' perspectives of AAC users. *Exceptional Parent, 18*(4), 32-33.

Huer, M. B., & Lloyd, L. L. (1988b). Perspectives of AAC users. *Communication Outlook, 9*(3), 10-18.

Huer, M. B., & Lloyd, L. L. (1990). AAC users' perspectives on augmentative and alternative communication. *Augmentative and Alternative Communication, 6*, 242-249.

Huggins, J., & Kovacs, T. (2018). Brain-computer interfaces for augmentative and alternative communication: Separating the reality from the hype. *Perspectives on Augmentative and Alternative Communication, 3*, 13-23.

Hughes, C. (1991). Independent performance among individuals with mental retardation: Promoting generalization through self-instruction. *Progress in Behavior Modification, 27*, 7-35.

Hughes, M. J. (1979). Sequencing of visual and auditory stimuli in teaching words and Blissymbols to the mentally retarded. *Australian Journal of Mental Retardation, 5*, 298-302.

Hull, R. H. (2014). *Introduction to aural rehabilitation* (2nd ed.). Plural Publishing.

Hunston, S. (2002). *Corpora in applied linguistics.* Cambridge University Press.

Huo, X., & Ghovanloo, M. (2012). Tongue drive: A wireless tongue-operated means for people with severe disabilities to communicate their intentions. *Communications Magazine IEEE, 50*(10), 128-135.

Hurlbut, B., Iwata, B., & Green, J. (1982). Nonvocal language acquisition in adolescents with severe physical disabilities: Blissymbol versus iconic stimulus formats. *Journal of Applied Behavior Analysis, 15*, 241-258.

Hurtig, R. R., Alper, R., Altschuler, T., Gendreau, S., Gormley, J., Marshall, S., Santiago, R., & Scibilia, S. (2020). Improving outcomes for hospitalized patients pre- and post-COVID-19. *Perspectives of the ASHA Special Interest Groups, 5*, 1577-1586.

Hurtig, R. R., Alper, R. M., & Berkowitz, B. (2018). The cost of not addressing the communication barriers faced by hospitalized patients. *Perspectives of the ASHA Special Interest Groups, 3*(12), 99-112.

Hurtig, R. R., Czerniejewski, E., Bohnenkamp, L., & Na, J. (2013). Meeting the needs of limited English proficiency patients. *Perspectives on Augmentative and Alternative Communication, 22*(2), 91-101.

Hurtig, R. R., & Downey, D. A. (2009). *Augmentative and alternative communication in acute and critical care settings.* Plural Publishing.

Hurtig, R. R., Nilsen, M., Happ, E. B., & Blackstone, S. (2015). Acute care/hospital/ICU-adults. In S. Blackstone, D. R. Beukelman, & K. Yorkston (Eds.), *Patient provider communication in health care settings: Roles for speech-language pathologists and other professionals.* Plural Publishing.

Hurtig, R. R., & Slayman, B. (2016, November). *Supporting medical decision making and end-of-life communication needs.* Presentation at the ALSA Clinical Conference.

Hustad, K. C. (2001). Unfamiliar listeners' evaluation of speech supplementation strategies for improving the effectiveness of severely dysarthric speech. *Augmentative and Alternative Communication, 17*, 213-220.

Hustad, K. C. (2005). Effects of speech supplementation strategies on intelligibility and listener attitudes for a speaker with mild dysarthria. *Augmentative and Alternative Communication, 21*, 256-263.

Hustad, K. C., Allison, K. M., Sakash, A., McFadd, E., Broman, A. T., & Rathouz, P. J. (2017). Longitudinal development of communication in children with cerebral palsy between 24 and 53 months: Predicting speech outcomes. *Developmental Neurorehabilitation, 20*(6), 323-330.

Hustad, K. C., & Beukelman, D. R. (2000). Integrating AAC strategies with natural speech in adults. In D. R. Beukelman, K. M. Yorkston, & J. Reichle (Eds.), *Augmentative and alternative communication for adults with acquired neurologic disorders* (pp. 83-106). Paul H. Brookes Publishing Co.

Hustad, K. C., Dardis, C. M., & Kramper, A. J. (2011). Use of listening strategies for the speech of individuals with dysarthria and cerebral palsy. *Augmentative and Alternative Communication, 27*(1), 5-15.

Hustad, K. C., Morehouse, T., & Gutmann, M. (2002). AAC strategies for enhancing the usefulness of natural speech in children with severe intelligibility challenges. In J. Reichle, D. R. Beukelman, & J. Light (Eds.), *Exemplary practices for beginning communicators: Implications for AAC* (pp. 433-474). Paul H. Brookes Publishing Co.

Hutchins, T. L., & Prelock, P. A. (2014). Using communication to reduce challenging behaviors in individuals with autism spectrum disorders and intellectual disability. *Child and Adolescent Psychiatric Clinics of North America, 23*, 41-55.

Hux, K., Knollman-Porter, K. P., Brown, J., & Wallace, S. E. (2017). Comprehension of synthetic speech and digitized natural speech by adults with aphasia. *Journal of Communication Disorders, 69*, 15-26.

Hwa-Froelich, D., & Vigil, D. C. (2004). Three aspects of cultural influence on communication: A literature review. *Communication Disorders Quarterly, 25*(3), 107-118.

Hymes, D. (1971). Competence and performance in linguistic theory. In R. Huxley and E. Ingram (Eds.), *Language acquisition: Models and methods* (pp. 3-28). Academic Press.

Hynan, A., Goldbart, J., & Murray, J. (2015). A grounded theory of internet and social media use by young people who use augmentative and alternative communication (AAC). *Disability Rehabilitation, 37*(17), 1559-1575.

Hyter, Y. D., & Salas-Provance, M. B. (2019). *Culturally responsive practice in speech, language and hearing science.* Plural Publishing.

Iacono, T. (2002). Words. *Augmentative and Alternative Communication, 18*(4), 215-216.

Iacono, T. (2019). Personal communication via email, February 4, 2019.

Iacono, T., Mirenda, P., & Beukelman, D. R. (1993). Comparison of unimodal and multimodal AAC techniques for children with intellectual disabilities. *Augmentative and Alternative Communication, 9*, 83-94.

Iacono, T., Trembath, D., & Erickson, S. (2016). The role of augmentative and alternative communication for children with autism: Current status and future trends. *Neuropsychiatric Disease and Treatment, 12*, 2349-2361.

Illingworth, R. (1967). The development of the infant and young child [book review]. *American Journal of the Medical Sciences, 253*, 501.

Individuals with Disabilities Education Improvement Act. (2004). Retrieved from https://sites.ed.gov/idea/

Induruwa, I., Constantinescu, C., & Gran, B. (2012). Fatigue in multiple sclerosis: A brief review. *Journal of Neurological Science, 323*, 9-15.

Institute of Medicine and National Research Council. (2001). *Musculoskeletal disorders and the workplace: Low back and upper extremities.* The National Academies Press.

International Communication Learning Institute. (1986). *Introducing visual phonics* [videotape]. Author.

International Society for Augmentative and Alternative Communication (ISAAC). (2013). The International Society for Augmentative and Alternative Communication. Retrieved from https://www.isaac-online.org/english/home/

Isaacson, M. D. (2017). Personal communication, June 14, 2017.

Isaacson, M. D., & Lloyd, L. L. (2013). A computerized procedure for teaching the relationship between graphic symbols and their referents. *Assistive Technology, 25*, 127-136.

Isaacson, M. D., & Lloyd, L. L. (2015). A tactile communication system based on Blissymbolics: An efficacy study. *Developmental Neurorehabilitation, 18*, 47-58.

Isaacson, M. D., Supalo, C., Michaels, M., & Roth, A. (2016). An examination of accessible hands-on science learning experiences: Self-confidence in one's capacity to function in the sciences, and motivation and interest in scientific studies and careers. *Journal of Science Education for Students with Disabilities, 19*(1), Article 7.

Iverson, J. M., & Goldin-Meadow, S. (2005). Gesture paves the way for language development. *Psychological Society, 16*(5), 367-371.

Iverson, J. M., & Thal, D. (1998). Communication transitions: There's more to the hand than meets the eye. In A. Wetherby, S. Warren, & J. Reichle (Eds.), *Transitions to prelinguistic communication* (pp. 59-86). Paul H. Brookes Publishing Co.

Iwata, B. A., DeLeon, I. G., & Roscoe, E. M. (2013). Reliability and validity of the Functional Analysis Screening Tool. *Journal of Applied Behavior Analysis, 46,* 271-284.

Iwata, B. A, Dorsey, M. F., Slifer, K. J., Bauman, K. E., & Richman, G. S. (1982). Toward a functional analysis of self-injury. *Analysis and Intervention in Developmental Disabilities, 2,* 3-20.

Jacoby, L. L. (1978). On interpreting the effects of repetition: Solving a problem versus remembering a solution. *Journal of Verbal Learning and Verbal Behavior, 17,* 649-667.

Jaffe, J., Beebe, B., Feldstein, S., Crown, C. L., Jasnow, M. D., Rochat, P., & Stern, D. N. (2001). Rhythms of dialogue in infancy: Coordinated timing in development. *Monographs of the Society for Research in Child Development, 66,* 1-132.

Jagaroo, V., & Wilkinson, K. (2008). Further considerations of visual cognitive neuroscience in aided AAC: The potential role of motion perception systems in maximizing design display. *Augmentative and Alternative Communication, 24*(1), 29-42.

Jahoda, A., Wilson, A., Stalker, K., & Cairney, A. (2010). Living with stigma and the self-perceptions of people with mild intellectual disabilities. *Journal of Social Issues, 66,* 521-534.

James, J. T. (2013). A new, evidence-based estimate of patient harms associated with hospital care. *Journal of Patient Safety, 9,* 122-128.

Jan, J. E., & Groenveld, M. (1993). Visual behaviors and adaptations associated with cortical and ocular impairments in children. *Journal of Visual Impairment and Blindness, 87,* 101-105.

Janssen, M., & Rødbroe, I. (2007). *Communication and congenital deafblindness: Contact and social interaction* (Vol. 2). VCDBF/Viataal.

Jeffree, D. (1981). A bandage between pictures and print. *Special Education Forward Trends, 8,* 28-31.

Joffee, E., & Rikhye, C. H. (1991). Orientation and mobility for students with severe visual and multiple impairments: A new perspective. *Journal of Visual Impairment and Blindness, 85,* 211-216.

Johns, J. (2005). *Basic reading inventory.* Kendall/Hunt.

Johnson, C. E. (2012). *Introduction to auditory rehabilitation: A contemporary issues approach.* Pearson.

Johnson, J. M., Inglebret, E., Jones, C., & Ray, J. (2006). Perspectives of speech language pathologists regarding success versus abandonment of AAC. *Augmentative and Alternative Communication, 22*(2), 85-99.

Johnson, R. K. (1985). *The picture communication symbols—Book II.* Mayer-Johnson Co.

Johnson, R. K., & Prebor, J. (2019). Update on preservice training in augmentative and alternative communication for speech-language pathologists. *American Journal of Speech-Language Pathology, 28,* 536-549.

Johnston, S. S., & Reichle, J. (1993). Designing and implementing interventions to decrease challenging behavior. *Language, Speech, and Hearing Services in Schools, 24,* 225-235.

Johnston, S. S., Reichle, J., Feeley, K. M., & Jones, E. A. (2012). *AAC strategies for individuals with moderate to severe disabilities.* Paul H. Brookes Publishing Co.

Joint Committee on Infant Hearing. (2007). Year 2007 position statement: Principles and guidelines for early hearing detection and intervention programs. *American Academy of Pediatrics, 120*(4), 898-921.

Jones, J. (1979). A rebus system of non-fade visual language. *Child Care, Health, and Development, 5,* 1-7.

Jones, K. R. (1972). Rebus materials in pre-school playgroups. In Teachers' Research Groups Journal. Bristol, England Research Unit, School of Education, University of Bristol.

Jones, K. R. (1976). The development of pre-reading procedures based upon the reading of rebus materials. In A. Cashdan (Ed.), *The content of reading.* Ward Look Educational.

Jones, M., & Gray, S. (2005). Assistive technology: Positioning and mobility. In S. K. Effgen (Ed.), *Meeting the physical therapy needs of children* (pp. 621-633). F. A. Davis Company.

Jones, P. R. & Cregan, A. (1986). *Sign and symbol communication for mentally handicapped people.* Croom Helm.

Judge, S., & Colven, D. (2006). Switch access to technology: A comprehensive guide. The ACE Centre, 92 Windmill Road Headington Oxford OX3 7DR. Retrieved from http://eprints.whiterose.ac.uk/10291/

Judge, S., & Townsend, G. (2013). Perceptions of the design of voice output communication aids. *International Journal of Language and Communication Disorders, 48*(3), 366-381.

Kagan, A. (1998). Supported conversation for adults with aphasia: Methods and resources for training conversation partners. *Aphasiology, 12*(9), 816-830.

Kagan, A., Black, S. E., Duchan, J. F., Simmons-Mackie, N., & Square, P. (2001). Training volunteers as conversation partners using "Supported Conversation for Adults with Aphasia" (SCA). *Journal of Speech, Language, and Hearing Research, 44,* 624-638.

Kalyanpur, M., & Harry, B. (1999). *Culture in special education: Building reciprocal family-professional relationships.* Paul H. Brookes Publishing Co.

Kalyanpur, M., Harry, B., & Skrtic, T. (2000). Equity and advocacy expectations of culturally diverse families' participation in special education. *International Journal of Disability, Development, and Education, 47*(2), 119-136.

Kambanaros, M., Pampoulou, E., Charalambous, M., & Georgiou, A. (2019). *Modification of the SAQoL tool to promote understanding for people with aphasia.* Conference Proceedings, Communication Matters.

Kamps, D., Mason, R., Thiemann-Bourque, K., Feldmiller, S., Turcotte, A., & Miller, L. (2014). The use of peer networks to increase communicative acts of students with autism spectrum disorders. *Focus on Autism and Other Developmental Disabilities, 29,* 230-245.

Kamps, D., Thiemann-Bourque, K., Heitzman-Powell, L., Schwartz, I., Rosen, N., Mason, R., & Cox, S. (2015). A comprehensive peer network intervention to improve the social communication of children with autism spectrum disorders: A randomized trial in kindergarten and first grade. *Journal of Autism and Developmental Disorders, 45,* 1809-1824.

Kane, S. K., Linam-Church, B., Althoff, K., & McCall, D. (2012). What we talk about: Designing a context-aware communication tool for people with aphasia. In *Proceedings of the 14th international ACM SIGACCESS conference on computers and accessibility* (pp. 49-56).

Kane, S. K., Morris, M. R., Perkins, A. Z., Wigdor, D., Ladner, R. E., & Wobbrock, J. O. (2011). Access overlays: Improving nonvisual access to large touch screens for blind users. In *Proceedings of the User Interface Software and Technology (UIST 2011) Conference* (pp. 273-282).

Kangas, K. A., & Lloyd, L. L. (1988). Early cognitive skills as prerequisites to augmentative and alternative communication use: What are we waiting for? *Augmentative and Alternative Communication, 4*(4), 211-221.

Kaplan, E., Goodglass, H., Weintraub, S., & Segal, O. (2001). *Boston naming test* (2nd ed.). Lippincott Williams & Wilkins.

Karlan, G. R., & Lloyd, L. L. (1983). Considerations in the planning of communication intervention: Selecting a lexicon. *Journal of the Association for Persons with Severe Handicaps, 8,* 13-25.

Karlsson, P., Allsop, A., Dee-Price, B. J., & Wallen, M. (2018). Eye-gaze control technology for children, adolescents and adults with cerebral palsy with significant physical disability: Findings from a systematic review. *Developmental Neurorehabilitation, 21*(8), 497-505.

Kates, B., & McNaughton, S. (1975). *The first application of Blissymbolics as a communication medium for nonspeaking children: History and development, 1971-1974.* Easter Seals Communication Institute.

Katz, J. (2015). *Handbook of clinical audiology* (7th ed.). Wolters Kluwer.

Katz, R., & Wertz, R. (1997). The efficacy of computer-provided reading treatment for chronic aphasic adults. *Journal of Speech, Language, and Hearing Research, 40*(3), 493-507.

Kawachi, I. (2019). Neuropathological features of "non-motor" symptoms in multiple sclerosis and neuromyelitis optica. *Clinical and Experimental Neuroimmunology, 10*, 161-168.

Kay, D. (2014). Holistic approach to physical motor access assessment in pediatric AAC. *Perspectives on Augmentative and Alternative Communication, 23*, 84-90.

Kearney, C. A. (1994). Interrater reliability of the Motivation Assessment Scale: Another closer look. *Journal of the Association for Persons with Severe Handicaps, 2*, 139-142.

Keen, D., Meadan, H., Brady, N. C., & Halle, J. W. (2016). *Prelinguistic and minimally verbal communicators on the autism spectrum.* Springer Nature.

Keith, R. W. (1999). Treatment for central auditory processing disorders - Clinical issues in central auditory processing disorders. *Language Speech and Hearing Services in Schools, 30*(4), 339-344.

Kelford-Smith, A., Thurston, S., Light, J., Parnes, P., & O'Keefe, B. (1989). The form and use of written communication produced by physically disabled individuals using microcomputers. *Augmentative and Alternative Communication, 5*, 115-124.

Kelley, P., Davidson, R., & Sanspree, M. J. (1993). Vision and orientation and mobility consultation for children with severe multiple disabilities. *Journal of Visual Impairment and Blindness, 87*, 7-9.

Keltner, D. (2010, September). *Hands on research: The science of touch.* Greater Good Magazine: Science-Based Insights for a Meaningful Life.

Kemp, C., & Parette, H. (2000). Barriers to minority family involvement in assistive technology decision-making processes. *Education and Training in Mental Retardation and Developmental Disabilities, 4*, 211-221.

Kennard, G., Grove, T., & Hall, L. (1992). *Signalong* (2nd ed.). The Signalong Group.

Kent, R. (1992). *Intelligibility in speech disorders: Theory, measurement and management.* John Benjamins Publishing Company.

Kent-Walsh, J., & McNaughton, D. (2005). Communication partner instruction in AAC: Present practices and future directions. *Augmentative and Alternative Communication, 21*(3), 195-204.

Keogh, B., & Reichle, J. (1985). Communication intervention for the "difficult-to-teach" severely handicapped. In S. Warren & A. Rogers-Warren (Eds.), *Teaching functional language* (pp. 157-196). Pro-Ed.

Kerzner, H. (2017). *Project management: A systems approach to planning, scheduling, and controlling.* John Wiley & Sons.

Kevan, F. (2003). Challenging behaviour and communication difficulties. *British Journal of Learning Disabilities, 31*, 75-80.

Kiernan, C. C., Reid, B., & Jones, L. (1982). *Signs and symbols: A review of literature and survey of the use of non-vocal communication.* Heinemann Educational Books.

Kiese-Himmel, C. (2002). Unilateral sensorineural hearing impairment in childhood: Analysis of 31 consecutive cases. *International Journal of Audiology, 41*(1), 57-63.

Kiese-Himmel, C., & Ohlwein, S. (2003). Characteristics of children with permanent mild hearing impairment. *Folia Phoniatrica et Logopaedica, 55*(2), 70-79.

Kilgarriff, A., Charalabopoulou, F., Gavrilidou, M., Johannessen, J. B., Khalil, S., Kokkinakis, S. J., Lew, R., Sharoff, S., Vadlapudi, R., & Volodina, E. (2014). Corpus-based vocabulary lists for language learners for nine languages. *Language Resources and Evaluation, 48*, 121-163.

Kim, J. S., & Kim, C. H. (2014). A review of assistive listening device and digital wireless technology for hearing instruments. *Korean Journal of Audiology, 18*(3), 105-111.

Kim, J., Park, H., Bruce, J., Rowles, D., Holbrook, J., Nardone, B., West, D. P., Laumann, A. E., Roth, E., Veledar, E., & Ghovanloo, M. (2014). Qualitative assessment of a tongue drive system by people with high-level spinal cord injury. *Journal of Rehabilitation Research and Development, 51*(3), 451-465.

Kimura, D. (1990). How special is language? *Sign Language Studies, 66*, 79-84.

King, M., Ward, H., Soto, G., & Barrett, T. (2022). Supporting emergent bilinguals who use augmentative and alternative communication and their families: Lessons in telepractice from the COVID-19 pandemic. *American Journal of Speech-Language Pathology, 31*(5), 2004-2021.

King, T. W. (1999). *Assistive technology: Essential human factors.* Allyn & Bacon.

King-DeBaun, P. (1990). *Storytime: Stories, symbols, and emergent literacy activities for young, special needs children.* Author.

Kingdom, F. A. A., & Prins, N. (2016). *Psychophysics: A practical introduction* (2nd ed.). Academic Press.

Kiresuk, T., & Sherman, R. (1968). Goal attainment scaling: A general method for evaluating comprehensive mental health programmed. *Community Mental Health Journal, 4*, 443-453.

Kirkwood, S., Su, J., Conneally, P., & Foroud, T. (2001). Progression of symptoms in the early and middle stages of Huntington disease. *Archives of Neurology, 58*(2), 273-278.

Klasner, E. R., & Yorkston, K. M. (2000). AAC for Huntington's disease and Parkinson's disease. In D. R. Beukelman, K. M. Yorkston, & J. Reichle (Eds.), *Augmentative and alternative communication for adults with acquired neurologic disorders* (pp. 233-270). Paul H. Brookes Publishing Co.

Klasner, E. R., & Yorkston, K. M. (2001). Linguistic and cognitive supplementation strategies as augmentative and alternative communication techniques in HD. *Augmentative and Alternative Communication, 17*(3), 154-160.

Klatt, D. H. (1987). Review of text-to-speech conversion for English. *The Journal of the Acoustical Society of America, 82*(3), 737-793.

Kleiman, L. (2003). *Functional communication profile, revised.* LinguiSystems.

Klein, C. (2016). Overcoming barriers with cerebral palsy [web log post]. Retrieved from https://helphopelive.org/breaking-barriers-with-cerebral-palsy/

Kleinert, H. L., Browder, D. M., & Towles-Reeves, E. A. (2009). Models of cognition for students with significant cognitive disabilities: Implications for assessment. *Review of Educational Research, 79*, 301-326.

Klima, E., & Bellugi, U. (1979). *The signs of language.* Harvard University Press.

Kluger, B., Krupp, L., & Enoka, R. (2013). Fatigue and fatigability in neurologic illnesses: Proposal for a unified taxonomy. *Neurology, 80*(4), 409-416.

Knight, V., Sartini, E., & Spriggs, A. D. (2015). Evaluating visual activity schedules as evidence-based practice for individuals with autism spectrum disorders. *Journal of Autism and Developmental Disorders, 45*, 157-178.

Kochkin, S., & Rogin, C. M. (2002). Quantifying the obvious: The impact of hearing instruments on quality of life. *The Hearing Review.* Retrieved from https://pdfs.semanticscholar.org/44ca/4bd1d9007aab 0e75ea61f104c0fe7c9e1cf9.pdf

Koczur, E. L., Strine, C. E., Peischl, D., Lytton, R., Rahman, T., & Alexander, M. A. (2015). Orthotics and assistive devices. In M. A. Alexander & D. J. Matthews (Eds.), *Pediatric rehabilitation: Principles and practice* (5th ed., Ch. 8, pp. 170-195). Demos Medical Publishing.

Koehler, L., Lloyd, L. L., & Swanson, L. (1994). Visual similarity between manual and printed alphabet letters. *Augmentative and Alternative Communication, 10,* 87-95.

Koenigsfeld, A. S., Beukelman, D. R., & Stoefen-Fisher, J. M. (1993). Attitudes of severely hearing-impaired persons towards augmentative communication characteristics. *The Volta Review, 95*(Spring), 109-124.

Koester, H. H., & Levine, S. P. (1994). Learning and performance of able-bodied individuals using scanning systems with and without word prediction. *Assistive Technology, 6,* 42-53.

Koester, H. H., & Simpson, R. C. (2017). Effectiveness and usability of scanning wizard software: A tool for enhancing switch scanning. *Disability and Rehabilitation: Assistive Technology, 24,* 1-11.

Kohl, F. L. (1981). The effects of motor requirements on the acquisition of manual sign responses by severely handicapped students. *American Journal of Mental Deficiency, 85,* 396-403.

Kohn, L. T., Corrigan, J. M., & Donaldson, M. S. (Eds.). (2000). *To err is human: Building a safer health system: A report of the Committee on Quality of Health Care in America.* National Academic Press.

Kohnert, K. (2010). Bilingual children with primary language impairment: Issues, evidence and implications for clinical actions. *Journal of Communication Disorders, 43*(6), 456-473.

Kohnert, K. (2013a). *Language disorders in bilingual children and adults* (2nd ed.). Plural Publishing.

Kohnert, K. (2013b). One insider's reflections on white privilege, race and their professional relevance. *Perspectives on Communication Disorders and Sciences in Culturally and Linguistically Diverse Populations, 20*(2), 41-48.

Kohnert, K., & Medina, A. (2009). Bilingual children and communication disorders: A 30-year research retrospective. *Seminars in Speech and Language, 30*(4), 219-233.

Konstantareas, M. M. (1984). Sign language as a communication prosthesis with language-impaired children. *Journal of Autism and Developmental Disorders, 14,* 9-23.

Konstantareas, M. M., Oxman, J., & Webster, C. D. (1978). Iconicity: Effects on the acquisition of sign language by autistic and other severely dysfunctional children. In P. Siple (Ed.), *Understanding language through sign language research* (pp. 213-237). Academic Press.

Kopchick, G., & Lloyd, L. L. (1976). Total communication programming for the severely language impaired: A 24-hour approach. In L. L. Lloyd (Ed.), *Communication assessment and intervention strategies* (pp. 501-521). University Park Press.

Koppenhaver, D. A., Coleman, P. P., Kalman, S. L., & Yoder, D. E. (1991). The implications of emergent literacy research for children with developmental disabilities. *American Journal of Speech-Language Pathology, 1*(1), 38-44.

Koppenhaver, D. A., Evans, D., & Yoder, D. E. (1991). Childhood reading and writing experiences of literate adults with severe speech and motor impairments. *Augmentative and Alternative Communication, 7,* 20-33.

Koppenhaver, D. A., & Yoder, D. E. (1993). Classroom literacy instruction for children with severe speech and physical impairments (SSPI): What is and what might be. *Topics in Language Disorders, 13*(2), 1-15.

Körner, S., Sieniawski, M., Kollewe, K., Rath, K. J., Krampfl, K., Zapf, A., Dengler, R., & Petri, S. (2013). Speech therapy and communication devices: Impact on quality of life and mood in patients with amyotrophic lateral sclerosis. *Amyotrophic Lateral Sclerosis and Frontotemporal Degeneration, 14*(1), 20-25.

Korsten, J. (2011). AAC: Systemic change for individual success, Jane Farrell Consulting, QIAT Listserv 4th April. [Electronic mailing list message]. Retrieved from http://www.janefarrall.com/aac-systemic-change-for-individual-success/

Koul, R. K. (Ed.). (2011). *Augmentative and alternative communication for adults with aphasia: Science and clinical practice.* Emerald Group Publishing Limited.

Koul, R. K., & Corwin, M. (2003). Efficacy of AAC intervention in individuals with chronic severe aphasia. In R.W. Schlosser (Ed.), *The efficacy of augmentative and alternative communication: Toward evidence-based practice* (pp. 449-470). Elsevier Science.

Koul, R. K., Corwin, M., & Hayes, S. (2005). Production of graphic symbol sentences by individuals with aphasia: Efficacy of a computer-based augmentative and alternative communication intervention. *Brain and Language, 92*(1), 58-77.

Koul, R. K., Corwin, M., Nigam, R., & Oetzel, S. (2008). Training individuals with chronic severe Broca's aphasia to produce sentences using graphic symbols: Implications for AAC intervention. *Journal of Assistive Technologies, 2*(1), 23-34.

Koul, R. K., & Harding, R. (1998). Identification and production of graphic symbols by individuals with aphasia: Efficacy of a software application. *Augmentative and Alternative Communication, 14*(1), 11-24.

Koul, R. K., & Lloyd, L. L. (1994). Survey of professional preparation in augmentative and alternative communication (AAC) in speech-language pathology and special education programs. *American Journal of Speech-Language Pathology, 3,* 13-22.

Koul, R. K., Petroi, D., & Schlosser, R. (2010). Systematic review of speech generating devices for aphasia. In *Computer synthesized speech technologies: Tools for aiding impairment* (pp. 148-160). IGI Global.

Kouremenos, D., Ntalianis, K., & Kollias, S. (2018). A novel rule based machine translation scheme from Greek to Greek Sign Language: Production of different types of large corpora and language models evaluation. *Computer Speech and Language, 51,* 110-135.

Kouri, T. A. (1988). Effects of simultaneous communication in a child-directed treatment approach with preschoolers with severe disabilities. *Augmentative and Alternative Communication, 4,* 222-232.

Kovach, T. M. (2009). *Augmentative and alternative communication profile: A continuum of learning.* LinguiSystems.

Kraat, A. (1990). Augmentative and alternative communication: Does it have a future in aphasia rehabilitation? *Aphasiology, 4*(4), 321-338.

Królak, A., & Strumiłło, P. (2012). Eye-blink detection system for human-computer interaction. *Universal Access in the Information Society, 11,* 409-419.

Kulkarni, S. S., & Parmar, J. (2017). Culturally and linguistically diverse student and family perspectives of AAC. *Augmentative and Alternative Communication, 33*(3), 170-180.

Kummerer, S. (2012). Promising strategies for collaborating with Hispanic parents during family-centered speech-language intervention. *Communication Disorders Quarterly, 33*(2), 84-95.

Kuntz, J. B. (1975). *A nonvocal communication program for severely retarded children.* (Doctoral dissertation, Kansas State University, 1974), Dissertation Abstracts International, 36, 219A.

Kyle, J. G., & Woll, B. (1985). *Sign language: The study of deaf people and their language.* Cambridge University Press.

Laing, S. P., & Kamhi, A. G. (2003). Alternative assessment of language and literacy in culturally and linguistically diverse populations. *Language, Speech, and Hearing Services in Schools, 34,* 44-55.

Lalli, J. S., & Goh, H. L. (1993). Naturalistic observations in community settings. In J. Reichle & D. P. Wacker (Eds.), *Communicative alternatives to challenging behavior: Integrating functional assessment and intervention strategies* (pp. 11-40). Paul H. Brookes Publishing Co.

Lancioni, G. E., O'Reilly, M. F., Cuvo, A. J., Singh, N. N., Sigafoos, J., & Didden, R. (2007). PECS and VOCAs to enable students with developmental disabilities to make requests: An overview of the literature. *Research in Developmental Disabilities, 28,* 468-488.

Lancioni, G. E., Singh, N. N., O'Reilly, M. F., Sigafoss, J., & Didden, R. (2012). Functions of challenging behaviors. In J. L. Matson (Ed.), *Functional assessment for challenging behaviors* (pp. 45-64). Springer.

Landman, C., & Schaeffler, C. (1986). Object communication boards. *Communication Outlook, 8,* 7-8.

Landrigan, C. P., Parry, G. J., Bones, C. B., Hackbarth, A. D., Goldmann, D. A., & Sharek, P. J. (2010). Temporal trends in rates of patient harm resulting from medical care. *New England Journal of Medicine, 363,* 2124-2134.

Lane, H. (1984). *When the mind hears: A history of the deaf.* Random House.

Lang, M. L. (2018). Power mobility: Alternative access methods. In M. L. Lang & J. L. Minkel (Eds.), *Seating and wheeled mobility: A clinical resource guide* (pp. 179-198). SLACK Incorporated.

Langdon, D. W. (2011). Cognition in multiple sclerosis. *Current Opinion in Neurology, 24*(3), 244-249.

Langdon, H. W. (2008). *Assessment and intervention for communication disorders in culturally and linguistically diverse populations.* Thomson Delmar.

Langdon, H. W., & Saenz, T. I. (2016). *Working with interpreters and translators: A guide for speech-language pathologists and audiologists.* Plural Publishing.

Lanzi, A., Burshnic, V., & Bourgeois, M. S. (2017). Person-centered memory and communication strategies for adults with dementia. *Topics in Language Disorders, 37*(4), 361-374.

Larson, J., McMorris Rodgers, C., Cassidy, B., & Klobuchar, A. (2017). Steve Gleason Enduring Voices Act. Retrieved from https://www.medicareadvocacy.org/steve-gleason-enduring-voices-act-introduced/

Laska, A. C., Hellblom, A., Murray, V., Kahan, T., & Von Arbin, M. (2001). Aphasia in acute stroke and relation to outcome. *Journal of Internal Medicine, 249*(5), 413-422.

Lasker, J. P. (2008). AAC language assessment: Considerations for adults with aphasia. *Perspectives on Augmentative and Alternative Communication, 17*(3), 105-112.

Lasker, J. P., & Bedrosian, J. (2001). Promoting acceptance of augmentative and alternative communication by adults with acquired communication disorders. *Augmentative and Alternative Communication, 17,* 141-153.

Lasker, J. P., & Beukelman, D. R. (1999). Peers' perception of storytelling by an adult with aphasia. *Aphasiology, 13*(9-11), 857-869.

Lasker, J. P., & Garrett, K. (2006). Using the Multimodal Communication Screening Test for Persons with Aphasia (MCST-A) to guide the selection of alternative communication strategies for people with aphasia. *Aphasiology, 20*(02-04), 217-232.

Lasker, J. P., Garrett, K., & Fox, L. (2007a). AAC—Aphasia needs assessment. In D. R. Beukelman, K. L. Garrett, & K. M. Yorkston (Eds.), *Augmentative communication strategies for adults with acute or chronic medical conditions* (Form 6.2 on accompanying CD-ROM). Paul H. Brookes Publishing Co.

Lasker, J. P., Garrett, K., & Fox, L. (2007b). Severe aphasia. In D. Beukelman, K. Garrett, & K. Yorkston (Eds.), *Augmentative communication strategies for adults with acute or chronic medical conditions* (pp. 163-206). Paul H. Brookes Publishing Co.

Lasker, J. P., Hux, K., Garrett, K., Moncrief, E., & Eischeid, T. (1997). Variations on the written choice communication strategy for individuals with severe aphasia. *Augmentative and Alternative Communication, 13*(2), 108-116.

Lazarou, I., Nikolopoulos, S., Petrantonakis, P. C., Kompatsiaris, I., & Tsolaki, M. (2018). EEG-based brain–computer interfaces for communication and rehabilitation of people with motor impairment: A novel approach of the 21st century. *Frontiers in Human Neuroscience.* Retrieved at https://www.ncbi.nlm.nih.gov/pmc/articles/PMC5810272/

Leathart, A. (1994). Communication and socialization (1): An exploratory study and explanation for nurse patient communication in an ICU. *Intensive and Critical Care Nursing, 10,* 93-104.

LeBlanc, K. E., & LeBlanc, L. L. (2010). Musculoskeletal disorders. *Primary Care Clinical Office Practice, 37,* 389-406.

Lee, C. Y., & Cherner, T. S. (2015). A comprehensive evaluation rubric for assessing instructional apps. *Journal of Information Technology Education: Research, 14,* 21-53.

Lee, C. Y., Jeong, S. W., & Kim, L. S. (2013). AAC intervention using a VOCA for deaf children with multiple disabilities who received cochlear implantation. *International Journal of Pediatric Otorhinolaryngology, 77*(12), 2008-2013.

Leighton, J. A. (2015). Collaboration in this environment of mobile technology and change: One clinician's perspective. *Perspectives on Augmentative and Alternative Communication, 24*(1), 12-18.

Leonhart, W., & Maharaj, S. (1979). A comparison of initial recognition and rate of acquisition of Pictogram Ideogram Communication (PIC) and Bliss symbols with institutionalized severely retarded adults. Unpublished manuscript.

Lequia, J., Machalicek, W., & Rispoli, M. J. (2012). Effects of activity schedules on challenging behavior exhibited in children with autism spectrum disorders: A systematic review. *Research in Autism Spectrum Disorders, 6,* 480-492.

Lesher, G. W., Rinkus, G. J., Moulton, B. J., & Higginbotham, D. J. (2000). Logging and analysis of augmentative communication. In *Proceedings of the RESNA 2000 Annual Conference* (pp. 82-85). RESNA Press.

Leslie, L., & Caldwell, J. A. (2017). *Qualitative reading inventory* (6th ed.). Pearson.

Leslie, P., Xia, B., & Yoo, J. (2021). It's not such a small world after all: The intersection of food, identity, and the speech-language pathologist. *Perspectives of the ASHA Special Interest Groups, 6,* 876-884.

Levelt, W. J. M. (1989). *Speaking: From intention to articulation.* MIT Press.

Levelt, W. J. M. (1993). *Speaking: From intention to articulation* (2nd ed.). MIT Press.

Levesque, K. C., Breadmore, H. L., & Deacon, S. H. (2021). How morphology impacts reading and spelling: Advancing the role of morphology in models of literacy development. *Journal of Research in Reading, 44*(1), 10-26.

Levine, S. P., Gauger, J. R. D., Bowers, L. D., & Khan, K. J. (1986). A comparison of mouthstick and Morse code text inputs. *Augmentative and Alternative Communication, 2,* 51-55.

Levinson, D. R. (2010). *Adverse events in hospitals: National incidence among Medicare beneficiaries.* Department of Health and Human Services Office of Inspector General.

Levinson, R. B. (1967). *A Plato reader.* Houghton Mifflin College Division.

Liang, C. A., Braddock, B. A, Heithaus, J., Christensen, K., Braddock, S. R., & Carey, J. C. (2013). Reported communication ability of persons with trisomy 18 and trisomy 13. *Developmental Neurorehabilitation, 18,* 322-329.

Liang, J., & Liu, H. (2013). Noun distribution in natural languages. *Poznan Studies in Contemporary Linguistics, 49,* 509-529.

Liao, Y., Loures, E. R., Deschamps, F., Brezinski, G., & Venâncio, A. (2017). The impact of the fourth industrial revolution: A cross-country/region comparison. *Production, 28,* e20180061.

Liberoff, M. (1992). *Comunicacion augmentativa: PCP programa de comunicacion pictogrdfico.* Marymar.

Light, J. C. (1988). Interaction involving individuals using augmentative and alternative communication systems: State of the art and future directions. *Augmentative and Alternative Communication, 4,* 66-82.

Light, J. C. (1989). Toward a definition of communicative competence for individuals using augmentative and alternative communication systems. *Augmentative and Alternative Communication, 5*(2), 137-144.

Light, J. C. (1997a). "Communication is the essence of human life:" Reflections on communicative competence for individuals using augmentative and alternative communication systems. *Augmentative and Alternative Communication, 13,* 61-70.

Light, J. C. (1997b). "Let's go star fishing:" Reflections on the contexts of language learning for children who use aided AAC. *Augmentative and Alternative Communication, 13*(3), 158-171.

Light, J. C. (2003). Shattering the silence: Development of communicative competence by individuals who use AAC. In J. C. Light, D. R. Beukelman, & J. Reichle (Eds.), *Communicative competence for individuals who use AAC: From research to effective practice* (pp. 3-38). Paul H. Brookes Publishing Co.

Light, J. C., Beukelman, D. R., & Reichle, J. (2003). *Communicative competence for individuals who use AAC: From research to effective practice.* Paul H. Brookes Publishing Co.

Light, J. C., Binger, C., & Smith, A. K. (1994). Story reading interactions between preschoolers who use AAC and their mothers. *Augmentative and Alternative Communication, 10*(4), 255-268.

Light, J. C., Collier, B., & Parnes, P. (1985). Communicative interaction between young nonspeaking physically disabled children and their primary caregivers: Part II—Communicative function. *Augmentative and Alternative Communication, 1*(3), 98-107.

Light, J. C., & Drager, K. (2007). AAC technologies for young children with complex communication needs: State of the science and future research directions. *Augmentative and Alternative Communication, 23*(3), 204-216.

Light, J. C., & Kent-Walsh, J. (2003). Fostering emergent literacy for children who require AAC. *The ASHA Leader, 8*(10), 4-5, 28-29.

Light, J. C., & Lindsay, P. (1991). Cognitive science and augmentative and alternative communication. *Augmentative and Alternative Communication, 7,* 186-203.

Light, J. C., & McNaughton, D. (2012a). Supporting the communication, language, and literacy development of children with complex communication needs: State of the science and future research priorities. *Assistive Technology, 24*(1), 34-44.

Light, J. C., & McNaughton, D. (2012b). The changing face of augmentative and alternative communication: Past, present, and future challenges. *Augmentative and Alternative Communication, 28*(4), 197-204.

Light, J. C., & McNaughton, D. (2013). Putting people first: Re-thinking the role of technology in augmentative and alternative communication intervention. *Augmentative and Alternative Communication, 29*(4), 299-309.

Light, J. C., & McNaughton, D. (2014a). Communicative competence for individuals who require augmentative and alternative communication: A new definition for a new era of communication? *Augmentative and Alternative Communication, 30*(1), 1-18.

Light, J. C., & McNaughton, D. (2014b). From basic to applied research to improve outcomes for individuals who require augmentative and alternative communication: Potential contributions of eye tracking research methods. *Augmentative and Alternative Communication, 30*(2), 99-105.

Light, J. C., & McNaughton, D. (2015). Designing AAC research and intervention to improve outcomes for individuals with complex communication needs. *Augmentative and Alternative Communication, 31*(2), 85-96.

Light, J. C., McNaughton, D., Weyer, M., & Karg, L. (2008). Evidence-based literacy instruction for individuals who require augmentative and alternative communication: A case study of a student with multiple disabilities. *Seminars in Speech and Language, 29*(2), 120-132.

Light, J. C., Page, R., Curran, J., & Pitkin, L. (2007). Children's ideas for the design of AAC assistive technologies for young children with complex communication needs. *Augmentative and Alternative Communication, 23*(4), 274-287.

Lilienfeld, M., & Alant, E. (2005). The social interaction of an adolescent who uses AAC: The evaluation of a peer-training program. *Augmentative and Alternative Communication, 21*(4), 278-294.

Lillo, P., Mioshi, E., & Hodges, J. P. (2012). Caregiver burden in amyotrophic lateral sclerosis is more dependent on patients' behavioral changes than physical disability: A comparative study. *BMC Neurology, 12.* Retrieved from https://www.ncbi.nlm.nih.gov/pubmed/23216745

Lillo, P., Savage, S., Mioshi, E., Kiernan, M. C., & Hodges, J. R. (2012). Amyotrophic lateral sclerosis and frontotemporal dementia: A behavioral and cognitive continuum. *Amyotrophic Lateral Sclerosis, 13*(1), 102-109.

Lin, F. R., Niparko, J. K., & Ferrucci, L. (2011). Hearing loss prevalence in the United States. *Archives of Internal Medicine, 171*(20), 1851-1852.

Liu, Q., Feng, G., Shang, Y., Wang, S., & Gao, Z. (2018). Vibrant soundbridge implantation: Floating mass transducer coupled with the stapes head and embedded in fat. *Journal for Oto-Rhino-Laryngology and Its Related Specialties, 80*(2), 59-64.

Lloyd, L. L. (1976). *Communication assessment and intervention strategies.* University Park Press.

Lloyd, L. L. (1985). *Comments on terminology. Augmentative and Alternative Communication, 1*(3), 95-97.

Lloyd, L. L. (1986). Editorial. *Augmentative and Alternative Communication, 2,* 67-68.

Lloyd, L. L. (1993). Editorial. *Augmentative and Alternative Communication, 9,* 227-228.

Lloyd, L. L., & Belfiore, P. J. (1994). The academic infrastructure needed to encourage scholarship on employment for the AAC community. In R. V. Conti & C. Jenkins-Odorisio (Eds.), *Proceedings of the 2nd annual Pittsburgh employment conference for augmented communicators* (pp. 109-118). SHOUT Press.

Lloyd, L. L., & Blischak, D. M. (1992). AAC terminology policy and issues update. *Augmentative and Alternative Communication, 8,* 104-109.

Lloyd, L. L., & Cox, B. P. (1972). Programming for the audiologic aspects of mental retardation. *Mental Retardation, 10*(2), 22-26.

Lloyd, L. L., & Daniloff, J. K. (1983). Issues in using Amer-Ind code with retarded persons. In T. Gallagher & C. Prutting (Eds.), *Pragmatic issues: Assessment and intervention.* College-Hill Press.

Lloyd, L. L., & Doherty, J. (1983). The influence of production mode on recall of signs in normal adult subjects. *Journal of Speech and Hearing Research, 26,* 595-600.

Lloyd, L. L., & Fuller, D. R. (1986). Toward an augmentative and alternative communication symbol taxonomy: A proposed superordinate classification. *Augmentative and Alternative Communication, 2*(4), 165-171.

Lloyd, L. L., & Fuller, D. R. (1990). The role of iconicity in augmentative and alternative communication symbol learning. In W. I. Fraser (Ed.), *Key issues in mental retardation research* (pp. 295-306). Routledge.

Lloyd, L. L., Fuller, D. R., & Arvidson, H. H. (1997). *Augmentative and alternative communication: A handbook of principles and practices.* Allyn & Bacon.

Lloyd, L. L., & Kangas, K. A. (1988). Unaided and aided alternative and augmentative communication. In D. E. Yoder & R. D. Kent (Eds.), *Decision making in speech-language pathology* (pp. 78-81). B.C. Decker.

Lloyd, L. L., & Kangas, K. A. (1994). Augmentative and alternative communication. In G. H. Shames, E. H. Wiig, & W. A. Secord (Eds.), *Human communication disorders* (4th ed., pp. 606-657). Merrill/Macmillan Publishing.

Lloyd, L. L., & Karlan, G. R. (1983). Nonspeech communication symbol selection considerations. In *Proceedings of the XIX Congress of the International Association of Logopaedics and Phoniatrics* (Vol III, pp. 1155-1160). University of Edinburgh.

Lloyd, L. L., & Karlan, G. R. (1984). Nonspeech communication symbols and systems: Where have we been and where are we going? *Journal of Mental Deficiency Research, 28,* 3-20.

Lloyd, L. L., Quist, R. W., & Windsor, J. (1990). A proposed augmentative and alternative communication model. *Augmentative and Alternative Communication, 6,* 172-183.

Lobentanz, I. S., Asenbaum, S., Vass, K., Sauter, C., Klösch, G., Kollegger, H., Kristoferitsch, W., & Zeitlhofer, J. (2004). Factors influencing quality of life in multiple sclerosis patients: Disability, depressive mood, fatigue and sleep quality. *Acta Neurologica Scandinavia, 110,* 6-13.

Locke, P. A., & Mirenda, P. (1988). A computer-supported communication approach for a nonspeaking child with severe visual and cognitive impairments: A case study. *Augmentative and Alternative Communication, 4,* 15-22.

Lomen-Hoerth, C., Anderson, T., & Miller, B. (2002). The overlap of amyotrophic lateral sclerosis and frontotemporal dementia. *Neurology, 59*, 1077-1079.

Loncke, F. (2014). *Augmentative and alternative communication: Models and applications for educators, speech-language pathologists, psychologists, caregivers and users.* Plural Publishing.

Loncke, F., Vander Beken, K., & Lloyd, L. L. (1997). Toward a theoretical model of symbol processing and use. In E. Biorck-Akesson & P. Lindsay (Eds.), *Theoretical and methodological issues in augmentative and alternative communication.* Proceedings of the fourth ISAAC research symposium, Vancouver, Canada, August 1996. Malardalen University Press.

Longmore, P. K., & Goldberger, D. (2000). The league of the physically handicapped and the great depression: A case study in the new disability history. *The Journal of American History, 87*(3), 888-922.

Lorah, E. R., Parnell, A., Whitby, P. S., & Hantula, D. (2015). A systematic review of tablet computers and portable media players as speech generating devices for individuals with autism spectrum disorder. *Journal of Autism and Developmental Disorders, 45*, 3792-3804.

Lorah, E. R., Tincani, M., Dodge, J., Gilroy, S., Hickey, A., & Hantula, D. (2013). Evaluating picture exchange and the iPad as a speech generating device to teach communication to young children with autism. *Journal of Developmental and Physical Disabilities, 25*, 637-650.

Lord, C., Rutter, M., DiLavore, P. C., Risi, S., Gotham, K., & Bishop, S. L. (2012). *Autism Diagnostic Observation Schedule* (2nd ed.) (ADOD-2) manual (part I): Modules 1-4. Western Psychological Services.

Lovaas, I., Newsom, C., & Hickman, C. (1987). Self-stimulatory behavior and perceptual reinforcement. *Journal of Applied Behavior Analysis, 20*, 45-68.

Luckner, J. L., Bruce, S. M., & Ferrell, K. A. (2016). A summary of the communication and literacy evidence-based practices for students who are deaf or hard-of-hearing, visually impaired, and deafblind. *Communication Disorders Quarterly, 37*(4), 225-241.

Luetke-Stahlman, B., & Milburn, W. O. (1996). A history of Seeing Essential English (SEE-I). *American Annals of the Deaf, 141*, 29-33.

Luftig, R. L., & Bersani, H. A., Jr. (1985). An investigation of two variables influencing Blissymbol learnability with nonhandicapped adults. *Augmentative and Alternative Communication, 1*, 32-37.

Luftig, R. L., & Lloyd, L. L. (1981). Manual sign translucency and referential concreteness in the learning of signs. *Sign Language Studies, 30*, 49-60.

Lund, S. K., Quach, W., Weissling, K., McKelvey, M., & Dietz, A. (2017). Assessment with children who need augmentative and alternative communication (AAC): Clinical decisions of AAC specialists. *Language, Speech, and Hearing Services in Schools, 48*(1), 56-68.

Lund, S. K., & Troha, J. M. (2008). Teaching young people who are blind and have autism to make requests using a variation on the Picture Exchange Communication System with tactile symbols: A preliminary investigation. *Journal of Autism and Developmental Disorders, 38*, 719-730.

Lund, S. K., Weissling, K., Quach, W., & McKelvey, M. (2021). Finding a voice for individuals with ASD who are minimally verbal through comprehensive communication assessment. *Perspectives of the ASHA Special Interest Groups, 6*(2), 306-314.

Lundälv, M., Derbring, S., Mühlenbock, K. H., Brännström, A., Farre, B., & Nordberg, L. (2014). Inclusive AAC: Multi-modal and multilingual language support for all. *Technology and Disability, 26*(2-3), 93-103.

Lundman, M. (1978). *Technical aids for the speech-impaired: An international survey on research and development projects.* The Swedish Institute for the Handicapped.

Luqman, H., & Mahmoud, S. A. (2018). Automatic translation of Arabic text-to-Arabic sign language. *Universal Access in the Information Society, 18*(4), 1-13.

Luterman, D. (2008). *Counseling persons with communication disorders and their families* (5th ed.). Pro-Ed.

Lynch, G. T. (2016). AAC for individuals with autism spectrum disorder: Assessment and establishing treatment goals. In T. A. Cardon (Ed.), *Technology and the treatment of children with autism spectrum disorder* (pp. 3-25). Springer Publishing.

Lyon, J. G. (1995). Drawing: Its value as a communication aid for adults with aphasia. *Aphasiology, 9*(1), 33-50.

Lyon, J. G., & Helm-Estabrooks, N. (1987). Drawing: Its communicative significance for expressively restricted aphasic adults. *Topics in Language Disorders, 8*(1), 61-71.

Mace, F. C., & Roberts, M. L. (1993). Factors affecting selection of behavioral interventions. In J. Reichle & D. P. Wacker (Eds.), *Communicative alternatives to challenging behavior: Integrating functional assessment and intervention strategies* (pp. 113-133). Paul H. Brookes Publishing Co.

MacFarland, S. Z. C. (1995). Teaching strategies of the van Dijk curricular approach. *Journal of Visual Impairment and Blindness, 89*, 222-228.

Machado, J. M. (2016). *Early childhood experiences in language arts: Early literacy* (11th ed.). Cengage Learning.

Machalicek, W., Sanford, A., Lang, R., Rispoli, M., Molfenter, N., & Mbeseha, M. (2009). Literacy interventions for students with physical and developmental disabilities who use aided AAC devices: A systematic review. *Journal of Developmental and Physical Disabilities, 22*(3), 219-240.

Macht, J. (1971). Operant measurement of subjective visual acuity in nonverbal children. *Journal of Applied Behavior Analysis, 4*, 23-36.

Maclean, W. E., & Dornbush, K. (2012). Self-injury in a statewide sample of young children with developmental disabilities. *Journal of Mental Health Research in Intellectual Disabilities, 5*(3), 236-245.

Magnus, V. S., & Turkington, L. (2006). Communication interaction in ICU—Patient and staff experiences and perceptions. *Intensive and Critical Care Nursing, 22*(3), 167-180.

Maier, H., Lenarz, T., Agha-Mir-Salim, P., Agterberg, M. J., Anagiotos, A., Arndt, S., ... & Snik, A. (2022). Consensus statement on bone conduction devices and active middle ear implants in conductive and mixed hearing loss. *Otology & Neurotology, 43*, 1-17.

Majaranta, P., & Räihä, K. J. (2002). Twenty years of eye typing: Systems and design issues. *Eye Tracking Research and Applications, 2*, 15-22.

Makkonen, T., Ruottinen, H., Puhto, R., Helminen, M., & Palmio, J. (2018). Speech deterioration in amyotrophic lateral sclerosis (ALS) after manifestation of bulbar symptoms. *International Journal of Language and Communication Disorders, 53*(2), 385-392.

Malandraki, G., & Okalidou, A. (2007). The application of PECS in a deaf child with autism: A case study. *Focus on Autism and Other Developmental Disabilities, 22*(1), 23-32.

Malloy, P., & Bruce, S. (2008). Path to symbolism. *Practice Perspectives—Highlighting Information on Deaf-Blindness, 3*, 1-7.

Malone, J. (1962). The larger aspects of spelling reform. *Elementary English, 39*, 435-445.

Mandak, K., & Light, J. C. (2018). Family-centered services for children with complex communication needs: The practices and beliefs of school-based speech-language pathologists. *Augmentative and Alternative Communication, 34*(2), 130-142.

Mandel, M. (1977). Iconic devices in American Sign Language. In L. Friedman (Ed.), *On the other hand: New perspectives in American Sign Language* (pp. 57-108). Academic Press

Mandewill, T. F. (1994). KWLA: Linking the affective and cognitive domains. *Reading Teacher, 47*(8), 679.

Manjaly, Z. M., Harrison, N. A., Critchley, H. D., Do, C. T., Stefanics, G., Wenderoth, N., Lutterotti, A., Müller, A., & Stephan, K. E. (2019). Pathophysiological and cognitive mechanisms of fatigue in multiple sclerosis. *Journal of Neurology Neurosurgery and Psychiatry, 90*, 642-651.

Manjaly, Z. R., Scott, K. M., Abhinav, K., Wijesekera, L., Ganesalingam, J., Goldstein, L. H., Janssen, A., Dougherty, A., Willey, E., Stanton, B. R., Turner, M. R., Ampong, M. A., Sakel, M., Orrell, R. W., Howard, R., Shaw, C. E., Leigh, P. N., & Al-Chalabi, A. (2010). The sex ratio in amyotrophic lateral sclerosis: A population based study. *Amyotrophic Lateral Sclerosis, 11(5)*, 439-442.

Mann, W. C., Hurren, D., Karuza, K., & Bentley, D. W. (1993). Needs of home-based older visually impaired persons for assistive devices. *Journal of Visual Impairment and Blindness, 87*, 106-110.

Manurung, R., Ritchie, G., Pain, H., Waller, A., O'Mara, D., & Black, R. (2008). The construction of a pun generator for language skills development. *Applied Artificial Intelligence, 22(9)*, 841-869.

Marko, K. (1967). Symbol accentuation: Applications to classroom instruction of retardates. In *Proceedings of the First Congress of the International Association for the Scientific Study of Mental Deficiency* (pp. 773-775). IASSMD.

Marschark, M., Sapere, P., Convertino, C., & Pelz, J. (2008). Learning via direct and mediated instruction by deaf students. *Journal of Deaf Studies and Deaf Education, 13*, 546-561.

Marshall, P. (1990). Augmentative communication: The call of one's life. *Communicating Together, 8(2)*, 5-6.

Marshall, S., & Hurtig, S. S. (2019). Developing a culture of successful communication in acute care settings: Part I. Solving patient-specific issues. *Perspectives of the ASHA Special Interest Groups (SIG 12), 4(5)* 1028-1036.

Martin, J. A., Messacar, K., Yang, M. L., Maloney, J. A., Lindwall, J., Carry, T., Kenyon, P., Sillau, S. H., Oleszek, J., Tyler, K. L., Dominguez, S. R., & Schreiner, T. L. (2017). Outcomes of Colorado children with acute flaccid myelitis at 1 year. *Neurology, 89(2)*, 129-137.

Martin, M. (2010). Low-income minorities with disabilities see services disparity. *NPR Health*. Retrieved from https://www.npr.org/templates/transcript/transcript.php?storyId=128932141

Marvin, C., Beukelman, D., & Bilyeu, D. (1994). Vocabulary-use patterns in preschool children: Effects of context and time sampling. *Augmentative and Alternative Communication, 10*, 224-236.

Marvin, C. A., & Ogden, N. J. (2002). A home literacy inventory: Assessing young children's contexts for emergent literacy. *Young Exceptional Children, 5(2)*, 2-10.

Masuda, T., & Nisbett, R. E. (2001). Attending holistically versus analytically: Comparing the context sensitivity of Japanese and Americans. *Journal of Personality and Social Psychology, 81*, 922-934.

Matas, J., Mathy-Laikko, P., Beukelman, D. R., & Legresley, K. (1985). Identifying the nonspeaking population: A demographic study. *Augmentative and Alternative Communication, 1*, 17-31.

Mathews, M. (1966). *Teaching to read, historically considered*. University of Chicago Press.

Matosin, N., Frank, E., Engel, M., Lum, J. S., & Newell, K. A. (2014). Negativity towards negative results: A discussion of the disconnect between scientific worth and scientific culture. *Disease Models and Mechanisms, 7*, 171-173.

Matson, J. L. (2009). Aggression and tantrums in children with autism: A review of behavioral treatments and maintaining variables. *Journal of Mental Health Research in Intellectual Disabilities, 2*, 167-187.

Matson, J. L., Boisjoli, J., & Mahan, S. (2009). The relation of communication and challenging behaviors in infants and toddlers with autism spectrum disorders. *Journal of Developmental and Physical Disabilities, 21*, 253-261.

Matson, J. L., Dixon, D. R., & Matson, M. L. (2005). Assessing and treating aggression in children and adolescents with developmental disabilities: A 20-year overview. *Educational Psychology, 25*, 151-181.

Matson, J. L., Hess, J. A., & Mahan, S. (2010). Moderating effects of challenging behaviors and communication deficits on social skills in children diagnosed with an autism spectrum disorder. *Research in Autism Spectrum Disorders, 7*, 23-28.

Maxwell, M., Bernstein, M. E., & Mear, K. M. (1991). Bimodal language production. In P. Siple & S. Fischer (Eds.), *Theoretical issues in sign language research. Volume 2: Psychology* (pp. 171-190). University of Chicago Press.

May, S. (1999). Critical multiculturalism and cultural difference: Avoiding essentialism. In S. May (Ed.), *Critical multiculturalism: Rethinking multicultural and antiracist education*. Falmer Press.

May, S., & Sleeter, C. E. (Eds.). (2010). *Critical multiculturalism: Theory and praxis*. Routledge.

Mayer, J. F., Mitchinson, S. I., & Murray, L. L. (2017). Addressing concomitant executive dysfunction and aphasia: Previous approaches and the new brain budget protocol. *Aphasiology, 31(7)*, 837-860.

Mayerson, A. (1991). The Americans with Disabilities Act—An historic overview. *Labor Law, 7*, 1.

Mayo Clinic. (2017a). Cytomegalovirus (CMV) infection. Retrieved from https://www.mayoclinic.org/diseases-conditions/cmv/symptoms-causes/syc-20355358

Mayo Clinic. (2017b). Premature birth. Retrieved from https://www.mayo-clinic.org/diseases-conditions/premature-birth/symptoms-causes/syc-20376730

McBride, D. (2011). AAC evaluations and new mobile technologies: Asking and answering the right questions. *Perspectives on Augmentative and Alternative Communication, 20*, 9-16.

McBride-Chang, C., Tardif, T., Cho, J. R., Shu, H., Fletcher, P., Stokes, S. F., Wong, A., & Leung, K. (2008). What's in a word? Morphological awareness and vocabulary knowledge in three languages. *Applied Psycholinguistics, 29*, 437-462.

McCall, D. (2012). Steps to success with technology for individuals with aphasia. *Seminars in Speech and Language, 33(3)*, 234-242.

McCarthy, J. W., & Dietz, A. (2015). *Augmentative and alternative communication: An interactive clinical casebook*. Plural Publishing.

McLean, L. K., Brady, N. C., McLean, J. E., & Behrens, G. A. (1999). Communication forms and functions of children and adults with severe mental retardation in community and institutional settings. *Journal of Speech, Language, and Hearing Research, 42(1)*, 231-240.

McClintock, K., Hall, S., & Oliver, C. (2003). Risk markers associated with challenging behaviours in people with intellectual disabilities: A meta-analytic study. *Journal of Intellectual Disability Research, 47*, 405-416.

McClure, M. J, & Rush, E. (2007). *Selecting symbols sets: Implications for AAC users, clinicians, and researchers*. ASHA.

McCord, S. M., & Soto, G. (2004). Perceptions of AAC: An ethnographic investigation of Mexican-American families. *Augmentative and Alternative Communication, 20(4)*, 209-277.

McEwen, I. R., & Lloyd, L. L. (1990). Positioning students with cerebral palsy to use augmentative and alternative communication. *Language, Speech, and Hearing Services in Schools, 21*, 15-21.

McGinnis, J., & Beukelman, D. (1989). Vocabulary requirements for writing activities for the academically mainstreamed student with disabilities. *Augmentative and Alternative Communication, 5*, 183-191.

McInnes, J. M. (1993). Educational services: Reaction. In J. W. Reiman & P. A. Johnson (Eds.), *Proceedings from the National Symposium on Children and Youth Who Are Deaf-Blind* (pp. 221-230). Teaching Research Publications.

McKelvey, M., Dietz, A., Hux, K., Weissling, K., & Beukelman, D. R. (2007). Performance of a person with chronic aphasia using personal and contextual pictures in a visual scene display prototype. *Journal of Medical Speech-Language Pathology, 15(3)*, 305-317.

McKelvey, M., Hux, K., Dietz, A., & Beukelman, D. R. (2010). Impact of personal relevance and contextualization on comprehension by people with chronic aphasia. *American Journal of Speech-Language Pathology, 19*, 22-33.

McKelvey, M., Weissling, K., Quach, W., & Lund S. K. (2018, November). *Augmentative and alternative communication clinical assessment project: Protocol for assessment of individuals with ALS*. Seminar presented at the Annual Convention of the American Speech-Language-Hearing Association.

McLaughlin, K., & Cascella, P. W. (2008). Eliciting a distal gesture via dynamic assessment among students with moderate to severe intellectual disability. *Communication Disorders Quarterly, 29*(2), 75-81.

McLean, J. E., McLean, L. K., Brady, N. C., & Etter, R. (1991). Communication profiles of two types of gesture using nonverbal persons with severe to profound mental retardation. *Journal of Speech and Hearing Research, 34,* 294-308.

McLean, L. K., Brady, N. C., McLean, J. E., & Behrens, G. A. (1999). Communication forms and functions of children and adults with severe mental retardation in community and institutional settings. *Journal of Speech, Language, and Hearing Research, 42*(1), 231-240.

McNairn, P., & Smith, Y. (1996, March). *AAC feature match software.* Paper presented at the CSUN Conference. (Software copyright by Doug Dodgen & Associates).

McNamara, L., & Casey, J. (2007). Seat inclinations affect the function of children with cerebral palsy: A review of the effect of different seat inclines. *Disability Rehabilitation Assistive Technology, 2*(6), 309-318.

McNaughton, D., & Bryen, D. N. (2007). AAC technologies to enhance participation and access to meaningful societal roles for adolescents and adults with developmental disabilities who require AAC. *Augmentative and Alternative Communication, 23*(3), 217-229.

McNaughton, D., & Light, J. C. (2013). The iPad and mobile technology revolution: Benefits and challenges for individuals who require augmentative and alternative communication. *Augmentative and Alternative Communication, 29*(2), 107-116.

McNaughton, D., & Light, J. C. (2015). What we write about when we write about AAC: The past 30 years of research and future directions. *Augmentative and Alternative Communication, 31*(4), 261-270.

McNaughton, D., Light, J. C., & Arnold, K. (2002). 'Getting your wheel in the door:' Successful full-time employment experiences of individuals with cerebral palsy who use augmentative and alternative communication. *Augmentative and Alternative Communication, 18*(2), 59-76.

McNaughton, D., & Tawney, J. (1993). Comparison of two spelling instruction techniques for adults who use augmentative and alternative communication. *Augmentative and Alternative Communication, 9,* 72-82.

McNaughton, D., Rackensperger, T., Benedek-Wood, E., Krezman, C., Williams, M. B., & Light, J. (2008). "A child needs to be given a chance to succeed:" Parents of individuals who use AAC describe the benefits and challenges of learning AAC technologies. *Augmentative and Alternative Communication, 24*(1), 43-55.

McNaughton, S. (1974). Mr. Symbol Man. *National Film Board of Canada.* Retrieved from https://archive.org/details/mrsymbolman

McNaughton, S. (1976). Blissymbols: An alternate symbol system for the non-verbal pre-reading child. In G. C. Vanderheiden & K. Grilley (Eds.), *Non-vocal communication techniques and aids for the severely physically handicapped* (pp. 85-104). University Park Press.

McNaughton, S. (Ed.). (1985). *Communicating with Blissymbolics.* Blissymbolics Communication Institute.

McNaughton, S. (1990). Gaining the most from AAC's growing years. *Augmentative and Alternative Communication, 6,* 2-14.

McNaughton, S., & Kates, B (1980). The application of Blissymbolics. In R. L. Schiefelbusch (Ed.), *Nonspeech language and communication: Analysis and intervention* (pp. 303-321). University Park Press.

McNaughton, S., & Lindsay, P. (1995). Approaching literacy with AAC graphics. *Augmentative and Alternative Communication, 11,* 212-218.

McNaughton, S., & Warrick A. (1984). Picture your Blissymbols. *The Canadian Journal of Mental Retardation, 34,* 1-9.

McNeill, D. (1985). Do you think gestures are nonverbal? *Psychological Review, 92,* 350-371.

McNeill, D. (1992). *Hand and mind: What gestures reveal about thought.* University of Chicago Press.

McNeill, D. (1993). The circle from gesture to sign. In M. Marshark & M. D. Clark (Eds.), *Psychological perspectives on deafness* (pp. 153-183). Lawrence Erlbaum Associates.

Meador, D. M., Rumbaugh, D. M., Tribble, M., & Thompson, S. (1984). Facilitating visual discrimination learning of moderately and severely mentally retarded children through illumination of stimuli. *American Journal of Mental Deficiency, 89,* 313-316.

Meder, A. M., & Wegner, J. R. (2015). iPads, mobile technologies, and communication applications: A survey of family wants, needs, and preferences. *Perspectives on Augmentative and Alternative Communication, 31*(1), 27-36.

MedicineNet. (n.d.). Microcephaly. Retrieved from https://www.medicinenet.com/microcephaly/article.htm#microcephaly_facts

Meinzen-Derr, J. (2018). Augmentative and alternative communication: Optimizing language learning of children with hearing loss. *The Hearing Journal, 73*(3), 22-26.

Meinzen-Derr, J., Sheldon, R., Altaye, M., Lane, L., Mays, L., & Wiley, S. (2021). A technology-assisted language intervention for children who are deaf or hard of hearing: A randomized clinical trial. *Pediatrics, 147*(2), 1-10.

Meinzen-Derr, J., Sheldon, R., Grether, S., Altaye, M., Smith, L., Choo, D.I., & Wiley, S. (2018). Language underperformance in young children who are deaf or hard-of-hearing: Are the expectations too low? *Journal of Developmental and Behavioral Pediatrics, 39*(2), 116-125.

Meinzen-Derr, J., Sheldon, R., Henry, S., Grether, S. M., Smith, L. F., Mays, L., Riddle, I., Altaye, M., & Wiley, S. (2019). Enhancing language in children who are deaf/hard-of-hearing using augmentative and alternative communication technology strategies. *International Journal of Pediatric Otorhinolaryngology, 125,* 23-31.

Meinzen-Derr, J., Wiley, S., McAuley, R., Smith, L., & Grether, S. (2017). Technology-assisted language intervention for children who are deaf or hard-of-hearing: A pilot study of augmentative and alternative communication for enhancing language development. *Disability and Rehabilitation: Assistive Technology, 12*(8), 808-815.

Memarian, N., Blain-Moraes, S., & Chau, T. (2014). Towards a physiological signal-based access solution for a non-verbal adolescent with severe and multiple disabilities. *Developmental Neurorehabilitation, 17*(4), 270-277.

Mental retardation: Past and present. (1977). Retrieved from https://www.acf.hhs.gov/sites/default/files/add/gm_1976.pdf

Merriam-Webster. (n.d.). Retrieved from https://www.merriam-webster.com/dictionary/model

Merriam-Webster's Collegiate Dictionary (10th ed.). (1999). Author.

Mesibov, G., Shea, V., & Schopler, E. (2006). Foundations of the TEACCH structured teaching approach. In *The TEACCH approach to autism spectrum disorders* (pp. 33-49). Springer.

Mgenge, F. (2012). Listen to our voice: Can you imagine what life can be without our voice? *The Fofa Voice* (1st ed.), 1-2.

Miles, B., & Riggio, M. (1999). *Remarkable conversations: A guide to developing meaningful communication with children and young adults who are deafblind.* Perkins School for the Blind.

Millar, D. C., Light, J. C., & Schlosser, R. W. (1999, November). *The impact of augmentative and alternative communication (AAC) on natural speech development: A meta-analysis.* Poster presented at the American Speech-Language-Hearing Association Annual Convention.

Millar, D. C., Light, J. C., & Schlosser, R. W. (2006). The impact of augmentative and alternative communication intervention on the speech production of individuals with developmental disabilities: A research review. *Journal of Speech, Language, & Hearing Research, 49,* 248-264.

Miller, A. (1967). Symbol accentuation. Outgrowth of theory and experiment. In E. Meshorer (Chair), *A new approach to language development with retardates.* Symposium presented at the First International Congress on the Scientific Study of Mental Deficiency.

Miller, A. (1968). *Symbol accentuation—A new approach to reading.* Doubleday Multimedia.

Miller, A., & Miller, E. K. (1968). Symbol accentuation. The perceptual transfer of meaning from spoken to printed words. *American Journal of Mental Deficiency, 73,* 202-208.

Miller, A., & Miller, E. K. (1971). Symbol accentuation, single-track functioning, and early reading. *American Journal of Mental Deficiency, 76,* 110-117.

Miller, E. K., Swanson, L. A., Steele, N. K., Thelin, S. J., & Thelin, J. W. (2011). Forms and functions in communication. In T. S. Hartshorne, M. A. Hefner, S. L. H. Davenport & J. W. Thelin (Eds.), *CHARGE syndrome* (pp. 295-313). Plural Publishing.

Miller, J. (2010). The difference between ASL and English signs: Signing savvy. Retrieved from https://www.signingsavvy.com/blog/45/The+difference+between+ASL+and+English+signs

Miller, J., & Allaire, J. (1987). Augmentative communication. In *Systematic instruction of persons with severe handicaps* (3rd ed., pp. 273-296). Merrill.

Miller J., & Chapman, R. (1985). *Systematic analysis of language transcripts: User's manual.* University of Wisconsin.

Mills, T., Bunnell, H., & Patel, R. (2014). Towards personalized speech synthesis for augmentative and alternative communication. *Augmentative and Alternative Communication, 30,* 226-236.

Miltenberger, R. G. (2008). *Behavior modification: Principles and procedures* (4th ed.). Thompson Wadsworth.

Mindel, M. (2020). Talk like me: Supporting students who are African American using augmentative and alternative communication. *Perspectives of the ASHA Special Interest Groups, 5,* 1586-1592.

Mindel, M., & John, J. (2018). Bridging the school and home divide for culturally and linguistically diverse families using augementative and alternative communication systems. *Perspectives of the ASHA Special Interest Groups: SIG 12, 3*(12), 154-163.

Mindel, M., & John, J. (2021). *AAC for all: Culturally and linguistically responsive practice.* Plural Publishing.

Mineo, B., Peischl, D., & Pennington, C. (2008). Moving targets: The effect of animation on identification of action word representations. *Augmentative and Alternative Communication, 24*(2), 162-173.

Minnesota DeafBlind Project. (n.d.). Usher syndrome coalition. Retrieved from https://www.dbproject.mn.org/Families/resources.html

Mirenda, P. (1985). Designing pictorial communication systems for physically able-bodied students with severe handicaps. *Augmentative and Alternative Communication, 1,* 58-64.

Mirenda, P. (1997). Supporting individuals with challenging behavior through functional communication training and AAC: Research review. *Augmentative and Alternative Communication, 13,* 207-225.

Mirenda, P. (1998). Educational inclusion of AAC users. *Augmentative and Alternative Communication, 2,* 391-424.

Mirenda, P. (1999). Augmentative and alternative communication techniques. In J. E. Downing (Ed.), *Teaching communication skills to students with severe disabilities* (pp. 119-138). Paul H. Brookes Publishing Co.

Mirenda, P. (2003). Toward functional augmentative and alternative communication for students with autism: Manual signs, graphic symbols, and voice output communication aids. *Language, Speech, and Hearing Services in Schools, 34,* 203-216.

Mirenda, P. (2009). Introduction to AAC for individuals with autism spectrum disorders. In P. Mirenda & T. Iacono (Eds.), *Autism spectrum disorders and AAC* (pp. 3-22). Paul H. Brookes Publishing Co.

Mirenda, P., & Brown, K. (2007). Supporting individuals with autism and problem behavior using AAC. *Augmentative and Alternative Communication, 16*(2), 26-31.

Mirenda, P., & Erickson, K. (2000). Augmentative communication and literacy. In A. Wetherby & B. Prizant (Eds.), *Autism spectrum disorders: A transactional developmental perspective* (pp. 333-367). Paul H. Brookes Publishing Co.

Mirenda, P., & Locke, P. A. (1989). A comparison of symbol transparency in nonspeaking persons with intellectual disabilities. *Journal of Speech and Hearing Disorders, 54,* 131-140.

Mirenda, P., & Santogrossi, J. (1985). A prompt-free strategy to teach pictorial communication system use. *Augmentative and Alternative Communication, 1,* 143-150.

Mitchell, A., Benito-Leon, J., Morales Gonzalez, J., & Rivera-Navarro, J. (2005). Quality of life and its assessment in multiple sclerosis: Integrating physical and psychological components of wellbeing. *Lancet Neurology, 4,* 556-566.

Mitchell, P. R., & Alvares, R. (2015). Facilitating family and client involvement in the SGD evaluation and decision process. *Perspectives on Augmentative and Alternative Communication, 24,* 135-141.

Mitchell, R. E., & Karchmer, M. A. (2004). Chasing the mythical ten percent: Parental hearing status of deaf and hard of hearing students in the United States. *Sign Language Studies, 4*(2), 138-163.

Mizuko, M. I. (1987). Transparency and ease of learning symbols represented by Blissymbols, PCS, and PICSYMS. *Augmentative and Alternative Communication, 3,* 129-136.

Mizuko, M. I., & Reichle, J. (1989). Transparency and recall of symbols among intellectually handicapped adults. *Journal of Speech and Hearing Disorders, 54*(4), 627-633.

Mizuko, M. I., Reichle, J., Ratcliff, A., & Esser, J. (1994). Effects of selection techniques and array sizes on short-term visual memory. *Augmentative and Alternative Communication, 10,* 237-244.

Mngomezulu, J., Tönsing, K. M., Dada, S., & Bokaba, N. B. (2019). Determining a Zulu core vocabulary for children who use augmentative and alternative communication. *Augmentative and Alternative Communication,* 1-11.

Moe, A. J., Hopkins, C. J., & Rush, R. T. (1982). *The vocabulary of first-grade children.* Charles C. Thomas Publishing.

Moeller, M. P. (2000). Early intervention and language development in children who are deaf and hard-of-hearing. *Pediatrics, 106*(3), e43-e43.

Moeller, M. P., Osberger, M. J., & Morford, J. A. (1987). Speech-language assessment and intervention with preschool hearing impaired children. In J. G. Alpmer & P. A. McCarthy (Eds.), *Rehabilitative audiology children and adults* (pp. 163-187). Williams & Wilkins.

Moghaddam Tabrizi, F., & Radfar, M. (2015). Fatigue, sleep quality, and disability in relation to quality of life in multiple sclerosis. *International Journal of Multiple Sclerosis Care, 17,* 268-274.

Moller, C. (2003). Deafblindness: Living with sensory deprivation. *The Lancet, 362,* 46-47.

Moms, S. A. S. (1986). *Transparency of two representational systems: PICSYMS and Picture Communication Symbols.* Unpublished master's thesis, Western Carolina University, Cullowhee, NC.

Mondelli, M. F. C. G., Mariano, T. C. B., Honório, H. M., & Brito, R. V. De. (2016). Vibrant soundbridge and bone conduction hearing aid in patients with bilateral malformation of external ear. *International Archives of Otorhinolaryngology, 20*(1), 34-38.

Monetta, L., & Pell, M. (2007). Effects of verbal working memory deficits on metaphor comprehension in patients with Parkinson's disease. *Brain and Language, 101,* 80-89.

Moores, D. (1978). *Educating the deaf.* Houghton Mifflin.

Mora, G. (1997). The American Psychiatric Association, 1844-1994: International perspectives. *History of Psychiatry, 8*(29), 121-148.

Morin, K. L., Ganz, J. B., Gregori, E. V., Foster, M. J., Gerow, S. L., Genç-Tosun, D., & Hong, E. R. (2018). A systematic quality review of high-tech AAC interventions as an evidence-based practice. *Augmentative and Alternative Communication, 34*(2), 104-117.

Morris, M. A., Dudgeon, B. J., & Yorkston, K. (2013). A qualitative study of adult AAC users' experiences communicating with medical providers. *Disability and Rehabilitation: Assistive Technology, 8*(6), 472-481.

Morris, M. W., & Peng, K. (1994). Culture and cause: American and Chinese attributions for social physical events. *Journal of Personality and Social Psychology, 67,* 949-971.

Morse, M. T. (1990). Cortical visual impairment in young children with multiple disabilities. *Journal of Visual Impairment and Blindness, 84,* 200-203.

Morse, M. T. (1992). Augmenting assessment procedure for children with severe multiple handicaps and sensory impairments. *Journal of Visual Impairment and Blindness, 86,* 73-77.

Mosby, I. (2017). *Mosby's dictionary of medicine, nursing and health professions* [E-book]. Mosby.

Mucha, A., Collins, M. W., Elbin, R. J., Furman, J. M., Troutman-Enseki, C., DeWolf, R. M., Marchetti, G., Kontos, A. P. (2014). A brief vestibular/ocular motor screening (VOMS) assessment to evaluate concussions: Preliminary findings. *American Journal of Sports Medicine, 42*(10), 2479-2486.

Mühlenbock, K. H., & Lundälv, M. (2011, July). *Using lexical and corpus resources for augmenting the AAC lexicon.* Paper presented at the Second Workshop on Speech and Language Processing for Assistive Technologies.

Mukhopadhyay, S. (2008). *Understanding autism through rapid prompting method.* Outskirts Press.

Mukhopadhyay, S. (2018). Helping autism through learning and outreach [HALO]. Retrieved from https://www.halo-soma.org/

Munoz, M., Hoffman, L., & Brimo, D. (2013). Be smarter than your phone: A framework for using apps in clinical practice. *Contemporary Issues in Communication Sciences and Disorders, 40*, 138-150.

Munroe, S. (2001). *Developing a national volunteer registry for persons with deafblindness in Canada. Results from the study, 1999-2001.* Canadian Deafblind and Rubella Association.

Murphy, J. (2000). Enabling people with aphasia to discuss quality of life. *British Journal of Therapy and Rehabilitation, 7*(11), 454-457.

Murphy, J., Factor-Litvack, P., Goetz, R., Lomen-Hoerth, C., Nagy, P., Hupf, J., . . . Mitsumoto, H. (2016). Cognitive-behavioral screening reveals prevalent impairment in a large multicenter ALS cohort. *Neurology, 86*, 813-820.

Murphy, J., Gray, C., & Cox, S. (2007). Talking Mats: The effectiveness of a low technology communication framework to help people with dementia express their views. *Journal of Assistive Technologies, 1*(2), 30-34.

Murphy, J., Gray, C., van Achterberg, T., Wyke, S., & Cox, S. (2010). The effectiveness of the Talking Mats framework in helping people with dementia to express their views on well-being. *Dementia, 94*(4), 454-472.

Murphy, J., Markova, I., Moodie, E., Scott, J., & Boa, S. (1995). Augmentative and alternative communication systems used by people with cerebral palsy in Scotland: Demographic survey. *Augmentative and Alternative Communication, 11*, 26-36.

Murphy, J., & Oliver, T. M. (2013). The use of Talking Mats to support people with dementia and their carers to make decisions together. *Health and Social Care in the Community, 2*(12), 171-180.

Murray, L. L. (2000). Spoken language production in Huntington's and Parkinson's diseases. *Journal of Speech, Language, and Hearing Research, 43*, 1350-1366.

Murray, L. L. (2012). Attention and other cognitive deficits in aphasia: Presence and relation to language and communication measures. *American Journal of Speech-Language Pathology, 21*, 51-64.

Murray, L. L., & Stout, J. C. (1999). Discourse comprehension in Huntington's disease and Parkinson's disease. *American Journal of Speech-Language Pathology, 8*, 137-148.

Murray, M., Popelka, G. R., & Miller, R. (2011). Efficacy and safety of an in-the-mouth bone conduction device for single-sided deafness. *Otology and Neurotology, 32*(3), 437-443.

Murray-Branch, J., Udavan-Solner, A., & Bailey, B. (1991). Textured communication systems for individuals with severe intellectual and dual sensory impairments. *Language, Speech, and Hearing Services in Schools, 22*, 260-268.

Murray-Branch, J., & Bailey, B. R. (1998). *Textures as communication symbols.* Blumberg Center for Interdisciplinary Studies in Special Education, Indiana State University.

Musselwhite, C. R. (1982). *A comparison of three symbolic communication systems.* Unpublished doctoral dissertation, West Virginia University.

Musselwhite, C. R. (1985). *Songbook: Signs and symbols for children.* Don Johnston Incorporated.

Musselwhite, C. R. (1986). *Adaptive play for special needs children: Strategies to enhance communication and learning.* College-Hill Press.

Musselwhite, C. R., & Ruscello, D. (1984). Transparency of three communication symbol systems. *Journal of Speech and Hearing Research, 27*, 436-443.

Musselwhite, C. R., & St. Louis, K. W. (1988). *Communication programming for persons with severe handicaps: Vocal and augmentative strategies* (2nd ed.). College-Hill Press.

Mustafa, E., & Dimopoulos, K. (2014). *Sign language interpretation using Kinect.* Unpublished Master's thesis, University of Sheffield, UK. Retrieved from https://www.researchgate.net/publication/266144236_Sign_Language_Recognition_using_Kinect

Mylander, C., & Goldin-Meadow, S. (1991). Home sign systems in deaf children: The development of morphology without a conventional model. In P. Siple & S. Fischer (Eds.), *Theoretical issues in sign language research. Volume 2: Psychology* (pp. 41-63). University of Chicago Press.

Naguib Bedwani, M. A., Bruck, S., & Costley, D. (2015). Augmentative and alternative communication for children with autism spectrum disorder: An evidence-based evaluation of the Language Acquisition through Motor Planning (LAMP) programme. *Cogent Education, 2*, 1-25.

Nagy, W., & Anderson, R. C. (1984). How many words are there in printed school English? *Reading Research Quarterly, 19*, 304-330.

Nail-Chiwetalu, B. J. (1992). The influence of symbol and learner factors on the learnability of Blissymbols by students with mental retardation, (Doctoral dissertation, Purdue University, 1991). *Dissertation Abstracts International, 53*, 1125A.

Nam, S., & Hwang, Y. (2016). Evaluating acquisition of picture exchange-based vs. signed mands and implications to teach functional communication skills to children with autism. *The Journal of Special Education Apprenticeship, 5*, 1-23.

Nam, S., Kim, J., & Sparks, S. (2018). An overview of review studies on effectiveness of major AAC systems for individuals with developmental disabilities including autism. *The Journal of Special Education Apprenticeship, 7*, 1-14.

Namy, L. L., Campbell, A. L., & Tomasello, M. (2004). The changing role of iconicity in non-verbal symbol learning: A U-shaped trajectory in the acquisition of arbitrary gestures. *Journal of Cognition and Development, 5*, 37-57.

Nash, B., Clark, A. K., & Karvonen, M. (2015). First contact: A census report on the characteristics of students eligible to take alternate assessments (Technical Report No. 16-01). University of Kansas, Center for Educational Testing and Evaluation. Retrieved from https://dynamiclearningmaps.org/sites/default/files/documents/publication/First_Contact_Census_2016.pdf

Nasreddine, Z. S., Phillips, N. A., Bédirian, V., Charbonneau, S., Whitehead, V., Collin, I., Cummings, J. L., & Chertkow, H. (2005). The Montreal Cognitive Assessment, MoCA: A brief screening tool for mild cognitive impairment. *Journal of the American Geriatrics Society, 53*, 695-699.

National Aphasia Association. (n.d.a). Aphasia. Retrieved March 6, 2019, from https://www.aphasia.org/aphasia-definitions/

National Aphasia Association. (n.d.b). Apraxia. Retrieved from https://www.aphasia.org/aphasia-resources/apraxia/

National Association of State Directors of Special Education. (2006). *Meeting the needs of students who are deaf or hard of hearing: Educational services guidelines.* Author.

National Autism Center. (2015). Findings and conclusions: National standards project, phase 2. Retrieved from http://www.nationalautismcenter.org/national-standards-project/results-reports/

National Center on Birth Defects and Developmental Disabilities, Centers for Disease Control and Prevention. (2015). Developmental disabilities. Retrieved from https://www.cdc.gov/ncbddd/developmentaldisabilities/index.html

National Center on Deaf-Blindness. (2017). 2016 national child count of children and youth who are deaf-blind report. Retrieved from http://nationaldb.org/reports/national-child-count-2016/etiologies

National Center on Deaf-Blindness. (2020). 2019 national child count of children and youth who are deaf-blind report. Retrieved from https://www.nationaldb.org/products/national-child-count/report-2019/etiologies/

National Consortium on Deaf-Blindness. (2013). Definition of intervener services and interveners in educational settings technical report. Retrieved from https://files.eric.ed.gov/fulltext/ED545215.pdf

National Development Center on Autism Spectrum Disorder. (2010). Steps for implementation: Functional communication training. Retrieved from https://autismpdc.fpg.unc.edu/sites/autismpdc.fpg.unc.edu/files/FCT_Steps_0.pdf

National Institute of Neurological Disorders and Stroke. (2019). Hydrocephalus fact sheet. Retrieved from https://www.ninds.nih.gov/disorders/patient-caregiver-education/fact-sheets/hydrocephalus-fact-sheet#3125_5

National Institute of Neurological Disorders and Stroke. (n.d.). Spinal muscular atrophy fact sheet. Retrieved from https://www.ninds.nih.gov/Disorders/Patient-Caregiver-Education/Fact-Sheets/Spinal-Muscular-Atrophy-Fact-Sheet

National Institutes of Health. (2010). Fact sheet: Intellectual and developmental disabilities. Retrieved from https://archives.nih.gov/asites/report/09-09-2019/report.nih.gov/nihfactsheets/ViewFactSheet34ef.html?csid=100&key=I#I

National Institutes of Health—Genetic and Rare Diseases Information Center. (2015). Trisomy 13. Retrieved from https://rarediseases.info.nih.gov/diseases/7341/trisomy-13

National Joint Committee for the Communicative Needs of Persons With Severe Disabilities. (1992). Guidelines for meeting the communication needs of persons with severe disabilities. *ASHA, 34*(Suppl. 7), 2-3.

National Joint Committee for the Communication Needs of Persons with Severe Disabilities. (2003). Position statement on access to communication services and supports: Concerns regarding the application of restrictive "eligibility" policies [position statement]. Retrieved from https://www.asha.org/policy/PS2003-00227/

National Library of Medicine—National Institutes of Health. (n.d.). Introduction to the musculoskeletal system. Retrieved from https://www.ncbi.nlm.nih.gov/pmc/articles/PMC1271013/

National Organization for Rare Disorders. (2007). Rare disease database: Hydrocephalus. Retrieved from https://rarediseases.org/rare-diseases/hydrocephalus/

Neale, G., Woloshynowych, M., & Vincent, C. (2001). Exploring the causes of adverse events in NHS hospital practice. *Journal of the Royal Society of Medicine, 94*, 322-330.

Neel, R. S., Billingsley, F. F., McCarty, F., Symonds, D., Lambert, C., Lewis-Smith, N., & Hanashiro, R. (1983). Innovative model program for autistic children and their teachers. Unpublished manuscript, University of Washington.

Neidert, P. L., Rooker, G. W., Bayles, M. W., & Miller, J. R. (2013). Functional analysis of problem behavior. In D. D. Reed, F. D. DiGennaro, & J. K. Luiselli (Eds.), *Issues in clinical child psychology: Handbook of crisis intervention and developmental disabilities* (pp. 147-167). Springer.

Nelson, L. B., Ehrlick, S., Calhoun, J. H., Matteucci, T., & Finnegan, L. P. (1987). Occurrence of strabismus in infants born to drug-dependent women. *American Journal of Diseases of Childhood, 141*, 175-178.

Nelson, N. W. (1992). Performance is the prize: Language competence and performance among AAC users. *Augmentative and Alternative Communication, 8*(1), 3-18.

Newell, A. F., Arnott, J. L., Booth, L., Beattie, W., Brophy, B., & Ricketts, I. W. (1992). Effect of the "PAL" word prediction system on the quality and quantity of text generation. *Augmentative and Alternative Communication, 8*(4), 304-311.

Newport, E. L., & Meier, R. P. (1985). The acquisition of American Sign Language. In D. I. Slobin (Ed.), *The crosslinguistic study of language acquisition* (Vol. 1. The data; Vol. 2. Theoretical issues [pp. 881-938]). Lawrence Erlbaum Associates, Inc.

Nicholas, J. G., & Geers, A. E. (2006). Effects of early auditory experience on the spoken language of deaf children at 3 years of age. *Ear and Hearing, 27*(3), 286-298.

Nicholas, M., & Connor, L. (2017). People with aphasia using AAC: Are executive functions important? *Aphasiology, 31*(7), 819-836.

Nicholas, M., Sinotte, M. P., & Helm-Estabrooks, N. (2011). C-Speak aphasia alternative communication program for people with severe aphasia: Importance of executive functioning and semantic knowledge. *Neuropsychological Rehabilitation, 21*(3), 322-366.

Nielsen, J., & Molich, R. (1990). Heuristic evaluation of user interfaces. In J. Carrasco-Chew & J. Whiteside (Eds.), *Proceedings of the SIGCHI Conference on Human Factors in Computing Systems* (CHI '90, pp. 249-256). ACM.

Nietupski, J., & Hamre-Nietupski, S. (1979). Teaching auxiliary communication skills to severely handicapped students. *AAESPH Review, 4*, 107-124.

Nigam, R., & Karlan, G. R. (1994, November). *Cultural validation of Picture Communication Symbols set for Asian-Indian children.* Poster session presented at the Annual Convention of the American Speech-Language-Hearing Association.

Nip, I. S. B. (2017). Interarticulator coordination in children with and without cerebral palsy. *Developmental Neurorehabilitation, 20*, 1-13.

Nordness, A. S., & Beukelman, D. R. (2017). Supporting patient provider communication across medical settings. *Topics in Language Disorders, 37*(4), 334-347.

Norrie, C. S., Waller, A., & Hannah, E. F. S. (2021). Establishing context: AAC device adoption and support in a special-education setting. *ACM Transactions on Computer-Human Interaction, 28*(2), 1-30.

Norrie, C. S., Waller, A., & Zhang, J. (2018). Developing a novel system to support age acquisition in children with CCN: An ethnographic study. *Communication Matters, 32*(2), 8-10.

Northern, J. L., & Downs, M. P. (2014). *Hearing in children* (6th ed.). Plural Publishing.

Northup, J., Wacker, D., Sasso, G , Steege, M., Cigrand, K., Cook, J., & DeRaad, A. (1991). A brief functional analysis of aggressive and alternative behavior in an outclinic setting. *Journal of Applied Behavior Analysis, 24*, 509-522.

Noyes, J. M., & Frankish, C. R. (1992). Speech recognition technology for individuals with disabilities. *Augmentative and Alternative Communication, 8*, 297-303.

O'Brien, E. (2020). Here's a list of prepositions. Retrieved from http://www.english-grammar-revolution.com/list-of-prepositions.html

O'Dell, C. D., Harshaw, K., & Boothe, R. G. (1993). Vision screening of individuals with severe or profound mental retardation. *Mental Retardation, 31*, 154-160.

Ogletree, B. T. (2010). A causal relationship between pre-treatment matching or motor imitation skills and later acquisition of manual signing or picture exchange communication in children with ASD remains to be established. *Evidence-Based Communication Assessment and Intervention, 4*, 105-108.

Ogletree, B. T. (2017). Addressing the communication and other needs of persons with severe disabilities through engaged interprofessional teams: Introduction to a clinical forum. *American Journal of Speech-Language Pathology, 26*, 157-161.

Ogletree, B. T., McMurry, S., Schmidt, M., & Evans, K. (2018). The changing world of augmentative and alternative communication (AAC): Examining three realities faced by today's AAC provider. *Perspectives of the ASHA Special Interest Groups: SIG 12, 3*, 113-122.

Ohio Department of Education. (2017). Orthopedic impairment. Retrieved from http://education.ohio.gov/Topics/Special-Education/Students-with-Disabilities/Orthopedic-Impairment

Olin, A. R., Reichle, J., Johnson, L., & Monn, E. (2010). Examining dynamic visual scene displays: Implications for arranging and teaching symbol selection. *American Journal of Speech-Language Pathology, 19*, 284-297.

Olusanya, B. O., Neumann, K. J., & Saunders, J. E. (2014). The global burden of disabling hearing impairment: A call to action. *Bulletin World Health Organization, 92*(5), 367-373.

O'Neill, R. E., Horner, R. H., Albin, R. W., Sprague, J. R., Storey, K., & Newton, J. S. (1990). *Functional assessment and program development for problem behavior*. Brooks/Cole Publishing.

O'Neill, R. E., & Reichle, J. (1993). Addressing socially motivated challenging behavior by establishing communicative alternatives: Basics of a general-case approach. In J. Reichle & D. P. Wacker (Eds.), *Communicative alternatives to challenging behavior: Integrating functional assessment and intervention strategies* (pp. 205-235). Paul H. Brookes Publishing Co.

O'Neill, T., Light, J. C., & Pope, L. (2018). Effects of interventions that include aided augmentative and alternative communication input on the communication of individuals with complex communication needs: A meta-analysis. *Journal of Speech, Language, and Hearing Research, 61*(7), 1743 1765.

Ong-Dean, C. (2009). *Distinguishing disability: Parents, privilege, and special education*. The University of Chicago Press.

Ong-Dean, C., Daly, A. J., & Park, V. (2011). Privileged advocates: Disability and education policy. *Policy Futures in Education, 9*(3), 392-405.

Ooi, Y. P., Tan, Z. J., Lim, C. X., Goh, T. J., & Sung, M. (2011). Prevalence of behavioural and emotional problems in children with high-functioning autism spectrum disorders. *Australian and New Zealand Journal of Psychiatry, 45*, 370-375.

Oosthuizen, I., Dada, S., Bornman, J., & Koul, R. (2018). Message banking: Perceptions of persons with motor neuron disease, significant others and clinicians. *International Journal of Speech-Language Pathology, 20*, 756-765.

Orel-Bixler, D. (1999). Clinical vision assessment for infants. In D. Chen (Ed.), *Essential elements in early intervention* (pp. 107-156). AFB Press.

Orlando, A., & Ruppar, A. (2016). *Literacy instruction for students with multiple and severe disabilities who use augmentative/alternative communication* (Document No. IC-16). University of Florida, Collaboration for Effective Educator, Development, Accountability, and Reform Center. Retrieved from https://ceedar.education.ufl.edu/wp-content/uploads/2016/10/IC-Literacy-multiple-severe-disabilities.pdf

O'Sullivan, S. B., Schmitz, T. J., & Fulk, G. (2014). *Physical rehabilitation* (6th ed.). F.A. Davis.

Owen, A. (2004). Cognitive dysfunction in Parkinson's disease: The role of frontostriatal circuitry. *Neuroscientist, 10*(6), 525-537.

Owens, R. E., Jr. (2010). *Language disorders: A functional approach to assessment and intervention*. Pearson.

Owens, R. E., Jr., & House, L. I. (1984). Decision-making processes in augmentative communication. *Journal of Speech and Hearing Disorders, 49*, 18-25.

Oyiborhoro, J. M. A. (2005). *Aural rehabilitation for people with disabilities*. Elsevier.

Padula, W. V., & Shapiro, J. B. (1993). Head injury and the post trauma vision syndrome. *Review, 24*, 153-158.

Paget Gorman Sign System. (n.d.). Paget Gorman sign system. Retrieved August 29, 2022, from https://www.wikiwant.com/en/Paget_Gorman_Sign_System

Pampoulou, E. (2006). *Graphic symbol set selection considerations by speech and language therapists: A pilot study*. Unpublished thesis, King's College London.

Pampoulou, E. (2015). *The use of graphic symbols in inclusive primary schools: An exploration of teachers' and speech and language therapists' experiences of graphic symbols*. Unpublished thesis, King's College London.

Pampoulou, E. (2016). Collaboration between speech and language therapists and school staff when working with graphic symbols. *Journal of Child Language Teaching and Therapy, 20*, 33-54.

Pampoulou, E. (2017). Exploring speech and language therapists' and teachers' experiences when choosing graphic symbol set(s) for their students in inclusive primary schools in England and Cyprus. *Journal of Enabling Technologies, 11*(2), 49-58.

Pampoulou, E. (2018). Speech and language therapists' views about AAC system acceptance by people with acquired communication disorders. *Disability and Rehabilitation: Assistive Technology, 18*(1), 1-8.

Pampoulou, E., & Detheridge, C. (2007). The role of symbols in the mainstream to access literacy. *Journal of Assistive Technologies, 1*(1), 15-21.

Pampoulou, E., & Fuller, D. R. (2020). Exploring AAC graphic symbol choices: A preliminary study. *Journal of Enabling Technologies, 14*(3), 171-185.

Pampoulou, E., & Fuller, D. R. (2021). Introduction of a new AAC symbol classification system: The multidimensional quaternary symbol continuum (MQSC). *Journal of Enabling Technologies, 15*(4), 252-267.

Parette, H. P., Brotherson, M. J., & Huer, M. B. (2000). Giving families a voice in augmentative and alternative communication decision-making. *Education and Training in Mental Retardation and Developmental Disabilities, 35*(2), 177-190.

Parette, H. P., Hourcade, J. J., & VanBiervliet, A. (1993). Selection of appropriate technology for children with disabilities. *Teaching Exceptional Children, 25*, 18-22.

Parette, H. P., VanBiervliet, A., & Hourcade, J. J. (2000). Family-centered decision making in assistive technology. *Journal of Special Education Technology, 15*, 45-55.

Parker, A. T., Banda, D. R., Davisson, R. C., & Liu-Gitz, L. (2010). Adapting the picture communication system for a student with visual impairment and autism: A case study. *AER Journal Research and Practice in Visual Impairment and Blindness, 3*, 2-11.

Parker, R. (2013). PrAACtical thoughts on challenging behavior: Things to think about. Retrieved from https://praacticalaac.org/praactical/praactical-thoughts-on-challenging-behavior-things-to-think-about/

Parliamentary and Health Service Ombudsman. (n.d.). Introduction to the social and medical models of disability. Retrieved from https://www.ombudsman.org.uk/sites/default/files/FDN-218144_Introduction_to_the_Social_and_Medical_Models_of_Disability.pdf

Parton, B. S. (2006). Sign language recognition and translation: A multidisciplined approach from the field of artificial intelligence. *Journal of Deaf Studies and Deaf Education, 11*(1), 94-101.

Paul, D. R., Blosser, J., & Jakubowitz, M. D. (2006). Principles and challenges for forming successful literacy partnerships. *Topics in Language Disorders, 26*(1), 5-23.

Paul, R., & Norbury, C. F. (2012). *Language disorders from infancy through adolescence*. Elsevier Health Sciences.

Pautasso, M. (2010). Worsening file-drawer problem in the abstracts of natural, medical and social science databases. *Scientometrics, 85*, 193-202.

Peirce, C. S. (1931). In C. Hartshorne, P. Weiss & A. W. Burks (Eds.), *Collected papers of Charles Sanders Peirce* (Vol. 2). Harvard University Press.

Pelka, F. (1997). *The ABC-CLIO companion to the disability rights movement*. Abc-Clio Incorporated.

Pell, M., Cheang, H., & Leonard, C. (2006). The impact of Parkinson's disease on vocal-prosodic communication from the perspective of listeners. *Brain and Language, 97*, 123-134.

Pell, M., & Leonard, C. (2005). Facial expression decoding in early Parkinson's disease. *Cognitive Brain Research, 23*, 327-340.

Pell, M., & Monetta, L. (2008). How Parkinson's disease affects non-verbal communication and language processing. *Language and Linguistics Compass, 2*(5), 739-759.

Peltokorpi, S., & Huttunen, K. (2008). Communication in the early stage of language development in children with CHARGE syndrome. *The British Journal of Visual Impairment, 26*(1), 24-49.

Pennington, G., Karlan, G. R., & Lloyd, L. L. (1986). Considerations in selection of sign systems and initial lexica. In D. Ellis (Ed.), *Sensory impairments in mentally handicapped people* (pp. 383-407). College Hill Press.

Pennington, L., Marshall, J., & Goldbart, J. (2007). Describing participants in AAC research and their communicative environments: Guidelines for research and practice. *Disability and Rehabilitation, 29*(7), 521-535.

Penrod, J. P. (1985). Speech discrimination testing. In J. Katz (Ed.), *Handbook of clinical audiology* (3rd ed., pp. 235-255). Williams & Wilkins.

Perez, M. (2015, March). *Choosing the iPad as a dedicated AAC device.* Paper presented at the Texas Speech-Language-Hearing Association Convention.

Périer, O., Charlier, B., Hage, C., & Alegria, J. (1990). Evaluation of the effects of prolonged cued speech practice upon the reception of spoken language. *Cued Speech Journal, 4,* 47-59.

Perrin, M., Robillard, M., & Roy-Charland, A. (2017). Observing eye movements and the influence of cognition during a symbol search task: A comparison across three age groups. *Augmentative and Alternative Communication, 33*(4), 249-259.

Pester, E. J., Petrosko, J. M., & Poppe, K. J. (1994). Optimizing size and spacing for introducing blind adults to the Braille code. *Review, 26,* 15-22.

Peters, S. J. (2003). *Inclusive education: Achieving education for all by including those with disabilities and special education needs.* The World Bank.

Peterson, M. E., & Bell, T. S. (2008). *Foundations of audiology: A practical approach.* Pearson.

Petit, L. K., Tonsing, K. M., & Dada, S. (2016). The perspectives of adults with aphasia and their team members regarding the importance of nine life areas for rehabilitation: A pilot investigation. *Topics in Stroke Rehabilitation, 1,* 1-8.

Petroi, D., Koul, R. K., & Corwin, M. (2014). Effect of number of graphic symbols, levels, and listening conditions on symbol identification and latency in persons with aphasia. *Augmentative and Alternative Communication, 30*(1), 40-54.

Petry, P., Polli, J. B., Mattos, V. F., Rosa, R. C. M., Zen, P. R. G., Graziadio, C., & Rosa, R. F. M. (2013). Clinical features and prognosis of a sample of patients with trisomy 13 (Patau syndrome) from Brazil. *American Journal of Medical Genetics, 161A,* 1278-1283.

Petscher, E. S., Rey, C., & Bailey, J. S. (2009). A review of empirical support for differential reinforcement of alternative behavior. *Research in Developmental Disabilities, 30,* 409-425.

Philip, S. S., & Dutton, G. N. (2014). Identifying and characterising cerebral visual impairment in children: A review. *Clinical and Experimental Optometry, 97,* 196-208.

Piccin, T. B., & Waxman, S. R. (2007). Why nouns trump verbs in word learning: New evidence from children and adults in the human simulation paradigm. *Language Learning and Development, 3,* 295-323.

Piché, L., & Reichle, J. (1991). Teaching scanning selection techniques. In J. Reichle, J. York, & J. Sigafoos (Eds.), *Implementing augmentative and alternative communication: Strategies for learners with severe disabilities* (pp. 257-274) Paul H. Brookes Publishing Co.

Pickering, J., & Embry, E. (2013). So long, silos. Interprofessional care benefits patients but teaching future clinicians how to provide it can be challenging. Follow these guidelines to "de-silo" your academic program. *The ASHA Leader, 18*(6), 38-45.

Pickl, G. (2011). Communication intervention in children with severe disabilities and multilingual backgrounds: Perceptions of pedagogues and parents. *Augmentative and Alternative Communication, 27*(4), 229-244.

Pierce, P. L., & McWilliam, P. J. (1993). Emerging literacy and children with severe speech and physical impairments (SSPI): Issues and possible intervention strategies. *Topics in Language Disorders, 13*(2), 47-57.

Pindiprolu, S. (2012). A review of naturalistic interventions with young children with autism. *The Journal of International Association of Special Education, 12,* 69-78.

Pinker, S. (1994). *The language instinct: The new science of language and mind.* Allan Lane.

Pistorius, M. (2013). *Ghost boy: The miraculous escape of a misdiagnosed boy trapped inside his own body.* Nelson Books.

Polzer, K. R.., Wankoff, L. L., & Wollner, S. G. (1979, April). *The acquisition of arbitrary and iconic signs: Imitation vs. comprehension.* Paper presented at New York State Speech and Hearing Association.

Ponchillia, S. V. (1993). Complications of diabetes and their implication for service providers. *Journal of Visual Impairment and Blindness, 87,* 354-358.

Pope, L., Light, J., & Franklin, A. (2022). Black children with developmental disabilities receive less augmentative and alternative communication intervention than their white peers: Preliminary evidence of racial disparities from a secondary data analysis. *American Journal of Speech-Language Pathology, 31*(5), 2159-2174.

Porayska-Pomsta, K., Alcorn, A. M., Avramides, K., Beale, S., Bernadini, S., Foster, M. E., Frauenberger, C., Good, J., Guldberg, K., Keay-Bright, W., Kossyvaki, L., Lemon, O., Mademtzi, M., Menzies, R., Pain, H., Rajendran, G., Waller, A., Wass, S., & Smith, T. J. (2018). Blending human and artificial intelligence to support autistic children's social communication skills. *ACM Transactions on Computer-Human Interaction, 25*(6), 1-35.

Porter, G., & Cafiero, J. M. (2009). Pragmatic organization dynamic display (PODD) communication books: A promising practice for individuals with autism spectrum disorders. *Perspectives on Augmentative and Alternative Communication, 18*(4), 121-129.

Porter, P. (1989). Intervention in end stage multiple sclerosis: A case study. *Augmentative and Alternative Communication, 5,* 125-127.

Porter, P., Carter, S., Goolsby, E., Martin, N., Reed, M., Stowers, S., & Wurth, B. (1985). *Prerequisites to the use of augmentative communication.* Division for Disorders of Development and Learning.

Potenski, D. H. (1993). Use of blacklight as visual for people with profound mental and multiple handicaps. *Mental Retardation, 31,* 111-115.

Pottgen, J., Dziobek, I., Reh, S., Heesen, C., & Gold, S. (2013). Impaired social cognition in multiple sclerosis. *Journal of Neurology, Neurosurgery and Psychiatry, 84,* 523-528.

Power, M. R., Power, D., & Horstmanshof, L. (2006). Deaf people communicating via SMS, TTY relay service, fax, and computers in Australia. *Journal of Deaf Studies and Deaf Education, 12,* 80-92.

Prakash, R., Snook, E., Lewis, J., Motl, R., & Kramer, R. (2008). Cognitive impairment in relapsing-remitting multiple sclerosis: A meta-analysis. *Multiple Sclerosis, 14,* 1250-1261.

Prentke Romich Company. (2014). Realize language [computer software]. Retrieved from https://realizelanguage.com/

Priest Erhardt, R. (1974). Sequential levels in development of prehension. *The American Journal of Occupational Therapy, 28,* 592-596.

Pringsheim, T., Wiltshire, K., Day, L., Dykeman, J., Steeves, T., & Jette, N. (2012). The incidence and prevalence of Huntington's disease: A systematic review and meta-analysis. *Movement Disorders, 27*(9), 1083-1091.

Prior, S., Waller, A., & Kroll, T. (2013). Focus groups as a requirement gathering method with adults with severe speech and physical impairments. *Behavior and Information Technology, 32*(8), 752-760.

PL 93-112. (1973). *Rehabilitation act of 1973.* U.S. Congress.

PL 94-142. (1975). *Education for all handicapped children act of 1975.* U.S. Congress.

PL 100-407. (2004). *Technology-related assistance for individuals with disabilities act.* U.S. Congress.

PL 101-336. (1990). *Americans with disabilities act of 1990.* U.S. Congress.

PL 110-325. (2008). *Americans with disabilities act amendments of 2008.* U.S. Congress.

Pufpaff, L. A. (2008). Barriers to participation in kindergarten literacy instruction for a student with augmentative and alternative communication needs. *Psychology in the Schools, 45,* 582-599.

Pumfrey, P. D., & Reason, R. (1991). *Specific learning difficulties: Challenges and responses.* NFER-Nelson.

Purdy, M. (2002). Executive function ability in persons with aphasia. *Aphasiology, 16*(4-6), 549-557.

Purdy, M., & Dietz, A. (2010). Factors influencing AAC usage by individuals with aphasia. *Perspectives on Augmentative and Alternative Communication 19*(3), 70-78.

Purdy, M., & Wallace, S. E. (2016). Intensive multimodal communication treatment for people with chronic aphasia. *Aphasiology, 30*(10), 1071-1093.

Quach, W., Lund, S., McKelvey, M., & Weissling, K. (2018, November). *Augmentative and alternative communication clinical assessment project: Protocol for assessment of children with cerebral palsy.* Seminar at the Annual Convention of the American Speech-Language-Hearing Association.

Quick, N., Erickson, K., & McCright, J. (2019). The most frequently used words: Comparing child-directed speech and young children's speech to inform vocabulary selection for aided input. *Augmentative and Alternative Communication, 35,* 120-131.

Quist, R. W., & Lloyd, L. L. (1990, May). *A comparison of two teaching approaches as they relate to the learning of Blissymbols by cognitively impaired individuals: A preliminary report.* Paper presented at the Annual Meeting of the American Association on Mental Retardation.

Quist, R. W., & Lloyd, L. L. (1997). Principles and uses of technology. In L. L. Lloyd, D. R. Fuller, & H. H. Arvidson (Eds.), *Augmentative and alternative communication: A handbook of principles and practices* (pp. 107-126). Allyn & Bacon.

Raban, B. (1987). *The spoken vocabulary of five-year-old children.* The Reading and Language Information Centre.

Radtke, J., Tate, J., & Happ, M. (2012). Nurses' perceptions of communication training in the ICU. *Intensive and Critical Care Nursing, 28,* 16-25.

Raghavendra, P., & Fristoe, M. (1990). "A spinach with a V on it." What 3-year-olds see in standard and enhanced Blissymbolics. *Journal of Speech and Hearing Disorders, 55,* 149-159.

Raghavendra, P., Olsson, C., Sampson, J., Mcinerney, R., & Connell, T. (2012). School participation and social networks of children with complex communication needs, physical disabilities, and typically developing peers. *Augmentative and Alternative Communication, 28*(1), 33-43.

Rainforth, B., & England, J. (1997). Collaborations for inclusion. *Education and Treatment of Children, 20*(1), 85-104.

Rainforth, B., & York-Barr, J. (1997). *Collaborative teams for students with severe disabilities: Integrating therapy and educational services* (2nd ed.). Paul H. Brookes Publishing Co.

Rajaram, P., Alant, E., & Dada, S. (2012). Application of the self-generation effect to the learning of Blissymbols by persons presenting with a severe aphasia. *Augmentative and Alternative Communication, 28*(2), 64-73.

Randolph, C., Tierney, M., Mohr, E., & Chase, T. (1998). The Repeatable Battery for the Assessment of Neuropsychological Status (RBANS): Preliminary clinical validity. *Journal of Clinical and Experimental Neuropsychology, 20*(3), 310-319.

Rankin, J., Harwood, K., & Mirenda, P. (1994). Influence of graphic symbol use on reading comprehension. *Augmentative and Alternative Communication, 10,* 269-281.

Rao, P. (1995). Drawing and gesture as communication options in a person with severe aphasia. *Topics in Stroke Rehabilitation, 2*(1), 49-56.

Ratcliff, A. (1987). *A comparison of two message selection techniques used in augmentative communication systems by normal children with differing cognitive styles.* Unpublished doctoral dissertation, University of Wisconsin.

Ratcliff, A. (1994). Comparison of relative demands implicated in direct selection and scanning: Considerations from normal children. *Augmentative Alternative Communication, 10,* 67-74.

Ratcliff, A., & Beukelman, D. R. (1995). Preprofessional preparation in augmentative and alternative communication: State of the art report. *Augmentative and Alternative Communication, 11,* 61-73.

Ratcliff, A., Koul, R., & Lloyd, L. L. (2008). Preparation in augmentative and alternative communication: An update for speech-language pathology training. *American Journal of Speech-Language Pathology, 17*(1), 48-59.

Reade, A., & Sayko, S. (2017). *Learning about your child's reading development: Improving literacy brief for parents and families.* Washington, DC: U.S. Department of Education, Office of Elementary and Secondary Education, Office of Special Education Programs, National Center on Improving Literacy. Retrieved from http://improvingliteracy.org

Records, N. L., & Tomblin, J. B. (1994). Clinical decision making: Describing the decision rules of practicing speech-language pathologists. *Journal of Speech, Language, and Hearing Research, 37*(1), 144-156.

Reed, C. M., Durlach, N. I., Braida, L. D., & Schultz, M. C. (1989). Analytic study of the Tadoma method: Effects of hand position on segmental speech perception. *Journal of Speech and Hearing Research, 32,* 921-929.

Reed, V. A. (2018). *An introduction to children with language disorders* (5th ed.). Pearson.

Regenbogen, L. S., & Coscas, G. C. (1985). *Oculo-auditory syndromes.* Masson Publishing.

Rehabilitation Engineering and Assistive Technology Society of North America (RESNA). (2019). Retrieved from: https://www.resna.org/professional-development/volunteer-and-leadership-opportunities/special-interest-groups/special

Rehabilitation Engineering Research Center on Communication Enhancement. (2011). Mobile devices and communication apps: An AAC-RERC White Paper. Retrieved from http://aac-rerc.psu.edu/index.php/pages/show/id/46

Reichle, J. (1991). Defining the decision involved in designing and implementing augmentative and alternative communication systems. In J. Reichle, J. York, & J. Sigafoos (Eds.), *Implementing augmentative and alternative communication: Strategies for learners with severe disabilities* (pp. 39-60). Paul H. Brookes Publishing Co.

Reichle, J., Beukelman, D. R., & Light, J. C. (2002). *Exemplary practices for beginning communicators: Implications for AAC.* Paul H. Brookes Publishing Co.

Reichle, J., & Brown, L. (1986). Teaching the use of a multi-page direct selection communication board to an adult with autism. *Journal of the Association for Persons with Severe Handicaps, 11,* 68-73.

Reichle, J., & Yoder, D. (1985). Communication board use in severely handicapped learners. *Language, Speech, and Hearing Services in Schools, 16,* 146-157.

Reichle, J., York, J., & Sigafoos, J. (1991). *Implementing augmentative and alternative communication: Strategies for learners with severe disabilities.* Paul H. Brookes Publishing Co.

Renaud, S., Mohamed-Said, L., & Macoir, J. (2016). Language disorders in multiple sclerosis: A systematic review. *Multiple Sclerosis and Related Disorders, 10,* 103-111.

Reppen, R. (2010). *Using corpora in the language classroom.* Cambridge University Press.

Resnick, M. B., Armstrong, S., & Carter, R. L. (1988). Developmental intervention program for high-risk premature infants: Effects on development and parent-infant interactions. *Journal of Developmental and Behavioral Pediatrics, 9*(2), 73-78.

Reuss, V. (1991). Die akzeptanz von BLISS in der umwelt. In H. Becker, M. Gangkofer, & E. Schroeder (Eds.), *Kom-munizieren mit BLISS. sprechen ueber BLISS: Doku-mente der ersten Bremer BLISS-Tagung (Communicating with Bliss speaking about Bliss. Documents of the first Bremer Bliss conference)* (pp. 42-56). Selbstverlag des Pantaetischen Bildungswerks.

Richardson, K., Sussman, J., Stathopoulos, E., & Huber, J. (2014). The effect of increased vocal intensity on interarticulator timing in speakers with Parkinson's disease: A preliminary analysis. *Journal of Communication Disorders, 52,* 44-64.

Richter, M., Ball, L., Beukelman, D., Lasker, J., & Ullman, C. (2003). Attitudes toward communication modes and message formulation techniques used for storytelling by people with amyotrophic lateral sclerosis. *Augmentative and Alternative Communication, 19*(3), 170-186.

Ricks, M. D., & Wing, L. (1975). Language, communication, and the use of symbols in normal and autistic children. *Journal of Autism and Childhood Schizophrenia, 5*(3), 191-221.

Riggio, M., & McLetchie, B. (Eds.). (2008). *Deafblindness: Educational service guidelines.* Perkins School for the Blind.

Rincover, A., & Devany, J. (1982). The application of sensory extinction procedures to self-injury. *Analysis and Intervention in Developmental Disabilities, 2,* 67-81.

Ringdahl, J. E., Falcomata, T. S., Christensen, T. J., Bass-Ringdahl, S. M., Lentz, A., Dutt, A., & Schuh-Claus, J. (2009). Evaluation of a pre-treatment assessment to select mand topographies for functional communication training. *Research in Developmental Disabilities, 30,* 330-341.

Ringholz, G. M., Appel, S. H., Bradshaw, M., Cooke, N. A., Mosnik, D. M., & Schulz, P. E. (2005). Prevalence and patterns of cognitive impairment in sporadic ALS. *Neurology, 65*(4), 586-590.

Ripat, J., & Woodgate, R. (2011). The intersection of culture, disability and assistive technology. *Disability and Rehabilitation: Assistive Technology, 6*(2), 87-96.

Rispoli, M. J., Franco, J., Van Der Meer, L., Lang, R., & Camargo, S. P. H. (2010). The use of speech generating devices in communication interventions for individuals with developmental disabilities: A review of the literature. *Developmental Neurorehabilitation, 13*(4), 276-293.

Roalf, D. R., Moore, T. M., Wolk, D. A., Arnold, S. E., Mechanic-Hamilton, D., Rick, J., Kabadi, S., Ruparel, K., Chen-Plotkin, A. S., Chahine, L. M., Dahodwala, N. A., Duda, J. E., Weintraub, D. A., & Moberg, P. J. (2016). Defining and validating a short form Montreal Cognitive Assessment (s-MoCA) for use in neurodegenerative disease. *Journal of Neurology Neurosurgery and Psychiatry, 87,* 1303-1310.

Robillard, M., Mayer-Crittenden, C., Minor-Corriveau, M., & Bélanger, R. (2014). Monolingual and bilingual children with and without primary language impairment: Core vocabulary comparison. *Augmentative and Alternative Communication, 30,* 267-278.

Rocca, M. A., Amato, M. P., De Stefano, N., Enzinger, C., Geurts, J. J., Penner I. K., Rovira, A., Sumowski, J. F., Valsasina, P., Filippi, M., & MAGNIMS Study Group. (2015). Clinical and imaging assessment of cognitive dysfunction in multiple sclerosis. *The Lancet Neurology, 14*(3), 302-317.

Roche, L., Sigafoos, J., Lancioni, G. E., O'Reilly, M. F., Green, V. A., Sutherland, D., van der Meer, L., Schlosser, R. W., Marschik, P. B., & Edrisinha, C. D. (2014). Tangible symbols as an AAC option for individuals with developmental disabilities: A systematic review of intervention studies. *Augmentative and Alternative Communication, 30*(1), 28-39.

Rødbroe, I., & Janssen, M. (2006). Communication and congenital deafblindness: Congenital deafblindness and the core principles of intervention (Vol. 1). Perkins School for the Blind.

Rodriguez, C. S., Rowe, M., Thomas, L., Shuster, J., Koeppel, B., & Cairns, P. (2016). Enhancing the communication of suddenly speechless critical care patients. *American Journal of Critical Care, 25*(3), e40-e46.

Roeser, R. J., Valente, M., & Hosford-Dunn, H. (2007). *Audiology diagnosis* (2nd ed.). Thieme Medical Publishers Inc.

Rohner, T. (1966). *Fonetic English spelling.* Fonetic English Spelling Associates.

Römer, U. (2011). Corpus research applications in second language teaching. *Annual Review of Applied Linguistics, 31,* 205-225.

Romich, B., Hill, K., Seagull, A., Ahmad, N., Strecker, J., & Gotla, K. (2003). AAC performance report tool. In *Proceedings of the RESNA 2001 Annual Conference.* RESNA Press.

Romski, M. A., & Sevcik, R. A. (1988). Augmentative and alternative communication systems: Considerations for individuals with severe intellectual disabilities. *Augmentative and Alternative Communication, 4,* 83-93.

Romski, M. A., & Sevcik, R. A. (1993). Language learning through augmented means: The process and its products. In A. P. Kaiser & D. B. Gray (Eds.), *Enhancing children's communication: Research foundations for intervention* (pp. 85-104). Paul H. Brookes Publishing Co.

Romski, M. A., & Sevcik, R. A. (1996). *Breaking the speech barrier: Language development through augmented means.* Paul H. Brookes Publishing Co.

Romski, M. A., & Sevcik, R. A. (2005). Augmentative communication and early intervention: Myths and realities. *Infants and Young Children, 18*(3), 174-185.

Romski, M. A., Sevcik, R. A., Adamson, L. B., Cheslock, M., Smith, A., Barker, R. M., & Bakeman, R. (2010). Randomized comparison of augmented and nonaugmented language interventions for toddlers with developmental delays and their parents. *Journal of Speech, Language, and Hearing Research, 53,* 350-364.

Romski, M. A., Sevcik, R. A., Barton-Hulsey, A., & Whitmore, A. S. (2015). Early intervention and AAC: What a difference 30 years makes. *Augmentative and Alternative Communication, 31,* 181-202.

Romski, M. A., Sevcik, R. A., & Pate, J. L. (1988). Establishment of symbolic communication in persons with severe retardation. *Journal of Speech and Hearing Disorders, 53*(1), 94-107.

Romski, M. A., Sevcik, R. A., Pate, J. L., & Rumbaugh, D. (1985). Discrimination of lexigrams and traditional orthography by non-speaking severely mentally retarded persons. *American Journal of Mental Deficiency, 90,* 185-189.

Rose, T., Worrall, L., & McKenna, K. (2003). The effectiveness of aphasia-friendly principles for printed health education materials for people with aphasia following stroke. *Aphasiology, 17,* 947-963.

Rose, V., Trembath, D., Keen, D., & Paynter, J. (2016). The proportion of minimally verbal children with autism spectrum disorder in a community-based early intervention programme. *Journal of Intellectual Disability Research, 60*(5), 464-477.

Rosen, D. R., Siddique, T., Patterson, D., Figlewicz, D. A., Sapp, P., Hentati, A., Donaldson, D., Goto, J., O'Regan, J. P., Den, H. X., Rahmani, Z., Krizus, A., McKenna-Yasek, D., Cayabyab, A., Gaston, S. M., Berger, R., Tanzi, R. E., Halperin, J. J., Herzfeldt, B., … Brown, R. H. Jr. (1993). Mutations in Cu/Zn superoxide dismutase gene are associated with familial amyotrophic lateral sclerosis. *Nature, 362,* 59-62.

Rosenthal, J. L. (1993). Special problems of people with diabetes and visual impairment. *Journal of Visual Impairment and Blindness, 87,* 331-333.

Rosenthal, R. (1979). The file drawer problem and tolerance for null results. *Psychological Bulletin, 86,* 638-641.

Rosenthal, R. (2002). The Pygmalion effect and its mediating mechanism. In J. Aronson (Ed.), *Improving academic achievement: Impact of psychological factors on education* (pp. 26-36). Academic Press.

Ross, M., & Lerman, J. (1970). A picture identification test for hearing impaired children. *Journal of Speech and Hearing Research, 13,* 44-53.

Rotholz, D. A., Berkowitz, S. F., & Burberry, J. (1989). Functionality of two modes of communication in the community by students with developmental disabilities: A comparison of signing and communication books. *Journal of the Association for Persons with Severe Handicaps, 14,* 227-233.

Roush, J., & Wilson, K. (2013). Interdisciplinary assessment of children with hearing loss and multiple disabilities. *Perspectives on Hearing and Hearing Disorders in Childhood, 23*(1), 13.

Rowland, C. (1990). Communication in the classroom for children with dual sensory impairments: Studies of teacher and child behavior. *Augmentative and Alternative Communication, 6,* 262-274.

Rowland, C. (2011a). Communication Matrix [assessment instrument]. Retrieved from http://communicationmatrix.org

Rowland, C. (2011b). Using the Communication Matrix to assess expressive skills in early communicators. *Communication Disorders Quarterly, 32*(3), 190-201.

Rowland, C. (2013). *Handbook: Online Communication Matrix.* Oregon Institute on Disability and Development.

Rowland, C., & Fried-Oken, M. (2010). Communication Matrix: A clinical and research assessment tool targeting children with severe communication disorders. *Journal of Pediatric Rehabilitation Medicine, 3*(4), 319-329.

Rowland, C., Fried-Oken, M., Bowser, G., Granlund, M., Lollar, D., Phelps, R., Simeonsson, R. J., & Steiner, S. A. M. (2016). Communication Supports Inventory-Children & Youth (CSI-CY): A new instrument based on the ICF-CY. *Disability and Rehabilitation, 38*(19), 1909-1917.

Rowland, C., & Schweigert, P. D. (1989a). Tangible symbols: Symbolic communication for individuals with multisensory impairments. *Augmentative and Alternative Communication, 5,* 226-234.

Rowland, C., & Schweigert, P. D. (1989b). Tangible symbol systems for individuals with multisensory impairments [videotape and manual]. Communication Skill Builders.

Rowland, C., & Schweigert, P. D. (1990). *Tangible symbol systems. Symbolic communication for individuals with multisensory impairments.* Communication Skill Builders.

Rowland, C., & Schweigert, P. D. (2000a). Tangible symbols: Tangible outcomes. *Augmentative and Alternative Communication, 16*(2), 61-78.

Rowland, C., & Schweigert, P. D. (2000b). *Tangible symbol systems: Making the right to communicate a reality for individuals with severe disabilities* (2nd ed.). Oregon Health Science University.

Rowland, C., & Schweigert, P. D. (2003). Cognitive skills and AAC. In J. C. Light, D.R. Beukelman, & J. Reichle (Eds.), *Communicative competence for individuals who use AAC: From research to effective practice* (pp. 241-275). Paul H. Brookes Publishing Co.

Rowland, C., Schweigert, P. D., Sacks, S., & Silberman, R. K. (1998). Enhancing the acquisition of functional language and communication. In S. Sacks & R. Silberman (Eds.), *Educating students who have visual impairments and other disabilities.* Paul H. Brookes Publishing Co.

Ruberl, A., & Franklin, H. (2006). *Cued speech: Myths and facts. National Cued Speech Association fact sheet.* National Cued Speech Association.

Ruet, A., Deloire, M., Charré-Morin, J., Hamel, D., & Brochet, B. (2013). Cognitive impairment differs between primary progressive and relapsing-remitting MS. *Neurology, 80*(16), 1501-1508.

Rumbaugh, D. M. (Ed.). (1977). *Language learning by a chimpanzee: The LANA project.* Academic Press.

Ruppar, A. L., Dymond, S. K., & Gaffney, J. S. (2011). Teachers' perspectives on literacy instruction for students with severe disabilities who use augmentative and alternative communication. *Research and Practice for Persons with Severe Disabilities, 36,* 100-111.

Rupprecht, S., Beukelman, D., & Vrtiska, H. (1995). Comparative intelligibility of five synthesized voices. *Augmentative and Alternative Communication, 11*(4), 244-248.

Rush, E. L., & Helling, C. R. (2012, November). *Evidence-based AAC assessment: Integrating new protocols and existing best practice.* Paper presented at the American Speech-Language-Hearing Association Convention.

Russo, M., Prodan, V., Meda, N., Carcavallo, L., Muracioli, A., Sabe, L., Bonamico, L., Allegri, R. F., & Olmos, L. (2017). High-technology augmentative communication for adults with post-stroke aphasia: A systematic review. *Expert Review of Medical Devices, 14*(5), 355-370.

Ryan, C. (2013). Language use in the United States: 2011. US Census Bureau, American Community Survey Reports, ACS-22.

Sacks, H., Goren, L. & Burke, L. (1991). Ophthalmologic screening of adults with mental retardation. *American Journal on Mental Retardation, 95,* 571-574

Saji, E., Arakawa, M., Yanagawa, K., Toyoshima, Y., Yokoseki, A., Okamoto, K., Otsuki, M., Akazawa, K., Kakita, A., Takahashi, H., Nishizawa, M., & Kawachi, I. (2013). Cognitive impairment and cortical degeneration in neuromyelitis optica. *Annals of Neurology, 73*(1), 65-76.

Sakurada, T., Nakajima, T., Morita, M., Hirai, M., & Watanabe, E. (2017). Improved motor performance in patients with acute stroke using the optimal individual attentional strategy. *Scientific Reports, 7,* Article number 40592.

Samuels, S. J. (1967). Attentional processes in reading: The effects of pictures on the acquisition of reading responses. *Journal of Educational Psychology, 58,* 337-342.

Sanders, D. A. (1971). *Aural rehabilitation.* Prentice-Hall.

Sanders, D. A. (1976). A model for communication. In L. L. Lloyd (Ed.), *Communication assessment and intervention strategies* (pp. 1-32). University Park Press.

Sanders, D. A. (1982). *Aural rehabilitation* (2nd ed.). Prentice-Hall.

Santangelo, G., Altieri, M., Gallo, A., & Trojano, L. (2019). Does cognitive reserve play any role in multiple sclerosis? A meta-analytic study. *Multiple Sclerosis and Related Disorders, 30,* 265-276.

Saunders, R. J., & Solman, R. R. (1984). The effect of pictures on the acquisition of a small vocabulary of similar sight words. *British Journal of Educational Psychology, 54,* 265-275.

Savage, R. D., Evans, L., & Savage, J. F. (1981). *Psychology and communication in deaf children.* Grune & Stratton.

Schaeffer, B., Kolinzas, G., Musil, A., & McDowell, P. (1977). Spontaneous verbal language for autistic children through signed speech. *Sign Language Studies, 17,* 287-328.

Scherer, M., & Craddock, G. (2002). Matching person and technology (MPT) assessment process. *Technology and Disability, 14,* 125-131.

Scherer, M., Jutai, J., Fuhrer, M., Demers, L., & DeRuyter, F. (2007). A framework for modelling the selection of assistive technology devices (ATDs). *Disability and Rehabilitation: Assistive Technology, 2*(1), 1-8.

Scherz, J., Dutton, L., Steiner, H., & Trost, J. (2010, November). *Smartphone applications useful in communication disorders.* Presentation at the Annual Convention of the American Speech-Language-Hearing Association.

Schiefelbusch, R. L. (Ed.). (1977). *Non-speech language and communication: Analysis and intervention.* University Park Press.

Schiefelbusch, R. L., & Lloyd, L. L. (1974). *Language perspectives— Acquisition, retardation, and intervention.* University Park Press.

Schlosser, R. W. (1992, November). *Nomenclature and category levels in graphic MC symbol sets and systems.* Paper presented at the Annual Convention of the American Speech-Language-Hearing Association.

Schlosser, R. W. (1995). Effectiveness of three teaching strategies on Blissymbol learning, retention, generalization, and use. (Doctoral dissertation, Purdue University, 1994). *Dissertation Abstracts International, 56,* (03) 892A.

Schlosser, R. W. (1997a). Nomenclature and category levels in graphic AAC symbols. Part I. Is a flower a flower a flower? *Augmentative and Alternative Communication, 13,* 4-13.

Schlosser, R. W. (1997b). Nomenclature of category levels in graphic AAC symbols. Part II. Role of similarity in categorization. *Augmentative and Alternative Communication, 13,* 14-19.

Schlosser, R. W., Balandin, S., Hemsley, B., Iacono, T., Probst, P., & von Tetzchner, S. (2014). Facilitated communication and authorship: A systematic review. *Augmentative and Alternative Communication, 30*(4), 359-368.

Schlosser, R. W., Belfiore, P. J., Nigam, R., Blischak, D., & Hetzroni, O. (1995). The effects of speech output technology in the learning of graphic symbols. *Journal of Applied Behavior Analysis, 28,* 537-549.

Schlosser, R. W., & Goetze, H. (1992). Effectiveness and treatment validity of interventions addressing self-injurious behavior: From narrative reviews to meta-analyses. In T. E. Scruggs & M. A. Mastropieri (Eds.), *Advances in learning and behavioral disabilities* (Vol 7, pp. 135-175). JAI Press.

Schlosser, R. W., Koul, R., Shane, H., Sorce, J., Brock, K., Harmon, A., & Hearn, E. (2014). Effects of animation on naming and identification across two graphic symbol sets representing verbs and prepositions. *Journal of Speech, Language, and Hearing Research, 57*(5), 1779-1791.

Schlosser, R. W., & Lee, D. (2000). Promoting generalization and maintenance in augmentative and alternative communication: A meta-analysis of 20 years of effectiveness research. *Augmentative and Alternative Communication, 16*(4), 208-226.

Schlosser, R. W., & Lloyd, L. L. (1993). Effects of initial element teaching in a storytelling context on Blissymbol acquisition and generalization. *Journal of Speech and Hearing Research, 36*, 979-995.

Schlosser, R. W., & Lloyd, L. L. (1997). Effects of paired-associated learning versus symbol explanations on Blissymbol comprehension and production. *Augmentative and Alternative Communication, 13*, 226-238.

Schlosser, R. W., Lloyd, L. L., & Quist, R. (1991, November). *Effects of initial element teaching on Blissymbol learning and generalization.* Paper presented at the Annual Convention of the American Speech-Language-Hearing Association.

Schlosser, R. W., & Raghavendra, P. (2004). Evidence-based practice in augmentative and alternative communication. *Augmentative and Alternative Communication, 20*, 1-21.

Schlosser, R. W., Shane, H., Sorce, J., Koul, R., & Bloomfield, E. (2011). Identifying performing and underperforming graphic symbols for verbs and prepositions in animated and static formats: A research note. *Augmentative and Alternative Communication, 27*(3), 205-214.

Schlosser, R. W., & Sigafoos, J. (2002). Selecting graphic symbols for an initial request lexicon: Integrative review. *Augmentative and Alternative Communication, 18*(2), 102-123.

Schoenborn, C. A., & Heyman, K. (2008). Health disparities among adults with hearing loss: United States, 2000-2006. Health E-Stats, National Center for Health Statistics.

Schow, R. L., & Nerbonne, M. A. (2013). *Introduction to audiologic rehabilitation* (6th ed.). Pearson.

Schroeder, M. R. (1993). A brief history of synthetic speech. *Speech Communication, 13*(1-2), 231-237.

Schulte-Sasse, H. (1991) Lesen und BLISS Frau S. lernt lesen (Reading and Bliss: Mrs. S learns how to read). In H. Becker, M. Gangkofer, & E. Schroeder (Eds.), *Kommunizieren mit BLISS. Sprechen ueber BLISS. Dokumente der ersten Bremer BLISS -Tagung (Communicating with Bliss: Speaking about Bliss. Documents of the first Bremer Bliss conference)* (pp. 42-56). Selbstverlag des Pantaetischen Bildungswerks.

Schwab, K. (2016). The fourth industrial revolution: What is means, how to respond. World Economic Forum. Retrieved from www.weforum.org/agenda/2016/01/the-fourth-industrial-revolution-what-it-means-and-how-to-respond

Schwartz, J. B., & Nye, C. (2006). A systematic review, synthesis, and evaluation of the evidence for teaching sign language to children with autism. *Evidence-Based Practice Briefs, 1*, 1-17.

Schweigert, P., & Rowland, C. (1992). Early communication and microtechnology: Instructional sequence and case studies of children with severe multiple disabilities. *Augmentative and Alternative Communication, 8*(4), 273-286.

Seal, B., & Bonvillian, J. (1997). Sign language and motor functioning in students with autistic disorder. *Journal of Autism and Developmental Disorders, 27*, 437-466.

Seale, J. M., Garrett, K. L., & Figley, L. (2007, September). *Quantitative differences in aphasia interactions with visual scene AAC displays.* Poster presented at the 2007 Clinical AAC Research Conference.

Segalman, R. (2011). AAC, aging, and telephone relay access technology. *Disability Studies Quarterly, 31*(4). Retrieved from https://dsq-sds.org/article/view/1722/1770

Senner, J., & Baud, M. (2016). Pre-service training in AAC: Lessons from school staff instruction. *Perspectives on Augmentative and Alternative Communication, 1*, 24-31.

Sennott, S. C., Light, J. C., & McNaughton, D. (2016). AAC modeling intervention research review. *Research and Practice for Persons with Severe Disabilities, 41*, 101-115.

Sennott, S. C., & Niemeijer, D. (2008). Proloquo2Go [computer software]. Assistiveware.

Sense. (2019). Communicating using sign language. Retrieved from www.sense.org.uk/content/sign-systems-and-languages

Seton, E. T. (1918). *Sign talk of the Cheyenne Indians and other cultures.* Dover Publications.

Sevcik, R. A. (2006). Comprehension: An overlooked component in augmented language development. *Disability and Rehabilitation, 28*, 159-167.

Sevcik, R. A., Barton-Hulsey, A., Romski, M., & Hyatt Fonseca, A. (2018). Visual-graphic symbol acquisition in school age children with developmental and language delays. *Augmentative and Alternative Communication, 34*(4), 265-275.

Sevcik, R. A., & Romski, M. A. (1986). Representational matching skills of persons with severe retardation. *Augmentative and Alternative Communication, 2*, 160-164.

Sevcik, R. A., Romski, M. A., & Wilkinson, K. M. (1991). Role of graphic symbols in the language acquisition process for persons with severe cognitive disabilities. *Augmentative and Alternative Communication, 7*, 161-170.

Shadden, B. (2005). Aphasia as identity theft: Theory and practice. *Aphasiology, 19*(3-5), 211-223.

Shakila, D., Stockley, N., Wallace, S., & Koul, R. (2019). The effect of augmented input on the auditory comprehension for persons with aphasia: A pilot investigation. *Augmentative and Alternative Communication, 35*, 148-155.

Shane, H. C., Blackstone, S., Vanderheiden, G., Williams, M., & DeRuyter, F. (2012). Using AAC technology to access the world. *Assistive Technology, 24*(1), 3-13.

Shane, H. C., & Costello, J. (1994, November). *Augmentative communication assessment and feature matching process.* Mini-seminar presented at the Annual Convention of the American Speech-Language-Hearing Association.

Shane, H. C., & Kearns, K. (1994). An examination of the role of the facilitator in "facilitated communication." *American Journal of Speech-Language Pathology, 3*(3), 48-54.

Shane, H. C., Laubscher, C., Schlosser, R., Flynn, H., Sorce, R., & Abramson, W. (2012). Applying technology to visually support language and communication in individuals with autism spectrum disorders. *Journal of Autism and Developmental Disorders, 42*(6), 1228-1235.

Shannon, C. E., & Weaver, W. W. (1949). *The mathematical theory of communication.* University of Illinois.

Shattuck, P. T., Roux, A. M., Hudson, L. E., Taylor, J. L., Maenner, M. J., & Trani, J. F. (2012). Services for adults with an autism spectrum disorder. *The Canadian Journal of Psychiatry, 57*(5), 284-291.

Sheehy, K., & Duffy, H. (2009). Attitudes to Makaton in the ages on integration and inclusion. International *Journal of Special Education, 24*(2), 91-102.

Sheline, D. (n.d.). Guidelines for modifying books for students in phase I, II, and III. *Paths to Literacy for Students Who are Blind or Visually Impaired.* Retrieved from http://www.pathstoliteracy.org/guidelines-modifying-books-students-phases-i-ii-and-iii

Sherrill, C. (2010). Language matters: From "mental retardation" to "intellectual disabilities". *Palaestra, 25*(1), 54-56.

Shin, S., & Hill, K. (2016). Korean word frequency and commonality study for augmentative and alternative communication. *International Journal of Language and Communication Disorders, 51*, 415-429.

Shin, S., & Park, H. (2022). The effect of non-verbal working memory in graphic symbol selection. *Augmentative and Alternative Communication, 38*(2), 82-90.

Shojaei, E., Jafari, Z., & Gholami, M. (2016). Effect of early intervention on language development in hearing-impaired children. *Iranian Journal of Otorhinolaryngology, 28*(84), 13.

Shumway-Cook, A., & Woollacott, M. H. (2017). *Motor control: Translating research into clinical practice* (5th ed.). Lippincott Williams & Wilkins.

Sidman, M. (1994). *Equivalence relations and behavior: A research story.* Authors Cooperative, Inc.

Sidman, M. (2009). Equivalence relations and behavior: An introductory tutorial. *The Analysis of Verbal Behavior, 25*, 5-17.

Siegel, E., & Wetherby, A. (2000). Nonsymbolic communication. In M. Snell (Ed.), *Instruction of students with severe disabilities* (5th ed., pp. 409-451). Merrill.

Sienkiewicz-Mercer, R. (1995, June). *Acceptance: Key to the future.* Plenary session presented at the 119th Annual Meeting of the American Association on Mental Retardation.

Sienkiewicz-Mercer, R., & Kaplan, A. B. (1989). *I raise my eyes to say yes.* Whole Health Books.

Sigafoos, J., Doss, S., & Reichle, J. (1989). Developing mand and tact repertoires in persons with severe developmental disabilities using graphic symbols. *Research in Developmental Disabilities, 10*, 183-200.

Sigafoos, J., & Drasgow, E. (2001). Conditional use of aided and unaided AAC: A review and clinical case demonstration. *Focus on Autism and Other Developmental Disabilities, 16*, 152-161.

Sigafoos, J., & Mirenda, P. (2002). Strengthening communicative behaviors for gaining access to desired items and activities. In J. Reichle, D. R. Beukelman, & J. C. Light (Eds.), *Exemplary practices for beginning communicators: Implications for AAC* (pp. 123-156). Paul H. Brookes Publishing Co.

Sigafoos, J., O'Reilly, M. F., & Lancioni, G. E. (2009). Functional communication training and choice-making interventions for the treatment of problem behavior in individuals with autism spectrum disorders. In P. Mirenda & T. Iacono (Eds.) *Autism spectrum disorders and AAC* (pp. 333-354). Paul H. Brookes Publishing Co.

Sigafoos, J., & Reichle, J. (1992). Comparing explicit to generalized requesting in an augmentative communication mode. *Journal of Developmental and Physical Disabilities, 4*, 167-188.

Sigafoos, J., O'Reilly, M. F., Schlosser, R. W., & Lancioni, G. E. (2007). Communication intervention. In P. Sturmey & A. Fitzer (Eds.), *Autism spectrum disorders: Applied behavior analysis, evidence and practice* (pp. 151-185). Pro-Ed.

Sigafoos, J., Woodyatt, G., Deen, D., Tait, K., Tucker, M., Roberts-Pennell, D., & Pittendreigh, N. (2000). Identifying potential communicative acts in children with developmental and physical disabilities. *Communication Disorders Quarterly, 21*, 77-87.

Silverman, F. H. (1995). *Communication for the speechless* (3rd ed.). Allyn & Bacon.

Silverman, H., McNaughton, S., & Kates, B. (1978). *Handbook of Blissymbolics.* Blissymbolics Communication Institute.

Siminoff, L. A. (2013). Incorporating patient and family preferences into evidence-based medicine. *BioMed Central Medical Informatics and Decision Making, 13*(3), s6.

Simmons-Mackie, N., King, J. M., & Beukelman, D. R. (2013). *Supporting communication for adults with acute and chronic aphasia.* Paul H. Brookes Publishing Co.

Simone, R. (1995). *Iconicity in language (Current issues in linguistic theory).* J. Benjamins.

Simpson, K. L. (2013). Syndromes and inborn errors of metabolism. In M. L. Batshaw, N. J. Roizen, & G. R. Lotrecchiano (Eds.), *Children with disabilities* (7th ed., pp. 757-801). Paul H. Brookes Publishing Co.

Simpson, S., Blizzard, L., Otahal, P., Van der Mei, I., & Taylor, B. (2011). Latitude is significantly associated with the prevalence of multiple sclerosis: A meta-analysis. *Journal of Neurology, Neurosurgery, and Psychiatry, 82*, 1132-1141.

Singh, N. N., & Solman, R. T. (1990). A stimulus control analysis of the picture-word problem in children who are mentally retarded: The blocking effect. *Journal of Applied Behavior Analysis, 23*, 525-532.

Singson, M., Mahony, D., & Mann, V. (2000). The relation between reading ability and morphological skills: Evidence from derivational suffixes. *Reading and Writing, 12*, 219-252.

Skeat, W. W. (1958). *An etymological dictionary of the English language.* Clarendon Press.

Skelly, M. (1979). *Amer-Ind gestural code based on universal American Indian hand talk.* Elsevier.

Skelly, M., Schinsky, L., Smith, R. W., Donaldson, R. C., & Griffin, J. M. (1975). American Indian sign: A gestural communication system for the speechless. *Archives of Physical Medicine and Rehabilitation, 56*(4), 156-160.

Skinner, B. F. (1953). Some contributions of an experimental analysis of behavior to psychology as a whole. *American Psychologist, 8*(2), 69-78.

Slamecka, N. J., & Graf, P. (1978). The generation effect: Delineation of a phenomenon. *Journal of Experimental Psychology: Human Learning and Memory, 4*, 592-604.

Smith, A., Barker, R. M, Barton-Hulsey, A., Romski, M., & Sevcik, R. (2016). Augmented language interventions for children with severe disabilities. In R. A. Sevcik & M. Romski (Eds.), *Communication interventions for individuals with severe disabilities* (pp. 123-146). Paul H. Brookes Publishing Co.

Smith, F. (1982). *Understanding reading: A psycholinguistic analysis of reading and learning to read.* Holt, Rinehart and Winston.

Smith, K. G., Smith, I. M., & Blake, K. (2010). CHARGE syndrome: An educator's primer. *Education and Treatment of Children, 33*, 289-314.

Smith, M. M. (1994, July). *Comprehension of graphics vs. verbal signs in two children with severe speech and physical impairments.* Presentation at the 23rd International Congress of Applied Psychology, Madrid.

Smith, M. M. (2006). Speech, language and aided communication: Connections and questions in a developmental context. *Disability and Rehabilitation, 28*(3), 151-157.

Smith, T., Scahill L., Dawson G., Guthrie, D., Lord, C., Odom, S., Rogers, S., & Wagner, A. (2007). Designing research studies on psychosocial interventions in autism. *Journal of Autism and Developmental Disorders, 37*, 354-366.

Smith-Lewis, M. (1994). Discontinuity in the development of aided augmentative and alternative communication systems. *Augmentative and Alternative Communication, 10*, 14-26.

Smith-Lewis, M., & Ford, A. (1987). A user's perspective on augmentative communication. *Augmentative and Alternative Communication, 3*, 12-17.

Snapp, H. (2019). Nonsurgical management of single-sided deafness: Contralateral routing of signal. *Journal of Neurological Surgery Part B: Skull Base, 80*(2), 132-138.

Snell, M. (2002). Using a dynamic assessment with learners who communicate nonsymbolically. *Augmentative and Alternative Communication, 18*, 163-176.

Snell, M. E., Chen, L., & Hoover, K. (2006). Teaching augmentative and alternative communication to students with severe disabilities: A review of intervention research 1997-2003. *Research and Practice for Persons with Severe Disabilities, 31*, 203-214.

Snodgrass, M., Stoner, J., & Angell, M. (2013). Teaching conceptually referenced core vocabulary for initial augmentative and alternative communication. *Augmentative and Alternative Communication, 29*, 322-333.

Snow, C. E., Burns, M. S., & Griffin, P. (Eds.). (1998). *Preventing reading difficulties in young children.* The National Academy Press.

Snyder-McLean, L. (1978, November). *Functional stimulus and response variables in sign training with retarded subjects.* Paper presented at the Annual Convention of the American Speech-Language-Hearing Association.

Sobsey, D., & Wolf-Schein, E. G. (1996). Sensory impairments. In F. P. Orelove & D. Sobsey (Eds.), *Educating children with multiple disabilities: A transdisciplinary approach* (3rd ed., pp. 411-450). Paul H. Brookes Publishing Co.

Society for Disabilities Studies. (n.d.). Disability studies 101. Models of disability. Retrieved from https://disstudies101.com/perceptions/models-of-disability/

Sonksen, P. M., Petrie, A., & Drew, K. J. (1991). Promotion of visual development of severely visually impaired babies. *Developmental Medicine and Child Neurology, 33*, 320-335.

Soto, G. (2012). Training partners in AAC in culturally diverse families. *Perspectives on Augmentative and Alternative Communication, 21*(4), 144-150.

Soto, G. (2018). Introduction to the special issue on cultural and linguistic diversity and AAC. *Perspectives on Augmentative and Alternative Communication, 3,* 136-137.

Soto, G., Müller, E., Hunt, P., & Goetz, L. (2001). Critical issues in the inclusion of students who use augmentative and alternative communication: An educational team perspective. *Augmentative and Alternative Communication, 17*(2), 62-72.

Soto, G., & Yu, B. (2014). Considerations for the provision of services to bilingual children who use augmentative and alternative communication. *Augmentative and Alternative Communication, 30*(1), 83-92.

Soto, G., Yu, B., & Henneberry, S. (2007). Supporting the development of narrative skills of an eight-year old child who uses an augmentative and alternative communication device. *Child Language Teaching and Therapy, 23*(1), 27-45.

Soto, G., & Zangari, C. (Eds.) (2009). *Practically speaking: Language, literacy, and academic development for students with AAC needs.* Paul H. Brookes Publishing Co.

Souriau, J., Rødbroe, I., & Janssen, M. (Eds.). (2008). *Communication and congenital deafblindness: Meaning making.* Vol. 3. VCDBF/Viataal.

Souriau, J., Rødbroe, I., & Janssen, M. (Eds.). (2009). *Communication and congenital deafblindness: Transition to the cultural language.* Vol. 4. VCDBF/Viataal.

Sperber, D., & Wilson, D. (1986). *Relevance, communication and cognition.* Blackwell.

Spiegel, B., Benjamin, B. J., & Spiegel, S. (1993). One method to increase spontaneous use of an assistive communication device: A case study. *Augmentative and Alternative Communication, 9,* 111-117.

Spinal Muscular Atrophy Foundation. (n.d.). About SMA: Overview. Retrieved from http://www.smafoundation.org/about-sma/

Spirkovska, L. (2005). Summary of tactile user interface techniques and systems. *NASA Ames Research Center.* Retrieved from https://ti.arc.nasa.gov/m/pub-archive/905h/0905%20(Spirkovska)%20v2.pdf

Sriranjani, R., Reddy, M. R., & Umesh, S. (2015). Improved acoustic modeling for automatic dysarthric speech recognition. In *Proceedings of the Twenty-first National Conference on Communications (NCC),* 1-6.

Stanovich, K. (1986). Matthew effects in reading: Some consequences of individual differences in the acquisition of literacy. *Reading Research Quarterly, 21,* 360-407.

Stathopoulos, E. T., Huber, J. E., Richardson, K., Kamphaus, J., DeCicco, D., Darling, M., Fulcher, K., & Sussman, J. E. (2014). Increased vocal intensity due to the Lombard effect in speakers with Parkinson's disease: Simultaneous laryngeal and respiratory strategies. *Journal of Communication Disorders, 48,* 1-17.

Statista. (2007). Number of smartphone users worldwide from 2016 to 2021. Retrieved from https://www.statista.com/statistics/330695/number-of-smartphone-users-worldwide/

Steele, R., Weinrich, M., Wertz, R., Kleczewska, M., & Carlson, G. (1989). Computer-based visual communication in aphasia. *Neuropsychologia, 27*(4), 409-426.

Steelman, J. D., Pierce, P. L., & Koppenhaver, D. A. (1993). The role of computers in promoting literacy in children with severe speech and physical impairments (SSPI). *Topics in Language Disorders, 13*(2), 76-88.

Stern, Y. (2012). Cognitive reserve in ageing and Alzheimer's disease. *Lancet Neurology, 11,* 1006-1012.

Steve Gleason Enduring Voices Act. (2017). (Report 115-469, to accompany H.R. 2465). Retrieved from https://www.congress.gov/115/crpt/hrpt469/CRPT-115hrpt469.pdf

Stevens, G., Flaxman, S., Brunskill, E., Mascarenhas, M., & Mathers, C. D. (2011). Global and regional hearing impairment prevalence: An analysis of 42 studies in 29 countries. *European Journal of Public Health, 23*(1), 146-152.

Stevenson, J., & Richman, N. (1978). Behavior, language, and development in three-year-old children. *Journal of Autism and Childhood Schizophrenia, 8,* 299-313.

Stirnimann, N., N'Diaye, K., Le Jeune, F., Houvenaghel, J. F., Robert, G., Sophie, D., Drapier, D., Grandjean, D., Verin, M., & Peron, J. (2018). Hemispheric specialization of the basal ganglia during vocal emotion decoding evidence from asymmetric Parkinson's disease and 18 FDG-PET. *Neuropsychologia, 119,* 1-11.

Stokes, T. F., & Baer, D. M. (1977). An implicit technology of generalization. *Journal of Applied Behavior Analysis, 10,* 349-367.

Stokoe, W. (1960). *Sign language structure: An outline of the visual communication system of the American Deaf.* Gallaudet College.

Strauss, D. J., Shavelle, R. M., Rosenbloom, L., & Brooks, J. C. (2008). Life expectancy in cerebral palsy: An update. *Developmental Medicine and Child Neurology, 50,* 487-493.

Stredler-Brown, A. (2014). Development of listening and language skills in children who are deaf or hard-of-hearing. In R. H. Hull (Ed.), *Introduction to aural rehabilitation.* (2nd ed., pp. 153-178). Plural Publishing.

Stremel-Campbell, K., & Rowland, C. (1987). Prelinguistic communication intervention: Birth-to-2. *Topics in Early Childhood Special Education, 7*(2), 49-58.

Strobl, W. M. (2013). Seating. *Journal of Child Orthopedics, 7,* 395-399.

Strong, M. J., Abrahams, S., Goldstein, L. H., Woolley, S., McLaughlin, P., Snowden, J., Mioshi, E., Roberts-South, A., Benatar, M., HortobáGyi, T., Rosenfeld, J., Silani, V., Ince, P. G., & Turner, M. R. (2017). Amyotrophic lateral sclerosis—Frontotemporal spectrum disorder (ALS-FTSD): Revised diagnostic criteria. *Amyotrophic Lateral Sclerosis and Frontotemporal Degeneration, 18,* 153-174.

Stuart, S., Beukelman, D., & King, J. (1997). Vocabulary use during extended conversations by two cohorts of older adults. *Augmentative and Alternative Communication, 13*(1), 40-47.

Stuart, S., & Parette, H. P. (2002). Native Americans and augmentative and alternative communication issues. *Multiple Voices for Ethnically Diverse Exceptional Learners, 5*(1), 38-53.

Stuart, S., Vanderhoof, D., & Beukelman, D. (1993). Topic and vocabulary use patterns of elderly women. *Augmentative and Alternative Communication, 9,* 95-110.

Stubbs, M. (2010). Three concepts of keywords. In M. Bondi & M. Scott (Eds.), *Keyness in texts: Corpus linguistic investigations* (pp. 21-42). John Benjamins.

Sturken, M. (1997). *Tangled memories: The Vietnam War, the AIDS epidemic, and the politics of remembering.* University of California Press.

Sturm, J. M., Beukelman, D. R., & Mirenda, P. (1998). Literacy development of AAC users. In D. R. Beukleman & P. Mirenda (Eds.), *Augmentative and alternative communication: Management of severe communication disorders in children and adults* (2nd ed., pp. 355-390). Paul H. Brookes Publishing Co.

Sturm, J. M., & Clendon, S. A. (2004). Augmentative and alternative communication, language, and literacy: Fostering the relationship. *Topics in Language Disorders, 24*(1), 76-91.

Sturm, J. M., Spadorcia, S. A., Cunningham, J. W., Cali, K. S., Staples, A., Erickson, K., & Koppenhaver, D. A. (2006). What happens to reading between first and third grade? Implications for students who use AAC. *Augmentative and Alternative Communication, 22*(1), 21-36.

Sundberg, M. L., & Partington, J. W. (1998). *Teaching language to children with autism and other developmental disabilities.* Behavior Analysts, Inc.

Sutton, A., Gallagher, T., Morford, J., & Shahnaz, N. (2000). Relative clause sentence production using augmentative and alternative communication systems. *Applied Psycholinguistics, 21,* 473-486.

Sutton, A., Soto, G., & Blockberger, S. (2002). Grammatical issues in graphic symbol communication. *Augmentative and Alternative Communication, 18,* 192-204.

Suvagiya, P. H., Bhatt, C. M., & Patel, R. P. (2016). Indian Sign Language translator using Kinect. In *Proceedings of the International Conference on ICT for Sustainable Development: Advances in Intelligent Systems and Computing* (Vol. 408, pp. 15-23). Retrieved from https://link.springer.com/chapter/10.1007/978-981-10-0135-2_2

Svindt, V., Bona, J., & Hoffmann, I. (2019). Changes in temporal features of speech in secondary progressive multiple sclerosis (SPMS)-Case studies. *Clinical Linguistics and Phonetics, 25*, 1-18.

Swanson, L. A. (2011). Communication: The speech and language perspective. In T. S. Hartshorne, M. Hefner, S. Davenport, & J. W. Thelin (Eds.), *CHARGE syndrome* (pp. 253-273). Plural Publishing.

Swiffin, A., Arnott, J. L., Pickering, J. A., & Newell, A. (1987). Adaptive and predictive techniques in a communication prosthesis. *Augmentative and Alternative Communication, 3*(4), 181-191.

Tabak, J. (2006). *Significant gestures*. Praeger.

Tabe, N., & Jackson, M. (1989). Teaching sight word vocabulary to children with developmental disabilities. *Australia and New Zealand Journal of Developmental Disabilities, 15*, 27-39.

Talk English. (n.d.a). Top 1000 verbs. Retrieved from https://www.talk-english.com/vocabulary/top-1000-verbs.aspx

Talk English. (n.d.b). Top 1500 nouns. Retrieved from http://www.talk-english.com/vocabulary/top-1500-nouns.aspx

Talk English. (n.d.c). Top 250 adverbs. Retrieved from http://www.talk-english.com/vocabulary/top-250-adverbs.aspx

Talkington, L. W., Hall, S., & Altman, R. (1971). Communication deficits and aggression in the mentally retarded. *American Journal of Mental Deficiency, 76*, 235-237.

Tavernier, G. G. F. (1993). The improvement of vision by vision stimulation and training: A review of the literature. *Journal of Visual Impairment and Blindness, 87*, 143-148.

Taylor, S., Wallace, S., & Wallace, S. (2019). High-technology augmentative and alternative communication in post-stroke aphasia: A review of the factors that contribute to successful augmentative and alternative communication use. *Perspectives of the ASHA Special Interest Groups SIG 12, 4*, 464-473.

Taylor, S. V., & Sobel, D. M. (2011). *Culturally responsive pedagogy: Teaching like our students' lives matter*. Emerald Group Publishing.

Texas School for the Blind and Visually Impaired. (n.d.). A word about prematurity. Retrieved from https://www.tsbvi.edu/deaf-blind-project/1056-a-word-about-prematurity

Thal, D. J., & Tobias, S. (1992). Communicative gestures in children with delayed onset of oral expressive vocabulary. *Journal of Speech, Language, and Hearing Research, 35*, 1281-1289.

Tharpe, A. M. (2008). Unilateral and mild bilateral hearing loss in children: Past and current perspectives. *Trends in Amplification, 12*(1), 7-15.

The Joint Commission. (2010). *Advancing effective communication, cultural competence, and patient-and family-centered care: A roadmap for hospitals*. Author.

Thelin, J. W., & Fussner, J. C. (2005). Factors related to the development of communication in CHARGE syndrome. *American Journal of Medical Genetics, 133A*, 282-290.

Theodoros, D., Hill, A., & Russell, T. (2016). Clinical and quality of life of speech treatment for Parkinson's disease delivered to the home via telerehabilitation: A noninferiority randomized controlled trial. *American Journal of Speech-Language Pathology, 25*, 214-232.

Theodoros, D., & Ramig, L. (2011). Telepractice supported delivery of LSVT LOUD. *Perspectives on Neurophysiology and Neurogenic Speech and Language Disorders, 21*(3), 107-119.

Therrien, M. C., & Light, J. C. (2016). Using the iPad to facilitate interaction between preschool children who use AAC and their peers. *Augmentative and Alternative Communication, 32*(3), 163-174.

Thiessen, A., & Beukelman, D. R. (2019). Learning styles and motivations of individuals without prior exposure to augmentative and alternative communication. *Topics in Language Disorders, 39*(1), 104-114.

Thirumanickam, A., Raghavendra, P., & Olsson, C. (2011). Participation and social networks of school-age children with complex communication needs: A descriptive study. *Augmentative and Alternative Communication, 27*(3), 195-204.

Thistle, J. J., & Wilkinson, K. M. (2012). What are the attentional demands of aided AAC? *Perspectives on Augmentative and Alternative Communication, 21*, 17-22.

Thistle, J. J., & Wilkinson, K. M. (2013). Working memory demands of aided augmentative and alternative communication for individuals with developmental disabilities. *Perspectives on Augmentative and Alternative Communication, 29*, 235-245.

Thistle, J. J., & Wilkinson, K. M. (2015). Building evidence-based practice in AAC display design for young children: Current practices and future directions. *Augmentative and Alternative Communication, 31*(2), 124-136.

Thompson, D. (Ed.). (1995). *The concise Oxford dictionary*. Oxford University Press.

Thorslund, B. (2015). Effect of hearing loss on traffic safety and mobility. In H. A. Charlotte (Ed.), *Handbook of hearing disorders research*. Nova Science Publishers, Inc.

Thunberg, G., Johnson, E., Bornman, J., Öhlén, J., & Nilsson, S. (2022). Being heard—Supporting person-centred communication in paediatric care using augmentative and alternative communication as universal design: A position paper. *Nursing Inquiry, 29*(2), e12426.

Tincani, M. (2004). Comparing the Picture Exchange Communication System and sign language training for children with autism. *Focus on Autism and Other Developmental Disabilities, 19*, 152-163.

Tobii Dynavox. (2004-2019). Picture communication symbols (PCS). Retrieved from https://goboardmaker.com

Todman, J., Alm, N., Higginbotham, J., & File, P. (2008). Whole utterance approaches in AAC. *Augmentative and Alternative Communication, 24*(3), 235-254.

Tomasello, M. (1988). The role of joint attentional processes in early language development. *Language Sciences, 10*(1), 69-88.

Tomasello, M. (2003). *Constructing a language: A usage-based theory of language acquisition*. Harvard University Press.

Tomkins, W. (1969). *Indian sign language*. Dover Publications.

Tompkins, G. (2010). *Literacy for the 21st century: A balanced approach* (5th ed.). Allyn & Bacon.

Tong, X., Deacon, S. H., Kirby, J. R., Cain, K., & Parrila, R. (2011). Morphological awareness: A key to understanding poor reading comprehension in English. *Journal of Educational Psychology, 103*, 523-534.

Tönsing, K. M., Van Niekerk, K., Schlünz, G. I., & Wilken, I. (2018). AAC services for multilingual populations: South African service provider perspectives. *Journal of Communication Disorders, 73*, 62-76.

Tostanoski, A., Lang, R., Raulston, T., Carnett, A., & Davis, T. (2014). Voices from the past: Comparing the rapid prompting method and facilitated communication. *Developmental Neurorehabilitation, 17*, 219-223.

Trainor, A. A. (2010). Reexamining the promise of parent participation in special education: An analysis of cultural and social capital. *Anthropology and Education Quarterly, 41*, 245-263.

Traxler, C. B. (2000). The Stanford Achievement Test: National norming and performance standards for deaf and hard-of-hearing students. *Journal of Deaf Studies and Deaf Education, 5*(4), 337-339.

Trembath, D., Balandin, S., & Togher, L. (2007). Vocabulary selection for Australian children who use augmentative and alternative communication. *Journal of Intellectual and Developmental Disability, 32*, 291-301.

Treviranus, J. (1994). Mastering alternative computer access: The role of understanding, trust, and automaticity. *Assistive Technology, 6*, 26-41.

Treviranus, J., & Roberts, V. (2003). Supporting competent motor control of ACC systems. In J. C. Light, D. R. Beukelman, & J. Reichle (Eds.), *Communicative competence for individuals who use ACC* (pp. 107-145). Paul H. Brookes Publishing Co.

Trief, E. (2007). The use of tangible cues for children with multiple disabilities and visual impairment. *Journal of Visual Impairment and Blindness, 101,* 613-619.

Trief, E. (2013). *STACS: Standardized tactile augmentative communication symbols.* American Printing House for the Blind.

Trief, E., Bruce, S. M., & Cascella, P. W. (2010). The selection of tangible symbols by educators of students with multiple disabilities and visual impairment. *Journal of Visual Impairment and Blindness, 104,* 499-504.

Trief, E., Bruce, S. M., Cascella, P. W., & Ivy, S. (2009). The development of a universal tangible symbol system. *Journal of Visual Impairment and Blindness, 103,* 425-430.

Trief, E., Cascella, P. W., & Bruce, S. M. (2013). A field study of a standardized tangible symbol system for learners who are visually impaired and have multiple disabilities. *Journal of Visual Impairment and Blindness, 107,* 180-191.

Trief, E., Duckman, R., Morse, A. R., & Silberman, R. K. (1989). Retinopathy of prematurity. *Journal of Visual Impairment and Blindness, 83,* 500-504.

Trief, E., & Morse, A. R. (1988). Strabismus and amblyopia. *Journal of Visual Impairment and Blindness, 82,* 327-330.

Trottier, N., Kamp, L., & Mirenda, P. (2011). Effects of peer-mediated instruction to teach use of speech-generating devices to students with autism in social game routines. *Augmentative and Alternative Communication, 27*(1), 26-39.

Trudeau, N., Cleave, P., & Woelk, E. (2003). Using augmentative and alternative communication approaches to promote participation of preschoolers during book reading: A pilot study. *Child Language Teaching and Therapy, 19,* 181-210.

Trussell, J. W., & Easterbrooks, S. R. (2017). Morphological knowledge and students who are deaf or hard-of-hearing. *Communication Disorders Quarterly, 38*(2), 67-77.

Tuthill, J. (2014). Get real with visual scene displays: Use of real-life scenes adds appeal to AAC apps that clients use to communicate about everyday needs and situations. *The ASHA Leader, 19*(6), 34-35.

Tye-Murray, N. (2015). *Foundations of aural rehabilitation: Children, adults, and their family members* (4th ed.). Cengage Learning.

U.S. Commission on Civil Rights. (2009, December). *Minorities in special education: A briefing before the United States Commission on Civil Rights.* Author.

Udwin, O., & Yule, W. (1990). Augmentative communication systems taught to cerebral palsy children-A longitudinal study. 1: The acquisition of signs and symbols and syntactic aspects of their use over time. *British Journal of Disorders of Communication, 25,* 295-309.

Ulmer, E., Hux, K., Brown, J., Nelms, T., & Reeder, C. (2016). Using self-captured photographs to support the expressive communication of people with aphasia. *Aphasiology, 31*(10), 1-22.

U.S. Department of Health & Human Services. (2022, March). Autism and developmental disabilities monitoring (ADDM) network. *Centers for Disease Control and Prevention.* https://www.cdc.gov/ncbddd/autism/addm.html

Usher Syndrome Coalition. (2019). What is Usher syndrome? Retrieved from https://www.usher-syndrome.org/what-is-usher-syndrome/usher-syndrome.html

Uslan, M. M. (1992). Barriers to acquiring assistive technology: Cost and lack of information. *Journal of Visual Impairment and Blindness, 86,* 402-407.

Valente, M., Hosford-Dunn, H., & Roeser, R. J. (2008). *Audiology: Treatment* (2nd ed.). Thieme Medical Publishers Inc.

Valentic, V. (1991). Successful integration from a student's perspective. *Communicating Together, 9*(2), 8-9.

Vallila-Rohter, S., & Kiran, S. (2015). An examination of strategy implementation during abstract nonlinguistic category learning in aphasia. *Journal of Speech, Language, and Hearing Research, 58*(4), 1195-1209.

Vallotton, C. D. (2009). Do infants influence their quality of care? Infants' communicative gestures predict caregivers' responsiveness. *Infant Behavior and Development, 32*(4), 351-365.

Van Balkom, H., & Verhoeven, L. (2010). Literacy learning in users in AAC: A neurocognitive perspective. *Augmentative and Alternative Communication, 26*(3), 149-157.

Van Balkom, H., & Welle Donker-Gimbrere, M. (1985). *Kiezen voor communicatie: Van mensen met een motorische of meervoudige handicap (Choosing for communication: A handbook about the communication of motoric and multiple handicapped children).* ThiemeMeulenhoff bv.

Van den Berg, J. P., Kalmijn, S., Lindeman, E., Veldink, J. H., de Visser, M., Van der Graaff, M. M., Wokke, J. H. J., & Van den Berg, L. H. (2005). Multidisciplinary ALS care improves quality of life in patients with ALS. *Neurology, 65*(8), 1264-1267.

Vanderah, T. W., & Gould, D. J. (2015). *Nolte's the human brain: An introduction to its functional anatomy* (7th ed.). Elsevier.

Vanderheiden, G. C. (2003). A journey through early augmentative communication and computer access. *Journal of Rehabilitation Research and Development, 39*(6; Suppl.), 39-53.

Vanderheiden, G. C., & Harris-Vanderheiden, D. (1976). Communication techniques and aids for the nonvocal severely handicapped. In L. L. Lloyd (Ed.), *Communication assessment and intervention strategies* (pp. 607-652). University Park Press.

Vanderheiden, G. C., & Kelso, D. (1987). Comparative analysis of fixed-vocabulary communication acceleration techniques. *Augmentative and Alternative Communication, 3,* 196-206.

Vanderheiden, G. C., & Lloyd, L. L. (1986). Communication systems and their components. In S. Blackstone (Ed.), *Augmentative communication: An introduction* (pp. 49-161). American Speech-Language-Hearing Association.

Vanderheiden, G. C., & Treviranus, J. (2011). Creating a global public inclusive infrastructure. In C. Stephanidis (Ed.), *Universal access in human-computer interaction: Design for all and inclusion. UAHCI 2011. Lecture Notes in Computer Science* (Vol. 6765, pp. 517-526). Springer.

Vanderheiden, G. C., & Yoder, D. E. (1986). Overview. In S. W. Blackstone (Ed.), *Augmentative communication: An introduction* (pp. 1-28). American Speech-Language-Hearing Association.

van der Meer, L., Kagohara, D., Achmadi, D., O'Reilly, M. F., Lancioni, G. E., Sutherland, D., & Sigafoos, J. (2012). Speech-generating devices versus manual signing for children with developmental disabilities. *Research in Developmental Disabilities, 33,* 1658-1669.

van der Meer, L., Sigafoos, J., O'Reilly, M. F., & Lancioni, G. E. (2011). Assessing preferences for AAC options in communication interventions for individuals with developmental disabilities: A review of the literature. *Research in Developmental Disabilities, 32,* 1422-1431.

Van de Sandt-Koenderman, M. (2004). High-tech AAC and aphasia: Widening horizons? *Aphasiology, 18*(3), 245-263.

van de Sandt-Koenderman, M., Weigers, J., & Hardy, P. (2005). A computerised communication aid for people with aphasia. *Disability and Rehabilitation, 27*(9), 529-533. https://doi.org/10.1080/09638280400018635

van de Sandt-Koenderman, M., Wiegers, J., Wielaert, S., Duivenvoorden, H., & Ribbers, G. (2007). A computerised communication aid in severe aphasia: An exploratory study. *Disability and Rehabilitation, 29*(22), 1701-1709. https://doi.org/10.1080/09638280601056178

Van Dijk, J. V. (1966). The first steps of the blind child toward language. *The International Journal for the Education of the Blind, 15,* 112-114.

Van Genderen, M., Dekker, M., Pilon, F., & Bals, I. (2012). Diagnosing cerebral visual impairment in children with good visual acuity. *Strabismus, 2,* 78-83.

Van Hedel-Van Grinsven, R. (1989). Communication and language development in a child with severe visual and auditory impairments: A case study and discussion of multiple modalities. *Review, 26,* 153-162.

Van Niekerk, K., Dada, S., & Tönsing, K. (2019). Influences on selection of assistive technology for young children in South Africa: Perspectives from rehabilitation professionals. *Disability and Rehabilitation, 41*(8), 912-925.

Van Niekerk, K., Dada, S., Tönsing, K., & Boshoff, K. (2017). Factors perceived by rehabilitation professionals to influence the provision of assistive technology to children: A systematic review. *Physical and Occupational Therapy in Pediatrics, 38*(2), 168-189.

van Oosterom, J., & Devereux, K. (1982). REBUS at Rees Thomas School. *Special Education Forward Trends, 9,* 31-33.

van Oosterom, J., & Devereux, K. (1985). *Learning with rebuses.* EARO, The Resource Centre.

van Sluis, K. E., van der Molen, L., van Son, R. J. J. H., Hilgers, F. J. M., Bhairosing, P. A., & van den Brekel, M. W. M. (2018). Objective and subjective voice outcomes after total laryngectomy: A systematic review. *European Archives of Oto-Rhino-Laryngology, 275*(1), 11-26.

Van Tatenhove, G. (1979, November). *Augmentative communication board development: A response training protocol.* Paper presented at the Annual Convention of the American Speech-Language-Hearing Association.

Van Tatenhove, G. (2009). Building language competence with students using AAC devices: Six challenges. *Perspectives on Augmentative and Alternative Communication, 18*(2), 38-47.

Van Tatenhove, G. (2014a). AAC needs assessment checklist. Retrieved from https://praacticalaac.org/praactical/aac-assessment-forms/

Van Tatenhove, G. (2014b). Issues in language sample collection and analysis with children using AAC. *Perspectives on Augmentative and Alternative Communication, 23,* 65-74.

Van Tatenhove, G. (2016). Normal language development, generative language and AAC. Retrieved from https://www.texasat.net/Assets/1--normal-language--aac.pdf

Van Tilborg, A., & Deckers, S. R. J. M. (2016). Vocabulary selection in AAC: Application of core vocabulary in atypical populations. *Perspectives of the ASHA Special Interest Groups SIG 12, 1*(12), 125-138.

Venkatagiri, H. S. (1993). Efficiency of lexical prediction as a communication acceleration technique. *Augmentative and Alternative Communication, 9,* 161-167.

Venkatagiri, H. S. (2002). Clinical implications of an augmentative and alternative communication taxonomy. *Augmentative and Alternative Communication, 18*(1), 1-24.

Ventura, L. O., Ventura, C. V., Lawrence, L., van der Linden, V., van der Linden, A., Gois, A. L., Cavalcanti, M. M., Barros, E. A., Dias, N. C., Berrocal, A. M., & Miller, M. T. (2017). Visual impairment in children with congenital Zika syndrome. *Journal of American Association for Pediatric Ophthalmology and Strabismus, 21*(4), 295-299.

Verma, V. K., & Srivastava, S. (2018). Toward machine translation linguistic issues of Indian Sign Language. In S. Agrawal, A. Devi, R. Wason, & P. Bansal (Eds.), *Speech and language processing for human-machine communications: Advances in intelligent systems and computing* (Vol. 664, pp. 129-135). Springer.

Vertanen, K., Fletcher, C., Gaines, D., Gould, J., & Kristensson, P. O. (2018). The impact of word, multiple word, and sentence input on virtual keyboard decoding performance. *ACM Conference on Human Factors in Computing Systems Proceedings, 4*(21-26), 626.

Vicker, B. (Ed.). (1974). *Nonoral communication system project 1964/1973.* Campus Stores.

Villegas, A. M., & Lucas, T. (2002). Preparing culturally responsive teachers: Rethinking the curriculum. *Journal of Teacher Education, 53*(1), 20-32.

Villegas, A. M., Strom, K., & Lucas, T. (2012). Closing the racial/ethnic gap between students of colors and their teachers: An elusive goal. *Equity and Excellence in Education, 45*(2), 283-301.

Vinson, B. P. (2001). *Essentials for speech-language pathologists.* Singular Thomson Learning.

Vision Council, The. (2015). *U.S. optical overview and outlook: December 2015.* Author.

Vitter, D. (2015). Steve Gleason Act of 2015. Retrieved from https://www.congress.gov/bill/114th-congress/senate-bill/984

Vogt, S., & Kauschke, C. (2017). Observing iconic gestures enhances word learning in typically developing children and children with specific language impairment. *Journal of Child Language, 44*(6), 1458-1484.

von Tetzchner, S. (1985). Words and chips: Pragmatics and pidginization of computer-aided communication. *Child Language Teaching and Therapy, 1,* 298-305.

von Tetzchner, S., Grove, N., Loncke, F., Barnett, S., Woll, B., & Clibbens, J. (1996). Preliminaries to a comprehensive model of augmentative and alternative communication. In S. von Tetzchner & M. H. Jensen (Eds.), *European perspectives on augmentative and alternative communication* (pp. 19-36). Whurr.

Wacker, D. P., Steege, M. W., Northup, J., Sasso, G., Berg, W., Reimers, T., Cooper, L., Cigrand, K., & Donn, L. (1990). A component analysis of functional communication training across three topographies of severe behavior problems. *Journal of Applied Behavior Analysis, 23,* 417-429.

Waddington, H., Sigafoos, J., Lancioni, G. E., O'Reilly, M. F., van der Meer, L., Carnett, A., Stevens, M., Roche, L., Hodis, F., Green, V. A., Sutherland, D., Lang, R., & Marschik, P. B. (2014). Three children with autism spectrum disorder learn to perform a three-step communication sequence using an iPad-based speech-generating device. *International Journal of Developmental Neuroscience, 39,* 59-67.

Wagner, B. T., & Jackson, H. M. (2006). Developmental memory capacity resources of typical children receiving picture communication symbols using direct selection and visual linear scanning with fixed communication displays. *Journal of Speech, Language, and Hearing Research, 49*(1), 113-126.

Wagner, B. T., & Shaffer, L. A. (2015). Identifying, locating, and sequencing picture communication symbols: Contributions from developmental visuospatial and temporal memory. *Evidence-Based Communication Assessment and Intervention, 9*(1), 21-42.

Wagner, B. T., Shaffer, L. A., & Swim, O. A. (2012). Identifying, locating, and sequencing visual-graphic symbols: A perspective on the role of visuospatial and temporal memory. *Perspectives on Augmentative and Alternative Communication, 21,* 23-29.

Walker, H. K., Hall, W. D., & Hurst, J. W. (1990). *Clinical methods: The history, physical, and laboratory examinations* (3rd ed.). Butterworth.

Walker, M. (1973). *An experimental evaluation of the success of a system of communication for the deaf mentally handicapped.* Unpublished master's thesis, University of London.

Walker, M. (1977). Teaching sign language to deaf mentally handicapped adults. (Institute of Mental Subnormality Conference Proceedings). *Language and the Mentally Handicapped, 3,* 3-25.

Walker, M., Mitha, S., & Riddington, C. (2019). Cultural issues in developing and using signs within the Makaton Language Programme in different countries. In N. Grove & K. Launonen (Eds.), *Manual sign acquisition in children with developmental disabilities* (Chapter 20). Nova Science.

Walker, M., Parsons, F., Cousins, S., Henderson, R., & Carpenter, B. (1985). *Symbols for Makaton.* Makaton Vocabulary Development Project.

Walker, V. L., & Snell, M. E. (2013). Effects of augmentative and alternative communication on challenging behavior: A meta-analysis. *Augmentative and Alternative Communication, 29,* 117-131.

Wallace, S., & Diehl, S. (2017). Multimodal communication program for adults: Cognitive considerations. *Perspectives on Augmentative and Alternative Communication, 2*(12), 4-12.

Wallace, S., & Hux, K. (2014). Effect of two layouts on high technology AAC navigation and content location by people with aphasia. *Disability and Rehabilitation: Assistive Technology, 9*(2), 173-182.

Waller, A. (2006). Communication access to conversational narrative. *Topics in Language Disorders, 26*(3), 221-239.

Waller, A. (2009). Interpersonal communication. In C. Stephanidis (Ed.), *The universal access handbook.* CRC Press Taylor and Francis Group.

Waller, A. (2019). Telling tales: Unlocking the potential of AAC technologies. *International Journal of Language and Communication Disorders, 54*(2), 159-169.

Waller, A., Balandin, S. A., O'Mara, D. A., & Judson, A. D. (2005, August). *Training AAC users in user-centred design.* Paper presented at the Accessible Design in the Digital World Conference.

Waller, A., & Black, R. (2012). Personal storytelling for children who use augmentative and alternative communication. In N. Grove (Ed.), *Using storytelling to support children and adults with special needs* (pp. 111-119). Routledge.

Waller, A., Black, R., O'Mara, D. A., Pain, H., Ritchie, G., & Manurung, R. (2009). Evaluating the STANDUP pun generating software with children with cerebral palsy. *Association for Computing Machinery Transactions on Accessible Computing, 1*(3), 16.

Waller, A., Dennis, F., Brodie, J., & Cairns, A. (1998). Evaluating the use of the TalksBac, a predictive communication device for nonfluent adults with aphasia. *International Journal of Language and Communication Disorders, 33*(1), 45-70.

Wan, M. W., Green, J., Elsabbagh, M., Johnson, M., Charman, T., Plummer, F., & BASIS Team. (2012). Parent–infant interaction in infant siblings at risk of autism. *Research in Developmental Disabilities, 33*(3), 924-932.

Wang, T. N., Howe, T. H., Hinojosa, J., & Weinberg, S. L. (2011). Relationship between postural control and fine motor skills in preterm infants at 6 and 12 months adjusted age. *American Journal of Occupational Therapy, 65*, 695-701.

Wang, Z., Li, Y., & Liu, Z. (2014). Birth weight and gestational age on retinopathy of prematurity in discordant twins in China. *International Journal of Ophthalmology, 7*(4), 663-667.

Warburg, M. (2001). Visual impairment in adult people with intellectual disability: Literature review. *Journal of Intellectual Disability Research, 45*(5), 424-438.

Warren, S. F., Bredin-Oja, S., Fairchild-Escalante, M., Finestack, L., Fey, M., & Brady, N. (2006). Responsivity education/prelinguistic milieu teaching. In R. McCauley & M. Fey (Eds.), *Treatment of language disorders in children* (pp. 47-77). Paul H. Brookes Publishing Co.

Warren, S. F., & Yoder, P. J. (1998). Facilitating the transition from preintentional to intentional communication. In A. Wetherby, S. Warren, & J. Reichle (Eds.), *Transitions in prelinguistic communication* (Vol. 7, pp. 365-385). Paul H. Brookes Publishing Co.

Washburn, A. (1983). SEE-I: The development and use of a sign system over two decades. In *Teaching English to Deaf and second-language students*. Department of English, Gallaudet University.

Wasson, C. A., Arvidson, H. H., & Lloyd, L. L. (1997). Low technology. In L. L. Lloyd, D. R. Fuller, & H. H. Arvidson (Eds.), *Augmentative and alternative communication: A handbook of principles and practices* (pp. 127-136). Allyn & Bacon.

Wasson, P., Tynan, T., & Gardiner, P. (1981). *Test adaptations for the handicapped.* Education Service Center.

Watt, N., Wetherby, A., & Shumway, S. (2006). Prelinguistic predictors of language outcome at 3 years of age. *Journal of Speech, Language, and Hearing Research, 49*, 1224-1237.

Webster, J. (2019). Contingency: The important relationship between behavior and reinforcement. Retrieved from https://www.thoughtco.com/contingency-behavior-and-reinforcement-3110376

Wegner, J. W. (1983). The antidiscrimination model reconsidered: Ensuring equal opportunity without respect to handicap under section 504 of the Rehabilitation Act of 1973. *Cornell Law Review, 69*, 401.

Weinberg, B., & Bosma, J. F. (1970). Similarities between glossopharyngeal breathing and injection methods of air intake for esophageal speech. *Journal of Speech and Hearing Disorders, 35*, 25-32.

Weinrich, M. (1991). Computerized visual communication as an alternative communication system and therapeutic tool. *Journal of Neurolinguistics, 6*(2), 159-176.

Weissling, K., McKelvey, M., Lund, S., & Quach, W. (2017, November). *An AAC assessment protocol for aphasia: Presentation of the validated product.* Seminar presented at the ASHA Convention.

Weissling, K., & Prentice, C. (2010). The timing of remediation and compensation rehabilitation programs for individuals with acquired brain injuries: Opening the conversation. *Perspectives on Augmentative and Alternative Communication, 19*(3), 87-96.

Wendon, L. (1979). Exploring the scope of a picture code system for teaching reading and spelling. *Remedial Education, 7*, 33-42.

Wendt, O., & Lloyd, L. L. (2011). Definitions, history, and legal aspects of augmentative and alternative communication and assistive technology. In O. Wendt, R. W. Quist, & L. L. Lloyd (Eds.), *Assistive technology: Principles and applications for communication disorders and special education* (pp. 1-22). Emerald Publishing.

Wendt, O., Quist, R. W., & Lloyd, L. L. (Eds.) (2011). *Assistive technology: Principles and applications for communication disorders and special education.* Emerald Publishing.

Wepener, C., Johnson, E., & Bornman, J. (2021). Text messaging "helps me to chat": Exploring the interactional aspects of text messaging using mobile phones for youth with complex communication needs. *Augmentative and Alternative Communication, 37*(2), 75-86.

Werner, H., & Kaplan, B. (1988). On developmental changes in the symbolic process. In M. Franklin & S. Barten (Eds.), *Child language: A reader* (pp. 7-9). Oxford University Press.

Westby, C., Burda, A., & Mehta, Z. (2003). Asking the right questions in the right ways: Strategies for ethnographic interviewing. *The ASHA Leader, 8*(8), 4-17.

Wetherby, A. M. (2014, April). *Engaging families of children with developmental disabilities in early detection, early intervention, and prevention.* Keynote presentation at the National Academy of Sciences' Workshop on "Strategies for Scaling Tested and Effective Family-Focused Preventive Interventions to Promote Children's Cognitive, Affective, and Behavioral Health."

Whitehurst, G. J., & Lonigan, C. J. (1998). Child development and emergent literacy. *Child Development, 69*(3), 848-872.

Wiggins, G., & McTighe, J. (1998). Backward design. In *Understanding by design* (pp. 13-34). ASCD.

Wilkinson, K. M., & Hennig, S. C. (2007). The state of research and practice in augmentative and alternative communication for children with developmental/intellectual disabilities. *Mental Retardation and Developmental Disabilities Research Reviews, 13*(1), 58-69.

Wilkinson, K. M., & Hennig, S. C. (2009). Considerations of cognitive, attentional, and motivational demands in the construction and use of aided AAC systems. In G. Soto & C. Zangari (Eds.), *Practically speaking: Language, literacy, and academic development for students with AAC needs* (pp. 313-334). Paul H. Brookes Publishing Co.

Wilkinson, K. M., Light, J. C., & Drager, K. D. (2012). Considerations for the composition of visual scene displays: Potential contributions of information from visual and cognitive sciences. *Augmentative and Alternative Communication, 28*(3), 137-147.

Wilkinson, K. M., & Wolf, S. J. (2021). An in-depth case description of gaze patterns of an individual with cortical visual impairment to stimuli of varying complexity: Implications for augmentative and alternative communication design. *Perspectives of the ASHA Special Interest Groups, 6*(6), 1591-1602.

Williams, B. (2000). More than an exception to the rule. In M. Fried-Oken & H. A. Bersani (Eds.), *Speaking up and spelling it out: Personal essays on augmentative and alternative communication* (pp. 245-254). Paul H. Brookes Publishing Co.

Williams-Gray, C. H., Foltynie, T., Brayne, C. E. G., Robbins, T. W., & Barker, R. A. (2007). Evolution of cognitive dysfunction in an incident Parkinson's disease cohort. *Brain, 130*(7), 1787-1798.

Willoughby, D. M. (1995). When people ask, "How much can you see?" In B. Cheadle (Ed.), *Future reflections special issue: The National Federation of the Blind Magazine for Parents and Teachers of Blind Children, 14*(2), 2.

Wilson, P. E, & Kishner, S. (2016). Seating evaluation and wheelchair prescription. *Medscape*. Retrieved from http://emedicine.medscape.com/article/318092-overview3a2

Wilson, R., Rochon, E., Mihaildis, A., & Leonard, C. (2012). Examining success of communication strategies used by formal caregivers assisting individuals with Alzheimer's disease during an activity of daily living. *Journal of Speech, Language, and Hearing Research, 55*(2), 328-341.

Winborn-Kemmerer, L., Ringdahl, J. E., Wacker, D. P., & Kitsukawa, K. (2009). A demonstration of individual preference for novel mands during functional communication training. *Journal of Applied Behavior Analysis, 42*, 185-189.

Winborn-Kemmerer, L., Wacker, D. P., Harding, J., Boelter, E., Berg, W., & Lee, J. (2010). A randomized comparison of the effect of two prelinguistic communication interventions on the acquisition of spoken communication in pre-schoolers with ASD. *Journal of Speech, Language and Hearing Research, 49*, 698-711.

Windsor, J., & Fristoe, M. (1991). Key word signing: Perceived and acoustic differences between signed and spoken narratives. *Journal of Speech and Hearing Research, 34*, 260-268.

Wingert, J. R., Burton, H., Sinclair, R. J., Brunstrom, J. E., & Damiano, D. L. (2009). Joint-position sense and kinesthesia in cerebral palsy. *Archive Physical Medicine Rehabilitation, 90*(3), 447-453.

Witchalls, J., Blanch, P., Waddington, G., & Adams, R. (2012). Intrinsic functional deficits associated with increased risk of ankle injuries: A systematic review with meta-analysis. *British Journal of Sports Medicine, 46*(7), 515-523.

Witkowski, D., & Baker, B. (2012). Addressing the content vocabulary with core: Theory and practice for nonliterate or emerging literate students. *Perspectives on Augmentative and Alternative Communication, 21*, 74-81.

Wodlinger-Cohen, R. (1991). The manual representation of speech by deaf children, their mothers, and their teachers. In P. Siple & S. Fischer (Eds.), *Theoretical issues in sign language research. Volume 2: Psychology* (pp. 149-169). University of Chicago Press.

Wolf-Nelson, N. (2010). *Language and literacy disorders: Infancy through adolescence*. Pearson.

Woll, B., & Barnett, S. (1998). Toward a sociolinguistic perspective on augmentative and alternative communication. *Augmentative and Alternative Communication, 14*(4), 200-211.

Wolter, J. A., & Green, L. (2013). Morphological awareness intervention in school-age children with language and literacy deficits: A case study. *Topics in Language Disorders, 33*, 27-41.

Wong, C., Odom, S. L., Hume, K. A., Cox, A. W., Fettig, A., Kucharczyk, S., Brock, M. E., Plavnick, J. B., Fleury, V. P., & Schultz, T. R. (2015). Evidence-based practices for children, youth, and young adults with autism spectrum disorder: A comprehensive review. *Journal of Autism and Developmental Disorders, 45*(7), 1951-1966.

Wood, C., Appleget, A., & Hart, S. (2016). Core vocabulary in written personal narratives of school-age children. *Augmentative and Alternative Communication, 32*, 198-207.

Wood, C., Storr, J., & Reich, P. A. (Eds.). (1992). *Blissymbol reference guide*. Blissymbolics Communication International.

Woodcock, R. W. (Ed.). (1965). *The rebus reading series*. Institute on Mental Retardation and Intellectual Development, George Peabody College, Vanderbilt University.

Woodcock, R. W. (1968). *Rebuses as a medium in beginning reading instruction*. Institute on Mental Retardation and Intellectual Development, George Peabody College, Vanderbilt University.

Woodcock, R. W., Clark, C. R., & Davies, C. O. (1968). *Peabody rebus reading program*. American Guidance Service.

Woods, J., Kashinath, S., & Goldstein, H. (2004). Effects of embedding caregiver-implemented teaching strategies in daily routines on children's communication outcomes. *Journal of Early Intervention, 26*, 175-193.

Woodson, E. A., Reiss, L. A. J., Turner, C. W., Gfeller, K., & Gantz, B. J. (2010). The hybrid cochlear implant: A review. *Advances in Otorhinolaryngology, 67*, 125-134.

Woolley, S., York, M., Moore, D., Strutt, A., Murphy, J., Schultz, P., & Katz, J. (2010). Detecting frontotemporal dysfunction in ALS: Utility of the ALS Cognitive Behavioral Screen (ALS-CBS). *Amyotrophic Lateral Sclerosis and Frontotemporal Degeneration, 11*, 303-311.

World Health Organization. (2001). *International classification of functioning, disability and health: ICF*. Author.

World Health Organization (2008). *Guidelines on the provision of manual wheelchairs in less resourced settings*. Author.

World Health Organization and World Bank. (2011). *World report on disability*. Author.

Worrall, L., Rose, T., Howe, T., Brennan, A., Egan, J., Oxenham, D., & McKenna, K. (2005). Access to written information for people with aphasia. *Aphasiology, 19*, 923-929.

Wortman, P. M., & Greenberg, L. D., (1971). Coding, recoding, and decoding of hierarchal information in long-term memory. *Journal of Verbal Learning and Verbal Behavior, 10*, 234-243.

Wright, J. (2003). Forced choice reinforce assessment: Guidelines. *Intervention Central*. Retrieved from https://www.interventioncentral.org/behavioral-interventions/special-needs/forced-choice-reinforcer-assessment-guidelines

Wu, A. W., Boyle, D. J. Wallace, G., & Mazor, K. M. (2013). Disclosure of adverse events in the United States and Canada: An update and a proposed framework for improvement. *Journal of Public Health Research, 2*(32), 186-193.

Yaida, J., & Reuben, S. E. (1992). Job roles of assistive technology service providers in the United States. *Journal of Rehabilitation Research, 15*, 277-287.

Yamagishi, J., Veaux, C., King, S., & Renals, S. (2012). Speech synthesis technologies for individuals with vocal disabilities: Voice banking and reconstruction. *Acoustical Science and Technology, 33*, 1-5.

Yell, M. L., Rogers, D., & Rogers, E. L. (1998). The legal history of special education: What a long, strange trip it's been! *Remedial and Special Education, 19*(4), 219-228.

Yılmaz, E., & Soruç, A. (2015). The use of concordance for teaching vocabulary: A data-driven learning approach. *Procedia - Social and Behavioral Sciences, 191*, 2626-2630.

Yoder, D. E. (1980). Communication systems for non-speech children. *New Directions for Exceptional Children, 2*, 63-78.

Yoder, D. E., & Kraat, A. (1993). Intervention issues in nonspeech communication. In D. E. Yoder & R. Schiefelbusch (Eds.), *Contemporary issues in language intervention* (ASHA Reports 12, pp. 27-51). American Speech-Language-Hearing Association.

Yoder, P. J., Kaiser, A. P., & Alpert, C. L. (1991). An exploratory study of the interactions between language teaching methods and child characteristics. *Journal of Speech and Hearing Research, 34*, 155-167.

Yoder, P. J., McCathren, R., Warren, S., & Watson, A. (2001). Important distinctions in measuring maternal responses to communication in prelinguistic children with disabilities. *Communication Disorders Quarterly, 22*, 135-147.

Yorganci, R., Kindiroglu, A. A., & Kose, H. (n.d.). Avatar-based sign language training interface for primary school education. Retrieved from https://pdfs.semanticscholar.org/82ad/413a6b5dba026478b1dc9f61c8bbdf22aeb6.pdf

Yorkston, K. M., & Beukelman, D. R. (2007). AAC intervention for progressive conditions. In D. Beukelman, K. Garrett, & K. Yorkston (Eds.), *Augmentative communication strategies for adults with acute or chronic medical conditions* (pp. 317-345). Paul H. Brookes Publishing Co.

Yorkston, K. M., Beukelman, D. R., Hakel, M., & Dorsey, M. (2007). *Speech intelligibility test for Windows*. Madonna Rehabilitation Hospital.

Yorkston, K. M., Johnson, K. L., & Klasner, E. R. (2005). Taking part in life: Enhancing participation in multiple sclerosis. *Physical Medicine and Rehabilitation Clinics of North America, 16*, 583-594.

Yorkston, K. M., & Karlan, G. R. (1986). Assessment procedures. In S. Blackstone (Ed.), *Augmentative communication: An introduction* (pp. 163-196). American Speech-Language-Hearing Association.

Yorkston, K. M., Klasner, E., & Swanson, K. (2001). Communication in context: A qualitative study of the experiences of individuals with multiple sclerosis. *American Journal of Speech-Language Pathology, 10*, 126-137.

Yorkston, K. M., Miller, R., Strand, E., & Britton, D. (2013). *Management of speech and swallowing disorders in degenerative diseases* (3rd ed.). Pro-Ed.

Yorkston, K. M., Strand, E., Miller, R., Hillel, A., & Smith, K. (1993). Speech deterioration in amyotrophic lateral sclerosis: Implications for the timing of intervention. *Journal of Medical Speech-Language Pathology, 1*, 35-46.

Yoshinaga-Itano, C. (2003). From screening to early identification and intervention: Discovering predictors to successful outcomes for children with significant hearing loss. *Journal of Deaf Studies and Deaf Education, 8*(1), 11-30.

Young, C. V. (1986). Developmental disabilities. In J. Katz (Ed.), *Handbook of clinical audiology* (3rd ed., pp. 689-706). Williams & Wilkins.

Yovetich, W. S., & Paivio, A. (1980, August). *Cognitive processing of Bliss-like symbols by normal populations: A report on four studies.* Presentation at the European Association for Special Education.

Zabala, J. (2010). The SETT framework: Straight from the horse's mouth. Retrieved from http://joyzabala.com/uploads/CA_Kananaskis__SETT_Horses_Mouth.pdf

Zahnert, T. (2011). The differential diagnosis of hearing loss. *Deutsches Aerzteblatt International, 108*(25), 433-445.

Zakzanis, K. (1998). The subcortical dementia of Huntington's disease. *Journal of Clinical and Experimental Neuropsychology, 20*(4), 565-578.

Zangari, C. (2016a). AAC apps and devices: Thoughts on conducting AAC trials [blog post]. Retrieved from http://praacticalaac.org/praactical/aac-apps-and-devices-thoughts-on-conducting-aac-trials/

Zangari, C. (2016b). Selecting AAC apps and devices: A handful of reasons not to skip the trial period [blog post]. Retrieved from http://praacticalaac.org/praactical/selecting-aac-apps-devices-a-handful-of-reasons-not-to-skip-the-trial-period/

Zangari, C. (2021). PrAACtical questions: "What does a robust AAC system look like? Retrieved from https://praacticalaac.org/praactical/praactical-questions-what-does-a-robust-aac-system-look-like/

Zangari, C., Lloyd, L., & Vicker, B. (1994). Augmentative and alternative communication: An historic perspective. *Augmentative and Alternative Communication, 10*(1), 27-59.

Zangari, C., & Proctor, L. (2009). Language assessment for students who use AAC. In G. Soto & C. Zangari (Eds.), *Practically speaking: Language, literacy, and academic development for students with AAC needs* (Ch. 3, pp. 47-69). Paul H. Brookes Publishing Co.

Zangari, C., & Van Tatenhove, G. (2009). Supporting more advanced linguistic communicators in the classroom. In C. Zangari & G. M. Soto (Eds.), *Practically speaking: Language, literacy, and academic development for students with AAC needs* (pp. 173-194). Paul H. Brookes Publishing Co.

Zavalani, T. S. (1995). *CyberGlyphs: A pictographic communication system.* Author.

Zeno, S. M., Ivens, S. H., Millard, R. T., & Duvvuri, R. (1995). *The educator's word frequency guide.* Touchstone Applied Science Associates.

Zgaljardic, D., Borod, J., Foldi, N., Mattis, P., Gordon, M., Feigin, A., & Eidelberg, D. (2006). An examination of executive dysfunction associated with frontostriatal circuitry in Parkinson's disease. *Journal of Clinical and Experimental Neuropsychology, 28*(7), 1127-1144.

Zgaljardic, D., Foldi, N., & Borod, J. (2004). Cognitive and behavioral dysfunction in Parkinson's disease: Neurochemical and clinicopathological contributions. *Journal of Neural Transmission, 111*, 1287-1301.

Zhai, S., & Kristensson, P. O. (2012). The word-gesture keyboard: Reimagining keyboard interaction. *Communications of the Association for Computing Machinery, 55*(9), 91-101.

Ziegler, W., & Ackermann, H. (2013). Neuromotor speech impairment: It's all in the talking. *Folia Phoniatrica et Logopaedica, 65*(2), 55-67.

Zimmerman, G., & Vanderheiden, G. (2008). Accessible design and testing in the application development process: Considerations for an integrated approach. *Universal Access in the Information Society, 7*(1-2), 117-128.

Zipf, G. (1936). *The psychobiology of language.* Routledge.

Zubow, L., & Hurtig, R. (2013). A demographic study of AAC/AT needs in hospitalized patients. *Perspectives on Augmentative and Alternative Communication, 22*(2), 79-90.

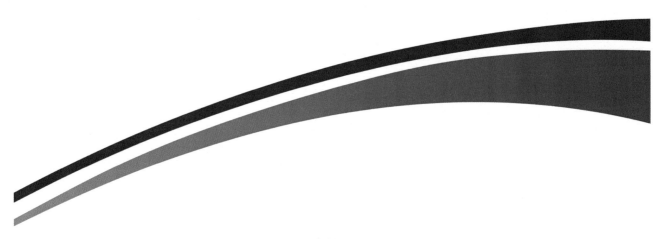

Financial Disclosures

Dr. Erna Alant has no financial or proprietary interest in the materials presented herein.

Dr. Meher H. Banajee has no financial or proprietary interest in the materials presented herein.

Dr. Susan M. Bashinski has no financial or proprietary interest in the materials presented herein.

Lisa Beccera-Walker has no financial or proprietary interest in the materials presented herein.

Dr. Juan Bornman has no financial or proprietary interest in the materials presented herein.

Dr. Barbara A. Braddock has no financial or proprietary interest in the materials presented herein.

Dr. Donna R. Brooks has no financial or proprietary interest in the materials presented herein.

Janie Cirlot-New contracts with the Center for AAC and Autism, PRC-Saltillo to provide trainings. She also receives equipment for use in trainings.

Russell T. Cross has no financial or proprietary interest in the materials presented herein.

Dr. Ruth Crutchfield has no financial or proprietary interest in the materials presented herein.

Krista Davidson has no financial or proprietary interest in the materials presented herein.

Dr. Aimee Dietz has no financial or proprietary interest in the materials presented herein.

Dr. Debora Downey has no financial or proprietary interest in the materials presented herein.

Dr. Karen A. Erickson has no financial or proprietary interest in the materials presented herein.

Dr. Donald R. Fuller has no financial or proprietary interest in the materials presented herein.

Dr. Lori A. Geist has no financial or proprietary interest in the materials presented herein.

Lewis Golinker has no financial or proprietary interest in the materials presented herein.

Dr. Michelle L. Gutmann has not disclosed any financial or proprietary interest in the materials presented herein.

Cindy Halloran is an employee owner of PRC-Saltillo and an author/developer of Language Acquisition through Motor Planning.

John Halloran is an employee owner of PRC-Saltillo and an author/developer of Language Acquisition through Motor Planning.

Dr. Elizabeth K. Hanson has no financial or proprietary interest in the materials presented herein.

Dr. Penny Hatch has no financial or proprietary interest in the materials presented herein.

Amanda Hettenhausen is employed by PRC-Saltillo.

Dr. Richard Hurtig is the Founder and Chief Scientific Officer of Voxello. He developed the Voxello system.

Dr. Mick Isaacson has not disclosed any financial or proprietary interest in the materials presented herein.

Dr. Rajinder Koul has no financial or proprietary interest in the materials presented herein.

Annette Loring has no financial or proprietary interest in the materials presented herein.

Dr. John Luna has no financial or proprietary interest in the materials presented herein.

Dr. Georgina Lynch has no financial or proprietary interest in the materials presented herein.

Chitrali Mamlekar has no financial or proprietary interest in the materials presented herein.

Dr. Samuel N. Mathew has no financial or proprietary interest in the materials presented herein.

Dr. Miechelle McKelvey has no financial or proprietary interest in the materials presented herein.

Dr. Katrina E. Miller has no financial or proprietary interest in the materials presented herein.

Dr. Eliada Pampoulou has no financial or proprietary interest in the materials presented herein.

Erin Colone Peabody has no financial or proprietary interest in the materials presented herein.

Dr. Vineetha S. Philip has no financial or proprietary interest in the materials presented herein.

Jack Ruelas has no financial or proprietary interest in the materials presented herein.

Sayda E. Ruelas has no financial or proprietary interest in the materials presented herein.

Lin Sun has no financial or proprietary interest in the materials presented herein.

Gail M. Van Tatenhove has no financial or proprietary interest in the materials presented herein.

Dr. Annalu Waller has no financial or proprietary interest in the materials presented herein.

Dr. Kristy S. E. Weissling is the Vice President of the Nebraska Stroke Association. She has also conducted a Medbridge presentation on augmentative and alternative communication.

Dr. Shirley Wells has no financial or proprietary interest in the materials presented herein.

Dr. Oliver Wendt has no financial or proprietary interest in the materials presented herein.

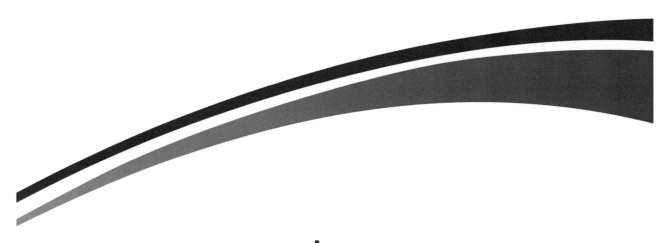

INDEX

Printed in the United States
by Baker & Taylor Publisher Services